Encyclopedia of Trauma Care

Peter J. Papadakos • Mark L. Gestring
Editors

Encyclopedia of Trauma Care

Volume 1

A–K

With 398 Figures and 146 Tables

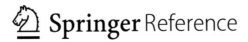
Springer Reference

Editors

Peter J. Papadakos
Departments of Anesthesiology
Surgery and Neurosurgery
University of Rochester Medical Center
Rochester, NY, USA

Mark L. Gestring
Department of Surgery
Emergency Medicine and Pediatrics
University of Rochester
School of Medicine
Rochester, New York, USA

ISBN 978-3-642-29611-6   ISBN 978-3-642-29613-0 (eBook)
ISBN 978-3-642-29612-3 (print and electronic bundle)
DOI 10.1007/ 978-3-642-29613-0

Library of Congress Control Number: 2015941451

Springer Heidelberg New York Dordrecht London
© Springer-Verlag Berlin Heidelberg 2015

Printed on acid-free paper

Springer-Verlag GmbH Berlin Heidelberg is part of Springer Science+Business Media
(www.springer.com)

This work is dedicated to my children, Matthew and Sarah, and to my wife, Holly, for their consistent and unwavering support. It is also dedicated to my parents, Gidon and Anne, and to my brothers, Craig and Brian, for a lifetime's worth of advice, direction, and guidance.

Mark L. Gestring

A work cannot move forward without the support of one's family, and in this, I am very grateful to my wife Susan and my children Yanni and Ava. I could not have done this project without your help, love, and, of course, your understanding. This work is also dedicated to the many teachers of medicine and surgery who taught me both the art and science of this wonderful profession and to the many generations of students, residents, and fellows. I am in your debt for keeping me sharp, up to date and in focus all these years. I also have a special thanks to my administrative assistant Shari, who, over the years, has typed hundreds of papers and chapters, contacted authors and collaborators throughout the world, and kept me on schedule.

Peter J. Papadakos

Foreword

When I reflect on the last 25 years of progress in trauma care, it is overwhelming to consider the explosion of data that has emerged and transformed our management approach to patients across a broad spectrum of injury patterns and severity. With the emergence of new technology, better understanding of the physiology of shock and resuscitation, more judicious use of operative approaches, vigilant intensivist-driven bedside critical care, and a focus on achieving optimal outcomes for injured patients, the challenge of staying current in best practice has become monumental. Moreover, the focus of care provision has shifted from rapid *recall* of information to rapid *retrieval* of information for immediate integration and application into the patient care setting.

While a whole host of modalities have surfaced to assist the clinician in meeting this challenge, the *Encyclopedia of Trauma Care* stands as a seminal compendium of works that provide easily accessible, easily abstracted information at the ready. The scope of the material is expansive, the organization of the content is outstanding, and the structure of each review is systematic and consistent allowing the reader to hone in on key areas of interest without an undue amount of filtering and culling. The broad range of material and the easy alphabetical order of subject areas constitute a comprehensive yet convenient "first-stop" on the way to understanding straightforward approaches to not-so-straightforward clinical problems of interest.

The contributors to this two-volume set represent a "Who's Who" in international trauma care and their perspectives, based on their in-depth knowledge and years of experience in managing injured patients, are invaluable to the reader. It becomes immediately apparent on review of the text that this sort of expertise across a broad spectrum of trauma problems is a significant advantage in sorting the conundrums that complex injury patterns present to the working clinician. In over 1,200 pages replete with numerous tables and illustrations, the authors provide the most current and practical information available on topics such as airway emergencies, strategies in shock resuscitation, salvage modes of mechanical ventilation, prolonged open abdomen, mass casualty management, and teamwork in trauma care. Certainly, working knowledge of the material covered herein is of paramount importance in daily practice. Conveniently enough, it also serves as an exceptional review tool in preparation for examinations at every level.

Papadakos and Gestring have done a masterful job as editors of this text. They bring to the process a balanced approach due to their diverse backgrounds. While both share a passion for surgical critical care, Peter Papadakos is an anesthesiologist by training and brings this viewpoint and expertise to the work. Mark Gestring, an accomplished trauma surgeon, adds perspective that flavors the encyclopedia throughout. The work will be applicable and useful as an outstanding source of information for a broad range of physicians from many specialties, students, residents, fellows, nurses, advanced practice provides as well as scientists from bench top to bedside. This places the *Encyclopedia of Trauma Care* in a unique category of references; compiled in multidisciplinary fashion it offers great value to the readership.

Michael F. Rotondo
Department of Surgery
University of Rochester
Rochester, NY, USA

Acknowledgements

We both have an insurmountable debt to Springer for allowing us to develop this project. We wish to especially thank two highly dedicated individuals in the Springer family, Barbara Wolf and Esther Niederhammer, who shepherded us in bringing this book to print; without their devoted guidance and support, such a massive project would never come to completion. Their hundreds of e-mails to authors and section editors were the fuel that kept the train moving forward.

About the Editors

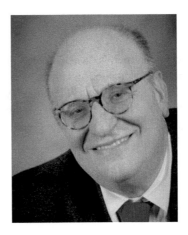

Peter J. Papadakos is Professor of Anesthesiology and Surgery, Neurosurgery and of Neurology as well as Director of the Division of Critical Care at the University of Rochester Medical Center in New York. He is also Professor of Respiratory Care and Medical Director at the State University of New York at Genesee Community College. Professor Papadakos is the author of numerous original papers, reviews, book chapters, and monographs and serves on a number of editorial boards and state and national committees.

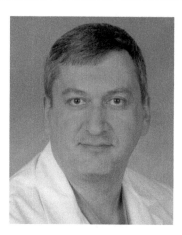

Mark L. Gestring serves as the Medical Director of the Kessler Trauma Center at Strong Memorial Hospital in Rochester, New York, where he holds the rank of Associate Professor of Surgery, Emergency Medicine, and Pediatrics at the University of Rochester, School of Medicine. Dr. Gestring has authored numerous papers and serves on both regional and national committees dedicated to the field of trauma care.

Section Editors

Joshua Brown University of Pittsburgh, Pittsburgh, PA, USA

Imaging in the Trauma Patient

Roy H. Constantine St. Francis Hospital – The Heart Center, Roslyn, NY, USA

Midlevel Providers in Trauma Care

Bryan A. Cotton Department of Surgery, Division of Acute Care Surgery, Trauma and Critical Care, University of Texas Health Science Center at Houston, The University of Texas Medical School at Houston, Houston, TX, USA

Blood Replacement Following Injury

Edward T. Dickinson Department of Emergency Medicine, Perelman School of Medicine, Hospital of the University of Pennsylvania, Philadelphia, PA, USA

Blunt Trauma Mechanisms of Injury

Mirsad Dupanovic Department of Anesthesiology, Kansas University Medical Center, The University of Kansas Hospital, Kansas City, KS, USA

Trauma Anesthesia

Thomas J. Esposito Loyola University Medical Center, Maywood, IL, USA

Injury Epidemiology and Prevention

Douglas Fetkenhour Department of Physical Medicine and Rehabilitation, University of Rochester School of Medicine, Rochester, NY, USA

Rehabilitation Following Injury

John T. Gorczyca Division of Orthopaedic Trauma, Department of Orthopedic Surgery, University of Rochester School of Medicine, Rochester, NY, USA

Musculoskeletal Injury

Oscar D. Guillamondegui Surgery, Division of Trauma and Surgical Critical Care, Department of Surgery, Vanderbilt University Medical Center, Nashville, TN, USA

Head Injury

Elliot Haut School of Medicine, The Johns Hopkins University, Baltimore, MD, USA

Neck and Cervical Spine Injury

Donald H. Jenkins Department of Surgery, Division of Trauma, Critical Care and Emergency General Surgery, Saint Marys Hospital, Rochester, MN, USA
Mayo Clinic, Rochester, MN, USA

Military Trauma Care

Michael Kamali School of Medicine, University of Rochester, Rochester, NY, USA

Airway Management in the Trauma Patient

Patrick K. Kim Division of Traumatology, Surgical Critical Care and Emergency Surgery, Department of Surgery, Perelman School of Medicine at the University of Pennsylvania, Philadelphia, PA, USA

Abdominal Injury

Younsuck Koh Department of Pulmonary and Critical Care Medicine, Asan Medical Center, University of Ulsan College of Medicine, Seoul, South Korea

Ethics in Trauma Care

Stanley J. Kurek Department of Surgery, University of South Florida Morsani College of Medicine, Lawnwood Regional Medical Center, Ft. Pierce, FL, USA

Complications Associated with Trauma Care

Stephen E. Lapinsky Interdepartmental Division of Critical Care, University of Toronto, Toronto, ON, Canada

General Critical Care Topics in the Trauma ICU

Manjunath Markandaya Department of Neurosurgery, University of Rochester Medical Center, Rochester, NY, USA

Neurocritical Care in the Trauma Unit

Barto Nascimento Trauma Program, Department of Surgery, Sunnybrook Health Sciences Centre, University of Toronto, Toronto, ON, Canada

Blood Product Use in the Trauma ICU

Peter J. Papadakos Departments of Anesthesiology, Surgery and Neurosurgery, University of Rochester, Rochester, NY, USA

Safety

Jignesh H. Patel Department of Pharmacy, University of Rochester Medical Center, Strong Memorial Hospital, Rochester, NY, USA

Trauma Pharmacology

Tarek Razek McGill University, Montreal, QC, Canada

Chest Injury

Sandro Rizoli Trauma & Acute Care Surgery, Departments of Critical Care & Surgery, St.Michael's Hospital, University of Toronto, Toronto, Ontario, Canada

Blood Product Use in the Trauma ICU

Nicole Stassen University of Rochester, Rochester, NY, USA

Damage Control and Open Abdomen Management

Contributors

Sara J. Aberle Department of Emergency Medicine, Mayo School of Graduate Medical Education – Mayo Clinic, Rochester, MN, USA

Nicole M. Acquisto Department of Emergency Medicine, University of Rochester School of Medicine and Dentistry, Rochester, NY, USA

Department of Pharmacy, University of Rochester Medical Center, Rochester, NY, USA

Kayode Adeniji Department of Critical Care, Queen Alexandra Hospital, Portsmouth, UK

Sarah M. Adriance Department of Pharmacy, The Ohio State University Wexner Medical Center, Columbus, OH, USA

Vikas Agarwal Department of Radiology, Neuroradiology Division, University of Pittsburgh Medical Center, Pittsburgh, PA, USA

Akira Akabayashi Department of Biomedical Ethics, The University of Tokyo Graduate School of Medicine, Tokyo, Japan

Ariful Alam Department of General Surgery, Staten Island University Hospital, Staten Island, NY, USA

Nelson Nicolás Algarra Department of Anesthesiology, University of Florida, Gainesville, FL, USA

Steven R. Allen Department of Traumatology, Surgical Critical Care and Emergency Surgery, Hospital of the University of Pennsylvania, Philadelphia, PA, USA

Dennis Allin Department of Emergency Medicine, University of Kansas School of Medicine, Kansas City, KS, USA

Jalal Alowais Department of Surgery, Al Imam Mohammad Ibn Saud University, Riyadh, Saudi Arabia

Rona Altaras Division of Acute Surgery/Trauma/Surgical Critical Care, Lawnwood Regional Medical Center, Fort Pierce, FL, USA

Katrina B. Altenhofen Iowa Department of Public Health-Bureau of EMS, Washington, IA, USA

Mohammad Alzghari Trauma, Critical Care and General Surgery Department, Mayo Clinic, Rochester, MN, USA

Mahmoud A. Amr Division of Trauma, Critical Care, and General Surgery, Mayo Clinic, Rochester, MN, USA

Rahul Anand Department of Surgery, Division of Trauma, Critical Care and Emergency Surgery, Virginia Commonwealth University, Richmond, VA, USA

Staci A. Anderson Department of Pharmacy, Community Regional Medical Center, Fresno, CA, USA

Penny Andrews Department of Surgical Critical Care, R Adams Cowley Shock Trauma Center/University of Maryland Medical Center, Baltimore, MD, USA

Arun Aneja Department of Orthopaedic Surgery and Rehabilitation Medicine, University of Chicago Medicine & Biological Sciences, Chicago, IL, USA

Hitoshi Arima Graduate School of Urban Social and Cultural Studies, Yokohama City University, Yokohama, Japan

Ani Aydin Shock Trauma Center, University of Maryland Medical Center, Baltimore, MD, USA

Sean M. Bagshaw Division of Critical Care Medicine, Faculty of Medicine and Dentistry, University of Alberta, Edmonton, AB, Canada

Julian E. Bailes Department of Neurosurgery, NorthShore University Health System, Evanston, IL, USA

Anthony J. Baldea Loyola University Medical Center, Maywood, IL, USA

Roger A. Band Department of Emergency Medicine, Perelman School of Medicine, University of Pennsylvania, Philadelphia, PA, USA

Michael P. Bannon Department of Surgery, Division of Trauma, Critical Care, and General Surgery, Mayo Clinic, Rochester, MN, USA

Timothy J. Barreiro Ohio University Heritage College of Osteopathic Medicine, Athens, OH, USA

Department of Medicine, Northeast Ohio Medical University, Rootstown, OH, USA

Department of Internal Medicine, Pulmonary Health and Research, St. Elizabeth Health Center, Youngstown, OH, USA

Craig Bartlett Department of Orthopaedics and Rehabilitation, University of Vermont/Fletcher Allen Healthcare, Burlington, VT, USA

Thomas J. Bayuk Department of Medicine, Neurology Section, San Antonio Military Medical Center, Fort Sam Houston, TX, USA

Christopher E. Beck Department of Anesthesiology, University of Kansas, Kansas City, KS, USA

Gina M. Berg Trauma Research, Wesley Medical Center, Wichita, KS, USA

Department of Preventive Medicine and Public Health, University of Kansas School of Medicine – Wichita, Wichita, KS, USA

Kristina Bermas Department of Trauma and General Surgery, University of Pittsburgh Medical Center, Pittsburgh, PA, USA

Stepheny Berry Department of Surgery, The University of Kansas Medical Center, Kansas City, KS, USA

Avinash Bhakta Department of General Surgery, General Surgery Resident, Albany Medical College, Albany, NY, USA

Archana Bhaskaran Division of Infectious Diseases and Multi-Organ Transplantation, University Health Network/University of Toronto, Toronto, ON, Canada

Gregory M. Blanton Department of Emergency Medicine, University of Rochester, Rochester, NY, USA

Phil Blazar Department of Orthopedics, Brigham and Women's Hospital, Boston, MA, USA

Ryan P. Bodkin Department of Emergency Medicine, University of Rochester School of Medicine and Dentistry, Rochester, NY, USA

Colin D. Booth Orthopaedic Surgery Resident, Atlanta Medical Center, Atlanta, GA, USA

Bjug Borgundvaag Schwartz/Reisman Emergency Medicine Institute, Department of Family and Community Medicine, Mount Sinai Hospital, University of Toronto, Toronto, ON, Canada

Zana Borovcanin Department of Anesthesiology, University of Rochester, School of Medicine and Dentistry, Rochester, NY, USA

Amy O. Bowles Department of Brain Injury Rehabilitation, San Antonio Military Medical Center, Fort Sam Houston, TX, USA

John Bracken Department of Anesthesiology, University of Kansas Medical Center, Kansas City, KS, USA

Matthew J. Bradley R. Adams Cowley Shock Trauma Center, University of Maryland Medical Center, Baltimore, MD, USA

Mary-Margaret Brandt St. Joseph Mercy Hospital, Ann Arbor, MI, USA

Patrick Braun Department of Anesthesiology and Critical Care Medicine, Innsbruck Medical University, Innsbruck, Austria

Edward E. Braun Department of Anesthesiology, University of Kansas Medical Center, Kansas City, KS, USA

Andrew S. Brock Division of Gastroenterology and Hepatology, Medical University of South Carolina, Charleston, SC, USA

Imad Btaiche Department of Pharmacy Practice, School of Pharmacy, Lebanese American University, Byblos, Lebanon

Lisa D. Burry Department of Pharmacy, Mount Sinai Hospital, Toronto, ON, Canada

Frank K. Butler Department of the Army, Committee on Tactical Combat Casualty Care, U.S. Army Institute of Surgical Research, Fort Sam Houston, TX, USA

Department of the Army, Prehospital Trauma Care, Joint Trauma System, U.S. Army Institute of Surgical Research, Fort Sam Houston, TX, USA

Maureen Byrne St. Francis Hospital-The Heart Center, Roslyn, NY, USA

Nahit Çakar Istanbul Medical Faculty Anesthesiology and Intensive Care, Istanbul, Turkey

Xzabia A. Caliste University of Rochester Medical Center, Rochester, NY, USA

Jeannie L. Callum Sunnybrook Health Sciences Centre and Department of Laboratory Medicine, Department of Clinical Pathology, University of Toronto, Toronto, ON, Canada

Stephen M. Campbell Department of Anesthesiology, University of Kansas Medical Center, Kansas City, KS, USA

Leopoldo C. Cancio Medical Corps, U.S. Army, U.S. Army Institute of Surgical Research, Fort Sam Houston, TX, USA

Elena Cecilia Capello Dipartimento di Anestesiologia e Rianimazione, Università di Torino, Azienda Ospedaliera Città della Salute e della Scienza, Torino, Italy

Robert Cartotto Ross Tilley Burn Centre, Sunnybrook Health Sciences Centre and Department of Surgery, University of Toronto, Toronto, ON, Canada

Diana Catalina Casas Lopez Faculty of Medicine, Department of Anesthesiology and Interdepartmental, Division of Critical Care Medicine, Toronto General Hospital, University of Toronto, Toronto, ON, Canada

Davide Cattano Department of Anesthesiology, Memorial Hermann Hospital-TMC, The University of Texas Medical School at Houston, Houston, TX, USA

Martin Chapman Department of Critical Care, Sunnybrook Health Sciences Centre and Department of Anesthesia, University of Toronto, Toronto, ON, Canada

Jean Charchaflieh Department of Anesthesiology, Yale University School of Medicine, New Haven, CT, USA

Albert Chi Department of Surgery, The Johns Hopkins Hospital, Baltimore, MD, USA

Jacqueline J. L. Chin Centre for Biomedical Ethics, Yong Loo Lin School of Medicine, National University of Singapore, Singapore, Singapore

Kyoung Hyo Choi Department of Rehabilitation Medicine, Asan Medical Center, University of Ulsan College of Medicine, Seoul, South Korea

Kevin K. Chung Medical Corps, U.S. Army, U.S. Army Institute of Surgical Research, Fort Sam Houston, TX, USA

Sarah J. Clutter University of Kansas Medical Center, Kansas City, Kansas, USA

Torry Grantham Cobb Dartmouth–Hitchcock Medical Center, Lebanon, NH, USA

St. Francis University, Loretto, PA, USA

Peter A. Cole Department of Orthopaedics, University of Minnesota-Regions Hospital, St. Paul, MN, USA

Jamie J. Coleman Department of Surgery, Indiana University School of Medicine, Indianapolis, IN, USA

Philip N. Collis Department of Orthopaedic Surgery, University of Louisville School of Medicine, Louisville, KY, USA

Roy H. Constantine St. Francis Hospital – The Heart Center, Roslyn, NY, USA

Bianca Conti Trauma Anesthesia, R Adams Cowley Shock Trauma Center, Baltimore, MD, USA

Maya Contreras Department of Anesthesia, Keenan Research Centre for Biomedical Science, St. Michael's Hospital and University of Toronto, Toronto, ON, Canada

P. Christopher Cook University of Rochester Medical Center and Golisano Children's Hospital, Rochester, NY, USA

Ruggero M. Corso Department of Emergency, Division of Anesthesia and Intensive Care, G.B. Morgagni-L. Pierantoni Hospital, Forlì, Italy

Bryan A. Cotton Department of Surgery, Division of Acute Care Surgery, Trauma and Critical Care, University of Texas Health Science Center at Houston, The University of Texas Medical School at Houston, Houston, TX, USA

Marie Crandall Department of Surgery, Northwestern University Feinberg School of Medicine, Chicago, IL, USA

Christine Cserti-Gazdewich Department of Laboratory Hematology (Blood Transfusion Laboratory), University Health Network, Toronto, ON, Canada

Nicola S. Curry NHS Blood & Transplant, Oxford University Hospitals NHS Trust, Headington, Oxford, UK

Marcelo Cypel Surgical Director ECLS Program at UHN, Canada Research Chair in Lung Transplantation, Assistant Professor of Surgery, Division of Thoracic Surgery, University of Toronto, Toronto, ON, Canada

Katarzyna H. Czerniecka Department of Neurosurgery, University of Rochester Medical Center, Rochester, NY, USA

Dima Danovich Department of General Surgery, Staten Island University Hospital, Statent Island, NY, USA

Matthew L. Dashnaw Department of Neurosurgery, University of Rochester Medical Center, Rochester, NY, USA

Colleen O. Davis Departments of Emergency Medicine and Pediatrics, University of Rochester Medical Center, Rochester, NY, USA

William Bradley Davis Department of Anesthesiology, University of Rochester, Rochester, NY, USA

Martin De Ruyter Department of Anesthesiology, University of Kansas Medical Center, Kansas City, KS, USA

Dan L. Deckelbaum Division of Trauma Surgery and Critical Care Medicine, Centre for Global surgery, The Montreal General Hospital – Room L9-411, Montreal, QC, Canada

Michael J. Desborough NHS Blood & Transplant, Oxford Radcliffe Hospitals Trust John Radcliffe Hospital, Headington, Oxford, UK

Ravneet Dhillon Department of Emergency Medicine, St Joseph's Hospital Health Center, Syracuse, NY, USA

Edward T. Dickinson Department of Emergency Medicine, Perelman School of Medicine, Hospital of the University of Pennsylvania, Philadelphia, PA, USA

Charles J. DiMaggio Department of Anesthesiology and Epidemiology, Mailman School of Public Health, Columbia University, New York, NY, USA

Joseph Dooley Department of Anesthesiology, University of Rochester, Rochester, NY, USA

Paul Dougherty Department of Orthopedic Surgery, University of Michigan, Ann Arbor, MI, USA

Anahita Dua Department of Surgery, Center for Translational Injury Research (CeTIR), University of Houston Health Science Center, Houston, TX, USA

Iris Dupanović University of Missouri, Kansas City, MO, USA

Mirsad Dupanovic Department of Anesthesiology, Kansas University Medical Center, The University of Kansas Hospital, Kansas City, KS, USA

Michael Eaton Department of Anesthesiology, University of Rochester, Rochester, NY, USA

Issam Eid Department of Otolaryngology and Communicative Sciences, University of Mississippi Medical Center, Jackson, MS, USA

John Elfar Department of Orthopaedics, University of Rochester, Rochester, NY, USA

Thomas J. Esposito Loyola University Medical Center, Maywood, IL, USA

Sarah Fabiano Department of Emergency Medicine, University of South Carolina Medical School, Greenville, SC, USA

Jennifer Falvey Department of Pharmacy, University of Rochester Medical Center, Rochester, NY, USA

J. Christopher Farmer Department of Critical Care, Mayo Clinic - Phoenix Campus, AZ, USA

Paula Ferrada Department of Surgery, Division of Trauma, Critical Care and Emergency Surgery, Virginia Commonwealth University, Richmond, VA, USA

Lorenzo E. Ferri Department of Thoracic Surgery, McGill University Health Centre, The Montreal General Hospital – Room L9-512, Montreal, QC, Canada

Douglas Fetkenhour Department of Physical Medicine and Rehabilitation, University of Rochester School of Medicine, Rochester, NY, USA

Ryan P. Ficco Department of Orthopaedic Surgery, Erlanger Hospital, University of Tennessee College of Medicine-Chattanooga, Chattanooga, TN, USA

Ryan T. Fitzgerald Department of Radiology, Neuroradiology Division, University of Arkansas for Medical Sciences, Little Rock, AR, USA

John M. Flynn Division of Orthopaedic Surgery, The Children's Hospital of Philadelphia, Philadelphia, PA, USA

Jeffrey J. Fong School of Pharmacy Worcester/Manchester, MCPHS University, Worcester, MA, USA

Daniel Forsberg Department of Surgery, Forest Hills Hospital, New York, NY, USA

Robert A. Fowler Departments of Medicine and Critical Care Medicine, Sunnybrook Hospital, University of Toronto, Toronto, ON, Canada

Kenneth Foxx Department of Neurosurgery, Strong Memorial Hospital, University of Rochester Medical Center, Rochester, NY, USA

Dietmar Fries Department for General and Surgical Critical Care Medicine, Medical University Innsbruck, Innsbruck, Austria

Charles A. Frosolone Medical Department, USS Nimitz CVN-68, Everett, WA, USA

Eric C. Fu Department of Orthopaedic Surgery, Massachusetts General Hospital, Harvard Medical School, Boston, MA, USA

Catherine L. Gaines Emergency Medical Associates, Southeastern Regional Medical Center, Lumberton, NC, USA

Christopher P. Gallati Department of Neurosurgery, School of Medicine and Dentistry, University of Rochester, Rochester, NY, USA

Michael Gardam Infection Prevention and Control, University Health Network, Toronto, ON, Canada

Lesli T. Giglio The Heart Center, St Francis Hospital, Roslyn, NY, USA

Jan Gillespie Trauma Program Manager, Loyola University Medical Center, Maywood, IL, USA

Laurent G. Glance Department of Anesthesiology, University of Rochester School of Medicine and Dentistry, Rochester, NY, USA

Shannon Goddard Sunnybrook Health Sciences Centre, University of Toronto, Toronto, ON, Canada

John T. Gorczyca Division of Orthopaedic Trauma, Department of Orthopedic Surgery, University of Rochester School of Medicine, Rochester, NY, USA

Stephen D. Gowing Department of Thoracic Surgery, McGill University Health Centre The Montreal General Hospital – Room L9-112, Montreal, QC, Canada

Robert Grabenkort Emory Center for Critical Care, Atlanta, GA, USA

John Graffeo York College Physician Assistant Program, City University of New York, Jamaica, NY, USA

John Granton Division of Respirology at University Health Network, Mount Sinai Hospital and Women's College Hospital, Toronto, ON, Canada

Department of Medicine, and Interdepartmental, Division of Critical Care, Faculty of Medicine, University of Toronto, Toronto, ON, Canada

Matt L. Graves Department of Orthopaedic Surgery, Division of Trauma, University of Mississippi Medical Center, Jackson, MS, USA

Karla Greco Trauma Anesthesia, R Adams Cowley Shock Trauma Center, Baltimore, MD, USA

Cesare Gregoretti Dipartimento di Anestesiologiae Rianimazione, Universita' di Torino, Azienda Ospedaliera Citta'della Salute e della Scienza, Torino, Italy

Erin Griffeth The University of Kansas Medical Center, Department of Anesthesiology and Pain Medicine, Kansas City, KS, USA

Emmanouil Grigoriou Division of Orthopaedic Surgery, The Children's Hospital of Philadelphia, Philadelphia, PA, USA

Gary Gronseth Department of Neurology, University of Kansas Medical Center, Kansas City, KS, USA

Mari L. Groves Department of Neurosurgery, The Johns Hopkins University School of Medicine, Baltimore, MA, USA

Oscar D. Guillamondegui Surgery, Division of Trauma and Surgical Critical Care, Department of Surgery, Vanderbilt University Medical Center, Nashville, TN, USA

Sundeep Guliani Department of Vascular Surgery, Medical College of Virginia, Richmond, VA, USA

Barbara Haas Department of Surgery, University of Toronto, Toronto, ON, Canada

Daniel Haase Department of Emergency Medicine, R Adams Cowley Shock Trauma Center, University of Maryland Medical Center, Baltimore, MD, USA

Nader Habashi Department of Surgical Critical Care, R Adams Cowley Shock Trauma Center/University of Maryland Medical Center, Baltimore, MD, USA

Malik A. Hamid Department of Anesthesiology, University of Kansas Medical Center, Kansas City, KS, USA

Warren C. Hammert Department of Orthopaedic Surgery, University of Rochester Medical Center, Rochester, NY, USA

Waël C. Hanna Division of Thoracic Surgery, McMaster University - St. Joseph's Healthcare – Room T2105, Hamilton, ON, Canada

Jennifer K. Hansen Department of Anesthesiology, University of Kansas Medical Center, Kansas City, KS, USA

Brett Hartman Department of Surgery, Division of Plastic and Reconstructive Surgery, Indiana University, Indianapolis, IN, USA

Patrick Harvey Department of Emergency Medicine, Hospital of the University of Pennsylvania, Philadelphia, PA, USA

Virginia Harvey Department of Emergency Medicine, University of Pennsylvania, Philadelphia, PA, USA

Patti L. Hass Department of Brain Injury Rehabilitation, San Antonio Military Medical Center, Fort Sam Houston, TX, USA

Harvey G. Hawes Department of Surgery, Division of Acute Care Surgery, Trauma and Critical Care, University of Texas Health Science Center at Houston, The University of Texas Medical School at Houston, Houston, TX, USA

Mark Hawk Adult–Gerontology Acute Care Nurse Practitioner Speciality (Retired), School of Nursing University of California, San Francisco, CA, USA

Trauma Nurse Practitioner (Retired), San Francisco General Hospital, San Francisco, CA, USA

Matthew T. Heller Department of Radiology, Division of Abdominal Imaging, University of Pittsburgh Medical Center, Pittsburgh, PA, USA

Gina Hendren Department of Anesthesia, University of Kansas, Kansas City, KS, USA

Margaret Herridge Department of Medicine, University of Toronto, Toronto, ON, Canada

Beth Hochman Division of Traumatology, Surgical Critical Care, and Emergency Surgery, Hospital of the University of Pennsylvania, Philadelphia, PA, USA

Amie Hoefnagel Department of Anesthesiology, University of Rochester Medical Center, Rochester, NY, USA

John B. Holcomb Department of Surgery, Center for Translational Injury Research (CeTIR), University of Houston Health Science Center, Houston, TX, USA

Robert Holloway Department of Neurology, Strong Memorial Hospital, University of Rochester, Rochester, NY, USA

Jin Pyo Hong Department of Psychiatry, University of Ulsan College of Medicine, Seoul, Republic of Korea

Jonathan R. Van Horn Legacy Emanuel Hospital and Randall Children's Hospital, Portland, OR, USA

Jason H. Huang FACS Baylor Scott and White Healthcare 2401 S, TX, USA

Huayong Hu Department of Anesthesiology, University of Rochester Medical Center, Rochester, NY, USA

Catherine Humphrey Department of Orthopaedics and Rehabilitation, University of Rochester Medical Center, Rochester, NY, USA

Shahid Husain Division of Infectious Diseases and Multi-Organ Transplantation, University Health Network/University of Toronto, Toronto, ON, Canada

Barbara Imhoff Stanford Hospital and Clinics, Stanford, CA, USA

Venesa Ingold Department of Anesthesiology, Kansas University Medical Center, The University of Kansas Hospital, Kansas City, KS, USA

Terence Ip Interdepartmental Division of Critical Care, University of Toronto, Toronto, ON, Canada

MariaLisa Itzoe Department of Neurosurgery, The Johns Hopkins University School of Medicine, Baltimore, MD, USA

J. Seth Jacob Department of Anesthesiology, Kansas University Medical Center, Kansas City, KS, USA

Babak S. Jahromi Department of Neurosurgery, School of Medicine and Dentistry, University of Rochester, Rochester, NY, USA

Ashika Jain Trauma Critical Care, Emergency Ultrasound, Department of Emergency Medicine, Kings County Hospital Center, SUNY Downstate Medical Center, Brooklyn, NY, USA

Jan O. Jansen Departments of Surgery & Intensive Care Medicine, Aberdeen Royal Infirmary, Aberdeen, UK

Donald H. Jenkins Department of Surgery, Division of Trauma, Critical Care and Emergency General Surgery, Saint Marys Hospital, Rochester, MN, USA

Mayo Clinic, Rochester, MN, USA

Richard Jenkinson Division of Orthopaedic Surgery, MSK Trauma Section, Sunnybrook Health Sciences Centre, University of Toronto, Toronto, ON, Canada

Mary P. Johnson Columbia University School of Nursing, New York, NY, USA

Nicholas J. Johnson Department of Emergency Medicine, Perelman School of Medicine, University of Pennsylvania, Philadelphia, PA, USA

Caitlin A. Jolda R Adams Cowley Shock Trauma Center, University of Maryland School of Medicine, Baltimore, MD, USA

Mary L. Jones Department of Brain Injury Rehabilitation, San Antonio Military Medical Center, Fort Sam Houston, TX, USA

Bellal Joseph Division of Trauma, Critical Care, Burns and Emergency Surgery, The University of Arizona, Tucson, AZ, USA

Manjari Joshi R Adams Cowley Shock Trauma Center, Section of Infectious Diseases, University of Maryland Medical Center, Baltimore, MD, USA

Gavin M. Joynt Department of Anaesthesia and Intensive Care, The Chinese University of Hong Kong, Hong Kong, China

Marko Jukić Department of Anesthesiology, University of Split, Split, Dalmatia, Croatia

Steven Kahn Division of Trauma and Surgical Critical Care, Department of Surgery, Vanderbilt University Medical Center, Nashville, TN, USA

Myoung Sheen Kang Department of Dental Hygiene, College of Dentistry, Gangneung-Wonju National University, Gangneung City, Gangwon Province, Republic of Korea

Stamatis Kantartzis Department of Radiology, University of Pittsburgh Medical Center, Pittsburgh, PA, USA

Marcin K. Karcz Department of Anesthesiology, University of Rochester, Rochester, NY, USA

Kevin A. Kaucher Departments of Pharmacy and Emergency Medicine, Denver Health Medical Center, Denver, CO, USA

Brian P. Kavanagh Departments of Anesthesia and Critical Care Medicine, Hospital for Sick Children, and University of Toronto, Toronto, ON, Canada

Natasha Keric Banner Good Samaritan Medical Center, Phoenix, AZ, USA

John P. Ketz University of Rochester, Strong Memorial Hospital, Rochester, NY, USA

Mansoor Khan Consultant Esophagogastric and Acute Care Surgeon, Doncaster Royal Infirmary, Doncaster, South Yorkshire, UK

Talal W. Khan Department of Anesthesiology, University of Kansas Medical Center, Kansas City, KS, USA

Kosar Khwaja Departments of Surgery and Critical Care Medicine, McGill University Health Centre, Montreal, QC, Canada

Brian D. Kim Division of Trauma, Critical Care & General Surgery, Mayo Clinic, Rochester, MN, USA

Patrick K. Kim Division of Traumatology, Surgical Critical Care and Emergency Surgery, Department of Surgery, Perelman School of Medicine at the University of Pennsylvania, Philadelphia, PA, USA

Katarzyna Kimborowicz Department of Pharmacy, Morristown Medical Center, Morristown, NJ, USA

Kristopher Kimmell University of Rochester Medical Center, Rochester, NY, USA

James D. Kindscher Department of Anesthesiology, University of Kansas Medical Center, Kansas City, KS, USA

Ruth M. Kleinpell Department of Adult Health and Gerontology, Rush University Medical Center, Chicago, IL, USA

Jennifer Knight Department of Surgery, West Virginia University, Morgantown, WV, USA

Younsuck Koh Department of Pulmonary and Critical Care Medicine, Asan Medical Center, University of Ulsan College of Medicine, Seoul, South Korea

Anthony L. Kovac Kasumi Arakawa Professor of Anesthesiology, Department of Anesthesiology, University of Kansas Medical Center, Kansas City, KS, USA

Colleen Kovach Department of Emergency Medicine, Strong Memorial Hospital, Rochester, NY, USA

Hans J. Kreder Orthopaedic Surgery and Health Policy Evaluation and Management, Division of Orthopaedic Surgery, Sunnybrook Health Sciences Centre, University of Toronto, Toronto, ON, Canada

Corry Jeb Kucik Navy Bureau of Medicine and Surgery (M5), Falls Church, VA, USA

Navy Trauma Training Center, Los Angeles, CA, USA

John G. Laffey Departments of Anesthesia and Critical Care, Keenan Research Centre for Biomedical Science, St. Michael's Hospital, and University of Toronto, Toronto, ON, Canada

Stephen E. Lapinsky Interdepartmental Division of Critical Care, University of Toronto, Toronto, ON, Canada

Brenton J. LaRiccia Division of Trauma and Acute Care Surgery, Department of Surgery, University of Rochester Medical Center, Strong Memorial Hospital, Rochester, Rochester, NY, USA

Adriana Laser Department of General Surgery, University of Maryland Medical Center, Baltimore, MD, USA

Loren L. Latta Department of Orthopaedics, University of Miami, School of Medicine, Miami, FL, USA

Department of Industrial Engineering, University of Miami, College of Engineering, Coral Gables, FL, USA

Max Biedermann Institute for Biomechanics Research, Mount Sinai Medical Center, Miami Beach, FL, USA

Neil M. Lazar Department of Medicine and Interdepartmental Division of Critical Care, University Health Network, University of Toronto, Toronto, ON, Canada

Christie Lee Interdepartmental Division of Critical Care, Department of Medicine, Mount Sinai Hospital and University Health Network, Toronto, ON, Canada

Cook-John Lee Trauma Service, Department of Surgery, Ajou Trauma Center, School of Medicine, Ajou University, Suwon, South Korea

Abhijit Lele Department of Anesthesiology, Neurology and Neurosurgery, University of Kansas Medical Center, Kansas City, KS, USA

Penelope C. Lema Department of Emergency Medicine, State University of New York University at Buffalo, Buffalo, NY, USA

Alex Lesiak Department of Orthopaedics and Rehabilitation, University of Vermont/Fletcher Allen Healthcare, Burlington, VT, USA

Yulia Lin Department of Clinical Pathology, Sunnybrook Health Sciences Centre, Toronto, ON, Canada

Department of Laboratory Medicine and Pathobiology, University of Toronto, Toronto, ON, Canada

Pamela Lipsett Department of Surgery, The Johns Hopkins Hospital, Baltimore, MD, USA

Peter C. W. Loke Centre for BioMedical Ethics, National University Hospital System, Singapore, Singapore

Mint Medical Centre, Singapore, Singapore

Resolvers Pte Ltd, Singapore, Singapore

George T. Loo Department of Epidemiology and Biostatistics, School of Public Health, University at Albany, Rensselaer, NY, USA

Erica A. Loomis Trauma, Critical Care, General Surgery, Mayo Clinic, Rochester, MN, USA

Fred A. Luchette Department of Surgery, Stritch School of Medicine, Loyola University Medical Center, Maywood, IL, USA

Stephanie Lueckel Department of Trauma Surgery and Critical Care, Rhode Island Hospital and Warren Alpert Medical School, Providence, RI, USA

James K. Lukan Department of Surgery, State University of New York, Buffalo, NY, USA

Xuan Luo Harvard Combined Orthopedic Residency Program, Massachusetts General Hospital, Boston, MA, USA

Kristen MacEachern Intensive Care Unit, Mount Sinai Hospital, Toronto, ON, Canada

Michael Maceroli Department of Orthopaedics and Rehabilitation, University of Rochester, Rochester, NY, USA

John E. Mack Surgical Physician Assistant Service, Health Quest Medical Practice, PC, Poughkeepsie, NY, USA

Michael Mackowski Department of Surgery, University of Louisville, Louisville, KY, USA

Zoë Maher The Trauma Center at Penn, University of Pennsylvania, Philadelphia, PA, USA

H. S. Jeffrey Man Division of Respirology, and Interdepartmental Division of Critical Care Medicine, Department of Medicine, University Health Network and Mount Sinai Hospital, University of Toronto, Toronto, ON, Canada

Paul E. Marik Division of Pulmonary and Critical Care Medicine, Eastern Virginia Medical School, Norfolk, VA, USA

Manjunath Markandaya Department of Neurosurgery, University of Rochester Medical Center, Rochester, NY, USA

Department of Neurology, School of Medicine and Dentistry, University of Rochester Medical Center, Rochester, NY, USA

Joshua A. Marks Division of Traumatology, Surgical Critical Care and Emergency Surgery, Department of Surgery, Perelman School of Medicine at the University of Pennsylvania, Philadelphia, PA, USA

Scott A. Marshall Department of Medicine, Neurology Section, San Antonio Military Medical Center, Fort Sam Houston, TX, USA

Department of Medicine, Critical Care Section, San Antonio Military Medical Center, Fort Sam Houston, TX, USA

Kathleen R. Marzluf University of Kansas Medical Center, Kansas City, Kansas, USA

Adrian Matioc Department of Anesthesiology, University of Wisconsin School of Medicine and Public Health, W.S. Middleton VA Medical Center, Madison, WI, USA

Joshua Matthias Department of Anesthesiology, University of Kansas Medical Center, Kansas City, KS, USA

Michael L. McCartney Department of Anesthesiology, University of Missouri-Kansas City, Kansas City, MO, USA

Laura A. McElroy Department of Anesthesiology, Critical Care Medicine, University of Rochester Medical Center, Rochester, NY, USA

Leslie L. McIntyre-Spatar Department of Internal Medicine, Pulmonary Health and Research, St. Elizabeth Health Center, Youngstown, OH, USA

Daniel C. Medina Department of General Surgery, University of Maryland Medical Center, Baltimore, MD, USA

Dawn M. Miller Department of Clinical Pharmacy, St. Elizabeth Health Center, Youngstown, OH, USA

Northeast Ohio Medical University, Rootstown, OH, USA

James T. Miller Department of Pharmacy Services, University of Michigan Hospitals and Health Centers and University of Michigan College of Pharmacy, Ann Arbor, MI, USA

Amrendra Miranpuri Department of Neurosurgery, School of Medicine and Dentistry, University of Rochester, Rochester, NY, USA

Derek Mitchell Department of Anesthesiology, University of Rochester Medical Center, Rochester, NY, USA

Bryan Monier Department of Orthopaedics and Rehabilitation, University of Vermont/Fletcher Allen Healthcare, Burlington, VT, USA

Simone P. Montoya Department of Neurosurgery, University of Rochester Medical Center, School of Medicine and Dentistry, Rochester, NY, USA

Jason Moore Department of Surgery, Lawnwood Regional Medical Center, Fort Pierce, FL, USA

Martin Morales Physician Assistant Services, North Shore – LIJ Health System, Great Neck, NY, USA

Andrew M. Morris Department of Medicine, Mount Sinai Hospital, University Health Network and University of Toronto, Toronto, ON, Canada

David S. Morris Division of Trauma, Critical Care, and General Surgery, Mayo Clinic, Rochester, MN, USA

Jonathan J. Morrison The Academic Department of Military Surgery & Trauma, Royal Centre for Defence Medicine, Birmingham, UK

Michael J. Mosier Department of Surgery, Loyola University Medical Center, Maywood, IL, USA

William A. Mosier Wright State University, Dayton, OH, USA

Jeanne Mueller Department of Surgery, Trauma, Loyola University Medical Center, Maywood, IL, USA

Indraneil Mukherjee Department of General Surgery, Staten Island University Hospital, Staten Island, NY, USA

The Southeastern Center for Digestive Disorders & Pancreatic Cancer, Advanced Minimally Invasive & Robotic Surgery, Florida Hospital Tampa, Tampa, FL, USA

David S. Mulder Division of Thoracic Surgery, McGill University Health Centre, The Montreal General Hospital – Room L9-512, Montreal, QC, Canada

Laveena Munshi Clinical Associate, Critical Care, Mount Sinai Hospital and University Health Network, University of Toronto, Toronto, Canada

Claire V. Murphy Department of Pharmacy, The Ohio State University Wexner Medical Center, Columbus, OH, USA

Sarah Murthi Department of Surgery, R Adams Cowley Shock Trauma Center, University of Maryland Medical Center, Baltimore, MD, USA

John Muscedere The Critical Care Program and Department of Medicine, Queen's University, Kingston, ON, Canada

Lejla Music-Aplenc Children's Mercy Hospital, University of Missouri, Kansas City, MO, USA

John Nachtigal Department of Anesthesiology, University of Kansas Medical Center, Kansas City, KS, USA

Khanjan H. Nagarsheth R Adams Cowley Shock Trauma Center, University of Maryland School of Medicine, Baltimore, MD, USA

Mayur Narayan R Adams Cowley Shock Trauma Center, University of Maryland School of Medicine, Baltimore, MD, USA

Barto Nascimento Trauma Program, Department of Surgery, Sunnybrook Health Sciences Centre, University of Toronto, Toronto, Ontario, Canada

Catherine Nelson Division of Acute Care Surgery and Trauma, University of Rochester Medical Center, Rochester, NY, USA

Norman Nicolson Northwestern University Feinberg School of Medicine, Chicago, IL, USA

Anthony Noto Department of Neurology, Strong Memorial Hospital, University of Rochester, Rochester, NY, USA

Peter J. Nowotarski Department of Orthopaedic Surgery, Erlanger Hospital, University of Tennessee College of Medicine-Chattanooga, Chattanooga, TN, USA

Sue M. Nyberg Department of Physician Assistant, Wichita State University, Wichita, KS, USA

Department of Trauma/Critical Care, Wesley Medical Center, Wichita, KS, USA

James V. O'Connor Shock Trauma Center, University of Maryland Medical Center, Baltimore, MD, USA

Patrick Offner Department of Surgery, St Anthony Hospital, Lakewood, CO, USA

Ryan O'Gowan Surgical Critical Care, St. Francis Hospital, Hartford, CO, USA

Jason S. Oh Shock Trauma Center, University of Maryland Medical Center, Baltimore, MD, USA

Lindsay O'Meara Shock Trauma Center, University of Maryland Medical Center, Baltimore, MD, USA

Ellen C. Omi Division of Trauma and Critical Care, Department of Surgery, Advocate Christ Medical Center, Oak Lawn, IL, USA

Division of Critical Care, Department of Surgery, The University of Illinois, Chicago, IL, USA

Michael Orland Department of Emergency Medicine, University of Pennsylvania, Philadelphia, PA, USA

Amy Ortman Department of Anesthesiology, University of Kansas Hospital, Kansas City, KS, USA

James Osorio Department of Anesthesiology, New York Presbyterian Hospital Weill Cornell Medical College, New York, NY, USA

Tao Ouyang Department of Radiology, Penn State Milton S. Hershey Medical Center, Hershey, PA, USA

Paul M. Palevsky Renal Section, VA Pittsburgh Healthcare System, Pittsburgh, PA, USA

Renal–Electrolyte Division, University of Pittsburgh School of Medicine, Pittsburgh, PA, USA

Katherine Palmieri Department of Anesthesiology, University of Kansas School of Medicine, Kansas City, KS, USA

Peter J. Papadakos Departments of Anesthesiology, Surgery and Neurosurgery, University of Rochester Medical Center, Rochester, NY, USA

Subin Park Department of Psychiatry, Seoul National Hospital, Seoul, Republic of Korea

Kellie Park Department of Anesthesiology, Yale University School of Medicine, New Haven, CT, USA

Mayur B. Patel Veterans Affairs (VA) Tennessee Valley Healthcare System, Nashville VA Medical Center, Surgical Service, Nashville, TN, USA

Surgery, Division of Trauma and Surgical Critical Care, Department of Surgery, Vanderbilt University Medical Center, Nashville, TN, USA

Jignesh H. Patel Department of Pharmacy, University of Rochester Medical Center, Strong Memorial Hospital, Rochester, NY, USA

Tara Paterson Department of Anesthesiology Critical Care, University of Maryland Medical Center, Baltimore, MD, USA

Anthony L. Petraglia Department of Neurosurgery, Rochester Regional Health System, Rochester, NY, USA

Herb A. Phelan Division of Burns/Trauma/Critical Care, Department of Surgery, UT Southwestern Medical Center, Dallas, TX, USA

Alberto Piacentini Department of Emergency, Division of Anesthesiology and Intensive Care, SSuEm118, Sant'Anna Hospital, San Fermo della Battaglia, CO, Italy

Amy M. Pichoff Department of Anesthesiology, University of Kansas Hospital, Kansas City, KS, USA

Melissa R. Pleva Department of Pharmacy Services, University of Michigan Hospitals and Health Centers and University of Michigan College of Pharmacy, Ann Arbor, MI, USA

Jennifer K. Plichta Department of Surgery, Loyola University Medical Center, Maywood, IL, USA

Russell Plowman The University of Kansas School of Medical, Kansas City, KS, USA

Nathaniel Poulin Department of Surgery, Brody School of Medicine East Carolina University, Greenville, NC, USA

Elizabeth K. Powell Department of Emergency Medicine, Hospital of the University of Pennsylvania, Philadelphia, PA, USA

Ipshita Prakash Resident, General Surgery, McGill University Health Centre, Montreal, QC, Canada

Alicia Privette Department of Surgery, Medical University of South Carolina, Charleston, SC, USA

Ronald Rabinowitz R Adams Cowley Shock Trauma Center, Section of Infectious Diseases, University of Maryland Medical Center, Baltimore, MD, USA

Timothy Rainer Accident and Emergency Department, Prince of Wales Hospital, The Chinese University of Hong Kong, Shatin, Hong Kong, China

Maureen C. Regan Winthrop University Hospital, Mineola, NY, USA

Melissa A. Reger Department of Pharmacy, Community Regional Medical Center, Fresno, CA, USA

Oleksa Rewa Department of Critical Care Medicine, Faculty of Medicine, University of Toronto, Toronto, ON, Canada

The Critical Care Program and Department of Medicine, Queen's University, Kingston, ON, Canada

Peter Rhee Division of Trauma, Critical Care, Burns and Emergency Surgery, The University of Arizona, Tucson, AZ, USA

W. Lee Richardson Department of Orthopaedics, University of Rochester, Rochester, NY, USA

Robert M. A. Richardson Division of Nephrology, University of Toronto, University Health Network, Toronto, ON, Canada

Michael de Riesthal Hearing and Speech Sciences, Vanderbilt University, Nashville, TN, USA

David Ring Department of Orthopaedic Surgery, Massachusetts General Hospital, Harvard Medical School, Boston, MA, USA

Amir R. Rizkala Department of Orthopaedics, University of Minnesota-Regions Hospital, St. Paul, MN, USA

Sandro Rizoli Trauma & Acute Care Surgery, Departments of Critical Care & Surgery, St. Michael's Hospital, University of Toronto, Toronto, Ontario, Canada

Craig S. Roberts Department of Orthopaedic Surgery, University of Louisville School of Medicine, Louisville, KY, USA

Michael W. Robertson Department of Orthopaedic Surgery, MetroHealth Medical Center, Affiliated with Case Western Reserve University, Cleveland, OH, USA

Andrew Y. Robinson Department of Medicine, Neurology Section, San Antonio Military Medical Center, Fort Sam Houston, TX, USA

Melissa Rockford Department of Anesthesiology, University of Kansas Medical Center, Kansas City, KS, USA

Joseph Romagnuolo Division of Gastroenterology and Hepatology, Medical University of South Carolina, Charleston, SC, USA

Louise Rose Lawrence S. Bloomberg Faculty of Nursing, University of Toronto, Toronto, ON, Canada

Michael F. Rotondo Department of Surgery, University of Rochester, Rochester, NY, USA

Milton Lee (Chip) Jr Routt University of Texas (Houston) Medical School – Memorial Hermann Medical Center, Houston, TX, USA

Ju Seok Ryu Department of Rehabilitation Medicine, Seoul National University Bundang Hospital, Seoul National University College of Medicine, Seongnam, South Korea

Erin Sabolick Department of Emergency Medicine, Drexel University College of Medicine, Philadelphia, PA, USA

Moheb S. Said Department of General Surgery, Staten Island University Hospital, Staten Island, NY, USA

Noelle Saillant Division of Traumatology, Department of Surgery, Critical Care and Acute Care Surgery, University of Pennsylvania, Philadelphia, PA, USA

Joseph V. Sakran Department of Surgery, Medical University of South Carolina, Charleston, SC, USA

James O. Sanders Department of Orthopaedics and Rehabilitation, School of Medicine and Dentistry, University of Rochester, Rochester, NY, USA

Stephen Sandwell Department of Neurosurgery, University of Rochester, Rochester, NY, USA

Arthur P. Sanford Department for General and Surgical Critical Care Medicine, Stritch School of Medicine, Loyola University Medical Center, Maywood, IL, USA

Claudia C. dos Santos Interdepartmental Division of Critical Care, St. Michael's Hospital/University of Toronto, The Keenan Research Centre of the Li Ka Shing Knowledge Institute, Toronto, ON, Canada

Augusto Sarmiento Department of Orthopaedics, University of Miami, School of Medicine, Miami, FL, USA

Department of Orthopaedics, University of Southern California, Los Angeles, California, USA

Dawood Sayed The University of Kansas Medical Center, Department of Anesthesiology and Pain Medicine, Kansas City, KS, USA

Dane Scantling Philadelphia College of Osteopathic Medicine, Philadelphia, PA, USA

Tyler Schmidt University of Rochester Medical Center, Rochester, NY, USA

Annabel L. Schumaker Department of Pharmacy, San Antonio Military Medical Center, Fort Sam Houston, TX, USA

Department of Medicine, Critical Care Section, San Antonio Military Medical Center, Fort Sam Houston, TX, USA

David Schwaiberger Department of Anesthesiology and Intensive Care Medicine, Campus Charité Mitte and Campus Virchow-Klinikum, Charité - University Medicine Berlin, Berlin, Germany

Daniel M. Sciubba Department of Neurosurgery, The Johns Hopkins University School of Medicine, Baltimore, MA, USA

Evren Şentürk Istanbul Medical Faculty Anesthesiology and Intensive Care, Istanbul, Turkey

Nazia Selzner University of Toronto, Toronto, ON, Canada

Fernando Serna Orthopedic Trauma Surgeon, Department of Orthopedics, Mayo Clinic Health System, Eau Claire, WI, USA

Ashish Seth The Heart Center, St. Francis Hospital, Roslyn, NY, USA

Abha A. Shah Department of Anesthesiology, University of Kansas Medical Center, Kansas City, KS, USA

Aakash A. Shah Department of Orthopedic Surgery, Menorah Medical Center, Overland Park, KS, USA

Nadine Shehata Departments of Medicine and Pathology and Laboratory Medicine, Mount Sinai Hospital, Institute of Health Policy Management and Evaluation, Li Ka Shing Knowledge Institute University of Toronto, Toronto, ON, Canada

Erin L. Sherer Emergency Medicine, Columbia University Medical Center, New York, NY, USA

Jodi Siegel Department of Orthopaedics, UMass Memorial Medical Center, University of Massachusetts Medical School, Worcester, MA, USA

Howard J. Silberstein Department of Neurosurgery, University of Rochester School of Medicine and Dentistry, Rochester, NY, USA

Craig D. Silverton Department of Orthopedic Surgery, Henry Ford Hospital, Detroit, MI, USA

Inga Simning Department of Speech Pathology, University of Rochester School of Medicine, Rochester, NY, USA

Gerald T. Simons Weill Cornell Graduate School of Medical Science Physician Assistant Program, New York, NY, USA

Southampton Hospital, Southampton, NY, USA

Jeffrey M. Singh Critical Care Medicine, University Health Network and Assistant Professor, Division of Critical Care, University of Toronto, Toronto, ON, Canada

Michael J. Singh University of Pittsburgh Medical Center, Pittsburgh, PA, USA

Nina Singh-Radcliff Department of Anesthesiology, AtlantiCare Regional Medical Center, Pomona, NJ, USA

Galloway Township, NJ, USA

David J. Skarupa Division of Acute Care Surgery, Department of Surgery, University of Florida College of Medicine, Jacksonville, FL, USA

Jason W. Smith Department of Surgery, University of Louisville, Louisville, KY, USA

Wade R. Smith Department of Orthopaedics, Swedish Medical Center, Englewood, CO, USA

Brian P. Smith Perelman School of Medicine, University of Pennsylvania, Philadelphia, PA, USA

Gillian L. S. Soles Department of Orthopaedics and Rehabilitation, University of Rochester, Rochester, NY, USA

Jason Sperry Department of Trauma and General Surgery, University of Pittsburgh Medical Center, Pittsburgh, PA, USA

Jonathan D. Spicer Division of Thoracic Surgery, McGill University Health Centre, The Montreal General Hospital – Room L9-512, Montreal, QC, Canada

Mary Ann Spott U.S. Army Institute of Surgical Research, JBSA Fort Sam Houston, TX, USA

Srilata Kavita Sridhar Department of Emergency Medicine and Critical Care, Lakeridge Health, Bowmanville, ON, Canada

Jocelyn A. Srigley University of Toronto, Toronto, ON, Canada

Vasisht Srinivasan Department of Neurosurgery, University of Rochester Medical Center, Rochester, NY, USA

James Stannard Department of Orthopaedics, Missouri Orthopaedic Institute, University Hospital, University of Missouri, Columbia, SC, USA

Simon J. Stanworth NHS Blood & Transplant, Oxford University Hospitals NHS Trust, Headington, Oxford, UK

Shaun Fay Steeby Department of Orthopaedics, Missouri Orthopaedic Institute, University Hospital, University of Missouri, Columbia, SC, USA

Andrew C. Steel Faculty of Medicine, Department of Anesthesiology and Interdepartmental, Division of Critical Care Medicine, Toronto General Hospital, University of Toronto, Toronto, ON, Canada

Robert J. Steffner Department of Orthopedic Surgery, University of California-Davis Medical Center, Sacramento, CA, USA

Jonathan J. Stone School of Medicine, Department of Neurosurgery, Neurosurgery University of Rochester Medical Center, Rochester, NY, USA

Maude St-Onge Clinical Pharmacology and Toxicology, University of Toronto, Toronto, ON, Canada

Tarun J. Subrahmanian Department of Anesthesiology, Emory University School of Medicine, Atlanta, GA, USA

Georgia Anesthesiologists, Marietta, GA, USA

Sachin Sud Department of Medicine, Trillium Hospital, Mississauga, ON, Canada

Marcel Tafen Department of General Surgery, Section of Trauma and Surgical Critical Care, Albany Medical College, Albany, NY, USA

Robert D. Teasdall Department of Orthopaedic Surgery, Wake Forest Baptist Health, Winston-Salem, NC, USA

Subarna Thirugnanam Department of Medicine, Scarborough General Hospital, Toronto, ON, Canada

Zachariah Thomas Department of Pharmacy Practice and Administration, Ernest Mario School of Pharmacy Rutgers, the State University of New Jersey, Piscataway, NJ, USA

Glen H. Tinkoff Department of Surgery, Christiana Care Health System, Newark, DE, USA

Svjetlana Tisma-Dupanovic Department of Cardiology, Children's Mercy Hospital, University of Missouri, Kansas City, MO, USA

Christopher Tolleson Department of Neurology, Vanderbilt University, Nashville, TN, USA

Ashita J. Tolwani Division of Nephrology, University of Alabama at Birmingham, Birmingham, AL, USA

Ronald Torline Department of Anesthesiology, University of Kansas Medical Center, Kansas City, KS, USA

Paul III Tornetta Department of Orthopaedic Surgery, Boston University Medical Center, Boston, MA, USA

Jennifer L. Y. Tsang Department of Medicine (Critical Care Medicine), Niagara Health System, ON, Canada

Ben Usatch Department of Emergency Medicine, Lankenau Hospital, Wynneood, PA, USA

Emily C. Vafek Department of Orthopaedic Surgery, Wake Forest Baptist Health, Winston-Salem, NC, USA

Heather A. Vallier Department of Orthopaedic Surgery, MetroHealth Medical Center, Affiliated with Case Western Reserve University, Cleveland, OH, USA

Srinivasan Vasisht Department of Neurosurgery, University of Rochester Medical Center, Rochester, NY, USA

Daniel T. Vetrosky Department of Physician Assistant Studies, University of South Alabama, Mobile, AL, USA

Mark S. Vrahas Harvard Orthopaedic Trauma Initiative, Brigham and Women's Hospital and Massachusetts General Hospital, Boston, MA, USA

Corey T. Walker Department of Neurosurgery, University of Rochester Medical Center, Rochester, NY, USA

Michael J. Weaver Harvard Orthopaedic Trauma Initiative, Brigham and Women's Hospital and Massachusetts General Hospital, Boston, MA, USA

Kathleen Webster Department of Pediatric Critical Care, Loyola University Medical Center, Maywood, IL, USA

Adam S. Weltz R. Adams Cowley Shock Trauma Center, University of Maryland Medical Center, Baltimore, MD, USA

M. Elizabeth Wilcox Interdepartmental Division of Critical Care, University Health Network, Toronto, ON, Canada

Kristine C. Willett School of Pharmacy Worcester/Manchester, MCPHS University, Manchester, NH, USA

Alison Wilson Department of Surgery, West Virginia University, Morgantown, WV, USA

Carla J. Wittenberg University of California, San Francisco Medical Center, San Francisco, CA, USA

Mary M. Wolfe Department of Surgery, Community Regional Medical Center, Fresno, CA, USA

Philip R. Wolinsky Department of Orthopedic Surgery, University of California-Davis Medical Center, Sacramento, CA, USA

Franklin Wright Division of Trauma, Surgical Critical Care and Burns, Department of Surgery, Stritch School of Medicine, Loyola University Medical Center, Maywood, IL, USA

Michael Wright Department of Orthopaedics and Rehabilitation, University of Vermont/Fletcher Allen Healthcare, Burlington, VT, USA

Raymond D. Jr Wright Department of Orthopaedic Surgery and Sports Medicine, University of Kentucky Chandler Medical Center, Lexington, KY, USA

Young Ho Yun Department of Medicine, Seoul National University College of Medicine, Seoul, South Korea

Patricia L. Zadnik Department of Neurosurgery, The Johns Hopkins University School of Medicine, Baltimore, MD, USA

Dun Yuan Zhou Interdepartmental Division of Critical Care, Institute of Medical Sciences, University of Toronto, Toronto, ON, Canada

Martin D. Zielinski Department of Surgery, Mayo Clinic, Rochester, MN, USA

Bruce H. Ziran Orthopaedic Trauma Surgery, The Hughston Clinic at Gwinnett Medical Center, Lawrenceville, GA, USA

Navid M. Ziran Department of Orthopaedics, Hip and Pelvis Institute, Saint John's Health Center, Santa Monica, CA, USA

Martin P. Zomaya Department of General Surgery, Staten Island University Hospital, Staten Island, NY, USA

A

Abbreviated Laparotomy

▶ Damage Control Surgery

Abbreviated Laparotomy Outcomes

▶ Damage Control Surgery: Outcomes of the Open Abdomen

ABCDE of Trauma Care

Mirsad Dupanovic
Department of Anesthesiology, Kansas
University Medical Center, The University of
Kansas Hospital, Kansas City, KS, USA

Synonyms

Initial trauma assessment; Initial trauma evaluation; Initial trauma resuscitation; Primary trauma survey; The "golden" hour of trauma care

Definition

The ABCDE of trauma care represents a systematic approach to goal-oriented initial evaluation and resuscitation of injured patients. It is a five-step sequence:

- **A**... Airway must be either maintained or secured while protecting the cervical spine
- **B**... Breathing must be either supported or controlled while oxygen is delivered
- **C**... Circulation is supported and hemorrhage contained
- **D**... Disability is assessed and the risk of secondary injury is restricted
- **E**... Exposure helps evaluate the full extent of obvious injuries/Environmental control helps minimize or prevent hypothermia

The ABCDE sequence is usually performed in a coordinated team effort. The primary survey is followed by a more detailed secondary survey. The "golden" hour of trauma care refers to the entire initial period of trauma assessment and resuscitation that plays the crucial role in trauma outcomes. Advanced Trauma Life Support® (ATLS®) represents the foundation of the ABCDE procedure.

Preexisting Condition

The epidemic of trauma has massively increased the need for field responses and hospital treatment of injured patients in the modern era. Injury is a disease that can affect any body system; it may lead to quick deterioration of vital functions, and

© Springer-Verlag Berlin Heidelberg 2015
P.J. Papadakos, M.L. Gestring (eds.), *Encyclopedia of Trauma Care*,
DOI 10.1007/978-3-642-29613-0

an instantaneous or early death. Conversely, consequences of a contained trauma may lead to long-term disease, disability, and late death. It has been emphasized "that injury kills in certain reproducible time frames" and that the greatest threat to life should be recognized and treated first (ATLS 2008). Thus, the purpose of the ABCDE approach is to highlight the effective sequence of evaluation and resuscitation in trauma. The primary survey must never be delayed in order to obtain a detailed medical history. The lack of definitive diagnosis should never impede the application of an indicated treatment.

There are three peaks of death caused by or related to trauma. The tallest peak occurs within 1 hour of injury. Severe traumatic brain injuries and high spinal cord injuries may result in apnea while rupture of the heart or injury of large blood vessels may lead to rapid exsanguination. Rapid physiologic deterioration due to apnea, exsanguination, or both may cause death within minutes of such severe trauma. The second peak occurs within first 24 h of injury (typically within first few hours) as a consequence of concealed hemorrhage within the intracranial, thoracic, abdominal, and pelvic cavities, or hemorrhages at multiple sites. Once the threshold of physiologic decompensation of a vital organ is reached, life-threatening neurologic, respiratory, or hemodynamic deterioration may occur. The third peak of trauma-related death occurs a few weeks subsequent to injury. These late deaths are usually caused by sepsis or multiple organ failure. However, the distribution of deaths may differ between various trauma systems, e.g., urban vs. rural systems. Advanced medical care has improved survival in modern trauma systems, and it has modified the classic trimodal distribution of trauma-related deaths to bimodal distribution. The first peak still occurs within the first hour, while the second peak occurs 24–48 h subsequent to trauma (Demetriades et al. 2005). However, there is no discernible peak of trauma-related death after the 48 h period. The mechanism of injury, the body area affected by the major impact of the mechanical force, and age of the injured patient are the most important determinants of trauma outcome. Severe head injuries do not

follow described temporal distribution of death (Demetriades et al. 2005). In general, penetrating injuries cause more early deaths than blunt injuries. However, blunt trauma may be more difficult to diagnose and treat than penetrating trauma. Assessment is more difficult because the symptoms and signs of internal injuries may be still subclinical and thus the pathologic process not easy to diagnose. Additionally, multiple concurrent injuries may have opposing physiologic resuscitation goals, e.g., coexisting traumatic brain injury vs. intraabdominal hemorrhage. The severity of total body injury in case of multitrauma is related to the number of injuries and to the severity of every individual injury present.

Only injury prevention can significantly reduce the number of instantaneous deaths caused by trauma. This is a major public health problem especially among adolescents and young adults. On the other hand, early recognition of concealed hemorrhage(s) that represent significant threat to life or a vital organ function may help reduce the number of early deaths. Since injuries kill in reproducible time frames and a successful surgical intervention provides a definitive treatment, this initial time period is often referred to as "the golden hour of trauma care." Triage may be necessary in case of multiple persons injured as well as in case of disasters in order to prioritize care based on severity of injuries, make rational decisions about transport, and the most optimal use of available medical resources.

Application

Primary Survey

In order to achieve necessary rapidity and completeness of trauma evaluation and resuscitation, primary survey is usually a team effort. The ABCDE sequence is a process repeated at different levels of care until definitive trauma care can be provided. It starts at the site of injury and it continues on a transport vehicle by the prehospital team. The primary survey is then performed in the emergency room by the hospital team. The initial trauma assessment and resuscitation involves coordinated participation of multiple medical professionals with a team leader facilitating active communication, directing, and supervising procedures. Close communication between the prehospital team and the hospital team is important. On one hand the assistance may be provided to the prehospital team, while on the other hand admitting team's preparation and consequently the trauma patient's resuscitation may be facilitated by such communication. Sometimes, if it is obvious or highly suspected that a potentially lifesaving immediate surgical intervention is unavoidable, the team leader, usually a trauma surgeon, may decide to transfer a trauma victim directly from the emergency room to the operating room. Otherwise the primary survey is followed by the secondary survey, laboratory, and imaging investigations.

Airway

Airway Assessment

Due to the rapidity of hypoxic brain injury, death may be imminent without an immediate intervention in cases of severe airway obstruction or significant ventilatory compromise. Thus, ensuring airway patency, while protecting the cervical spine, is the first resuscitation priority in trauma care. Patient's ability to produce normal voice is a reassuring sign about preserved patency of the upper airway. However, the extent and the mechanism of injury may point toward the potential for development of a progressive and potentially fatal respiratory failure. Progressive airway edema as a consequence of a severe inhalational injury or blunt neck trauma may exemplify such risk. On the other hand, compromise of ventilation is frequent with tension pneumothorax or massive hemothorax. Thus, securing the airway by performing a prophylactic tracheal intubation will prevent the potential for loss of the airway or ventilatory failure under such clinical circumstances.

Airway evaluation is performed simultaneously with administration of supplemental oxygen, assessment of the efficacy of spontaneous ventilation, and measurement of arterial hemoglobin saturation using the pulse oximeter. If airway patency is preserved, spontaneous ventilation is maintained, and an imminent or progressive airway compromise is not anticipated, administration of supplemental oxygen and close monitoring of such trauma victim may be sufficient. Otherwise, airway must be secured while protecting the cervical spine. The patency of a compromised airway may be attained by chin-lift, jaw-thrust, and bag-valve-mask ventilation. Placement of a supraglottic, glottic, or infraglottic airway may follow depending on the initial assessment of the trauma victim, expertise of resuscitators, availability of drugs, and the airway equipment. Any cervical spine movement must be minimized while performing airway rescue procedures either by applying manual inline immobilization or by maintaining cervical collar in place.

Airway Maintenance

Due to multiple circumstantial factors, tracheal intubation in the field may be very challenging, incidence of hypoxia is frequent, and thus risks and benefits of placing an artificial airway, when muscle paralysis is required, must be cautiously considered. This is especially true in medical systems where prehospital trauma care is provided by less experienced providers and risks of intubation failure may be high (Cobas et al. 2009). Hypoxia of significant degree and duration may be especially damaging to patients with traumatic brain injury. Maintenance of normocapnia is another important factor that determines the outcome of brain injured patients (Davis et al. 2004; Boer et al. 2012). Thus, in order to avoid potential devastating risks of muscle paralysis and hypoxia one should always carefully consider feasibility of airway maintenance as an airway management option under difficult trauma circumstances.

Bag-valve-mask ventilation is the first step in maintenance of the airway and it has two goals: (a) assessing its efficacy as a temporary airway maintenance tool and (b) increasing lung oxygen reserve in order to ensure maximal length of the safe apnea time following anesthetic induction. Effective application of bag-valve-mask ventilation may prove difficult in patients having any of the following seven findings: beard, obesity, no dentition, elderly (older than 55), history of snoring, Mallampati class III or IV, and abnormal mandibular protrusion test (El-Orbany and Woehlck 2009). Clinicians often refer to the first five findings by using their initial letters and constructing the mnemonic BONES. Because of frequent difficulty with patient cooperation, assessment of the Mallampati class and mandibular protrusion may be impossible under trauma circumstances. Difficult mask ventilation may be managed by insertion a supraglottic airway as a rescue ventilatory device or as a bridging ventilatory device until a definitive airway can be placed (Dupanovic et al. 2010). Other rescue options include use of an esophageal airway or an esophageal-tracheal tube.

Definitive Airway

Rapid-sequence intubation (RSI) represents a standard approach in attaining and securing the airway. This procedure may be performed in the field, on a transport vehicle, in the emergency room, or in the operating room. Some of the indications for RSI in trauma are apnea, hypoxia, hypercarbia, obtundation, coma, Glasgow Coma Scale ≤8, shock, and severe inhalation injury. Performance of the RSI in the field or on a transport vehicle is much more challenging than in the controlled setting of an emergency room or the operating room. Thus, careful consideration of physical exam findings, vital signs, injuries, and distance to the hospital is necessary before making a decision about the RSI. Preventing additional harm exemplified in hypoxic brain injury or pulmonary aspiration is the highest priority. A trauma victim that requires intravenous drug administration, which will cause apnea, also requires a rapid airway assessment. The mnemonic LEMON (look, evaluate, Mallampati, obstruction, neck mobility) is easy to remember and may be useful in assessment of potential tracheal intubation difficulty. However, there are inherent problems with the validity of airway assessment in general patient population and especially in trauma victims. The Mallampati score has only moderate sensitivity and slightly better specificity. Additionally, a trauma victim may not be cooperative enough to allow oropharyngeal evaluation. Thus, simply looking and evaluating the face, the neck, the ability of the trauma victim to open the mouth, and to produce voice may provide clues about risks of drug-induced apnea. If physical clues pointing toward a difficult tracheal intubation are present and the specific circumstances allow the RSI to be postponed, this should be done until the personnel capable of creating a surgical airway is present and equipment is available (Dupanovic et al. 2010). Since the cervical spine must be protected, manual in-line stabilization will be routinely applied during the RSI in order to reduce neck mobility and restrict the risk of secondary cervical spine injury. However, this protective maneuver may result in increased difficulty of laryngeal visualization, increased pressure of the laryngoscope blade, and potential for pathologic craniocervical motion (Santoni et al. 2009; Aziz 2013). The other feasible protective option that can be used during RSI is leaving the cervical collar in place and using a video laryngoscope for tracheal intubation.

Breathing

Airway patency is only a prerequisite for adequate ventilation, which will depend on proper function of the entire respiratory system. In trauma situations, this particularly means intact function of the chest wall, diaphragm, and lungs. Physical assessment of these components is accomplished by inspection, palpation, and auscultation. Inspection may detect signs of respiratory distress or a penetrating chest wall injury. Palpation of the chest may detect subcutaneous emphysema or rib fractures. Auscultation will evaluate for presence and quality of breath sounds. Pulse oxymetry will provide a quick assessment of oxygenation. Severe chest injuries such as tension pneumothorax or massive hemothorax may compromise gas exchange, hemodynamic status, and may require immediate interventions. These conditions should be diagnosed during the primary survey. Chest X-ray will help diagnose lung or chest wall injuries that have compromised ventilatory function to a lesser degree and have not been diagnosed during the primary survey. However, it should be also noted that tracheal intubation and vigorous ventilation can uncover and exacerbate a subclinical pneumothorax. Thus, chest X-ray should be obtained as soon as practical following tracheal intubation.

Circulation

The shock represents inadequate vital organ perfusion and oxygen delivery due to circulatory failure. The hypovolemic shock is almost the norm in severe trauma and is most commonly due to hemorrhage. The chance of survival of a bleeding trauma victim will mostly depend on its location and severity. The first priority in restoring adequate circulation is stopping the bleeding, while the second priority is replacing the intravascular volume. On the other hand, hypovolemic shock caused by loss of fluid and plasma with extensive burns should be aggressively treated with crystalloids and colloids as indicated. Obstructive shock may be a consequence of a tension pneumothorax and traumatic pericardial tamponade. Neurogenic shock may be a consequence of spinal cord injury.

External hemorrhage should be identified and contained during the initial assessment. Major body cavities are the main areas of concealed blood loss: the chest, abdominal cavity, retroperitoneal space, and pelvis. Pneumatic antishock garments can decrease bleeding in the abdomen, pelvis, and lower extremities. Bleeding in the abdominal cavity may tamponade itself and may allow time for completion of necessary diagnostic evaluation. Bleeding from intercostals arteries often slows or stops following chest tube placement and lung expansion. However, if severe cavitary injury is not amenable to the above resuscitative measures and is causing rapid hemodynamic deterioration, an emergent surgical exploration may be necessary based just on the clinical assessment during the primary survey.

Basic hemodynamic assessment includes inspection and palpation of skin (color and temperature of extremities as well as capillary refill), pulse palpation (the rate, regularity, and strength), and assessment of patient's level of consciousness. Jugular venous distension may be a presenting sign of the obstructive shock. Noninvasive blood pressure measurements and ECG may provide additional information if available. Signs of poor circulation include pale, cyanotic, cool extremities with delayed capillary refill, tachycardia, weak peripheral pulses, altered level of consciousness, and hypotension. However, different age groups may have different physiologic reserves and different responses to hemorrhage. Children and well-trained athletes may have large physiologic reserves and tachycardia and/or hypotension may be a late sign of hypovolemia. Once these signs become apparent, hemodynamic deterioration may occur very rapidly. On the other hand, elderly patients may have a limited physiologic reserve and their hemodynamic deterioration as a response to hemorrhage may occur much sooner. Additionally, administration of beta-blockers or other cardiotropic medications may further modify patient's hemodynamic response. A comprehensive evaluation, anticipation based on the mechanism of injury, and frequent reevaluation are necessary in order to avoid missed injuries and rapid deterioration of hemodynamic status because of under resuscitation.

Disability

A rapid neurologic evaluation as a component of the primary survey establishes the patient's level of consciousness, pupillary size and reaction, and signs of spinal cord injury. Glasgow Coma Scale (GCS) should be performed to evaluate motor response (1–6), verbal response (1–5), and eye response (1–4). The minimum GCS is 3 points and the maximum is 15 points. The GCS is predictive of patient neurologic outcome. An altered level of consciousness requires reevaluation of ABCs. Drug abuse and hypoglycemia should also be considered. If these factors are excluded, traumatic brain injury should be considered until proven otherwise. The GCS 13–14 represents mild impairment, 9–12 moderate, and 3–8 represents severe neurologic impairment.

Exposure/Environmental Control

Undressing the patient facilitates assessment of the extent of injury. However, this should take place in a warm environment in order to prevent unnecessary and potentially harmful heat loss. With the same goal in mind, the patient should be covered with warm blankets after completion of the assessment. Additionally, pre-warming of crystalloids and warming all other intravenous fluids and blood products during their administration is another important strategy in preventing perioperative hypothermia in trauma care.

Cross-References

▶ Abdominal Major Vascular Injury, Anesthesia for
▶ Burn Anesthesia
▶ Cardiac and Aortic Trauma, Anesthesia for
▶ Diaphragmatic Injuries
▶ Head Injury
▶ Hemorrhage
▶ Hemorrhagic Shock
▶ Hypothermia, Trauma, and Anesthetic Management
▶ Pediatric Trauma, Assessment, and Anesthetic Management
▶ Pneumothorax
▶ Pulmonary Contusion
▶ Trauma Patient Evaluation
▶ Shock
▶ Spinal Shock

References

American College of Surgeons Committee on Trauma (2008) Advanced Trauma Life Support® for Doctors (ATLS®) Student Course Manual, 8th edn. American College of Surgeons Committee on Trauma, Chicago
Aziz M (2013) Use of video-assisted intubation devices in the management of patients with trauma. Anesthesiol Clin 31:157–166
Boer C, Franschman G, Loer AS (2012) Prehospital management of severe traumatic brain injury: concepts and ongoing controversies. Curr Opin Anesthesiol 25:556–562
Cobas MA, De la Pena MA, Manning R et al (2009) Prehospital intubations and mortality; a level 1 trauma center perspective. Anesth Analg 109:489–493
Davis DP, Dunford JV, Poste JC et al (2004) The impact of hypoxia and hyperventilation on outcome after paramedic rapid sequence intubation of severely head-injured patients. J Trauma 57:1–10
Demetriades D, Kimbrell B, Salim A et al (2005) Trauma death in a mature trauma urban system: is "trimodal" distribution a valid concept? J Am Coll Surg 201:343–348
Dupanovic M, Fox H, Kovac A (2010) Management of the airway in multitrauma. Curr Opin Anesthesiol 23:276–282
El-Orbany M, Woehlck AJ (2009) Difficult mask ventilation. Anesth Analg 109:1870–1880
Santoni BG, Hindman BJ, Puttlitz CM et al (2009) Manual in-line stabilization increases pressures applied by the laryngoscope blade during direct laryngoscopy and orotracheal intubation. Anesthesiology 110:24–31

Abdominal Aorta Injury

▶ Abdominal Major Vascular Injury, Anesthesia for

Abdominal Compartment Syndrome as a Complication of Care

Khanjan H. Nagarsheth
R Adams Cowley Shock Trauma Center, University of Maryland School of Medicine, Baltimore, MD, USA

Synonyms

Abdominal compartment syndrome; Intra-abdominal hypertension

Definition

Introduction

Intra-abdominal hypertension (IAH) and abdominal compartment syndrome (ACS) are causes of morbidity and mortality in critically ill patients. It is important to realize that IAH and ACS may affect almost every organ system (Cheatham 2011).

Intra-abdominal pressure (IAP) is normally 5–7 mmHg in adults. IAH is as sustained or repeated pathologic elevation of IAP of 12 mmHg or greater. This is further subdivided into four grades based on pressure value. ACS is sustained IAP greater than 20 mmHg associated with new organ dysfunction/failure (Cheatham 2011). Causes of IAH and ACS include, but are not limited to, intra-abdominal hemorrhage, pneumoperitoneum from perforated viscus, and, most importantly in the trauma patient, third spacing of fluid during massive resuscitation.

Preexisting Condition

Physiology

Cardiovascular
Cardiac dysfunction is seen in patients with IAH and ACS due to increased intrathoracic pressure (ITP) from upward displacement of the diaphragm. This increased ITP causes decreased venous return to the heart, thereby reducing cardiac output. When treating patients with IAH or ACS, there is an association between intra-abdominal pressure (IAP) and ITP (Wauters et al. 2007). Fifty percent of the IAP is transmitted and affects the ITP. Cheatham and colleagues point out that catheter-based hemodynamic measures such as pulmonary artery occlusion pressure and central venous pressure, therefore, have significant limitations as indices of volume status in the face of IAH. Volumetric measurements such as end-diastolic volume index can aid in directing adequate resuscitation in these patients. Knowing this transmitted relationship and using volume indexes for estimation of preload could help to prevent inadequate resuscitation and inappropriate use of vasoactive agents in patients with IAH or ACS. Resuscitation efforts geared towards a right ventricular end-diastolic volume index (RVEDVI) goal-directed model have been shown in the literature to result in reduction of multiple organ failure (MOF) and death (Cheatham et al. 1999). Using cardiac echo and ultrasonography as a way of guiding resuscitation efforts in a patient with IAH and ACS can help to avoid the dreaded complications of these disease processes.

Respiratory
IAH results in increased ITP by decreasing chest wall compliance and pulmonary parenchymal compression. Pulmonary compression causes increased pulmonary intravascular pressure and pulmonary hypertension. In order to overcome the alveolar compression and atelectasis, PEEP is increased or added, in order to maintain oxygenation and ventilation. Aggressive PEEP can result in not only opening up atelectatic areas of the lung but also overdistending the normal lung and also inhibiting adequate ventilation (Cheatham 2011).

Renal
One of the first signs of end-organ hypoperfusion associated with IAH and ACS is decreased urine output. Renal dysfunction due to IAH usually presents with oliguria at 15 mmHg and anuria at 30 mmHg in euvolemic patients with no underlying renal disease. This is believed to be due to compression of the renal parenchyma and renal vein along with decreased renal perfusion pressures. This leads to renal microcirculatory dysfunction and decreased urine output. Urine output is dependent on the renal filtration gradient (FG) or the glomerular filtration pressure (GFP) minus the proximal tubular pressure (PTP) that can be estimated as mean arterial pressure (MAP) minus two times the IAP (Cheatham 2011):

$$FG = GFP - PTP = MAP - 2 \times IAP$$

Application

Assessment of Intra-Abdominal Hypertension and Abdominal Compartment Syndrome.

Intravesicular Pressure
Measurements are performed using a bladder pressure monitor at the end of expiration in a supine position with the transducer zeroed at the iliac crest in the midaxillary line using 25 mL of saline instilled into the bladder.

The measurement is taken in mmHg between 30 and 60 s after the saline is instilled and catheter clamped. A caveat is that all abdominal muscle contractions should be absent during the measurement (Cheatham et al. 2006).

Intragastric Pressure

Intragastric pressure (IGP) monitoring has been used in place of bladder pressure monitoring in some experimental models to obtain an abdominal pressure reading (Decramer et al. 1984). There is a close relationship between IAP and IGP with potential for inaccuracy in patients with ileus and in those who are being enterally fed.

Abdominal Sonography in the Diagnosis of IAH and ACS

Cavaliere and associates described the use of ultrasound to measure changes in abdominal vein dimension in the setting of simulated increased abdominal pressure in normal volunteers as a marker of ACS. The authors used a pelvic binder to create external compression, inducing mild IAH (Cavaliere et al. 2011). They used a Doppler to measure peak blood flow velocities at the end of expiration and also measured the diameter of the inferior vena cava (IVC) below the renal veins, the right suprahepatic vein, the portal vein (PV), the right external iliac vein, and the segmental branches of the right renal artery. Statistically significant changes in IVC and PV diameters were noted. There was no significant change noted in peak velocities through any of the vessels noted above, although there was significant variability between individuals. There is evidence based on CT scan studies that reveal certain findings such as distorted IVC shape and decreased AP diameter as well as flattening of renal vasculature (Patel et al. 2007). It is reasonable, based on the data presented by Cavaliere's group, to extrapolate that these findings would hold true on US in patients with a diagnosis of IAH or ACS.

Renal Duplex Ultrasound

Renal duplex ultrasonography has been used in patients with many different kidney diseases to determine their renal resistive index (RI which correlates with renal function (Tublin et al. 2003). The RI is defined as (peak systolic velocity – end-diastolic velocity)/peak systolic velocity. The method for obtaining the images as described in the literature involves obtaining a pulse wave Doppler sampling of the vessel at a 60° angle to the US beam. Signals are obtained from the interlobar arteries along the border of the medullary pyramids. Typically one will obtain images and measurements at multiple points in the organ and average these values to calculate the RI. The normal mean value for the RI is about 0.60 for patients without underlying renal disease (Keogan et al. 1996). Cavaliere's group also looked at the renal microvasculature with Duplex ultrasonography and calculated the RI in their subjects. The RI was found to be higher in the subjects with mild IAH. Although there has been some controversy as to the usefulness of RI in patients with vascular-interstitial diseases, there may be a role for its use in helping to identify ACS at the renal microvascular level.

Focused Transthoracic Echocardiography

The purpose of using transthoracic echocardiography (TTE) in patients with IAH and ACS is to determine cardiac function, intraventricular filling, and intravascular volume status quickly and in a noninvasive manner. TTE can then be a tool utilized by the clinician to garner information and then base resuscitation efforts on volumetric measurements (Cheatham et al. 1999). Classical methods of assessing cardiac function and fluid status include the use of pulmonary artery catheters and obtaining a pulmonary artery occlusion pressure (PAOP) measurement. There have been several studies that have shown no survival benefit to employing this invasive technique. Therefore using TTE to assess cardiac function and assess volume status is a reasonable alternative in people with IAH and ACS as it is noninvasive and poses less potential risk to the patient.

Treatment of Abdominal Compartment Syndrome

Decompressive laparotomy (DL) is the definitive treatment of ACS. A recent meta-analysis of

18 studies published between 1972 and 2004 looked at the effects of DL on patients with ACS (De Waele et al. 2006). These 18 studies yielded a total of 250 patients that had been treated for ACS with DL. Of the 250 patients noted, 161 were found to have before and after IAP recorded in relation to their DL. As expected there was a statistically significant drop in IAP from a mean of 34.6 mmHg to a mean of 15.5 mmHg. They also noted that the mortality in these studies, after DL, ranged from 22 % to 100 % with a mean of 49.2 %. This meta-analysis noted that there were some improvements noted in cardiac output, urine output, and respiratory function as evidenced by improved PaO_2/FiO_2.

Nonoperative management of IAH and ACS includes five alternate therapies, all aimed at reduction of IAP. These therapies include the following: (1) evacuation of intraluminal contents, (2) evacuation of intra-abdominal space-occupying lesions, (3) improvement of abdominal wall compliance, (4) optimization of fluid administration, and (5) optimization of systemic and regional tissue perfusion (Cheatham 2009). Each of these five therapies consists of escalating interventions, from noninvasive to more invasive with the final step consisting of DL.

In looking more closely at the second therapy listed, the graded management algorithm put forth by Dr. Cheatham involves first obtaining an abdominal ultrasound to identify the space-occupying lesion or fluid collection. Hemoperitoneum, ascites, intra-abdominal abscess, retroperitoneal hemorrhage, and free air can all be space-occupying lesions that can raise the IAP. A recent review of results of percutaneous drainage for the treatment of IAH/ACS revealed a success rate of 81 % (25/31) in avoiding a DL (Cheatham and Safcsak 2011). This same group found that successful management of IAH/ACS with percutaneous drainage was associated with drainage of greater than 1,000 mL of fluid or decrease in IAP by greater than 9 mmHg in the first 4 h after placement of the drain. They recommended that in patients with significant IAH (which they defined as IAP 20–25 mmHg) or patients with ACS, bedside ultrasound should be performed to confirm the presence of free intra-abdominal fluid or blood. If a sufficient fluid pocket is identified which would allow for safe placement of a drainage catheter, this should be performed. Of course, a caveat is in using US to decompress someone who is actively bleeding and needs to be in the operating room or in an interventional radiology/angiography suite to address it, apart from the ACS.

Cross-References

▶ Acute Abdominal Compartment Syndrome in Trauma

References

Cavaliere F, Cina A, Biasucci D, Costa R et al (2011) Sonographic assessment of abdominal vein dimensional and hemodynamic changes induced in human volunteers by a model of abdominal hypertension. Crit Care Med 32(2):344–348

Cheatham ML (2009) Nonoperative management of intraabdominal hypertension and abdominal compartment syndrome. World J Surg 33:1116–1122

Cheatham ML, Safcsak K (2011) Percutaneous catheter decompression in the treatment of elevated intraabdominal pressure. Chest 140:1428–1435

Cheatham M, Safcsak K, Block E et al (1999) Preload assessment in patients with an open abdomen. J Trauma 46(1):16–22

Cheatham ML, Malbrain ML, Kirkpatrick A et al (2006) Results from the international conference of experts on intra-abdominal hypertension and abdominal compartment syndrome. I. Definitions. Intensive Care Med 32(11):1722–1732

Cheatham ML, Malbrain ML, Kirkpatrick A et al (2011) Definitions and pathophysiological implications of intra-abdominal hypertension and abdominal compartment syndrome. Am Surg 77(Suppl 1):S6–S11

De Waele JJ, Hoste EA, Malbrain ML (2006) Decompressive laparotomy for abdominal compartment syndrome—a critical analysis. Crit Care 10:R51

Decramer M, De Troyer A, Kelly S et al (1984) Regional differences in abdominal pressure swings in dogs. J Appl Physiol 57:1682–1687

Keogan M, Kliewer M, Hertzberg B, DeLong DM, Tupler RH, Carroll BA (1996) Renal resistive indexes: variability in Doppler US measurement in a healthy population. Radiology 199:165–169

Patel A, Lall CG, Jennings SG et al (2007) Abdominal compartment syndrome. AJR Am J Roentgenol 189:1037–1043

Tublin ME, Bude RO, Platt JF (2003) The resistive index in renal doppler sonography: where do we stand? Am J Roentgenol 180:885–892
Wauters J, Wilmer A, Valenza F (2007) Abdomino-thoracic transmission during ACS: facts and figures. Acta Clin Belg Suppl 1:200–205

Suggested Reading

Cheatham ML, Malbrain ML (2007) Cardiovascular implications of abdominal compartment syndrome. Acta Clin Belg Suppl 62:98–112
Papavramidis TS, Marinis AD, Pliakos I, Kesisoglou I, Papavramidou N (2011) Abdominal compartment syndrome – intra-abdominal hypertension: defining, diagnosing, and managing. J Emerg Trauma Shock 4:279–291
Richard C, Warszawski J, Anguel N et al (2003) Early use of the pulmonary artery catheter and outcomes in patients with shock and acute respiratory distress syndrome: a randomized controlled trial. JAMA 290(20):2713–2720

Abdominal Compartment Syndrome

Jennifer Knight
Department of Surgery, West Virginia University, Morgantown, WV, USA

Synonyms

Elevated intra-abdominal pressure; Intra-abdominal hypertension

Definition

Abdominal compartment syndrome is a disease process in critically ill patients from an elevation of intra-abdominal pressures that results in multisystem organ dysfunction or failure.

Preexisting Condition

Causes of Abdominal Compartment Syndrome

Abdominal compartment syndrome (ACS) and intra-abdominal hypertension result from increase intra-abdominal pressures within the confines of the abdominal cavity. This elevation in pressure leads to impairment of the cardiac, pulmonary, renal, gastrointestinal, hepatic, and central nervous system function. There are both surgical and nonsurgical causes of abdominal compartment syndrome, and it is increasingly recognized as a potential complication in critically ill patients.

Abdominal compartment syndrome can occur from acute or chronic problems as listed in the following table (Table 1). ACS can also be classified by primary abdominal pathologies or secondary to non-abdominal causes (Papavramidis et al. 2011).

Pathophysiology of Abdominal Compartment Syndrome

The abdominal compartment is a closed space involving the diaphragm, pelvis, spine, and abdominal wall musculature. While there is some elasticity to this compartment, the overall pressure within this space is at a steady state. Should the volume of any of the contents of this space increase, the pressure within the space will increase as well. The resting pressure within the abdomen is 0 mm Hg in a normal patient and 5–7 mm Hg in critical illness. Abdominal perfusion pressure is calculated as the mean arterial pressure minus the intra-abdominal pressure (IAP). Increases in IAP can result in compromise of venous and arterial blood flow within the abdomen.

The World Society of the Abdominal Compartment Syndrome (https://www.wsacs.org) has defined intra-abdominal hypertension as a graded disease process – Grade I: IAP 12–15 mm Hg, Grade II: 16–20 mm Hg, Grade III: 21–25 mm Hg, and Grade IV: IAP > 25 mm Hg. Abdominal compartment syndrome is further subclassified as hyperacute, acute, subacute, and chronic based on the time the elevated pressure is maintained.

End-organ dysfunction that results from ACS can affect many organ systems (Papavramidis et al. 2011). Cardiovascular effects involve compression of the intra-abdominal vessels and result in decreased preload of the heart due to vena cava compression and increased afterload due to increased systemic vascular resistance from compression of the abdominal aorta. As pressure is transmitted across the diaphragm to the chest,

Abdominal Compartment Syndrome, Table 1 Causes of abdominal compartment syndrome

Acute causes of abdominal compartment syndrome	Chronic causes of abdominal compartment syndrome	Secondary causes of abdominal compartment syndrome
Hemorrhage – intra-abdominal or retroperitoneal	Intra-abdominal or retroperitoneal tumor	Respiratory failure requiring high positive end expiratory pressure
Peritonitis or intra-abdominal abscess	Ascites from liver failure or malignancy	Massive fluid resuscitation
Pancreatitis	Pregnancy	Prone positioning
Bowel distension from ileus, obstruction, pseudo-obstruction	Obesity	Peritoneal dialysis
Abdominal surgery with tight fascial closure		
Repair or reduction of large hernia		
Insufflation with laparoscopic surgery		
Burns		

respiratory failure will worsen as tidal volumes decrease and intrathoracic pressures increase. Renal perfusion will be compromised resulting in decreased urine output. Gastrointestinal absorption and motility are impaired. Liver function is decreased and direct hepatocellular damage can occur.

Application

Diagnosis of Abdominal Compartment Syndrome

The diagnosis of abdominal compartment syndrome is not always straightforward. The combination of elevated intra-abdominal pressures and its consequence on organ function that make the diagnosis (An and West 2008).

Signs and symptoms may be limited subjectively due to this process being present in critically ill patients. Physical exam findings that suggest elevated intra-abdominal pressures include abdominal distention or peritonitis with guarding or rigidity. Other signs may be increased need for ventilator support either by the need for increased pressure or volume needed depending on the mode of ventilation being used. Poor urine output and feeding intolerance may also be early signs of organ dysfunction.

There is no imaging study that can reliably diagnose ACS. Plain x-ray may show distended bowel loops. Ultrasonography may show the presence or

an increase of abdominal free fluid. CT imaging can show abdominal pathologies that may lead to or be a result of increased abdominal pressures such as bowel edema or ischemia, or flattening of the vena cava. None of these diagnose ACS; they may add, however, to the information needed to make the diagnosis in a critically ill patient.

Measurement of intra-abdominal pressures remains the most accurate means of diagnosing ACS as physical exam and radiographs have poor sensitivity and specificity. IAP monitoring can be performed directly or indirectly, intermittently or continuously, and is safe and inexpensive. IAP measurements from the bladder or foley are most commonly used; however, nasogastric or direct measurement through an intraperitoneal catheter is an alternative if the foley cannot be used.

Abdominal compartment syndrome results from the end-organ dysfunction that results from prolonged elevated intra-abdominal hypertension and is defined as a pathologic state caused by IAP > 20–25 mm Hg, the presence of end-organ dysfunction with the need for abdominal decompression.

Treatment/Decompression of Abdominal Compartment Syndrome

Preventative efforts are the first line options for treatment of ACS. Fluid overload in the setting of intra-abdominal sepsis, bowel obstruction, or hemorrhage control are the lead causes of elevated intra-abdominal pressures. Early detection

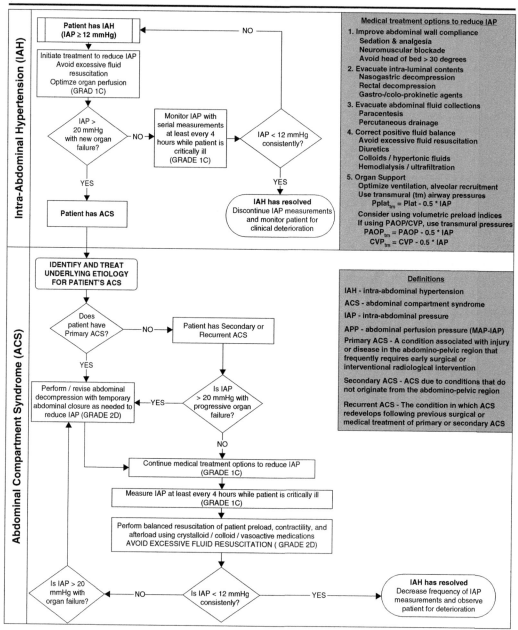

Abdominal Compartment Syndrome, Fig. 1 Intra-abdominal hypertension/abdominal compartment syndrome management algorithm

of elevated pressures can prevent progression to end-organ dysfunction.

The World Society of the Abdominal Compartment syndrome published an updated intra-abdominal hypertension and abdominal compartment syndrome consensus defintion and clinical practice guideline in 2013. The WSACS's most recent recommendations for the clinical practice guidelines are listed in Figs. 1 and 2. A summary of management recommendations

IAH / ACS MEDICAL MANAGEMENT ALGORITHM

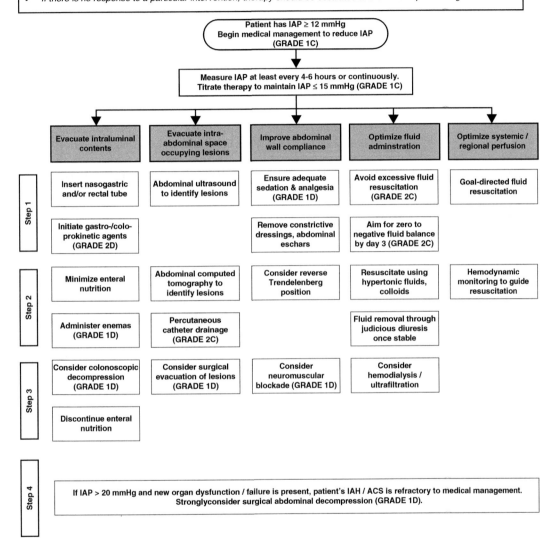

- The choice (and success of the medical management strategies listed below is strongly related to both the etiology of the patient's IAH / ACS and the patient's clinical situation. The aproriateness of each intervention should always be considered prior to implementing these interventions in any individual patient.
- The invterventions should be applied in a stepwise fashion until the patient's intra-abdominal pressure (IAP) decreases.
- If there is no response to a particular intervention, therapy should be escalated to the next step in the algorithm.

Patient has IAP ≥ 12 mmHg
Begin medical management to reduce IAP
(GRADE 1C)

Measure IAP at least every 4-6 hours or continuously.
Titrate therapy to maintain IAP ≤ 15 mmHg (GRADE 1C)

| Evacuate intraluminal contents | Evacuate intra-abdominal space occupying lesions | Improve abdominal wall compliance | Optimize fluid adminstration | Optimize systemic / regional perfusion |

Step 1

| Insert nasogastric and/or rectal tube | Abdominal ultrasound to identify lesions | Ensure adequate sedation & analgesia (GRADE 1D) | Avoid excessive fluid resuscitation (GRADE 2C) | Goal-directed fluid resuscitation |
| Initiate gastro-/colo-prokinetic agents (GRADE 2D) | | Remove constrictive dressings, abdominal eschars | Aim for zero to negative fluid balance by day 3 (GRADE 2C) | |

Step 2

| Minimize enteral nutrition | Abdominal computed tomography to identify lesions | Consider reverse Trendelenberg position | Resuscitate using hypertonic fluids, colloids | Hemodynamic monitoring to guide resuscitation |
| Administer enemas (GRADE 1D) | Percutaneous catheter drainage (GRADE 2C) | | Fluid removal through judicious diuresis once stable | |

Step 3

| Consider colonoscopic decompression (GRADE 1D) | Consider surgical evacuation of lesions (GRADE 1D) | Consider neuromuscular blockade (GRADE 1D) | Consider hemodialysis / ultrafiltration | |
| Discontinue enteral nutrition | | | | |

Step 4

If IAP > 20 mmHg and new organ dysfunction / failure is present, patient's IAH / ACS is refractory to medical management. Stronglyconsider surgical abdominal decompression (GRADE 1D).

Abdominal Compartment Syndrome, Fig. 2 Intra-abdominal hypertension/abdominal compartment syndrome medical management algorithm

for noninvasive and minimally invasive treatment is listed in the following table (Table 2).

It should be noted that while the WSACS makes no recommendations for diuretics, renal replacement therapies, or albumin use, this statement is made because no randomized controlled trials exist.

Multiple review articles still list these therapies as viable options for medical treatment of ACS.

It is recommended that patients with ACS with an intra-abdominal pressure of greater than 20 mm Hg and signs of organ dysfunction (abdominal distention, decompensating cardiac, pulmonary,

Abdominal Compartment Syndrome, Table 2 Summary of recommendations from the WSACS (Kirkpatrick et al. 2013)

Noninvasive and minimally invasive treatment	Recommended (yes or no or suggest)	Comments
Sedation and analgesia	Suggest	Suggest that optimal pain and anxiety relief be achieved
Neuromuscular blockade	Suggest	Brief trials as a temporizing measure
Body positioning	Suggest	Some body positions may elevate IAP
Nasogastric/colonic decompression	Suggest	Liberal use when the stomach or colon is dilated in the presence of IAH/ACS
Promotility agents	Suggest	Neostigmine be used for the treatment of established colonic ileus not responsive to simple measures
Negative or neutral fluid balance	Suggest	A protocol to avoid positive accumulative fluid balance
Diuretics	No recommendation	There is lack of evidence to support this intervention
Renal replacement therapies	No recommendation	There is lack of evidence to support this intervention
Albumin	No recommendation	There is lack of evidence to support this intervention
Damage control resuscitation	Suggest	Use of enhanced ration of plasma/packed red blood cells for massive hemorrhage
Paracentesis	Suggest	May be useful when obvious intraperitoneal fluid is present and is preventing decompressive laparotomy

and renal dysfunction) should undergo emergent or urgent decompressive laparotomy. Laparotomy should be considered in acute increased intra-abdominal pressure of greater than 25 mm Hg without organ dysfunction.

When preparing for decompressive laparotomy, it is important to ensure that the patient is adequately resuscitated. The acute drop in intra-abdominal pressure that occurs with decompression significantly lowers preload and will result in hypotension or perhaps cardiac arrest. Communication with the anesthesiologist at the time of operation is essential.

Once decompression has occurred, the open abdomen should be managed with negative pressure wound therapy. Primary fascial closure should be achieved during the same hospital stay as this decreases morbidity and improves quality of life for these patients.

Complications of Abdominal Compartment Syndrome

Death is the worst complication that can occur from abdominal compartment syndrome, either as a direct result of ACS or the process that caused the ACS. Prevention, early detection, and aggressive treatment are all measures to decrease mortality from ACS.

Primary fascial closure is the goal for definitive closure of the abdomen once the underlying process is resolved and the patient is more stable. The success rate of primary fascial closure varies greatly across institutions. When primary fascial closure is not achieved, multiple options are available for definitive closure, but all of these require more surgical operations. Enterocutaneous or entero-atmospheric fistulas may result. The morbidity and decrease in quality of life is increased if primary fascial closure cannot be achieved at the time of initial hospitalization (Diaz et al. 2010).

The multisystem organ failure that accompanies abdominal compartment syndrome may be transient or could become permanent. Renal failure requiring dialysis and respiratory failure requiring tracheostomy are all possible complications from ACS.

Cross-References

References

An G, West M (2008) Abdominal compartment syndrome: a concise clinical review. Crit Care Med 36:1304–1310

Diaz J, Cullinane D, Dutton W, Jerome R, Bagdonas R, Bilaniuk J, Collier B, Como J, Cummin J, Griffen M, Gunter O, Kirby J, Lottenburg L, Mowery N, Riodan W, Martin N, Platz J, Stassen N, Winston E (2010) The management of the open abdomen in trauma and emergency general surgery: part 1 – damage control. J Traum 68:1424–1438

https://www.wsacs.org. Accessed 27 Jan 2014

Kirkpatrick A, Roberts D, Waele J, Jaeschke R, Malbrain M, Keulenaer B, Duchesnes J, Bjorck M, Leppaniemi A, Ejike J, Sugrue M, Cheatham M, Ivatury R, Ball C, Blaser A, Regli A, Balogh Z, D'Amours S, Debergh D, Kaplan M, Kimball E, Olvera C (2013) Intra-abdominal hypertension and the abdominal compartment syndrome: updated consensus definitions and clinical practice guidelines from the World Society of the Abdominal Compartment Syndrome. Intensive Care Med 39:1190–1206

Papavramidis T, Marinis A, Pilakos I, Kesisoglou I, Papavramidou N (2011) Abdominal compartment syndrome – intra-abdominal hypertension: defining, diagnosis, and managing. J Emerg Trauma Shock 4:279–291

Abdominal Major Vascular Injury, Anesthesia for

A

Zana Borovcanin
Department of Anesthesiology, University of Rochester School of Medicine and Dentistry, Rochester, NY, USA

Synonyms

Abdominal aorta injury; Celiac artery injury; Iliac vascular injury; Inferior vena cava injury; Mesenteric artery injury; Renovascular injury

Definition

The abdominal major vascular injuries are usually caused by penetrating abdominal traumas, gunshot wounds, or stab wounds. The blunt abdominal trauma may also cause major vascular injuries by rapid deceleration mechanism, direct anteroposterior crushing, or direct laceration. In a prospective study of vascular abdominal trauma caused by gunshot injuries in 217 patients who underwent exploratory laparotomy, the incidence of vascular trauma was 14.3 % (Demetriades et al. 1997). The incidence of vascular injuries in patients undergoing laparotomy for stab wounds was 10 % (Feliciano et al. 2000). In a review of 302 abdominal vascular injuries, the most commonly injured abdominal vessel was the inferior vena cava (accounted for 25 % of injuries), followed by aorta (21 %), the iliac arteries (20 %), the iliac veins (17 %), the superior mesenteric vein (11 %), and the superior mesenteric artery (10 %) (Asensio et al. 2000).

Preexisting Conditions

For major vascular trauma purposes, the abdomen is conventionally divided in four anatomic areas (Fig. 1).

Abdominal Major Vascular Injury, Anesthesia for, Fig. 1 Retroperitoneal vascular zones

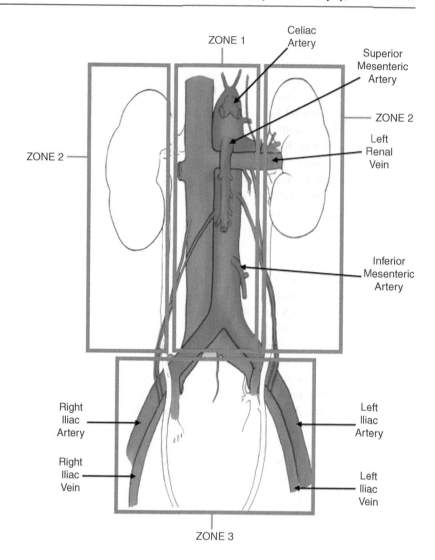

Zone 1 (upper, central box) is the upper midline retroperitoneum, from the aortic hiatus to the aortic bifurcation longitudinally and laterally from renal hilum to renal hilum. This zone is subdivided into supramesocolic and inframesocolic regions. It contains the midline vessels, the aorta, the celiac artery, the superior and inferior mesenteric arteries and veins, the renal arteries and veins, as well as the inferior vena cava.

Zone 2 (upper left and right boxes) is the lateral perinephric area, encompassing the upper lateral retroperitoneum from the renal hilum laterally. It contains the renal vessels.

Zone 3 (lower box) is the pelvic retroperitoneum from the aortic bifurcation inferiorly. It contains the iliac vessels.

Zone 4 is the perihepatic area, which contains the hepatic artery and veins, the portal vein, and the retrohepatic inferior vena cava.

Anatomic Location of Hemorrhage

Midline supramesocolic hemorrhage or hematoma (superior to the transverse mesocolon) is usually caused by injury to the suprarenal aorta, the celiac axis, the proximal superior mesenteric artery, or the proximal renal artery. Midline inframesocolic hemorrhage or hematoma results from infrarenal aorta or inferior vena cava injury. Lateral perirenal hematoma or hemorrhage suggests injury to the renal vessels or kidneys. Lateral pelvic hematoma or hemorrhage indicates injury to the iliac artery, the iliac vein, or both. Hepatoduodenal ligament hematoma or hemorrhage indicates injury to the portal vein, the hepatic artery, or both. Injury of the aorta above or involving superior mesenteric artery will produce abdominal pain, pararenal involvement may lead to hematuria, or injury to the infrarenal aorta may manifest as unilateral or bilateral lower extremity ischemia.

Resuscitation

Patients sustaining major vascular injury usually present with severe physiologic derangements due to hemorrhage, tissue hypoxia, and the sequelae of anaerobic metabolism. Severe hemorrhage may lead to "lethal triad" of trauma: hypothermia, coagulopathy, and acidosis. Patients require massive transfusion, generally defined as requiring greater than twenty units of packed red blood cells (PRBCs) within 24 h or more than 4–5 units within an hour. Many current prehospital resuscitation protocols recommend insertion of peripheral intravenous lines and resuscitation with isotonic crystalloid solution as soon as possible following trauma. On arrival to the emergency department the patient should have inserted a minimum of two large caliber intravenous lines (if not already placed in prehospital setting) and an arterial line inserted in the upper extremities. If adequate peripheral intravenous access is not possible to obtain, central line should be inserted at thoracic inlet (internal jugular or subclavian veins). The access site should be above the diaphragm in any patient with possibility of abdominal or pelvic bleeding. At the time of line insertion, blood should be drawn for type and crossmatch, arterial blood gas, and laboratory studies (CBC, chemistry, and coagulation). Blood bank should be contacted and massive transfusion protocol should be activated. Monitoring used during the resuscitation phase includes electrocardiography, blood pressure monitoring, pulse oximetry, and capnography in intubated patient. Placement of urinary and nasogastric catheters is also considered part of the resuscitation phase. Diagnostic testing, radiologic examination, and essential laboratory tests should not delay patient's resuscitation and transfer to the operating room as indicated.

Trauma room preparation should include setting up all equipment necessary for the management of major trauma: rapid transfusion device, fluid warmers, autologous cell saver device, difficult intubation cart, equipment necessary for the placement of invasive monitors, and infusion pumps as necessary. The operating room environment should be maintained as warm as possible, and the infused fluid should be prewarmed to 40–42 °C. Blood and blood products should be immediately available in the operating room. If patient is hemodynamically unstable and crossmatched blood is not available, blood transfusion should be initiated with uncrossmatched blood (O Rh negative PRBC). If uncrossmatched blood transfusion was initiated, transfusion should be converted to type-specific blood as soon as that one becomes available. Serial measurement of hematocrit, ionized calcium, and coagulation parameters is necessary for guiding transfusion of blood products (PRBC, fresh frozen plasma, platelets, and cryoprecipitate).

Application

Anesthetic Management

Monitoring
Besides the American Society of Anesthesiologists standard monitoring, invasive monitoring is necessary for abdominal major vascular injury cases: arterial line, central venous pressure, and potentially transesophageal echocardiography. Arterial line is important for hemodynamic management on induction and during maintenance of anesthesia and should be placed prior to induction of anesthesia.

Induction of Anesthesia
These patients are considered "full stomach" with high risk of aspiration. An adequate

preoxygenation, rapid sequence induction and intubation with cricoid pressure, and in-line stabilization of cervical spine are recommended approaches for the endotracheal tube placement. Airway management may take place in the emergency department or the operating room (if not already performed in the prehospital setting). Capnography is the most reliable method for confirmation of endotracheal tube placement.

Etomidate and ketamine are the preferred induction agents in hypotensive patients with major abdominal vascular injury. Etomidate (0.1–0.2 mg/kg) has the advantage of inducing less hemodynamic changes in comparison to other induction agents. Ketamine (0.25–1.0 mg/kg) may cause hypertension and tachycardia from endogenous catecholamine release, which may be advantageous in patients with hemorrhagic shock. It is important to recognize that both induction agents can cause hypotension and decrease in cardiac output in trauma patients; thus, conventional dosages should be reduced. Succinylcholine (1.0–1.5 mg/kg) is a neuromuscular blocker of choice for rapid sequence induction, due to its rapid onset (less than 1 min) and short duration (5–10 min). If succinylcholine is contraindicated, rocuronium (1.0–1.2 mg/kg) is recommended neuromuscular-blocking agent for rapid sequence induction. Cricoid pressure should be applied throughout induction and attempts at intubation. However, cricoid pressure can be released to ease intubation or insertion of laryngeal mask airway if necessary. Waking up the patient is not the choice in patient with abdominal vascular injury, and trauma team should be ready to rapidly proceed with invasive airway in the case of unsuccessful intubation and "cannot intubate, cannot ventilate" scenario.

The patients with major abdominal vascular injury have high abdominal pressure from hemoperitoneum. Thus, patient's abdomen and thorax should be "prepped and draped" before the induction of anesthesia because the latter is often associated with rapid hemodynamic decompensation in this patient group. After rapid sequence induction and intubation, a rapid midline incision is made to enter the abdomen. Intraperitoneal blood is evacuated and abdomen is rapidly packed in all four quadrants with laparotomy pads. The surgery is then temporarily suspended to allow anesthesia team to catch up with the patient's resuscitation as needed. Once the patient is sufficiently hemodynamically stable, a systemic exploration of the entire abdomen is accomplished. Proximal and distal control should be obtained for any vascular injury.

Maintenance of Anesthesia

It is often very challenging to meet all objectives of anesthetic maintenance and to provide adequate depth of general anesthesia in a hemodynamically unstable patient such as a patient with major abdominal vascular injury. General anesthesia is usually maintained with a combination of volatile agent, benzodiazepines, and narcotics. Isoflurane, sevoflurane, and desflurane all decrease arterial blood pressure through reduction in systemic vascular resistance. Thus, in hypotensive bleeding patient, minimum alveolar concentration (MAC) of volatile agent must be decreased, and the anesthetic agent titrated to maintain minimum necessary blood pressure and adequate tissue perfusion. MAC of 0.3–0.5 is often used in addition to midazolam to prevent recall of intraoperative events. Small boluses of midazolam may be administered repeatedly throughout the surgery to assure amnesia. Fentanyl is another adjuvant anesthetic and is usually administered in increments throughout the procedure. However, fentanyl alone does not guarantee amnesia.

Aortic Cross-Clamping and Unclamping

Temporary clamping of the abdominal aorta may be required during the surgery for abdominal major vascular injuries, and adequate preparation is essential to prevent severe hemodynamic changes and decompensation. Application of aortic cross-clamp results in a sudden increase in afterload and systemic blood pressure. Increased afterload results in increased left ventricular end-systolic wall stress. These changes are accompanied with decrease in cardiac output. A sudden increase in afterload can lead to left ventricular failure, especially in patients with noncompliant left ventricle. All these changes are more profound in the case of a supraceliac cross-clamp placement. The addition of inotrope may be necessary in the case of left ventricular failure. After the removal of aortic cross-clamp, systemic vascular resistance and arterial blood pressure decrease dramatically, as a result of peripheral vasodilation. Vasodilation can become systemic as the lactic acid is washed out of the extremities into central circulation. In order to minimize hypotensive response, volume loading prior to cross-clamp release is necessary to raise filling pressures to slightly above normal. Acidosis should be corrected and calcium replaced immediately after the removal of aortic cross-clamp (Gelman 1995). The patient may require temporary pharmacologic support to achieve an acceptable blood pressure. Ephedrine, an indirect alpha- and beta-receptor-stimulating agent can be used. Other options include appropriate dosing of direct alpha- and beta-receptor agonists such as epinephrine, norepinephrine, and dopamine. Phenylephrine, a pure alpha$_1$ receptor agonist, can be also used to increase patient's blood pressure. However, phenylephrine has not been shown to improve end-organ perfusion and may result in end-organ ischemia, especially bowel ischemia, in hypovolemic patients (Thiele et al. 2011). Transesophageal echocardiography can be useful in differentiating between myocardial ischemia and cardiac failure versus continuous hemorrhage and consequent hypovolemia. Myocardial ischemia or cardiac failure results in elevated filling pressures, while hemorrhage results in low filling pressures.

Damage Control Surgery (DCS)

DCS refers to a limited surgical procedure or set of procedures with very discrete, life-saving goals and the intent to defer more definitive repair until resuscitation has occurred (Sagraves et al. 2006). The basic principles of DCS include rapid surgical control of bleeding, control of sources of contamination, and deferral of definitive procedure until patient is more stable. Patients with major abdominal vascular injuries may benefit from early damage control and definitive reconstruction at a later stage after resuscitation and stabilization in the ICU. Damage control approach

should be considered before the patient becomes severely hypotensive and coagulopathic. With the damage control approach, any large vessel bleeding should be surgically controlled and repaired in an expeditious fashion. Any source of contamination, such as injury of gastrointestinal tract, should be controlled as well. If possible, vascular continuity should be restored by either expeditious definitive repair or temporizing measure such as vascular shunt. The abdomen is closed temporarily with vacuum dressing techniques in order to prevent abdominal compartment syndrome. The damage control strategy has been shown to lead to better than expected survival rates for abdominal trauma.

Abdominal Compartment Syndrome (ACS)

All patients with severe abdominal trauma, especially vascular trauma, are at risk of developing ACS. Major risk factors include massive blood transfusion, prolonged hypotension, hypothermia, aortic cross-clamping, damage control procedures, and tight closure of abdominal wall. ACS is characterized by a tense abdomen, tachycardia with or without hypotension, respiratory dysfunction with high peak inspiratory pressure in mechanically ventilated patients, and oliguria. After damage control procedures, the abdominal wall should never be closed under tension because postoperative bowel edema results in ACS in most patients. When the bowel edema improves, usually within 2–3 days, the patient is returned to the operating room for definitive vascular repair and abdominal wall closure. Knowledge of ACS is important, and necessary measures for prevention of this complication should be undertaken whenever possible.

Cross-References

▶ Abdominal Compartment Syndrome as a Complication of Care
▶ Abdominal Solid Organ Injury, Anesthesia for
▶ Acid-Base Management in Trauma Anesthesia
▶ Acute Abdominal Compartment Syndrome in Trauma

▶ Acute Coagulopathy of Trauma
▶ Awareness and Trauma Anesthesia
▶ Cardiac and Aortic Trauma, Anesthesia for
▶ Compartment Syndrome, Acute
▶ Compartment Syndrome: Complication of Care in ICU
▶ Damage Control Procedure
▶ Damage Control Resuscitation
▶ Damage Control Resuscitation, Military Trauma
▶ Damage Control Surgery
▶ General Anesthesia for Major Trauma
▶ Hemodynamic Management in Trauma Anesthesia
▶ Hemorrhage
▶ Hemorrhagic Shock
▶ Massive Transfusion
▶ Massive Transfusion Protocols in Trauma
▶ Monitoring of Trauma Patients during Anesthesia
▶ Open Abdomen
▶ Open Abdomen, Temporary Abdominal Closure
▶ Operating Room Setup for Trauma Anesthesia
▶ Pharmacologic Strategies in Adult Trauma Anesthesia
▶ Prehospital Emergency Preparedness
▶ Rapid Sequence Intubation
▶ Resuscitation Goals in Trauma Patients
▶ Shock Management in Trauma
▶ Thoracic Vascular Injuries
▶ Transfusion Strategy in Trauma: What Is the Evidence?
▶ Vascular Access in Trauma Patients

References

Asensio JA, Chahwan S, Hanpeter D et al (2000) Operative management and outcome of 302 abdominal vascular injuries. Am J Surg 180:528–534
Demetriades D, Velmahos G, Cornwell EE et al (1997) Selective nonoperative management of gunshot wounds of the anterior abdomen. Arch Surg 132:178–183
Feliciano DV, Burch JM, Graham JM (2000) Abdominal vascular injury. In: Mattox KL, Feliciano DV, Moore EE (eds) Trauma, 4th edn. McGraw-Hill, New York, pp 783–806
Gelman S (1995) The pathophysiology of aortic cross-clamping and unclamping. Anesthesiology 82:1026–1060
Sagraves SG, Toschlog EA, Rotondo MF (2006) Damage control surgery – the intensivist's role. J Intensive Care Med 21:5–16
Thiele RH, Nemergut EC, Lynch C (2011) The clinical implications of isolated alpha$_1$ adrenergic stimulation. Anesth Analg 113:297–304

Abdominal Solid Organ Injury, Anesthesia for

Gina Hendren
Department of Anesthesia, University of Kansas, Kansas City, KS, USA

Synonyms

Damage control surgery; Kidney injury; Kidney insult; Liver contusion; Liver injury; Liver laceration; Nephrectomy; Pancreatic injury; Pancreatic insult; Splenic injury; Splenic laceration; Splenic rupture

Definition

Traumatic force to the abdomen may be blunt or penetrating. Solid organs of the abdomen are different in their size, structure, and anatomic positions. These factors along with the mechanism of injury will be the main determinants of the type and severity of abdominal solid organ injury. The propensity for profuse bleeding requiring surgical intervention occurs most often with injury to the liver and spleen.

Preexisting Condition

Liver

The liver is one of the most commonly injured organs in abdominal trauma (Polanco et al. 2008). Both low- and high-grade injuries of the liver due to blunt and penetrating trauma can be successfully managed nonoperatively in the hemodynamically stable patient (Ahmed and Vernick 2011).

The grade of the liver injury, although important, should not dictate the decision to proceed to the operative suite. The patient's hemodynamics in the field or emergency room should remain of primary importance regarding the decision to proceed directly to the operating room or interventional radiology suite. For the stable patient, imaging studies including focused assessment by ultrasound for trauma (FAST) and computed tomography (CT) scans remain the diagnostic modalities of choice to further clarify and classify liver injuries (Ahmed and Vernick 2011) before the operating room. The FAST scan is not designed to identify the degree of organ injury but is useful in assessing for blood in the abdomen. If available, a CT scan provides details of the organ injuries and can show active bleeding by extravasation of contrast. Knowing the anatomic location of the injury or injuries allows the anesthesiologist to anticipate the amount of blood loss and the scope and magnitude of the surgery and allows for thoughtful placement of intravenous lines and arterial access.

Spleen

The spleen is more commonly injured than other hollow, viscous structures of the abdomen following blunt trauma. It is second only to the liver in injuries sustained in blunt abdominal trauma (Wilson et al. 1999). These patients will often present in the trauma bay or emergency room after sustaining an injury to the left thorax or abdominal wall. Spleen injuries requiring operative intervention often present with hypotension due to hemorrhage but should be suspected in any trauma patient who complains of left upper quadrant tenderness or left shoulder pain. Any patient who undergoes a splenectomy should be vaccinated against pneumococcal infections postoperatively.

Kidney

Renal injury occurs in approximately 1–5 % of all traumas (Shoobridge et al. 2011). The kidney is frequently injured by a deceleration mechanism as seen in motor vehicle accidents. Current management of hemodynamically stable patients with kidney injuries is watchful waiting with serial abdominal exams, trending of hemoglobin, and CT scans. Heme identified on Foley catheter placement or flank pain may suggest a renal injury. Indications for exploration in renal trauma include hemorrhage, renal pedicle avulsion, or retroperitoneal hematoma (Shoobridge et al. 2011). Although at some centers it is possible to salvage the injured kidney, often a nephrectomy is performed (Kuan et al. 2006).

Pancreas

Injuries to the pancreas rarely occur in isolation in the abdominal trauma patient. Injury to the pancreas and duodenum is reported to be approximately 5 % of all abdominal injuries (Choi et al. 2012). The pancreas can be injured by compression against the spinal column in an anterior-posterior mechanism that can be seen with motor vehicle accidents. The patient presents often with upper abdominal and back pain. Major ductal injury is the main determinant for outcome with pancreatic injury (Choi et al. 2012). Patients with disruption of the major pancreatic duct typically require surgery.

Once a trauma victim arrives in the emergency room, an initial history from either the patient or EMS personnel is obtained. This history should focus on the mechanism of injury as well as other associated injuries including seatbelt imprint or hematoma, lumbar spine fractures, rib fractures, pelvic fractures, or chest or head injuries. Patients with multiple injuries have increased incidence of intra-abdominal injuries requiring surgery (Wilson et al. 1999). If the ABCDE assessment determines that the abdominal injury is a penetrating injury, urgent surgical intervention may be required. A hemodynamically stable with a blunt abdominal injury with suspected solid organ injury will likely undergo additional assessment. The patient should have a cursory set of labs drawn in the emergency room including serum chemistry, hemoglobin, and coagulation studies. The patient should also have an arterial blood gas drawn to assess ventilation, oxygenation, and base deficit. A type and cross for blood products should also be sent.

Application

The unstable or deteriorating patient in the trauma bay should be expedited to the operating room or radiology suite within 15 min (Ahmed and Vernick 2011). The patient should have blood products including packed red blood cells, fresh frozen plasma, and platelets available. Also, if the hospital has a massive transfusion protocol (MTP), it should be activated in the emergency room to have the products available as soon as possible in the operating room. Early activation of the MTP has been shown to reduce mortality (Kozar and McNutt 2010) in the trauma patient. In addition to the standard ASA monitors, two large-bore intravenous catheters should be obtained. Since a significant abdominal venous injury is possible, obtaining IV access on lower extremities should be avoided if possible. Intravenous access placed on either the upper extremities or neck is more desirable. The patient should also have an arterial line placed and rapid transfusion system started.

Induction

If the patient is not yet intubated, induction of anesthesia should be achieved with careful titration of medication to prevent profound hypotension. Induction can be achieved with etomidate, propofol, or ketamine. Although all can be used safely, it is important to appreciate that dosage adjustments may be required in the hypovolemic trauma patient to avoid worsening any preexisting hypotension. During the "prep and drape" period, a significant amount of crystalloids and colloids may need to be administered in order to increase preload and minimize the severity of hypotension post- laparotomy. Before surgical incision a broad-spectrum antibiotic covering both gram-positive and gram-negative bacteria should be given. An orogastric tube should also be placed to decompress the stomach.

Maintenance

The surgeon will proceed with the standard open exploratory laparotomy incision, xyphoid process to pubic symphysis. Once this incision is made, an increase in bleeding from the abdominal wounds may be noted since the tamponade effect of the abdominal wall will be released. The anesthetic goal at this time is to maintain near-normal hemodynamics by treating hypotension first with warm fluid or blood products dependent on the patient's laboratory data and temporizing only with vasopressors until fluid and product administration can catch up. During this dynamic time, the anesthesiologist should be reevaluating the patient's condition continually, including checking vital signs, additional hemodynamic monitors (pressure control variation and central venous pressure), urine output, and laboratory data with point of care testing if available. If the blood pressure remains adequate throughout this time, other anesthetic agents can be added including narcotic pain medication and inhalational anesthetics. Muscle relaxants are titrated to achieve maximum surgical exposure. Depending on the patient's critical nature, tolerance to anesthetic agents may be minimal. These patients should be given a benzodiazepine to decrease the risk of recall and awareness during surgery. The surgeon's initial goal will be four-quadrant packing, direct bleeding compression, and control of fecal contamination. The surgeon will assess the liver as well as the spleen. If the patient has injury to the hepatic artery or portal vein, the surgeon may use the Pringle maneuver. The Pringle maneuver is used to isolate and control rapid blood loss associated with severe hepatic injury. Hemodynamic changes associated with the Pringle maneuver include hypotension due to decreased venous return. If .hepatic bleeding is not controlled with this Pringle maneuver and packing, there is concern for retrohepatic vena cava or hepatic vein injury.

Fluids and blood products should be administered according to the patient's needs to help prevent excess fluid administration and subsequent bowel edema. If blood loss at any point becomes excessive, communication with the surgeon asking for abdominal packing allowing a catch-up time for product administration may be needed. In addition frequently monitored temperature, hemoglobin, calcium, coagulation studies, and platelets help to minimize coagulopathic bleeding. Cell saver technique using salvaged blood is also a viable option for blood administration. If at any point in the operative course the patient develops the triad of acidosis, coagulopathy, and hypothermia, the operative repair should be focused on damage control surgery.

Trauma patients are prone to hypothermia. The environment in which the patient was injured and transfusion of unwarmed IV fluids and blood products can further exacerbate hypothermia in the trauma patient. The patient undergoing an anesthetic also has skin exposure and loss of normal physiological heat conservation such as vasoconstriction and shivering. The hypothermic patient has increased risk of coagulopathic bleeding and ventricular ectopy as well as decreased drug metabolism.

Pediatric Considerations

Blunt trauma is much more common than penetrating trauma in the pediatric population. Children have proportionally larger intra-abdominal organs than adults; the organs are closer together, and the abdominal wall and cartilaginous rib cage are weaker. These anatomical factors result in higher risk of severe and/or multiple organ injuries. The liver and spleen are the most frequently injured solid organs in children (Loy 2008). Most of these injuries may be managed nonoperatively. Hemodynamic instability despite adequate fluid and blood resuscitation (30–40 ml/kg) will be the indicator of the need for urgent surgical repair. Tachycardia is the most sensitive indicator of hypovolemic shock in children.

Damage Control Surgery

If the decision by the surgeon is to proceed with damage control surgery, the primary surgical management goal changes from definitive surgical management to control of hemorrhage, abdominal packing, and temporary abdominal closure (Dutton 2012). The patient is then taken to the intensive care unit for continued resuscitation, optimization of hemodynamics, and correction of coagulation status before being brought back to the operating room suite for definitive repair of the intra-abdominal injuries. Good communication with the surgery team regarding vital signs and laboratory data helps the entire trauma team decide if damage control is a more viable option before the patient is severely acidotic, hypothermic, and coagulopathic.

Cross-References

▶ ABCDE of Trauma Care
▶ Acute Abdominal Compartment Syndrome in Trauma
▶ Acute Coagulopathy of Trauma
▶ Awareness and Trauma Anesthesia
▶ Blood Volume
▶ Coagulopathy in Trauma: Underlying Mechanisms
▶ Damage Control Resuscitation
▶ Damage Control Surgery
▶ Exsanguination Transfusion
▶ Fluid, Electrolytes, and Nutrition in Trauma Patients
▶ General Anesthesia for Major Trauma
▶ Hemodynamic Management in Trauma Anesthesia
▶ Hemodynamic Monitoring
▶ Hypothermia, Trauma, and Anesthetic Management
▶ Massive Transfusion Protocols in Trauma
▶ Methods of Containment of the Open Abdomen, Overview
▶ Shock Management in Trauma
▶ Thoracic Vascular Injuries

References

Ahmed N, Vernick J (2011) Management of liver trauma in adults. J Emerg Trauma Shock 4(1):114–119

Choi SB, Jiyoung Y, Choi SY (2012) A case of traumatic pancreaticoduodenal injury: a simple and an organ-preserving approach as damage control surgery. JOP 13(1):76–79

Dutton RP (2012) Resuscitative strategies to maintain homeostasis during damage control surgery. Br J Surg 99(Suppl 1):21–28

Kozar RA, McNutt M (2010) Management of adult blunt hepatic trauma. Curr Opin Crit Care 16(6):596–601

Kuan JK, Wright JL, Nathens AB, Rivara FP, Wessells H (2006) American Association for the Surgery of Trauma Organ injury Scale for kidney injuries predicts nephrectomy, dialysis, and death in patients with blunt injury and nephrectomy for penetrating injuries. J Trauma 60(2):351–356

Loy J (2008) Pediatric trauma and anesthesia in trauma anesthesia. Cambridge University Press, New York

Polanco P, Leon S, Pineda J, Puyana JC, Ochoa JB, Alarcon L, Harbrecht BG, Geller D, Peitzman AB (2008) Hepatic resection in the management of complex injury to the liver. J Trauma 65(6):1264–1270

Shoobridge K, Corcoran N, Martin K, Koukounaras J, Royce P, Bultitude M (2011) Contemporary management of renal trauma. Rev Urol 13(2):65–72

Wilson W, Patel N, Hoyt D, Murphy M (1999) Perioperative anesthetic management of patients with abdominal trauma. Anesthesiol Clin North Am 17(1):211–236

Abdominal Wall Defect

▶ Repair of the Open Abdomen Hernia, Scope of the Problem

Ability

▶ Competency

Absolute Stability

▶ Principles of Internal Fixation of Fractures

Absorbable Mesh Temporary Abdominal Closure

▶ Mesh Temporary Closure

Absorption

▶ Pharmacokinetic and Pharmacodynamic Alterations in Critical Illness

ABThera Wound Dressing

▶ Open Abdomen, Vacuum Dressing

Abuse

▶ Interpersonal Violence

Academic Programs in Trauma Care

William A. Mosier
Wright State University, Dayton, OH, USA

Synonyms

Burn and plastics trauma fellowship; Emergency and trauma care education programs; Masters degree in trauma sciences (M.Sc.); Orthopedic trauma fellowship; Trauma and critical care electives; Trauma anesthesia fellowship; Trauma care fellowship; Trauma, critical care, and acute care surgery fellowship; Trauma radiology fellowship; Trauma research fellowship; Trauma surgery and critical care fellowship; Trauma surgery fellowship

Definition

Trauma care refers to medical interventions occurring in a timely manner shortly after the injury causing body damage due to a physical impact (such as damage caused by a motor vehicle accident, explosion, or military combat). The World Health Organization and other international and national trauma groups provide guidelines for injury management. Academic programs related to trauma care, emergency medicine, critical care, and trauma surgery have adopted these treatment standards and seek to provide residency and fellowship training opportunities for health-care providers pursuing graduate-level education at locations throughout the United States and parts of Europe.

The trauma.org database lists fellowships, lectureships and research positions that focus on trauma care. Additional information regarding trauma education can be found through the American Association for the Surgery of Trauma (www.aast.org), the Eastern Association for the Surgery of Trauma (www.east.org) and the Orthopaedic Trauma Association (www.ota.org).

Cross-References

▶ Burn and Plastics Trauma Fellowship
▶ Orthopedic Trauma Fellowship
▶ Trauma Anesthesia Fellowship
▶ Trauma Care Fellowship
▶ Trauma Radiology Fellowship
▶ Trauma Surgery

Acalculous Cholecystitis

Lindsay O'Meara[1] and Khanjan H. Nagarsheth[2]
[1]Shock Trauma Center, University of Maryland Medical Center, Baltimore, MD, USA
[2]R Adams Cowley Shock Trauma Center, University of Maryland School of Medicine, Baltimore, MD, USA

Synonyms

Cholecystitis

Definition

Acalculous cholecystitis (ACC) was first reported in 1844 in a patient who just underwent a femoral hernia repair. It is a rare, yet severe, and potentially fatal condition affecting critically ill and trauma patients. ACC is defined as inflammation of the gallbladder without calculi (Crichlow et al. 2012). Ultrasound examination of the abdomen has been shown to be the most accurate diagnosis of ACC in critically ill patients. Thickening of the gallbladder wall to 3 mm has 90 % specificity, and 100 % sensitivity while a wall thickness of 3.5 mm has 98.5 % specificity and 80 % sensitivity. The other major criteria for identifying ACC include gallbladder wall edema, sonographic murphy's sign (which may be difficult if the patient is obtunded), pericholecystic fluid, mucosal sloughing, and intramural gas. Sludge, nonshadowing stones, cholesterolosis, hypoalbuminemia, or ascites can mimic a thickened gallbladder causing a false-positive reading (Barie and Eachempati 2010).

Preexisting Condition

The incidence of ACC in critically ill trauma patients has been reported to occur between 0.5 % and 18 % (Hamp et al. 2009), with a mortality rate as high as 30 %. Multiple risk factors have been shown to increase the risk of developing ACC. Studies have demonstrated that the higher the injury severity score (ISS) the more likely the trauma patient is to develop ACC. The ISS is the only risk factor that is considered an independent variable (Pelinka et al. 2003). However, dependent variables such as shock, requirements of blood transfusions, duration of ventilatory support, use of total parenteral nutrition (TPN), opioid therapy, and tachycardia have also been identified as risk factors for the development of ACC. Critically ill trauma patients often experience episodes of low cardiac output. This results in the release of vasopressin and epinepherine, which interact synergistically causing splanchnic vasoconstriction and hypoxia. When the splanchnic bed experiences vasoconstriction secondary to shock or the use of opioids, the celiac trunk, which is the gallbladder's blood supply, is restricted, resulting in hypoxia. The hypoxic effects lead to decreased mucin secretion. Mucin helps to protect the gallbladder lining from bile salts and acids. The build-up of irritants and the lack of blood flow can lead to necrosis or irreversible cell injury (Sanda 2008). The use of opioids and TPN can result in impaired gallbladder motility and emptying, leading to a distended gallbladder. The lack of emptying allows for irritants to accumulate, leading to further necrosis (Hamp et al. 2009). Much research has demonstrated that majority of these risk factors correlate with, and trigger, one another. The risk factors a patient may have are determined by their preexisting condition and severity.

Application

It is often very difficult to diagnosis ACC. Sedation, a low Glasgow Coma Scale, and distracting injuries can make it difficult for a patient to relay right upper quadrant abdominal pain and tenderness. Laboratory data may not be useful in a critically ill patient as their labs are often already abnormal (Hamp et al. 2009). Fevers and tachycardia, along with a generalized septic-like deterioration, are often the only signs a clinician may have to help identify ACC. Rapid and accurate diagnosis of ACC is essential because gallbladder ischemia can quickly progress to gangrene, perforation, and death (Barie and Eachempati 2010). Once identified, the treatment of ACC is dependent upon the provider and the patient's presentation. Some studies have shown that immediate cholecystectomy should be performed in order to decrease mortality from the disease and improve outcomes. However, an invasive option is often difficult in an unstable trauma patient or a patient who has undergone recent abdominal surgery. Other studies have supported the use of a percutaneous cholecystostomy tube to be beneficial in the treatment of ACC. The timing of removal of the percutaneous cholecystostomy tube or if an interval cholecystectomy is necessary once the patient has stabilized has not been fully studied.

ACC continues to be a severe condition that is difficult to diagnose. Critically ill trauma patients who remain or become unstable despite intervention should have ACC considered as part of their differential diagnosis. Early identification of the disease can help to reduce mortality and improve outcomes in the trauma patient.

Cross-References

▶ Nutritional Deficiency/Starvation
▶ Nutritional Support

References

Barie P, Eachempati S (2010) Acute acalculous cholecystitis. Gastroenterol Clin N Am 39:343–357
Crichlow L, Walcott-Sapp S, Major J et al (2012) Acute acalculous cholecystitis after gastrointestional surgery. Am Surg 78:220–224
Hamp T, Fridrich P, Mauritz W et al (2009) Cholecystitis after trauma. J Trauma 66(2):400–406
Pelinka L, Schmidhammer R, Hamid L et al (2003) Acute acalculous cholecystitis after trauma: a prospective study. J Trauma 55(2):323–329
Sanda R (2008) Acute acalculous cholecystitis after trauma: the role of microcirculatory failure and cellular hypoxia. South Med J 101(11):1087–1088

Accident Surgery

▶ Traumatology

Accidental Hypothermia

▶ Hypothermia

Accidental Strangulation

▶ Strangulation and Hanging

Accomplishment

▶ Competency

Acetabulum Fracture-Dislocation

▶ Hip Dislocations and Fracture-Dislocations

Acetabulum Fractures

Milton Lee (Chip) Routt Jr
University of Texas (Houston) Medical
School – Memorial Hermann Medical Center,
Houston, TX, USA

Synonyms

Hip socket fracture

Definition

Acetabular fractures are injuries that involve the
hip socket region of the pelvis, usually due to
a traumatic event that abnormally loads the proximal femur and femoral head within the socket to
cause the fracture (Fig. 1).

Epidemiology

Acetabular fracture patterns are determined by
the hip position at impact, the local bone quality,
and the magnitude of the applied load. As the
load is further transmitted, the acetabular fracture
displaces, and the femoral head may dislocate
from the hip joint. These fractures commonly
occur in a bimodal age distribution. Older
patients have poor bone quality and sustain
them after a fall from standing. Young patients
have better bone quality and are also more
exposed to high-energy traumatic events such as
car and motorcycle crashes.

Osteology

Normal pelvic osteology is complex and confusing, and displaced acetabular fractures are even
more challenging to thoroughly comprehend.
The acetabulum is a hemisphere-shaped recess
located between the ilium, ischium, and pubis. It
develops from the triradiate cartilage and matures
into the adult acetabulum. The acetabular surface
is concave and is mostly covered by hyaline cartilage. The fossa acetabuli is a recessed area in the
center of the acetabulum that contains fat and the
ligamentum teres. The acetabular labrum is
attached to the acetabular wall perimeter and the
hip capsule.

The Inverted Y Structural Concept

The structural acetabular concept describes it as
being located between the limbs of two boney
supports or "columns" shaped as an inverted Y.
The anterior column is comprised of the superior
pubic ramus, anterior acetabular wall, and the anterior portion of the ilium and quadrilateral surface.

Acetabulum Fractures,
Fig. 1 Excessive loading
of the proximal femur
through the femoral head
causes the acetabulum to
fracture. In this example,
the left-sided unstable
acetabular fracture
fragments are displaced
significantly as the
proximal femur intrudes
medially into the pelvis

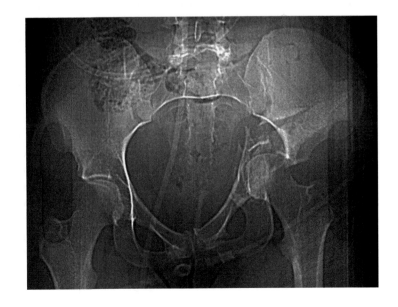

Acetabulum Fractures, Fig. 2 These two medial and lateral hemipelvis illustrations demonstrate the structural anterior and posterior acetabular columns. The anterior wall area is a part of the anterior column just as the posterior wall area is a part of the posterior column

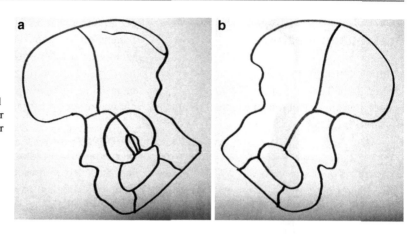

The posterior column is comprised of the greater and lesser sciatic notches, posterior acetabular wall, and the posterior half of the quadrilateral surface. The two-column structural model was intended to simplify the acetabular osseous architecture so that clinicians could better understand the injury patterns (Fig. 2).

Radiology

Acetabular fracture diagnosis and classification schemes are based on the radiographic findings and the two-column acetabular concept (Judet et al. 1964). The normal radiographic markers represent bony cortical surfaces and edges revealed by tangential X-ray beams. These cortical lines include the peripheral edges of both the anterior and posterior walls; the dense line representing the pelvic brim and superior pubic ramus' posterior cranial edge (iliopectineal line); the dense line representing the pelvic brim and quadrilateral surface (ilioischial line); the dome region's subchondral arc (sourcil); and the acetabular "teardrop" representing the fossa acetabuli, obturator sulcus, and a portion of the quadrilateral surface. These six radiographic markers help clinicians to better understand and mark the two walls, the two supporting columns, the weight-bearing dome, and the caudal joint. Oblique acetabular imaging is accomplished by rolling the patient 45° toward each side so the fracture is seen in biplanar views. A pelvic computed tomogram (CT) scan uses axial, sagittal, and coronal images to further reveal the osseous and soft tissue details related to the injury.

Surface-rendered three-dimensional images are created from the CT information to further identify the specific fracture sites and displacements (Fig. 3). Other imaging modalities may be indicated for certain patients, for example, a hemodynamically unstable patient with fracture involving the greater sciatic notch may benefit from pelvic angiography to assess the superior gluteal artery. These angiographic images can be used for diagnostic means and surgical planning also.

Classification

Acetabular fractures are classified into two broad categories, elementary and associated patterns. The elementary patterns have a singular primary fracture plane. Four of the five elementary patterns involve a single wall or a single column – these are the posterior wall, posterior column, anterior wall, and anterior column patterns. Unlike the other elementary patterns, transverse acetabular fractures involve the two walls and the two columns but are included in the elementary group because transverse patterns have a singular fracture plane. The associated patterns have several primary fracture planes combined together rendering the fracture more complex than the elementary fractures. Four of the associated patterns involve anterior and posterior acetabular areas, while the posterior column with associated posterior wall fracture is limited to the posterior acetabular column and posterior wall areas only. The other four associated patterns that involve the anterior and

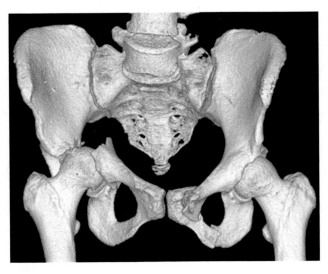

Acetabulum Fractures, Fig. 3 Three-dimensional surface-rendered images generated from CT data are helpful when planning the surgical treatment of a displaced acetabular fracture. In this example, the right-sided transverse acetabular fracture is seen to divide the joint into two separate halves. The caudal fragment is displaced medially from the intact and stable cranial portion, and the proximal femur remains in association with the displaced caudal fragment. The 3D image also demonstrates a left-sided sacroiliac joint disruption and pubic ramus fracture

Acetabulum Fractures, Table 1 Acetabular fracture groups and specific injury patterns

Elementary	Associated
Posterior wall	Transverse/posterior wall
Posterior column	T-type
Anterior wall	Anterior column/posterior hemitransverse
Anterior column	Both column
Transverse	Posterior column/posterior wall

posterior acetabular areas are the transverse with associated posterior wall, T-type, anterior column with associated posterior hemitransverse, and associated both-column patterns. The associated both-column pattern is unique in that no articular cartilage remains on the intact, stable fragment (Table 1).

Initial Management

Patients with these fractures may present in a variety of manners depending usually on the mechanism of injury. Each patient is resuscitated according to ATLS protocols, and plain pelvic radiographs are obtained once the patient has been stabilized. Fracture-dislocations are reduced urgently once the fracture pattern details are understood. Posteriorly directed dislocations are usually associated with posterior wall, posterior column/posterior wall, and transverse/posterior wall acetabular fracture patterns. Medial dislocations are usually noted with associated both-column, transverse, T-type, anterior column/posterior hemitransverse, and posterior column fracture patterns. Prior to closed reduction, the treating physician should carefully assess the femoral neck area on the X-rays for fracture. Adequate muscle relaxation is mandatory prior to the manipulative reduction attempt and can be achieved using a variety of techniques. The dislocated femoral head is then manipulated so that it can be held beneath the area of the weight-bearing dome. Skeletal traction may be needed to secure this reduction.

Once the patient and the fracture have been stabilized, secondary and tertiary repeat evaluations are indicated to identify other injuries that were initially missed. Pelvic imaging is then obtained so the treatment can be planned.

Some dislocations are obstructed by bone debris in the joint or misplaced soft tissue

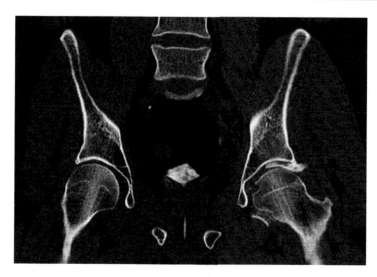

Acetabulum Fractures, Fig. 4 This pelvic coronal CT image identifies a displaced posterior wall fracture fragment that is located between the femoral head and acetabular dome causing a nonconcentric reduction. This was one of five separate displaced posterior wall fracture fragments that were noted to be within the joint. An open reduction was indicated and performed urgently. The displaced fracture fragments were first removed from the hip joint so the femoral head could be congruent with the acetabular dome. Then the individual fragments were reduced and stabilized with two supporting plates

structures such as the piriformis muscle tendon due to the injury rendering it irreducible via closed manipulation. These rare patients require urgent open reduction (Fig. 4).

Nonoperative Treatment

For patients with stable and minimally displaced acetabular fractures, nonoperative management is recommended, consisting of protected weight bearing on the injured extremity for 6–12 weeks after injury. Serial weekly plain pelvic radiographs are recommended for 1–3 weeks after injury to assure that further fracture displacement is not occurring and that the hip joint remains congruent when nonoperative management is chosen. Skeletal traction is used when the fracture is unstable but the patient is a poor candidate for surgery and the fracture reduction is sufficient in traction. Usually ten pounds of traction is applied through a distal femoral traction pin and simple pulley system attached to the foot of the bed. When traction is chosen, the head of the patient's bed should be elevated to decrease the risk of aspiration, especially in elderly patients.

Operative Treatment

Displaced and unstable acetabular fractures are treated operatively (Letournel 1993; Helfet et al. 1992). Open anatomical reduction with stable internal fixation (ORIF) is recommended for the majority of patients with these articular injuries. Anatomical reduction restores the articular surfaces and lowers the risk of post-traumatic arthritis formation. Access to the fracture fragments allows the surgeon to directly clean the fracture surfaces of organized hematoma and small bone fragments that can obstruct the reduction and physically manipulate the fracture fragments into a reduced position. Clamps, wires, lag screws, and other devices are routinely used to temporarily maintain the reduction while the definitive fixation is applied to the bone. The Kocher-Langenbeck surgical exposure is used for posterior acetabular injuries, and the ilioinguinal surgical exposure provides access to anterior acetabular fractures. For patients with more complex fracture patterns, the two exposures can be used in sequence either at the same anesthesia or at a subsequent anesthesia. Some recommend using the two exposures

A

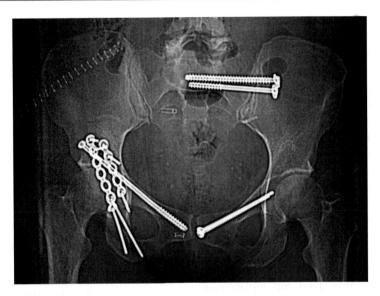

Acetabulum Fractures, Fig. 5 This patient (previously seen in Fig. 3) had a right transverse acetabular fracture-dislocation as well as left pubic ramus fracture and SI joint disruption. The acetabular fracture was treated operatively using a posterior Kocher-Langenbeck exposure. The reduction was accomplished after cleaning the fracture surfaces and then clamping the transverse fracture. A cancellous lag screw was inserted percutaneously in the superior pubic ramus, and then two malleable plates were applied posteriorly to stabilize the transverse fracture. The SI joint injury and pubic ramus fracture were treated with closed reduction and then screw fixation. An initial iliosacral cancellous lag screw compressed the SI joint, and the subsequent fully threaded cancellous screw provided additional support. The acetabular lag screw, iliosacral screws, and the retrograde superior pubic ramus screw were all inserted percutaneously using biplanar fluoroscopic imaging

simultaneously (Routt and Swiontkowski 1990). The extended iliofemoral and several other more extensive surgical exposures have also been advocated for difficult fracture patterns (Siebenrock et al. 2002). Each surgical exposure and patient positioning for surgery has associated risks. When the lateral patient position is chosen, the patient must be securely positioned on the operating table, usually using a vacuum beanbag and obstructing posts. In the lateral decubitus position, the uninjured side is at risk to pressure points particularly at the axilla, hip, and knee. Medially displaced fracture fragments and instability are much more difficult to accurately correct in the lateral position. Prone patient positioning risks blindness if hypotensive anesthesia is used and the eye regions are not relieved of pressure. The airway access, upper extremities, and male genitalia are also at risk while the patient is prone. When positioned prone, supporting chest rolls suspend the abdomen to facilitate mechanical ventilation during surgery.

The foundation for stable fixation is a well-reduced fracture. In surgery, bone clamps are initially positioned to hold the reduced fracture fragments, and then lag screws and plates link and stabilize the acetabular fracture fragments together. Malleable plates are contoured precisely to match the cortical surfaces so the implant functions best (Qureshi et al. 2004). Long-length medullary screws are often used in both the anterior and posterior columns to stabilize the fractures (Fig. 5).

Manipulative reduction of the fracture fragments with percutaneous fixation is another operative treatment method. These techniques usually are reserved for patients who are unable to withstand a routine open reduction due to their overall clinical condition and those fractures that are minimally or essentially non-displaced and do not involve the acetabular dome. In these patients, simple traction maneuvers realign the major fracture fragments so that medullary columnar screws are inserted to stabilize the fracture.

This technique may also be useful for morbidly obese patients or those with soft tissue injuries that preclude open procedures.

Arthroplasty has been used sparingly as a primary treatment for certain patients with acetabular fractures (Herscovici et al. 2010). Usually this technique is reserved for older patients with preexisting arthritis and extensive articular damage such that the fracture cannot be reduced accurately. Reduction and stable fixation of the displaced column and wall components of the fracture are still required initially so the replacement cup can be securely placed into stabilized acetabular fracture fragments. Patients with acute acetabular fractures are not as medically optimized as those with degenerative conditions scheduled for elective total hip replacement. A patient with acute acetabular fractures may have other injuries or complications due to their overall condition after trauma that threatens the hip arthroplasty success.

Rehabilitation

Rehabilitation after acetabular fracture repair consists of protected weight bearing on the injured side using crutches or a walker for 12 weeks after surgery. During the initial 6 weeks, the amount of pressure applied to the injured side is limited to the weight of the extremity. Isometric muscle exercises and active range of motion activities are allowed. During the second 6-week time period, muscle strengthening exercises are instituted along with gradual progression of load applied to the injured limb. The goal of independent ambulation at week 13 is achieved for most patients.

Complications

Deep venous thrombosis (DVT), infection, and symptomatic ectopic bone formation are several of the complications associated with acetabular fractures (Russell et al. 2001). A variety of techniques such as early surgery, anticoagulation, and sequential compression devices have been advocated for DVT prophylaxis. Deep wound infections are unusual but demand early and aggressive surgical debridement along with appropriate intravenous antibiotics. Indomethacin,

targeted low dose irradiation, and muscle debridement have been recommended to decrease the incidence and extent of heterotopic ossification (Rath et al. 2002; Moore et al. 1998).

Cross-References

▶ ABCDE of Trauma Care
▶ Acute Respiratory Distress Syndrome (ARDS), General
▶ Anticoagulation/Antiplatelet Agents and Trauma
▶ Avascular Necrosis of the Femoral Head
▶ Catheter-Related Infections
▶ Compartment Syndrome of the Leg
▶ Damage Control Orthopedics
▶ DVT, as a Complication
▶ Falls
▶ Geriatric Trauma
▶ Heterotopic Ossification
▶ Imaging of Abdominal and Pelvic Injuries
▶ Imaging of Spine and Bony Pelvis Injuries
▶ Monitoring of Trauma Patients during Anesthesia
▶ Motor Vehicle Crash (MVC), Side Impact
▶ Pedestrian Injuries
▶ Teamwork and Trauma Care
▶ Venous Thromboembolism (VTE)
▶ Venous Thromboembolism Prophylaxis and Treatment Following Trauma

References

Helfet DL, Borrelli J Jr, DiPasquale T, Sanders R (1992) Stabilization of acetabular fractures in elderly patients. J Bone Joint Surg Am 74(5):753–765
Herscovici D Jr, Lindvall E, Bolhofner B, Scaduto JM (2010) The combined hip procedure: open reduction internal fixation combined with total hip arthroplasty for the management of acetabular fractures in the elderly. J Orthop Trauma 24(5):291–296
Judet R, Judet J, Letournel E (1964) Fractures of the acetabulum: classification and surgical approaches for open reduction. Preliminary report. J Bone Joint Surg Am 46:1615–1646
Letournel E (1993) The treatment of acetabular fractures through the ilioinguinal approach. Clin Orthop Relat Res 292:62–76

Moore KD, Goss K, Anglen JO (1998) Indomethacin versus radiation therapy for prophylaxis against heterotopic ossification in acetabular fractures: a randomised prospective study. J Bone Joint Surg Br 80(2):259–263

Qureshi AA, Archdeacon MT, Jenkins MA, Infante A, DiPasquale T, Bolhofner BR (2004) Infrapectineal plating for acetabular fractures: a technical adjunct to internal fixation. J Orthop Trauma 18(3):175–178

Rath EM, Russell GV Jr, Washington WJ, Routt ML Jr (2002) Gluteus minimus necrotic muscle debridement diminishes heterotopic ossification after acetabular fracture fixation. Injury 33(9):751–756

Routt ML Jr, Swiontkowski MF (1990) Operative treatment of complex acetabular fractures. Combined anterior and posterior exposures during the same procedure. J Bone Joint Surg Am 72(6):897–904

Russell GV Jr, Nork SE, Chip Routt ML Jr (2001) Perioperative complications associated with operative treatment of acetabular fractures. J Trauma 51(6):1098–1103

Siebenrock KA, Gautier E, Woo AK, Ganz R (2002) Surgical dislocation of the femoral head for joint debridement and accurate reduction of fractures of the acetabulum. J Orthop Trauma 16(8):543–552

Aching

▶ Pain

Acid Burns

▶ Chemical Burns

Acid-Base Management in Trauma Anesthesia

Kellie Park and Jean Charchaflieh
Department of Anesthesiology, Yale University
School of Medicine, New Haven, CT, USA

Synonyms

Acidosis, academia (respiratory versus metabolic); Alkalosis, alkalemia (respiratory versus metabolic)

Definition

1. Acidosis is defined as an overabundance of acid in body fluids (Seifter 2011). It occurs when there is an accumulation of acid (hydrogen ion, H^+) or loss of base (primarily bicarbonate ion, HCO_3^-). Acidosis can be respiratory, metabolic, or mixed. Respiratory acidosis develops when carbon dioxide (CO_2) accumulates due to hypoventilation or increased production. Metabolic acidosis develops with accumulation of acids, (ketones, lactate, uric acid, or ingested acids), loss of HCO_3^- through the kidneys (renal tubular acidosis [RTA]) or the intestines (diarrhea) or dilution of serum HCO_3^- (hyperchloremic metabolic acidosis)

2. Alkalosis is defined as an overabundance of base (alkali) in body fluids (Seifter 2011). It occurs when there is an accumulation of (HCO_3^-) or a decrease in acid (primarily CO_2). Alkalosis can be respiratory or metabolic. Respiratory alkalosis occurs with hyperventilation. Metabolic alkalosis occurs secondary to loss of hydrogen (H^+), chloride (Cl^-), potassium (K^+), sodium (Na^+), or free water (H_2O), due to vomiting, diarrhea, diuretic or antacid use, and endocrine disorders.

Preexisting Condition

In trauma patients, bleeding and hypoperfusion can lead to lactic metabolic acidosis. Massive bleeding is the second most common cause of death in the trauma (after head injury), and about 3–5 % of trauma patients require massive transfusion (more than one blood volume) (Nunez et al. 2010).[2] Fluid resuscitation with few liters of NaCl can lead to hyperchloremic metabolic acidosis. Hypoventilation due to traumatic brain injury (TBI) or analgesic/hypnotic drugs can lead to respiratory acidosis. Alternatively, pain and anxiety can lead to hyperventilation and respiratory alkalosis. Preexisting medical conditions such as diabetes mellitus (DM) can be exacerbated with the stress of trauma and lead to diabetic keto-acidosis (DKA) or hyperosmolar non-keto-acidosis (HONK). Preexisting pulmonary, renal, or hepatic disease impairs the body's ability to handle trauma-induced acid-base disturbances, such as impaired ability of the liver to clear lactate through metabolism to bicarbonate. Impaired cardiac function and/or autonomic dysfunction can impair the ability of the cardiovascular system to compensate for hypovolemic shock. It is likely that the acid-base disturbance found in trauma patients be of mixed nature and multifactorial (Morris and Low 2008).

Application

Pathophysiology

The maintenance of a stable acid-base balance is essential to life. The concentration of hydrogen ion ($[H^+]$) is expressed as pH, which is the negative logarithm (to the base of 10) of the H^+ concentration (mol/L) where a change of 1 unit of pH expresses a 10-fold change in the opposite direction of H^+ concentration. A state of acid-base balance is a state where the number of $[H^+]$ and $[OH^-]$ ions is equal, and has a pH value of 7, which is the pH of water at 25 °C. Under normal physiologic conditions, human plasma has a pH of 7.4 (slightly alkalotic). This physiologic pH is maintained by the functions of buffer systems that have the capacity to either bind or release $[H^+]$ ions. These buffers system are: (1) bicarbonate (H_2CO_3/HCO_3^-), (2) hemoglobin (HbH/Hb^-), (3) proteins (PrH/Pr^-), (4) phosphates ($H_2PO_4^-/HPO_4^{2-}$), and (5) ammonia ($NH3/NH4+$) (Corey 2005). Bicarbonate is the most important buffer in plasma, Hb is important in blood, proteins are important intracellularly, while phosphate and ammonia are important in the urine.

Diagnosis

Diagnosis of acid-base disturbances consists of two steps: first measuring serum pH to detect the degree and direction of imbalance, and second measuring carbon dioxide partial pressure (pCO_2)

and HCO_3^- concentration to perform a differential diagnosis of the etiology of the disturbance. Additional measurements such as the concentrations of Na^+, K^+, Cl^-, lactate, ketones, suspected drugs, or toxic substances are measured in the plasma and/or urine as well plasma osmolality to further elucidate the etiology of the disturbance.

These measurements are facilitated by the presence of arterial catheter, which allows accurate, continuous measurement of blood pressure (BP) as well as frequent blood sampling for serial ABGs and other measurements. Currently available point-of-care devices allow for instant ABGs and measurements of other substances. In the absence of ABGs, venous blood gases (VBGs) may be used as substitute since they do correlate with ABGs, BE, and lactate levels (Kruse et al. 2011). Furthermore, in shock, central VBGs may more accurately reflect tissue pH levels than ABGs and elevated lactate levels may indicate hypoperfusion, even in the presence of normal BP and heart rate (HR).

A stepwise approach to diagnosis of acid-base disturbance may consist of the following:

1. Blood pH is used to detect acidosis or alkalosis based on deviation from 7.40 ± 0.05.
2. $PaCO_2$ is used to determine if the derangement is respiratory acidosis or alkalosis.
3. HCO_3^- and BE values are used to determine if the derangement is metabolic acidosis or alkalosis.
4. Change in pH is compared with changes in $paCO_2$ and HCO_3^- to determine whether the primary problem is respiratory or metabolic.
5. In metabolic disorders, the predicted $paCO_2$ is calculated to detect a coexisting respiratory component if the measured $paCO_2$ falls outside the predicted value, as follows:
    (a) Metabolic acidosis: Predicted $paCO_2$ should be $= 1.5 ([HCO_3^-]) + 8$.
    (b) Metabolic alkalosis: Predicted $paCO_2$ should be $= 40 + 0.6 (\Delta[HCO_3^-])$.
6. In metabolic acidosis, the anion gap (AG) is calculated to differentiate between high AG

metabolic acidosis (HAGMA) and normal AG metabolic acidosis (NAGMA), as follows:

(a) AG = [Na$^+$] − ([Cl$^-$] + [HCO$_3$$^-$]) (should be ≤12)

(b) AG is corrected down by 2 for every 1 g/dl decrease in serum albumin.

7. HAGMA can be due to accumulation of ketones, lactates, aspirins, or alcohols.

8. In HAGMA, the serum osmolar gap (OG) is calculated to detect the presence of uncharged acidic osmolar substances, as follows:

(a) OG = calculated osmolality–measured osmolality (should be ≤10)

(b) Calculated osmolality = 2(Na$^+$) + glucose/18 + BUN/2.8

9. NAGMA can be due to loss of HCO$_3$$^-$ from intestines (diarrhea) or urine (RTA), dilution of serum HCO$_3$$^-$ (hyperchloremic metabolic acidosis) or ingestion of HCl.

10. In NAGMA, serum potassium is used to differentiate hyperkalemic (≥5.5 mEq/l) NAGMA from hypokalemic (≤3.5 mEq/l) NAGMA.

11. Hyperkalemic NAGMA can be due to ingestion of HCl or RTA type IV.

12. In hypokalemic NAGMA, the urine anion gap (UAG) is calculated to differentiate RTA type I and II (positive UAG) from intestinal loss of HCO$_3$$^-$ (negative UAG), as follows:

UAG = urine [K$^+$] + urine [Na$^+$] − urine [Cl$^-$]

13. In metabolic alkalosis, urine [Cl$^-$] is used to differentiate between low urinary chloride metabolic alkalosis (LUCMA) and high (≥40 mEq/l) urinary chloride metabolic alkalosis (HUCMA).

(a) LUCMA is more common and can be due to volume depletion, vomiting, or nasogastric (NG) suction.

(b) HUCMA can be due to corticosteroids, mineralocorticoids, diuretics. or excessive NaHCO$_3$$^-$ administration.

14. In metabolic disorders, the delta:delta is calculated to detect further hidden metabolic disorders, as follows:

(a) Delta:delta = (ΔAG: Δ[HCO$_3$$^-$])

(b) ΔAG = measured AG − 12

(c) Δ[HCO$_3$$^-$] = normal [HCO$_3$$^-$] − measured [HCO$_3$$^-$]

(d) ΔAG + measured [HCO$_3$$^-$] should be = 24 (normal [HCO$_3$$^-$])

(e) if ΔAG + measured [HCO$_3$$^-$] < 24 → there is further NAGMA hidden

(f) if ΔAG + measured [HCO$_3$$^-$] > 24 → there is further metabolic acidosis hidden

Complications

Acidosis is part of the self-perpetuating lethal triad of trauma of hypothermia, acidosis, and coagulopathy, where each element in the triad can contribute to the development of other elements and perpetuates the cycle. Acidosis contributes to the development of coagulopathy by impairing platelet function, protease function, and thrombin generation (Curry and Davis 2012). Acidosis contributes to the development of hypothermia by vasodilation and impairing vascular response to endogenous and exogenous catecholamines. Acidosis contributes to the development of further acidosis by worsening hypoperfusion through decreased cardiac contractility, increased cardiac irritability and predisposition to arrhythmias, impaired vasoactive response to shock, and decreased response to endogenous and exogenous catecholamines.

Hypoperfusion-induced lactic acidosis in trauma has been found to be of diagnostic value (correlates with degree of tissue hypoxia), therapeutic value (response to resuscitative measures), and prognostic value (likelihood of organ failure and death) (Manikis et al. 1996).

Treatment

Treatment of acid-base disorders depends on the underlying causes. It is likely that acid-base imbalance in trauma is of mixed nature and multifactorial. Treatment of life-threatening acid-base imbalance should be initiated while search for the cause is ongoing. Hypoperfusion-induced lactic acidosis should be suspected in most cases of bleeding. Massive bleeding requires the initiation of massive transfusion protocol (MTP), which refers to replacement of an entire blood volume within 24 h, transfusion of 10 units of packed red blood cells (PRBCs) in 24 h, or transfusion of 4 units of PRBCs in 1 h with ongoing needs (Curry and Davis 2012).

Early transfusion of blood products facilitates maintaining oxygen delivery and hemostatic function as well as reducing tissue ischemia and acid-base imbalance. The concept of hemostatic resuscitation allows for some degree of mild hypotension in order to decrease dilutional coagulopathy, while it emphasizes early and aggressive use of blood products. Recent recommendations call for a transfusion ratio of 1:1:1 for PRBCs, fresh frozen plasma (FFPs), and platelets (Shere-Wolfe and Fouche 2012, and Dutton 2012). Transfusion at a rate greater than 1 unit/5 min can lead to citrate toxicity manifesting as metabolic alkalosis and hypocalemia.

Serial measurements of ABGs, pH, and lactate levels can gauge the adequacy of resuscitation. Initial serum lactate levels ≥ 4 mEq/L are associated with higher mortality (Manikis et al. 1996). Reducing lactate levels by ≥ 5 % within the first hour of resuscitation is associated with better prognosis.

Administration of sodium bicarbonate to treat severe acidosis should be accompanied by increasing minute ventilation to clear the associated increase in CO_2 production.

When end-tidal CO_2 ($EtCO_2$) levels are measured, the gradient of $EtCO_2$ to $PaCO_2$ should guide adjusting minute ventilation to avoid hypoventilation and worsening acidosis.

Prophylactic hyperventilation ($PaCO_2 \leq 25$ mmHg) is not recommended in traumatic brain injury (TBI) because the resulting vasoconstriction may worsen brain ischemia. Instead, hyperventilation is only recommended as a temporizing measure to lower intracranial pressure (ICP) briefly during emergency craniotomy for intracranial blood evacuation. Often, the respiratory alkalosis that is caused by briefly lowering $PaCO_2$ is balanced by the hyperchloremia metabolic acidosis that develops with isotonic normal saline administration.

Prognosis

The ability to control acid-base disorders depends on the ability to diagnose and treat the underlying causes. In trauma patients, initial blood lactate levels were found to differentiate survivors (average 2.8 mEq/L) from non-survivors (average 4.0 mEq/l), with mortality risk reaching 95 % with lactate level being (>10 mEq/l), while persistent elevation of lactate levels was found to correlate with increased risk of organ failure (Manikis et al. 1996). These findings support the recommendation of admitting trauma patients with blood lactate level >2.5 mEq/L with serial monitoring of lactate levels during resuscitation until the trend is reversed or serum lactates are cleared.

Cross-References

► Blood Component Transfusion
► Damage Control Resuscitation
► Electrolyte and Acid-Base Abnormalities
► Fluid, Electrolytes, and Nutrition in Trauma Patients
► Hemodynamic Management in Trauma Anesthesia
► Massive Transfusion
► Monitoring of Trauma Patients During Anesthesia
► Transfusion Strategy in Trauma: What Is the Evidence?

References

Corey HE (2005) Bench-to-bedside review: fundamental principles of acid-base physiology. Crit Care 9:184–192
Curry N, Davis PW (2012) What's new in resuscitation strategies for the patient with multiple trauma? Injury. Int J Care Inj 43:1021–1028
Dutton R (2012) Blood component therapy and trauma coagulopathy. In: Varon AJ, Smith CE (eds) Essentials of trauma anesthesia. Cambridge University Press, Cambridge, pp 66–75
Kruse O, Grunnet N, Barfod C (2011) Blood lactate as a predictor for in-hospital mortality in patients

admitted acutely to hospital: a systematic review. Scand J Trauma Resusc Emerg Med 19:74–86

Manikis P, Jankowski S, Zhang H, Kahn R, Vincent J-L (1996) Correlation of serial blood lactate levels to organ failure and mortality after trauma. Am J Emerg Med 13:619–622

Morris CG, Low J (2008) Metabolic acidosis in the critically ill: Part 1. Classification and pathophysiology. Anaesthesia 63:294–301

Nunez TC, Young PP, Holcomb JB, Cotton BA (2010) Creation, implementation, and maturation of a massive transfusion protocol for the exsanguinating trauma patient. J Trauma 68(6):1498–1505

Seifter JL (2011) Acid-base disorders. In: Goldman L, Schafer AI (eds) Cecil medicine, 24th edn. Saunders Elsevier, Philadelphia

Shere-Wolfe R, Fouche Y (2012) Shock, resuscitation, and fluid therapy. In: Varon AJ, Smith CE (eds) Essentials of trauma anesthesia. Cambridge University Press, Cambridge, pp 43–54

Recommended Reading

Gindi M, Sattler S, Hoos K, Matei M, Paulus C, Yens D (2007) Can venous blood gas samples replace arterial blood gas samples for measurement of base excess in severely injured trauma patients? N Y Med J 2(2)

Hayter MA, Pavenski K, Baker J (2012) Massive transfusion in the trauma patient: continuing professional development. J Can Anesth 59:1130–1145

Kraut JA, Madias NE (2012) Treatment of acute metabolic acidosis: a pathophysiologic approach. Nat Rev Nephrol 8:589–601

Povlishock JT (ed) (2000) Guidelines for the management of severe traumatic brain injury. J Neurotrauma 17:449–554

Severinghaus JW, Astrup PB (1985) History of blood gas analysis II: pH and acid-base balance measurements. J Clin Monit 1:259–277

Sihler KC, Napolitano LM (2009) Massive transfusion: new insights. Chest 136:1654–1667

Wilson M, Davis DP, Coimbra R (2003) Diagnosis and monitoring of hemorrhagic shock during the initial resuscitation of multiple trauma patients: a review. J Emerg Med 24:413–422

Acid-Citrate-Dextrose, ACD

▶ Citrate-Dextrose Solutions

Acidosis, Academia (Respiratory Versus Metabolic)

▶ Acid-Base Management in Trauma Anesthesia

ACOT

▶ Acute Coagulopathy of Trauma

ACOTS

▶ Acute Coagulopathy of Trauma

Acquired Brain Injury

▶ Neurotrauma, Anesthesia Management

Activated Partial Thromboplastin Time

▶ Partial Thromboplastin Time

Activated Recombinant Human Blood Coagulation Factor VII

▶ Adjuncts to Transfusion: Recombinant Factor VIIa, Factor XIII, and Calcium

Activity Restrictions

Douglas Fetkenhour
Department of Physical Medicine and Rehabilitation, University of Rochester School of Medicine, Rochester, NY, USA

Synonyms

Weight bearing restrictions

Definition

Physician guided limitations to weight bearing or range of motion to facilitate proper healing.

Trauma often results in injury to bone and soft tissue to a degree that its structural integrity is compromised. Fractures of load bearing bones can no longer accept full weight without risk of non-union. Areas of denuded skin that require skin grafting may also be at risk of 'not taking' if the region bears weight or is put through range of motion. Restriction of specific activities is often necessary to allow proper healing.

The duration of activity restrictions depends on the nature of the injury. Non-weight bearing status for fractures of load bearing bones may be necessary until callous formation occurs, typically 12 weeks. Range of motion restrictions for a soft tissue injury may require 1 or 2 weeks to allow the tissue to heal.

Activity restrictions will impact the trauma patient's functional activity. NWB of the lower limbs will affect the ability to ambulate and upper limb non weight bearing may create difficulties with bed mobility and self care tasks. Restrictions on range of motion will affect both mobility and self care. Physical and Occupational therapists are instrumental in teaching the trauma patient compensatory techniques to allow them to function within the limits of their activity restrictions.

Cross-References

▶ Occupational Therapist
▶ Physical Therapist

References

JeMe Cioppa-Mosca, Janet B. Cahill, Carmen Young Tucker (8 June 2006) Postsurgical rehabilitation guidelines for the orthopedic clinician. Elsevier Health Sciences

Acute Abdominal Compartment Syndrome in Trauma

Charles A. Frosolone
Medical Department, USS Nimitz CVN-68, Everett, WA, USA

Synonyms

Abdominal compartment syndrome; Intra-abdominal hypertension with organ dysfunction

Definition

Abdominal compartment syndrome (ACS) is characterized by critical organ dysfunction within and beyond the abdomen resulting from intra-abdominal hypertension (IAH).

Prevention

Particularly at risk is the trauma patient requiring large-volume resuscitation and emergent abdominal surgery as seen in battlefield trauma (Kozar et al. 2008). It also can be seen in burn patients or others requiring large-volume resuscitation. Prevention can be accomplished by use of temporary abdominal closure techniques for patients who are at risk for development of ACS or to closely monitor those at risk and intervene early. This is a scenario often seen in battlefield injuries necessitating damage control surgery, and these types of victims generally have their abdomens left open, utilizing some type of temporary abdominal closure.

Diagnosis

In a patient who is at risk of ACS, look for findings that can be cardiopulmonary, gastrointestinal, renal, and central nervous system in nature and are consistent with IAH (Corbridge and Wood 2005). First, look for a distended, tense abdomen in a patient who has had a major blood loss and/or fluid resuscitation. Elevation of the diaphragm by IAH decreases pulmonary compliance and increases work of breathing. IAH decreases venous return to the heart by compression on the inferior vena cava and worsening of ventricular compliance and contractility. IAH decreases gut perfusion and can result in gut ischemia and bacterial translocation. IAH causes decreasing renal function, decreased urine output, and anuria untreated. IAH can also cause an increase in intracranial pressures and decreased cerebral perfusion pressures (Ameloot et al. 2012). Intra-abdominal pressure (IAP) is easily measured at the level of the symphysis pubis through a saline column (50–100 mL) previously injected into an empty bladder and connected to a pressure transducer or manometer. IAP of 25 mmHg is an indicator to decompress the abdomen (Cothren et al. 2010).

Treatment

Once ACS is identified, neuromuscular blockers may decrease IAP, but decompressive laparotomy with temporary abdominal closure or revising a patient's temporary abdominal closure if the abdomen is already open should be done. There are many described methods of temporary abdominal closure from towel clip or suture closure of the skin to temporary silos.

Later in the patient's course as midgut edema resolves, and the risk of recurrent ACS has passed, the open abdomen is closed and techniques range from delayed fascial closure to planned ventral hernia.

Cross-References

▶ Abdominal Compartment Syndrome as a Complication of Care
▶ ABThera Wound Dressing
▶ Bogota Bag
▶ Mesh Temporary Closure

▶ Methods of Containment of the Open Abdomen, Overview
▶ Open Abdomen
▶ Open Abdomen, Temporary Abdominal Closure
▶ Towel Clip Closure

References

Ameloot K, Gillebert C, Desie N, Manu LNG (2012) Hypoperfusion, shock states, and Abdominal Compartment Syndrome (ACS). Surg Clin N Am 92:207–220
Corbridge T, Wood LD (2005) Restrictive disease of the respiratory system and the abdominal compartment syndrome. In: Hall JB, Schmidt GA, Wood LD (eds) Principles of critical care. McGraw Hill, New York, Chapter 42. 3e
Cothren CC, Biffl WL, Moore EE (2010) Trauma. In: Brunicardi FC, Andersen DK, Billiar TR, Dunn DL, Hunter JG, Matthews JB, Pollock RE (eds) Schwartz's principles of surgery. McGraw Hill, New York, Chapter 7. 9e
Kozar RA, Weisbrodt NW, Moore FA (2008) Gastrointestinal failure. In: Moore EE, Feliciano DV, Mattox KL (eds) Trauma. McGraw Hill, New York, Chapter 64. 6e

Acute Blood Loss Anemia

▶ Hemorrhage

Acute Brain Dysfunction

▶ Delirium as a Complication of ICU Care
▶ Preventing Delirium in the Intensive Care Unit

Acute Care Nurse Practitioner

▶ Nurse Practitioners in Trauma Care

Acute Coagulopathy of Trauma

Bryan A. Cotton[1] and Laura A. McElroy[2]
[1]Department of Surgery, Division of Acute Care
Surgery, Trauma and Critical Care, University of
Texas Health Science Center at Houston, The
University of Texas Medical School at Houston,
Houston, TX, USA
[2]Department of Anesthesiology, Critical Care
Medicine, University of Rochester Medical
Center, Rochester, NY, USA

Synonyms

ACOT; ACOTS; ATC; COT; Early trauma-
associated coagulopathy; TAC; TIC

Definition

Acute coagulopathy of trauma (ACOT) is an early
post-injury endogenous hypocoagulability that
occurs in severely injured trauma patients (Frith
et al. 2010). Approximately 25 % of trauma
patients arrive to the hospital with clinical and
biochemical evidence of impaired clot formation
and early clot lysis (Brohi et al. 2003). ACOT has
been strongly associated with hemorrhagic shock
states and is associated with a significantly worse
overall prognosis. Initial standard coagulations
studies, including international normalized ratio
of prothrombin time (PT) and partial thromboplastin time (PTT), are insensitive, while viscoelastic
tests of clot strength such as thromboelastography
(Holcomb et al. 2012) can detect coagulation
defects early and can be used to guide resuscitation
of the coagulation system (Schochl et al. 2013).

The etiology of ACOT is at present unclear but
likely involves aspects of shock, coagulation factor depletion (Rizoli et al. 2011; Cohen et al.
2013), activation of protein C, enthusiastic thrombolysis, and platelet and endothelial dysfunction
(Frith et al. 2010). Current treatment includes limiting exacerbating factors, such as the minimization of crystalloid fluids (Cotton et al. 2012), and
avoidance of hypothermia and acidosis, in tandem
with prompt surgical control of hemorrhage; early
correction to normal coagulability with plasma,
cryoprecipitate, and platelet transfusion; and
selective use of antifibrinolytics.

There is some debate about whether ACOT is
a distinct coagulopathic entity or a subset of
disseminated intravascular coagulopathy with
a fibrinolytic phenotype (Gando et al. 2012;
Yanagida et al. 2013). Due to the heterogeneity
of timing and types of blood samples taken in
individual studies, more standardized research is
needed to elucidate the full range of pathophysiologic changes that occur after trauma.

Cross-References

▶ Coagulopathy
▶ Coagulopathy in Trauma: Underlying
   Mechanisms
▶ International Normalized Ratio
▶ Partial Thromboplastin Time
▶ Prothrombin Time

References

Brohi K, Singh J, Heron M et al (2003) Acute trauma
    coagulopathy. J Trauma 54(6):1127–1130
Cohen MJ, Kutcher M, Redick B et al (2013) Clinical and
    mechanistic drivers of acute traumatic coagulopathy.
    J Trauma Acute Care Surg 75(Suppl 1):1
Cotton BA, Harvin JA, Kostousouv V et al
    (2012) Hyperfibrinolysis at admission is an uncommon
    but highly lethal event associated with shock and
    prehospital fluid administration. J Trauma Acute
    Care Surg 73(2):365–370
Frith D, Goslings JC, Gaarder C (2010) Definition and
    drivers of acute trauma coagulopathy: clinical and
    experimental drivers. J Thromb Haemost 8:1919–1925
Gando S, Wada H, Kim HK et al (2012) Scientific and
    standardization committee on DIC of the international
    society on thrombosis and haemostasis official com-
    munications. Comparison of disseminated intravascu-
    lar coagulation (DIC) in trauma with coagulopathy of
    trauma/acute coagulopathy of trauma-shock (COT/
    ACOTS). J Thromb Haemost 10:2593–2595
Holcomb JB, Minei KM, Scerbo ML et al (2012) Admis-
    sion rapid thromboelastography can replace conven-
    tional coagulation tests in the emergency department:
    experience with 1974 consecutive trauma patients.
    Ann Surg 256:476–486

Rizoli SB, Scarpelini S, Callum J et al (2011) Clotting factor deficiency in early trauma-associated coagulopathy. J Trauma 71(5 Suppl 1):S441–S447. doi:10.1097/TA.0b013e318232e688

Schochl H, Voelckel W, Grassetto A, Schlimp CJ (2013) Practical application of point-of-care coagulation testing to guide treatment decisions in trauma. J Trauma Acute Care Surg 74:1587–1598

Yanagida Y, Gando S, Sawamura A et al (2013) Normal prothrombinase activity, increased systemic thrombin activity, and lower antithrombin levels in patients with disseminated intravascular coagulation at an early phase of trauma: comparison with acute coagulopathy of trauma-shock. Surgery 154:48–57

Acute Compartment Syndrome

▶ Compartment Syndrome of the Forearm

Acute Confusion

▶ Delirium as a Complication of ICU Care

Acute Confusional State

▶ Preventing Delirium in the Intensive Care Unit

Acute Kidney Injury

Oleksa Rewa[1] and Sean M. Bagshaw[2]
[1]Department of Critical Care Medicine, Faculty of Medicine, University of Toronto, Toronto, ON, Canada
[2]Division of Critical Care Medicine, Faculty of Medicine and Dentistry, University of Alberta, Edmonton, AB, Canada

Synonyms

Acute renal failure; AKI; ARF; Kidney failure; Renal insufficiency

Introduction

Acute kidney injury (AKI), which represents an abrupt deterioration of kidney function, is a frequently encountered phenomenon in hospitalized patients. The impact of AKI is most profound among patients admitted to intensive care units (ICU). The frequency of AKI among critically ill patients is increasing, such that AKI now complicates the course in an estimated two-thirds of critically ill patients. This is likely attributable to the growing prevalence of older patients and more comorbid illness, including preexisting chronic kidney disease (CKD), diabetes mellitus, and cardiovascular disease. For critically ill patients with more severe forms of AKI, an estimated 50–70 % will require support with acute dialysis (i.e., also known as renal replacement therapy (RRT)), which represents a small (4–8 %) but important group of all critically ill patients. For these individuals, RRT initiation often results in a considerable escalation in both the complexity and associated costs of care. Moreover, these critically ill patients also experience substantial morbidity, including non-recovery of kidney function and dialysis dependence, as well as excess mortality, with hospital mortality rates commonly exceeding 60 %. Thus, AKI remains a frequently encountered entity in the ICU and is an important therapeutic hurdle that deserves important consideration when dealing with its consequences and managing its various complications.

Definition

AKI, previously referred to as acute renal failure, is a complex syndrome characterized by the acute loss of renal excretory function, resulting in the accumulation of nitrogenous end products of metabolism and fluid. It is typically diagnosed by the retention of markers of kidney function (i.e., urea and creatinine) and oligo-anuria.

Traditionally, there has been a wide spectrum of definitions for AKI used in the literature. These definitions have used a range of conventional surrogates of kidney function (i.e., urea, serum

Acute Kidney Injury, Table 1 RIFLE classification

	Change in serum creatinine	Change in estimated glomerular filtration rate	Urine output criteria
R – risk of kidney dysfunction	Increase × 1.5	Decrease >25 %	< 0.5 ml/kg/h for >6 h
I – injury	Increase × 2	Decrease >50 %	<0.5 ml/kg/h for >12 h
F – failure of the kidney	Increase × 3 **or** Cr ≥ 354 µmol/L (acute rise >44 µmol/L)	Decrease >75 %	< 0.5 ml/kg/h for >24 h or anuria for >12 h
L – loss of kidney function	Loss of kidney function, which requires dialysis, for longer than 4 weeks		
E – end-stage kidney disease	Loss of kidney function, which requires dialysis, for longer than 3 months		

The RIFLE classification includes biochemical as well as clinical parameters as outlined above. The worst of any of the three parameters is considered when determining stage of renal injury

creatinine (sCr), urine output, or a combination of these) to describe the presence and severity of function loss. This heterogeneity has presented significant challenges for clinical investigation, epidemiology, and therapeutic trials and likely held up scientific progress in AKI research. In 2004, a consensus definition was published by Acute Dialysis Quality Initiative (ADQI) group, referred to as the RIFLE classification system (acronym: *r*isk, *i*njury, *f*ailure, *l*oss, and *e*nd-stage renal disease) (Table 1). The classification defined three grades of AKI severity (risk, injury, failure) based on relative changes to sCr and/or absolute changes in urine output. The outcome classes (*l*oss and *e*nd-stage kidney disease) are based on the duration of RRT. This novel classification scheme has been shown to have value across a range of clinical studies for identifying/classifying AKI, along with robust prediction for clinical outcomes, and has been widely integrated into the medical literature. The RIFLE definition was later refined by the Acute Kidney Injury Network (AKIN), a consortium uniting representatives from all major nephrology and critical care societies (Table 2). This new definition recognized that changes in glomerular filtration rate (GFR) may be inaccurate for the detection of early kidney injury, and thus only sCr and urine criteria were included. It also specified that acute changes in kidney function should occur in less than 48 h to qualify as AKI. Finally, it simplified the AKI

Acute Kidney Injury, Table 2 The AKIN classification

Stage	Serum creatinine criteria	Urine output criteria
1	Increase in sCr ≥26.4 µmol/L **or** increase sCr to ≥150–200 %	<0.5 ml/kg/h for >6 h
2	Increase in sCr to >200–300 %	<0.5 ml/kg/h for >12 h
3	Increase in sCr >300 % **or** Cr ≥354 µmol/L (acute rise >44 µmol/L) **or** on RRT	<0.3 ml/kg/h for 24 h **or** Anuria >12 h

The AKIN classification includes both biochemical and clinical criteria. It is important to note that these need to occur over a maximal 48-h period to be considered acute. As for the RIFLE classification system, the stage is based on the most severe parameter

sCr serum creatinine, *RRT* renal replacement therapy

staging to three stages – the first two being progressive stages of renal dysfunction and the third stage encompassing kidney failure. These three stages were deemed to be successively progressive along the continuum of kidney injury ending in overt renal failure and have now been consolidated into the KDIGO guidelines for AKI (Kellum and Lameire 2012).

While the development of a consensus classification scheme for AKI has been an important landmark for AKI research, these classification schemes have notable limitations. In particular, they still use surrogate markers of kidney function rather than specific biomarkers for kidney damage; they rely on a known "baseline" creatinine for diagnosis, which is often unknown; and they still diagnose AKI relatively "late" after the injury stimulus has occurred. These limitations will likely result in these consensus definitions being modified over time as new knowledge is gained. However, the majority of studies now use the RIFLE and/or AKIN definition for the diagnosis and classification of AKI. This has improved generalizability and comparisons across epidemiologic investigations. Novel biomarkers of kidney damage, such as neutrophil gelatinase-associated lipocalin (NGAL), are increasingly being characterized and may provide incremental benefit for the early detection of kidney damage and enable earlier triage to interventions, prior to decline or overt failure of kidney function, beyond currently available conventional measures.

Preexisting Condition

Scope of Clinical Problem

As aforementioned, AKI is common in critically ill patients and may impact 2–50 % of major trauma patients admitted to ICU, depending on the definition of AKI used for diagnosis (Bagshaw et al. 2008). Several observational studies have found that the development of AKI in major trauma is independently associated with a dose–response increase in risk for hospital mortality (Table 3). These data have also shown AKI contributes to increased risk for development of multiorgan dysfunction and prolonged duration of ICU stay. A number of non-modifiable and potentially

Acute Kidney Injury, Table 3 Observational studies examining AKI in trauma

Author	Year	Design	N	Incidence	Risk factors	Outcome
Shashaty MG	2012	Single center prospective	400	36.8 % (AKIN)	African American, BMI > 30, DM, major abdominal injury, unmatched packed RBC transfusion	Mortality
Wohlauer MV	2012	Single center retrospective	2,157	2.13 % (Denver MOF score – sCr > 159)	Older age, shock, massive RBC transfusion, thrombocytopenia	MOF, mortality
De Abreu KL	2010	Single center retrospective	129	40.3 % (RIFLE)	Abdominal trauma, furosemide use, sepsis, hypotension	Mortality
Gomes E	2010	Single center retrospective	436	50.0 % (RIFLE)	Illness severity	ICU LOS
Moore EM	2010	Multicenter retrospective	207 (TBI)	9.2 % (RIFLE)	Older age, illness severity	–
Bihorac A	2010	Multicenter prospective	982 (blunt)	26.0 % (RIFLE)	Older age, female, obesity, CKD, illness severity	Mortality, ICU LOS
Costantini TW	2009	Single center retrospective	541	29.8 % (AKIN)	Older age, illness severity, ICU length of stay	MOF, ICU LOS, mortality
Bagshaw SM	2008	Multicenter retrospective	9,449	18.1 % (RIFLE)	Older age, female, comorbid illness, illness severity	Mortality
Brandt MM	2007	Single center retrospective	1,033	23.8 % (RIFLE)	Older age, ICU length of stay, ventilator days	Mortality, ICU LOS, cost

Risk factors are those determined significant for the development of AKI, and the outcomes included below are only those found to be significantly increased with the development of AKI
MOF multiple organ failure, *RBC* red blood cell, *LOS* length of stay

Acute Kidney Injury, Table 4 Causes of AKI in trauma

Non-modifiable	Trauma related	Iatrogenic
Older age	Arterial underfilling (hemorrhage/hypovolemia)	HES
Female sex	Anemia	Contrast dyes
Race	Rhabdomyolysis/myoglobinemia	ACS
Obesity	Renal contusion/infarction	Fluid accumulation
Comorbid illness	Intra-abdominal trauma	Medications
Cardiovascular disease	Vascular dissections/thrombosis	Major surgery
Chronic kidney disease	Retroperitoneal hematoma	Sepsis
Diabetes mellitus		Transfusion

Abdominal compartment syndrome is listed as an iatrogenic cause as it is often due to fluid administration. Medications commonly associated with AKI include NSAIDs, aminoglycosides, vancomycin, metformin, and ACE inhibitors
HES hydroxyethyl starch, *ACS* abdominal compartment syndrome

modifiable factors have been shown to be associated with development of AKI in trauma, including older age, female sex, African American, obesity, and preexisting comorbid illnesses (i.e., chronic kidney disease, diabetes mellitus), along with severity of illness, abdominal trauma, shock, sepsis, use of furosemide, thrombocytopenia, transfusions of unmatched blood, as well as massive blood transfusions. Table 4 summarizes the scope of potential contributing factors for AKI in trauma.

Application

General Principles of Acute Kidney Injury Prevention and Management

Accordingly, strategies to prevent or mitigate AKI should be individualized while avoiding further exposure to kidney insults and mitigating the complications associated with kidney failure. In general, the overarching tenets for *ALL*

potentially susceptible patients should consider the following:

1. Consider the early use of invasive/functional hemodynamic monitoring (i.e., arterial catheter, central venous pressure, echocardiography, pulmonary artery catheter, or methods to measure stroke or pulse pressure variation, abdominal compartment pressures) where available to guide resuscitation. The physiologic endpoints should be to ensure adequate intravascular volume repletion, preservation of cardiac output, mean arterial pressure, and maintenance of oxygen carrying capacity (i.e., hemoglobin).

2. Monitor and maintain fluid and electrolyte homeostasis, including the use of balanced crystalloid solutions when available to mitigate the risk of iatrogenic hyperchloremic acidosis during large volume resuscitation. Avoid the use of nephrotoxic synthetic colloids, such as hydroxyethyl starch (HES) in those at high risk for or with early evidence of AKI.

3. Remove and avoid all nonessential and potentially nephrotoxic exposures. When selected investigations (i.e., contrast-enhanced computerized tomography) and medications are considered vital (i.e., antimicrobials in sepsis), there must be careful attention to minimizing exposure, applying techniques to mitigate the risk of AKI, and appropriate therapeutic monitoring and dose-adjustment based on changes to kidney function.

4. Review whether there are context- and/or syndrome-specific interventions available, such as in contrast media-associated AKI (CA-AKI), rhabdomyolysis, sepsis-associated AKI, or abdominal compartment syndrome (ACS).

5. Mitigate the risk of complications of over kidney failure, with particular attention to life-threatening complications including hyperkalemia, hypocalcaemia, metabolic acidosis and diuretic-resistant intravascular fluid overload, and pulmonary edema, and when indicated, plan appropriately for initiation of RRT.

General Therapies

Fluid Therapy

One of the first principles of therapy for AKI involves appropriate fluid resuscitation and restoration of adequate intravascular circulation volume. There is no consensus on the type of fluid used; however, recent data have suggested that HES may contribute to and/or exacerbate AKI and should be avoided (Schortgen et al. 2001). Typically a crystalloid (either 0.9 % normal saline or balanced Ringer's lactate) is normally chosen, and boluses of 10–20 mL/kg are given to reestablish intravascular volume. If a specific etiology of hypovolemia is determined, such as hemorrhage, resuscitation with blood products is indicated. In all cases, resuscitation should ideally be guided by invasive functional hemodynamic monitoring targeted to physiologic endpoints, with attention to and avoidance of unnecessary fluid accumulation.

Diuretics

The role of diuretic therapy in the management of patients with AKI is controversial; however, diuretics remain a key therapy for excessive fluid accumulation and/or intravascular volume overload. Most studies to date have not shown definitive benefit for diuretic therapy to treat AKI, with some suggesting potential for harm (de Abreu et al. 2010). Diuretics have been utilized to convert "oliguric" to "non-oliguric" AKI, and this may delay or ameliorate the need for RRT; however, improvements in survival or kidney recovery have not been shown. Of note, in a subgroup analysis of the FACCT (Grams et al. 2011) trial which focused on acute lung injury patients whose course was complicated by AKI (only 8 % had primary lung injury attributable to trauma), those who received a greater cumulative dose of furosemide were found to have lower mortality, while those with greater fluid accumulation had higher mortality. Moreover, there was no observed threshold of furosemide dose beyond which mortality was shown to increase. These data would imply, in a cohort of critically ill patients with AKI, that the selective use of furosemide is likely effective and safe, in particular when confronted by fluid accumulation and overload; however, further randomized trials are needed.

Specific Trauma-Related Syndromes

Contrast Media-Associated AKI (CA-AKI)

CA-AKI is a leading cause of iatrogenic kidney injury following diagnostic and interventional procedures. The pathophysiology of CA-AKI remains incompletely understood; however, it is believed to involve a combination of renal vasoconstriction, corticomedullary ischemia, direct tubular toxicity, and tubular cast formation/obstruction. Strategies for prevention have generally included inducing a forced diuresis and high urine flow rates, inducing renal vasodilatation, and attenuation of oxidative stress and inflammation (Wong et al. 2012). CA-AKI has been shown to occur in 3.0–7.7 % of patients with major trauma. Among critically ill patients, CA-AKI occurs in approximately 15 % of cases receiving contrast media with imaging procedures. Risk factors for the occurrence of this condition include preexisting, diabetes mellitus, older age, atherosclerotic disease, and impaired cardiac function (Wong et al. 2012). Studies have also found that acute anemia, transfusions, and increased injury severity score also modify the risk of CA-AKI in trauma patients. The presence of proteinuria may also predict increased susceptibility to CA-AKI in major trauma. The majority of preventative interventions studied to date, with the exception of hydration, have been shown either ineffective or inconsistent, including forced diuresis, N-acetylcysteine, sodium bicarbonate, and prophylactic hemofiltration. For most major trauma patients, the benefits of CT diagnostic/therapeutic imaging outweigh the risks of developing CA-AKI; however, whenever possible, this risk should be minimized by ensuring adequate volume repletion, avoiding concomitant nephrotoxins, using the minimum volume of contrast media, avoiding repeated contrast media exposure, and in high-risk patients, when necessary, planning for the potential of need for RRT initiation.

A

Rhabdomyolysis and Myoglobinuria

Rhabdomyolysis is characterized by the breakdown of skeletal muscle resulting in the release of myoglobin and other muscle constituents into the extracellular fluid. Rhabdomyolysis may develop due to disruption of substrate and/or oxygen metabolism, impaired cellular energy production, and increased intracellular calcium influx. In trauma, disruption of substrate/oxygen supply for metabolism due to crush injury, secondary compartment syndrome, and muscle ischemia are the most common precipitating factors for rhabdomyolysis. This may be accompanied by concomitant intravascular volume depletion due to fluid sequestration in the injured muscle resulting in arterial under filling and kidney hypoperfusion. There can be direct tubular injury from heme-pigment cast formation as well as uric acid crystallization and obstruction. Secondary kidney damage may result from oxidative stress from iron-mediated free radical production and myoglobin-induced nitric oxide scavenging and finally from the circulation of inflammatory mediators and activation of the innate immune system (Malinoski and Slater 2004).

The cornerstone for the prevention and treatment of rhabdomyolysis and myoglobinuric AKI remains aggressive volume resuscitation. This is achieved initially with crystalloid fluid infusion (10–15 mL/kg/h) titrated to achieve urine outputs of 200–300 mL/h. Following initial resuscitation, bicarbonate may be added (50–100 mEg/L) and titrated to achieve a urine pH > 6.5 to increase the solubility and renal excretion of tubular myoglobin and uric acid as well as attenuation of acidosis, hyperkalemia, and release of free iron from myoglobin. However, if urine alkalization is ineffective, bicarbonate containing solutions should be discontinued to avoid development of symptomatic hypocalcaemia (Bosch et al. 2009). There are theoretical benefits for the use of mannitol to provoke an osmotic diuresis to flush intratubular myoglobin deposition and cast formation and to remove sequestered water from injured muscle and prevent compartment syndromes, but this is currently not supported by evidence from randomized trials. Other controversial strategies include allopurinol

Acute Kidney Injury, Table 5 Classification of intra-abdominal hypertension

Grade	Intra-abdominal pressure
I	12–15 mmHg
II	16–20 mmHg
III	21–25 mmHg
IV	>25 mmHg

Abdominal compartment syndrome is generally defined as abdominal hypertension (grade III or IV) with the presence of end-organ dysfunction

to reduce uric acid production, use of pentoxifylline to improve microcirculatory blood flow, reducing oxidant injury with glutathione, chelation of free iron with deferoxamine, and dantrolene to reduce intracellular calcium, but these are also not supported by data from randomized trials. When AKI progresses to overt kidney failure, no specific therapy is available, and patients should be supported by the timely initiation of RRT. For those with severe rhabdomyolysis and increased risk for myoglobinuric AKI, consideration can be given to accelerate myoglobin clearance with extracorporeal support with high-flux or super high-flux hemofiltration.

Abdominal Compartment Syndrome (ACS)

Intra-abdominal injury, large volume fluid resuscitation, and postoperative factors may all contribute to the development of intra-abdominal hypertension (IAH) and abdominal compartment syndrome (ACS) (Table 5). ACS has been shown to occur in 13–26 % of critically ill patients with major trauma (De Waele et al. 2011). With IAH/ACS, AKI occurs in response to impaired renal blood flow and reduced renal perfusion pressure. IAH/ACS may also lead to increased renal venous pressures contributing to reduce renal perfusion pressure. In addition, as the kidneys are encapsulated organs, renal parenchymal edema may contribute to a phenomenal known as "renal compartment syndrome" and AKI. This concept is supported by observations of improved kidney function following release of the renal capsule. In theory, ACS could contribute to post-obstructive AKI; however, recent data have suggested that placement of ureteral stents has not resulted in immediate resolution of AKI

(De Waele et al. 2011). Clinical apparent changes to kidney function typically begin to occur with an intra-abdominal pressure of ≥15 mmHg manifesting with the development of oliguria and at pressures ≥30 mmHg, overt anuria. The primary treatment of AKI occurring in ACS is to reverse the ACS with either appropriate medical or surgical therapy. Medical therapy may include removal of intra-abdominal contents (i.e., nasogastric/rectal drainage to reduce bowel distension), paracentesis for hemoperitoneum or ascites, and diuresis for fluid accumulation. If these conservative measures fail, surgical decompression in the form of a laparotomy and releasing of abdominal contents is necessary.

Sepsis

Sepsis is the most common contributing factor for AKI in critically ill patients and represents an important late precipitate for patients with major trauma. The pathophysiology of sepsis-related AKI remains poorly understood, but it associated with a higher risk of poor clinical outcomes. Early sepsis may be due to wound contamination (i.e., open fractures, abrasions, or lacerations), intra-abdominal/pelvic injury, and contamination or aspiration at time of injury. Late sepsis is more often the result of nosocomial infections such as surgical site infections, nosocomial and ventilator-associated pneumonias, and catheter-related bloodstream infections (CRBSIs) in those patients with lines in situ. Delays in the initiation of appropriate antimicrobial therapy have resulted in worsening AKI, and mortality is increased in conjunction with more severe stages of AKI (Bagshaw et al. 2009). Early wound decontamination, timely surgical management when necessary, and adherence to appropriate care bundles to prevent nosocomial infections are also all part of the general care package to prevent sepsis and subsequent AKI in trauma patients.

Conclusion

AKI is commonly encountered in trauma patients and portends a significant increase in morbidity and mortality. Numerous non-modifiable and modifiable (i.e., potentially iatrogenic) factors contribute to AKI in trauma. In addition to the general principles for preventing and treating AKI, attention should also be given to precipitants with interventions supported by evidence such as avoidance of unnecessary and/or repeated contrast media exposure, early resuscitation in myoglobinuria, early surveillance for and management of IAH/ACS, and sepsis. Finally, in those trauma patients who develop overt kidney failure, complications should be anticipated, and patients should be supported early with RRT when indicated.

Cross-References

▶ Abdominal Compartment Syndrome as a Complication of Care
▶ Crush Injuries
▶ Dialysis
▶ Electrolyte and Acid-Base Abnormalities
▶ Fluid, Electrolytes, and Nutrition in Trauma Patients
▶ Renal Failure as a Complication, Acute

References

Bagshaw SM, George C, Gibney RTN, Bellomo R (2008) A multi-center evaluation of early acute kidney injury in critically ill trauma patients. Ren Fail 30(6):581–589

Bosch X, Poch E, Grau JM (2009) Rhabdomyolysis and acute kidney injury. N Engl J Med 361(1):62–72

de Abreu KS, Silva GB, Barreto AG, Melo FM, Oliveira BB, Mota RM, Rocha NA, Silva SL, Araújo SM, Daher EF (2010) Acute kidney injury after trauma: prevalence, clinical characteristics and RIFLE classification. Indian J Crit Care Med 14:121–128

De Waele JJ, De Laet I, Kirkpatrick AW, Hoste E (2011) Intra-abdominal hypertension and abdominal compartment syndrome. Am J Kidney Dis 57(1):159–169

Grams ME, Estrella MM, Coresh J, Brower RG, Liu KD (2011) Fluid balance, diuretic use, and mortality in acute kidney injury. Clin J Am Soc Nephrol 6:966–973

Kellum JA, Lameire N (2012) KDIGO clinical practice guideline for acute kidney injury. Kidney Int Suppl 2(1):1–141

Malinoski DJ, Slater MS (2004) Crush injury and rhabdomyolysis. Crit Care Clin 20:171–192

Schortgen F, Lacherade J-C, Bruneel F et al (2001) Effects of hydroxyethylstarch and gelatin on renal function in severe sepsis: a multicentre randomised study. Lancet 357(9260):911–916

A

The Cooperative Antimicrobial Therapy of Septic Shock (CATSS) Database Research Group, Bagshaw SM, Lapinsky S et al (2009) Acute kidney injury in septic shock: clinical outcomes and impact of duration of hypotension prior to initiation of antimicrobial therapy. Intensive Care Med 35(5):871–881

Wong PCY, Li Z, Guo J, Zhang A (2012) Pathophysiology of contrast-induced nephropathy. Int J Cardiol 158(2):186–192

Acute Kidney Injury (AKI)

▶ Renal Failure as a Complication, Acute

Acute Liver Failure

▶ Hepatic Failure

Acute Lung Injury

▶ Acute Respiratory Distress Syndrome (ARDS), General
▶ ARDS, Complication of Trauma

Acute Normovolemic Hemodilution

▶ Autologous Donation

Acute Pain Management in Trauma

Edward E. Braun, Talal W. Khan and Stephen M. Campbell
Department of Anesthesiology, University of Kansas Medical Center, Kansas City, KS, USA

Synonyms

Pain management in acute injury state

Definition

The International Association for the Study of Pain defines pain as "an unpleasant sensory and emotional experience associated with actual or potential tissue damage or described in terms of such damage." Pain can be identified as either acute or chronic. Acute pain is a predicted response to a noxious mechanical, thermal, or chemical stimulus such as trauma or surgery and is often responsive to appropriately adjusted analgesics (Nicholson 2003) Pain is defined as "chronic" when it persists for at least 3 months or lasts longer than healing would normally occur (Nicholson 2003).

Preexisting Condition

Trauma

Physical trauma is an injury to the body as a result of blunt force, penetrating trauma, or controlled trauma such as that resulting from surgery. Unintentional injury is the leading cause of death for those below the age of 45 according to the Centers for Disease Control and Prevention. About 75 % of those who suffer physical trauma will experience moderate-to-severe pain during the course of their recovery. More than 60 % of patients suffering from major trauma report at least moderately severe pain at 1-year postinjury (Rivara et al. 2008).

Untreated Trauma Pain

The consequences of untreated pain in the acute trauma setting can be severe due to the associated stress response. Trauma results in sympathetic activation, leading to increased catabolism. This causes mobilization of substrates to provide energy sources for healing and also retention of salt and water for maintenance of fluid volume and cardiovascular homeostasis. Myocardial oxygen demand is increased, while myocardial oxygen supply is reduced, causing cardiac arrhythmias and myocardial ischemia. Trauma-related pain can result in hypoventilation and atelectasis. This respiratory dysfunction results in decreased functional residual capacity, vital capacity, and atelectasis. (Hedderich and Ness 1999) Increased sympathetic tone from trauma causes decreased gastrointestinal motility which can lead to ileus, nausea, and vomiting (Malchow and Black 2008). Furthermore acute phase reactants develop following traumatic injury leading to increased coagulability and venous thromboembolism risk. Immune function is impaired and risk of infection is increased (Hedderich and Ness 1999).

Failure to treat pain adequately can contribute to development of psychological comorbidities including: anxiety, sleep disturbance, and depression. Early treatment of pain following injury can help to reduce the stress-induced sympathetic activation and catabolism that occurs following trauma and reduce the incidence of cardiac, pulmonary, gastrointestinal, immunologic, hematologic, renal, and psychological complications in the acute setting (Keene et al. 2011).

Approximately one third of patients hospitalized for major trauma go on to develop posttraumatic stress disorder (PTSD) and major depression. PTSD is more likely to occur following assault-related injury as opposed to accidental injury. If PTSD occurs, quality of life and functional impairments are altered beyond the scope of injury severity (Malchow and Black 2008). Effective analgesia in the acute setting can reduce the incidence of PTSD and depression following major trauma. Chronic pain is one of the leading causes of health care consumption and worker disability in the developed world. Uncontrolled postoperative pain can negatively impact surgical recovery and may induce changes in the central nervous system which causes pain to transition to a chronic state (Kehlet et al. 2006).

Application

Preemptive Analgesia

Preemptive analgesia is pain treatment given before tissue injury to prevent establishment of altered central processing of afferent input from sites of injury, and thereby prevent development of pain hypersensitivity. While preemptive analgesia is not possible in the setting of unanticipated trauma, it may reduce the magnitude and duration of postoperative pain following surgery for trauma. Emphasizing the importance of measures to reduce postoperative pain is the observation that patients with high intensity of acute postoperative pain scores demonstrate a higher risk of developing a chronic pain state (Moiniche et al. 2002). Preemptive analgesia can be established with local infiltration of incisions sites, peripheral nerve block, central neuraxial blockade, and pharmacologic therapy.

Assessment

Pain is subjective, and the most reliable indicator for the presence and severity of pain is the patient's self-report. Particularly in the setting of trauma, the therapeutic plan should not be based entirely on the patient's ability to communicate. The visual analog pain scale is usually presented as a 10-cm line anchored by verbal descriptors and is useful in detecting changes in pain level (Jamison et al. 2002). For nonverbal patients, observation of behavior is the most effective tool for pain assessment. For noncommunicative patients, scales such as the Faces Pain Scale Revised (FPS-R), Verbal Descriptor Scale (VDS), Numeric Rating Scale (NRS), and Iowa Pain Thermometer (IPT) have been validated for pain assessment (Herr et al. 2007).

Pain Therapies

Treatment of posttraumatic pain can be optimized through implementation of a stepwise algorithm approach. Assessment of the patient and injury type will guide early management of pain (Fig. 1).

The World Health Organization (WHO) developed a stepwise approach for treatment of pain consisting of a three-step analgesic ladder.

This method has been validated in studies and found to be extremely effective in pain management. The steps of this analgesic ladder advocate choosing analgesics primarily based upon pain intensity. According to the ladder, a patient with mild pain should be started on acetaminophen, aspirin, or one of the NSAIDs. Moderate pain can be treated with low potency opioids

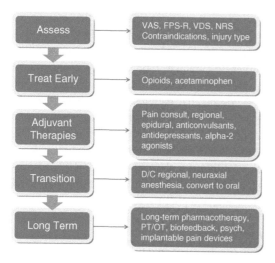

Acute Pain Management in Trauma, Fig. 1 Flow Diagram in the Management of Acute Pain in the Trauma Patient. *VAS* Visual Analog Scale, *FPS-R* Faces Pain Scale Revised, *VDS* Visual Descriptor Scale, *NRS* Numeric Rating Scale

including codeine and hydrocodone. Those with severe pain can receive potent opioids such as morphine or hydromorphone. Adjuvant medications such as antidepressants and anticonvulsants can be added at each step of the ladder, if indicated.

Opioids

Opioids are the mainstay of pharmacologic treatment of moderate-to-severe pain in trauma. Opioids can be administered by oral, intravenous, cutaneous, epidural, intrathecal, and caudal routes. Common side effects of opioid therapy include sedation, respiratory depression, nausea or vomiting, mental confusion, dizziness and mood changes, nightmares, and sleep disorders. Bolus doses of narcotics can lead to chest wall rigidity which may make ventilation difficult during resuscitation as well as intubation.

Trauma patients may vary greatly in their intraoperative and postoperative opioid requirements. Patients with a history of chronic opioid use often become opioid tolerant, creating a situation where standard treatment dosages need to be exceeded. Patients with a history of chronic opioid use tend to report higher pain scores.

A barrier to effective management of posttraumatic and postoperative pain is the concern that opioid use will result in addiction. Physician or patient fear of opioid addiction in the acute trauma setting may prevent needed treatment of pain. In the absence of history of addiction, it is rare to develop opioid addiction in the context of acute pain treatment.

Parenteral administration of opioid analgesics via IV PCA for treatment of acute pain improves efficacy of pain control and patient satisfaction. Patients who have the opportunity for self-administration of analgesics report improved satisfaction compared with nurse-administered analgesia as needed (Hudcova et al. 2006). Choice of opioid does not appear to affect patient satisfaction.

Acetaminophen

In 2010, the FDA approved intravenous acetaminophen (Ofirmev) for use in adults and children >2 years of age. Plasma and CSF levels are significantly higher when compared to oral acetaminophen dosing as the intravenous form avoids hepatic first-pass metabolism. Ofirmev should be avoided in patients with suspected hepatic impairment, renal insufficiency, or severe hypovolemia. Ofirmev may prove to be a useful adjunct to opioids and reduce opioid consumption and adverse side effects when used in the appropriate patient population (Jahr et al. 2010).

NSAIDs

NSAIDs have a limited role in treatment of acute pain in the trauma setting. Potential complications of NSAID use include hemorrhage secondary to impairment of platelet function, renal insufficiency, and acute gastric ulceration. Situations with a high risk of bleeding in confined spaces, or where it cannot be easily controlled such as traumatic brain injury, are contraindications to NSAID use. In the limited situations during trauma when contraindications do not exist, NSAIDs are powerful adjuvant analgesic agents to opioids and can improve pain control and reduce opioid requirements and opioid adverse effects.

Anticonvulsants

Gabapentin and pregabalin are anticonvulsant medications active at the alpha-2 delta subunit of the presynaptic voltage gated calcium channel used primarily in the treatment of neuropathic pain, but may be helpful in the treatment of acute inflammatory pain in burn patients and acute nociceptive pain (Wiffen et al. 2005).

Alpha-2 agonists

Clonidine and dexmedetomidine are centrally acting alpha agonists that produce analgesia and sedation. They can be useful adjuncts to opioid therapy that can reduce opioid consumption. Clonidine has the side effect of hypotension and bradycardia without respiratory depression and should be avoided in patients who are not hemodynamically stable. Dexmedetomidine is a shorter acting alpha-2 agonist approved by the FDA for short-term ICU sedation that may be useful in reducing postoperative opioid requirements (Tobias 2007).

Antidepressants

Tricyclic antidepressants (TCAs) such as amitriptyline and nortriptyline have been used to treat neuropathic pain by inhibiting reuptake of norepinephrine and serotonin. Early use of these medications in acute traumatic pain may have a role in preventing the progression of acute to chronic pain.

Other agents

Ketamine is unique in that it can provide analgesia, amnesia, and sedation without depressing the sympathetic nervous system. Ketamine causes an increase in sympathetic outflow through the inhibition of uptake of endogenous catecholamines. Caution should be exercised when using ketamine in trauma in the setting of shock. Ketamine acts as a direct myocardial depressant and can cause hemodynamic collapse when used in catecholamine-depleted patients (Weiskopf et al. 1984). Contraindications to ketamine use are age <3 months, psychosis, globe injury and other causes of increased intraocular pressure, myocardial ischemia or infarction, hypertension, intracranial mass or hemorrhage secondary to transient increases in intracranial pressure.

Regional Anesthetic Techniques

Techniques for delivery of regional anesthesia include epidural catheters, wound infiltration, and peripheral nerve blocks (PNBs). Use of peripheral nerve catheters has increased both in the perioperative setting and by the military to address combat-related injuries. Advantages of the use of peripheral nerve blocks are the rapid establishment of analgesia, reduction of opioid consumption and associated side effects, and improved perioperative pain control. Use of ultrasound guidance for needle and catheter placement may decrease block latency and improve sensory and motor block efficacy.

Use of regional anesthesia in traumatic injury is controversial because it has the potential to obscure pain from a compartment syndrome. The most common injuries associated with compartment syndrome are upper and lower extremity fractures and crush injuries. Proponents argue that parenteral analgesia also has the potential to obscure pain as an early warning sign of impending limb compromise. Evidence also exists that effective regional analgesia can be employed without concealing symptoms of limb compromise (Wu et al. 2011).

Rib fractures are the most common injury following blunt chest trauma Increasing number of rib fractures correlates directly with morbidity and mortality. Patients suffering from rib fractures can be treated with intercostal nerve blocks, paravertebral blocks, epidural anesthesia, or POPs (posterior, paramedian, subrhomboidal) block. Intercostal nerve blocks can be easily performed with the patient in the lateral position. Thoracic epidural analgesia is the preferred technique and can reduce the splinting and atelectasis associated with hypoventilation. Risks of nerve injury from hematoma formation need to be weighed against the risk of respiratory compromise.

Outcomes

Poorly controlled postoperative pain increases morbidity and mortality, and decreases quality of life. Potential benefits of providing adequate pain relief following trauma include reduced postoperative morbidity and mortality, shorter hospital stay, and improved patient comfort.

Factors contributing to patient satisfaction with pain management following trauma include how seriously the medical staff takes the complaint of pain, the frequency of breakthrough pain episodes, and actual pain intensity. Response to requests for analgesics correlates more strongly with patient satisfaction than pain intensity. Use of regional techniques, including involvement of an acute pain service, appears to improve patient reports of satisfaction with their pain management (Wu et al. 2011).

Cross-References

▶ Awareness and Trauma Anesthesia
▶ Complex Regional Pain Syndrome and Trauma
▶ Crush Injuries
▶ Fasciotomy
▶ Military Trauma, Anesthesia for
▶ Phantom Limb Pain
▶ Regional Anesthesia in Trauma
▶ Sedation and Analgesia
▶ Sedation, Analgesia, Neuromuscular Blockade in the ICU

References

Hedderich R, Ness TJ (1999) Analgesia for trauma and burns. Crit Care Clin 15(1):167–184
Herr K, Spratt KF, Garand L, Li L (2007) Evaluation of the Iowa pain thermometer and other selected pain intensity scales in younger and older adult cohorts using controlled clinical pain: a preliminary study. Pain Med 8(7):585–600
Hudcova J, McNicol E, Quah C, Lau J, Carr DB (2006) Patient controlled opioid analgesia versus conventional opioid analgesia for postoperative pain. Cochrane Database Syst Rev (4):CD003348
Jahr JS, et al. (2010) Intravenous acetaminophen. Anesthesiol Clin 28(4):619–645
Jamison RN, Gracely RH, Raymond SA, Levine JG, Marino B, Herrmann TJ, Daly M, Fram D, Katz NP (2002) Comparative study of electronic vs. paper VAS ratings: a randomized, crossover trial using healthy volunteers. Pain 99(1–2):341–347
Keene DD, Rea WE, Aldington D (2011) Acute pain management in trauma. Trauma 13(3):167–179
Kehlet H, Jensen TS, Woolf CJ (2006) Persistent postsurgical pain: risk factors and prevention. Lancet 367(9522):1618–1625
Malchow RJ, Black IH (2008) The evolution of pain management in the critically ill trauma patient: emerging concepts from the global war on terrorism. Crit Care Med 36(Suppl 7):S346–S357
Moiniche S, Kehlet H, Dahl JB (2002) A qualitative and quantitative systematic review of preemptive analgesia for postoperative pain relief: the role of timing of analgesia. Anesthesiology 96(3):725–741
Nicholson B (2003) Responsible prescribing of opioids for the management of chronic pain. Drugs 63(1):17–32
Rivara FP, Mackenzie EJ, Jurkovich GJ, Nathens AB, Wang J, Scharfstein DO (2008) Prevalence of pain in patients 1 year after major trauma. Arch Surg 143(3):282–287; discussion 288
Tobias J (2007) Dexmedetomidine in trauma anesthesiology and critical care. International TraumaCare (ITACCS) 17(1):1–7
Weiskopf RB, Bogetz MS, Roizen MF, Reid IA (1984) Cardiovascular and metabolic sequelae of inducing anesthesia with ketamine or thiopental in hypovolemic swine. Anesthesiology 60(3):214–219
Wiffen P, Collins S, McQuay H, Carroll D, Jadad A, Moore A (2005) Anticonvulsant drugs for acute and chronic pain. Cochrane Database Syst Rev (3):CD001133
Wu J, Lollo L, Grabinsky A (2011) Regional anesthesia in trauma medicine. Anesthesiol Res Pract 2011:1–7

Acute Renal Failure

▶ Acute Kidney Injury

Acute Renal Injury

▶ Renal Failure as a Complication, Acute

Acute Renal Insufficiency

▶ Renal Failure as a Complication, Acute

Acute Respiratory Distress Syndrome

▶ ARDS, Complication of Trauma

Acute Respiratory Distress Syndrome (ARDS), General

Jason S. Oh[1] and Khanjan H. Nagarsheth[2]
[1]Shock Trauma Center, University of Maryland Medical Center, Baltimore, MD, USA
[2]R Adams Cowley Shock Trauma Center, University of Maryland School of Medicine, Baltimore, MD, USA

Synonyms

Acute lung injury; Adult respiratory distress syndrome; Diffuse alveolar damage; Diffuse alveolar injury; Noncardiogenic pulmonary edema; Severe acute respiratory syndrome; Ventilator-associated lung injury

Definition

Respiratory failure is a common complication in the critically ill patient, particularly the critically ill trauma patient. Hypoxemia as a cause of respiratory failure is often a primary result of the trauma as in pulmonary contusion, pneumothorax, or hemothorax. It can also result from a delayed secondary effect of trauma as is seen with the development of acute respiratory distress syndrome (ARDS).

The American-European Consensus Conference (AECC) set the original definition of ARDS in 1994. It defined ARDS as acute hypoxemia with a PaO_2/FiO_2 (P/F ratio) ≤ 200, bilateral infiltrates on frontal chest radiograph, and no evidence of left atrial hypertension. Acute lung injury (ALI) was the descriptor if the P/F ratio ≤ 300 with the other parameters being met. This definition did not take into account CT imaging compared to traditional radiography, required the measurement of PCWP to rule out left atrial hypertension, and did not consider a standard PEEP level when evaluating the P/F ratio.

This older definition of ARDS was recently modified to describe a continuum of disease including acute lung injury (ALI) and included parameters to account for the prior deficiencies. The newer Berlin definition describes ARDS as occurring within 1 week of a known clinical insult or new/worsening respiratory symptoms; bilateral opacities on imaging not fully explained by effusions, lobar/lung collapse, or nodules; and respiratory failure not fully explained by cardiac failure or fluid overload (if no risk factor present, need objective assessment to exclude hydrostatic edema) (The ARDS Definition Task Force 2012). The degree of hypoxemia grades the severity of ARDS: P/F ratio 201–300 mmHg with PEEP/CPAP ≥ 5 cm H_2O is mild, 100–200 mmHg with PEEP/CPAP ≥ 5 cm H_2O is moderate, and if P/F ratio < 100 mmHg with PEEP/CPAP ≥ 5 cm H_2O, severe ARDS is present.

At the core of the definition is the development of noncardiogenic pulmonary edema due to inflammation from various etiologies. Direct injury (aspiration, inhalation, pulmonary contusion) and indirect causes such as sepsis, transfusion, ischemia/reperfusion syndromes, fat emboli, and missed distant injuries are among the causes of ARDS.

Increased cytokines from an inflammatory state cause changes at the alveolar-capillary endothelial interface resulting in deficiencies in hemostasis, immune function, and gas exchange. Neutrophils migrate to the lung in response to proinflammatory cytokines such as TNF-alpha, IL-6, and IL-8. When recruited, they release toxic mediators that damage the capillary endothelium and alveolar epithelium. Leakage of protein rich fluid overwhelms the clearance capacity of the lymphatics leading to pulmonary edema, increased lung weight with decreased compliance, and poor diffusion capacity. Surfactant is also lost resulting in alveolar collapse. This is known as the acute exudative stage. As the inflammatory cause resolves and healing begins (alveolar fluid is cleared, damaged alveolar-capillary cells are replaced, collagen is laid down), remodeling occurs. This is the proliferative stage. Some recover to near premorbid function, while others progress to the fibrotic stage with a change in lung architecture leading to poor pulmonary function.

Preexisting Condition

ARDS is a syndrome with many different causes that increase the inflammatory cascade. Predisposing factors for ARDS include sepsis, trauma, aspiration, and transfusions (Garber et al. 1996). In the trauma population, the risk factors most commonly associated with ARDS in blunt trauma are an injury severity scale (ISS) >25, pulmonary contusion, age >65 years, hypotension on admission, and 24-h transfusion requirement >10 units (Miller et al. 2002). Interestingly, ARDS associated with trauma does not seem to independently increase mortality and may have a better prognosis than non-trauma-related ARDS (Calfee et al. 2007).

Any proinflammatory process may place an individual at a higher risk of developing ARDS.

Application

The mortality from ARDS is 25–35 %, and 50 % of survivors are on the ventilator 3 weeks after onset (Sloane et al. 1992). Given this severity, it is prudent that we find ways to prevent ARDS but also ways to treat it once it is present. To date, only ventilator support utilizing lung protective strategies has been shown to decrease mortality after ARDS has developed.

Ventilator support is utilized to improve oxygenation in the hypoxemic ARDS patient. Despite improvements in ventilation and oxygenation, ventilator support can actually worsen ARDS and increase lung injury if used improperly. Lung protective ventilation refers to lower tidal volumes and airway pressures to minimize and hopefully prevent lung injury.

The ideal pressure and volume changes during ventilator support to avoid significant barotrauma, volutrauma, and atelecti-trauma are hypothesized to be between the upper and lower inflection points of the pressure-volume curve. While any individual patient's pressure-volume curve in a given instant is different from the next patient, the ARMA trial showed a tidal volume and plateau pressure goal that would

benefit most patients if set at 6 ml/kg of ideal body weight and <30 cm H_2O, respectively (The Acute Respiratory Distress Syndrome Network 2000). Critics of the study argue that the 12 ml/kg of ideal body of tidal volume in the control group was not the standard of care at the time of the study, although this group did have a similar mortality as described in the literature when compared to the standard conventional ventilation of the time.

Other therapies are more controversial as they have been investigated without any proven mortality benefit. These include steroids, ketoconazole, surfactant, inhaled nitric oxide, recruitment maneuvers, and prone positioning. Inverse ratio pressure control ventilation, airway pressure release ventilation (APRV), high-frequency oscillatory ventilation (HFOV), and extracorporeal membranous oxygenation (ECMO) are additional therapies utilized when conventional ventilatory support fails to provide adequate oxygenation. Early neuromuscular blockade may improve mortality (Papazian et al. 2010).

A conservative fluid strategy is also an approach to management that is often employed to decrease the time to ventilator liberation and ICU length of stay. Unfortunately this approach of diuresis based on CVP does not improve mortality (The National Heart, Lung, and Blood Institute Acute Respiratory Distress Syndrome (ARDS) Clinical Trials Network 2006).

ARDS is serious condition that occurs from various causes due to increased inflammation. It can affect any critically ill patient and prolong length of stay in the hospital and intensive care unit. Despite advances in research and medical technology, the only known therapy that improves survival is lung protective ventilation and possibly early neuromuscular blockade. Other therapies are either ineffective or not recommended as first-line therapy.

Cross-References

▶ Ventilatory Management of Trauma Patients
▶ Ventilator-Associated Pneumonia

References

Calfee CS, Eisner MD, Ware LB et al (2007) Trauma-associated lung injury differs clinically and biologically from acute lung injury due to other clinical disorders. Crit Care Med 35:2243

Garber BG, Hébert PC, Yelle JD et al (1996) Adult respiratory distress syndrome: a systemic overview of incidence and risk factors. Crit Care Med 24(4):687–695

Miller PR, Croce MA, Kilgo PD et al (2002) Acute respiratory distress syndrome in blunt trauma: identification of independent risk factors. Am Surg 68(10):845–850

Papazian L, Forel J, Gacouin A et al (2010) Neuromuscular blockers in early acute respiratory distress syndrome. N Engl J Med 363(12):1107–1116

Sloane PJ, Gee MH, Gottlieb JE et al (1992) A multi-center registry of patients with acute respiratory distress syndrome. Physiology and outcome. Am Rev Respir Dis 146(2):419–426

The Acute Respiratory Distress Syndrome Network (2000) Ventilation with lower tidal volumes as compared with traditional tidal volumes for acute lung injury and the acute respiratory distress syndrome. N Engl J Med 342(18):1301

The ARDS Definition Task Force (2012) Acute respiratory distress syndrome the Berlin definition. JAMA 307(23):2526–2533

The National Heart, Lung, and Blood Institute Acute Respiratory Distress Syndrome (ARDS) Clinical Trials Network (2006) Comparison of two fluid-management strategies in acute lung injury. N Engl J Med 354(24):2564–2575

Recommended Reading

Adhikari NK, Burns KE, Friedrich JO et al (2007) Effect of nitric oxide on oxygenation and mortality in acute lung injury: systematic review and meta-analysis. BMJ 334(7597):779

Dellinger RP, Zimmerman JL, Taylor RW et al (1998) Effects of inhaled nitric oxide in patients with acute respiratory distress syndrome; results of randomized phase II trial. Inhaled nitric oxide in ARDS study group. Crit Care Med 26(1):15–23

Derdak S (2002) High-frequency oscillatory ventilation for acute respiratory distress syndrome in adults: a randomized, controlled trial. Am J Respir Crit Care Med 166(6):801–808

Gattinoni L, Tognoni G, Pesenti A et al (2001) Effect of prone positioning on the survival of patients with acute respiratory failure. N Engl J Med 345:568–573

Gattinoni L, Caironi P, Cressoni M et al (2006) Lung recruitment in patients with the acute respiratory distress syndrome. N Engl J Med 354(17):1775–1786

González M, Arroliga AC, Frutos-Vivar F et al (2010) Airway pressure release ventilation versus assist-control ventilation: a comparative propensity score and international cohort study. Intensive Care Med 36(5):817–827

Hirshberg E, Miller RR 3rd, Morris AH (2013) Extracorporeal membrane oxygenation in adults with acute respiratory distress syndrome. Curr Opin Crit Care. 19(1):38–43

Jones A, Barrett N, Scales D et al (2010) Ventilatory support versus ECMO for severe adult respiratory failure. Lancet 375(9714):550–551

Maxwell RA, Green JM, Waldrop J et al (2010) A randomized prospective trial of airway pressure release ventilation and low tidal volume ventilation in adult trauma patients with acute respiratory failure. J Trauma 69(3):501–510

Morris AH, Wallace CJ, Menlove RL et al (1994) Randomized clinical trial of pressure-controlled inverse ratio ventilation and extracorporeal CO_2 removal for adult respiratory distress syndrome. Am J Respir Crit Care Med 149(2 Pt 1):295–305

Papazian L, Gainnier M, Marin V et al (2005) Comparison of prone positioning and high-frequency oscillatory ventilation in patients with acute respiratory distress syndrome. Crit Care Med 33(10):2162–2171

Peek GJ, Mugford M, Tiruvoipati R et al (2009) Efficacy and economic assessment of conventional ventilatory support versus extracorporeal membrane oxygenation for severe adult respiratory failure (CESAR): a multicentre randomised controlled trial. Lancet 374:1351–1363

Steinberg KP, Hudson LD, Goodman RB et al (2006) Efficacy and safety of corticosteroids for persistent acute respiratory distress syndrome. N Engl J Med 354(16):1671–1684

Sundar KM, Thaut P, Nielsen DB et al (2012) Clinical course of ICU patients with severe pandemic 2009 influenza a (H1N1) pneumonia: single center experience with proning and pressure release ventilation. J Intensive Care Med 27(3):184–190

Taccone P, Pesenti A, Latini R et al (2009) Prone positioning in patients with moderate and severe acute respiratory distress syndrome: a randomized controlled trial. JAMA 302(18):1977–1984

The Acute Respiratory Distress Syndrome Network (2000) Ketoconazole for early treatment of acute lung injury and acute respiratory distress syndrome: a randomized controlled trial. JAMA 283:1995–2002

Acute Stress Disorder

▶ Post Traumatic Stress Disorder

Acute Traumatic

▶ Coagulopathy in Trauma: Underlying Mechanisms

Adaptive Equipment

Douglas Fetkenhour
Department of Physical Medicine and
Rehabilitation, University of Rochester School of
Medicine, Rochester, NY, USA

Synonyms

Assistive device; Orthotic

Definition

Adaptive equipment is a device that is used to assist with mobility and activities of daily living.

The physiatrist and physical therapist will recommend adaptive equipment to improve mobility. Examples include wheelchairs, walkers, and adjustable beds that help the trauma rehab patient maximize their independence. Manual wheelchairs are essential for a patient that has significant lower limb weakness or weight-bearing restrictions. An individual with three or four limb weakness may need a power wheelchair as they will be unable to propel a manual wheelchair. Patients with limited function in one lower limb from fracture may be able to ambulate with a rolling walker or axillary crutches. Canes provide stability for those who can ambulate with both lower limbs. Beds that can be raised and lowered allow for easier transfers in and out of bed. Ramps to traverse steps for home access are another form of adaptive equipment. The trauma patient who requires a wheelchair may need to ramp steps to get into their home. The ratio of ramp length to stair height is 9:1 to meet building code and ideally 12:1 to allow an individual in a manual wheelchair to ascend and descend the ramp independently.

Adaptive equipment to simplify ADLs is recommended by the physician and occupational therapist. Tub transfer benches, reachers, and built-up handled utensils are examples. For the patient who has hip precautions limiting range of motion or abdominal incision pain, a reacher allows for manipulation of clothing and shoes at the distal lower limbs. A patient with severely limited hand function from burns or cervical spinal cord injury may be able to independently feed themselves with a large-handled fork and knife. The occupational therapist may also make recommendations for home modifications that will make activity in the kitchen and bathroom easier. Examples include lower countertops, roll-in showers, and minimum turning space for a wheelchair.

Cross-References

▶ Occupational Therapist
▶ Physical Therapist

Recommended Reading

web.alsa.org/site/DocServer/chapter_6_web_ready.pdf

Adeptness

▶ Competency

Adjuncts to Damage Control Laparotomy: Endovascular Therapies

James K. Lukan
Department of Surgery, State University of
New York, Buffalo, NY, USA

Synonyms

Angioembolization; Balloon occlusion; Covered stenting; Embolization; Stent graft; Stenting

Definition

Endovascular modalities may be used in the context of damage control in a number of ways. While the field has now expanded to include many options, perhaps the most commonly employed include embolization, covered stenting, and temporary balloon occlusion. The goal of endovascular therapy in the unstable patient ranges from temporary control of hemorrhage as a bridge to definitive open repair to definitive restoration of flow with exclusion of bleeding.

Preexisting Condition

Endovascular methods are employed in conjunction with standard damage control techniques in situations in which the patient's condition demands rapid control of bleeding and maintenance of perfusion of the extremities and vital organs. The decision to pursue endovascular treatment may be made in the emergency department based upon injury patterns and patient condition, after imaging studies have been obtained, or after an open surgery has begun.

Application

When endovascular techniques were first introduced to the field of trauma surgery, one had to decide upon whether open or endovascular repair would be pursued, while today we realize that each may be complementary to the other. The advent of hybrid operating suites in which open surgery and advanced endovascular techniques may be employed simultaneously has greatly expanded, simplifying the decision tree and streamlining care (D'Amours et al. 2013). While the hybrid suite offers simplicity of logistics, certainly excellent endovascular care can be achieved in a dedicated angiography suite in conjunction with care in the operating room. Such care requires more planning and forethought as to priorities but can be done quite effectively.

If the intervention is undertaken in the angiography suite, close attention is paid to resuscitative efforts as described elsewhere in the encyclopedia. It is the goal that conditions will be as conducive to resuscitation, if not more so, than would occur in the trauma intensive care unit. In short, attention must be paid to the provision of high-level nursing staff, warmed ambient room temperature, a heated water blanket beneath the patient, and two air warmers over the patient with only the access site exposed. Fluid warmers are obviously used as well. If needed, additional large bore femoral access is added for resuscitation simultaneous with arterial access. Standard resuscitative techniques as 1:1 transfusion and permissive hypotension are routine. It is important to alter the approach from procedures that may be undertaken in the interventional suite on a more routine basis and to emphasize to all involved staff the goals of the intervention. In addition it is important to monitor the duration of the procedure to be sure one does not become too involved in a complex endovascular treatment if a simpler, albeit less desirable, option exists.

In considering endovascular options for the unstable patient, it may be useful to consider not only the various modalities available but also the various anatomic locations where they may be employed. Broadly speaking, the anatomic locations where such options may be used include the abdomen and pelvis, the thoracic cavity, the thoracic outlet, the head and neck, and the extremities.

Within the abdomen and pelvis, embolization is commonly employed for the control of hepatic and pelvic arterial bleeds. While splenic embolization is also used as an option to splenectomy, it plays little role in conjunction with damage control laparotomy. In these instances, splenectomy is generally a more expeditious option.

Packing of the liver to control venous hemorrhage and subsequent arterial embolization complement each other well. Certainly if a clear arterial hemorrhage is identified at laparotomy, ligation of the offending vessel should be performed. This is not always as easy as might be hoped and one should not waste too much time in this endeavor as hypothermia and coagulopathy worsen. Packing can be achieved quickly and effectively with subsequent embolization often more expeditious. Even the common hepatic artery can be embolized without significant adverse sequelae so long as perfusion is maintained. Packs should be removed as soon as possible if proximal embolization is performed so venous flow can maintain viability of hepatic parenchyma. Approach may be made from the common femoral artery, although we prefer the trans-brachial approach as it allows for rapid and secure entry to the celiac and superior mesenteric artery as needed.

Embolization of pelvic arterial bleeding is complementary to placement of a binder to close the pelvic volume and control venous bleeding. The chosen access site is based upon the injury and fracture pattern. Preferentially, the common femoral artery contralateral to the expected area of injury is chosen for percutaneous access. When necessary, both internal iliac arteries may be embolized without adverse events.

The opportunities to limit bleeding through embolization are considerable and, as mentioned earlier, extend far beyond the abdomen and pelvis. In proceeding one must always consider the sequelae of devascularization of the region or organ as balanced against open surgical options and the risks of continued uncontrolled bleeding. In applying this judgment to each clinical scenario, the field rapidly extends beyond the few examples provided above.

When bleeding would be difficult to control through an open approach and devascularization not tolerable, one should consider covered stenting for control of bleeding with maintenance of distal perfusion in the damage control setting. The question of patency rates when compared with autologous conduit bypass is often raised, but one must keep in mind the goal of damage control interventions. Issues of correction of metabolic abnormalities, speed, and limitation of ongoing blood and fluid losses must take precedence over other concerns. Considerable

judgment and experience is crucial in this regard. In employing such techniques, one accepts that subsequent interventions or even later bypasses may be necessary, with the understanding that they may be undertaken in a stable patient without hematoma and with the luxury of time.

With advances in endovascular devices, the profile of covered stents has diminished considerably. Currently a wide variety of covered self-expanding stents may be delivered through sheaths that range from 6 to 8 French for peripheral work and somewhat larger sheaths for central work. This has increased the safety and decreased access site complications. Furthermore, closure devices that can be employed to seal the access sites of larger sheaths are now quite reliable. Precision of placement is now very exacting. More sophisticated technology such as hybrid stents that combine covered stents with standard graft material extend the horizons of endovascular therapy well beyond where it began many years ago. Cost of such devices is considerable but should be interpreted in the context of the unstable multiply injured patient. If used judiciously, such devices may actually offer cost savings over the course of the patient's hospital stay.

The use of covered stent graft repair for thoracic injury is well described in the literature. Concerns over durability of repair seem to be fading with experience and improvements in available devices. Problems with stent graft conformation to the contour of the aortic arch that were evident with early devices have largely disappeared with evolution of the available technology. Considerable attention has been paid to the consequences of coverage of the left subclavian artery, but again with the precision of current devices, we are generally able to deploy the stent grafts distal to the takeoff of the left subclavian with good results. Certainly while endovascular repair can be achieved much more quickly and with less hemodynamic changes than open repair, one must consider whether even this repair should be pursued in the setting of true damage control trauma management. In general, most patients with aortic injuries that have reached the hospital can be managed with tight blood pressure control and endovascular repair when acute blood loss from other injuries is controlled and metabolic derangements corrected.

Stent grafting of anatomically challenging vessels such as the subclavian artery was one of the first to gain wide acceptance, as control can be obtained more quickly with less blood loss than open repair. One must be very aware of branch vessels such as the vertebral artery in such cases in order to reduce the risk of posterior stroke that could have devastating consequences (Du Toit et al. 2008; Cohen et al. 2008).

More recently, stenting of carotid and vertebral injuries when intervention is deemed necessary is becoming the preferred option and may be achieved quickly in the setting of damage control (Gaurav et al. 2013; Greer et al. 2013).

Stent grafting of peripheral injures should also be considered in the setting of damage control. While patency rates may be less than that of open autologous grafts, the time savings and reduction in blood loss may be considerable. Open revascularization can always be undertaken subsequently if needed in a more controlled setting (Trellopoulos et al. 2012).

As our experience grows, stent grafting of vessels such as the superior mesenteric artery can also be achieved with good success.

One of the primary limitations of stent grafting is the ability to cross the area of injury with a wire. In many blunt and penetrating injuries, complete disruption of the vessel may preclude crossing the injury with a wire. In these injuries, endovascular treatment is generally not possible. In some cases the wire may actually exit the proximal end of the vessel and reenter the distal segment. If this can be achieved, successful stenting can be achieved. In the setting of damage control, however, one should avoid excessive time wasted in attempting to cross such injuries. In these cases, with access already gained and a wire in position, a balloon should be inflated proximal to the injury to achieve proximal control before proceeding with open repair or shunting. This should result in a reduction of blood loss and more rapid improvement in metabolic derangements. Either compliant balloons or standard angioplasty balloons that are widely available may be used. One should use care in sizing balloons appropriately and avoiding overdistension to prevent additional iatrogenic injury. One should also be aware that migration of balloons may occur.

With improvements in technology such as hybrid stents, the rapid treatment of complete transections and blast injuries is likely to be possible in the near future.

Cross-References

References

Cohen JE, Rajz G et al (2008) Urgent endovascular stent-graft placement for traumatic penetrating subclavian artery injuries. J Neurol Sci 272:151–157

D'Amours SK, Rastogi P, Ball CG (2013) Utility of simultaneous interventional radiology and operative surgery in a dedicated suite for seriously injured patients. Curr Opin Crit Care 19:587–593

Du Toit DF, Lambrechts AV, Stark H, Warren BL (2008) Long-term results of stent graft treatment of subclavian artery injuries: management of choice for stable patients? J Vasc Surg 47:739–743

Gaurav J, Fortes M, Miller T, Scalea T, Ghandi D (2013) Endovascular stent repair of traumatic cervical internal carotid artery injuries. J Trauma 75:896–903

Greer LT, Reed KB et al (2013) Contemporary management of combat-related vertebral artery injuries. J Trauma 74:818–824

Trellopoulos G, Georgiadis GS et al (2012) Endovascular management of peripheral arterial trauma in patients presenting in hemorrhagic shock. J Cardiovasc Surg 53:495–506

Adjuncts to Damage Control Laparotomy: Vascular Shunts

James K. Lukan
Department of Surgery, State University of
New York, Buffalo, NY, USA

Synonyms

Temporary extra-anatomic bypass for trauma

Definition

The vascular shunt describes a temporary conduit that is designed to carry blood across an injured segment of a blood vessel. The conduit varies, most commonly being an adapted carotid shunt, such as a Javid or Pruitt-Inahara type. Alternatively, any type of available tubing may be used, including extension sets, suction catheters, or any suitable silastic tube. Once proximal and distal control of the injured vessel has been obtained with vessel loops or fine vascular clamps, the shunt may be inserted. The shunt is secured using ties, vessel loops, clamps, or, in the case of the Pruitt-Inahara, balloons. It is left in place to avoid ischemia to the affected limb or organ and to achieve relative hemostasis until systemic stabilization has been accomplished. Once the patient has been stabilized enough to allow definitive repair, the patient is returned to the operating room where repair or formal bypass can be performed after removal of the shunt.

One should be careful to differentiate a shunt from a stent as both are used in damage control situations, but have different goals. While a shunt offers a short-term bridge to definitive repair, the stent offers the opportunity to provide the definitive care in an expeditious fashion. As technology progresses, the lines are likely to blur somewhat.

Preexisting Condition

Use of a vascular shunt as a damage control strategy is applied in those instances in which definitive repair of an injured vessel would not be tolerated due to instability including hypothermia, acidosis, coagulopathy, or continued hypotension. It may be used as a temporizing procedure in civilian situations in which a vascular surgeon is unavailable to complete a repair and transport to tertiary care is required. The technique may be applied to cases of combined vascular and orthopedic trauma in which the shunt provides perfusion while the bony repair is completed. Subsequent vascular repair may be undertaken in a more careful fashion with the luxury of having a stable limb at appropriate length. Finally, it may be used in a military application in which a forward field hospital is designed to stabilize the injured patient in order to evacuate to a higher echelon facility where definitive repair is performed. While none of the latter of these applications refers to damage control strictly speaking, the technique of shunting is the same and the terms are often used interchangeably. One must be cautious in the interpretation of outcomes however, as injury severity scores, the degree of extremis and the total duration of stent placement may vary greatly.

Application

The initial modern descriptions of a type of shunt date to the early 1900s when Tuffier attempted this with a silver tube. The technique was attempted again in WWII with glass and plastic tubes, but was largely abandoned until 1971 when it was again described by Eger (Hancock et al. 2010; Eger et al. 1971). It has gained in popularity as recent conflicts have shown a fivefold increase in the number of extremity wounds over those of the past (Anahita et al. 2012). In addition, the wide application of tourniquets in the field has allowed better survival to forward hospitals where a shunt can be placed before the patient is evacuated to a hospital where a vascular surgeon can accomplish a definitive repair or bypass. This process, streamlined by the military has now filtered to civilian trauma systems.

Broadly speaking, the use of vascular shunting can be divided into central or peripheral types and either may be a part of the damage control process. Beginning with intra-abdominal uses, one should remember that many blood vessels such as the celiac, inferior mesenteric, internal iliac, and hepatic arteries can generally be ligated without consequence. A full consideration of ligation or embolization for trauma is outside the scope of this chapter, but it must be considered as an option before proceeding with shunt placement.

Endovascular repair must also be considered as an option for those arteries that have vital outflow. A more detailed discussion of this is provided elsewhere in the encyclopedia. Small injuries of vital arteries may often be repaired quickly, obviating the need for a shunt.

In cases where there the patient is not deemed stable for reconstruction, a shunt may be used for arteries such as the superior mesenteric artery with delayed reconstruction. This has been described in case reports as well as in animal studies in which an improvement in early survival in those shunted versus those undergoing immediate repair has been demonstrated in a pig model (Ding et al. 2010a). If such a shunt is used, it should be removed as soon as possible to prevent thrombosis which could be catastrophic (Ding et al. 2010b). The common and external iliac arteries may also be shunted in conjunction with the damage control laparotomy with significant reductions in amputation and mortality when compared with ligation (Ball and Feliciano 2010).

The technique of peripheral shunting has been described by many, most impressively in two large reports from the military in which shunts were placed with subsequent formal reconstruction. Patency rates for proximal shunts were up to 86 % with overall good results when used. The patency rate for distal shunts has been more disappointing. Fortunately, the indications are more limited, in that if a single vessel remains uninjured, the others may often be ligated without consequence. When all three infrapopliteal vessels have been injured, there is often such severe injury that the limb may not be salvageable. While some reports have been unable to show a significant reduction in amputation rates with shunt use, more recent reports have suggested an improvement (Anahita et al. 2012; Rasmussen et al. 2006; Gifford et al. 2009). It must be kept in mind that many of the shunts used in the military setting were in place for very short periods of time, on the order of two hours. This is a somewhat different experience then when the technique is used in a civilian damage control setting and as such, the excellent results may be difficult to reproduce.

The issue of anticoagulation for shunts has been debated, but is generally not thought to be necessary if the shunt is to be removed quickly and would be contraindicated in the multiply injured, unstable patient for whom the technique would generally be employed. In addition, many of these patients are already coagulopathic (Ding et al. 2008).

Potential complications of shunting include dislodgement, bleeding, thrombosis, infection, and intimal injury. Complication rates directly related to the shunts have been shown to be relatively low.

Cross-References

► Adjuncts to Damage Control Laparotomy: Endovascular Therapies
► Amputation
► Compressible Hemorrhage
► Damage Control Resuscitation, Military Trauma
► Extremity Injury
► Gunshot Wounds to the Extremity
► Knee Dislocations
► Noncompressible Hemorrhage
► Pelvis Fractures
► Thoracic Vascular Injuries
► Tracheoinnominate Fistula

References

Anahita D, Bhavin P et al (2012) Long term follow-up and amputation free survival in 497 casualties with combat-related injuries and damage-control resuscitation. J Trauma 73:1517–1524

Ball CG, Feliciano DV (2010) Damage control techniques for common and external iliac artery injuries: have temporary intravascular shunts replaced the need for ligation? J Vasc Surg 52:1112–1113

Ding W, Wu X, Li J (2008) Temporary intravascular shunts used as a damage control surgery adjunct in complex vascular injury: collective review. Injury 39:970–977

Ding W, Xingjang W et al (2010a) Temporary intravascular shunting improves survival in a hypothermic traumatic shock swine model with superior mesenteric artery injuries. Surgery 147:79–88

Ding W, Xingjang W et al (2010b) Time course study on the use of temporary intravascular shunts as a damage control adjunct in a superior mesenteric artery injury model. J Trauma 68:409–414

Eger M, Golcman L et al (1971) The use of a temporary shunt in the management of arterial vascular injuries. Surg Gynecol Obstet 132:67–70

Gifford SM, Aidinian G et al (2009) Effect of temporary shunting on extremity vascular injury: an outcome analysis from the global war on terror vascular injury initiative. J Vasc Surg 50:549–556

Hancock H, Rasmussen TE, Walker AF, Rich NM (2010) History of temporary intravascular shunts in the management of vascular injury. J Vasc Surg 52:1405–1409

Rasmussen T, Clouse DW et al (2006) The use of temporary vascular shunts as a damage control adjunct in the management of wartime vascular injury. J Trauma 61:8–15

Adjuncts to Transfusion: Antifibrinolytics

Jonathan J. Morrison[1] and Jan O. Jansen[2]
[1]The Academic Department of Military Surgery & Trauma, Royal Centre for Defence Medicine, Birmingham, UK
[2]Departments of Surgery & Intensive Care Medicine, Aberdeen Royal Infirmary, Aberdeen, UK

Definition

Antifibrinolytic agents are drugs which block the conversion of *plasminogen* to *plasmin*, which is the enzyme responsible for the degradation of fibrin clots, a process called fibrinolysis. These agents can be used in trauma patients who are at risk of hemorrhage, by reducing clot breakdown, which can become pathologically upregulated (hyperfibrinolysis) following traumatic injury and shock (Hess et al. 2008).

Antifibrinolytic Drugs

The two principal antifibrinolytic agents available are aminocaproic acid and tranexamic acid (TXA); both of which are derivatives of the amino acid lysine. Aminocaproic acid has not been reported as a hemostatic adjunct in trauma and will not be discussed further. TXA competitively inhibits the activation of plasminogen by blocking the lysine-binding site. It has a biological half-life of 3.1 h, with negligible plasma protein binding and is excreted via the kidneys (Astedt 1987).

The CRASH-2 trial enrolled 20,211 patients, who either had or were considered at risk of significant bleeding and randomized them to either TXA (1 g bolus, followed by a 1 g 8-h infusion) or placebo (CRASH-2 Collaborators 2010). The all-cause mortality was significantly reduced in the TXA arm compared to placebo (14.5 % vs. 16.0 %; RR 0.91 (95 % CI 0.85–0.97); $p = 0.004$). The relative risk (RR) of death due to bleeding was also significantly reduced in the TXA arm (RR 0.85, 95 % CI 0.76–0.96). The greatest benefit was identified in patients with a systolic blood pressure less than 75 mmHg (RR 0.87, 95 % CI 0.76–0.99).

A further analysis of the CRASH-2 data explored the effect of different times of administration. Administration within an hour of injury was associated with a significant reduction in the RR of death in the TXA arm (0.68, 0.57–0.82); however, the RR was found to be increased when TXA was administered after 3 h (1.44, 1.12–1.84) (CRASH-2 Collaborators 2011). A further important finding from the CRASH-2 dataset was that there was no increase in fatal or nonfatal vascular occlusive events between the treatment and placebo arms. However, the CRASH-2 trial has been criticized for several shortcomings relating to the lack of a standardized resuscitation algorithm and no measure of injury severity.

Some of these questions have been answered by the retrospective MATTERs study, which examined 896 patients requiring at least 1 unit of packed red blood cells (PRBCs) treated in a military field hospital in Afghanistan (Morrison et al. 2012). The study demonstrated a lower mortality in patients receiving TXA compared with those who did not (17.4 % vs. 23.9 %; $p = 0.03$) despite a greater injury severity in the TXA group (mean$\pm$sd ISS 25 $\pm$ 17 vs. 23 $\pm$ 19; $p < 0.001$). The greatest TXA mortality benefit was identified in patients requiring 10 units of PRBCs or more, within 24 h of admission (14.4 % vs. 28.1 %; $p = 0.004$), where TXA was also identified as an independent predictor of survival following multivariate analysis (OR 7.23, 95 % CI 3.02–17.32).

Overall, the administration of TXA is supported by level 1 evidence that demonstrates a reduction in hemorrhage-related mortality. TXA is most efficacious in hypotensive patients and when administered within 3 h of injury. There does not appear to be an increased risk of vascular occlusive events with the use of TXA in trauma patients.

Cross-References

▶ Coagulopathy

References

Astedt B (1987) Clinical pharmacology of Tranexamic acid. Scand J Gastroenterol Suppl 137:22–25

CRASH-2 Collaborators (2010) Effects of tranexamic acid on death, vascular occlusive events, and blood transfusion in trauma patients with significant haemorrhage (CRASH-2): a randomised, placebo-controlled trial. Lancet 376:23–32

CRASH-2 Collaborators (2011) The importance of early treatment with tranexamic acid in bleeding trauma patients: an exploratory analysis of the CRASH-2 randomised controlled trial. Lancet 377:1–6

Hess JR, Brohi K, Dutton RP, Hauser CJ, Holcomb JB, Kluger Y et al (2008) The coagulopathy of trauma: a review of mechanisms. J Trauma 65:748–754

Morrison JJ, DuBose JJ, Rasmussen TE, Midwinter MJ (2012) Military Application of Tranexamic acid in Trauma Emergency Resuscitation (MATTERs) study. Arch Surg 147(2):113–119

Adjuncts to Transfusion: Fibrinogen Concentrate

A

Dietmar Fries
Department for General and Surgical Critical Care Medicine, Medical University Innsbruck, Innsbruck, Austria

Synonyms

Clottafact®; Concentrated lyophilized protein; Factor I concentrate; Haemocomplettan®; Human fibrinogen concentrate; Lyophilized fibrinogen concentrate; RiaSTAP®

Definition

Fibrinogen concentrate is a lyophilized protein concentrate that is easily reconstituted within minutes. Compared to other fibrinogen sources like fresh frozen plasma (FFP) and cryoprecipitate, it is labeled with exact fibrinogen content. Fibrinogen concentrate is virus inactivated.

Preexisting Condition

Fibrinogen concentrate is registered in the United States and some European countries for congenital fibrinogen deficiency. Fibrinogen concentrate reduced blood loss in cardiovascular surgery as well as in urological surgery. Actually, two randomized controlled trials evaluate the efficacy of fibrinogen concentrate in trauma.

Application

Coagulopathy kills trauma patients! In patients with identical Injury Severity Scores (ISS), the mortality is virtually doubled if patients suffer from coagulopathy. The main goal of any hemostatic intervention is to promptly secure hemostasis, minimize blood loss, and avoid unnecessary transfusion of allogeneic blood products.

In the event of marked blood loss, fibrinogen reaches critical values as a function of its original concentration and as a rule more so than any other procoagulatory factor or thrombocytes (Fries and Martini 2010). Already small quantities of colloids (>1,000 ml) impair, first of all, fibrin polymerization and thus clot strength. The question of the critical threshold value is presently the subject of heated debate. Some old recommendations quote a threshold of 100 mg/dl as being soon enough, whereby this figure is based on the results of a study in which four out of four patients with a fibrinogen count of < 50 mg/dl were seen to have diffuse microvascular bleeding. By contrast, recent clinical data from peripartal hemorrhage, neurosurgery, and cardiac surgery show that at a fibrinogen count of <150–200 mg/dl, there is already an increased tendency to peri- and postoperative bleeding. As a general rule, it must be recognized that it is difficult to standardize the determination of high or very low fibrinogen plasma counts. Moreover, the presence of colloids, particularly HES, can cause these to be false high and not necessarily agree with functional measurement readings.

In many hospitals, the administration of FFP remains the standard therapy for the prevention and treatment of plasma coagulation disorders. Fresh frozen plasma has been available since the 1940s and was initially used as a volume expander. With the advent of synthetic volume expanders, the indication has shifted toward prevention of bleeding, treatment of coagulation disorders, and influencing pathological coagulation outcomes. But transfusion of FFP has considerable drawbacks (Sorensen and Fries 2012).

It is obvious that the administration of FFP is unavoidably associated with volume expansion (FFP corresponds to an 8.5 % protein solution) and that the concentration of critically decreased factors cannot be increased only by administration of 10–15 ml/kg BW of FFP. Consequently, large quantities of FFP are needed (>30 ml FFP/kg) to achieve a clinically meaningful rise in coagulation factor concentrations in the presence of a deficit and ongoing loss. In a coagulopathic but normovolemic patient, the resulting volume overload can lead to the clinical situation of transfusion-associated cardiac overload (TACO), particularly in patients with cardiac failure, renal impairment, and liver disorders. Furthermore, a series of retrospective studies showed that the rate of severe infections and respiratory complications was distinctly increased in patients who received FFP (Innerhofer et al. 2013). This effect was also proven to be dose dependent. Another concern with FFP transfusion is the risk of TRALI, which is now one of the most common fatal side effect of blood transfusion and can be triggered, among other things, by an interaction with donor-specific leukocyte antibodies. Because of the logistics involved, there is also a delay of 35–45 min until requested units of FFP are obtained. This means either that FFP must be ordered early on suspicion and administered "prophylactically" – a practice which many specialist societies flatly reject – or that they are actually received and administered too late, particularly when massive bleeding and coagulopathy is present. With regard to the quantity or the ratio of erythrocyte concentrate/FFP transfused, the literature contains a highly diverse array of recommendations which describe institution-related algorithms but which do not refer to prospectively collected data (Görlinger et al. 2012).

Compared to FFP, coagulation factor concentrates are immediately available, contain a defined concentration of the relevant factors, can be administered without volume overload, and may be regarded safe in relation to the transmission of viral diseases and induction of TRALI and TACO.

The data on the efficacy of administering fibrinogen concentrate to treat acquired fibrinogen deficiency are presently limited but growing in volume (Sorensen and Fries 2012). In vitro studies and experimental studies, observational reports following administration, initial prospective clinical studies, and retrospective analyses have shown that following administration of fibrinogen concentrate, there is an increase in fibrinogen concentration and clot strength, the majority of bleeding episodes were stopped, and further transfusion requirement was reduced. A retrospective study correlated the amount of fibrinogen administered (as cryoprecipitate and fresh frozen plasma) with survival.

Based on current evidence and decades of empirical experience with POC-guided coagulation management algorithm, future treatment of trauma-induced coagulopathy can be based on systemic antifibrinolytics, local hemostatics, and individualized point-of-care-guided rational including the use of coagulation factor concentrates such as fibrinogen concentrate. Timely and rational use of coagulation factor concentrates will be more efficacious and safer than ratio-driven use of transfusion packages of allogeneic blood products. Massive transfusion protocols are unlikely to be suitable to all kinds of bleeding. Nevertheless, prospective randomized controlled trials are necessary to prove this hypothesis.

Summary

High fibrinogen counts exert a protective effect with regard to the amount of blood loss. In multiple-traumatized patients, priority must be given to early and effective correction of impaired fibrin polymerization by administering fibrinogen concentrate. Because of the timely delay and imprecision involved in measuring plasma count, measurement of fibrin polymerization by ROTEM®/TEG® is preferred to estimate the need for fibrinogen administration. If the maximum clot firmness (MCF) in the FIBTEM® analysis is <10–12 mm and/or the 10-min value is <7 mm, administration of 50 mg/kg fibrinogen concentrate is recommended. If ROTEM®/TEG® monitoring is not possible, fibrinogen should be maintained at minimum 150–200 mg/dl.

If no fibrinogen concentrate is available, fresh frozen plasma (minimum 30 ml/kg) must be transfused.

Cross-References

▶ Acute Coagulopathy of Trauma
▶ Adjuncts to Transfusion: Antifibrinolytics
▶ Adjuncts to Transfusion: Prothrombin Complex Concentrate
▶ Adjuncts to Transfusion: Recombinant Factor VIIa, Factor XIII, and Calcium

References

Fries D (2012) Coagulation monitoring under bleeding conditions: time to reconsider basic principles for our clinical decisions! Minerva Anestesiol 78(5):517–518

Fries D, Martini WZ (2010) Role of fibrinogen in trauma-induced coagulopathy. Br J Anaesth 105(2):116–121

Görlinger K, Fries D, Dirkmann D, Weber CF, Hanke AA, Schöchl H (2012) Reduction of fresh frozen plasma requirements by perioperative point-of-care coagulation management with early calculated goal-directed therapy. Transfus Med Hemother 39(2):104–113

Innerhofer P, Westermann I, Tauber H, Breitkopf R, Fries D, Kastenberger T, El Attal R, Strasak A, Mittermayr M (2013) The exclusive use of coagulation factor concentrates enables reversal of coagulopathy and decreases transfusion rates in patients with major blunt trauma. Injury 44(2):209–216

Sorensen B, Fries D (2012) Emerging treatment strategies for trauma-induced coagulopathy. Br J Surg 99(Suppl 1):40–50

Adjuncts to Transfusion: Prothrombin Complex Concentrate

Bellal Joseph and Peter Rhee
Division of Trauma, Critical Care, Burns and Emergency Surgery, The University of Arizona, Tucson, AZ, USA

Synonyms

Factor IX complex concentrate; Prothrombin complex concentrate

Definition

Coagulopathy perpetuates bleeding. Trauma triggers systemic inflammation with subsequent extensive activation of the coagulation cascade resulting in the rapid consumption and depletion of the coagulation factors.

Damage control resuscitation (DCR) focuses on rapid reversal of acidosis, prevention of hypothermia, and rapid reversal of coagulopathy. Principles of DCR include permissive hypotension, minimization of crystalloids, liberal use of blood products, and use of drugs to reverse coagulopathy.

Prothrombin complex concentrate (PCC) which contains vitamin K-dependent clotting factors (II, VII, IX, and X) is reserved for correction of coagulopathy. PCC formulations provided are liable and fast alternative to fresh frozen plasma for the reversal of both medication-induced coagulopathy and the coagulopathy of trauma (Holcomb 2007).

Composition and Dosage

PCC is available in two compositions: four-factor PCC and three-factor PCC. Three-factor PCC contains all four factors but is defined three factor by the minimal quantities of factor VII (35 units of FVII/100 units of PCC) (Holland et al. 2009). Only three-factor PCC formulations are available in the USA. Four-factor PCC is available in Europe and is currently being tested for efficacy and safety so that they can get FDA approval for use in the USA.

A standard dose of 25 units per kilogram is recommended for all patients irrespective of pre-injury anticoagulation. Because PCC is concentrated, it delivers a much higher dose of vitamin K-dependent factors than the same volume of FFP (McSwain and Barbeau 2011). Half-life ranges from 3 to 6 h with time to peak effect ranging from 10 to 30 min after intravenous administration. All patients who receive PCC should be given vitamin K 10 mg IV as an infusion over 15 min. Failure to administer

vitamin K may result in a rebound increase in INR after 6 h (Franchini and Lippi 2010).

Indications of Use

The FDA-approved indication for PCC is for patients with factor IX deficiency due to hemophilia B. However, the use of PCC has been expanding beyond its use in bleeding disorders. PCC is the current standard of treatment for the reversal of warfarin in the emergency setting (Spahn et al. 2007). The European and The American College of Chest Physician guidelines recommend the use of PCC as primary treatment of rapid anticoagulation reversal in patients with life-threatening bleedings and increased INR.

PCC has shown to be effective in rapid correction of INR, decreasing hemorrhage, and correction of coagulopathy of trauma (Joseph et al. 2012) and traumatic brain injury (Joseph et al. 2013) (Table 1).

Safety

PCC has a better safety profile than FFP because the PCC preparations undergo viral inactivation steps to minimize the risk of transmission of a variety of infective agents. The risk of TRALI (transfusion-associated acute lung injury) is minimal with the use of PCC, as the responsible antibodies are removed during manufacturing (Franchini and Lippi 2010).

Adverse effects include immediate allergic reactions, heparin-induced thrombocytopenia, and thromboembolic complications. The primary safety concern has been its association with stroke, myocardial infarction, pulmonary embolism, and deep vein thrombosis (Samama 2008).

Summary

PCC is well defined as first-line therapy for reversal of bleeding emergency patients with medically induced coagulopathy. The use of PCC for the treatment of the coagulopathy of

Adjuncts to Transfusion: Prothrombin Complex Concentrate, Table 1 PCC studies in trauma

Study	Results	Conclusion
Joseph B PCC in trauma	INR and PRBC administration reduced in both the non-warfarin and warfarin patients	PCC rapidly and effectively treats coagulopathy of trauma
Joseph B PCC vs. factor 7	INR and PRBC administration reduced in traumatic brain injury (TBI) patients	PCC rapidly and effectively treats TBI coagulopathy
Dikneite G PCC vs. FFP	PCC shortened the time to hemostasis after trauma and reduced the volume of blood lost	PCC was effective in correcting dilutional coagulopathy
Dikneite G PCC vs. factor 7	Peak thrombin generation time was greater in PCC group with shorter time to hemostasis	PCC promotes thrombin regeneration faster than factor 7

trauma is novel. PCC is an important hemostatic adjunct in DCR of trauma patients and allows for rapid correction of INR and life-threatening hemorrhage. PCC should be considered as an effective tool to treat acute coagulopathy of trauma.

Cross-References

▶ Acute Coagulopathy of Trauma
▶ Massive Transfusion Protocols in Trauma

References

Dickneite G, Pragst I (2009) Prothrombin complex concentrate vs fresh frozen plasma for reversal of dilutional coagulopathy in a porcine trauma model. British journal of anaesthesia 102(3):345–354

Dickneite G, Dörr B, Kaspereit F, Tanaka KA (2010) Prothrombin complex concentrate versus recombinant factor VIIa for reversal of hemodilutional coagulopathy in a porcine trauma model. The Journal of Trauma and Acute Care Surgery 68(5):1151–1157

Franchini M, Lippi G (2010) Prothrombin complex concentrates: an update. Blood Transfus 8(3):149–154

Holcomb JB (2007) Damage control resuscitation. J Trauma 62(Suppl 6):S36–S37

Holland L, Warkentin TE, Refaai M (2009) Suboptimal effect of a three-factor Prothrombin complex concentrate (Profilnine-SD) in correcting supratherapeutic international normalized ratio due to warfarin overdose. Transfusion 49(6):1171–1177

Joseph B, Amini A, Friese RS (2012) Factor IX complex for the correction of traumatic coagulopathy. J Trauma Acute Care Surg 72(4):828–834

Joseph B, Hadjizacharia P, Aziz H (2013) Prothrombin complex concentrate: an effective therapy in reversing the coagulopathy of traumatic brain injury. J Trauma Acute Care Surg 74(1):248–253

McSwain N Jr, Barbeau J (2011) Potential use of Prothrombin complex concentrate in trauma resuscitation. J Trauma 70(5 Suppl):S53–S56

Samama CM (2008) Prothrombin complex concentrates: a brief review. Eur J Anaesthesiol 25(10):784–789

Spahn DR, Cerny V, Coats TJ et al (2007) Task Force for Advanced Bleeding Care in Trauma Management of bleeding following major trauma: a European guideline. Crit Care 11:R17

Adjuncts to Transfusion: Recombinant Factor VIIa, Factor XIII, and Calcium

Yulia Lin
Department of Clinical Pathology, Sunnybrook Health Sciences Centre, Toronto, ON, Canada
Department of Laboratory Medicine and Pathobiology, University of Toronto, Toronto, ON, Canada

Synonyms

Activated recombinant human blood coagulation factor VII; Calcium; Chemical element "Ca^{2+}"; Coagulation "factor IV"; Corifact™ (coagulation factor XIII made from pooled human plasma); Eptacog alfa (activated); Factor XIII; Fibrin stabilizing factor; Fibrogammin®-P (coagulation factor XIII made from pooled human plasma); Niastase RT®; NovoSeven®RT; Recombinant coagulation factor XIII ($rFXIII-A_2$); Recombinant Factor VIIa

Definitions

Recombinant Factor VIIa

Recombinant factor VIIa (rFVIIa) acts through two mechanisms. The first is a tissue factor-dependent mechanism whereby rFVIIa binds tissue factor at the site of injury to activate factor X to Xa, generating small amounts of thrombin. Secondly, once activated, rFVIIa can act directly on the surface of platelets to produce a thrombin burst which converts fibrinogen to fibrin (Hedner and Lee 2011).

Factor XIII

Factor XIII (FXIII) is converted to activated factor XIII (FXIIIa) by thrombin and calcium. FXIIIa then catalyzes calcium-dependent fibrin polymerization through cross-linking, stabilizing fibrin, and protecting it from fibrinolysis (Levy and Greenberg 2013).

Calcium

Calcium is a key element required for coagulation and has been described as coagulation "factor IV." It enables interaction between the negatively charged vitamin K-dependent factors II, VII, IX, and X and the endothelium as well as phospholipids on the surfaces of platelets. Calcium also plays a role by binding to fibrinogen protecting it from proteolysis and in the stabilization of fibrin polymerization. All platelet activities and platelet incorporation into the thrombus require adequate concentrations of intracellular calcium. Pathways that inhibit coagulation such as the activation of protein C and fibrinolysis are also dependent on calcium (Lier et al. 2008).

Preexisting Condition

Recombinant Factor VIIa

Recombinant factor VIIa (Niastase RT®, NovoSeven®RT, NovoNordisk) is currently licensed for the treatment of bleeding episodes in hemophilia A or B patients with inhibitors in Canada and the United States. However, initial reports of the hemostatic success of rFVIIa

outside of the setting of hemophilia in 1999 were soon followed by more case reports and observational studies reporting its benefit in off-label use. Fortunately, two randomized controlled trials (RCT) were published examining the effect of rFVIIa in the specific setting of trauma (Boffard et al. 2005; Hauser et al. 2010). Both publications included patients with blunt and penetrating trauma. Boffard et al. conducted the first multicenter study and randomized 301 patients with severe trauma to rFVIIa (200 mcg/kg intravenously followed by 100 mcg/kg at 1 h and 3 h after the first dose) or placebo administered after the transfusion of the eighth red blood cell (RBC) unit. There was no difference in the primary outcome of number of RBC units transfused during the first 48 h after treatment or in the secondary outcomes of 48-h or 30-day mortality. A post-hoc analysis considering only blunt trauma patients alive at 48 h showed that the median number of RBC units was 7.0 in the rFVIIa group compared to 7.5 in the placebo group with a statistically significant reduction of 2.6 RBC units (90 % CI, 0.7–4.6) favoring the rFVIIa-treated group ($P = 0.02$). Hauser et al. followed with a phase 3 multicenter RCT where 573 patients were randomized to rFVIIa (same dosing as Boffard et al.) or placebo after the transfusion of the fourth RBC unit but before receiving the eighth RBC unit. There was no difference in the primary outcome of 30-day mortality. The study was terminated early due to a high likelihood of futility in demonstrating benefit of rFVIIa. In a systematic review of these two trials, there was no benefit in mortality nor was there an increase in thromboembolic complications. However, a decrease in the risk of acute respiratory distress syndrome was observed (RD −0.05; 95 % CI, −0.02 to −0.08) (Yank et al. 2011). Given the lack of mortality benefit, rFVIIa is not recommended in the treatment of patients with blunt or penetrating trauma.

Factor XIII

In 2011, plasma-derived human FXIII concentrate (Corifact™, Fibrogammin®-P, CSL Behring) was approved for use in the prophylactic treatment of congenital FXIII deficiency.

Recombinant FXIII (rFXIII, NovoNordisk) has not yet been licensed. Neither product has been assessed in the setting of trauma.

In surgical settings outside of congenital FXIII deficiency, decreases in the level of FXIII to below 60–70 % have been associated with increased bleeding. Godje et al. conducted a small preliminary RCT in the setting of cardiopulmonary bypass (CPB) surgery using plasma-derived human FXIII, Fibrogammin (Godje et al. 2006). Seventy-five patients were randomized to one of three arms: placebo, 1,250 units or 2,500 units of plasma-derived human FXIII administered immediately after administration of protamine. The first observation was that FXIII levels fell from normal preoperative values to their lowest levels (30–50 % below normal) at 30 min after onset of the extracorporeal circulation circuit in all three groups. The second observation was a dose-dependent decrease in bleeding, but this was not statistically different between any of the groups. Finally, the authors noted that a FXIII level below 70 % was associated with a statistically significant increase in drain loss and transfusion requirements compared to a level of 70 % and above. The authors concluded that after cardiac surgery, particularly in settings of prolonged diffuse bleeding, FXIII levels should be tested and the use of FXIII replacement is justified if levels are below 70 %.

Another preliminary RCT evaluated the safety and pharmacokinetics of recombinant FXIII (rFXIII-A_2, NovoNordisk) in cardiac surgery (Levy et al. 2009). Thirty-five patients were randomized to receive a single dose of rFXIII-A_2 at doses of 11.9, 25, 35, or 50 IU/kg post-CPB after protamine reversal of heparin compared to eight patients receiving placebo. As noted previously, FXIII levels decreased post-cardiopulmonary bypass. Doses of 25–50 IU/kg of rFXIII-A2 restored levels to preoperative levels. Optimal dosing was concluded to be 35 IU/kg as doses of 50 IU/kg tended to raise levels to above preoperative levels. One myocardial infarction occurred in a patient receiving 35 IU/kg rFXIII-A2. No other thromboembolic events were seen.

Calcium

Hypocalcemia occurs frequently in the trauma setting. In a prospective study of 212 consecutive severe trauma patients on admission who had been resuscitated in the prehospital phase without blood transfusion, 74 % had hypocalcemia as defined by an ionized calcium of <1.15 mmol/L, and 10 % had severe hypocalcemia (ionized calcium (iCa) < 0.9 mmol/L) (Vivien et al. 2005). In a cohort study of 353 patients receiving massive transfusion, the frequency of severe hypocalcemia (iCa < 0.8 mmol/L) climbed to 52 % in the 24-h period following massive transfusion (Ho and Leonard 2011). In a study of 941 patients in the intensive care unit (ICU), Hastbacka et al. found that 85 % had hypocalcemia (iCa < 1.16 mmol/L) at some point during their ICU stay (Hastbacka and Pettila 2003). Not only was hypocalcemia common, but admission hypocalcemia was associated with increased mortality, with hazard ratios of 5.1 for severe (<0.9 mmol/L) and 1.8 for mild ionized hypocalcemia (0.90–1.15 mmol/L). However, hypocalcemia was a poor predictor of mortality and, in multivariate regression analysis, not found to be an independent predictor of 30-day mortality. Whether hypocalcemia is more a sign of severity of injury or illness rather than a contributor to poor outcome is not clear.

The mechanism of hypocalcemia in trauma is multifactorial. In the study by Vivien et al., hypocalcemia on trauma admission was associated with resuscitation with colloids, but not crystalloids and low arterial pH (Vivien et al. 2005). The authors conducted an in vitro binding study demonstrating that lactate could bind calcium. Therefore, lactic acidosis could contribute to hypocalcemia. Another mechanism could be intracellular influx of calcium from ischemia and reperfusion. In another study, acidosis and amount of FFP transfused were important risk factors (Ho and Leonard 2011). Transfusion, particularly massive transfusion, may exacerbate hypocalcemia because citrate (which binds calcium) is the anticoagulant used in blood components. Liver dysfunction or poor liver perfusion may compound the issue further as the liver is the primary site of citrate metabolism.

Hypocalcemia has important potential consequences, namely, coagulopathy and cardiac function. As calcium plays such a critical role in hemostasis, hypocalcemia can contribute to coagulopathy. Hemostasis is impaired at values below 0.6–0.7 mmol/L. Acidosis may worsen coagulopathy as the affinity of the coagulation factors' calcium-binding sites is reduced under acidic conditions. Hypocalcemia may also adversely affect cardiac function at levels below 0.8–0.9 mmol/L. Prolonged QT and cardiac failure can occur at ionized calcium levels of 0.5 mmol/L (Lier et al. 2008). Other symptoms and signs of hypocalcemia include perioral and acral paresthesias, carpopedal spasm, tetany, Chvostek's sign (contraction of ipsilateral facial muscle elicited by tapping the facial nerve), laryngospasm, hypotension, narrow pulse pressure, and arrhythmias.

Application

Recombinant Factor VIIa

It should be noted that rFVIIa has been used as a "last ditch" treatment in the management of "refractory bleeding." No RCTs have been conducted in this setting; observational reports of such use may be prone to patient selection bias and observer bias as the treatment is not masked. The determination of whether rFVIIa is effective in such situations is further hampered by the complex coagulopathy that exists and the multiple blood components and other hemostatic therapies that may have also been simultaneously given to the patient. It is critical to recognize that the hemostatic effect of rFVIIa may be negated by hypothermia and acidosis. Knudson et al. reviewed 380 civilian trauma patients and found that severe acidosis, thrombocytopenia, and hypotension were associated with decreased survival despite rFVIIa (Knudson et al. 2011), implying correction of these abnormalities prior to consideration of rFVIIa use. Platelets, fibrinogen, and calcium are all critical for hemostasis and must be replaced prior to rFVIIa administration. Finally, clinicians should be aware of the potential thromboembolic complications; an increased risk of arterial thrombosis has been described with the use of rFVIIa,

particularly for patients 65 years or older, and most RCTs have excluded patients with a history of thrombosis (Levi et al. 2010).

Factor XIII

At this time, it is not clear if and how FXIII replacement should be used in the clinical setting of trauma and ongoing bleeding and whether its use impacts on clinical outcomes such as decreasing transfusion requirements and, more importantly, bleeding. Hopefully, future clinical trials will shed more light on this area.

Calcium

The management of hypocalcemia requires prompt identification with frequent laboratory assessment of calcium included with regular blood work during trauma resuscitation. Two compounds may be used: 10 % calcium gluconate contains 9.3 mg elemental calcium per mL and 10 % calcium chloride contains 27 mg elemental calcium per mL. Typical doses are 1 g (10 mL) IV over 10–20 min. This should be infused through a separate line from blood components to avoid chelation with citrate. Ionized calcium should be maintained at least above 0.9 mmol/L (Lier et al. 2008). Because of cardiac effects, magnesium levels should also be assessed. It is not known whether hypocalcemia is a consequence of the underlying severity of trauma or a contributing factor to its severity. As there are little downsides, it is reasonable to replace calcium in hypocalcemic patients who are actively bleeding.

Cross-References

▶ Anticoagulation/Antiplatelet Agents and Trauma
▶ Blood Bank
▶ Blood Component Transfusion
▶ Citrate-Dextrose Solutions
▶ Coagulopathy
▶ Damage Control Resuscitation
▶ Damage Control Resuscitation, Military Trauma
▶ Electrolyte and Acid-base Abnormalities
▶ Exsanguination Transfusion

▶ Factor I Concentrate

▶ Factor VIIa

▶ Fluid, Electrolytes, and Nutrition in Trauma Patients

▶ Hemostatic Adjunct

▶ Massive Transfusion

▶ Massive Transfusion Protocols in Trauma

▶ Transfusion Strategy in Trauma: What Is the Evidence?

▶ Trauma Intensive Care Management

▶ Trauma Operating Room Management

References

Boffard KD, Riou B, Warren B, Choong PI, Rizoli S, Rossaint R, Axelsen M, Kluger Y, NovoSeven Trauma Study Group (2005) Recombinant factor VIIa as adjunctive therapy for bleeding control in severely injured trauma patients: two parallel randomized, placebo-controlled, double-blind clinical trials. J Trauma 59:8–15, discussion 15–8

Godje O, Gallmeier U, Schelian M, Grunewald M, Mair H (2006) Coagulation factor XIII reduces postoperative bleeding after coronary surgery with extracorporeal circulation. Thorac Cardiovasc Surg 54:26–33

Hastbacka J, Pettila V (2003) Prevalence and predictive value of ionized hypocalcemia among critically ill patients. Acta Anaesthesiol Scand 47:1264–1269

Hauser CJ, Boffard K, Dutton R, Bernard GR, Croce MA, Holcomb JB, Leppaniemi A, Parr M, Vincent JL, Tortella BJ, Dimsits J, Bouillon B, CONTROL Study Group (2010) Results of the CONTROL trial: efficacy and safety of recombinant activated factor VII in the management of refractory traumatic hemorrhage. J Trauma 69:489–500

Hedner U, Lee CA (2011) First 20 years with recombinant FVIIa (NovoSeven). Haemophilia : Off J World Fed Hemophilia 17:e172–e182

Ho KM, Leonard AD (2011) Concentration-dependent effect of hypocalcaemia on mortality of patients with critical bleeding requiring massive transfusion: a cohort study. Anaesth Intensive Care 39:46–54

Knudson MM, Cohen MJ, Reidy R, Jaeger S, Bacchetti P, Jin C, Wade CE, Holcomb JB (2011) Trauma, transfusions, and use of recombinant factor VIIa: a multicenter case registry report of 380 patients from the western trauma association. J Am Coll Surg 212:87–95

Levi M, Levy JH, Andersen HF, Truloff D (2010) Safety of recombinant activated factor VII in randomized clinical trials. N Engl J Med 363:1791–1800

Levy JH, Greenberg C (2013) Biology of factor XIII and clinical manifestations of factor XIII deficiency. Transfusion 53:1120–1131

Levy JH, Gill R, Nussmeier NA, Olsen PS, Andersen HF, Booth FV, Jespersen CM (2009) Repletion of factor XIII following cardiopulmonary bypass using a recombinant A-subunit homodimer. Thromb Haemost 102:765–771, A preliminary report

Lier H, Krep H, Schroeder S, Stuber F (2008) Preconditions of hemostasis in trauma: a review. The influence of acidosis, hypocalcemia, anemia, and hypothermia on functional hemostasis in trauma. J Trauma 65:951–960

Vivien B, Langeron O, Morell E, Devilliers C, Carli PA, Coriat P, Riou B (2005) Early hypocalcemia in severe trauma. Crit Care Med 33:1946–1952

Yank V, Tuohy CV, Logan AC, Bravata DM, Staudenmayer K, Eisenhut R, Sundaram V, McMahon D, Olkin I, McDonald KM, Owens DK, Stafford RS (2011) Systematic review: benefits and harms of in-hospital use of recombinant factor VIIa for off-label indications. Ann Intern Med 154:529–540

Adolescent Trauma

▶ Pediatric Trauma, Assessment, and Anesthetic Management

Adrenal Failure

▶ Adrenal Insufficiency

Adrenal Insufficiency

Paul E. Marik
Division of Pulmonary and Critical Care Medicine, Eastern Virginia Medical School, Norfolk, VA, USA

Synonyms

Adrenal failure; Corticosteroid insufficiency

Definition

Critical Illness-Related Corticosteroid Insufficiency (CIRCI)

There has recently been a great deal of interest regarding the assessment of "adrenal function" and the indications for corticosteroid therapy in critically ill patients. While the use of high-dose corticosteroid (10,000–40,000 mg of hydrocortisone equivalent over 24 h) in patients with severe sepsis and ARDS failed to improve outcome and was associated with increased complications (Annane et al. 2004), an extended course of "stress-dose" corticosteroids (200–350 mg hydrocortisone equivalent/day for up to 21 days) has been demonstrated to increase ventilator- and hospital-free days and improve short-term survival in select groups of ICU patients (Annane et al. 2004). These patients typically have an exaggerated pro-inflammatory response and are considered to be "relatively" corticosteroid insufficient. Until recently the exaggerated pro-inflammatory response that characterizes patients with systemic inflammation has focused on suppression of the HPA axis and "adrenal failure." However, experimental and clinical data suggest that corticosteroid tissue resistance may also play an important role. This complex syndrome is referred to as *Critical Illness-Related Corticosteroid Insufficiency* (CIRCI) (Marik and Varon 2008). CIRCI is defined as inadequate corticosteroid activity for the severity of the patient's illness. CIRCI manifests with insufficient corticosteroid-mediated downregulation of inflammatory transcription factors.

Preexisting Condition

Exposure of the host to diverse noxious stimuli results in a stereotypic and coordinated response, referred to by Hans Selye as the *general adaption syndrome* (or stress response) which serves to restore homeostasis and enhance survival. The stress response is mediated primarily by the hypothalamic-pituitary-adrenal (HPA) axis as well as the sympathoadrenal system (SAS). Activation of the HPA axis results in increased secretion from the paraventricular nucleus of the hypothalamus of corticotropin-releasing hormone (CRH) and arginine vasopressin (AVP). CRH plays a pivotal integrative role in the response to stress. CRH stimulates the production

of ACTH by the anterior pituitary, causing the zona fasciculata of the adrenal cortex to produce more glucocorticoids (cortisol in humans). The increase in cortisol production results in multiple effects (metabolic, cardiovascular, and immune) aimed at restoring homeostasis during stress. In addition, the HPA axis and immune system are closely integrated in multiple positive and negative feedback loops (see Fig. 1).

Cortisol Physiology

Cortisol (hydrocortisone) is the major endogenous glucocorticoid secreted by the adrenal cortex. Over 90 % of circulating cortisol is bound to corticosteroid-binding globulin (CBG) with less than 10 % in the free, biologically active form. CBG is the predominant binding protein with albumin binding a lesser amount. During acute illness, including trauma and sepsis, CBG levels fall by as much as 50 %, resulting in a significant increase in the percentage of free cortisol. The circulating half-life of cortisol varies from 70 to 120 min, with a biological half-life of about 6–8 h. The adrenal gland does not store cortisol; increased secretion arises due to increased synthesis under the control of ACTH. Cholesterol is the principal precursor for steroid biosynthesis in steroidogenic tissue. At rest and during stress, about 80 % of circulating cortisol is derived from plasma cholesterol, the remaining 20 % being synthesized in situ from acetate and other precursors. High-density lipoprotein (HDL) is the preferred cholesterol source of steroidogenic substrate in the adrenal gland.

The activity of glucocorticoids is mediated by both the glucocorticoid receptor (GR) and mineralocorticoid receptor (MR). At low basal levels, cortisol binds to the high-affinity, low-capacity mineralocorticoid receptor (MR). However, with increased cortisol secretion, the MR is saturated, and cortisol then binds to the low-affinity, high-capacity glucocorticoid receptor (GR).

Cortisol diffuses rapidly across cell membranes binding to the GR. Through the association and disassociation of chaperone molecules, the glucocorticoid-GR-α complex moves into the nucleus where it binds as a homodimer to DNA

Adrenal Insufficiency,
Fig. 1 Activation of the
hypothalamic-pituitary-
adrenal axis (HPA) and the
interaction with the
inflammatory response.
ACTH
adrenocorticotrophic
hormone, *CRH*
corticotrophin, *IL-6*
interleukin-6, *IL-11*
interleukin-11,
LIF leukemia inhibitory
factor, *POMC*
pro-opiomelanocortin,
TGF-beta transforming
growth factor-beta,
TNF tumor necrosis factor
(Reproduced with
permission from
Lippincott, Williams, and
Wilkens (Marik and Varon
2008))

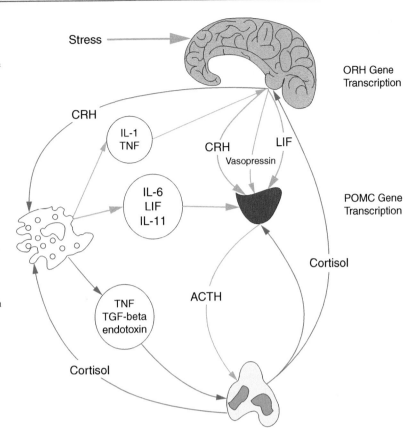

sequences called glucocorticoid-responsive elements (GREs) located in the promoter regions of target genes which then activate or repress transcription of the associated genes (see Fig. 2). In addition, the cortisol-GR complex may affect cellular function indirectly by binding to and modulating the transcriptional activity of other nuclear transcription factors such as nuclear factor κB (NF-κB) and activator protein-1 (AP-1). Overall, glucocorticoids affect the transcription of thousands of genes in every cell of the body. It has been estimated that glucocorticoids affect 20 % of the genome of mononuclear blood cells.

Trauma-, Surgery-, and Stress-Induced Immuno-paresis

Classic teaching suggests that tissue injury from trauma and surgery results in a systemic inflammatory response syndrome (SIRS) with "unbridled inflammation" which after a few days/weeks evolves into an immuno-paretic phase known as

the compensated anti-inflammatory response syndrome (CARS). However, multiple reports over the last two decades have indicated that the proliferative response to T-cell mitogens is significantly impaired in patients and experimental animals immediately after traumatic or thermal injury (Marik and Flemmer 2012). The T-cell dysfunction after traumatic stress is characterized by a decrease in T-cell proliferation, an aberrant cytokine profile, decreased T-cell monocyte interactions, and attenuated expression of the T-cell receptor complex (TCR). Furthermore, surgical stress induces a shift in the T-helper (Th)1/Th2 balance resulting in impaired cell-mediated immunity. While the Th1 cytokines may be increased following trauma and surgery, these cytokines do not reach the levels seen in patients with sepsis, and unlike patients with sepsis, the Th2 response predominates. Activation of the HPA and SAS is believed to be responsible for the Th1/Th2 imbalance that

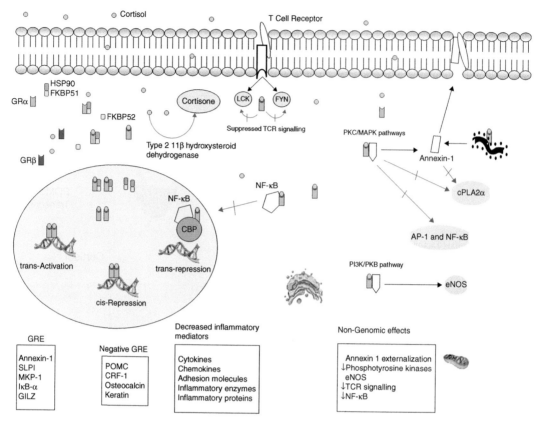

Adrenal Insufficiency, Fig. 2 An overview of the mechanisms of action of glucocorticoids. *SLP1* secretory leukoprotease inhibitor, *GILZ* glucocorticoid-induced leucine zipper protein, *eNOS* endothelial nitric oxide synthetase, *PI3K* phosphatidylinositol 3-kinase, *PKB* protein kinase B, *PKC* protein kinase C, *MAPK* mitogen-activated protein kinases, *LCK* lymphocyte-specific protein tyrosine kinase, *FYN* FYN oncogene-related kinase, *MKP-1* MAPK phosphatase 1, *HSP90* heat shock protein 90, *FKBP51/52* FK-binding protein 51/52, *POMC* pro-opiomelanocortin, *CRH* corticotropin-releasing hormone, *NF-κB* nuclear factor kappa B, *cPLA2α* cytosolic phospholipase A2 alpha, *CBP* cyclic AMP response element binding [CREB] binding protein, *GRα* glucocorticoid receptor-α, *Grβ* glucocorticoid receptor-β (Reproduced with permission from American College of Chest Physicians (Marik 2009))

occurs following tissue damage and trauma (Fig. 3) (Marik and Flemmer 2012). Epinephrine released predominantly by the adrenal medulla and norepinephrine released by the postganglionic nerve terminals act synergistically with glucocorticoids to induce a Th2 shift. Epinephrine and norepinephrine inhibit the production of IL-12 and enhance the production of IL-10. These effects are mediated by stimulation of β-adrenergic receptors. Glucocorticoids shift the Th1/Th2 balance by decreasing the synthesis of type 1 cytokines and increasing the synthesis of type 2 cytokines, by acting directly on CD4+ T cells, and indirectly by inhibiting IL-12 production by monocytes.

It would appear that the role of glucocorticoids as part of the stress response is to enhance the local clearance of foreign antigens, toxins, micro-organisms, and dead cells while at the same time preventing an overexuberant pro-inflammatory response. Glucocorticoids enhance opsonization and macrophage phagocytotic ability. Macrophage inhibitory factor (MIF) is an important pro-inflammatory cytokine whose secretion is enhanced by glucocorticoids. Toll-like receptor (TLR)-4 expression is increased by MIF which underscores the role of MIF in the macrophage response to endotoxins and gram-negative bacteria.

Adrenal Insufficiency, Fig. 3 Postulated mechanism involved in T-helper 2 pathways and arginine deficiency after physical trauma and surgery. *iNOS* inducible nitric oxide synthetase, *CMI* cell-mediated immunity, *CRH* corticotropin-releasing hormone, *DAMPs* damage-associated molecular patterns, *HPA* hypothalamic-pituitary-adrenal axis, *PGE2* prostaglandin E2, *Th1* T-helper 1, *Th2* T-helper 2, *IL-1* interleukin-1, *TNF* tumor necrosis factor, *INF* interferon, *MDSC* myeloid-derived suppressor cell, *Treg* regulatory T cell

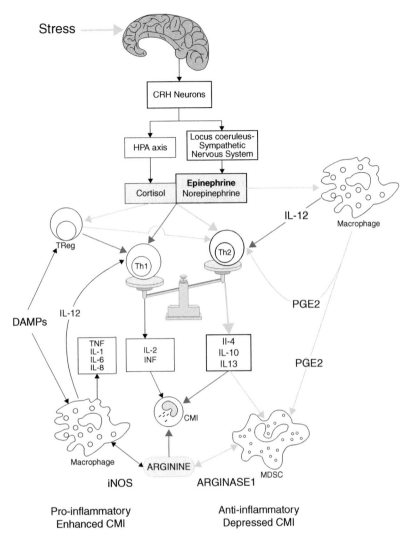

Clinical Manifestations of CIRCI

Patients with chronic adrenal insufficiency (Addison's disease) usually present with a history of weakness, weight loss, anorexia, and lethargy with some patients complaining of nausea, vomiting, abdominal pain, and diarrhea. Clinical signs include orthostatic hypotension and hyperpigmentation (primary adrenal insufficiency). Laboratory testing may demonstrate hyponatremia, hyperkalemia, hypoglycemia, and a normocytic anemia. This presentation contrasts with the features of CIRCI. The clinical manifestations of CIRCI are consequent upon an exaggerated pro-inflammatory immune response.

Hypotension refractory to fluids and requiring vasopressors is a common manifestation of CIRCI. CIRCI should therefore be considered in all ICU patients requiring vasopressor support as well as those with severe progressive ARDS. Patients usually have a hyperdynamic circulation which may compound the hyperdynamic profile of the patient with sepsis/systemic inflammation. However, the systemic vascular resistance, cardiac output, and pulmonary capillary wedge pressure can be low, normal, or high. The variability in hemodynamics reflects the combination of CIRCI and the underlying disease. CIRCI should also be considered in patients with progressive ALI.

Laboratory assessment may demonstrate eosinophilia and hypoglycemia. Hyponatremia and hyperkalemia are uncommon.

Diagnosis of Adrenal Insufficiency and CIRCI

The diagnosis of adrenal insufficiency in the critically ill is fraught with difficulties. Furthermore, we have no test that quantifies corticosteroid activity at the tissue level. Traditionally the diagnosis of adrenal insufficiency in the critically ill has been based on the measurement of a random total serum cortisol ("stress" cortisol level) or the change in the serum cortisol in response to 250 ug of synthetic ACTH (cosyntropin), the so-called delta cortisol. Both of these tests have significant limitations in the critically ill. Commercially available cortisol assays measure the total hormone concentration rather than the biologically active free cortisol concentration. Furthermore, the timing of cortisol measurements may be important as large hourly variations in cortisol have been reported. Despite these limitations, Annane and colleagues have reported that a delta cortisol of less than 9 mg/dl was the best predictor of adrenal insufficiency (as determined by metyrapone testing) in patients with severe sepsis/septic shock (Annane et al. 2006). A cortisol of less than 10 mg/dl was also highly predictive of adrenal insufficiency (PPV of 0.93); however, the sensitivity of the test was poor (0.19).

Application

The Use of Glucocorticoids in Patients with Sepsis and ARDS

Over the last three decades, approximately 20 randomized controlled trials (RCTs) have been conducted evaluating the role of glucocorticoids in patients with sepsis, severe sepsis, septic shock, and ARDS. Varying doses (37.5–40,000 mg/hydrocortisone eq/day), dosing strategies (single bolus/repeat boluses/continuous infusion/dose taper), and duration of therapy (1–32 days) were used in these studies (Annane et al. 2004). Despite multiple guidelines

and over 20 meta-analyses, the use of glucocorticoids in patients with sepsis remains extremely controversial with conflicting recommendations. Furthermore, while there are large geographic variations in the prescription of glucocorticoids for sepsis, up to 50 % of ICU patients receive such therapy. While it is difficult to make strong evidence-based recommendations at this time, an evidence-based review of this literature allows one to make the following conclusions:

1. Sepsis and ARDS cause complex alterations of the HPA axis and glucocorticoid signaling.
2. Short-course high-dose glucocorticoids are not beneficial in the treatment of severe sepsis/septic shock and ARDS.
3. Treatment of septic shock with moderate-dose glucocorticoids for 7 days significantly reduces vasopressor dependency (ACTH responders and nonresponders) and ICU length of stay.
4. Glucocorticoids do not increase the risk of superinfections.
5. Glucocorticoids may reduce mortality in subgroups of patients with septic shock.
6. Glucocorticoids appear to be of no benefit in patients with sepsis who are at a low risk of dying.
7. In patients with progressive early (<72 h) ARDS, glucocorticoids significantly increase the number of ventilator, ICU, and hospital-free days with a reduction in the risk of death.

CIRCI in Patients with Trauma

Clinical data suggests that in the absence of severe sepsis or the prior use of corticosteroids, patients who sustain traumatic injuries have heightened activation of the HPA axis with appropriate circulating levels of cortisol. However, hypothalamic-pituitary dysfunction following blunt head trauma may lead to the development of adrenal insufficiency. There is, however, limited data in the literature regarding the incidence of adrenal insufficiency following blunt head trauma. In a 5-year retrospective study of 2,100 trauma patients admitted to an ICU, the incidence of CIRCI was only 3.3 % (Walker et al. 2011). Similarly, in an analysis of 1,795 intubated trauma patients, 82 (4.5 %) were diagnosed with adrenal insufficiency (Guillamondegui et al. 2009). Fann and colleagues performed statistical modeling to predict adrenal insufficiency in trauma patients (Fann et al. 2007). In this study 3.3 % of patients admitted to the ICU were diagnosed with adrenal insufficiency. These authors reported 10 clinical variables to be predictive of adrenal insufficiency, the most important being endotracheal intubation, the use of vasopressor agents, a large positive fluid balance, and head injury. This data suggests that the incidence of CIRCI is generally low in trauma patients. However, the use of corticosteroids in trauma patients is a controversial topic. This controversy is largely fuelled by the use of etomidate for rapid-sequence intubation. Etomidate reversely inhibits cortisol production for up to 72 h. Roquilly and colleagues randomized 149 multi-trauma patients to receive a continuous infusion of hydrocortisone (200 mg/day for 5 days, followed by 100 mg on day 6 and 50 mg on day 7) or placebo (the HYPOLYTE study) (Roquilly et al. 2011). The primary end point of this study was hospital-acquired pneumonia within 28 days. In the intention to treat analysis, 35 % of the patients treated with hydrocortisone and 51 % of those treated with placebo developed pneumonia ($p = 0.007$). Most of the benefit of hydrocortisone appeared to be in the subgroup of patients with associated head injury. In this study 63 % of patients received etomidate on average 22 h prior to enrollment. The incidence of CIRCI at enrollment was 84 % in those who received etomidate compared to 62 % who had not received etomidate ($p = 0.01$). After controlling for the use of etomidate, the risk of hospital-acquired pneumonia still appeared to be lower in the hydrocortisone group ($p = 0.02$). In a follow-up publication of this study, these authors reported that etomidate was an independent risk factor for the development of hospital-acquired pneumonia. The results of this study are difficult to interpret due to the confounding effect of etomidate. This study, however, dispels an important myth, in that many believe that corticosteroids (even in stress doses) increase the risk of infectious complications in critically ill and injured patients.

The findings of the HYPOLYTE study stand in stark contrast to the Medical Research Council (MRC) CRASH trial. The CRASH trial randomized 100,008 adults with head injury and a Glasgow Coma Scale of 14 or less to a 48 h infusion of methylprednisolone or placebo (Anon 2004). Compared with placebo, the risk of death from all causes within 2 weeks and death or disability at 6 months was higher in the group allocated corticosteroids. It should however be noted that patients in the methylprednisolone group received a massive pharmacologic dose of corticosteroid (equivalent to 106,000 mg hydrocortisone over 48 h). This dose is similar to the dose of corticosteroids used to treat acute organ rejection after transplantation and results in profound immune suppression. Whether stress-dose corticosteroids improve the outcome of patients following blunt head trauma who do not have "adrenal insufficiency" is unclear at this time. Stress-dose corticosteroids may reduce the secondary inflammatory damage following head injury. The inflammatory response is an important component of traumatic brain injuries, particularly surrounding contusions and micro-hemorrhages. Cytokines are released from microglia, astrocytes, and polymorphonuclear cells within hours after traumatic brain injuries, leading to opening of the blood–brain barrier, complement-mediated activation of cell death, and the triggering of apoptosis. Although the inflammatory response may be beneficial in order to clean up cellular debris after injury, in excess it may promote secondary neuronal injury.

The complications associated with the use of corticosteroids are dependent upon the dose, the dosing strategy, and the duration of therapy. In the ICU setting (short-term treatment of CIRCI), the most important complications include immune suppression, hyperglycemia, and HPA axis and GR suppression. The effect of glucocorticoids on immune suppression is critically dose dependent. It is well known from the organ transplant experience that high-dose corticosteroids effectively abolish T-cell-mediated immune responsiveness and are very effective in preventing/treating graft rejection. However, while stress doses of corticosteroids inhibit systemic inflammation with decreased transcription of pro-inflammatory mediators, they maintain innate and acquired immune responsiveness and do not increase the risk of secondary infections. Corticosteroids should, however, be avoided in critically ill ICU patients who have progressed to CARS with generalized immuno-paresis. While myopathy is common in patients treated with high-dose corticosteroids, this complication is uncommon with stress-dose corticosteroids (Annane et al. 2004). Similarly, while high-dose corticosteroids may impair wound healing, this complication does not occur with stress-dose corticosteroids.

Perioperative Corticosteroids in Patients on Chronic Corticosteroids

Corticosteroids are prescribed for patients with a wide variety of autoimmune and inflammatory diseases, for patients with chronic obstructive pulmonary disease (COPD) and asthma, as well as recipients of organ transplants. Due to their chronic medical conditions, these patients frequently require both elective and emergency surgical procedures. It is generally believed that patients taking long-term glucocorticoids require perioperative "stress doses" of corticosteroids due to the presumed suppression of the hypothalamic-pituitary-adrenal (HPA) axis. Furthermore, it is believed that failure to provide supplemental perioperative corticosteroids will result in "adrenal crisis."

We performed a systematic review of prospective and cohort studies which specifically investigated the necessity for perioperative corticosteroids in patients receiving chronic corticosteroids (duration >2 weeks) (Marik et al. 2008). This study suggested that patients receiving therapeutic doses of corticosteroids who undergo a surgical procedure do not routinely require stress doses of corticosteroids so long as they continue to receive their usual daily dose of corticosteroid. Adrenal function testing is not required in these patients, as the test is overly sensitive and does not predict which patients will develop an adrenal crisis. However, the anesthesiologist, surgeon, and intensivist must be aware that the patient was receiving suppressive doses of corticosteroids, necessitating close perioperative hemodynamic monitoring and the use of stress doses of hydrocortisone in patients with volume refractory hypotension (a serum cortisol should be measured in these patients prior to initiating treatment). These recommendations do not apply to patients who receive physiologic replacement doses of corticosteroids due to primary dysfunction of the HPA axis, e.g., patients with primary adrenal failure due to Addison's disease and congenital adrenal hyperplasia, or patients with secondary adrenal insufficiency due to hypopituitarism. It is likely that these latter patients are unable to increase endogenous cortisol production in the face of stress. These patients require adjustment of their glucocorticoid dose during surgical stress under all circumstances.

In summary, the risk/benefit ratio of glucocorticoids should be determined in each patient. A course (7–10 days) of low-dose hydrocortisone (200 mg/day) should be considered in vasopressor-dependent patients (dosage of norepinephrine or equivalent >0.1 ug/kg/min) within 12 h of the onset of shock (Marik 2009). Steroids should be stopped in patients whose vasopressor dependency has not improved with 2 days of glucocorticoids. While the outcome benefit of low-dose glucocorticoids remains to be determined, such a strategy decreases vasopressor dependency and appears to be safe (no excess mortality, superinfections, or acute myopathy). At this time glucocorticoids appear to have a limited role in patients with sepsis or severe sepsis who are at a low risk of dying. A more "prolonged" course (21 days) of low-dose corticosteroids is recommended in patients with early progressive ARDS. Infection surveillance is critical in patients treated with corticosteroids, and to prevent the rebound phenomenon, the drug should be weaned slowly.

Cross-References

▶ Shock

References

Annane D, Bellissant E, Bollaert PE, Briegel J, Keh D, Kupfer Y (2004) Corticosteroids for severe sepsis and septic shock: a systematic review and meta-analysis. Br Med J 329:480–489

Annane D, Maxime V, Ibrahim F, Alvarez JC, Abe E, Boudou P (2006) Diagnosis of adrenal insufficiency in severe sepsis and septic shock. Am J Respir Crit Care Med 174:1319–1326

Anon (2004) Effect of intravenous corticosteroids on death within 14 days in 10 008 adults with clinically significant head injury (MRC CRASH trial): randomised placebo-controlled trial. Lancet 364:1321–1328

Fann SA, Kosciusko RD, Yost MJ, Brizendine JB, Blevins WA, Sixta SL, Morrison JE, Bynoe RP (2007) The use of prognostic indicators in the development of a statistical model predictive for adrenal insufficiency in trauma patients. Am Surg 73:210–214

Guillamondegui OD, Gunter OL, Patel S, Fleming S, Cotton BA, Morris JA Jr (2009) Acute adrenal insufficiency may affect outcome in the trauma patient. Am Surg 75:287–290

Marik PE (2009) Critical illness related corticosteroid insufficiency. Chest 135:181–193

Marik PE, Flemmer MC (2012) The immune response to surgery and trauma: implications for treatment. J Trauma Acute Care Surg 73:801–808

Marik PE, Varon J (2008) Requirement of perioperative stress doses of corticosteroids. A systematic review of the literature. Arch Surg 143:1222–1226

Marik PE, Pastores SM, Annane D, Meduri GU, Arlt W, Sprung CL, Keh D, Briegel J, Beishuizen A, Dimopoulou I, Tsagarakis S, Singer M, Chrousos GP, Zaloga G, Bokhari F, Vogeser M (2008) Recommendations for the diagnosis and management of corticosteroid insufficiency in critically ill adult patients: consensus statements from an international task force by the American College of Critical Care Medicine. Crit Care Med 36:1937–1949

Roquilly A, Mahe PJ, Seguin P, Guitton C, Floch H, Tellier AC, Merson L, Renard B, Malledant Y, Flet L, Volteau C (2011) Hydrocortisone therapy for corticosteroid insufficiency related to trauma. The HYPOLYT study. JAMA 305:1201–1209

Walker ML, Owen PS, Sampson C, Marshall J, Pounds T, Henderson VJ (2011) Incidence and outcomes of critical illness-related corticosteroid insufficiency in trauma patients. Am Surg 77:579–585

Adrenal Insufficiency in Trauma and Sepsis

A

Katarzyna Kimborowicz[2] and Zachariah Thomas[1]
[1]Department of Pharmacy Practice and Administration, Ernest Mario School of Pharmacy Rutgers, The State University of New Jersey, Piscataway, NJ, USA
[2]Department of Pharmacy, Morristown Medical Center, Morristown, NJ, USA

Synonyms

Critical illness-related corticosteroid insufficiency; Relative adrenal insufficiency

Definition

Adrenal insufficiency in the context of critical illness is defined as inadequate cellular corticosteroid activity for the severity of the patient's illness. Adrenal insufficiency during critical illness is usually transient.

Preexisting Condition

Both trauma and sepsis are proinflammatory conditions. Inflammatory cytokines are potent activators of cortisol secretion but also have inhibitory effects on the hypothalamic-pituitary-adrenal (HPA) axis. A variety of drugs that are commonly administered to trauma patients have important inhibitory effects on the adrenal system as well. These include etomidate, opiates, benzodiazepines, phenytoin, anticoagulants, and glucocorticoids (Thomas et al. 2010). Additional factors that have been associated with adrenal insufficiency are gram-negative bacteremia and hemodynamic instability. Among trauma patients, specific risk factors for adrenal insufficiency include younger age, greater injury severity, early ischemic insults, and the use of etomidate and metabolic suppressive agents (Cohan et al. 2005).

Application

Pathophysiology
Appropriate activation of the HPA axis is essential in surviving severe injury and surgical stress (Molina 2005). Although controversial, several studies have noted a positive correlation between the severity of trauma as indicated by the Injury Severity Score and cortisol concentrations. Pain, blood loss, and inflammatory cytokines are among the most important activators of the HPA axis in trauma patients (Burchard 2001). These stimuli and others result in the release of corticotropin-releasing hormone from the hypothalamus which stimulates adrenocorticotropin hormone (ACTH) release by the pituitary gland. ACTH-stimulated cortisol production occurs primarily in the zona fasciculata of the adrenal gland.

The pathophysiology of adrenal insufficiency in trauma is not completely understood. However, there is general agreement that the inflammatory response to trauma is thought to play a key role in the pathogenesis of adrenal insufficiency. Severe trauma is oftentimes associated with large increases in serum inflammatory cytokines such as IL-6 (Hoen et al. 2002). Several clinical and laboratory studies have demonstrated that higher concentrations and/or prolonged exposure to proinflammatory cytokines are associated with adrenal insufficiency. In addition to providing a potent inflammatory stimulus, hemorrhagic shock may also result in ischemia and necrosis of the adrenal glands thus resulting in primary adrenal insufficiency (Rushing et al. 2006). In traumatically brain-injured patients, direct injury to the hypothalamus and/or pituitary gland may result in secondary adrenal insufficiency (Bernard et al. 2006).

Diagnosis
The diagnosis of adrenal insufficiency in the critically ill is controversial. Various biochemical definitions have been used that rely upon either ACTH-stimulated or random cortisol concentrations. The diagnosis and prevalence of adrenal insufficiency will be highly dependent upon the definition used to characterize appropriate adrenal function. Guidelines published by the Society of Critical Care Medicine (SCCM) state that adrenal insufficiency in critical illness is best diagnosed by a delta cortisol (after 250 μg cosyntropin) of less than 9 μg/dL or a random total cortisol of less than 10 μg/dL (Marik et al. 2008). However, the utility of a biochemical definition is diminished in the critically ill due to hourly variations in serum cortisol concentrations and the presence of bias in routinely available assays for serum cortisol. Although these definitions have been extrapolated to trauma patients, no clear evidence supports these diagnostic values in patients without septic shock. A clinical diagnosis of adrenal insufficiency should be considered in critically ill patients who are poorly responsive to fluids and vasopressors. Unfortunately, no definitive recommendations are available to clearly delineate "poorly responsive."

Clinical Implications of Adrenal Insufficiency
In septic shock, adrenal insufficiency as defined by the SCCM criteria has been associated with a variety of harmful effects including refractory hypotension and increased mortality (Annane et al. 2002). The consequences of adrenal insufficiency in trauma patients are not as well studied. There are some data to suggest that adrenal insufficiency may increase the likelihood of vasopressor dependence (Dimopoulou et al. 2004), but the mortality impact of transient adrenal insufficiency in trauma patients is uncertain. However, it should be noted that prolonged pharmacologic adrenal suppression secondary to etomidate infusion has been shown to significantly increase mortality in trauma patients (Ledingham and Watt 1983).

The Role of Corticosteroids
Corticosteroids have been studied in sepsis for more than 50 years. Despite this, much uncertainty exists regarding their role. The historic approach of using short-course, high-dose

steroids in an attempt to blunt the inflammatory cascade has been abandoned due to inefficacy and possible immunosuppressant effects. Currently, moderate-dose corticosteroids (200–300 mg per day of hydrocortisone) are recommended in the treatment of septic shock in patients who are poorly responsive to fluid resuscitation and vasopressor therapy (Marik et al. 2008). Patients with severe sepsis not in shock or patients with septic shock stabilized with fluid and vasopressor therapy should not receive corticosteroid therapy.

There are few data to guide the role of corticosteroids in trauma patients. Results from the CRASH trial have definitively shown that short-course, high-dose corticosteroids (methylprednisolone 2 g bolus followed by 0.4 g per hour for 48 h) are harmful in the setting of traumatic brain injury (Roberts et al. 2004). In the multicenter HYPOLYTE study, moderate-dose corticosteroids (hydrocortisone 200 mg daily for 5 days, followed by 100 mg on day 6 and 50 mg on day 7) reduced the incidence of pneumonia and duration of mechanical ventilation in trauma patients with adrenal insufficiency (defined as a delta cortisol less than 9 μg/dL or random cortisol less than 15 μg/dL) (Roquilly et al. 2011). Despite these positive findings, this practice cannot be implemented until a larger confirmatory trial is conducted.

Adverse Effects of Corticosteroids

Corticosteroids have been associated with hyperglycemia, impaired wound healing, psychosis, an increased number of infectious complications, and myopathy. Corticosteroid-induced hyperglycemia is caused by impaired insulin-dependent glucose uptake in the periphery and enhanced gluconeogenesis in the liver. Hyperglycemia has been associated with increased mortality in critically ill patients, and early hyperglycemia can also result in poor outcomes in trauma and brain-injured patients (Laird et al. 2004). Therefore, glucose control is recommended in trauma patients. Corticosteroids affect many aspects of wound healing such as delaying the appearance of inflammatory cells and fibroblasts. Researchers suggest that supplementation with vitamin A may reverse the inhibitory effect of cortisone on wound healing; however, the majority of the published literature is based on animal models. An increased risk of bacterial and fungal infections has been reported with the use of corticosteroids. Behavioral disturbances such as mania, depression, memory loss, and psychosis are also of concern after corticosteroid administration. The relationship between corticosteroids and gastrointestinal bleeding remains an area of controversy. Risk factors related to an increased incidence of peptic ulceration in patients prescribed corticosteroids include total dose of corticosteroid, previous history of peptic ulceration, advanced malignant disease, and concurrent use of nonsteroidal anti-inflammatory drugs.

Future Research

In the near future, more definitive recommendations regarding the role of steroids in sepsis should be available from the Adjunctive Corticosteroid Treatment in Critically Ill Patients with Septic Shock (ADRENAL) study. The planned enrollment for this study (N = 3800) far exceeds the sample size of the largest study to date (N = 499) and, in fact, exceeds the totals of all patients included in recent meta-analyses. Thus, a more precise estimate of the risks and benefits of steroids are expected. Another ongoing study, Corticotherapy for traumatic brain-injured Patients – the Corti-TC trial, is examining the role of stress dose steroids in patients with traumatic brain injury who have a biochemical diagnosis of adrenal insufficiency (Asehnoune et al. 2011). The primary objectives are to determine whether hydrocortisone reduces the risk of pneumonia and improves long-term recovery.

Cross-References

► Brain Injury
► Sepsis, Treatment of
► Shock
► Ventilator-Associated Pneumonia

References

Annane D, Sébille V, Charpentier C et al (2002) Effect of treatment with low doses of hydrocortisone and fludrocortisone on mortality in patients with septic shock. JAMA 288:862–871

Asehnoune K, Roquilly A, Sebille V (2011) Corticotherapy for traumatic brain-injured patients–the Corti-TC trial: study protocol for a randomized controlled trial. Trials 12:228

Bernard F, Outtrim J, Menon DK, Matta BF (2006) Incidence of adrenal insufficiency after severe traumatic brain injury varies according to definition used: clinical implications. Br J Anaesth 96:72–76

Burchard K (2001) A review of the adrenal cortex and severe inflammation: quest of the "eucorticoid" state. J Trauma 51:800–801

Cohan P, Wang C, McArthur DL et al (2005) Acute secondary adrenal insufficiency after traumatic brain injury: a prospective study. Crit Care Med 33:2358–2366

Dimopoulou I, Tsagarakis S, Kouyialis AT et al (2004) Hypothalamic-pituitary-adrenal axis dysfunction in critically ill patients with traumatic brain injury: incidence, pathophysiology, and relationship to vasopressor dependence and peripheral interleukin-6 levels. Crit Care Med 32:404–408

Hoen S, Asehnoune K, Brailly-Tabard S et al (2002) Cortisol response to corticotropin stimulation in trauma patients: influence of hemorrhagic shock. Anesthesiology 97:807–813

Laird AM, Miller PR, Kilgo PD et al (2004) Relationship of early hyperglycemia to mortality in trauma patients. J Trauma 56:1058–1062

Ledingham IM, Watt I (1983) Influence of sedation on mortality in critically ill multiple trauma patients. Lancet 1:1270. http://www.ncbi.nlm.nih.gov/pubmed/6134053

Marik PE, Pastores SM, Annane D et al (2008) Recommendations for the diagnosis and management of corticosteroid insufficiency in critically ill adult patients: consensus statements from an international task force by the American College of Critical Care Medicine. Crit Care Med 36:1937–1949

Molina PE (2005) Neurobiology of the stress response: contribution of the sympathetic nervous system to the neuroimmune axis in traumatic injury. Shock 24:3–10

Roberts I, Yates D, Sandercock P et al (2004) Effect of intravenous corticosteroids on death within 14 days in 10008 adults with clinically significant head injury (MRC CRASH trial): randomised placebo-controlled trial. Lancet 364:1321–1328

Roquilly A, Mahe PJ, Seguin P et al (2011) Hydrocortisone therapy for patients with multiple trauma: a randomized controlled HYPOLYTE study. JAMA 305:1201–1209

Rushing GD, Britt RC, Britt LD (2006) Effects of hemorrhagic shock on adrenal response in a rat model. Ann Surg 243:652–654, discussion 654–6

Thomas Z, Bandali F, McCowen K, Malhotra A (2010) Drug-induced endocrine disorders in the intensive care unit. Crit Care Med 38:S219–S230

Adult Respiratory Distress Syndrome

▶ Acute Respiratory Distress Syndrome (ARDS), General
▶ ARDS, Complication of Trauma

Advance Directive

Hitoshi Arima[1] and Akira Akabayashi[2]
[1]Graduate School of Urban Social and Cultural Studies, Yokohama City University, Yokohama, Japan
[2]Department of Biomedical Ethics, The University of Tokyo Graduate School of Medicine, Tokyo, Japan

Synonyms

Advance health-care directive; Medical directive

Definition

Advance directives are statements conceived by competent individuals to express medical preferences in the event they become incapacitated. There are two main types of advance directives. One, called a living will, provides specific instructions on which treatment options the individual should receive or forego. The other, called a durable power of attorney, designates a surrogate for decision-making when the individual is declared incompetent.

Background

Legal Status in the United States

Both types of advance directives are legally recognized in the USA. All 50 states have enacted a living will statute, by virtue of which medical practitioners are immune from legal sanctions if they hasten death by implementing a patient's living will instructions in good faith.

The constitutionality of these statutes is guaranteed by the landmark Supreme Court decision for Cruzan case (1990), in which the father of a young woman in a persistent vegetative state petitioned for feeding tube removal so that she could die a natural death. The Supreme Court declared that the Constitution recognized a patient's right to decline treatment and the feeding tube could be removed as long as there is clear and convincing evidence that the patient had desired it.

A living will statute typically specifies the conditions under which the individual's instructions become effective. For example, California's Natural Death Act, the nation's first living will legislation, requires the following: that the patient be 18 years of age or older and of sound mind when signing the document, that two physicians certify that the patient is either terminally ill or permanently unconscious, and that the patient be too incompetent to make decisions. It should be noted that many of these statutes, or standard formats created in conjunction with various state legislations, maintain the instructions be activated only when the patient becomes terminally ill; several also set limits on the type of treatments a patient can decline. By contrast, benchmark American court decisions on this issue, such as the Cruzan, the Quinlan (1976), and the Bouvia (1986), are all clear that a patient need not be terminally ill in order to decline life-sustaining treatments. These decisions also agree that a patient may refuse any treatment, including artificial nutrition and hydration.

Each American state also has a durable power of attorney statute, which allows an individual to name a decision-maker for their affairs should that individual become incapacitated. These statutes were originally and principally pertinent to decisions regarding financial matters, but no court has denied that these laws should also apply to designation of proxies for health-care issues. Some states, including New York and Massachusetts, have an additional durable power of attorney statute that specifically deals with health-care issues (Annas 1991).

A durable power of attorney statute typically provides two sets of standards for the designated proxy to follow when making decisions for an incompetent patient, namely, the substituted judgment standard and the best interest standard. Substituted judgment requires that a proxy makes decisions based on the patient's wishes and beliefs pertaining to the situation. Since the incompetent patient's wishes or beliefs are not often specifically known, the proxy must make a decision based on conjecture as to what the patient, as a person still possessing some abstract pattern of desires, would have chosen had they been capable. The best interest standard is generally understood to apply when a patient's wishes or beliefs pertaining to the present situation are completely unknown. In these cases, the proxy should make decisions they believe will best promote the interests of the patient.

These advance directive statutes, which were first created independently in each state, were buttressed at the federal level in 1990, when Congress passed the Patient Self-Determination Act (PSDA). The PSDA targets all American health-care institutions that accept Medicare patients with the aim to secure a patient's right to make their own medical decisions, including the right to draft a living will and durable power of attorney. The institutions are obliged to notify patients of their right to draft an advance directive, to set a policy for keeping records of patients' directives, and to educate their staff and local citizens about advance directives.

Advance Directives in Other Countries and International Regions

The established legal status that advance directives have in the USA becomes a rare exception when turning to other parts of the world. Recent comparative studies suggest that the advance directive has either no role at all or only an unstable legal status with health practices in the vast majority of countries and regions around the world. Countries where an advance directive is reported to have no legal basis include Brazil, China, India, Kenya, and Turkey (Blank 2011). (*Bioethics*, Vol.24, no.3, 2010 is a special issue collecting six papers under the title of "Advance directive from a cross-cultural perspective." Robert H. Blank and Janna C. Merrick's book

(Blank and Merrick 2005) also contains 14 articles all on this topic. See also (Blank 2011) for a useful, concise summary of the topic and an update).

In some nations, while there are no formal laws recognizing its authority, advance directive may nonetheless have a binding force in practice due to the fact that its validity is underscored by guidelines issued from each nation's health-care authorities. Various government and professional bodies in Japan, including the Ministry of Health, Labor and Welfare, Japanese Medical Association, All Japan Hospital Association, and a few academic medical associations, successively but independently published guidelines in the late 2000s on the ethics of terminal care. The disparate guidelines all agree that some life-sustaining treatments can be withdrawn or refused for terminally ill patients and that medical practitioners should honor the wishes of a patient declared incompetent who previously expressed a wish to refuse treatment. The Korean Medical Association's guidelines on withdrawing life-sustaining treatments, published in 2001, similarly bestow an advance directive with some binding force in South Korea (Kim et al. 2010).

Legal systems in a handful of countries and regions outside the USA recognize advance directives, including Western European countries such as Austria, Germany, and the United Kingdom. Along with Western Europe and North America, Taiwan also enacted a Natural Death Act in 2000, which allows terminally ill patients to create a living will and durable power of attorney (Chiu 2005). While the contents of the other countries' laws are more or less the same as that of the USA, a notable exception is an Austrian law that distinguishes two types of advance directives with different levels of compliance. Medical practitioners are obliged to honor only what is called a binding advance directive; to create this document, patients are required to obtain a physician's advice and notarization, which can cost a considerable amount of money. The other option, called a nonbinding advance directive, requires no advice or acknowledgement but only requests that the instructions are given due respect. Binding advance directives

expire after 5 years, at which point the document becomes a nonbinding directive; a patient would need to seek the same medical and legal advice again for renewal (Schaden et al. 2010).

Application

Moral Basis of Advance Directives

Two moral considerations render strong support to the claim that patients' advance directives should be honored. In the USA and many other societies, there is almost unanimous consensus that a competent patient should retain the right to choose their medical treatment. Individual self-determination as such is highly valued on its own and also deemed to have a great instrumental value in promoting the individual's best interests for the reasons that people are usually the best judge of their own needs. That same pair of values, individual self-determination and best interests, supports the binding authority of advance directives; if allowing patients to make choices regarding contemporaneous medical treatment promotes their self-determination and their best interests, allowing them to make choices regarding future treatment should apparently have the same effects (Buchanan and Brock 1990).

The absolute binding authority of the advance directive, however, has detractors. One group of objections points to the various pragmatic difficulties involved with effective implementation of an advance directive and promotion of the two previously mentioned values, self-determination and an individual's best interests. Another group notes that other values may conflict with these two, implying that patient self-determination should not always be privileged.

Pragmatic Concerns over Effective Implementation of Advance Directives

A number of pragmatic difficulties have been raised in relation to effective implementation of living wills. In order for a living will to in fact promote a patient's self-determination and best interests, many things need to be true in the first place. Above all else, the individual must have adequate knowledge of the living will and actually sign the form. A patient's real wishes must also be accurately reflected in their living will instructions. Finally, medical providers and family members must see the living will documents and honor them when patients become incapacitated. Anecdotal evidence suggests these conditions are seldom met.

It has long been lamented that most Americans lack an advance directive despite decades of education. This oversight may not simply be due to people's ignorance; instead, many may find it unpleasant to contemplate their own death (Mappes 1998). Most standard advance directive formats currently available are written with language too difficult for the average person to comprehend, which could also contribute to the low adoption rate (Otto and Hardie 1997).

Even if a person creates a living will, it may not accurately reflect their preferences. Drafting a living will necessitates the individual to have some sense of what a critical illness would be like. In particular, one would need to predict treatment options and preferences relevant to any possible medical situation. This speculation, however, is exceedingly difficult for lay people to contemplate, especially those who are young and healthy. Additionally, people's preferences may change over time. Even if an individual had confidence in the accuracy of their living will instructions when they drafted it, their preferences may be completely different by the time they are incapacitated. In addition, empirical evidence suggests that among those who have signed living will forms, the majority do not have the document with them when a relevant medical situation arises; many in fact receive treatments that are inconsistent with their living wills (Fagerlin and Schneider 2004).

A more important pragmatic concern discussed by many critics pertains to interpretation of living will instructions. A living will is often drafted with terms that have a broad meaning. For example, one might refuse any life-sustaining treatment when a meaningful quality of life could no longer be expected. Implementing this instruction, however, requires interpretation of what exactly is meant by the terms "life-sustaining treatment" and "meaningful quality of life." Depending on who reads the instruction, it could be understood that the patient refused more or even less treatment than they had in fact desired.

It may seem that some of these living will issues do not apply to durable power of attorney. The purpose of durable power of attorney is only to designate a proxy, so preparing the directive does not require precise predictions regarding one's own preferences for particular treatment options. Additionally, appointing a specific person is not a matter of ambiguity, and interpretation problems may therefore seem unlikely. However, a closer look reveals that durable power of attorney faces challenges similar to the living will. The two standards set to guide proxy decision-making invite difficulties. First, the substituted judgment standard requires the proxy to make decisions based on their surmise of what the incapacitated patient would want. This in turn requires discerning what the patient's abstract sense of values would dictate as a treatment of choice for the concrete medical problem at hand. The interpretation issue thus resurfaces, albeit in a slightly different manner from living wills. The best interest standard fares no better. A proxy is likely to have little clue to an incompetent patient's best interests, especially when their preferences and values are unknown. Some best interest standards maintain the proxy should make a decision that an average, rational person would if they were fully informed, but understanding what an average, rational person would prefer in concrete situations again calls for ambiguous interpretation.

These facts and considerations led some commentators to believe that an advance directive should have less authority than a competent patient's treatment decisions. Therefore, it has been claimed, when there is serious doubt about the accuracy of an advance directive in representing the patient's real preferences, medical providers should sometimes override the directive either on paternalistic grounds or to secure the interests of others (e.g., a distressed family who wants the patient to live longer despite the patient's expressed wish) (Brock 1991).

Others believe that the enormous financial costs involved in promotion of advance directives to the public under the PSDA are unjustifiable, given that advance directives have seldom proven effective (Fagerlin and Schneider 2004).

However, there are also reasons to believe that these pragmatic difficulties are at least surmountable to a significant degree. Efforts have been made to create a standard living will format that utilizes plainer and more precise terminology to eliminate, or at least reduce, the room for interpretation (Emanuel and Emanuel 1989). The format could also juxtapose various treatment options with a list of situations critically ill and incapacitated patients often face, so that one could simply cross out unacceptable treatment options. Education programs that focus on encouraging people to discuss their medical preferences with family or close friends while still competent would also help overcome interpretation concerns.

In addition, some recent studies indicate a shift in empirical trends related to the implementation of advance directives. Previous reports uniformly determined that the majority of Americans had not completed an advance directive form, but a suggested explanation is that these results were due to selection bias from an exclusive focus on patients who died in acute care hospital settings. A nationwide study was conducted more recently in 2000, comprising data from 1,587 patient deaths in 25 states in all medical settings. This survey revealed that over 70 % of patients who died that year completed one of the two types of advance directives while still competent (Teno et al. 2007). The results of another study, published in 2010, showed that the majority of patients who completed an advance directive received treatment consistent with their preferences; 83 % of those who requested limited treatment and 97 % of those who asked for comfort care received their choice (Silveira et al. 2010). Researchers conducting these studies in the USA believe there has been a great increase in the use of advance directives in recent years and that both patients' families and medical providers have started to acknowledge its value.

These findings, combined with efforts to create more readable and unambiguous formats, point toward a possibility that advance directives will reflect self-determination and the best interests of a large number of patients.

Conflicts in Values

The advance directive aims to promote the values of individual self-determination and the patient's best interests. The pragmatic difficulties mentioned earlier which hinder realization of these values throw doubt on the binding authority of the advance directive. However, even if all of these difficulties are overcome, some doubts will remain. Conflict arises when implementation of an advance directive realizes the aforementioned values but violates other values as well.

A loving family may regret that the living will of an incompetent patient demands that life-sustaining treatment be terminated. Honoring this patient's living will would cause them deep grief and violate the value of promoting a family's best interests. The moral task would then be to choose between the patient's and the family's competing values.

While scholars tend to agree that the patient's self-determination should prevail in this case (as seen above, however, some critics do believe the interests of third parties provide sufficient reason to trump an advance directive even in the above case, given that advance directives often represent the patient's real preferences inaccurately), a more controversial moral question arises when a patient's past decision conflicts with their current interests. Consider an individual who has drafted a living will stating that any life-preserving intervention must be withheld should she suffer a severe mental impairment. Suppose this person is later afflicted with Alzheimer's disease, loses her decision-making capacity altogether as the illness advances, and eventually becomes incapable of taking food orally, requiring a nasogastric feeding tube for survival. Suppose further that, despite these difficulties, the patient appears to experience no negative emotions and is entirely free of physical pain. The patient even appears to take pleasure in various activities including picture drawing and singing. It seems undeniable that this patient has interest in continued life, even though her living will explicitly states that she should die by termination of treatments. If the living will and self-determination of the formerly competent patient are honored, the best interests of the presently incompetent patient would have to be compromised. Some commentators see a serious moral problem with implementing a living will in such cases, even assuming that the living will was drafted in a way that it accurately reflects the patient's real preferences (Robertson 1991; Cantor 1993).

These cases, in which patients' past decisions conflict with others' interests or their own current interests, pose perplexing moral questions. Thus, they also provide a reason to consider whether advance directive should have absolute binding force or if not, how much authority it should be endowed with.

Cross-References

▶ Autonomy
▶ Competency
▶ End-of-Life Care Communication in Trauma Patients
▶ Evaluating a Patient's Decision-Making Capacity
▶ Informed Consent in Trauma
▶ Life Support, Withholding and Withdrawal of
▶ Surrogate, Role in Decision-Making
▶ Terminal Care
▶ Withdrawal of Life-Support
▶ Withholding and Withdrawal of Life-Sustaining Therapy

References

Annas G (1991) The health care proxy and the living will. N Engl J Med 34(17):1210–1213

Blank RH (2011) End-of-life decision making across cultures. J Law Med Ethics 39(2):201–214

Blank RH, Merrick JC (2005) End-of-life decision making: a cross-national study. MIT Press, Cambridge, MA

Bouvia (1986) v. Superior Court, 179 Cal App.3rd 1127, 225 Cal.Rpt. 297 (Cal App 2nd Dist 1986)

Brock D (1991) Trumping advance directives. Hastings Center Report, September/October : 5–6

Buchanan A, Brock D (1990) Deciding for others. Cambridge University Press, New York, NY, p 99

Cantor NL (1993) Advance directives and the pursuit of death with dignity. Indiana University Press, Bloomington, IN

Chiu T-Y (2005) End-of-life decision making in Taiwan in [Blank and Merrick 2005]

Cruzan (1990) v. Director, Missouri Dept. of Health, 497 U.S. 261, 110 S.Ct. 2481, 111 L.Ed.2d 224 (1990)

Emanuel LL, Emanuel EJ (1989) The medical directive: a new comprehensive advance care document. J Am Med Assoc 261:3290

Fagerlin A, Schneider CE (2004) Enough: the failure of the living will. Hastings Cent Rep 34(2):30–42

Kim S, Hahn K-H, Park HW, Kang HH, Sohn M (2010) A Korean perspective on developing a global policy for advance directive. Bioethics 24(3):113–117

Mappes T (1998) Some reflections on advance directive. Newsletter on Philosophy and Medicine, in APA Newsletter, 98(1) Fall : 106–111

Otto BB, Hardie TL (1997) Readability of advance directive documents. J Nurs Scholarsh 29(1):53–57

Quinlan (1976) Matter of, 70 N.J. 10, 355 A.2d 647(N.J. 1976)

Robertson J (1991) Second thoughts on living wills. Hastings Cent Rep 21:6–9

Schaden E, Herczeg P, Hacker S, Schopper A, Krenn CG (2010) The role of advance directives in end-of-life decisions in Austria: survey of intensive care physicians. BMC Med Ethics 11:19

Silveira MJ, Kim SYH, Langa KM (2010) Advance directives and outcomes of surrogate decision making before death. N Engl J Med 362(13):1211–1218

Teno JM, Gruneir A, Schwartz Z, Nanda A, Wetle T (2007) Association between advance directives and quality of end-of-life care: a national study. J Am Geriatr Soc 55:189–194

Advance Health-Care Directive

▶ Advance Directive

Advance Life Support

▶ Life Support Training

Advanced Cardiac Life Support (ACLS)

▶ Cardiopulmonary Resuscitation in Adult Trauma
▶ Life Support Training

Advanced Practice Nurse

▶ Nurse Practitioners in Trauma Care

Advanced Practice Provider Care Delivery Models

Ruth M. Kleinpell
Department of Adult Health and Gerontology,
Rush University Medical Center, Chicago,
IL, USA

Synonyms

Advanced practice providers (APPs); Nurse practitioners and physician assistants

Definition

Care delivery models are healthcare models that outline the composition and roles of healthcare providers to meet patient care needs.

Preexisting Condition

The healthcare team plays an important role in the management of the patient with trauma. The care needs of the trauma patient require a coordinated focused approach to resuscitation and management with each member of the healthcare team impacting patient care and patient outcomes. Nurse practitioners (NPs) and

physician assistants (PAs) are increasingly being assimilated into healthcare teams to meet patient care as well as workforce needs. Factors influencing the need for NPs and PAs, or advanced practice providers, include the aging of the population and increased complexity of care requirements due to comorbidities and severity of illness, increased number of acute and critically ill patients who seek hospital care, a shortage of intensivists, and in the United States, restrictions on the work hours of medical and surgical residents in training (Pastores et al. 2012).

Overall, care delivery models using NPs and PAs are most often classified as service based, with the practitioner involved in care management of patients on a specific service, or unit based, with the practitioner involved in care management of patients within a specific unit (Kleinpell et al. 2008). Staffing models and patterns of use of NPs and PAs vary depending on the availability of physician coverage, number of advanced practice providers hired, and patient care volume and care needs. Reports of advanced practice provider coverage for patient care have ranged from daytime, nighttime, or weekend coverage to 24-h-7-day-a-week coverage (Kleinpell et al. 2008).

To date, the published literature on care delivery models using NPs and PAs has been limited to single institutional experiences or specific staffing models in specialty units such as the ICU (Gershengorn et al. 2011; Thourani and Miller 2006).

NPs and PAs in Trauma Care
NPs and PAS are increasingly being utilized as clinicians in the surgical subspecialty of trauma care. In a recent survey to 454 directors of major trauma centers in the United States, of the 246 respondents, 53 % reported using NPs and PAs (Nyberg et al. 2010). Of those currently not utilizing advanced practice providers, 19 % indicated an intent to do so in the near future, indicating the potential for continued growth in the utilization of NPs and PAs in trauma care.

The literature on the use of NPs and PAs in trauma care has focused on descriptions of role development and impact of advanced practice provider care, rather than on descriptions of specific models of care (Sise et al. 2011; McManaway and Drewes 2010). However, a number of studies have demonstrated beneficial impact of integrating NPs and PAs in trauma care. In a landmark study in 1990, Spisso and colleagues (Spisso et al. 1990) reported on the use of NPs in a trauma unit and the impact on decreasing length of stay for seriously injured patients from 8.10 to 7.05 days. In addition, the use of NPs was found to reduce physician workload.

Additional studies have demonstrated significantly shorter length of stay and higher patient satisfaction rate for patients cared for by advanced practice providers to care provided by resident staff, shorter intensive care unit and overall hospital length of stay, improved discharge rounding, decreased length of stay and no significant missed injuries in a trauma emergency department, improved nutritional care and bowel management for trauma rehabilitation patients, reduced length of stay with comparable mortality outcomes compared to data from the National Trauma Data Bank, improved patient satisfaction, and patient and trauma service provider satisfaction (Haan et al. 2007; Gillard et al. 2011; Sole et al. 2001; Sherwood et al. 2009; Berg et al. 2012).

Application

The role of advanced practice providers in trauma care is most often focused on direct patient care management; however, additional role components also include education of staff, patients, families and residents, practice guideline implementation, research and quality assurance initiatives, promoting communication of the plan of care, and discharge planning and, in some circumstances, post discharge clinic follow-up (Table 1). As a result of these role components, the advanced practice provider role has been described as enhancing continuity of care (Kleinpell et al. 2008).

Advanced Practice Provider Care Delivery Models, Table 1 Roles of NPs and PAs in trauma care (Adapted from Kleinpell et al. (2008))

Patient care management
Rounding
History and physical examinations
Diagnosing and treating illnesses
Ordering and interpreting tests
Initiating orders, often under protocols
Prescribes and performs diagnostic, pharmacologic, and therapeutic interventions consistent with education, practice, and state regulations
Performs procedures (as credentialed and privileged – such as arterial line insertion, suturing, and chest tube insertion)
Assessing and implementation of nutrition
Collaborates and consults with the interdisciplinary team, patient, and family
Assisting in the operating room
Responder to trauma, rapid response team, or code blue team
Education
Staff, patients, and families
Medical/surgical resident training
Practice guideline implementation
Lead, monitor, and reinforce practice guidelines for unit patients (i.e., central line insertion procedures, infection prevention measures, and stress ulcer prophylaxis)
Research
Data collection
Enrollment of subjects
Research study management
Quality assurance
Lead QA initiatives such as VAP bundle, sepsis bundle, and rapid response team
Communication
Promote and enhance communication with unit staff, family members, and the multidisciplinary team
Discharge planning
Transfer and referral consultations
Patient and family education regarding anticipated plan of care
Clinic follow-up post discharge

It becomes evident that additional information is needed on specific models of care, role components, and staffing ratios of NPs and PAs in trauma care. The integration and optimal utilization of NPs and PAs in trauma care holds much potential to improve trauma care outcomes.

Cross-References

▶ Crisis Intervention
▶ Critical Care Air Transport Team (CCATT)
▶ Discharge Planning
▶ End-of-Life Care Communication in Trauma Patients
▶ Family Preparation for Organ Donation
▶ Interdisciplinary Team
▶ Nurse Practitioner
▶ Performance Improvement
▶ Physician Assistant
▶ Teamwork and Trauma Care
▶ Triage

References

Berg GM, Crowe RE, Nyberg S, Burdsal C (2012) Trauma patient satisfaction with physician assistants: testing a structural equation model. J Am Acad Phys Assist 25(5):42–43, 49–51

Gershengorn HB, Wunsch H, Wahab R et al (2011) Impact of non-physician staffing on outcomes in a medical intensive care unit. Chest 139:1347–1353

Gillard JN, Szoke A, Hoff WS et al (2011) Utilization of PAs and NPs at a level I trauma center: effect on outcomes. J Am Acad Phys Assist 24:34–43

Haan JM, Dutton RP, Willis M, Leone S, Kramer ME, Scalea TM (2007) Discharge rounds in 80-hour work-week: importance of the trauma nurse practitioner. J Trauma 63:339–343

Kleinpell RM, Ely EW, Grabenkort R (2008) Nurse practitioners and physician assistants in the ICU: an evidence based review. Crit Care Med 26:2888–2897

McManaway C, Drewes B (2010) The role of the nurse practitioner in level II trauma at Nationwide Children's Hospital. J Trauma Nurs 17(2):82–84

Nyberg SM, Keuter KR, Berg GM, Helton AM, Johnston AD (2010) Acceptance of physician assistants and nurse practitioners in trauma centers. J Am Acad Phys Assist 23(1):35–37, 41

Pastores SM, O'Connor MF, Kleinpell RM, Napolitano L, Ward N, Bailey H, Mollenkopf FP, Coopersmith CM (2012) The ACGME resident duty-hour new standards: history, changes, and impact on staffing of intensive care units. Crit Care Med 39:2540–2549

Sherwood KL, Price RR, White TW, Stevens MH, Van Boerum DH (2009) A role in trauma care for advanced practice clinicians. J Am Acad Phys Assist 22(6):33–36, 41

Sise CB, Sise MJ, Kelley DM, Walker SB, Calvo RY, Shackford SR, Osler TM (2011) Resource commitment to improve outcomes and increase value at

a Level 1 Trauma center. J TRAUMA Injury, Infect Crit Care 70:560–568

Sole ML, Hunkar-Huie AM, Schiller JS, Cheatham ML (2001) Comprehensive trauma patient care by nonphysician providers. AACN Clinical Issues 12:438–446

Spisso J, O'Callaghan C, McKennan M et al (1990) Improved quality of care and reduction of house staff workload using trauma nurse practitioners. J Trauma 30:660–665

Thourani VH, Miller JI (2006) Physician assistants in cardiothoracic surgery: a 30-year experience in a university center. Ann Thorac Surg 81(1):195–199

Recommended Reading

Christmas AB, Reynolds J, Hodges S et al (2005) Physician extenders impact trauma systems. J Trauma 58:917–920

D'Agostino RD, Pastores SM, Halpern NA (2012) The NP staffing model in the ICU at Memorial Sloan-Kettering Cancer Center. In: Kleinpell RM, Buchman T, Boyle WA (eds) Integrating nurse practitioners and physician assistants in the ICU: strategies for optimizing contributions to care. Society of Critical Care Medicine, IL, USA, pp 17–26

Fanta K, Falcone RA, Rickets C, Schweer L, Brown RL, Garcia VE (2006) Pediatric trauma nurse practitioners provide excellent care with superior patient satisfaction for injured children. J Pediatr Surg 41:277–281

Hormann BM, Bello SJ, Hartman AR, Jacobs M (2004) The effects of a full-time physician assistant staff on postoperative outcomes in the cardiothoracic ICU: 1-year results. Surg Phys Assist 10(10):38–41

Jarrett LA, Emmett M (2009) Using trauma nurse practitioners to decrease length of stay. J Trauma Nurs 16(2):68–72

Kapu AN, Thomson Smith C, Jones P (2012) NPs in the ICU. The Vanderbilt experience. Nurse Pract 37(8):46–52

Nyberg SM, Waswick W, Wynn T, Keuter K (2007) Midlevel providers in a Level I trauma service: experience at Wesley Medical Center. J Trauma Injury Infect & Crit Care 63(1):128–134

Sherwood K, Sugerman S, Bossart P, Bledsoe J, Barton E, Bernhisel K, Bess E, Madsen T (2011) EDOU staffing by PAs: what are the effects on patient outcomes? J AM Acad Phys Assist 24(8):31–34, 37

Advanced Practice Providers (APPs)

▶ Advanced Practice Provider Care Delivery Models
▶ Physician Assistant

Aerodigestive Injury

▶ Tracheal and Esophageal Injury

Affective Changes

▶ Traumatic Brain Injury, Neurological/Psychiatric Issues

Aftercare

▶ Discharge Planning

Aged Person Trauma

▶ Elderly Trauma, Anesthetic Considerations for

Agitation

▶ Delirium as a Complication of ICU Care
▶ Sedation, Analgesia, Neuromuscular Blockade in the ICU

Agitation of the Heart

▶ Cardiac and Aortic Trauma, Anesthesia for

Air Route

▶ Airway Anatomy

Air Transport

▶ Critical Care Air Transport Team (CCATT)

Airbag Injuries

Virginia Harvey
Department of Emergency Medicine, University of Pennsylvania, Philadelphia, PA, USA

Synonyms

Blunt chest trauma; Facial burn; Motor vehicle collision

Epidemiology

Since 1998, the US Department of Transportation has required all passenger cars be equipped with frontal airbags (U.S. Department of Transportation 1999). Such legislation has led to a dramatic decrease in the number motor vehicle collision (MVC) fatalities and serious nonfatal injuries, with an estimated 28,000 lives saved as of January 2009 (U.S. Department of Transportation 2009). There are, however, reports on injuries resulting directly from airbag use, particularly among high-powered, first-generation airbags.

In 1997, the National Highway Traffic Safety Administration (NHTSA) began allowing vehicle manufacturers to install airbags with reduced inflation powers ("depowered" airbags) in an attempt to decrease the likelihood of airbag injury during an MVC. Airbag-related morbidity and mortality have further been reduced by the advent of advanced frontal airbags, which are now mandatory in all vehicles manufactured after September 1, 2006. These airbags rely on sensor input (including data on occupant size, seat position, seatbelt use, and crash severity) to automatically determine if and with what level of power an airbag should deploy (US Department of Transportation 2012).

Side-impact airbags (SABs) are designed to protect occupants during side-impact MVCs, including rollover collisions. In 2005, the NHTSA attributed 9,200 MVC fatalities to side-impact collisions and determined that 300 lives and 400 serious injuries could be prevented

A

each year with the universal implementation of SABs. In 2007, the NHTSA issued a mandate that all passenger vehicles be equipped with side-impact protection by 2013.

Anatomy of Injury

An airbag injury is any traumatic injury secondary to the inflation of a vehicle's airbag. The mechanism of airbag deployment involves the rapid inflation of a balloon, stored either in a vehicle's steering wheel, dashboard, or side paneling, under high pressure to protect the occupant from collision with the vehicle's interior. During moderate to severe collisions, a deceleration sensor triggers the ignition of a solid propellant which creates an exothermic reaction to inflate the bag at high speed. Most injuries occur when an occupant collides with an actively inflating bag.

Head, neck, and face injuries are most common during frontal collisions involving an unrestrained driver or front-seat passenger with a first-generation airbag (Fig. 1). These may include facial fractures, mandibular injuries, decapitation, cervical spine fractures, and vascular injury. Ocular trauma (orbital fractures, retinal detachment, and lens rupture) are more severe in the presence of corrective lenses and in front-seated children (Lueder 2000). Airbag-related injuries to the chest have included rib fractures, pneumothorax, aortic transection, heart valve injury, cardiac rupture, and thoracolumbar spine injuries. Some studies have shown an increased incidence of upper extremity injuries from MVCs with airbag deployment vs. no airbag deployment (Richter et al. 2000). The lower extremities are usually spared from direct airbag trauma due to their location. Approximately 8 % of airbag-related trauma includes burns (either friction, chemical, or thermal) from the intense chemical reaction that occurs during airbag deployment (Tintinalli et al. 2004). Rare injuries have included acoustic trauma and premature rupture of membranes in the setting of pregnancy (Wallis and Greaves 2002).

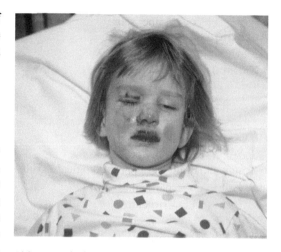

Airbag Injuries, Fig. 1 Facial injuries from first-generation airbag impact (Photo credit: Ed Dickinson, MD)

Special consideration should be given to airbag injuries in the pediatric population. There is good evidence that passenger airbags are associated with an increased risk of death in children. Specifically, infants in rear-facing child seats may sustain severe head and neck injury from airbag deployment. Forward-facing children who are improperly belted may have their heads in the airbag deployment area and are also at risk for severe injury. It is currently recommended that all children ages 12 and under ride in the back seat.

Clinical Impact

Trauma Triage Significance: It is best to assume an MVC resulting in airbag deployment involved sufficient forces to produce severe injury. Obvious head/neck trauma or changes in a patient's level of consciousness should prompt urgent triage to a trauma center. Similarly, because of the potential for torso damage, any chest wall or abdominal ecchymosis, deformity, or tenderness should raise the clinical suspicion for serious injury and should prompt responding personnel to direct these patients to the nearest trauma center.

Clinical Care/Care Caveats: The evaluation and care of airbag-protected crash victims follows the same ATLS algorithm as other blunt trauma patients. In the setting of face, head, and neck injury, airway management may be especially difficult. C-spine immobilization and assessment for vascular injury to the neck should be routine. Changes in hemodynamics or respiratory patterns should prompt emergent evaluation for serious chest and/or abdominal trauma. Occult abdominal injuries have also been reported (Augenstein et al. 1995). Careful screening should be performed for upper extremity injuries, particularly those that threaten major vascular structures. Ophthalmologic consultation may be needed for ocular trauma. A child who presents to the emergency department after an MVC should undergo a careful history regarding child seat placement and seatbelt usage. In such cases, a thorough physical exam and a high index of suspicion for head and neck trauma are paramount, particularly in the very young, preverbal patient.

Cross-References

▶ ABCDE of Trauma Care
▶ Chest Wall Injury
▶ Diaphragmatic Injuries
▶ Motor Vehicle Crash Injury
▶ Seatbelt Injuries
▶ Thoracic Vascular Injuries

References

Augenstein JS, Digges KH, Lombardo LV et al (1995) Occult abdominal injuries to airbag-protected crash victims: a challenge to trauma systems. J Trauma 38:502–8

Lueder GT (2000) Air bag-associated ocular trauma in children. Ophthalmology 107:1472–5

Richter M, Otte D, Jahanyar K et al (2000) Upper extremity fractures in restrained front-seat occupants. J Trauma 48:907–12

Safegcar.gov. US Department of Transportation. http://www.safercar.gov/Vehicle+Shoppers/Air+Bags/Advanced+Frontal+Air+Bags#7. Accessed 30 Nov 2012

Tintinalli JE, Kelen GD, Stapczynski JS (2004) Emergency medicine: a comprehensive study guide, 6th edn. American College of Emergency Physicians. McGraw-Hill, New York, p. 1230

U.S. Department of Transportation (1999) NHTSA federal motor vehicle safety standards (FMVSS). Standard No. 208. Washington. Revised March 1999

U.S. Department of Transportation (2009) NHTSA counts of frontal air bag related fatalities and seriously injured persons. Washington. January 2009

Wallis LA, Greaves I (2002) Injuries associated with airbag deployment. Emerg Med J 19:490–493

A

Airway Anatomy

Sarah Fabiano[1] and Penelope C. Lema[2]
[1]Department of Emergency Medicine, University of South Carolina Medical School, Greenville, SC, USA
[2]Department of Emergency Medicine, State University of New York University at Buffalo, Buffalo, NY, USA

Synonyms

Air route; Breathing passage; Respiratory tract; Ventilation passage

Definition

The passageway by which air enters and exits the lungs through the nares or oropharynx.

The airway is a continuous passageway but can be further categorized into the upper and lower airway. The upper airway begins from the nares and oropharynx to the vocal cords (Fig. 1a and b). The lower airway is located below the level of the vocal cords and extends distally.

Upper Airway Anatomy

Pharynx: The upper portion of the throat that consists of the *nasopharynx*, *oropharynx*, and *hypopharynx*. The *nasopharynx* is located at the base of the skull and extends to the soft palate. The *oropharynx* continues from the soft palate to the epiglottis. The *hypopharynx* includes the epiglottis to the cricoid ring and the piriform sinus (Kimoff 2005).

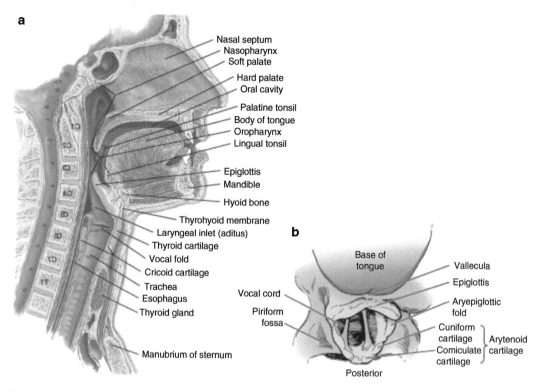

Airway Anatomy, Fig. 1 (**a**) Sagittal view of the upper airway anatomy. (**b**) Anatomy of the larynx and vocal cords as seen through laryngoscopy

Piriform sinus: Forms the recesses on both sides of the aryepiglottic folds and medial to the thyroid cartilage and thyrohyoid membrane. The inferior portion of each *piriform sinus* is called the piriform recess and is located at the level of the true vocal cord (Pawha et al. 2013).

Larynx: Contains the anterior structures of the throat, also called the voice box, from the tip of the epiglottis to the inferior border of the cricoid cartilage (Roberts 2004). The laryngeal soft tissue consists of the *thyroid, cricoid*, and *arytenoid cartilages* (Pawha et al. 2013).

Thyroid cartilage: Appears as an inverted V-shaped structure that is composed of two alae that merge in the midline and indents superiorly to form the superior thyroid notch. The *thyroid cartilage* articulates with the *cricoid cartilage* inferiorly at the cricothyroid joint. *Cricoid cartilage:* Located beneath the thyroid cartilage, forms a ring around

the trachea. *Laryngeal inlet:* The opening to the larynx. It is bordered by the epiglottis anterosuperiorly, the aryepiglottic folds laterally, and the arytenoid cartilage posteriorly (Roberts 2004).

Arytenoid cartilage: Located posterior to the laryngeal inlet, separates the glottis from the esophagus.

Glottis: The vocal apparatus of the larynx. It includes the true and false cords.

Vallecula: A groove located between the tongue base and the epiglottis (Roberts 2004).

Lower Airway Anatomy

Trachea: The "windpipe" travels and bifurcates at the carina, usually at the level of thoracic vertebrae (T5).

Bronchi: Right and left mainstem bronchi. The right side is shorter and straighter. The bronchi are lined with mucus cells and beta receptors. These further subdivide into secondary and tertiary bronchi.

Bronchioles: Mainly consists of smooth muscle and no cartilage. These further divide into alveolar ducts and sacs.

Alveoli: Small clusters, lined with surfactant, where gas exchange, ventilation, and perfusion occur.

Lungs: The right side has 3 lobes. The left side has two lobes.

Pleura: Visceral pleural covers the lungs, whereas the parietal pleura covers the inside of the pleural cavity which has pain receptors.

Pleural space: Located between the parietal and visceral pleura.

Vasculature

   Pulmonary arteries: Carry deoxygenated blood from the heart to the lungs.

   Capillary beds: Surround the alveoli where gas exchange occurs.

   Pulmonary veins: Return oxygenated blood to the heart (Finucane et al. 2011).

Preexisting Conditions

Trauma patients are unique since traumatic injuries often involve multiple organ systems and they must be stabilized and treated simultaneously. Hypoxia is one of the most common causes of morbidity and mortality in the trauma patient (Feliciano et al. 2004). If arterial blood levels of oxygen cannot be maintained due to hypoxia and desaturation ensues, this quickly leads to anoxic brain injury and mortality (Field et al. 2010). Direct injury or impairment of the lungs produces less hypoxia than airway obstruction itself. Despite the recent 2010 American Heart Association (AHA) changes in CPR from A-B-C to C-A-B, establishing a definitive airway is imperative (Field et al. 2010).

The trauma patient can pose challenges, while a definitive airway is being established or during attempts to ventilate. The patient may be obtunded, be comatose, have distorted airway anatomy, or be at risk of aspiration of secretions, blood, or gastric contents (Field et al. 2010). The patient may be on spine precautions with a cervical collar for possible spinal cord injury and remain on a backboard when an airway must be urgently established. With blunt or penetrating trauma, impending airway obstruction due to edema, hematoma, and muscle or nerve damage must be considered before the patient deteriorates. With penetrating trauma, the possibility of an air leak and vascular injury creates a different set of challenges when establishing an airway. The initial goal of the healthcare team is to establish an airway, ventilate, and oxygenate.

External Anatomy

A quick survey of the trauma patient's respiratory status and external anatomy can provide the team vital information. Auscultation provides additional information. This assessment may help predict a challenging or difficult airway. Studies have previously demonstrated that there are no real predictors of a difficult airway (Roberts 2004).

Face

Evaluation should include examination for facial deformities, avulsed or broken teeth (aspiration risk), foreign bodies, bleeding or hemorrhage, burns, soot in the nares or oropharynx, or simply loss of normal anatomy. Facial fractures and trauma are contraindications to nasotracheal intubation for risk of accidentally accessing the anterior cranial fossa. Extreme facial fractures and mandibular dislocations with the inability to directly visualize the airway may be an indication for cricothyroidotomy. Evaluation of the patient's anatomy, size, and position of teeth and chin may predict a more anterior and, perhaps, difficult airway. The trauma patient may require a nasopharyngeal airway (NPA) because of upper airway obstruction. If there are no contraindications after examination of the area, with identification of the septum for deviations and trauma, a NPA may be placed straight posteriorly, not upward, into the nose.

Neck

Look for obvious injury such as penetrating trauma to the zones of the neck and deformity (Fig. 2a and b). Palpation may reveal tracheal deviation. Bruising or an expanding hematoma may occur after blunt trauma. Evaluation of how the patient is breathing may help predict the patency of an airway. There may also be signs

A

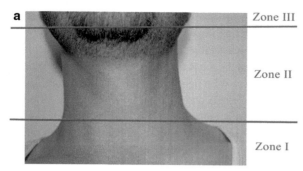
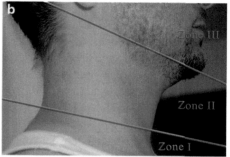

Airway Anatomy, Fig. 2 (**a**) Frontal view of the zones of the neck. (**b**) Right sagittal view of the zones of the neck. Zone 1 is the area from the clavicles to the cricoid cartilage, Zone 2 is the area from the cricoid cartilage to the angle of the mandible, and Zone 3 is the area above the angle of the mandible

of laryngotracheal injury. The patient with a short, thick neck may have a difficult airway. Look for normal anatomy landmarks, such as the cricoid and thyroid cartilages, which may be helpful during airway management.

Chest Wall

A quick evaluation of this area may reveal asymmetric chest rise, penetrating or sucking chest wounds, rib fractures, flail chest, or protrusion of tissue or bone. Ecchymosis, "seatbelt sign," or other blunt trauma may be a predictor of severe internal injury or an indication that the patient may eventually have problems with their airway or ventilation (Field et al. 2010). Palpation of the chest wall may reveal crepitus or deformities not appreciated by observation alone.

Internal Anatomy

Evaluation of the patient's internal anatomy is optimally performed by the physician performing the intubation. Direct visualization may reveal clues to underlying injury such as edema, mucosal disruption, hematoma, and vocal cord abnormalities (Field et al. 2010). Distortion of anatomy may make this assessment difficult and may complicate direct laryngoscopy attempts. Use of the GlideScope® (Verathon Inc., Bothwell, WA), fiberoptic intubation, bougie, or other airway assist devices may be necessary. The goal is to visualize the vocal cords, properly place the endotracheal tube, and secure the patient's airway.

Application

Special Populations

The pediatric population has anatomical differences in their airway. The pediatric airway is smaller and more compliant. The distance between the pharynx, vocal cords, and trachea is also shorter. There is more soft tissue in the pediatric pharynx than in adults. Also, children can have severe spinal cord damage in the setting of trauma without a cervical spine fracture. Therefore, it is imperative that spinal precautions are observed at all times. Pediatric patients also have a larger head compared to the rest of their body. Correct positioning of children is important in the trauma setting. The surgical airway is contraindicated in pediatric patients <1 year of age (Weathers 2010).

The patient with trisomy 21 (Down syndrome) can present a challenge with airway management. One study demonstrated that almost 45 % of these patients had obstructive sleep apnea, most relieved by tonsillectomy and adenoidectomy. Other important considerations are the midface hypotonia, glossoptosis, enlarged tonsils and adenoids, and increased secretions. These patients may have atlantoaxial instability caused by a congenital anomaly of the odontoid or laxity in transverse ligaments. Attempt a jaw thrust with c-spine stabilization if intubation or assisted respiration is needed (Marcus et al. 1991).

Positioning

The maintenance of cervical spine alignment during airway management is imperative in the trauma patient until spinal injuries have been ruled out. Removal of the cervical collar to manipulate the jaw is acceptable practice as long as in-line cervical spine stabilization is maintained. This differs from intubation in the non-trauma setting where extension of the head is accepted (Feliciano et al. 2004). When an obvious neck injury is present, especially with a penetrating injury, injury to the cervical spine and surrounding structures is highly likely (Field et al. 2010).

Last Resort

Despite excellent technique, proper positioning, experience, and special equipment, establishing a definitive airway can be difficult in the trauma situation. The key to the difficult airway is preparation, early recognition, and having alternate airway devices readily available. A surgical airway is the last resort. It is performed less frequently in the ED setting due to advances in technology and alternate airway techniques and devices. Identification of your normal external anatomy, such as the thyroid and cricoid cartilages and the cricothyroid membrane, is imperative to successful cricothyroidotomy (Gestring).

Pitfalls

Unfortunately in the setting of trauma, many external factors are out of the physician's control. Information regarding the patient's last meal and medications may be unknown. Patients may be anticoagulated. Patients may present with intractable emesis and profuse secretions or have severe facial injuries with a foreign body in the airway, all of which increase the risks aspiration. Accidental injury to the lips, teeth, or internal airway anatomy exists during any intubation attempt. Unforeseen esophageal intubation or right main stem intubation may occur.

Acknowledgements Ruth Fabiano and Scott Brzezinski for photography

Cross-References

▶ ABCDE of Trauma Care
▶ Airway Assessment
▶ Airway Exchange in Trauma Patients
▶ Airway Management in Trauma, Cricothyrotomy
▶ Airway Management in Trauma, Tracheostomy
▶ Airway Trauma, Management of
▶ Auto-PEEP
▶ Cardiopulmonary Resuscitation in Adult Trauma
▶ Cardiopulmonary Resuscitation in Pediatric Trauma
▶ Chest Wall Injury
▶ General Anesthesia for Major Trauma
▶ Hypoxemia, Severe
▶ Life Support Training
▶ Lung Injury
▶ Pediatric Airway Management
▶ Pediatric Trauma, Assessment, and Anesthetic Management
▶ Pneumothorax, Tension
▶ Pulmonary Trauma, Anesthetic Management for
▶ Rapid Sequence Intubation
▶ Strangulation and Hanging
▶ Tracheal and Esophageal Injury
▶ Trauma Emergency Department Management
▶ Trauma Patient Evaluation

References

Feliciano DV, Moore EE, Mattox KL (2004) Trauma, 5th edn. McGraw Hill, New York

Field JM et al (2010) American Heart Association guidelines for cardiopulmonary resuscitation and emergency cardiovascular care science. Circulation 122(18 suppl 3):S639

Finucane BT, Tsui Dip Eng BCH, Santora AH (2011) Principles of airway management. Springer, New York, pp 1–25

Gestring M, Difficult airway algorithm. University of rochester emergency medicine residents handbook

Kimoff RJ (2005) Physiology of the upper airways and upper airway obstruction in disease. In: Hamid O, Martin J, Shannon J (eds) Physiological basis of respiratory disease, 1st edn. People's Medical Publishing House, Hamilton, pp 581–596

A

Marcus CL et al (1991) Obstructive sleep apnea in children with Down syndrome. Pediatrics 88(1):132–139

Pawha P, Jiang N, Shpilberg K, Luttrull M, Govindaraj S (2013) Gross and radiographic anatomy. In: Levine AI, Govindaraj S, Demaria S (eds) Anesthesiology and otolaryngology, 1st edn. Springer, New York, pp 3–33

Roberts JR (2004) Clinical procedures in emergency medicine, 4th edn. W.B. Saunders, An Imprint of Elsevier, Philadelphia, pp 62–106

Weathers E (2010) The anatomy of the pediatric airway. RC Educational Consulting Services, Brockton, MA, pp 11–12

Airway Assessment

Colleen Kovach
Department of Emergency Medicine, Strong
Memorial Hospital, Rochester, NY, USA

Synonyms

LEMON; Mallampati

Definition

Assessment or evaluation of an airway or pathway from outside to the lungs in the setting of trauma.

The leisurely evaluation of an airway is not possible for ED physicians and trauma surgeons. Studies have suggested an intubation rate of 10 % in trauma patients within the initial 2 h of arrival with upwards of 10 % of those as difficult airway intubations. In addition, patients with severe traumatic injuries are at risk of developing airway obstruction or poor ventilation resulting in hypoxia, both of which (obstruction and hypoxia) have been linked to preventable acute trauma deaths (Sise et al. 2009; Hussain and Redmond 1994; Nolan 2006).

The initial airway assessment follows two different algorithms, depending on whether the patient is conscious or unconscious, stable or unstable.

In a conscious and stable trauma patient, the initial airway assessment can be completed by the observation and confirmation of the airway "ABCDs" (Mahadevan and Garmel 2005; Finucane and Santora 2003; American College of Surgeons 2008):

A – Airway: Check that the airway is open and patent; this can be done by having the patient answer a simple question, such as "What is your name?" An appropriate response shows that not only is the patient's mentation preserved but also he is protecting his airway appropriately at that time.

B – Breathing: Check that the breathing is present and adequate. Inspect the patient for any signs of respiratory difficulty, i.e., rate and pattern of inspiration, presence of stridor, use of accessory muscles, and movements of the chest wall.

C – Cavity (oral): Inspect for injuries to the oral cavity and teeth, foreign bodies, or possible obstructions. Be sure to note the presence or absence of the patient's dentition.

D – Damage (trauma): Inspect both the face and neck for any injuries; these may cause the patient to decompensate or lead to a difficult airway intubation. Examples of such injuries include lacerations, large hematomas, presence of subcutaneous crepitus, and facial fractures such as mandibular or Le Fort fractures, which may inhibit direct laryngoscopy. If a cervical collar is present, it may be necessary to temporarily remove the collar, while assuring that inline stabilization is maintained, to adequately assess the anterior neck for any injury.

The assessment of the airway in an unconscious patient varies from that of the conscious patient. If the patient is unstable, the establishment of a secure airway is expedited. If the patient is relatively stable, well oxygenated, and not in need of emergent intubation within the next few minutes, the advanced trauma life support guidelines support the assessment of the airway via a stepwise plan; this plan can be easily remembered by the mnemonic LEMON (American College of Surgeons 2008; Khan et al. 2011):

L – Look externally: External inspection for certain characteristics that are known to cause difficult ventilation and intubation – obesity, small mouth, short neck, foreign body, large tongue, small mandible, high-arched palate.

E – Evaluate the 3-3-2 rule:
- The distance between the patient's incisors is at least three finger breadths.
- The distance between the patient's hyoid bone and chin is at least three finger breadths.
- The distance from the patient's thyroid notch and floor of the mouth is at least three finger breadths.

This rule is based on the relation of the size of mouth opening and the mandible to the position of the larynx in the neck and the likelihood of appropriate visualization of the glottis with direct laryngoscopy (DL). Three keys that are taken into account for in this rule are:

1. Adequate visualization past the tongue is possible when both the endotracheal tube and laryngoscope blade are within the oral cavity.
2. The mandible is of sufficient size to allow for the displacement of the tongue.
3. The glottis is sufficiently distanced from the base of the tongue to allow for direct visualization of the cords from outside the mouth (Walls and Murphy 2008).

M – Mallampati score: This score is based on the relationship of the size of the tongue and proportion of the oropharynx it occupies with the difficulty of intubation. This is performed by having the patient sit upright and opening his mouth fully, and the examiner assesses the visibility of the hypopharynx with tongue maximally protruded (Finucane and Santora 2003). While it may not be possible to assess this in most trauma patients, an attempt should be made to see how easily the hypopharynx may be visualized (modified Mallampati score explained below):
- Class 1 – visibility of hard and soft palate, uvula, and tonsils
- Class 2 – visibility of hard and soft palate, uvula, and upper portion of tonsils
- Class 3 – visibility of hard and soft palate and base of uvula
- Class 4 – visibility of hard palate only

O – Obstruction: Any factor that may obstruct the airway, leading to difficulty with ventilation and/or laryngoscopy. Examples include abscess, hematoma, and edema.

N – Neck mobility: The ability to move the neck and adjust to assist with visualization of the cords helps to increase the likelihood of success. This is assessed by asking the patient to lift the chin to the chest and then extending the neck. Trauma patients who have a cervical collar in place and those who are on spine precautions have limited neck mobility, making intubation more difficult. In this subset of patients, the cervical collar should be removed, and another provider should be assisting to help maintain in-line stabilization.

Regardless of whether or not the trauma patient presents to the emergency department stable or unstable, conscious or unconscious, early preparation prior to the patient's arrival with an airway crash cart, including tools for the management of a difficult airway, can help assure proper and early airway intervention and decrease mortality.

Cross-References

▶ ABCDE of Trauma Care
▶ Airway Anatomy
▶ Airway Equipment
▶ Airway Management in Trauma, Cricothyrotomy
▶ Airway Management in Trauma, Nonsurgical
▶ Airway Management in Trauma, Tracheostomy
▶ Airway Trauma, Management of

References

American College of Surgeons Committee on Trauma (2008) Advanced trauma life support for doctors, student course manual, 8th edn. American College of Surgeons, Chicago

Finucane BT, Santora AH (2003) Principles of airway management. Springer, New Jersey, pp 126–139

Hussain LM, Redmond AD (1994) Are pre-hospital deaths from accidental injury preventable? BMJ 308(6936):1077

Khan RM et al (2011) Airway management in trauma. Indian J Anaesth 55(5):163–169

Mahadevan SV, Garmel GM (2005) An introduction to clinical emergency medicine. Cambridge University Press, New York, pp 21–28

Nolan J (2006) Airway management after major trauma, Continuing Education in Anaesthesia. Crit Care Pain 6(3):124–127

Sise MJ et al (2009) Early intubation in the management of trauma patients: indications and outcomes in 1,000 consecutive patients. J Trauma 66(1):32–39

Walls RM, Murphy MM (2008) Manual of emergency airway management, 3rd edn. Lippincott Williams & Wilkins, Philadelphia, pp 87–91

Airway Devices

▶ Airway Equipment

Airway Equipment

Gregory M. Blanton
Department of Emergency Medicine,
University of Rochester, Rochester, NY, USA

Synonyms

Airway devices; Airway rescue equipment

Definition

Airway equipment includes any device or tool used in the monitoring of respiratory function, in the assistance to a patient's own respiratory effort, and/or in the control of an unstable patient's respiratory system.

Pre-existing Condition

The trauma patient's respiratory function can range from normal to complete respiratory arrest.

Airway equipment must be flexible enough to provide support to or control of the patient's airway as his/her condition warrants. It would be the rare trauma patient who did not require some intervention with airway equipment or monitoring.

Application

Introduction

The first responsibility of a provider in trauma resuscitation is the airway. Providing definitive airway management begins with preparation, and preparation is not possible without the appropriate equipment. A provider must have access to equipment that runs the gamut from the most basic oxygen delivery and monitoring systems to the tools needed for surgical airways.

Organization and familiarity with devices is paramount. Prehospital providers should have a readily portable kit that includes the most essential airway equipment needed to stabilize a patient's airway with the goal being safe delivery to a facility with trauma support capabilities. Hospital providers should have an extensive, portable collection of all equipments needed for any airway contingency at hand.

A key to success in any life-saving management process is always to have backup equipment. A provider must be familiar with all primary and backup equipment and have plans for each step as success or failure occurs until, ultimately, a surgical airway either provides definitive management or the resuscitative effort has failed. Some of the most common devices and adjunct devices used in airway management in emergency and trauma patients are described in the following paragraphs.

Basic Oxygen Delivery and Monitoring

Often, passive oxygen delivery and diligent monitoring is sufficient to help stabilize a patient undergoing trauma resuscitation. A range of delivery systems are available. A **nasal cannula**, which consists of clear plastic tubing that is hooked to an oxygen source, is fitted over the patient's ears, and delivers oxygen through nasal prongs, will provide flow up to a 5–6 L/min efficiently. When available, high-flow nasal cannula devices can provide up to 60 L/min flow of warmed, humidified oxygen mixtures. **Face masks** also are used often in the trauma setting. Simple masks and **partial non-rebreathers** are most helpful. Simple masks, usually a plastic mask with an adjustable strap and nose-piece, placed over the nose and mouth, are similar to air-entrainment (or Venturi masks) but do not have adjustable flow valves. These can be used to deliver oxygen at higher flow rates than conventional nasal cannulae. Partial non-rebreathers and true **non-rebreathers** fit tightly over the nose and mouth and have one-way valves that allow exhaled air to escape the mask. These draw on attached reservoir bags that must be partially inflated for proper delivery. The latter can deliver high concentrations of oxygen and are important in providing passive delivery to unstable patients in the prehospital setting or during pre-oxygenation treatment before placement of invasive airways is performed.

Nearly as important as basic oxygen delivery, of course, is accurate monitoring of a patient's systemic oxygen saturation. **Continuous pulse oximetry** has become the standard noninvasive modality. Probes with sensors placed on digits or other areas of the body that provide access to waveforms produced by superficial arterial flow allow for transmission and analysis of light-frequency differences with conversion to saturation values. Similar devices, such as **CO oximeters** that provide carboxyhemaglobin levels, also can be useful for assessing trauma victims involved in fires or explosions.

Adjunct Devices for Passive Oxygen Delivery

Simple devices routinely are used to allow for more efficient and effective passive oxygen delivery by overcoming natural, anatomical obstructions. Generally, these devices are used in obtunded, unconscious, or chemically sedated and paralyzed patients, as they likely would be less tolerated by more alert individuals. **Oropharyngeal airway devices** are rigid and, when inserted, provide light traction on the posterior tongue to guard against closure over the glottis as

well as a small bite block anteriorly, which prevents obstruction by the lips and teeth. The device typically is inserted into the oral cavity upside-down (curved end pointing rostrally) and then rotated 180 at depth for seating. **Nasopharyngeal airway devices** are flexible tubes with a flared end. The tapered end is lubricated and inserted into a nare and is advanced until the flared end is flush with the nostril. Two devices may be placed side-by-side. They are much less likely to trigger a patient's gag reflex than an oropharyngeal airway. Nasopharyngeal airway devices are contraindicated in severe facial trauma or in patients with suspected basilar skull fractures. Positive pressure or active oxygen delivery, discussed next, also is better facilitated with these adjunct devices.

Positive Pressure Delivery

In the emergent setting, positive pressure delivery is administered when passive measures have failed to adequately oxygenate the patient. These can be used to ventilate the patient until more definitive measures can be undertaken. The major drawback to positive pressure delivery is unwanted pressure in the upper GI system, as forced air is not selective in its route. The simplest device is the **pocket mask** (or pocket airway mask or CPR mask), which simply allows a bystander or rescuer to deliver his/her own exhaled air to the patient without performing mouth-to-mouth resuscitation. An inflated mask fits over the patient's mouth and nose, and the rescuer breathes through a tube that inserts, usually via a one-way valve, into the interior mask from above. Some masks also are fitted with a port through which concentrated oxygen may be delivered, in addition to the rescuer breaths. A powerful delivery device is the **bag-valve mask**. With a patent airway, theoretically, a bag-valve mask can provide indefinite ventilation; however, the risk of aspiration as a consequence of GI distention and emesis must always be considered in prolonged positive pressure delivery. The bag-valve mask consists of a mask similar to the pocket mask, which is attached to a reservoir bag that can be squeezed by the rescuer to provide ventilation through a one-way valve. The mask can be removed to allow the bag and valve to connect to a more definitive airway, once inserted. The apparatus should be connected to a concentrated oxygen source, if available.

Temporizing Airway Devices

Temporizing airway devices are used when definitive control is not immediately possible due to lack of appropriate equipment, training, personnel, or simply due to circumstances. They can be inserted blindly. It must always be remembered that these devices are intended only to be a bridge to more definitive airway security. They should be exchanged for definitive airway control at the first possible opportunity, always keeping in mind the safety of the patient. Some examples follow:

A **laryngeal mask** consists of a distal, inflatable cuff that is shaped to seal off the esophagus after insertion and inflation at the level of the larynx. The cuff's pointed end projects into the proximal esophagus, allowing the inflated rim to act as a seal, separating the esophagus from the larynx and distal airway, therefore allowing ventilation through the tracheal opening via its main airway tube. This device is often used by anesthesiologists for shorter operative cases. Direct laryngoscopy is not necessary, as the device is inserted by hand and fed until seated and inflated.

A **Combitube** (brand name) is a dual-lumen, dual-balloon device that is inserted blindly to provide a temporizing airway. Two lumens are encased in an outer sheath. One continues through the device to the distal end, and the other terminates in a series of perforations mid-device. Normally, after insertion, the distal end of the device is seated in the esophagus. The distal balloon is inflated in the esophagus, and the proximal balloon in the pharynx. The perforations now are approximately at the supraglottic level, and ventilation may be accomplished, assuming the glottic opening and distal airways are patent. Should the distal end of the Combitube be inserted in the trachea via the glottic opening, ventilation may occur through the lumen that continues through the tube distally after balloon

inflation. This device provides a forgiving platform to prehospital providers. However, it must be remembered that this is not a definitive airway device; further, insertion and prolonged use can result in airway edema, which will make eventual definitive airway placement more difficult and dangerous. A carbon dioxide detector and/or esophageal intubation detector must be used in the algorithm to confirm placement and ventilation through the appropriate lumen. If normal placement is confirmed, a nasogastric tube may be dropped through the esophageal lumen to allow gastric decompression.

A **King airway device** (brand name) is similar to the Combitube, except only one inflation device and valve is used to inflate both balloons. Again, the device is inserted blindly, and nearly always, its distal end will be seated in the esophagus. This is even more likely with the King device, as it is more rigid and pre-formed with a curve to help prevent tracheal intubation. After the esophageal and oropharyngeal balloons are inflated respectively, perforations again provide ventilation at or just above the level of the glottic opening.

Definitive Airway Devices and Accessories

The **endotracheal tube** is the gold-standard for a definitive airway in the patient unable to maintain his/her native airway naturally. It may be inserted nasally (naso-tracheal intubation) or orally (oro-tracheal intubation). Modern endotracheal tubes usually are made of clear, semiflexible polymer material. They are manufactured in varying gauges (from pediatric to large adult patients) with varying corresponding lengths. Smaller tubes may be uncuffed, while most tubes intended for larger pediatric patients or adults are cuffed, or have an inflatable balloon near the distal end that seats the tube firmly in the trachea and provides a seal. The proximal end may be connected to any device that provides ventilation of room air or gas. Drugs may even be administered through the endotracheal tube, as indicated. While dual-lumen tubes have been designed to allow ventilation of single lungs during thoracic surgery, in the emergency or trauma setting, the single-lumen endotracheal tube is used.

Although it may be possible for an experienced provider to insert the endotracheal tube digitally in a comatose patient, direct visualization of insertion is always preferred. Various devices provide visualization of the glottic opening to facilitate insertion of the airway device. The basic **laryngoscope** usually consists of a handle with a hinged blade that includes a light source distally. The more common blades are either curved (MacIntosh) or straight (Miller). There are more esoteric variations, to include a blade with a levered tip that allows the provider to lift the epiglottis out of view to expose the glottic opening. **Fiber-optic or video-assisted scopes** provide visualization of the vocal cords when direct laryngoscopy has failed, or when patient anatomy or injuries make direct visualization difficult or impossible. Fiber-optic scopes may be inserted orally or nasally. Video-assisted scopes normally are inserted orally. A distal camera on the scope is connected via wire to a portable monitor, which the provider must view while guiding the endotracheal tube to the glottic opening.

Often, even with excellent visualization of the vocal cords, it may be difficult to pass an appropriately sized endotracheal tube through the opening. A provider must be prepared to utilize other methods to secure the patient's airway.

A **gum elastic bougie** or Eschmann stylet, is a semiflexible introducer, manufactured at varying lengths, usually with an upturned tip at one distal end, which aids in operator placement when direct view of the vocal cords is difficult or impossible, or when initial passage of the endotracheal tube cannot be accomplished. If the glottic opening cannot be visualized, anatomy is used as a guide. The upturned tip is aimed under the epiglottis and just superior to the interarytenoid notch, if visible. The diameter of most devices is around 5 mm, which facilitates introduction of endotracheal tubes over the introducer, once it has been advanced into the airway. This device may also be used for tube exchange, although it does not allow for continuous oxygen delivery during this maneuver, as an exchange catheter would.

An **exchange catheter** is a device that allows basic ventilation to continue as an endotracheal tube is removed in preparation for another to be introduced, such as occurs when one tube is damaged or occluded. The catheter is made of semiflexible material. It is inserted through the existing endotracheal tube to an appropriate depth, and a small internal lumen provides a passage for ventilation after removing the old tube over the catheter. Once the new tube slides down over the catheter and is secured, the exchange catheter may be withdrawn.

Final Resorts

In the vast majority of emergent cases, definitive airway management can be accomplished via endotracheal intubation, or even via less invasive airway management, depending on the stability of the patient. There are times, however, when ventilation and oxygenation cannot be accomplished by any of the above means, and a surgical airway is indicated to save the patient's life.

First, a cricothyroidotomy (or cricothyrotomy) may be indicated. This is accomplished by incising the skin anterior to the cricothyroid membrane and then the membrane itself, allowing the passage of an airway tube that can be secured, thereby enabling ventilation. Pre-packaged kits are available for this procedure, or trauma centers may assemble their own kits from available equipment. Common elements required to perform a cricothyroidotomy include: scalpel, tracheal hook, endotracheal tube, suture material, Seldinger needle, and wire (if Seldinger technique is to be used).

Second, a tracheotomy may be indicated, if an airway obstruction is at or below the level of the cricothyroid membrane. Similar equipment would be used for this procedure. However, a cricothyroidotomy is always preferred in the emergent setting, owing to less complications and obviating the need for extension of the neck, which is problematic in the undifferentiated and either comatose or nearly comatose trauma patient.

Finally, a temporizing surgical measure, percutaneous needle-guided jet insufflation, may provide a bridge to more definitive management, particularly in pediatric trauma patients. Once a large-bore needle and/or catheter has been used to puncture the midline trachea at any of various levels, the **jet insufflator** may be attached. This device consists of tubing and a valve, connected to an oxygen (or other gas) source. The valve can be activated by pushing a button, which will allow regular and periodic (i.e., not continuous, to allow for slow decompression of the lower airway, if obstructed) flow into the patient's airway. Again, this is only a temporizing measure, which may provide time (but certainly less than 1 h) for the provider to plan and conduct definitive airway management procedures.

Cross-References

▶ ABCDE of Trauma Care
▶ Airway Assessment
▶ Airway Exchange in Trauma Patients
▶ Airway Trauma, Management of
▶ Cardiopulmonary Resuscitation
▶ Hypoxemia, Severe
▶ Mechanical Ventilation
▶ Monitoring of Trauma Patients During Anesthesia
▶ Pediatric Airway Management
▶ Rapid Sequence Intubation

References

Recommended Reading

American Society of Anesthesiologists Task Force on Management of the Difficult Airway (2003) Practice guidelines for management of the difficult airway. Anesthesiology 98:1269–1277
Dupanovic M, Fox H, Kovac A (2010) Management of the airway in multitrauma. Curr Opin Anaesthesiol 23:276–282
Heidegger T, Gerig HJ, Henderson JJ (2005) Strategies and algorithms for the management of difficult airway. Best Pract Res Clin Anaesthesiol 19:661–674
Henderson JJ, Popat MT, Lotto IP, Pearce AC (2004) Difficult airway society guidelines for management of the unanticipated difficult intubation. Anaesthesia 59:675–694
Lecky F, Bryden D, Little R et al (2008) Emergency intubation for acutely ill and injured patients. Cochrane Database Syst Rev 2, CD001429
Mort TC (2005) Preoxygenation in critically ill patients requiring emergency tracheal intubation. Crit Care Med 33:2672–2675

Airway Exchange in Trauma Patients

Adrian Matioc
Department of Anesthesiology, University of Wisconsin School of Medicine and Public Health, W.S. Middleton VA Medical Center, Madison, WI, USA

Synonyms

Conversion of a dedicated airway into a definitive airway; Exchange of a supraglottic airway (or malfunctioning endotracheal tube) for an endotracheal tube

Definition

Airway exchange is an advanced airway management procedure that will convert a "temporary/ dedicated" airway, a supraglottic airway (SGA), or a defective endotracheal tube (ETT) into a "definitive" airway, an ETT, using an airway exchange catheter (AEC) or another technique. AEC is used to gain access to the trachea through the SGA or ETT and then to railroad an ETT into place. This exchange is needed for prolonged mechanical ventilation, airway protection, or general anesthesia.

Today's airway management algorithms emphasize oxygenation over intubation. Many prehospital programs use a SGA as their primary airway management device; similarly a SGA may be used in trauma in the hospital environment to salvage an unexpected difficult airway. Airway exchange in the trauma patient should be implemented in a timely manner and without complications (hypoxia, esophageal intubation, aspiration, cervical spine injury, and cardiovascular instability). Although there are no specific statistics for airway exchange in the nonelective trauma patient, airway management outside the operating room attributed morbidity and mortality is high.

Preexisting Condition

Airway management in general and airway exchange in trauma in particular are performed in the context of intrinsic and extrinsic variables. The *intrinsic* (patient-related) variables – specific pathology, airway trauma, full stomach, uncleared cervical spine, and uncooperative/unconscious patient – are addressed in trauma protocols. The trauma patient has limited physiologic reserves: increased oxygen consumption, hypoventilation (pneumothorax), anemia (acute or chronic), atelectasis, and abnormal cardiac performance. Airway management is challenging as the practitioner will face an unstable patient with previously instrumented and/or traumatized airway, no formal airway assessment, cricoid pressure and cervical spine precautions applied, and head in neutral position. The *extrinsic* variables are personnel related (experience, knowledge, and skill of the provider and support staff with an infrequently performed procedure) and environmental (available equipment, distracting events, ergonomics of the work space, light, functional intravenous line, disabled monitor alarms, access to the patient, bed height). An extreme situation is the airway exchange in the resuscitated trauma patient. Minimal interruption time for airway management during chest compression is now required.

Both the intrinsic and extrinsic variables may increase the difficulty and failure rate of the procedure and define the trauma airway in general and the airway exchange in particular as an "inherently difficult" or "critical" airway. The practitioner should be prepared to manage a "cannot ventilate-cannot intubate" situation with subglottic techniques (emergency cricothyroidotomy or tracheostomy).

Application

Airway exchange in trauma is a high-risk procedure and should be performed in a hospital environment (emergency room, operating room, intensive care unit) by trained personnel. This may be performed emergently (failing SGA or ETT) or semi-electively (functional SGA).

Although there is no solid evidence of benefit for any airway management strategy or algorithm, there is a strong agreement that a preplanned strategy may lead to improved outcome. It is accepted that increasing one's awareness of the risk can prevent the fixation error that is the root of many medical errors in critical situations. To optimize the first airway exchange attempt in a trauma patient, the practitioner should take the following steps:

- Assess the general status of the patient (communicate with the trauma team).
- Assess positive-pressure ventilation with the SGA (oxygenation, ventilation, stomach inflation, and if possible tidal volume and airway pressure) (Matioc and Wells 2006). A SGA inserted in the prehospital may be used for an extended period of time and may dislodge or malfunction. An overinflated SGA cuff may compromise venous drainage with tongue swelling complicating the airway exchange or reintubation. The cuff pressure may be checked using a manometer to keep it at maximum 60 cm H_2O. This is valid for all inflatable SGA except the Combitube that generates higher mucosal pressures at recommended inflation volumes.
- Insert an orogastric tube through the SGA gastric drain tube (when applicable) to empty the liquid and air content of the stomach. This may reduce the intragastric pressure (from positive-pressure bag valve mask and SGA ventilation), improve ventilation, and reduce the chances for aspiration during the exchange.
- Identify the cricothyroid membrane (neck scarring and morbid obesity may preclude subglottic techniques).

- Decide if the exchange is indicated and/or timely. If a (supraglottic) airway exchange is deemed unachievable, a subglottic technique may be considered.
- Share your conclusions and concerns with the trauma team. Discuss plan A, B, etc.
- Call for qualified help (including specialist for subglottic airway management).
- Decide if medication is needed to optimize instrumentation.
- Prepare for airway instrumentation: airway cart with fiberoptic scope (FOS), SGA, ETT position-verifying devices, suction, etc.
- Proceed with preoxygenation with 100 % O_2 through the functional SGA.
- Remove the anterior portion of the cervical collar and maintain in-line stabilization with the head in neutral position (if indicated).
- Be ready to apply cricoid pressure and suction.
- Perform the exchange.

Hypoventilation and low oxygenation due to the limited physiologic reserves and cardiovascular instability may result in severe hypoxemia within seconds after induction or airway instrumentation without ventilation. Removal of any functional SGA in the trauma patient may compromise ventilation and trigger an airway crisis.

There are many *SGA* available on the market used in trauma airway management:

- "LMA family" (cuffed perilaryngeal sealers): LMA Classic, LMA ProSeal, LMA Fastrach (LMA North America, San Diego, CA), air-Q disposable laryngeal mask and the air-Q blocker disposable laryngeal mask (Mercury Medical, Clearwater, FL), and Ambu AuraOnce (Ambu Inc.). The I-gel (Intersurgical Inc., Liverpool, NY, USA) is a noninflatable perilaryngeal sealer.
- "Combitube family" (cuffed pharyngeal sealers): Esophageal Tracheal Combitube (Covidien), EasyTube (Rusch), King Laryngeal Tube disposable (King Systems, Noblesville, IN), and King Laryngeal Tube Suction (King Systems, Noblesville, IN).

The I-gel, air-Q blocker disposable laryngeal mask, Esophageal Tracheal Combitube,

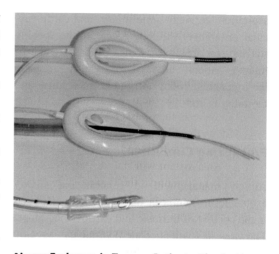

Airway Exchange in Trauma Patients, Fig. 1 Airway exchange catheters used with fiberoptic scopes. From the *top*: laryngeal mask airway with Aintree catheter over a fiberoptic scope; laryngeal mask airway with fiberoptic scope with protruding wire through the suction port; Parker endotracheal tube and Arndt exchange catheter over a wire

EasyTube, and King Laryngeal Tube Suction have a gastric drain tube to access stomach content.

AEC that need a FOS for tracheal positioning are the Aintree intubation catheter (Cook Critical Care, Bloomington, IN) and Arndt airway exchange catheter set (Cook Critical Care, Bloomington, IN). This technique applies to SGA in which passage of an adult size (>7) ETT through the ventilation port is problematic (Wong et al. 2012). Ventilation is maintained during the exchange by using a bronchoscope adapter connected to the resuscitator bag. Use of the pediatric size FOS in trauma airway management may be challenging, and the view may be easily obscured by blood or secretions.

The *Aintree* intubation catheter is a 19 Fr, 56 cm long disposable hollow catheter that allows a (4.5 mm) fiberoptic scope through its (4.7 mm) lumen leaving the distal 3–10 cm exposed at the tip (Fig. 1). This allows directing the FOS through the SGA ventilatory lumen then glottis into the trachea (step 1). Once the FOS and the SGA are removed (step 2), the Aintree is used to railroad the ETT into the trachea (step 3) (Wong et al. 2012).

The *Arndt* exchange catheter kit contains 8 or 14 Fr, 70 cm catheter with a tapered tip; multiple side ports; a 160 cm stiff wire guide with a flexible distal tip; and a Rapi-Fit adapter. The FOS is inserted through the SGA ventilatory lumen, the vocal cords, and into the trachea (step 1) (Fig. 1). The guidewire is then passed through the injection port of the fiberoptic scope and advanced until it is visualized beyond the tip of the scope (step 2). An assistant will stabilize the guidewire and will help to remove the FOS, and the Arndt AEC is passed over the wire approximately to the 30 cm mark (step 3) (Fig. 1). The wire and the AEC are maintained in position and the SGA removed (step 4). After the removal of the wire, the ETT is railroaded into the trachea (step 5) (Joffe et al. 2010). While the Arndt technique has more steps, it has the advantage that the FOS does not need to penetrate the glottis as the wire can be advanced into the trachea from a distance under visualization. This is helpful when the access is difficult to a poorly visualized or distorted glottis (by a suboptimally positioned SGA or edema).

The Combitube exchange raises specific challenges as the ventilation lumen has four small ports that cannot be penetrated by a pediatric FOS. If the Combitube is inserted into the trachea (rare occurrence), the exchange can be achieved using a wire or a small-diameter AEC with sufficient length (e.g., 11 Fr 100 cm soft-tipped AEC, Cook Critical Care, Bloomington, IN). If the Combitube is inserted in the esophagus, a decision should be made to remove it followed by a direct or indirect laryngoscopy or to leave it in place and deflate the large oropharyngeal cuff followed by the use of FOS, optical stylet, direct or indirect laryngoscopy, or retrograde technique. Considering that the removal of a rescue airway may lead to a "cannot intubate-cannot ventilate" situation, the second technique seems more controlled as the reinflation of the proximal cuff will allow oxygenation. However, this technique is cumbersome considering the large cuff and tube obstructing the oropharynx (Gaitini et al. 1999; Lam et al. 2009). The King LT can be exchanged using the same techniques as the Combitube inserted in the esophagus.

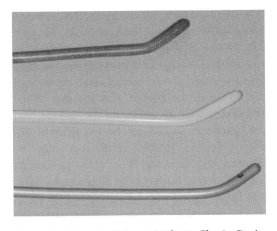

Airway Exchange in Trauma Patients, Fig. 2 Coude-tip airway exchange catheters. From the *top*: Eschmann "bougie" (reusable); Sun Medical Introducer (disposable); Frova Intubating Introducer (disposable, hollow, and with stiffening metallic cannula)

The hollow AEC is both a guide for reintubation and a safety system permitting administration of supplemental oxygen and CO_2 sampling. Supplemental oxygen can be administered as high-pressure jet ventilation (10–50 psi; using the Luer-Lok®adapter) or low-pressure variable-flow oxygen (1–10 l/min; 15 mm Rapi-Fit adapter). Jet ventilation is associated with a higher degree of complications (barotrauma, volutrauma, pneumothorax, pneumoperitoneum, subcutaneous emphysema, cardiovascular collapse, gastric rupture). Application of these rarely performed, time-consuming, and high-risk procedures assumes appropriate technical support and trained personnel (Benumof 1999; Duggan et al. 2011).

AEC that do not need FOS for positioning are used for "bougie-assisted" difficult direct and indirect laryngoscopies and for ETT exchange (Fig. 2).

These are distally angulated (coude)-tip catheters that are *reusable*, 60 cm *Eschmann*, "gum elastic bougie" (Portex Venn tracheal tube introducer, Smiths Industries Medical Systems, Keene, NH), and *disposable*, the 60-cm Portex "single-use bougie" (Portex tracheal tube introducer, SIMS Portex), the 15-Fr 70-cm Sun Medical (Sun Medical Largo, FL), and the 8- or 14-Fr hollow lumen 65-cm *Frova* Intubating Introducer

(Cook Critical Care, Bloomington, IN) packaged with a stiffening cannula and removable Rapi-Fit adapter that is able to facilitate jet ventilation/oxygenation (Janakiraman et al. 2009). The reusable Eschmann should be examined before use: the tip should be aligned with the axis of the introducer, with no cracks on the surface, and the introducer should not be too flexible. An overly flexible reusable introducer may be directed into the esophagus while railroading the ETT over it, leading to an esophageal intubation following a tracheal placement of the introducer. According to the manufacturer, the multiple-use AEC can be used five times.

The AEC coude tip is designed for the unexpected difficult direct intubation (to penetrate a poorly visualized glottis and to elicit the tracheal ring "clicks"). It may generate trauma when eliciting the "holdup" sign and when inserting the AEC more than 27 cm in men and 23 cm in women (distance to carina). This may be overcome for an ETT exchange by the 100-cm 11- or 14-Fr straight *soft-tipped* Cook Airway Exchange Catheter (Cook Critical Care, Bloomington, IN) designed for a double-lumen tube exchange that will generate the distal "holdup" sign without risk of trauma.

Maneuvers to facilitate the "blind" railroading of the ETT over the AEC and especially to avoid the holdup on periglottic structures and the right arytenoid are the following: the use of a curved laryngoscope, rotation of the ETT to 90° counterclockwise before reaching the glottis, and using a smaller ETT or a Parker Flex-Tip ETT (Parker Medical, CO). The Parker Flex-Tip ETT has two Murphy eyes and a pencil-point tip that leaves no gap between the ETT and the AEC, facilitating an unobstructed railroading. Both channeled and unchanneled videolaryngoscopes were used to transform a "blind" ETT exchange into an optimized procedure with "continuous glottic visualization" (Mort 2009). The combined use of an AEC or FOS with a direct or videolaryngoscope should be part of the armamentarium of any practitioner attempting airway exchange in a critical patient.

AEC complications stem primarily from the disposable (rigid) devices: inability to secure an airway ("cannot intubate-cannot ventilate"), esophageal intubation, tracheal or bronchial mucosal tears, pneumothorax, barotrauma, and perforation of the bronchi. In short series, life-threatening complication rate is high (Hames et al. 2003). Hypoxemia will occur quickly during trauma airway management of "iatrogenic" complications: esophageal intubation, regurgitation or aspiration, main stem bronchial intubation, and multiple unsuccessful intubation attempts.

There are SGA specifically designed for "blind" airway exchange *bypassing the need for AEC*: the intubating laryngeal mask airway (Fastrach, LMA North America, San Diego, CA) and the air-Q disposable laryngeal mask (Mercury Medical, Clearwater, FL). The former will be exchanged to a special, reinforced, silicone ETT (that may need further exchange for a generic ETT); the latter will accept a generic ETT.

Indirect intubation (videolaryngoscopy) may change the airway exchange strategy in general and in trauma patient in particular. Considering the complications associated with the use of AEC in critical patients, there are authors that prefer the use of indirect intubation or FOS instead of the standard AECs. Nevertheless, further studies will have to define the limitations of specific videolaryngoscopes. Indirect laryngoscopes are successfully used in the intubation of patients with rigid cervical collars, head in neutral position, suspected spine injuries, and difficult airways. However, any optical system can be easily compromised by secretions, blood, and debris. In a trauma situation, oropharyngeal suction should precede indirect laryngoscopy.

The exchange of an oral to a nasal ETT (and more rarely a nasal to an oral ETT) is usually a nonemergent procedure (unless the ETT in situ is failing) and is performed in the operating room (as a surgical indication) or in the ICU (for prolonged ventilation, facial trauma). There is no accepted standard technique and general principles should be followed: maintenance of oxygenation throughout the procedure, assured patient comfort (sedation or general anesthesia), monitoring, assessment of the airway and the clinical context prior to instrumentation, nasal mucosa preparation for instrumentation (e.g., phenylephrine nasal spray for vasoconstriction and 2 % lidocaine jelly for topical anesthesia and lubrication), communication of the airway management and pharmacologic plan with the team, and availability of instruments for plan A, B, etc. The pediatric population is particularly challenging considering the lack of cooperation, specific anatomy (adenoidal tissue, smaller choanae), and increased risk of bleeding. Each clinical situation needs a specific solution. Several techniques are described in the literature as case reports using different airway exchange catheters, (one or two) bougies, positioned with a flexible fiberoptic scope. The critical step is the exchange of the in situ (oral) ETT with the advancing (nasal) one. A safe approach is to maintain a viable access to the trachea, securing the in situ airway before ETT removal with an exchange airway catheter/wire. Videolaryngoscopes may be used preprocedure for airway assessment (glottic edema) and during instrumentation to visualize the critical advancement of the (nasal) ETT into the glottis. If performance of an ETT exchange appears very risky or potentially impossible, especially common in cases of neck trauma, a surgeon able to perform an immediate tracheostomy should be at the bedside. If risks for failure of the ETT exchange and potential loss of the airway appear to be too high or if performance of an urgent tracheostomy may be difficult, an elective tracheostomy should be performed instead of an ETT exchange.

Airway exchange in the trauma patient is a demanding task that needs appropriate preparation: personnel training and availability of airway management devices. It is the responsibility of the airway expert to become familiar with the specific SGA the hospital and afferent prehospital system is using and to master consequent airway exchange techniques. While the airway instrumentation depends on the experience of the provider, the airway exchange is not an individual effort in which the provider's expertise is expected to compensate for system failures (e.g., uncontrolled extrinsic variables). Critical airway management is at the crossroads of individual and collective responsibility.

Cross-References

▶ Airway Equipment
▶ Airway Management in Trauma, Nonsurgical

References

Benumof JL (1999) Airway exchange catheters. Anesthesiology 91:342–344

Duggan LV, Law A, Murphy MF (2011) Brief review: supplemental oxygen through an airway exchange catheter: efficacy, complications, and recommendations. Can J Anesth 58:560–568

Gaitini LA, Vaida SJ, Somri M, Fradis M, Ben-David B (1999) Fiberoptic-guided airway exchange of the esophageal tracheal Combitube in spontaneously breathing versus mechanically ventilated patients. Anesth Analg 88:103–106

Hames KC, Pandit JJ, Marfin AG, Popat MT, Yentis SM (2003) Use of bougie in simulated difficult intubation. Comparison of single use bougie with the fiberscope. Anaesthesia 58:846–851

Janakiraman C, Hodzovic I, Reddy S, Desai N, Wilkes AR, Latto IP (2009) Evaluation of tracheal tube introducers in simulated difficult intubation. Anaesthesia 64:309–314

Joffe AM, Arndt G, Willmann K (2010) Wire-guided catheter exchange after failed direct laryngoscopy in critically ill adults. J Clin Anesth 22:93–96

Lam NC, Hagberg CA, Bassili LM (2009) Use of the videolaryngoscopy for Combitube exchange in a difficult airway. J Clin Anesth 21:294–296

Matioc AA, Wells JA (2006) Positive pressure ventilation with the laryngeal mask airway in the operating room and prehospital: a practical review. J Trauma 60(6):1371–1376

Mort T (2009) Tracheal tube exchange: feasibility of continuous glottic viewing with advanced laryngoscopy assistance. Crit Care Trauma 108(4):1228–1231

Wong TD, Yang JJ, Mak HY, Jagannathan N (2012) Use of intubation introducers through a supraglottic airway to facilitate tracheal intubation: a brief review. Can J Anesth 59:704–715

Airway Injury

▶ Tracheal and Esophageal Injury

Airway Maintenance

▶ Airway Management in Trauma, Nonsurgical

Airway Management

▶ General Anesthesia for Major Trauma

Airway Management in Trauma, Cricothyrotomy

Steven Kahn
Division of Trauma and Surgical Critical Care,
Department of Surgery, Vanderbilt University
Medical Center, Nashville, TN, USA

Synonyms

Cricothyroidotomy

Definition

Cricothyrotomy is an invasive procedure that establishes a surgical opening in the airway through the cricothyroid membrane. This procedure is indicated in emergency scenarios when an airway cannot be established via less invasive methods. Cricothyrotomy differs from tracheostomy in the anatomic location of airway entry and is generally preferable in an emergent setting as it is generally quicker and relatively simplistic to perform (Flint 2010).

Preexisting Condition

Cricothyrotomy is generally performed to establish a definitive airway when it cannot be established by other means. Usually, this is when endotracheal or nasotracheal intubation (or cannot be performed) and mask-ventilation fails. Failure to establish an airway can result in hypoxemia, ischemic brain injury, and even death (Burkey et al. 1991; American Society of Anesthesiologists Task Force on Management of the Difficult Airway 2003). Cricothyrotomy is not generally a long-term airway solution.

After the patient has been stabilized, it should be converted to a more formal tracheostomy.

Application

Multiple methods of cricothyrotomy have been described (Flint 2010; Holmes et al. 1998). The approach that the author prefers is described below. In addition, some potential variations based upon what equipment is available. See Table 1 for list of equipment needed.

1. Identify the cricothyroid membrane and make a 2–3-cm vertical midline skin incision over the membrane with a #15 or a #20 blade scalpel.
   - The trachea should be stabilized between the first and third digits of the nondominant hand. The second digit can be used to locate the cricothyroid membrane or the soft, slightly depressed area between the thyroid and cricoid cartilages. The author recommends a midline vertical incision, especially for inexperienced providers – if the incision is not directly over the cricothyroid membrane, it can be extended in the appropriate direction to avoid making a second incision. In addition, it theoretically lessens the chance of injury to anterior jugular veins compared to a horizontal incision. If time permits, sterile gloves and antimicrobial skin prep should be used before making incision.
2. Make a 1.5 horizontal stab incision in the cricothyroid membrane. One must take care not to stab too deep and injure the posterior wall of the trachea with the scalpel.

Airway Management in Trauma, Cricothyrotomy, Table 1 Items needed for cricothyrotomy

Function of item	Item
Make incisions	#15 or #20 scalpel
Dilate incision	Kelly clamp, tracheal dilator, or blunt end of scalpel
Secure airway	#4 or #6 cuffed tracheostomy tube OR 5.–6.0 endotracheal tube
Misc	Sterile gloves, antimicrobial skin prep solution

3. Dilate the incision in the cricothyroid membrane.
   - If an emergency airway kit is available, a tracheal dilator can be used. If not, a Kelly clamp (or a hemostat) can be used. The clamp should be spread in a transverse direction. Do not spread in vertical direction. If not available, use the blunt end of the scalpel. The authors prefer the use of the Kelly clamp.
4. Insert either a #4 or #6 cuffed tracheostomy tube into the airway.
   - If a tracheostomy tube is not available, a 5.0, 5.5, or a 6.0 endotracheal tube (depending upon patient size) can be inserted instead. If available, a tracheal hook can be used to retract the surgically created opening to facilitate tube placement. If not, the blunt end of the scalpel can be rotated 90° to hold open the incision while the airway is placed.

Variation: For more experienced providers, a small, horizontal stab wound can initially be made through the skin and the cricothyroid membrane at once. This eliminates the need for two separate incisions. However, the user must be certain about anatomic landmarks and take care to avoid injury to anterior jugular veins, internal jugular veins, and carotid arteries.

Relative contraindications to cricothyrotomy include airway trauma (cricoid/thyroid cartilage fracture, laryngeal fracture, or disruption of the cricothyroid membrane). In addition, it should not be performed in pediatric patients (<12 year of age). In these patient populations, tracheostomy and percutaneous transcatheter ventilation are other options in a life-threatening situation (Wang and Yealy 2008).

Complications occur in 6–40 % of patients that undergo cricothyrotomy (Wright et al. 2003). These include hemorrhage, laryngeal fracture, cricothyroid fracture, esophageal perforation, and tracheal stenosis. Stenosis occurs when the tube is left in for a long period of time (cricothyrotomy is performed in a relatively narrow portion of the airway). Thus cricothyroidotomy should be converted to tracheostomy when the patient stabilizes in order to prevent stenosis (Flint 2010; Burkey et al. 1991; Wang and Yealy 2008; Wright et al. 2003).

Cross-References

▶ Airway Management in Trauma, Tracheostomy
▶ Airway Trauma, Management of
▶ Rapid Sequence Intubation

References

American Society of Anesthesiologists Task Force on Management of the Difficult Airway (2003) Practice guidelines for management of the difficult airway: an updated report by the American Society of Anesthesiologists Task Force on Management of the Difficult Airway. Anesthesiology 98(5):1269–1277

Burkey B, Esclamado R, Morganroth M (1991) The role of crycothyroidotomy in airway management. Clin Chest Med 12(3):561–571

Flint PW (2010) Cummings otolaryngology: head & neck surgery, 5th edn. Mosby, Philadelphia. An Imprint of Elsevier edited by Paul W. Flint

Holmes JF, Panacek EA, Sakles JC et al (1998) Comparison of 2 cricothyrotomy techniques: standard method versus rapid 4-step technique. Ann Emerg Med 32(4):442–446

Wang H, Yealy D (2008) Airway management. In: Peitzman A et al (eds) The trauma manual. Lipncott Williams and Wilkins, Philadephia, p 90

Wright MJ et al (2003) Surgical cricothyrotomy in trauma patients. South Med J 96(5):465–467

Airway Management in Trauma, Nonsurgical

Mirsad Dupanovic
Department of Anesthesiology, Kansas University Medical Center, The University of Kansas Hospital, Kansas City, KS, USA

Synonyms

Airway maintenance; Bag-mask ventilation; Definitive airway; Endotracheal intubation; Secured airway; Supraglottic airway

Definition

Nonsurgical airway management primarily involves establishing a reliable ventilation route with the purpose of oxygen delivery and carbon dioxide elimination. In addition, protection of cervical spine (C-spine) and lung protection are important primary objectives in trauma care. Airway maintenance devices usually provide adequate route for oxygenation and ventilation without reliable lung protection. Definitive nonsurgical airway represents the endotracheal tube (ETT) positioned with the cuff below the vocal cords. The ETT provides protection against pulmonary aspiration and can be secured from inadvertent dislodgement. Tracheostomy and cricothyrotomy are also types of a definitive airway and are discussed separately.

Preexisting Condition

Multiple clinical scenarios are possible under circumstances of obstructed airway and compromised ventilation. Hypoxemia resulting from a major traumatic insult may lead to rapid deterioration of vital organ functions, cardiac arrest, and death. Failure to establish an airway in survivable trauma will result not only in hypoxemia but also in hypercapnia and respiratory acidosis. Resultant adverse physiologic consequences may include decreasing myocardial function and worsening coagulopathy. Acidosis, coagulopathy, and hypothermia have been termed "the triad of death" in trauma. On the other hand, hypoxemia, hypercapnia, and hypotension are the major contributing factors to development of a secondary brain injury and poor outcomes in patients with traumatic brain injury (TBI). The above scenarios illustrate the importance of a timely and proper airway management for improved outcomes in trauma care.

The ABCDE approach highlights the effective sequence of evaluation and resuscitation in trauma (ATLS® 2012). Maintaining or securing the airway patency while protecting the C-spine, supporting or controlling the breathing, and delivering oxygen are the priorities. In general,

continuous monitoring of pulse oximetry and end-tidal CO_2 is essential. However, observing clinical signs is important as well. Independent of respiratory monitors, clinical signs may help in anticipation or recognition of a need for an intervention during initial airway evaluation and subsequent reevaluations. Patient's ability to talk is an important positive sign of airway patency and ability to maintain spontaneous ventilation. As long as the brain perfusion is adequate and the patient is able to talk effortlessly, the airway will be maintained. Hoarseness and subcutaneous emphysema of the neck may indicate laryngeal trauma and need further evaluation. Finding of stridor indicates partial upper airway obstruction and the etiology should be differentiated before induction of general anesthesia. A major inhalation injury will likely lead to a significant airway edema and will require prophylactic endotracheal intubation (ETI). Agitation and cyanosis usually indicate hypoxia while obtundation and poor respiratory effort may indicate hypercapnia. However, intoxicated patients and patients with TBI can be agitated or obtunded as well. Thus, these clinical problems may have multifactorial etiology. Ventilation can be compromised not only by depressed brain function, injury of the cervical spinal cord, and airway obstruction but also by chest injury causing altered mechanics of ventilation. Asymmetric chest movement and decreased breath sounds during auscultation suggest presence of thoracic injury and inadequate ventilation.

Application

In general, the difficult airway algorithm of the American Society of Anesthesiologists (Apfelbaum et al. 2013) is an important guide for airway management in elective cases; there is usually enough time for planning and performing airway procedures. However, time is often a limiting factor during airway management in acute trauma. Comprehensive guidelines for management of an acutely traumatized patient, including airway management in trauma, can be found in the Advanced Trauma Life

Support® manual (ATLS® 2012). Multiple basic airway management problems identified in these two publications should be considered when managing airway in acute trauma.

Patient cooperation is often challenging because of compromised brain function due to TBI, alcohol and/or drug intoxication, or all. Mask ventilation may be particularly inadequate in patients that have multiple of the following five characteristics: beard, obesity, no or few teeth, elderly, and history of snoring (BONES). It may be difficult to appropriately place a supraglottic airway in a patient with limited mouth opening, traumatic upper airway injury, or airway edema caused potentially by multiple attempts at intubation or by developing edema due to inhalation injury. It may be also risky to use a supraglottic airway to a patient that recently ingested a meal and thus has very high likelihood of regurgitation and pulmonary aspiration. Difficult laryngoscopy and difficult ETI may be related to unfavorable airway anatomy, airway edema or airway injury, the presence of C-collar, use of in-line cervical stabilization, application of cricoid pressure, time limitations dictated by suboptimal preoxygenation, and low tolerance to apnea in trauma patients. Difficult surgical airway may be related to increased size of the neck, enlarged thyroid gland, or neck hematoma. In general, airway management in patients with significant upper airway trauma may be difficult using available nonsurgical modalities, and thus surgical airway may be the primary airway management choice. In addition to all listed airway management problems in trauma time, to perform tracheal intubation procedure or to create a surgical airway is very limited. Functional reserve capacity and safe apnea time are particularly low in morbidly obese trauma patients that suffered chest injury and are splinting and/or have a pneumothorax or hemothorax. In addition to that, preoxygenation in trauma is usually suboptimal, patients are anemic with decreased blood oxygen content, and oxygen consumption is increased due to stress of trauma.

When considering basic airway management choices, awake fiberoptic ETI is not a frequently utilized option in acute trauma. There may be problems with patient cooperation, there is frequent presence of blood and secretions in the airway that limits the effect of topical airway anesthesia and makes fiberoptic visualization difficult, there is low respiratory reserve that limits the time available for passage of the fiberoptic scope into the trachea, and there may be "full stomach" considerations in patients that require intravenous sedation. In patients with suboptimal topical airway anesthesia that need strict cervical spine protection, coughing or bucking during fiberoptic scope-assisted ETI may potentially contribute to development of secondary neurologic injury. However, when properly performed, awake fiberoptic ETI is frequent in cooperative patients with C-spine injury and penetrating injury of the neck (Dupanovic et al. 2010).

Use of an airway maintenance device such as bag-mask ventilation or a supraglottic airway is generally a temporary airway management solution in trauma. Chin lift, jaw thrust, and placement of an oropharyngeal airway are all maneuvers used frequently to establish bag-mask ventilation. However, since excessive use of these maneuvers can produce secondary C-spine injury, their excess should be limited either by a hard neck collar left in place or by in-line C-spine immobilization. Supraglottic airways that have been investigated in trauma are laryngeal mask airway (LMA), laryngeal tube, and multilumen esophageal airway. Supraglottic airways are either used until the trauma patient is transported to a facility where a skilled personnel can place an endotracheal tube or in case of failed ETI until surgical airway is created. Preservation of spontaneous ventilation and use of assisted ventilation may be important to prevent unintended gastric insufflation during airway maintenance. In skilled hands supraglottic airway can be simultaneously used as a tool for maintenance of ventilation and as a channel for ETI. The LMA is the most feasible device to be used as a channel for intubation. The laryngeal tube airway can be used for the same purpose but the procedure is more complicated than with the LMA. Use of a supraglottic airway as a channel for ETI in trauma is the last option before decision for creation of a surgical airway because of high risk of pulmonary aspiration. If the risk for aspiration is very high, intubation should be abandoned, lungs ventilated through the supraglottic airway, and surgical airway created. If properly placed, multilumen esophageal airway provides protection from pulmonary aspiration of gastric contents, and it is a good supraglottic airway choice in rural areas where long time is needed for ground transport to the hospital. However, disadvantage of this airway is that it cannot be used as a channel for tracheal intubation. Either fiberoptic scope is placed in the hypopharynx, oropharyngeal cuff of the device deflated, and the scope passed into the larynx and trachea or the multilumen airway must be removed and trachea intubated using a laryngoscope.

The fastest option for securing the airway is laryngoscopic ETI with or without use of a video laryngoscope as an initial intubation choice. Surgical airway is typically a backup option to ETI. Indications for obtaining a definitive airway may be related to airway obstruction, inadequate ventilation, circulatory problems,

and disability (ABCD). Airway obstruction may be caused by blunt or penetrating maxillofacial or neck trauma and may be impending following inhalation injury. Induction of apnea and ETI may be very risky in these types of injuries and surgical team must be immediately present and ready to create a surgical airway. Inadequate respiratory effort may result in inadequate mask ventilation, intractable hypoxia, and hypercarbia and may require ETI. Hemorrhagic shock will result in inadequate cerebral perfusion, may result in unconsciousness, and apnea. Intubation will secure oxygenation and ventilation under such circumstances. TBI with GCS of ≤ 8 requires a definitive airway in order to ensure adequate oxygenation, ventilation, and prevention of secondary brain injury as well as protection from pulmonary aspiration. C-spine clearance should not delay ETI when clearly indicated. Rapid sequence induction with cricoid pressure is a standard technique. In-line immobilization of the C-spine is mandatory. Either direct laryngoscopy or video laryngoscopy is an acceptable technique. Video laryngoscopes provide better

Airway Management in Trauma, Nonsurgical, Table 1   Clinical airway management problems in acute trauma care

Clinical problem	Etiology	Clinical consequences
Agitated, obtunded, noncooperative patient	Traumatic brain injury; alcohol or illicit drug intoxication	Difficult preoxygenation, unfeasible awake intubation, high risk of pulmonary aspiration
Difficult mask ventilation	BONES (beard, obese, no teeth, elderly, snoring)	Hypoxia, hypercapnia, risk of secondary injury
Difficult/risky supraglottic airway placement	Limited mouth opening, upper airway injury or edema/"full stomach," alcohol intoxication	Limited airway management choices, hypoxia, hypercapnia/risk of regurgitation and aspiration
Difficult laryngoscopy/ difficult intubation	LEMON (look externally for abnormal airway anatomy, evaluate the 3-3-2 rule, Mallampati, obstruction of the airway, neck immobilization using the hard collar or in-line immobilization)	Limited airway management choices, high risk of hypoxia and hypercapnia, risk of secondary injury
Difficult surgical airway	Fat neck, enlarged thyroid gland, neck hematoma or emphysema	High risk of secondary injury, early planning of the surgical airway
Upper airway trauma	Maxillofacial trauma, laryngeal trauma, penetrating neck injuries, inhalation injury	Difficult nonsurgical airway management using multiple modalities
Injured cervical spine	Major blunt trauma, penetrating injury of the neck	Minimize neck movement, flexible fiberoptic scope or surgical airway
Time limitations	Low functional residual capacity (obesity, chest injury, COPD), poor preoxygenation, anemia, increased oxygen consumption	Hypoxia, hypercapnia, and high risk of secondary injury
Recent meal	Slowed gastric emptying due to stress of trauma	Risk of regurgitation, pulmonary aspiration, ARDS, and death

intubation success in inexperienced operators. Channeled video laryngoscopes significantly reduce movement of the cervical spine in elective intubations (Dupanovic et al. 2010). Gum-elastic bougie is an accessory device that can be placed into the trachea if direct placement of the ETT is difficult and then helps guide the ETT into the trachea (tracheal tube introducer). Unanticipated anatomic airway abnormalities, foreign material in the airway, and head and neck injuries are the most common causes of failed ETI (Table 1). If intubation fails after 2–3 optimal attempts by an experienced endoscopist, surgical airway should not be delayed. Paramedic prehospital teams have much higher incidence of ETI failure than physician-led prehospital teams. In-hospital performed ETI has success of 99.2–99.7 % (Dupanovic et al. 2010). Orotracheal intubation is preferred to nasotracheal intubation because of risks related to basilar skull fracture and potential brain injury.

Cross-References

- ▶ ABCDE of Trauma Care
- ▶ Airway Assessment
- ▶ Airway Equipment
- ▶ Airway Exchange in Trauma Patients
- ▶ Airway Management in Trauma, Cricothyrotomy
- ▶ Airway Management in Trauma, Tracheostomy
- ▶ Airway Trauma, Management of
- ▶ General Anesthesia for Major Trauma

References

American College of Surgeons Committee on Trauma (2012) Advanced Trauma Life Support® for Doctors (ATLS®) student course manual, 9th edn. American College of Surgeons Committee on Trauma, Chicago

Apfelbaum JL, Hagberg CA, Caplan RA et al (2013) Practice guidelines for management of the difficult airway; an updated report by the American Society of Anesthesiologists task force on management of the difficult airway. Anesthesiology 188:251–270

Dupanovic M, Fox H, Kovac A (2010) Management of the airway in multitrauma. Curr Opin Anesthesiol 23:276–282

Airway Management in Trauma, Tracheostomy

Issam Eid
Department of Otolaryngology and Communicative Sciences, University of Mississippi Medical Center, Jackson, MS, USA

Synonyms

Tracheostomy; Tracheotomy

Definition

Surgical management of the airway involves establishment of a direct opening into a trauma patient's airway. It is considered the definitive last resort for securing the airway. Tracheotomy traditionally refers to a temporary opening into the airway whereas tracheostomy refers to a permanent one; however, the terms are often used interchangeably. Cricothyrotomy differs from tracheostomy in that it involves a surgical airway through the cricothyroid membrane. Tracheostomy involves establishment of a surgical airway in the cervical trachea below the cricoid ring and can be performed as an open procedure or via percutaneous dilational tracheostomy (PDT).

Preexisting Condition

In the emergency and operating room setting, the need for a surgical airway arises in a patient who cannot be ventilated or intubated (Henderson 2010). Oral intubation remains the method of choice for securing the airway in trauma patients. When this cannot be established and alternative methods including laryngeal mask airway fail, a surgical method is sought for establishing ventilation. Tracheostomy is also indicated for patients who already have an established orotracheal or nasotracheal airway but need a more permanent airway in the critical care setting.

The list of conditions where the need for a tracheostomy arises includes the following:

1. Inability to mask ventilate or intubate
2. Maxillofacial or airway trauma preventing intubation
3. Upper airway obstruction or edema
4. High risk airway due to cervical fractures
5. Need for prolonged mechanical ventilation or prolonged inability to protect the airway (Gunter et al. 2012; Henderson 2010)

All patients who undergo emergent cricothyrotomy are usually taken to the operating room for conversion to a formalized tracheostomy once stabilized although the need for this is a matter of debate in the literature (Talving et al. 2010).

Two different settings for a surgical tracheostomy are presented here. The emergent setting which may be in the trauma bay or in the operating room (OR) and the more elective setting for tracheostomy in a trauma patient with an established endotracheal airway, which is usually in the critical care setting. For emergency tracheostomy, having a practitioner who is skilled in surgical airway management available is key for successful management of the airway.

Application

Securing the airway in a trauma patient is of paramount importance and remains the first priority in the ABCDE of trauma care. The first step to successful management of a surgical airway with tracheostomy is the recognition of the potential need for a surgical airway at the initial assessment of the patient. Preparation for a surgical airway involves having proper instrument tray for tracheostomy readily available in the trauma bay or OR. The timing for intervention with a tracheostomy is also critical. If efforts at orotracheal intubation are failing, a prompt decision should be taken to proceed as per the American Society of Anesthesiologists (ASA) algorithm for difficult airway in an expeditious manner.

Several factors can be a hindrance in the establishment of an emergent surgical airway and must be taken into consideration prior to proceeding.

The first factor is anatomy of the patient. Patients with large goiters or an obese neck can pose a tremendous challenge to obtaining an emergent surgical airway. Other factors include neck trauma or edema, prior neck surgery or scarring, and prior head and neck radiation therapy. Therefore, coordination between providers is essential in these situations for a favorable outcome and safely establishing an emergent surgical airway. Multidisciplinary approach to the airway with effective communication between the emergency room physician, anesthesiologist, and surgeon concerning the management plan is essential.

Emergency Tracheostomy

Emergent tracheotomy is the method of final resort of securing the airway according to the ASA algorithm for a difficult airway when all other methods of securing the airway and ventilation have been exhausted (Apfelbaum et al. 2013). Cricothyrotomy is the preferred method for securing a surgical airway by most providers in the trauma setting due to the simpler nature and increased familiarity of the procedure for nonsurgical providers. However, tracheostomy is a more definitive procedure and has been established as an equally effective method for securing a surgical airway in the emergency and trauma setting (Gillespie and Eisele 1999).

Technique

The setting of the emergent tracheostomy necessitates rapid access to the airway and part of the preparation measures may need to be omitted. The entire procedure can essentially be performed with a surgical blade. The preparation of the surgical site at the inferior central neck with povidone-iodine (Betadine) or chlorhexidine should be undertaken if time permits. Injection of this area with 1 % lidocaine with epinephrine is usually helpful for hemostasis as well as anesthesia and may be done in conjunction with attempts at obtaining orotracheal intubation in anticipation of a pending surgical airway. The incision is planned between the cricoid and the sternal notch. Extension of the neck will aid with the exposure of the trachea but the cervical spine precautions should be maintained if there is suspicion of cervical spine injury and C-collar should be maintained. The fastest way to enter the trachea in an emergent setting is through a vertical incision. The advantages of the vertical incision are the decreased incidence of bleeding, decreased risk of recurrent laryngeal nerve injury, and vascular injury compared to the usual horizontal incision that is generally used in elective tracheotomy. The cervical trachea immediately below the cricoid is grasped between the thumb and index finger and incision is made with a blade down through the skin and subdermal tissues as well as through the first 2–4 tracheal rings. Effort should be made to stay in the midline to decrease the chance of bleeding from the thyroid gland. The opening into the trachea should be made wide enough for placement of an appropriately sized endotracheal tube. Once ventilation is confirmed by presence of end-tidal carbon dioxide and bilateral lung breath sounds, the attention is turned to obtaining hemostasis with electrocautery, if available. If the procedure is done in the trauma bay, transfer to the OR should be considered for hemostasis, assuming the patient is hemodynamically stable. Once this is achieved, the endotracheal tube may be replaced by a tracheostomy tube of appropriate size and the tube is secured to the neck by ties and or suture (Fig. 1).

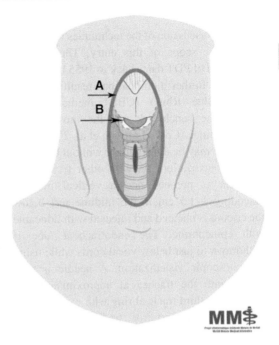

Airway Management in Trauma, Tracheostomy, Fig. 1 Anatomic landmarks of the neck. *A* thyroid cartilage. *B* cricoid cartilage and cricothyroid membrane. The thyroid is outlined below the cricoid cartilage (*dotted line*). The figure depicts the typical location of the tracheostomy tube placement, typically at the level of the second to fourth tracheal ring (Photo reproduced with permission from: Evolution of percutaneous dilation tracheostomy – a review of current techniques and their pitfalls (Cools-Lartigue et al. 2013))

Elective Tracheostomy

Although the timing of tracheostomy in the critically ill trauma patient is still debated, the consensus and practice has shifted toward early tracheostomy. Studies have shown a decrease in incidence of pneumonia, decreased duration of mechanical ventilation, and decreased ICU stay with early tracheostomy (Arabi et al. 2004 and Dunham and Ransom 2006). Once the need for prolonged mechanical ventilation is recognized, tracheostomy should ideally be performed within 7 days from endotracheal intubation. The two methods that remain widely accepted for elective tracheostomy are PDT and open surgical tracheostomy. Many studies have addressed the comparison of PDT to open tracheostomy. The techniques appear to have equivalent safety

(Dennis et al. 2013). The literature also shows equivalent risk of bleeding and mortality with a decrease in the rate of infection with PDT (Delaney et al. 2006).

PDT

PDT became commercially available in 1985 and has since become a widely accepted method for establishing tracheostomy. This procedure is usually done at the bedside in the ICU setting although it may also be performed in the OR. The safety of this method has been well established and extends to the obese population (Dennis et al. 2013). While the emergency setting has been traditionally a contraindication for PDT, there have been reports of use of this technique in the emergent tracheostomy setting (Davidson et al. 2012).

Technique

Extensive discussion of the techniques for PDT is beyond the scope of this entry. The original description of PDT dates back to 1955 by Ciaglia et al. with further modifications resulting in the Ciaglia Blue Rhino (CBR) method which remains the benchmark and the most widely used technique (Cools-Lartigue et al. 2013). The procedure may be done with or without broncho-scopic visualization. As with other techniques, the skin is prepped and a vertical incision extending 1–1.5 cm in the midline just below the cricoid is planned and injected with lidocaine with epinephrine. The endotracheal tube is withdrawn to just below vocal cords while using bronchoscopic visualization. A needle is then placed into the trachea at approximately the level of the third tracheal ring with care to avoid injury to the posterior tracheal wall. The confirmation of needle placement may be done by withdrawal of air or visualization with bronchoscope. A guide wire is then placed through the needle. The tract is dilated, and tracheostomy tube is then placed over the guide wire.

Open Surgical Tracheostomy

Open tracheostomy is usually performed in the operating room although the procedure can be performed in the ICU at the bedside with the proper equipment available (Hawkins et al. 1989).

Technique

Elective tracheostomy is usually performed with a horizontal incision as this will provide a more favorable scar upon removal of tracheostomy. In the elective setting, the skin is prepped and injec-tion should be undertaken with local anesthetic with epinephrine for hemostasis. The incision is fashioned between the sternal notch and the cri-coid cartilage, extending approximately 1–2 cm centered over trachea. Incision is made with a blade through the skin, and electrocautery is used to divide the subdermal layers down to the strap musculature. The musculature is then divided vertically in the midline raphe. The trachea is exposed by division of the thyroid isthmus or below the isthmus. Use of a cricoid

hook at this point allows better visualization by pulling up the cervical trachea into the wound. Coordination with the anesthesia team is critical at this point as the surgical team prepares to enter the airway. Horizontal incision is then made between tracheal rings. Creation of a Björk flap is optional and can be undertaken by making vertical cuts through the tracheal ring below the incision on either side of the trachea. This flap is then sutured to the lower skin inci-sion. Tracheostomy tube is then placed in the tracheal window, and adequate ventilation is verified.

Complications

Complications from emergent and elective tracheostomy can be divided into early and late complications. The complication rates for elective open tracheostomy and PDT vary in the literature and range from 0 % to 25 % (Delaney et al. 2006). Complication rates are significantly higher for emergency procedures and range from 13 % to 40 % (Gillespie and Eisele 1999). Early compli-cations include loss of airway, bleeding, cricoid cartilage injury, operating room fire, and wound infection. Late complications include poor scar formation on removal, subglottic/tracheal steno-sis, and persistent tracheocutaneous fistula.

Cross-References

▶ ABCDE of Trauma Care
▶ Airway Assessment
▶ Airway Equipment
▶ Airway Management in Trauma, Cricothyrotomy
▶ Airway Management in Trauma, Nonsurgical

References

Apfelbaum JL, Hagberg CA, Caplan RA, Blitt CD, Connis RT, Nickinovich DG, Hagberg CA, Caplan RA, Benumof JL, Berry FA, Blitt CD, Bode RH, Cheney FW, Connis RT, Guidry OF, Nickinovich DG, Ovassapian A (2013) Practice guidelines for manage-ment of the difficult airway: an updated report by the American Society of Anesthesiologists Task Force on

Management of the Difficult Airway. Anesthesiology 118(2):251–270

Arabi Y, Haddad S, Shirawi N, Al Shimemeri A (2004) Early tracheostomy in intensive care trauma patients improves resource utilization: a cohort study and literature review. Crit Care 8(5):R347–R352

Cools-Lartigue J, Aboalsaud A, Gill H, Ferri L (2013) Evolution of percutaneous dilatational tracheostomy – a review of current techniques and their pitfalls. World J Surg 37(7):1633–1646

Davidson SB, Blostein PA, Walsh J, Maltz SB, VandenBerg SL (2012) Percutaneous tracheostomy: a new approach to the emergency airway. J Trauma Acute Care Surg 73(2 Suppl 1):S83–S88

Delaney A, Bagshaw SM, Nalos M (2006) Percutaneous dilatational tracheostomy versus surgical tracheostomy in critically ill patients: a systematic review and meta-analysis. Crit Care 10(2):R55

Dennis BM, Eckert MJ, Gunter OL, Morris JA Jr, May AK (2013) Safety of bedside percutaneous tracheostomy in the critically ill: evaluation of more than 3,000 procedures. J Am Coll Surg 216(4):858–865; discussion 865–857

Dunham CM, Ransom KJ (2006) Assessment of early tracheostomy in trauma patients: a systematic review and meta-analysis. Am Surg 72(3):276–281

Gillespie MB, Eisele DW (1999) Outcomes of emergency surgical airway procedures in a hospital-wide setting. Laryngoscope 109:1766–1769

Gunter OL, Diaz JJ, May AK (2012) Bedside surgical procedures. In: Townsend CM (ed) Sabiston textbook of surgery: the biological basis of modern surgical practice, 19th edn. Elsevier Saunders, Philadelphia, pp 595–603

Hawkins ML, Burrus EP, Treat RC, Mansberger AR Jr (1989) Tracheostomy in the intensive care unit: a safe alternative to the operating room. South Med J 82(9):1096–1098

Henderson J (2010) Airway management in the Adult. In: Miller RD (ed) Miller's Anesthesia. Churchill Livingstone, Philadelphia, pp 1573–1608

Talving P, DuBose J, Inaba K, Demetriades D (2010) Conversion of emergent cricothyrotomy to tracheotomy in trauma patients. Arch Surg 145(1):87–91

Airway Rescue Equipment

▶ Airway Equipment

Airway Skills for Infants and Children

▶ Pediatric Airway Management

Airway Trauma, Management of

Davide Cattano[1] and Ruggero M. Corso[2]
[1]Department of Anesthesiology, Memorial Hermann Hospital-TMC, The University of Texas Medical School at Houston, Houston, TX, USA
[2]Department of Emergency, Division of Anesthesia and Intensive Care, G.B. Morgagni-L. Pierantoni Hospital, Forlì, Italy

Synonyms

Prehospital airway trauma; Traumatic airway injury

Definition

Airway trauma involves direct injury to the airway. Depending on the mechanism of trauma, the injury to the airway may be obvious or difficult to diagnose. Although seen in less than 1 % of trauma patients (Kummer et al. 2007), when present, the risk of patient morbidity and mortality is high due to the challenge involved with treating this condition.

Preexisting Condition

Types of Trauma

Airway trauma is categorized as either blunt, penetrating, or a combination of the two, and it can be either obvious or concealed.

Blunt trauma includes trauma to the airway where the mechanism of injury does not enter the patient's body. Examples of blunt airway trauma include, but are not limited to, manual strangulation (as in the case of choke holds), strangulation by a foreign object (e.g., rope), and direct blows to the neck (e.g., with a blunt object or with an appendage). The most common cause of blunt airway trauma is motor vehicle accidents where injury results from the neck coming into contact with the dashboard, steering wheel, or seatbelt. Research reports the incidence of trauma patients with blunt trauma to the airway between 0.4 % and 5 % (Kummer et al. 2007). Indications of this type of injury are hoarseness, stridor, laryngeal hematoma and/or laceration, difficulty or pain swallowing or talking, laryngeal edema and/or tenderness, loss of laryngeal landmarks, impaired vocal fold mobility, and cricoarytenoid dislocation.

Penetrating trauma includes trauma to the airway where the mechanism of injury pierces the skin and enters the patient's body. Examples of penetrating airway trauma include, but are not limited to, puncture wounds (e.g., made with sharp implements like knives) and projectile wounds (e.g., made with weapons such as guns or fragmentation grenades). Incidence rates for this type of trauma are reported at 4.5 % (Kummer et al. 2007). Indications of this type of injury are hoarseness, stridor, dyspnea, air leak, subcutaneous emphysema, dysphagia, and oronasopharyngeal bleeding.

The results of airway trauma range from airway occlusion, the most easily observed and rapidly fatal, to esophageal injuries, which may take as long as 24 h to diagnose.

Application

Securing the airway and providing adequate ventilation is the first priority in trauma patients, taking precedence over even management of bleeding. This task can be difficult in trauma patients but is further complicated by patients who have endured trauma directly to the airway.

Algorithms

Algorithms for the management of difficult airways have been developed by various scientific societies. The American Society of Anesthesiology (ASA) provides an algorithm, with a modified version for trauma (Wilson 2005). However, it is important to remember for what type of clinician and for what setting each algorithm is designed, as some may be ill suited for prehospital emergency use. A single comprehensive algorithm that includes all possible options is impossible and would have limited practical use if it did exist. Clinicians should familiarize themselves with a variety of different algorithms and construct an algorithm that best suits their own particular skills. Research found that when an emergency airway management algorithm is used in prehospital settings by trained personnel, failed intubations occur in only 0.1 % of cases (Combes et al. 2006).

Maxillofacial Trauma Associated Problems

The maxillofacial trauma patient often presents a problem of difficult mask ventilation and difficult intubation. Hutchinson et al. (1990) addressed six specific situations associated with maxillofacial trauma, which may adversely affect the airway:

1. Posteroinferior displacement of a fractured maxilla parallel to the inclined plane of the skull base may block the nasopharyngeal airway.
2. A bilateral fracture of the anterior mandible may cause the fractured symphysis to slide posteriorly along with the tongue attached to it via its anterior insertion. In the supine patient, the base of the tongue may drop back, thus blocking the oropharynx.
3. Fractured or exfoliated teeth, bone fragments, and vomitus and blood as well as foreign bodies – dentures, debris, shrapnel etc. – may block the airway anywhere along the upper aerodigestive tract.
4. Hemorrhage, either from distinct vessels in open wounds or severe nasal bleeding from complex blood supply of the nose, may also contribute to airway obstruction.
5. Soft tissue swelling and edema resulting from trauma to the head and neck may cause delayed airway compromise.
6. Trauma to the larynx and trachea may cause swelling and displacement of structures, such as the epiglottis, arytenoid cartilages, and vocal cords, thereby increasing the risk of cervical airway obstruction.

Zygoma or zygomatic arch fractures can impinge on the coronoid process of the mandibular ramus limiting mouth opening. Le Fort II and III fractures are associated with disruption of the cribriform plate, and nasally placed objects can enter the brain. Because disruption of the cribriform plate is very difficult to rule out in the acute setting, any evidence of a basal skull fracture or Le Fort II or III fracture [periorbital hematomas resembling "raccoon-eyes," hemotympanum, Battle's sign (ecchymosis overlying the mastoid process), or cerebral spinal fluid (CSF) rhinorrhea] should be presumed to involve cribriform plate disruption. Because of the possibility of causing meningitis or further brain injury by blindly forcing a nasally placed object into the cranial vault, blind manipulations are contraindicated. However, nasal intubations under FOB guidance are not universally held to be absolutely contraindicated. Furthermore, maxillofacial injury patients carry a statistically significant risk of also having both cervical spine and head injuries, strategies for airway management in these patients should therefore take account of these lesions. Even in life-threatening situations, a quick evaluation of airway must be performed; indeed, defining the exact difficulty involved could direct the physician to the best strategy to managing that airway.

Airway Assessment

For ease of remembrance, one is encouraged to use the following mnemonic for assessing the difficult airway in these patients: LEMON and BONES.

LEMON for assessing *difficult intubation*:

L – Look externally: For massive facial or neck trauma, receding mandible, and short neck (<3 finger breadth from sternal notch to thyroid cartilage).

E – Evaluate 3-3-2 rule: Mouth opening, submandibular space, and distance between the thyroid notch and the chin of less than 3, 3, and 2 fingers, respectively, suggest difficult intubation.

M – Mallampati grade: ≥2 should alert the operator for difficult laryngoscopy and tracheal intubation.

O – Obstruction: Obstruction to the airway may be fixed or rapidly changing as due to inhalation injury or faciomaxillary trauma.

N – Neck mobility: This may be fixed as in patients with cervical collar or halo frame.

Difficult mask ventilation may be anticipated if the patient has 2 or > of the following parameters in the Mnemonic **BONES**:

B   Beard
O   Obesity (BMI $> 26 \text{ kg/m}^2$)
N   No teeth
E   Elderly (age > 55 years)
S   Snorer

Laryngoscopic Techniques/Strategies

When ventilation or intubation is difficult in a patient, there are certain strategies that can be used to facilitate securing the airway. The airway itself or the device used to secure the airway can be manipulated.

There are four techniques that may be used to externally manipulate the airway to improve laryngeal visualization during intubation. Bimanual laryngoscopy (BL) consists of the laryngoscopist reaching around with his/her right hand to manipulate the larynx until the laryngeal view is optimized. At that point, an assistant provides pressure in place of the laryngoscopist, freeing him/her to secure the airway (Levitan et al. 2006). Optimal external laryngeal manipulation (OELM) is a modification of BL that involves the assistant manipulating the larynx from the beginning of the technique. The laryngoscopist directs the assistant's movements until an optimal view is achieved. Similar to OELM, the backward-upward-rightward pressure (BURP) technique involves an assistant applying BURP on the lower thyroid cartilage until the glottic view is improved or optimized. Cricoid pressure (also known as "Sellick's maneuver"), while often used to prevent regurgitation, may be used to improve visualization of the glottis during intubation (Levitan et al. 2006); however, this technique has the potential to distort visualization of the glottis and may even impede intubation in some cases.

Intubation/Ventilation Devices

Depending on the complexity of the airway encountered, there are a range of devices available to facilitate airway management.

Gum Elastic Bougie

Also known as a tracheal tube introducer, the gum elastic bougie is a simple yet highly effective adjunct for difficult intubations. A thin, semirigid tube that is twice the length of an endotracheal tube (ET), the bougie is passed through the laryngeal inlet when the glottic view is suboptimal. After insertion, the ET is loaded onto the bougie and advanced into the trachea. The narrow diameter (5 mm) provides easier visualization than a cuffed tracheal tube, and the bougie is not affected by blood and secretions. Successful placement is indicated by the feeling of clicks as the bent tip of the bougie hits the tracheal rings. In the case of penetrating trauma to the neck, the bougie can be used to introduce an ET directly into the trachea via an open wound or when performing a cricothyrotomy. Success rates for prehospital use of bougies are reported at 75–93 % for cases of difficult intubation (Jabre et al. 2005; Combes et al. 2006). However, care needs to be taken in their usage as they may worsen airway trauma. Failure rate of the GEB in the ED is higher than studies performed in the operating room. In a prospective observational study in emergency department, the GEB failure rate of the first laryngoscopist was 25/88 (28.4 %; 95 % CI 21.0–40.3 %), with the two most common reasons: inability to insert the bougie past the hypopharynx and inability to pass the endotracheal tube over the bougie. The Aintree Intubation Catheter (AIC) (Cook Medical, UK) is a modified GEB allowing to oxygenate and ventilate the patient during the intubation procedure. The AIC can be inserted into the trachea over a fiber-optic laryngoscope. It can also be positioned by passing it through a supraglottic airway, and an endotracheal tube can be railroaded over it, allowing endotracheal intubation (Berkow et al. 2011). Their use in combination with videolaryngoscopes has been reported.

Laryngeal Masks

When encountering the "cannot intubate/cannot ventilate" trauma patient, the laryngeal mask airway (LMA) is an excellent rescue device as it involves the use of an inflatable cuff to seal the airway. The most widely used and reported on example of the LM is the laryngeal mask airway (LMA; LMA North America, San Diego, CA, USA). The mask portion of the LMA is pushed through the oral cavity into the pharynx until the tip occupies the entire hypopharynx and the body of the mask rests against the upper esophageal sphincter behind the cricoid cartilage. The cuff is inflated to create an air-tight seal, allowing for ventilation of the patient. Although the potential for complication exists (e.g., over- or underinflation of cuff, mechanical obstruction caused by folding of mask tip), the success rates reported for use of the LMA as a primary and secondary device are high (87.4 % and 86.2 %, respectively) (Hubble et al. 2010). The LMA cannot however be considered a definitive airway, and in most acute maxillofacial trauma settings, it would be an inappropriate endpoint for airway management. Some evidence suggests that the LMA can produce significant movement of the cervical spine, which clearly may be clinically relevant in the maxillofacial trauma patient with possible neck injuries. Second-generation versions of LMAs exist which incorporate separate gastric channels into their design. Such devices are thought also to reduce the risk of aspiration by permitting regurgitant material to bypass the supraglottic area. The recently released national audit into airway complications (Cook et al. 2011) suggests that these second-generation supraglottic devices may be more appropriate than a standard LMA because of the separation of gastric and respiratory systems. Other single-use LMAs with an esophageal vent include the igel (Intersurgical UK). This supraglottic airway requires no cuff inflation and is designed to mould to the oropharynx, thereby creating a seal. Its use in trauma patients has been reported. The air-Q Disposable Laryngeal Mask Airway (Cookgas LLC, St. Louis, MO, USA) and the Intubating LMA (ILMA) are recent models that act as a conduit for intubation. The reported rapid learning curve of the ILMA and its successful use as a blind guide for intubation make it well suited for prehospital care. There are examples of the successful ILMAs use in patients suffering from maxillofacial trauma. These new models make laryngeal airways temporary devices used to ventilate patients while more permanent airway management is established.

Esophageal Airways

Esophageal airways are used to maintain ventilation in trauma patients suffering respiratory distress and are not meant for long-term airway control. Their chief benefits lie in the prevention of tongue obstruction, aspiration of gastric contents into the trachea, and air from entering the stomach. The perceived advantages over laryngeal masks are stability, ease of insertion, and stomach decompression. Because visualization of the trachea and manipulation of neck placement are unnecessary with this type of airway, it is particularly suited to trauma patients, but only those who are unconscious as conscious patients will reject the technique.

There are two types of esophageal airways, the esophageal obturator airway (EOA) and the esophageal gastric tube airway (EGTA), and they may be used only after a patent airway has been established. Use of either of these airways is indicated in adults only due to the unavailability of pediatric sizes. The EOA consists of an inflatable face mask which attaches to a tube with an inflatable cuff at the end. After insertion into the esophagus, the cuff is inflated, creating a seal that closes off gastric access and allows air to ventilate into the trachea. The EGTA is similar to the EOA except that the tube does not terminate at the inflatable cuff. The gastric tube has a valve that blocks off the esophagus and allows for ventilation of the patient. Reported success rates of EOG/EGTA use in prehospital settings by nonphysician clinicians are high at 92.6 % (Hubble et al. 2010).

Esophageal-Tracheal Tubes

Also known as the double-lumen airway, the esophageal-tracheal tube (ETT) is an alternative to esophageal airways. It is a blind insertion airway device used in emergency situations when visualization of the glottis is difficult or impossible. It consists of an inflatable cuff and a double-lumen tube that allows for ventilation of the patient even when one of the tubes has intubated the esophagus. While it allows for successful intubation of difficult airway patients, the ETT is used only in prehospital settings as it does not allow for long-term airway control. The Rüsch EasyTube (Teleflex Medical Inc., Durham, NC, USA) is one example of an ETT.

Another ETT device commonly used is the Esophageal-Tracheal Combitube (Kendall-Sheridan Catheter Corp., Argyle, NY, USA), generally referred to as the "Combitube." Its use is limited to adult patients as it does not come in pediatric sizes. Reported success rates are high when the Combitube is used as a primary or secondary airway device (85.4 % and 81.8 %, respectively) (Hubble et al. 2010).

The King laryngeal tube airway (King LT) is another widely used supraglottic airway device manufactured by King Systems Corp. (Noblesville, IN). Its design is simpler than the Combitube, and it is becoming increasingly used in prehospital settings. The King LT comes in single-lumen and double-lumen designs for ventilation and gastric access, respectively. Composed of two inflatable cuffs, the distal cuff inflates in the esophagus to isolate it from the laryngopharynx. The proximal cuff inflates at the base of the tongue and isolates the laryngopharynx from the oro- and nasopharynx. Although data is limited for the King LT, reported success rates are high when used by prehospital emergency clinicians (96.5 %) (Hubble et al. 2010).

Complications are often associated with the force of the blind insertion. In cases of unstable cervical spine injury, this may clearly be detrimental to neurological outcome. Other complications include a sore throat, dysphagia, and upper-airway hematoma. Esophageal rupture has been associated with use of Combitube, and it is relatively contraindicated in those with esophageal disease.

Lighted Stylets

Also called light wands, lighted stylets assist in placement of the ET by transilluminating the soft tissues of the neck. Available in adult and pediatric sizes, the flexible stylet has a light at the tip that, when placed in the esophagus instead of within the larynx, becomes diffuse. Contraindications include extremes in weight (i.e., obese and under-weight patients) and laryngopharyngeal trauma. Because the neck does not need to be hyperextended to use this device and it is not affected by blood and secretions, its use is well suited in trauma patients. Examples of lighted stylets include the Trachlight (Laerdal Medical Corp., Wappingers Falls, NY, USA), the Stylight (Omniglow, West Springfield, MA, USA), and the SurchLight (Aaron Medical Industries, St. Petersburg, FL, USA).

Fiber-Optic Stylets

These devices can be used to rescue situations after unanticipated difficult intubations and thereby improve the success rate of anticipated difficult tracheal intubation. Available in rigid and semirigid varieties, fiber-optic stylets incorporate the use of video technology to provide an indirect view of the glottis. Because the clinician utilizes the projected image to guide the intubating device into position, trauma patients can be intubated without adjusting neck position. Although this tool may be used by itself to intubate the patient, it may be used in conjunction with direct laryngoscopy. Semirigid models are more suited to austere conditions than rigid models because they are malleable enough to shape to fit challenging airway geometries. Examples of semirigid models include the Shikani Optical Stylet and Levitan FPS Scope (Clarus Medical, Minneapolis, MN, USA). Rigid models include the WuScope (Achi Corp., San Jose, CA, USA) and the Bonfils Retromolar Intubation Fiberscope (Karl Storz Endoscopy, Tuttlingen, Germany). Significant expertise is necessary for successful use of these devices, especially in trauma situations.

Videolaryngoscopy

A lens placed at the tip of the laryngoscopic blade transmits an image to a monitor, giving the clinician an indirect view of the glottis and facilitating placement of the intubating device.

Videolaryngoscopes are well suited for patients in which trauma has distorted airway anatomy, making it difficult or impossible to view the glottis directly using direct laryngoscopy. Of further value is the magnified, wide-angle image that the camera transmits, providing a superior view than what would be seen with the naked eye. The GlideScope (Verathon, Bothell, WA, USA) is a well-known example of a videolaryngoscope as it was the first commercially available one. Videolaryngoscopes are available in channeled and non-channeled models. Examples of channeled models are the AirTraq Optical Laryngoscope (AirTraq LLC, Fenton, MO, USA) and the PENTAX Airway Scope (Ambu, Ballerup, Denmark). The new King Vision Video Laryngoscope (King Systems, Noblesville, IN, USA) comes in both channeled and non-channeled versions.

Recently, portable models have been developed. Their portability makes them more suited to prehospital conditions. The monitor to which the glottic view is transmitted is built into the handles of these models, and they operate on battery power. The McGrath Portable Video Laryngoscope (Aircraft Medical Ltd., Edinburgh, UK), the GlideScope Ranger (Verathon, Bothell, WA, USA), and the C-MAC Video Laryngoscope (Karl Storz Endoscope, Tuttlingen, Germany) are examples of portable videolaryngoscopes. Their use in trauma patients has been described in few reports (Trimmel et al. 2011), and it has to be studied more extensively.

However, limitations of mouth opening, presence of blood, and distorted anatomy can make their use difficult or impossible. The combined use with a flexible fiberscope is a promising approach to manage very difficult airway.

Surgical Airways

All the above devices require access of the larynx from above. Most, potentially apart from nasal intubation, require some degree of mouth opening. In maxillofacial trauma, however, significant upper-airway distortion may occur. This may cause airway obstruction and make it impossible to access the larynx from above. Then, early consideration be given to direct tracheal access via surgical or percutaneous tracheostomy or needle or surgical cricothyroidotomy.

Cricothyrotomy remains the preferred procedure for establishing an emergency surgical airway and has a reported success rate of 90.5 % (Hubble et al. 2010). Used when trauma to the airway is too severe to allow passage of an intubating device or when there is an airway obstruction, a cricothyrotomy is performed by creating an incision through the cricothyroid membrane, followed by the placement of a tube. The materials needed are the use of a finger, a scalpel, and a tube (for insertion after incision).

A percutaneous cricothyrotomy (also known as Seldinger's technique) is a type of cricothyrotomy that uses a needle with a dilator, a guide wire, and a cannula. Instead of surgically opening the cricothyroid membrane, a needle is inserted into it and the opening is dilated, allowing for the insertion of a cannula. Kits, such as the Rüsch QuickTrach (Teleflex Medical, Durham, NC, USA) and the Portex Cricothyrotomy kit (Smiths Medical, Dublin, OH, USA), are sold that provide the materials needed for this procedure.

An alternative to a surgical cricothyrotomy is the needle cricothyrotomy, where a needle is inserted instead of an incision made. A large catheter is placed over the needle afterward. The procedure is limited in that it provides little airflow and cannot clear waste carbon dioxide. Its reported success rate is also low at 65.8 % (Hubble et al. 2010). This technique is not recommended due to the severity of its limitations and potential for complications.

Similar to a cricothyrotomy, a tracheostomy involves the creation of surgical airway in the cervical trachea, followed by the insertion of a tracheostomy tube. A tracheostomy must be done under anesthesia and is indicated for long-term use, whereas a cricothyrotomy is used in emergent situations.

The use of percutaneous tracheostomy in emergency has been reported (Davidson et al. 2012).

Reported complication rates of cricothyroidotomy vary from 0 % to 52 %, depending on the technique, the experience level of the operator, the patient population, and the clinical situation. The main complication is initial misplacement (e.g., paratracheal, superior or inferior to the cricothyroid membrane, or through the posterior tracheal wall) and is the principal cause of failure. Some complications are technique related. Narrow bore cannula techniques are associated with ventilation-related complications such as barotraumas (e.g., subcutaneous emphysema, pneumothorax, pneumomediastinum, and circulatory arrest due to impaired venous return) and cannula obstruction due to kinking. Kinking of the guidewire is a common problem peculiar to the Seldinger technique and increases the risk of tube misplacement. The surgical method is associated with complications of tube insertion (e.g., bleeding, laryngeal fracture). Damage to the larynx is normally a consequence of excessive pressure during device insertion and is reduced by use of small tubes and gentle technique. Long-term complications are subglottic stenosis, scarring, and voice changes. The recently released fourth National Audit Project suggests that surgical cricothyroidotomy has a higher success rate than the needle techniques and that anesthetic departments should consider when to use and how to train staff in these techniques.

For patients with maxillofacial trauma who do not require long-term ventilation, an alternative approach is the submental intubation. Submental intubation was first described by Hernandez in 1986 and was designed to eliminate the morbidity of tracheostomy in patients undergoing maxillofacial surgery. The patient is first intubated orally with a reinforced endotracheal tube. The original description places an incision within the submandibular triangle, parallel to and one finger's breadth below the mandibular border. The side opposite anybody or angle fractures is chosen if possible. Incisions below the mandibular angle and within the midline have also been described. Dissection is then carried bluntly through the mylohyoid and along the inner mandibular cortex. The floor of mouth mucosa is then incised over the dissecting instrument. The pilot balloon and endotracheal tube without connector are pulled through the incision while the tube is stabilized. Its use in acute trauma patients with difficult airway is limited by the fact that the endotracheal intubation has to be achieved before (Jundt et al. 2012).

Special Challenges

Training in the use of multiple advanced airway devices is essential for the success of personnel treating airway trauma. Research into the effect of education on emergency services personnel documented an association between cognitive knowledge and field performance; a statistically significant correlation ($p = 0.02$, chi-square) was found between personnel passing a cognitive examination and passing a field simulation of emergency airway scenarios (Sudnek et al. 2011). The implementation of a difficult airway program in one hospital significantly ($p < 0.0001$) reduced the use of surgical airways to almost half of the number performed preprogram (Berkow et al. 2009). Due to the variety of indications, both obvious and subtle, a high awareness of symptoms is also a prerequisite for success in the field.

Cross-References

► ABCDE of Trauma Care
► Airway Assessment
► Airway Equipment
► Airway Exchange in Trauma Patients
► Airway Management in Trauma, Cricothyrotomy
► Airway Management in Trauma, Nonsurgical
► Airway Management in Trauma, Tracheostomy

References

Berkow LC, Greenberg RS, Kan KH, Colantuoni E, Mark LJ, Flint PW, Corridore M, Bhatti N, Heitmiller ES (2009) Need for emergency surgical airway reduced by a comprehensive difficult airway program. Anesth Anal 109:1860–1869

Berkow LC, Schwartz JM, Kan K, Corridore M, Heitmiller ES (2011) Use of the Laryngeal Mask Airway-Aintree Intubating Catheter-fiberoptic bronchoscope technique for difficult intubation. J Clin Anesth 23(7):534–539

Combes X, Jabre P, Jbeili C, Leroux B, Bastuji-Garin S, Margenet A, Adnet F, Dhonneur G (2006) Prehospital standardization of medical airway management: incidence and risk factors of difficult airway. Acad Emerg Med 13:828–834

Cook TM, Woodall N, Frerk C (2011) Major complications of airway management in the UK: results of the fourth National Audit Project of the Royal College of Anaesthetists and the Difficult Airway Society. Part 2: intensive care and emergency departments. Br J Anaesth 106:632e42

Davidson SB, Blostein PA, Walsh J, Maltz SB, Vandenberg SL (2012) Percutaneous tracheostomy: a new approach to the emergency airway. J Trauma Acute Care Surg 73(2 Suppl 1):S83–S88

Hubble MW, Wilfong DA, Brown LH, Hertelendy A, Benner RW (2010) A meta-analysis of prehospital airway control techniques part II: alternative airway devices and cricothyrotomy success rates. Prehosp Emerg Care 14(4):515–530

Hutchison I, Lawlor M, Skinner D (1990) ABC of major trauma. Major maxillofacial injuries. BMJ 301:595–599

Jabre P, Combes X, Leroux B, Aaron E, Auger H, Margenet A, Dhonneur G (2005) Use of gum elastic bougie for prehospital difficult intubation. Am J Emerg Med 23:552–555

Jundt JS, Cattano D, Hagberg CA, Wilson JW (2012) Submental intubation: a literature review. Int J Oral Maxillofac Surg 41(1):46–54

Kummer C, Netto FS, Rizoli S, Yee D (2007) A review of traumatic airway injuries: potential implications for airway assessment and management. Injury (Int J Care Injured) 38:27–33

Levitan R, Kinkle W, Levin W, Everett W (2006) Laryngeal view during laryngoscopy: a randomized trial comparing cricoid pressure, backward-upward-rightward pressure, and bimanual laryngoscopy. Ann Emerg Med 47(6):548–555

Sudnek JR, Fernandez AR, Shimberg B, Garifo M, Correll M (2011) The association between emergency services field performance assessed by high-fidelity simulation and the cognitive knowledge of practicing paramedics. Acad Emerg Med 18:1177–1185

Trimmel H, Kreutziger J, Fertsak G, Fitzka R, Dittrich M, Voelckel WG (2011) Use of the Airtraq laryngoscope for emergency intubation in the prehospital setting: a randomized control trial. Crit Care Med 39(3):489–493

Wilson WC (2005) Trauma: airway management. ASA difficult airway algorithm modified for trauma—and five common trauma intubation scenarios. ASA Newsl 69(11):10

AKI

► Acute Kidney Injury

Alcohol

▶ Toxicology

Alcohol (ETOH) Withdrawal and Management

Brenton J. LaRiccia[1] and Jignesh H. Patel[2]
[1]Division of Trauma and Acute Care Surgery, Department of Surgery, University of Rochester Medical Center, Strong Memorial Hospital, Rochester, Rochester, NY, USA
[2]Department of Pharmacy, University of Rochester Medical Center, Strong Memorial Hospital, Rochester, NY, USA

Synonyms

Alcohol dependence; Alcoholic hallucinosis; Alcohol intoxication; Alcohol withdrawal delirium; Delirium tremens; ETOH withdrawal

Definition

Alcohol withdrawal syndrome (AWS) is the result of long-term, heavy, consistent alcohol consumption and is accompanied by clinical abnormalities when there is a significant decrease or cessation in consumption of alcohol (Brailowsky and Garcia 1999).

Preexisting Condition

Alcohol abuse and misuse is the most common form of addiction throughout the world. According to the National Institute on Alcohol Abuse and Alcoholism (NIAAA), alcohol-related diagnoses are significant contributors to emergency department visits and hospitalizations. Alcohol misuse is also associated with a significant number of traumatic injuries leading to admission to intensive care unit. For many patients, this institutionalization leads to an abrupt discontinuation of alcohol which can potentiate acute withdrawal syndromes. AWS is the result of long-term, heavy, consistent alcohol consumption and is accompanied by clinical abnormalities when there is a significant decrease or cessation in consumption of alcohol (Brailowsky and Garcia 1999). It has been estimated that 7 % of the population of the United States is dependent on or abuses alcohol (Stehman and Mycyk 2013). Some evidence indicates that up to 50 % of trauma patients chronically abuse alcohol (Heymann et al. 2002).

Alcohol withdrawal adds significant morbidity to trauma patients. In one study, patients who developed AWS had more ventilator days, intensive care unit (ICU) days, hospital days, increased pneumonia, respiratory failure, and urinary tract infections and underwent more tracheostomy and percutaneous endoscopic gastrostomy placement than those who did not have AWS (Bard et al. 2006).

Application

Physiology
Ethanol affects both the inhibitory and excitatory neurotransmitter receptor systems in the central nervous system, mainly the γ-aminobutyric acid (GABA) and glutamatergic receptors, respectively. Ethanol acts to increase GABA, a receptor-mediated inhibition, and also to reduce glutamatergic (NMDA) activity (Stehman and Mycyk 2013). Prolonged use of ethanol causes GABA receptor downregulation as well as noradrenergic hyperactivity (Maldonando 2010). These neurobiological changes in chronic ethanol users cause AWS when the stimulus is removed.

Symptoms
The symptoms of AWS include alcohol craving, tremors, irritability, fear, nausea, sleep disturbance, hypertension, tachycardia, sweating, perceptual distortion, delirium tremens, seizures, and death (Brailowsky and Garcia 1999; Sarff and Gold 2010). Delirium tremens manifests itself as the most severe form of alcohol

withdrawal (Stehman and Mycyk 2013). These symptoms can be divided into several time periods. Early withdrawal begins around 16–24 h after significant reduction or abstinence from alcohol and is evidenced by tremors, nausea, vomiting, and adrenergic symptoms. Alcohol withdrawal seizures can also begin on day 1, whereby up to 25 % can be grand mal seizures and up to 2 % of patients develop status epilepticus. Alcoholic hallucinosis consists of audiovisual hallucinations. Delirium tremens (DTs) has an onset of 1–3 days and usually peaks on days 4 and 5. The mortality of DTs can be as high as 15–20 % if untreated. DTs primary manifestation is delirium (as defined by DSM IV manual) as well as autonomic symptoms (Maldonando 2010).

Diagnosis

AWS is diagnosed by patient history and physical examination for signs and symptoms of withdrawal. When a patient is diagnosed with AWS, several objective tools are available to determine its severity. The most commonly utilized tool is the Clinical Institute Withdrawal Assessment for Alcohol-Revised (CIWA-Ar). Other tools such as the Alcohol Withdrawal Syndrome Scale (AWSS) are also used to determine severity of illness. Mild withdrawal is categorized as CIWA-Ar ≤ 8 or AWSS <5, moderate withdrawal is categorized as CIWA-Ar 9–15 or AWSS 6–9, and severe withdrawal is categorized as CIWA-Ar >15 or AWSS >9 (Maldonando 2010).

Treatment

Treatment of AWS typically utilizes GABAergic agents, classically benzodiazepines (GABA-a subtype), but can also include barbiturates, propofol, beta-blockers, and clonidine (Brailowsky and Garcia 1999). Mild withdrawal may not require treatment, with the exception of low dose, as-needed benzodiazepines (BZDs). Moderate and severe withdrawals are typically treated with an alcohol withdrawal management protocol based on the CIWA-Ar or AWSS score. Protocols vary by institution but typically include as-needed BZD administration for lower scores

(symptom triggered method) and a loading dose with scheduled BZDs for higher scores with additional as-needed BZDs for breakthrough agitation. Long-acting BZDs such as diazepam and chlordiazepoxide are typically used for loading and scheduled dosing, and short-acting BZDs such as midazolam should be used for breakthrough agitation. Barbiturates, particularly phenobarbital, have also shown benefit in the treatment of AWS. Severe agitation resistant to standard treatment may be treated with antipsychotics such as haloperidol, quetiapine, risperidone, and olanzapine; however, these agents do not possess GABAergic activity; therefore, their role is secondary to BZDs and other GABAergic agents (Maldonando 2010).

Alternative Agents for Treatment of AWS

Barbiturates are GABAergic and also inhibit stimulatory glutamate receptors, which are upregulated in AWS. There are many medications in the barbiturates class, but phenobarbital in particular has shown benefit in the treatment of AWS. Barbiturates are desirable for treatment due to its sedative and anticonvulsant properties. The main limitations however of barbiturates use are a narrow therapeutic window, long half-life, and potential to induce respiratory depression (Gold et al. 2007; Mariani et al. 2006).

Propofol can also be utilized in select cases of ventilated patients who are resistant to other sedative-hypnotics, due to its GABAergic affect and inhibition of N-methyl-D-aspartate (NMDA)-mediated neuroexcitation. Its use may be limited by the need for continuous infusion and close hemodynamic monitoring. Beta-blockers and clonidine are also sometimes used, in conjunction with other agents, to modulate autonomic signs of AWS (tachycardia and hypertension) (Gold et al. 2007).

The use of α_2-adrenergic agonist agents in AWS is increasing. The use of clonidine and, more recently, dexmedetomidine, for control of autonomic signs of AWS, has been shown to be efficacious. In addition, the use of these agents also reduces the anxiety, agitation, and irritability associated with AWS. These agents are being used with increased frequency as adjunctive methods of managing AWS (Maldonando 2010; Frazee et al. 2013). Using dexmedetomidine as an adjunct therapy to BZDs has been shown to decrease heart rate, blood pressure, and overall BZD usage in patients with severe AWS (Frazee et al. 2013). However, similar to propofol, its use may be limited by the need for continuous infusion and close hemodynamic monitoring.

Other agents that have been studied in the management of AWS include baclofen (through its GABA-b receptor modulation), carbamazepine, pregabalin, phenytoin, and gabapentin (Maldonando 2010; Mariani et al. 2006; Chabria 2008; Ait-Daoud et al. 2006; Leggio et al. 2008).

In addition to pharmacologic treatment of AWS, supportive care is also important. Severe cases should be admitted to the ICU for protective monitoring. These patients may be dehydrated from their symptoms, so fluid and electrolyte replacement should be performed as needed. Administration of thiamine 100 mg, folate 1 mg, and a multivitamin should be started on admission and given for 7–14 days, to correct folate and thiamine deficiency. Thiamine should be administered prior to giving glucose containing fluids to prevent precipitation of Wernicke-Korsakoff syndrome (Walker et al. 2013).

AWS Prophylaxis

Ethanol intravenous infusions have been used for alcohol withdrawal prophylaxis and treatment in the ICU setting; however, evidence has not shown superiority in efficacy or adverse sedative effects when compared to benzodiazepine use in AWS prophylaxis (Weinberg et al. 2009).'

Cross-References

▶ Alcohol Withdrawal
▶ ICU Management
▶ Preventing Delirium in the Intensive Care Unit
▶ Toxicology
▶ Trauma Intensive Care Management
▶ Trauma Patient Evaluation

References

Ait-Daoud N, Malcolm RJ Jr, Johnson BA (2006) An overview of medications for the treatment of alcohol withdrawal and alcohol dependence with an emphasis on the use of older and newer anticonvulsants. Addict Behav 31(9):1628–1649

Bard M, Goettler C, Toschlog E, Sagraves S, Schenarts P, Newell M, Fugate M, Rotondo M (2006) Alcohol withdrawal syndrome: turning minor injuries into a major problem. J Trauma 61:1441–1446

Brailowsky S, Garcia O (1999) Ethanol, GABA, and epilepsy. Arch Med Res 30:3–9

Chabria (2008) Inpatient management of alcohol withdrawal: a practical approach. Signae Vitae 3(1):24–29

Frazee E, N Personett H A, Leung J G, Nelson S, Dierkhising R A, and Bauer P R (2013) Influence of dexmedetomidine therapy on the management of severe alcohol withdrawal syndrome in critically ill patients. J Crit Care

Gold J, Rimal B, Nolan A, Nelson L (2007) A strategy of escalating doses of benzodiazepines and phenobarbital administration reduces the need for mechanical ventilation in delirium tremens. Crit Care Med 35:724–730

Heymann C, Langenkamp J, Dubisz N, Dossow V, Schaffartzik W, Kern H, Kox W, Spies C (2002) Posttraumatic immune modulation in chronic alcoholics is associated with multiple organ dysfunction syndrome. J Trauma 52:95–103

Leggio L, Kenna GA, Swift RM (2008) New developments for the pharmacological treatment of alcohol withdrawal syndrome. A focus on non-benzodiazepine GABAergic medications. Prog Neuro-Psychopharmacol Biol Psychiatry 32(5):1106–1117

Maldonando J (2010) An approach to the patient with substance use and abuse. Med Clin N Am 94:1169–1205

Mariani JJ, Rosenthal RN, Tross S, Singh P, Anand OP (2006) A randomized, open-label, controlled trial of gabapentin and phenobarbital in the treatment of alcohol withdrawal. Am J Addict 15(1):76–84

Sarff M, Gold J (2010) Alcohol withdrawal syndromes in the intensive care unit. Crit Care Med 38(Suppl): S494–S501

Stehman C, Mycyk M (2013) A rational approach to the treatment of alcohol withdrawal in the ED. Am J Emerg Med 31:734–742

Walker B, Anderson M, Hauser L, Werchan I (2013) Ethanol for alcohol withdrawal: the end of an era. J Trauma Acute Care Surg 74(3):926–931

Weinberg J, Magnotti L, Fischer P, Edwards N, Schroeppel T, Fabian T, Croce M (2009) Comparison of intravenous ethanol versus diazepam for alcohol withdrawal prophylaxis in the trauma ICU: results of a randomized trial. J Trauma 64:99–104

Alcohol Dependence

▶ Alcohol   (ETOH)   Withdrawal   and
Management

Alcohol Intoxication

▶ Alcohol   (ETOH)   Withdrawal   and
Management

Alcohol Withdrawal

Bjug Borgundvaag
Schwartz/Reisman Emergency Medicine
Institute, Department of Family and Community
Medicine, Mount Sinai Hospital, University
of Toronto, Toronto, ON, Canada

Synonyms

Delirium tremens; DTs; Withdrawal; Withdrawal
seizure

Definition

Ethyl alcohol (alcohol) is one of the most
commonly used mind-altering drugs worldwide.
Approximately 50 % of the population over
12 years of age drink alcohol regularly, and
estimates are that 10 % of these may be
considered alcoholics. Definitions of alcoholism
vary, but the condition can be broadly defined as:

1. Compulsive drinking despite evidence that
   doing so interferes with other aspects of life
2. The inability to moderate alcohol consumption
3. Physical dependence on alcohol (or the
   appearance of withdrawal symptoms upon
   reduction/cessation of consumption)

Excessive alcohol consumption is associated
with significant harm. It is estimated that between

10 % and 30 % of all emergency department
visits are associated with alcohol consumption
in some way. In the UK, data suggest that
between midnight and 5 a.m., 70 % of ED visits
are alcohol related (Studies IoA 2009). US statistics indicate that almost ½ of all traffic-related
fatalities are alcohol related (Centers for Disease
Control and Prevention (CDC) 1993). Individuals
who have been arrested for driving while
impaired are significantly more likely to die in
an alcohol-related motor vehicle collision, and
drunkenness is an important contributor to all
other types of fatal accidents (Brewer et al.
1994). Overall, it is estimated that alcohol is
linked to approximately 100,000 deaths/year in
the USA alone.

Many trauma and medical patients will end
up in hospital with unrecognized alcohol dependence and develop alcohol withdrawal (AW)
symptoms, which will complicate and prolong
their hospital stay. In one study (Foy et al. 1997),
8 % of all hospital admissions and 31 % of trauma
patients developed AW, a finding since confirmed
in other studies (Spies et al. 1996b). The development of AW in postsurgical and trauma patients
significantly complicates care and is associated
with a nearly threefold increase in mortality
(Spies et al. 1996a; Sonne and Tonnesen 1992).
Factors associated with increased risk of DT and
AW symptoms include age >70, seizure at the
time of admission, having been administered
a general anaesthetic, assisted ventilation, and
a delay of greater than 24 h before first assessment
for withdrawal symptoms (Foy et al. 1997).

Alcohol withdrawal is commonly diagnosed in
the Emergency Department, and undertreatment
of these patients results in significantly longer
and more complicated length of stay in the
ED compared to patients treated appropriately
(receiving adequate doses of benzodiazepines)
(Kahan et al. 2005).

Preexisting Condition

Alcohol withdrawal syndrome develops in
13–71 % of individuals who regularly consume
alcohol and then stop drinking and will develop

Alcohol Withdrawal, Table 1 Minor and major symptoms of alcohol withdrawal

Minor symptoms	Major symptoms
Craving for alcohol	Seizures
Tremor	Hallucinations
Anxiety	Delirium
Diaphoresis	
Irritability/agitation	
Insomnia	
Anorexia/nausea/vomiting	
Headache	

in a dose-dependent manner. Symptoms are related to the effects of regular alcohol intake on CNS neurotransmitter function, particularly that mediated by GABA and glutamate receptors, where alcohol potentiates GABA's inhibitory effects on CNS function and upregulates glutamate receptors (which are stimulatory). The net effect of these adaptations is the neuronal hyperexcitability that is characteristic of AW.

Symptoms can be categorized as minor or major as outlined in Table 1.

AW symptoms typically begin to appear within hours of stopping or lowering alcohol intake, with the typical progression of symptoms being (1) autonomic hyperactivity, (2) hallucinations, (3) neuronal excitation, and (4) delirium tremens. Major symptoms of withdrawal will typically develop within 1–4 days, and delirium tremens lasts 3–4 days. Both hallucinations and seizures may have an abrupt onset, and not necessarily be preceded by significant signs of withdrawal, making the diagnosis difficult. One of the key presenting symptoms of AW is tremor. AW tremor is characterized as an "intention tremor," that is to say, it is unmasked by purposeful movement. It may not be obvious in patients at rest, and quantitation requires some experience with evaluating patients in AW. Patients with moderately severe tremor will not be able to drink water from a cup without spilling the contents.

One important challenge of treating AW syndrome is identifying which patients are likely to require treatment. While most regular drinkers who suddenly stop consuming alcohol will experience some withdrawal symptoms, most of these will be minor. Various studies have demonstrated that seizures and DTs will occur in approximately 5–15 % of alcoholics (Saitz and O'Malley 1997; Sarff and Gold 2010). AW-related seizures are typically brief, are tonic-clonic in nature, and may recur in up to 60 % of individuals with subsequent episodes of withdrawal. Though multiple seizures with any episode of withdrawal are uncommon, AW is one of the most common causes of status epilepticus in the USA (Saitz 1998). Importantly, in chronically intoxicated individuals, seizures may occur while the patient has a blood alcohol level significantly exceeding the legal limit for intoxication.

Application

The management of AW will depend on the individual patient location in the hospital and personal circumstance. Experience suggests that it is a small minority of AW patients in the ED which will require hospital admission and most patients can be managed as outpatients. There are currently no clearly established guidelines to assist clinicians in determining which patients require hospitalization for detoxification/treatment of AW. Practically speaking, candidates for outpatient treatment should have no history of delirium, no medical or psychiatric condition which could complicate the withdrawal process, and should exhibit evidence of mild to moderate AW symptoms. In reality, many patients seen in the ED will present with AW seizures and if adequately treated in the ED, can be discharged safely. All AW patients should be given 100 mg of thiamine as soon as treatment begins to prevent the development of Wernicke's encephalopathy. Likewise, all patients require careful attention to, and correction of, other metabolic/electrolyte abnormalities.

Pharmacotherapeutic Choices

Numerous agents from a variety of drug classes have been investigated in the management of AW, including alpha-adrenergic agonists, barbiturates, benzodiazepines, beta-blocking agents, butyrophenones, calcium channel antagonists, gabapentin, propofol, and valproic acid. At the present time, evidence suggests that the treatment of choice are drugs in the benzodiazepine class. Notably, phenytoin has been shown to be no better than placebo in terms of treating AW-related seizures (Mayo-Smith 1997).

The effectiveness of benzodiazepines in the treatment of AW was first recognized over 40 years ago (Kaim et al. 1969), and their use in the management of AW syndrome has recently been extensively reviewed by the Cochrane Collaboration (Amato et al. 2010). Available evidence indicates that benzodiazepines are superior to placebo in preventing and treating seizures and delirium and are compared favorably to other treatments for the major manifestations of AW (more effective, less abuse potential, and a wider therapeutic index).

There is no current evidence to suggest that any one benzodiazepine is superior to another. The medication used in the initial studies of the treatment of AW was chlordiazepoxide. This agent, which is only available in oral formulation, has largely been replaced by diazepam, which can be administered orally or parenterally. The long half-life of diazepam is felt to produce a smoother withdrawal course. In elderly patients or those with significant hepatic dysfunction, shorter acting agents, which are renally cleared, such as lorazepam (also available in oral or parenteral formulations), may be preferable and are commonly used.

Traditionally, there have been two main approaches to the treatment of AW as follows:

1. In the **fixed-schedule model**, patients are treated with regular doses (front-end loaded, decreasing over time) of medication for a defined treatment period (typically 48–72 h). This approach was developed for use in inpatients, typically in the setting of a withdrawal treatment facility, and does not rely on any objective evaluation of symptom severity. The benefit of the fixed-schedule model is simplicity. Medications can be ordered in advance, subsequent evaluations are not required, and time-consuming reassessments are not required.

2. In the **symptom-driven therapy model**, patients are evaluated using a standardized assessment tool on a regular basis and treated according to severity of symptoms. The most commonly used assessment tool for this purpose is the CIWA-Ar (Sullivan et al. 1989). In two randomized controlled studies which assigned patients to a fixed-schedule model or symptom-driven therapy based on the CIWA-Ar, the symptom-driven approach was shown to be significantly better, with a significant decrease in both the duration of treatment and the total dose of benzodiazepine administered, with no difference in severity of withdrawal or incidence of seizures (Saitz et al. 1994; Daeppen et al. 2002).

Given that there is large variability in the treatment requirements for AW, with up to 40 % not requiring any treatment other than supportive care, an approach which guides therapy based on severity of withdrawal symptoms also has face validity.

ED Management of AW

The majority of patients seen in the ED with alcohol withdrawal can be treated in the ED and discharged to an outpatient detoxification program or to home with no further treatment required. This approach is made possible by the long half-life of diazepam and its metabolites. A typical protocol would require that severity of withdrawal be assessed using the CIWA-Ar hourly, with doses of benzodiazepine (10–20 mg diazepam, orally or intravenously) administered for a score of 10 or greater following each assessment. If a patient has had a CIWA of less than 10 for two sequential assessments, they are deemed to be fully treated, with the caveat that patients with a history of AW seizures receive a minimum of 60 mg of diazepam to prevent the development of seizures. Patients with an altered level of consciousness or clouded sensorium require further evaluation to rule out other causes of their symptomology and should be admitted to hospital for further investigation. It should be noted that alcoholic patients can be very tolerant to benzodiazepines, with many patients requiring in excess of 100 mg of diazepam to be administered over a relatively short time period. Following treatment, patients can be discharged with no further prescription for diazepam required.

Inpatient Management of AW

Once an inpatient has been identified as having symptoms of alcohol withdrawal, a similar approach may be taken. The key here appears to be early initiation of monitoring, as delays in the recognition and treatment of AW have been associated with complicated withdrawal. A similar assessment and treatment schedule can be undertaken on the ward, though patients admitted for other medical issues who develop AW may be able to have their assessments spaced out (e.g., to q 2 hourly) to facilitate nursing care. Appropriate and aggressive management of AW symptoms will likely lead to better compliance with other aspects of medical care and result in better outcomes overall, though further investigation is required in this area.

Cross-References

► Benzodiazepines
► Delirium as a Complication of ICU Care
► Drug abuse and Trauma Anesthesia
► Emergency Medical Services (EMS)
► Postoperative Management of Adult Trauma Patient
► Toxicology

References

Amato L, Minozzi S, Vecchi S et al (2010) Benzodiazepines for alcohol withdrawal. Cochrane Database Syst Rev 3(3):CD005063

Brewer RD, Morris PD, Cole TB et al (1994) The risk of dying in alcohol-related automobile crashes among habitual drunk drivers. New Engl J Med [Research Support, U.S. Gov't, P.H.S.] 331(8):513–517

Centers for Disease Control and Prevention (CDC) (1993) Reduction in alcohol-related traffic fatalities–United States, 1990–1992. MMWR Morb Mortal Wkly Rep 42(47):905–909

Daeppen JB, Gache P, Landry U et al (2002) Symptom-triggered vs fixed-schedule doses of benzodiazepine for alcohol withdrawal: a randomized treatment trial. Arch Intern Med 162(10):1117–1121

Foy A, Kay J, Taylor A (1997) The course of alcohol withdrawal in a general hospital. QJM 90(4):253–261

Kahan M, Borgundvaag B, Midmer D et al (2005) Treatment variability and outcome differences in the emergency department management of alcohol withdrawal. Can J Emerg Med 7(2):87–92

Kaim SC, Klett CJ, Rothfeld B (1969) Treatment of the acute alcohol withdrawal state: a comparison of four drugs. Am J Psychiatry 125(12):1640–1646

Mayo-Smith MF (1997) Pharmacological management of alcohol withdrawal. A meta-analysis and evidence-based practice guideline. JAMA 278:144–151

Saitz R (1998) Introduction to alcohol withdrawal. Alcohol Health Res World 22(1):5–12

Saitz R, O'Malley SS (1997) Pharmacotherapies for alcohol abuse. Withdrawal and treatment. Med Clin North Am 81(4):881–907

Saitz R, Mayo-Smith MF, Roberts MS et al (1994) Individualized treatment for alcohol withdrawal. A randomized double-blind controlled trial. JAMA 272(7):519–523

Sarff M, Gold JA (2010) Alcohol withdrawal syndromes in the intensive care unit. Crit Care Med 38(9 Suppl): S494–S501

Sonne NM, Tonnesen H (1992) The influence of alcoholism on outcome after evacuation of subdural haematoma. Br J Neurosurg 6(2):125–130

Spies CD, Nordmann A, Brummer G et al (1996a) Intensive care unit stay is prolonged in chronic alcoholic men following tumor resection of the upper digestive tract. Acta Anaesthesiol Scand 40(6):649–656

Spies CD, Dubisz N, Neumann T et al (1996b) Therapy of alcohol withdrawal syndrome in intensive care unit patients following trauma: results of a prospective, randomized trial. Crit Care Med 24(3):414–422

Studies IoA (2009) Alcohol and the NHS: the impact of alcohol on the National Health Service; admissions to hospital for alcohol related diagnoses. IAS Factsheet2009. Available from http://www.ias.org.uk/resources/factsheets/nhs.pdf

Sullivan JT, Sykora K, Schneiderman J et al (1989) Assessment of alcohol withdrawal: the revised clinical institute withdrawal assessment for alcohol scale (CIWA-Ar). Br J Addict 84(11):1353–1357

Alcohol Withdrawal Delirium

► Alcohol (ETOH) Withdrawal and Management

Alcoholic Hallucinosis

▶ Alcohol (ETOH) Withdrawal and Management

Alimentation

▶ Nutritional Support

Alkali Burns

▶ Chemical Burns

Alkalosis, Alkalemia (Respiratory Versus Metabolic)

▶ Acid-Base Management in Trauma Anesthesia

All-Terrain Vehicle

▶ ATV Injuries

Alterations in Volume of Distribution

▶ Pharmacologic Strategies in Adult Trauma Anesthesia

Ambulance Care

▶ Prehospital Emergency Preparedness

American College of Surgeons Committee on Trauma

▶ Trauma Registry

American Red Cross

▶ Prehospital Emergency Preparedness

AMICAR

▶ Aminocaproic Acid

Aminocaproic Acid

Harvey G. Hawes[1], Bryan A. Cotton[1] and Laura A. McElroy[2]
[1]Department of Surgery, Division of Acute Care Surgery, Trauma and Critical Care, University of Texas Health Science Center at Houston, The University of Texas Medical School at Houston, Houston, TX, USA
[2]Department of Anesthesiology, Critical Care Medicine, University of Rochester Medical Center, Rochester, NY, USA

Synonyms

AMICAR; EACA; e-Aminocaproic acid

Definition

Okamoto first descried both the antifibrinolytic drugs epsilon-aminocaproic acid (EACA) and tranexamic acid (TXA) in 1957. EACA is a lysine analogue that has acted as an antifibrinolytic by binding and inhibiting the actions of plasmin and plasminogen on fibrin and tissue plasminogen activator (Hardy and Belisle 1994). In acute settings EACA can also be used to counteract toxic effects or overdoses of tissue plasminogen activator (tPA) and strep-tokinase. EACA has been studied extensively in the coronary bypass literature as a means of reducing surgical bleeding, blood transfusion volume, the need for reoperation, and mortality

(Penta de Peppo et al. 1995; Dhir 2013) secondary to hyperfibrinolysis. Currently there is very little research on the use of EACA in trauma patients. Inferences are made from studies on the other lysine analogue, TXA, which has been extensively studied in a wide variety of clinical bleeding and was found to specifically reduce mortality in trauma patients during the CRASH-2 trial (Cap et al. 2011) when administered within 3 h of injury. By extension, EACA will likely have a role in treating hyperfibrinolytic states as identified clinically and by excessive clot lysis on thromboelastography (Levy 2010). EACA is only one tenth as potent as TXA. Though EACA and TXA exert similar action, there seems to be differences in their adverse events profile, with thrombosis and renal failure being of greatest concern (Ross and Salman 2012). Some reports in pediatric patients implicate TXA in increased incidence of seizures (Ortmann et al. 2013). Definitive causal evidence implicating EACA in any of these adverse effects is lacking.

Cross-References

▶ Fibrinogen (Test)
▶ Tranexamic Acid

References

Cap AP, Bauer DG, Orman JA et al (2011) Tranexamic acid for trauma patients: a critical review of the literature. J Trauma Inj Infect Crit Care 71:S9–S14
Dhir A (2013) Antifibrinolytics iin cardiac surgery. Ann Card Anaesth 16(2):117–125. doi:10.4103/0971-9784.109749
Hardy JF, Belisle S (1994) Natural and synthetic antifibrinolytics in adult cardiac surgery: efficacy, effectiveness, and efficiency. Can J Anaesth 41(11):1104–1112
Levy J (2010) Antifibrinolytic therapy: new data and new concepts. Lancet. doi:10.1016/S0140-6736(10)60939-7
Ortmann E, Besser MW, Klein AA (2013) Antifibrinolytic agents in current anaesthetic practice. Br J Anaesth 111(4):549–563
Penta de Peppo A, Pierri MD, Scafuri A et al (1995) Intraoperative antifibrinolysis and blood-saving techniques in cardiac surgery: prospective trial of 3 antifibrinolytic drugs. Tex Heart Inst J 22:231–236
Ross J, Salman RAS (2012) The frequency of thrombotic events among adults given antifibrinolytic drugs for spontaneous bleeding: systematic review and meta-analysis of observational studies and randomized trials. Curr Drug Saf 7:44–54

Ammunition

▶ Ballistics

Amputation

Douglas Fetkenhour
Department of Physical Medicine and Rehabilitation, University of Rochester School of Medicine, Rochester, NY, USA

Synonyms

Dismember; Limb loss

Definition

Significant trauma to a limb can result in soft tissue, neurovascular, and bony injury so severe that limb salvage may not be possible. This degree of injury can necessitate surgical amputation to prevent a life-threatening infection. Amputations are characterized by their site: transhumeral and transradial in the upper limb and transfemoral and transtibial in the lower limb. Lower limb amputations are often referred to as AKAs and BKAs (above- and below-knee amputations). Management of amputation is categorized into preprosthetic training and postprosthetic training.

Preprosthetic training involves pain management, wound care, maintenance of joint motion, strengthening, mobility, and ADLs. Following amputation, the patient is likely to have nociceptive pain at the surgical site. This type of pain often requires opiates initially, but can often be tapered to acetaminophen or ibuprofen as the site heals. Desensitization techniques can be used to improve the limb's acceptance of contact. Start with touching the limb with soft material such as cotton. As this becomes increasingly tolerable, more course material like terry cloth can be used. The patient is also encouraged to touch the residual limb with their hands to aid in desensitization and facilitate comfort in handling the limb. Nearly all patients with traumatic amputation will experience phantom sensations (1). 55 % of them will experience phantom pain (2). Phantom sensations such as buzzing or numbness rarely have clinical consequences, but phantom pain can significantly impact function. Phantom pain is a centrally mediated neuropathic process and responds well to treatment with GABAergic medications (gabapentin, pregabalin).

Wound care and residual limb shaping are important in the preprosthetic management of an amputation. The surgical wound should be monitored for signs of infection, wound dehiscence, and necrosis. Serosanguinous drainage is expected, but an increase in the amount of drainage or frank purulence should be treated with antibiotics. The presence of dehiscence will usually require surgical revision. Small amounts of soft tissue necrosis along the incision line or at the lateral margins will usually eschar and evolve without incident, but areas larger that have become boggy or draining may also require surgical revision. A dry dressing with a gauze roll is adequate for a healthy wound environment. If there are areas of open granular beds, a foam or hydrocolloid wound care product is appropriate to provide an optimal wound healing environment. Application of a "post-op sock" will provide a mild compressive force for control edema and begin shaping the limb. The ideal shape for an AKA is cylindrical and conical for a BKA.

Maintenance of range of motion and strengthening facilitates favorable functional outcome following amputation. A focus on forward flexion, abduction, and extension at the shoulder is important in a transhumeral amputation.

In a patient with a transradial amputation, the maintenance of elbow extension is important in addition to shoulder movement. Shoulder retraction is imperative for both transhumeral and transradial as this motion is what controls the terminal device in a typical cable-driven prosthesis. Resistance exercises for the deltoid, triceps, and biceps should be included depending on the location of the amputation. In the lower limb, flexion contracture at the hip can result from prolonged sitting up in bed. Hip extension can be maintained by lying prone for 5–10 min three times daily. If the individual has a BKA, focus should be on full extension at the knee and flexion to 90°. Pillows should not be placed under the knee as this leads to flexion contracture. Strengthening of the hip abductors is important in all lower limb amputations as is quadriceps strengthening for knee stabilization in a patient with a BKA.

Mobility and ADLs are impacted by limb loss so learning compensatory techniques for transfers, mobility, and self-care are important. Physical and occupational therapist will teach these techniques in the inpatient rehab setting. Wheelchairs are typically necessary for community distances and often for household distances. Safe transfers into and out of the wheelchair, the ability to manage footrests, and propulsion/steering are therefore important techniques to learn from the therapists. Having the capacity to independently perform self-care tasks in a seated position will allow the amputee to live in the community until they have a prosthesis.

Prosthetic fabrication can begin once the incision is well healed, sutures are removed, and the residual limb has undergone some initial shaping. A cast of the residual limb is taken that will be used to make the socket. Components are then added: the prosthetic elbows and knee for the above-joint amputations and terminal devices for below-joint amputations (hooks and feet).

Post-prosthetic training occurs in the outpatient setting and involves ongoing monitoring of the residual limb for skin breakdown from pressure points or shearing, pain management (usually neuropathic in nature), and learning to use the prosthesis for mobility. Regular follow-up with the prosthetist, rehabilitation physician, and physical therapist is therefore important for a favorable functional outcome in the trauma patient with amputation.

Cross-References

▶ Occupational Therapist
▶ Pain
▶ Physical Therapist
▶ Prosthetics

References

Warten S et al (1997) Phantom pain and sensation among British amputees. British J Anesth 78(6):652–659

Analgesia

▶ Sedation and Analgesia
▶ Sedation, Analgesia, Neuromuscular Blockade in the ICU

Anatomy, Cervical Spine

Patricia L. Zadnik and Daniel M. Sciubba
Department of Neurosurgery, The Johns Hopkins University School of Medicine, Baltimore, MD, USA

Definition

The occipitocervical junction is composed of two structurally distinct vertebrae: the atlas (C1) and axis (C2). C1 articulates directly with the inferior aspect of the occipital bone, and has no vertebral body. C2 has a protuberant vertebral body, the dens or odontoid process, which projects superiorly to articulate with the posterior aspect of the anterior arch of C1. This articulation is stabilized by the presence of a transverse ligament, (Fig. 1) as well as by the anterior and posterior atlantoaxial ligaments which continue inferiorly as the anterior and posterior longitudinal ligaments, respectively. The anterior and posterior longitudinal ligaments run longitudinally, adjacent to the anterior and posterior vertebral bodies, and the spinal interlaminar ligament runs posteriorly between the spinous processes. All cervical vertebral bodies have a foramen transversarium,

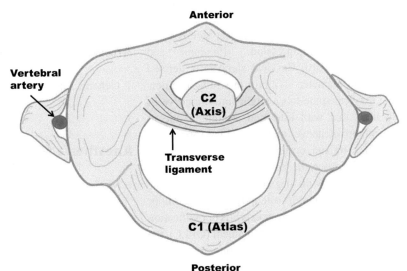

Anatomy, Cervical Spine, Fig. 1 The transverse ligament stabilizes the articulation of the odontoid process of *C2* (*axis*) with the posterior aspect of the anterior arch of *C1* (*atlas*). The vertebral artery is shown passing through the foramen transversarium

Anterior

Vertebral artery

C2 (Axis)

Transverse ligament

C1 (Atlas)

Posterior

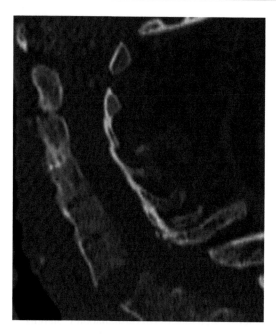

Anatomy, Cervical Spine, Fig. 2 Sagittal CT scan of a patient with ankylosing spondylitis demonstrating a displaced fracture at C5-C6 with a non-displaced fracture through the odontoid process of C2

through which the vertebral artery passes; however, the point of entry can be variable. (Fig. 1).

In the subaxial spine, C3-7, the uncinate process and uncus of adjacent cervical vertebral bodies articulate at the uncovertebral joints, or joints of Luschka. These joints decrease lateral flexion in the cervical spine. The spinal canal is widest at C1-C2 and considerably less spacious at C3-C7, predisposing this region to stenosis and spinal cord compression. (Pimentel and Diegelmann 2010) Cervical stenosis is defined as a canal diameter <12 mm in width. The normal cervical spine has a slight lordotic curve of 20–40 ° that with time can straighten due to degenerative changes and osteophyte formation.

When trauma occurs, the patient's age and anatomy impact the severity of the injury. In older patients with degenerative cervical spine disease with anterior osteophyte formation, or patients with ankylosing spondylitis or ossification of the posterior longitudinal ligament (OPLL), the anterior column is more brittle in resisting hyperflexion (Cusick and Yoganandan 2002) (Fig. 2). For patients with congenital stenosis of

the spinal column, any space-occupying mass (i.e., disk, bone fragment) or edema secondary to trauma will cause profound spinal cord compression.

Cross-References

▶ Clearance, Cervical Spine

References

Cusick JF, Yoganandan N (2002) Biomechanics of the cervical spine 4: major injuries. Clin Biomech (Bristol, Avon) 17(1):1–20

Pimentel L, Diegelmann L (2010) Evaluation and management of acute cervical spine trauma. Emerg Med Clin North Am 28(4):719–738

Anesthesia

▶ General Anesthesia for Major Trauma

Anesthesia Equipment Preparation

▶ Operating Room Setup for Trauma Anesthesia

Anesthesia Induction

▶ General Anesthesia for Major Trauma

Anesthesia Machine

▶ Mechanical Ventilation in the OR

Anesthesia Ventilator

▶ Mechanical Ventilation in the OR

Anesthesia Workstation

▶ Mechanical Ventilation in the OR

Anesthetic Drugs

▶ General Anesthesia for Major Trauma

Angioembolization

▶ Adjuncts to Damage Control Laparotomy: Endovascular Therapies

Angiography

▶ Imaging of Aortic and Thoracic Injuries

Ankle Bone

▶ Talus Fractures

Ankle Fractures

Jodi Siegel[1] and Paul III Tornetta[2]
[1]Department of Orthopaedics, UMass Memorial Medical Center, University of Massachusetts Medical School, Worcester, MA, USA
[2]Department of Orthopaedic Surgery, Boston University Medical Center, Boston, MA, USA

Synonyms

Broken ankle; Maisonneuve fracture; Malleolus fracture; Pilon fracture; Plafond fracture

Definition

An ankle fracture is a break in one or more of the bones that contribute to the ankle mortise. The most common type of ankle fracture is due to a low-energy, twisting injury. This mechanism often leads to a lateral malleolus (distal fibula) fracture near the joint (Fig. 1). There may be an associated fracture to the medial malleolus and/or the posterior malleolus of the distal tibia. Most of the weight-bearing surface of the distal tibia is spared. Less commonly, a rotational injury will result in a Maisonneuve (proximal fibula) fracture, which functionally is considered an ankle fracture. The determination of associated ligament disruptions determines whether a rotational ankle fracture is stable or unstable and therefore the treatment method (Davidovitch and Egol 2010).

Axial load injuries result in a more severe type of ankle fracture commonly referred to as tibial pilon or tibial plafond fracture. The higher energy and direction of the injury causes damage to the cartilage (weight-bearing surface) of the distal tibia (Fig. 2). Unlike rotational ankle fractures in which treatment is designed to realign the mortise, pilon fracture requires reconstruction of the joint surface (Barei 2010).

Preexisting Condition

The ankle joint is composed of three bones: the fibula, the tibia, and the talus. The articulation is created by the talus superiorly with the tibial plafond, laterally with the lateral malleolus of the distal fibula, posteriorly with the posterior malleolus of the distal tibia, and medially with the medial malleolus of the tibia. These bones join together to form the ankle mortise, which is the joint that allows dorsiflexion (moving your foot toward your head) and plantar flexion (pointing your toes downward) of your foot. The ankle joint is considered a saddle joint with the dome of the talus being wider anteriorly than posteriorly. The wedge-shaped talus creates a stable bony articulation when the foot is in dorsiflexion and a more mobile articulation,

Lauge-Hansen Classification

Supination · Adduction (SA)

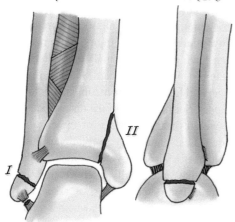

Pronation · Abduction (PA)

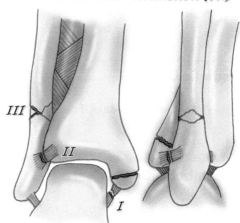

Supination · External Rotatioin (SER)

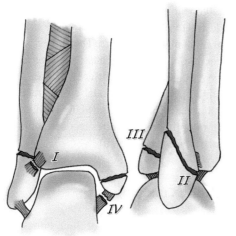

Pronation · External Rotation (PER)

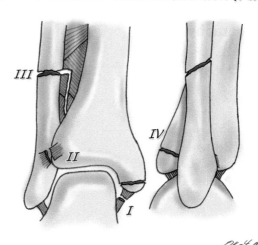

Ankle Fractures, Fig. 1 Schematic diagram of the Lauge-Hansen classification of rotational ankle fractures. The first part of the name indicates the position of the foot at the time of injury. The second part of the name describes the direction of the force applied to the foot (Credit Illustration by Louis Okafor)

requiring stability from the ankle ligaments, when the foot is in plantar flexion.

Understanding the ligamentous anatomy of the ankle is important for understanding rotational ankle fracture (Fig. 3). A lateral malleolus fracture can result in either a stable or an unstable ankle fracture (Lauge-Hansen 1950). This is determined by the competence of the medial structures. If the medial malleolus is not fractured, then the competence of the deltoid ligament determines the stability of the fractured ankle. An external rotation stress test performed under radiographic guidance allows dynamic examination of the mortise; if the deltoid ligament is intact, then the mortise will remain radiographically reduced with application of an external rotation moment. If the deltoid ligament is torn, the talus will subluxate laterally with stress, the medial clear space will widen, and an unstable ankle fracture is diagnosed.

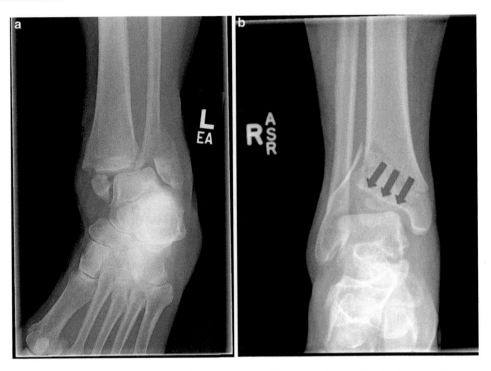

Ankle Fractures, Fig. 2 Anteroposterior radiographs of a bimalleolar, rotational ankle fracture (**a**) and an axial load tibial pilon type of ankle fracture (**b**). The higher-energy injury causes impaction of the articular (joint) surface (*arrows*)

The medial malleolus is composed of the anterior and posterior colliculi separated by the intercollicular groove. Medial malleolus fractures vary in size, and their effect on stability is determined based on fracture fragment size and the attachment sites of the deltoid ligament. The superficial deltoid ligament, which contributes minimally to ankle stability, attaches to the anterior colliculus, which is the most distal aspect of the medial malleolus. The deep deltoid ligament, which is the strongest and thickest component of the deltoid ligament complex, attaches to the posterior colliculus and the intercollicular groove. Supracollicular medial malleolus fractures, which render the deep deltoid ligament functionless, result in unstable ankle fractures. Likewise, an anterior colliculus fracture can be associated with a stable ankle facture if the deep deltoid ligament is not torn from the intact intercollicular groove.

The main ligamentous complex of the ankle is the syndesmosis, which is the distal tibiofibular articulation. It is stabilized by four ligaments that secure the fibula to the tibia. Rotational ankle fractures can be associated with injury to the syndesmosis, and a high index of suspicion is necessary to not miss these disruptions. Syndesmotic injuries require accurate reduction and stabilization, and they take a longer time to heal. Missed injuries are associated with poorer outcomes.

Injuries to the weight-bearing surface of the distal tibia typically are the result of high-energy, axial load mechanisms. The bony injury often includes significant articular comminution as the dome of the talus is driven into the tibial plafond (Reudi and Allgower 1969). Due to the viscoelastic properties of the bone, the energy of the mechanism is absorbed until failure. At failure, the energy is released into the surrounding soft tissue envelope resulting in significant swelling and blistering despite the lack of direct trauma. Although the differences in the bony injuries between rotational and axial load ankle fractures are radiographically apparent, it is this injury to the soft tissues that demands respect to avoid wound complications, soft tissue necrosis, and

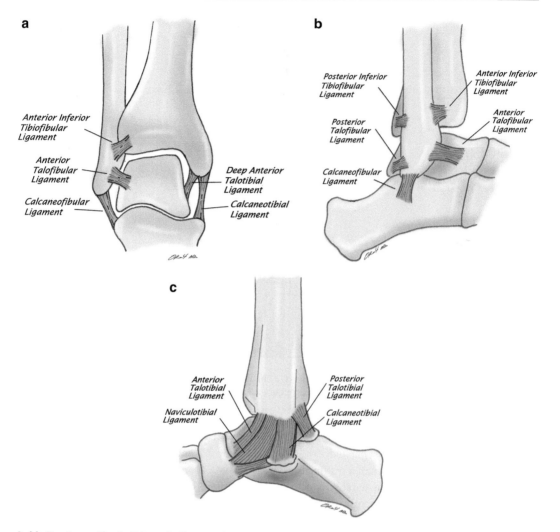

Ankle Fractures, Fig. 3 Schematic diagram of bony and ligamentous anatomy of the ankle. (**a**) Coronal view of ankle ligaments. (**b**) Lateral ankle ligaments. (**c**) Medial ligament complex (Credit Illustrations by Louis Okafor)

deep infection (Marsh et al. 2007). Although staged fixation, with temporizing spanning external fixators to maintain fracture length while allowing the soft tissues to heal before open reduction and internal fixation, has decreased soft tissue complications, consistently satisfactory outcomes still remains elusive.

Application

Evaluation

Successful treatment of patients with either rotational or axial load ankle fractures begins with an accurate diagnosis of the injury and an understanding of the patient. A thorough history and physical examination will identify mechanism and associated medial comorbidities that affect decision-making and overall care of the patient. Diabetes mellitus and cigarette smoking are known risk factors for complications and poor outcomes; discussing this with patients preoperatively may assist in behavior modification or surgical planning. Identification of various soft tissue issues including open wounds and exposed fractures determines surgical timing. Neurovascular compromise is important to discover and accurately document at the time of injury.

Radiographic evaluation includes plain films of the tibia, ankle, and foot. For rotational ankle fractures, this is often all that is required to make an accurate diagnosis of the injury. If the ankle mortise is well aligned, the decision as to whether to perform an external rotation stress test should be considered to determine ankle stability. Stress-negative lateral malleolus fractures can be treated with immediate weight-bearing. Unstable fractures with a widened mortise or a frank tibiotalar dislocation must be reduced, externally immobilized, and kept non-weight-bearing until definitive treatment options are determined.

Axial load, closed, tibial pilon fractures also require initial plain radiographs to obtain the bony diagnosis and external mobilization to stabilize the fracture and prevent any further soft tissue injury, but these fractures will often proceed to the operating theater within 6–12 h for a spanning external fixator to restore length to the fracture while providing bony and soft tissue stability. Once the fracture is out to length, then a CT scan is often obtained to allow for surgical planning of these complicated fractures.

Treatment

Most tibial pilon fractures and many ankle fractures that will be treated surgically are done so on a delayed basis. Patients will be required to adhere to strict elevation to allow resolution of swelling and healing of the soft tissues. Once adequate skin wrinkles are present, indicating decreased swelling, and any associated fracture blisters have healed, a safer surgical approach can be performed.

Unstable rotational ankle fractures that can be held with a reduced ankle mortise in a cast until fracture union can be successfully treated nonoperatively. If the mortise cannot be maintained with external immobilization, then surgical management is indicated. For lateral malleolus fractures, this typically means aligning the bone and holding it together with a plate and screws. Large medial malleolus fractures are frequently repaired with open reduction and screw-only fixation, with only certain fracture patterns requiring plate stabilization. If the distal tibiofibular syndesmosis is unstable, which is often determined at the time of surgery, it will also be reduced and stabilized with screws that cross from the fibula into the tibia. Postoperatively, patients will be immobilized for 2–6 weeks and weight-bearing will be limited for 6–12 weeks depending on bony healing and the status of the syndesmosis.

Definitive surgical management of tibial pilon fractures is delayed until the soft tissue envelope has healed and swelling has resolved so as to decrease wound complications. In some patients with closed injuries, the soft tissue injury is so severe that the skin never becomes amenable to safe internal fixation. In these patients, the fractures can be treated definitively in an external fixator. Either the temporary spanning frame can be used or the patient can return to the operating theater for conversion to a hybrid frame.

In those patients who have resolution of swelling, an open reduction and stabilization with plates and screws can be performed. Careful soft tissue handling intraoperatively is required to avoid additional surgical trauma to the tissues. Often the external fixator is removed and the patient is immobilized postoperatively in a splint or cast until the wounds have healed. Range of motion is started early to decrease stiffness and promote cartilage nutrition. Weight-bearing is limited for 8–12 weeks until bony union.

Outcomes

Infection rates are low with low-energy, rotational ankle fractures, ranging from 2 % to 5 % in the literature. Functional outcomes are known to continue to improve for up to a year after injury. Several recent long-term follow-up papers have reported good to excellent outcomes in 90 % of ankle fracture with a reduced mortise at bony union treated either surgically or nonsurgically. Alternatively, in patients with syndesmotic injuries, the outcomes are less favorable. Limited range of motion is a common long-term complaint. Accurate reduction of the fibula to the tibia can be challenging and should be done under direct visualization when there is any concern for malalignment. Multiple recent studies have shown that malreduction of the syndesmosis and a missed syndesmotic injury are known to have poorer outcomes.

Outcomes of tibial pilon fractures are often determined by the associated complications. Metaphyseal comminution and severe damage to the articular surface from the original injury make anatomic reconstruction difficult. Wound healing complications that can lead to deep infection are not uncommon when surgical management is performed through injured soft tissues. Malunion, posttraumatic arthrosis and scarring, and stiffness are not infrequent. Modern treatment techniques, including recognition of patient-specific factors, are aimed at reducing post-operative complications to optimize outcomes.

Acknowledgments The authors would like to thank Louis Okafor, M. D., for his skillful artwork used in this manuscript.

Cross-References

▶ Compartment Syndrome of the Leg
▶ External Fixation
▶ Falls from Height
▶ Open Fractures
▶ Principles of External Fixation

References

Barei D (2010) Pilon fractures. In: Rockwood and green's fractures in adults, 7th edn. Lippincott Williams Wilkins, Philadelphia, pp 1928–1974
Davidovitch R, Egol K (2010) Ankle Fractures. In: Rockwood and green's fractures in adults, 7th edn. Lippincott Williams Wilkins, Philadelphia, pp 1975–2021
Lauge-Hansen N (1950) Fractures of the ankle. II. Combined experimental-surgical and experimental-roentgenologic investigations. Arch Surg 60(5): 957–985
Marsh J, Borelli J, Dirschl D, Sirkin M (2007) Fractures of the tibial plafond. Instr Course Lect 56:331–352
Reudi T, Allgower M (1969) Fractures of the lower end of the tibia into the ankle-joint. Injury 1(2):92–99

Anoxic Hypoxia

▶ Hypoxemia, Severe

Anterior Cord Syndrome

MariaLisa Itzoe and Daniel M. Sciubba
Department of Neurosurgery, The Johns Hopkins University School of Medicine, Baltimore, MD, USA

Synonyms

Anterior spinal artery syndrome

Definition

Anterior cord syndrome (ACS), also known as anterior spinal artery syndrome, usually results from a hyperflexion injury or a horizontally oriented force that causes compression of the anterior artery which runs along the midline anterior to the spinal cord. Occlusion of the anterior spinal artery may result from trauma, disk herniation, osteophyte formation, iatrogenically induced surgical compression, or ligation of the anterior cord and its feeder vessels (Schneider 2010; Triggs and Beric 1992; Foo and Rossier 1983). Patients with damage to the anterior spinal cord frequently present with isolated motor deficits below the level of injury. Dissociated sensory loss can occur in which fine touch, pain and temperature sensation are compromised, but proprioception, joint position sense, and vibration sense are preserved (Foo and Rossier 1983). The extent of the motor deficit depends on the severity of damage and can range from paresis to complete muscle paralysis, affecting the lower extremities more than the upper extremities. Loss of bladder and bowel control have been known to occur in certain cases. Due to spinal shock, patients might initially present with flaccid paralysis and areflexia below the lesion. Dyesthesias can result in the development of muscle spacticity (Triggs and Beric 1992). Compression of the ventral (anterior) cord roots results in localized weakness in the muscles connected directly to injury sites, with subsequent atrophy of muscles unless compression is resolved. Small involuntary contractions or fasciculations of muscles may also be exhibited.

Patients with ACS injuries tend to require a protracted length of hospital stay compared to other SCI patients, and their prognosis is least favorable due to severe compromise of motor function. (McKinley et al. 2007) Only 10–15 % of patients demonstrate functional recovery; however, long-term outcomes are improved in cases where some pain or motor sensation below the lesion site is preserved (Foo and Rossier 1983). For example, patients with intact pin-prick sensation have been found to have significantly greater likelihood of regaining ambulation compared to those who retain only light touch sensation (Kirshblum and O'Connor 1998).

Cross-References

▶ Fractures
▶ Fracture, Flexion Injury

References

Foo D, Rossier AB (1983) Anterior spinal artery syndrome and its natural history. Paraplegia 21(1):1–10
Kirshblum SC, O'Connor KC (1998) Predicting neurologic recovery in traumatic cervical spinal cord injury. Arch Phys Med Rehabil 79(11):1456–1466
McKinley W, Santos K, Meade M, Brooke K (2007) Incidence and outcomes of spinal cord injury clinical syndromes. J Spinal Cord Med 30(3):215–224
Schneider GS (2010) Anterior spinal cord syndrome after initiation of treatment with atenolol. J Emerg Med 38(5):e49–e52
Triggs WJ, Beric A (1992) Sensory abnormalities and dysaesthesias in the anterior spinal artery syndrome. Brain 115(Pt 1):189–198

Anterior Spinal Artery Syndrome

▶ Anterior Cord Syndrome

Anterior Subluxation

▶ Fracture, Flexion Injury

Anti-A Antibody

▶ Blood Group Antibodies

Antiaggregants

▶ Anticoagulation/Antiplatelet Agents and Trauma

Anti-B Antibody

▶ Blood Group Antibodies

Antibiotic Therapy

Andrew M. Morris
Department of Medicine, Mount Sinai Hospital, University Health Network and University of Toronto, Toronto, ON, Canada

Synonyms

Antibiotic treatment; Anti-infective therapy; Antimicrobial therapy

Definition

Patients who have undergone trauma are at risk of infections related both to the trauma and to the sequelae of receiving trauma care (i.e., nosocomial infections). In this entry, I will explore antimicrobial (also known as antibiotic) therapy as it relates to these issues, with a focus on stewarding of antimicrobials in an era of drug resistance and an antimicrobial pipeline that is drying up.

Introduction

When Sir Alexander Fleming first discovered penicillin in 1929, it marked the realization that naturally occurring molds produced chemicals that could predictably (and reproducibly) counter bacterial infection. It took over a decade, however, for scientists at Pfizer to be able to mass-produce human-grade penicillin. Unfortunately, shortly after the introduction of penicillin into human clinical use in 1946, penicillin resistance appeared in staphylococci. The history of antimicrobial therapy since 1946 has been a consistent battle between antibiotic development and bacterial antibiotic resistance. Unfortunately, the last few decades have seen a dramatic decline in antimicrobial development, coinciding with an unprecedented increase (and appreciation) of antimicrobial-resistant organisms. For the traumatologist, the need to recognize the potential for drug-resistant organisms (making choosing empiric antimicrobial therapy a challenge) must be countered by the need to minimize unnecessary antimicrobials to prevent the growth of antimicrobial-resistant organisms.

Antibiotics are chemicals or medications that either kill or inhibit the growth of microorganisms. Traditionally, the term "antibiotic" was used by Selman Waksman to refer to a chemical produced by microorganisms to inhibit or kill the growth of competing microorganisms; the source of antibiotics are usually fungi. Nowadays, some chemicals in use are not produced by other microorganisms and, technically, are not antibiotics but remain under a more generic heading of "antimicrobial." The terms "antibiotic" and "antimicrobial" are generally used interchangeably.

Prophylaxis
Trauma-related infections arise, primarily, from penetrating wounds and animal bites. Applicable to the following discussion, it is important to recognize that antimicrobials should no longer be seen as a low-risk intervention. Globally, antimicrobial stewardship initiatives targeting the unnecessary use of antimicrobials have been gathering momentum, led by organizations such as the World Health Organization, the European Centre for Disease Prevention and Control, and the US Centers for Disease Control and Prevention. Complications resulting from antimicrobial use include adverse drug effects including allergies, drug-resistant organisms, and *C. difficile*. These consequences have been increasingly recognized in trauma centers, with prolonged and unnecessarily broad antimicrobials.

Tetanus
The most well-recognized such infection is tetanus, or "lockjaw," arising from the introduction of *Clostridium tetani* spores. Tetanus is a disease of global importance, with spores found widely in soil, feces, and dust. It is rare in developed countries (with approximately 30 cases annually in the United States or less than 1 case per million population), owing to the success of primary immunization schedules. In recent years, tetanus has been increasingly associated with injection drug use (Kretsinger et al. 2006).

Tetanus most commonly follows lacerations associated with necrotic tissue, although frequently occurs with blunt trauma. Clinical tetanus, generally occurring 3–21 days following inoculation, results from the production of a neurotoxin released from the replication of the bacterium that occurs in the presence of necrotic tissue.

Prophylaxis following trauma ("postexposure prophylaxis") is focused on cleaning the wound, debriding necrotic/devascularized tissue (to prevent spore production), and neutralizing toxin. The primary method of toxin neutralization is immunization, of which a detailed discussion is beyond the scope of this chapter. Most importantly, for patients in whom immunization is unknown, uncertain, or incomplete, tetanus immunoglobulin should be administered for all but clean, minor wounds.

There is no role for antimicrobial tetanus prophylaxis, as antimicrobials do not act on spores or the neurotoxin and are not delivered to devitalized tissue, the site of toxin production.

Open Fractures

Bony infection is a relatively frequent occurrence following trauma, when open fractures are present. In 1974, Patzakis demonstrated that prophylactic antimicrobial therapy for 10 days with cephalothin, a first-generation cephalosporin, following soft tissue trauma with bony exposure resulted in markedly fewer bony infections than placebo (2.3 % vs. 13.9 %); similar results were not seen with penicillin and streptomycin compared with placebo (9.7 % vs. 13.9 %). Subsequent studies have shown that short-course (i.e. single-dose pre-operative) antimicrobials are as effective as more prolonged courses. Coupled with the recognition that hand-trauma with open fractures rarely results in subsequent infection, it is reasonable to conclude that single-dose prophylaxis with a first-generation cephalosporin (usually cefazolin) is the most appropriate regimen.

Chest Trauma

Chest trauma is complicated by empyema and pneumonia in upwards of 7.6 % and 16 % of patients, respectively. Empyema tends to follow penetrating trauma, whereas pneumonia tends to follow blunt trauma. Observational studies have tended to report lower risks of infectious complications compared to randomized trials, and whether or not prophylactic antimicrobials are beneficial is a point of considerable debate. A meta-analysis of the available evidence, exploring 5 randomized, controlled trials, concluded that antimicrobial prophylaxis significantly reduced complications of empyema (RR = 0.19) and pneumonia (RR = 0.44) following chest trauma. In contradistinction to this, the largest trial performed in this area (which was included in the aforementioned meta-analysis) failed to show a benefit from cefazolin prophylaxis, with a 4.3 % absolute reduction in empyema but an accompanying 5 % increase in pneumonia. This may have been due to an underpowered study (the study was halted at 224 patients due to poor patient accrual), because of differences in proportion of blunt versus penetrating trauma in this study or because antimicrobial prophylaxis is ineffective. If antimicrobial prophylaxis is beneficial in chest trauma, then its benefit is most likely limited to penetrating rather than blunt trauma to reduce empyema. Cefazolin appears to be the most reasonable choice of agent.

Penetrating Abdominal Trauma

Antimicrobial prophylaxis following penetrating abdominal trauma has been practiced since the advent of antimicrobials, with the benefits of its use first being demonstrated during World War II. Subsequent studies demonstrated that antimicrobial prophylaxis was beneficial and that the prophylaxis required coverage of both aerobic and anaerobic bacteria. These studies also fairly conclusively demonstrated that the antimicrobials were beneficial when given preoperatively. However, more recently, the need for antimicrobial prophylaxis in this setting has been questioned, primarily where there is no fecal soiling of the peritoneum. In particular, some have questioned the ongoing necessity for antimicrobial prophylaxis when surgical asepsis and instrument sterilization standards are so high. Unfortunately, since the mid-1970s, there have been no placebo-controlled studies evaluating the utility of antimicrobial prophylaxis in penetrating abdominal trauma (Brand et al. 2009). We are left with guidelines that strongly advocate preoperative antimicrobial prophylaxis with aerobic and anaerobic activity in the setting of penetrating abdominal trauma and to continue the same antimicrobials for no more than 24 h in the setting of a perforated viscus. The ideal regimen is unclear. Indeed, there have been numerous studies in the 1980s and 1990s comparing different regimens. Cefazolin + metronidazole or a 3rd-generation cephalosporin (e.g., cefotaxime or ceftriaxone) + metronidazole seems the most prudent regimen, although clindamycin plus gentamicin or clindamycin plus a fluoroquinolone is acceptable in the setting of β-lactam allergy.

Human Bites

Human bites result in relatively minor trauma, most commonly involving the hand. Organisms most commonly isolated (in descending order of frequency) are *Streptococcus anginosus* (52 %), *Staphylococcus aureus* (30 %), *Eikenella corrodens* (30 %), *Fusobacterium nucleatum* (32 %), and *Prevotella melaninogenica* (22 %). Relatively frequent complications of clenched fist bite wounds include tenosynovitis, osteomyelitis, and septic arthritis. Because of this, most authorities recommend a short (approximately 3–5 day) course of antimicrobial "prophylaxis" targeting the most frequently identified organisms. Amoxicillin-clavulanic acid, moxifloxacin, and ciprofloxacin or levofloxacin plus metronidazole are all reasonable choices of agents.

Animal Bites

Trauma resulting from dog bites uncommonly get infected. When they do get infected, the most common causative organisms are *Pasteurella canis*, *Streptococcus* spp., *Staphylococcus* species, and anaerobes (Talan et al. 1999). Common practice has been not administer antimicrobial prophylaxis following dog bites. However, in a recent randomized controlled trial, 4 % of dog bites treated with placebo became infected, whereas no dog bites treated with 3 days of amoxicillin-clavulanic acid developed a subsequent infection by 2 weeks. On the basis of this information (with a number needed to treat of 25), it seems prudent to administer prophylaxis for dog bites with 3 days of amoxicillin-clavulanate. An equally acceptable regimen (in the setting of β-lactam allergy) would be moxifloxacin, or ciprofloxacin or levofloxacin plus metronidazole.

In contradistinction to dog bites, cat bites commonly get infected, with an infection rate as high as 80 %. The lower incisors of cats are the sharper of the biting teeth and commonly reach bone, especially in the hand. The spectrum of bacteria is fairly similar to dogs, apart from the fact that *Pasteurella multocida* is a causative agent in 75 % of cases (Talan et al. 1999). There have been no trials evaluating antimicrobial prophylaxis following cat bites. Regimens used in dog bites are equally acceptable.

Ventilator-Associated Pneumonia

Although a fuller discussion of ventilator-associated pneumonia is below (under **Nosocomial Infection**), it is worthwhile to discuss its prevention here. The pathogenesis of essentially all forms of bacterial pneumonia is colonization of the upper airway with potentially pathogenic organisms (perhaps originating from the digestive tract), followed by aspiration and subsequent replication of these bacteria in the lower respiratory tract. A recent approach to reducing the incidence of VAP has been selective decontamination of the digestive tract (SDD) and selective oropharyngeal decontamination (SOD) (de Smet et al. 2009). SDD uses a combination of systemic and nonabsorbable enteral antimicrobials to reduce the presence of pathogenic organisms in the digestive tract. SOD, on the other hand, uses topical oral antimicrobials to decontaminate the oropharynx. This approach has not been widely adopted, mainly due to concerns about the emergence of drug-resistant organisms in the ICU. In what would seem to have been a definitive trial on this approach to antimicrobial therapy (following numerous smaller studies, including one study in trauma patients), de Smet and colleagues demonstrated that SDD and SOD reduced overall mortality by 3.5 % and 2.9 %, respectively, while reducing the overall use of antimicrobials in treated patients in a cluster randomized trial in the Netherlands. Unfortunately, debate has continued, led by concerns of the emergence of drug-resistant organisms in the ICU.

Nosocomial Infection

Although there are myriad potential nosocomial infectious complications in patients admitted to hospital with trauma, aside from infection directly related to the trauma or surgical site, the majority of such infections are due to pneumonia, bloodstream infections, and urinary tract infection.

Ventilator-Associated Pneumonia

Ventilator-associated pneumonia (VAP) is generally defined as pneumonia acquired more than 48 h after being intubated. Numerous criteria for defining VAP (including the increasingly used clinical pulmonary infection score or CPIS) have been proposed, but most lack proper validation. Indeed, there is reasonable evidence that CPIS is not useful when used with trauma patients, lacking both sensitivity and specificity (Croce et al. 2006; Parks et al. 2012). In particular, CPIS appears to overdiagnose pneumonia and would result in overuse of antimicrobials. In response to many challenges that VAP definitions have posed, the US Centers for Disease Control have revised surveillance definitions for VAP. Further discussion of the challenges of the definition (and there are many) is beyond the scope of this chapter.

Treatment Once VAP has been diagnosed, the approach to therapy is equally complicated. Perhaps the most accurate statement is the simultaneously specific and vague statement that antimicrobial therapy should be targeted to the specific patient's pathogen, accounting for local resistance and susceptibility data. Despite this, what follows is a synopsis of the current available evidence for antimicrobial therapy in VAP:

(a) Initial treatment should be active against organisms circulating in your unit at the time and likely to colonize your patient. This demands close collaboration with the microbiology laboratory. Whether **all** potential organisms should be treated up-front is unclear at present, although few would question the need to cover **most** potential organisms.

(b) Therapy for 8 days is sufficient for most cases of VAP (and many centers assume 7 days would suffice). In a randomized controlled trial, patients with VAP due to *S. aureus* or non-lactose-fermenting agents (e.g., *Pseudomonas*) were more likely to have a recurrence with 8 days therapy compared with 15 days, but resistance was less and mortality was not different (Chastre et al. 2003).

(c) Patients who undergo bronchoalveolar lavage (BAL) with quantitative cultures can safely have treatment tailored to the culture results. Patients with negative cultures can have their antibiotics discontinued.

(d) If choosing to routinely use broad-spectrum empiric antimicrobials in patients at relatively low risk of drug-resistant organisms, there is no need to proceed to BAL: endotracheal tube sampling is sufficient guidance for therapy.

(e) Patients with a low risk of having VAP according to a clinical pulmonary infection score (CPIS) ≤ 6 can safely be treated with a short course (3 days) of antibiotics; withholding antibiotics altogether in this group may also be reasonable, although has not been formally evaluated.

(f) There are no clinical benefits apparent from combination antibiotic therapy compared to monotherapy for VAP, as long as the spectrum of activity closely mirrors the microbial ecology of the patients being treated (Heyland et al. 2008).

With regard to specific agents, there is limited reliable evidence guiding our therapeutic choices. One of the more common issues that have emerged has been the management of methicillin-resistant *S. aureus* (MRSA) pneumonia. Options for MRSA include trimethoprim-sulfamethoxazole (TMP-SMX), doxycycline, vancomycin, linezolid, and daptomycin. For MRSA VAP, daptomycin is not a therapeutic option because it is inactivated by surfactant. There is, unfortunately, little data in the way of TMP-SMX or doxycycline. On the other hand, a recent randomized trial compared linezolid with vancomycin for confirmed MRSA pneumonia. This trial randomized 448 patients to either linezolid or vancomycin. Mortality did not differ between treatment arms, nor did clinical cure according to intention-to-treat analysis.

Catheter-Related Bloodstream Infection

Catheter-related bloodstream infection (CRBI) is bacteremia or fungemia that originates from an intravascular catheter. For the purpose of this chapter, CRBI will be limited to catheters that are usually inserted and removed in trauma units (or emergency rooms) and will not include tunneled catheters or other long-term catheters. CRBI most commonly originates from the skin insertion site, with microorganisms traveling along the course of the vascular catheter into the bloodstream. Less often, organisms contaminate the catheter hub and travel intraluminally. The study of CRBI has been complicated by the lack of a definition that is both sensitive and specific. Fever and other clinical criteria are sensitive but nonspecific, whereas repeatedly positive blood cultures drawn from the periphery and vascular catheter with identical organisms in the presence of clinical signs of infection without other primary foci are specific but insensitive. For this reason, catheter-associated bloodstream infection is often measured, which identifies bacteremia in the presence of a vascular catheter, but may not be caused by the catheter.

Treatment of CRBI begins with removal of the vascular catheter when infection is suspected. In many cases, this proves curative, with fever abating and leukocytosis resolving without need for antimicrobials. Clearly, however, this requires further study. Optimal treatment of documented CRBI requires (a) removal of the catheter (where feasible) and (b) antimicrobial therapy.

Treatment Catheter removal for CRBI is always preferred; however, situations do occur when this is not feasible or desired. In such situations, options include *antibiotic lock therapy*, whereby an aliquot of antibiotic is left in the catheter hub and tubing continuously. This is only likely to be beneficial for patients with CRBI due to an intraluminal infection and is not supported by high-quality trials. Some experts recommend retaining the vascular catheter for CRBI due to coagulase-negative staphylococci, but the recurrence risk is high.

Empiric Therapy Empiric treatment for CRBI, as with all nosocomial infections, should be based on the likely organism coupled with severity of illness. For many such infections, patients will be hemodynamically stable, and treatment of the most likely pathogens (usually staphylococci) will suffice. In centers with a high prevalence of methicillin-resistant *S. aureus* (MRSA), vancomycin is likely an appropriate empiric therapy. However, it may be reasonable to consider a methicillin-like penicillin (e.g., cloxacillin) or 1st-generation cephalosporin in stable patients.

Pathogen-Specific Therapy Coagulase-negative staphylococci: Removal of the catheter is often sufficient, but many authorities recommend 5–7 days' therapy, unless there is no other medical hardware in situ, the vascular catheter has been removed, the patient is hemodynamically stable, and repeat blood cultures are negative. No approach has been formally evaluated with

randomized controlled trials. *S. lugdunensis* is a coagulase-negative staphylococcus that should be treated as *S. aureus*.

S. aureus: Treatment should be based on susceptibilities. The most effective therapy for methicillin-susceptible *S. aureus* is a ß-lactam, such as cloxacillin or cefazolin. However, in cases of severe allergy or resistance, vancomycin is a preferred agent. Recently, concerns have been raised regarding the effectiveness and safety of vancomycin, especially with the emergence of strains that are either resistant to or have reduced susceptibility to vancomycin. However, a recent open-label non-inferiority trial comparing linezolid with vancomycin for CRBI showed a trend favoring vancomycin in intention-to-treat analysis. Optimal duration of therapy for *S. aureus* CRBI is unclear. Although teaching for many years has maintained the axiom "treat for 2 weeks if a removable focus of infection, and it has been removed," recent studies have questioned this wisdom with the recognition that (a) infective endocarditis may complicate up to 13 % of catheter-associated bacteremia and (b) that infective endocarditis and other complications may be seen in approximately 6 % of cases of *S. aureus* CRBI treated with 2 weeks' therapy (compared with 4 weeks). I generally prefer 4 weeks of therapy unless a trans-esophageal echocardiogram is performed and is negative (making endocarditis highly unlikely), which is largely consistent with recent recommendations (Mermel et al. 2009).

Enterococci: The optimal treatment of enterococci is ampicillin; if unable to use ampicillin because of resistance or allergy, then vancomycin is the preferred agent. Linezolid or daptomycin are options for when ampicillin or vancomycin cannot be used, although there is limited experience with these agents. The duration of treatment for enterococcal bacteremia is unclear, although 7 days is usually sufficient (Havey et al. 2011). The risk of subsequent infective endocarditis is quite low, estimated at around 1 %.

Gram-negative bacilli: The optimal treatment of Gram-negative bacilli (GNB) is dependent on local susceptibilities. Empiric choices prior to speciation should cover the majority of possibilities and may include combination therapy (especially if the patient is neutropenic, severely ill, or known to be colonized with multidrug-resistant organisms). However, there is weak evidence supporting combination therapy once susceptibility is known, including therapy for non-lactose-fermenting agents such as *Pseudomonas aeruginosa*. The optimal duration of therapy is also unknown, although 7 days is usually sufficient (Havey et al. 2011).

Candida species: Candidemia is a frequent cause of CRBI in patients who have been receiving prolonged broad-spectrum antibacterial agents, as well as patients receiving total parenteral nutrition, or who have received solid organ or stem cell transplantation. Empiric therapy should be based on local data but may include amphotericin B, fluconazole, or an echinocandin. These appear to be equally efficacious, although azole resistance has been rising in centers with high azole use. For this reason, many have recommended echinocandin therapy to be the first-line treatment. Candidemia is generally treated with 2 weeks of effective therapy, with the first negative blood culture being considered day 1.

Urinary Tract Infection Catheter-associated urinary tract infection (CAUTI) is generally defined as bacteriuria or candiduria (of at least 10^3 cfu/ml) in association with a urinary catheter. The definition has remained problematic, as it is ignores a central tenet in the management of infections: differentiating colonization from infection. In patients without urinary catheters, pyuria is strongly associated with urinary tract infection, but such a criterion has poor predictive value for CAUTI. A preferred definition would be the symptoms and signs of urinary tract infection accompanied by pyuria and greater than 10^3 cfu/ml microorganisms in association with a urinary catheter. The diagnosis of a urinary tract infection in trauma patients, nonetheless, is associated with a worse prognosis.

Treatment There are few randomized trials evaluating management of CAUTI. A small trial of catheter-associated bacteriuria in women (not in the ICU) demonstrated that asymptomatic bacteriuria frequently progressed to symptomatic CAUTI and that single-dose antibiotic treatment was equivalent to a 10-day course of therapy. Another recent trial compared short-course (3 days) antibiotics and catheter change with standard care (i.e., no change, no antibiotics) for patients with asymptomatic catheter-associated bacteriuria and found no difference in meaningful outcomes, including the development of pyelonephritis. Similarly, treatment of candiduria with fluconazole in immunocompetent patients temporarily eradicated the candiduria but failed to offer any long-term benefit (Sobel et al. 2000).

We are therefore left with data from non-catheterized patients with pyelonephritis to guide our management of symptomatic infection (i.e., pyelonephritis). Although the data are relatively limited, there is an emerging consensus that antimicrobial for 7 days with a fluoroquinolone (if the cultured organism is susceptible) is sufficient therapy for even rather severe cases of pyelonephritis (Sandberg et al. 2012; Talan et al. 2000). Moxifloxacin is not a therapeutic option, however, because of its very low concentrations in the urinary tract. Alternatives to 7 days of fluoroquinolone therapy include penicillins, cephalosporins, carbapenems, and trimethoprim-sulfamethoxazole; however, the current evidence does not support a duration shorter than 14 days when using these agents for pyelonephritis.

Summary

Antimicrobial therapy for patients with trauma is most commonly used in the setting of prophylaxis or for common nosocomial infections such as pneumonia, bloodstream infections, and urinary tract infections. Treatment should always be targeted towards identified pathogens, and duration should be kept to a minimum which, for most scenarios, is approximately 7 days.

Cross-References

▶ Catheter Associated Urinary Tract Infection
▶ Catheter-Related Infections

▶ Central Line Associated Blood Stream
  Infection
▶ Fungal Infections
▶ Neurotrauma, Infectious Considerations
▶ Sepsis, Treatment of
▶ Surgical Site Infections
▶ Tetanus
▶ Ventilator-Associated Pneumonia

References

Brand M, Goosen J, Grieve A (2009) Prophylactic antibiotics for penetrating abdominal trauma. Cochrane
Database Syst Rev 4:CD007370, Epub 2009/10/13

Chastre J, Wolff M, Fagon JY, Chevret S, Thomas F,
Wermert D et al (2003) Comparison of 8 vs 15 days
of antibiotic therapy for ventilator-associated pneumonia in adults: a randomized trial. JAMA
290(19):2588–2598, Epub 2003/11/20

Croce MA, Swanson JM, Magnotti LJ, Claridge JA,
Weinberg JA, Wood GC et al (2006) The futility of the
clinical pulmonary infection score in trauma patients.
J Trauma 60(3):523–527; discussion 7–8. Epub 2006/
03/15

de Smet AM, Kluytmans JA, Cooper BS, Mascini EM,
Benus RF, van der Werf TS et al (2009) Decontamination of the digestive tract and oropharynx in ICU
patients. N Engl J Med 360(1):20–31, Epub 2009/01/02

Havey TC, Fowler RA, Daneman N (2011) Duration of
antibiotic therapy for bacteremia: a systematic review
and meta-analysis. Crit Care 15(6):R267, Epub 2011/
11/17

Heyland DK, Dodek P, Muscedere J, Day A, Cook D
(2008) Randomized trial of combination versus
monotherapy for the empiric treatment of suspected
ventilator-associated pneumonia. Crit Care Med
36(3):737–744, Epub 2007/12/20

Kretsinger K, Broder KR, Cortese MM, Joyce MP,
Ortega-Sanchez I, Lee GM et al (2006) Preventing
tetanus, diphtheria, and pertussis among adults: use
of tetanus toxoid, reduced diphtheria toxoid and acel-
lular pertussis vaccine recommendations of the Advisory Committee on Immunization Practices (ACIP)
and recommendation of ACIP, supported by the
Healthcare Infection Control Practices Advisory Committee (HICPAC), for use of Tdap among health-care
personnel. MMWR Recomm Rep 55(RR-17):1–37,
Epub 2006/12/15

Mermel LA, Allon M, Bouza E, Craven DE, Flynn P,
O'Grady NP et al (2009) Clinical practice guidelines
for the diagnosis and management of intravascular
catheter-related infection: 2009 update by the Infectious Diseases Society of America. Clin Infect Dis
49(1):1–45, Epub 2009/06/06

Parks NA, Magnotti LJ, Weinberg JA, Zarzaur BL,
Schroeppel TJ, Swanson JM et al (2012) Use of the
clinical pulmonary infection score to guide therapy for
ventilator-associated pneumonia risks antibiotic overex-
posure in patients with trauma. J Traumatol Acute Care
Surg 73(1):52–58; discussion 8–9. Epub 2012/06/30

Sandberg T, Skoog G, Hermansson AB, Kahlmeter G,
Kuylensterna N, Lannergard A et al (2012) Ciprofloxacin for 7 days versus 14 days in women with acute
pyelonephritis: a randomised, open-label and double-
blind, placebo-controlled, non-inferiority trial. Lancet
380(9840):484–490, Epub 2012/06/26

Sobel JD, Kauffman CA, McKinsey D, Zervos M,
Vazquez JA, Karchmer AW et al (2000) Candiduria:
a randomized, double-blind study of treatment with
fluconazole and placebo. The National Institute of
Allergy and Infectious Diseases (NIAID) Mycoses
study group. Clin Infect Dis 30(1):19–24

Talan DA, Citron DM, Abrahamian FM, Moran GJ, Goldstein EJ (1999) Bacteriologic analysis of infected dog
and cat bites. Emergency Medicine Animal Bite Infection Study Group. N Engl J Med 340(2):85–92, Epub
1999/01/14

Talan DA, Stamm WE, Hooton TM, Moran GJ, Burke T,
Iravani A et al (2000) Comparison of ciprofloxacin
(7 days) and trimethoprim-sulfamethoxazole
(14 days) for acute uncomplicated pyelonephritis in
women: a randomized trial. JAMA 283(12):
1583–1590, Epub 2000/03/29

Antibiotic Treatment

▶ Antibiotic Therapy

Antibody Screen

Harvey G. Hawes[1], Laura A. McElroy[2] and
Bryan A. Cotton[1]
[1]Department of Surgery, Division of Acute Care
Surgery, Trauma and Critical Care, University of
Texas Health Science Center at Houston, The
University of Texas Medical School at Houston,
Houston, TX, USA
[2]Department of Anesthesiology, Critical Care
Medicine, University of Rochester Medical
Center, Rochester, NY, USA

Synonyms

Type and screen

Definition

In transfusion medicine, an antibody screen refers to testing patient serum or plasma for unexpected alloantibodies to donor red cells. These IgG antibodies, which differ from antibodies to the ABO and Rh blood groups, are deemed clinically significant if they are known to cause transfusion reactions or hemolytic disease in newborns. An antibody screen, on top of blood type determination, makes up the standard "type and screen" and can correctly rule out clinically significant transfusion reaction over 99.94 % of the time (Reid 2010).

Donor plasma, as it is being processed, is tested to ensure no unexpected antibodies are transfused. Recipient plasma is tested against commercially prepared red blood cells (RBCs) in a warm agglutination reaction. These FDA-approved type O standard RBCs come from at least two donors and contain all of the common clinically significant D, C, E, c, e, M, N, S, s, P_1, Le^a, Le^b, K, k, Fy^a, Fy^b, Jk^a, and Jk^b antigens (Westhoff et al. 2012). A separate sample of the recipient's own red blood cells is run to check for potential autoantibodies.

The test, run in three phases, starts with a spin to exclude "nuisance" IgM antibodies, followed by an incubation at 37 °C and a Coombs test to check for agglutination of antibodies and red cells. A positive test will trigger further testing to elucidate the exact antibodies responsible and a further crossmatch (Reid 2010).

Cross-References

- ▶ Blood Group Antibodies
- ▶ Blood Type
- ▶ Crossmatch
- ▶ Rhesus Factor

References

Reid ME (2010) Erythrocyte antigens and antibodies, Chapter 137. In: Prchal JT, Kaushansky K, Lichtman MA, Kipps TJ, Seligsohn U (eds) Williams hematology, 8th edn. McGraw-Hill, New York

Westhoff C, Storry JR, Shaz BH (2012) Human blood group antigens and antibodies. Hematology: basic principles and practice, 6th edn. Churchill/Livingstone, London pp 1628–1641

Anticoagulation

- ▶ Neurotrauma, Anticoagulation Considerations
- ▶ Venous Thromboembolism Prophylaxis and Treatment Following Trauma

Anticoagulation/Antiplatelet Agents and Trauma

Davide Cattano[1] and Alberto Piacentini[2]
[1]Department of Anesthesiology, Memorial Hermann Hospital-TMC, The University of Texas Medical School at Houston, Houston, TX, USA
[2]Department of Emergency, Division of Anesthesiology and Intensive Care, SSuEm118, Sant'Anna Hospital, San Fermo della Battaglia, CO, Italy

Synonyms

Antiaggregants; Antiplatelet therapy; Antithrombotics; Blood thinners; Platelet aggregation inhibitors

Definition

Anticoagulation/antiplatelet agents are substances that hinder the clotting of blood by preventing the process of coagulation. Administered orally, subcutaneously, or intravenously, agents work in a variety of different ways. Anticoagulants interrupt blood coagulation pathways; antiplatelet therapy inhibits platelet aggregation or adhesion to vascular walls. Agents are used as primary or secondary prophylactics for cardiovascular and cerebrovascular disease, deep vein thrombosis, and pulmonary embolism.

Preexisting Condition

Anticoagulation Issues

Anticoagulation can be a temporary (i.e., intraoperatively for vascular surgery procedures) or chronic therapy for coexisting diseases such as:

- Atrial fibrillation
- Deep vein thrombosis
- Mechanical prosthetic heart valve

In the USA, the prevalence of atrial fibrillation (AF), a common arrhythmia, is close to 2.3 % of the population older than 40 and 5.9 % in patients above 65 years.

Antithrombotic Issues

Antiplatelet therapy is administered for conditions such as:

- Coronary artery disease (CAD)
- Cardiovascular disease (CVD)
- Coronary angioplasty/coronary stent placement
- Coronary ischemic event
- Vascular arterial disease (VAD)

Types of Therapies

Heparin

A commonly used anticoagulant, heparin functions by activating antithrombin III, which deactivates thrombin and other proteases, such as factor Xa. It can be given intravenously or subcutaneously, but not orally. Because there is a risk for heparin-induced thrombocytopenia, it is used primarily in hospitalized patients who can be observed by hospital staff. However, it is possible that patients can be prescribed injections of heparin on an outpatient basis. Due to heparin's short half-life, it is unlikely that trauma patients will have this drug in their systems unless they were recently discharged from the hospital.

Low-Molecular-Weight Heparin (LMWH)

Unlike naturally occurring heparin, which consists of molecular chains of varying lengths, low-molecular-weight heparin has a more uniform length of chains, and its effects are thus more predictable. Thus, LMWH can be administered subcutaneously with more predictable pharmacokinetics than natural heparin, and it can be used on an outpatient basis. A commonly prescribed LMWH is enoxaparin (Lovenox®). There is no effective or specific antidote to reverse rare but catastrophic bleeding complications that can occur with its use. Protamine sulfate only partially reverses the anticoagulant effects of LMWH and thus is not a reliable antidote. One mg of protamine could revert 1 mg LMWH. If APTT remains prolonged, a 2nd dose of 0.5 mg protamine per 1 mg LMWH may be given. Fresh frozen plasma (FFP), although a mainstay in UFH reversal, is a strategy which has been extrapolated to LMWH. Administration of large FFP volumes required to achieve normal hemostasis can lead increased intravascular volume and the potential development of congestive heart failure. Small "*off-label*" series demonstrated in clinical practice that in catastrophic bleeding secondary to LMWH use, rFVIIa concentrate at 20–30 mg/kg can restore hemostasis without precipitating additional thrombotic complications.

Warfarin (Coumadin®)

Warfarin is a vitamin K antagonist because it works by reducing the body's ability to produce vitamin K-dependent clotting factors. It is one of the most common oral anticoagulants prescribed. Great care must be taken when encountering patients on warfarin as research shows that the INR level of 56.2 % of trauma patients on warfarin is nontherapeutic (Anthony et al. 2011).

Hirudin

Hirudin is a proven potent thrombin inhibitor. It is an anticoagulant that, due to its limited supply in natural sources, is produced using recombinant technology.

Rivaroxaban (Xarelto®)

Rivaroxaban is an oral anticoagulant approved in Europe and the USA for prophylaxis of deep vein thrombosis and venous thromboembolism. An inhibitor of factor Xa, rivaroxaban has no measured effect on platelets or thrombin.

Dabigatran (Pradaxa®)

An oral anticoagulant used for prophylaxis of thromboembolic disease in patients who have undergone hip and knee surgery and strokes in patients with non-valvular atrial fibrillation, it functions by inhibiting thrombin development. Although preferred in some cases to warfarin due to its decreased risk of major bleeding events (Cotton et al. 2011b), dabigatran is irreversible. Despite initial enthusiasm for this agent, some concern emerged in acute injury patient: there is no readily available means for assessing the degree of anticoagulation with dabigatran. Today there is no readily available reversal strategy (antidote), and the only reversal option is emergency dialysis. Severely injured patients receiving dabigatran all demonstrated poor outcomes. Performing rapid dialysis in patients with bleeding whose condition is unstable or with expanding intracranial hemorrhage is practically impossible in local hospitals and an incredible challenge, even in a level 1 trauma centers. Despite normal screening coagulation laboratory test, rapid thromboelastography (r-TEG) at admission time can be altered. Activated clotting time on r-TEG (range, 86–118 s) is markedly prolonged.

Nonsteroidal Anti-inflammatory Drugs (NSAIDs)

The least potent of available antiplatelet therapies, NSAIDs prevent the clotting of blood by blocking the production of thromboxane A2 (TxA2) in platelets, which inhibits the platelets from clumping. NSAIDs accomplish this production by blocking cyclooxygenase-1 (COX 1), the enzyme that produces TxA2. Aspirin is the most commonly used NSAID because its effects last for days as opposed to the mere hours of other NSAIDs. It works on the adenosine diphosphate (ADP) channel, and a patient's responsiveness to it can be measured using platelet mapping assays.

Thienopyridines

This type of antiplatelet drug is an adenosine diphosphate (ADP) inhibitor which blocks the P2Y12 receptor on the platelet cell surface, thereby inhibiting the platelet clumping process. Examples of this type of drug include ticlopidine

(Ticlid) and clopidogrel (Plavix). In 2010, the Food and Drug Administration (FDA) released a warning on clopidogrel based on findings that patients with genetic differences in cytochrome P450 2C19 function may be unresponsive to therapy (Bansal et al. 2011). A large percentage of trauma patients (36.9 %) would be classified as clopidogrel resistant (Bansal et al. 2011). As the effectiveness of these drugs on a patient can be measured using platelet mapping assays that map the percent inhibition level of the arachidonic acid pathway, it is particularly important to test patients on clopidogrel to ascertain their level of responsiveness.

Glycoprotein IIb/IIIa Inhibitors

The most potent of available antiplatelet therapies, glycoproteins inhibit the stimulation response of platelets to clump by competing with the IIb and IIIa receptors on the platelet cell surface. Examples of this type of antiplatelet drug include abciximab (ReoPro), eptifibatide (Integrilin), and tirofiban (Aggrastat).

Dual-Antiplatelet Therapy

It is increasingly common for patients to be placed on dual-antiplatelet therapy (DAT) for increased protection against CVD and CAD. Combinations usually include a thienopyridine and aspirin.

Application

Therapy Effectiveness

Management decisions regarding patients on anticoagulation/antiplatelet agents are complicated by the variation in patient response to medications such as aspirin and clopidogrel (Cattano et al. 2013). Therefore, the use of point-of-care (POC) assays to measure platelet dysfunction is critical for guiding therapy in trauma patients where massive hemorrhage is a significant risk of mortality. The small sample size ($\approx$360 μL) and fast return of results ($\leq$15 min) are particularly advantageous for trauma patients, when loss of fluid volume is a concern and time is of the essence.

Prothrombin Time (PT)

Prothrombin time (PT) test is a test that measures how long it takes for blood to clot. PT measures factors I, II, V, VII, and X. Blood is drawn into a test tube that contains citrate, which binds the calcium in the sample. The mix is then placed in a centrifuge to separate the plasma from the blood cells. Tissue factor (factor III) is then added, and the time it takes for the sample to clot is measured by optical instruments.

Partial Thromboplastin Time (PTT)

Also known as the activated partial thromboplastin time (APTT), the PTT test evaluates blood's ability to clot. Often used in conjunction with the PT test, the PTT test uses different factors to check for bleeding irregularities. Blood samples are collected in tubes containing citrate and taken to a laboratory for testing. An activator and calcium are added to the sample, and the time it takes for a clot to form is measured. Coagulation factors I, II, V, VIII, IX, X, XI, and XII must be present in the sample for a normal PTT to result.

International Normalized Ratio (INR)

Because PT will differ according to the variations in manufacturers' tissue factor batches used in the reagent, the International Normalized Ratio (INR) was created to standardize times. By assigning an International Sensitivity Index (ISI) to every batch of tissue factor produced, each manufacturer identifies how closely each batch conforms to an international reference standard. The INR is obtained by dividing the patient's PT by the PT of a control sample and raising the dividend to the ISI of the tissue factor used (i.e., $INR = (PT_{Patient}/PT_{Control})^{ISI}$).

Activated Clotting Time (ACT)

Also known as activated coagulation time (ACT), this is a test of coagulation and is used to monitor the effects of heparin. It can also be used when the results of a PTT test are inconclusive or are taking too long to run.

Thromboelastography® (TEG®)

Trademarked by Haemoscope Corp. (Niles, IL, USA), thromboelastography (TEG) is a method for measuring coagulation that uses whole blood. A sample is taken from the patient and placed in an oscillating cuvette. If applicable, a thrombosis-inducing reagent (e.g., kaolin) is added to the cup and mixed by inversion immediately prior to testing. A piston is lowered into the cuvette, and a tracing is made based on the force the coagulating blood exerts on the piston. TEG provides patient overall percent inhibition level.

Rapid Thromboelastography® (r-TEG®)

A rapid thromboelastography (r-TEG) differs from a regular TEG because tissue factor, not kaolin, is added to the sample. The resulting reaction occurs much more rapidly than that of conventional TEG, and an analysis can therefore be made more quickly. The speed of returned early values has been documented at 5 min from drop-off of the specimen, making the r-TEG ideal for trauma patients (Cotton et al. 2011a).

Thromboelastography® with Platelet Mapping™ (TEG® with PM™)

In addition to providing the overall percent inhibition of a sample, TEG with Platelet Mapping (PM) also calculates the percent inhibition of the adenosine diphosphate (ADP) and arachidonic acid (AA) pathways. This information allows the determination of how responsive the patient is to antiplatelet therapy.

Rotational Thromboelastometry (ROTEM®)

Created by Tem Innovations GmbH (Munich, Germany), rotational thromboelastometry (ROTEM) functions similarly to TEG, except that the cuvette is stationary and it is the piston that rotates in ROTEM.

VerifyNow®

The VerifyNow-P2Y12 assay (Accumetrics, San Diego, CA, USA) has been validated to measure platelet inhibition in patients undergoing clopidogrel therapy as the combined use of aspirin does not affect it for tracking clopidogrel-induced platelet levels. A study by Bansal et al. (2011) recently found that a large percentage of trauma patients (36.9 %) would be classified as clopidogrel resistant. These results indicate that POC assays like the VerifyNow are essential in guiding the management of trauma patients who are on pre-injury anticoagulation/antiplatelet therapy.

Platelet Function Analyzer (PFA-100®)

Using whole blood, the platelet function analyzer (PFA-100) conducts a modified quantitative in vitro bleeding time under high-shear conditions.

Platelet Works®

A whole blood assay developed by Helena Laboratories (Beaumont, TX, USA), Platelet Works uses a Coulter counter to assess the platelet ratio of blood and determine platelet reactivity. Samples are placed in a standard ethylenediaminetetraacetic acid tube and a citrate tube, and their platelet counts are compared after activation with either ADP or collagen. Trauma patients can benefit from Platelet Works' ability to deliver results in 2 min. Because it provides the percent inhibition for the ADP and AA pathways, it is a useful tool for determining the level of response a patient has to antiplatelet therapy.

Multiplate®

The multiple platelet (Multiplate) function analyzer (Verum Diagnostica GmbH, Munich, Germay) is a whole blood assay that delivers results within 10 min. It provides the overall inhibition level of patients as well as the inhibition level of the ADP and AA pathways.

Management of Bleeding

For anticoagulant-related bleeding, prothrombin complex concentrates (PCCs) are recommended in both the USA and in Europe for emergency anticoagulant reversal. PCCs contain coagulation factor II, factor IX, factor X, and factor VII, which are the vitamin K-dependent clotting factors that anticoagulants disrupt. PCCs are preferred over fresh frozen plasma (FFP) because only a small volume is needed for infusion and their reversal of warfarin-induced anticoagulation is rapid. It has the added advantage of restoring overall thrombin generation and hemostasis.

FFP is used in conjunction with PCCs or when PCCs are unavailable. Less recommended is the use of recombinant activated factor VII (rFVIIa), which has been found to be less effective than PCCs (Dickneite 2007).

Challenges to Management of Bleeding

While there is much enthusiasm for newly developed drugs that have fewer complications than existing medications, their irreversibility should cause concern to emergency physicians and trauma service providers. Dabigatran, for example, is rapidly replacing warfarin as the anticoagulant of choice for patients with atrial fibrillation. Although the risk of bleeding is reduced with this drug and frequent monitoring is unnecessary while on it, physicians have reported worse patient outcomes for pre-injury medicated trauma patients on dabigatran than for those on warfarin (Cotton et al. 2011b). Similarly, prasugrel is a new thienopyridine antiplatelet agent that has been shown to be 10–100 times more potent than clopidogrel. While it is more effective than clopidogrel in preventing MI and stent thrombosis, its irreversibility and increased level of platelet aggregation increases the risk of morbidity and mortality in trauma patients (Hall and Mazer 2011).

Special Considerations

Acute traumatic coagulopathy (ATC) is an endogenous impairment that develops rapidly after trauma disrupts hemostatic equilibrium. Coagulopathy, metabolic acidosis (due to hypotension/hypoperfusion), and systemic hypothermia have often been related to "trauma's lethal triad" (Rotondo 1997). In patients with both severe tissue trauma and systemic hypoperfusion, ATC at clinical levels has been identified (Frith et al. 2012). As ATC has a confirmed negative impact on patient outcomes, it can exacerbate uncontrolled bleeding in patients already on anticoagulation/antiplatelet agents.

Deep vein thrombosis (DVT) prophylaxis is essential in trauma patients receiving anticoagulants as decreased levels of antithrombin III and the suppression of fibrinolysis, in addition to the effects of the anticoagulation/antiplatelet agents, may cause patients to become hypercoagulable.

Recently, the Centers for Disease Control and Prevention (CDC) has modified its guidelines regarding field triage of injured patients.

The panel highlighted the potential for rapid deterioration of patients on pre-injury anticoagulants that suffer head injuries as anticoagulants increase the risk for intracranial hemorrhage and longer hospital stays (Centers for Disease Control and Prevention (CDC) 2011).

Role of TEG in Trauma

Thromboelastography (TEG) is a time-sensitive dynamic assay of the viscoelastic properties of blood. It has been widely adopted for high-risk surgery like hepatic surgery, cardiac surgery, and organ transplantation (liver). TEG is becoming a key in management of "damage control resuscitation."

Keystones in Damage Control Resuscitation
- Early recognition of "trauma-induced coagulopathy"
- Massive transfusion protocol (MTP) activation policy (>10uPRBC/24 h, or now 6 h Kashuk and Moore)
- Minimize crystalloids use
- Early transfusion of RBC:FFP:PLTs in a 1:1:1 ratio
- Appropriate use of rFVIIa and fibrinogen-containing products such as cryoprecipitate
- When available: POC coagulation assays rapid thromboelastography (r-TEG) to guide administration of blood products

Interestingly most of current MTP underestimates the needed treatment to correct coagulopathy despite that simple scores have been developed to early predict need of transfusion: Assessment of Blood Consumption (ABC) score and Trauma-Associated Severe Hemorrhage score (TASH). There is no consensus when starting an MTP among different trauma centers. Different accepted "triggers" for MTP can be clinical only (operative bleeding), clinical and dynamical (prehospital and ED bleeding), and "triggers" plus TEG. TEG use in acute injury to monitor and target therapy in traumatic coagulopathy is modifying the classical approach and clinical management to acute posttraumatic bleeding and acquired bleeding disorders (patients on warfarin or LMWHs). TEG could close the gap in current recommendations

for resuscitation of the critically injured patient which are limited by a lack of point-of-care (POC) assessment of coagulation status. TEG should allow timely, goal-directed restoration of hemostasis via POC monitoring of coagulation status. Our current understanding of hemostasis should shift from a classic view, in which coagulation is considered a chain of catalytic enzyme reactions, to a cell-based model (CBM). CBM represents interaction between cellular and plasma components of clot formation. Another emerging role of POC TEG-based therapy and trauma patient management could be avoidance of allowed indiscriminant blood component administration. Typical post-injury coagulation status could be also monitored by TEG use avoiding complications resulting from overzealous component administration. Although thromboembolic events have been described shortly after injury, the time sequences of post-injury coagulation changes are unknown.

Possible Future Indications of "Early" TEG Analysis in Trauma Population from ED

1. Massive transfusion
2. TBI brain injury with bleeding
3. Unexplained continued surgical bleeding (use of anticoagulants)
4. Suspect of platelet dysfunction
5. Recombinant Factor VIIa use
6. Potential organ donor with coagulopathy
7. Identification of postoperative hypercoagulable patient

Cross-References

▶ Acute Coagulopathy of Trauma
▶ Adjuncts to Transfusion: Antifibrinolytics
▶ Adjuncts to Transfusion: Fibrinogen Concentrate
▶ Adjuncts to Transfusion: Prothrombin Complex Concentrate
▶ Adjuncts to Transfusion: Recombinant Factor VIIa, Factor XIII, and Calcium
▶ Blood Component Transfusion
▶ Coagulopathy
▶ FP24
▶ Platelets

References

Anthony CJ, Karim S, Ackroyd-Stolarz S, Fry A, Murphy NG, Christie R, Zed PJ (2011) Intensity of anticoagulation with warfarin and risk of adverse events in patients presenting to the emergency department. Ann Pharmacother 45:881–887

Bansal V, Forlage D, Lee J, Doucet J, Potenza B, Coimbra R (2011) A new clopidogrel (Plavix) point-of-care assay: rapid determination of antiplatelet activity in trauma patients. J Trauma 70:65–70

Cattano D, Altamirano AV, Kaynak HE, Seitan C, Paniccia R, Chen Z, Huang H, Prisco D, Hagberg CA, Pivalizza EG (2013) Perioperative assessment of platelet function by Thromboelastograph® Platelet Mapping™ in cardiovascular patients undergoing non-cardiac surgery. J Thromb Thrombolysis 35(1):23–30

Centers for Disease Control and Prevention (CDC) (2011) Guidelines for field triage of injured patients – recommendations of the national expert panel on field triage. Morb Mortal Wkly Rep 61:1–23

Cotton BA, Faz G, Hatch QM, Radwan ZA, Podbielski J, Wade C, Kozar RA, Holcomb JB (2011a) Rapid thromboelastography delivers real-time results that predict transfusion within 1 hour of admission. J Trauma 71:407–414

Cotton BA, McCarthy JJ, Holcomb JB (2011b) Acutely injured patients on dabigatran. N Engl J Med 365(21):2039–2040

Dickneite G (2007) Prothrombin complex concentrate versus recombinant factor VIIafor reversal of coumarin anticoagulation. Thromb Res 119:643–651

Frith D, Davenport R, Brohi K (2012) Acute traumatic coagulopathy. Curr Opin Anesthesiol 25:229–234

Hall R, Mazer CD (2011) Antiplatelet drugs: a review of their pharmacology and management in the perioperative period. Anesth Anal 112(2):292–318

Rotondo MZM (1997) The damage control sequence and underlying logic. Surg Clin North Am 77(4):761–777

Antihypertensives

▶ Vasoactive Agents in the ICU

Anti-infective Therapy

▶ Antibiotic Therapy

Antimicrobial Therapy

▶ Antibiotic Therapy

Antipersonnel Landmines

▶ IED (Improvised Explosive Device)

Antiplatelet

▶ Neurotrauma, Anticoagulation Considerations

Antiplatelet Therapy

▶ Anticoagulation/Antiplatelet Agents and Trauma

Anti-Rh Antibody

▶ Blood Group Antibodies

Antitank Landmines

▶ IED (Improvised Explosive Device)

Antithrombotics

▶ Anticoagulation/Antiplatelet Agents and Trauma

Anti-vehicle Landmines

▶ IED (Improvised Explosive Device)

Aortic Dissection: Aortic Tear

▶ Cardiac and Aortic Trauma, Anesthesia for

Apheresis Platelets

Harvey G. Hawes[1], Laura A. McElroy[2] and Bryan A. Cotton[1]

[1]Department of Surgery, Division of Acute Care Surgery, Trauma and Critical Care, University of Texas Health Science Center at Houston, The University of Texas Medical School at Houston, Houston, TX, USA
[2]Department of Anesthesiology, Critical Care Medicine, University of Rochester Medical Center, Rochester, NY, USA

Synonyms

Plateletpheresis;   Thrombapheresis;
Thrombocytapheresis

Definition

A method of obtaining large numbers of platelets from a single donor, apheresis (Latin: apherios – "to take from") platelets offer many advantages to both donor and recipient. Apheresis platelet preparations thus compare favorably to traditional whole blood-derived platelets (buffy coat and platelet-rich plasma methods), which due to decreased efficiency and platelet extraction are pooled products derived from multiple donors (Thiele et al. 2013).

Today, many automated apheresis systems exist and can extract 2–3 units of platelets at a single donation session lasting up to 2 h. A single or double puncture system may be utilized by either centrifugation, filtration, or a combination of both to allow for isolation of platelet products. The remaining blood components are either returned to the donor or further separated for multicomponent apheresis collection (Vassallo and Murphy 2006). Currently it is estimated that almost 80 % of all platelets transfused are obtained via apheresis.

Due to the large numbers of platelets extracted (a minimum of 3×10^{11}), a recipient may receive a therapeutic platelet dose from a single donor, increasing transfusion safety. There is a reduced risk of bacterial contamination and exposure to other blood-borne diseases, and the apheresis process allows for platelet crossmatching or HLA antigen matching in alloimmunized patients and leukocyte reduction (Vamvakas 2009). Advantages for donors include reduced adverse events from donation and the ability to donate more frequently, both a result of extracting only platelets and returning the remaining blood components to the donor. In fact, apheresis platelets have the added recipient benefit of being more likely to come from repeat donors, increasing their safety profile as first-time donors are twice as likely to test positive for infectious diseases (Heddle et al. 2008). Adverse events are generally less than seen with whole blood-derived platelet compounds for both donor and recipient (Schrezenmeter et al. 2007).

Cross-References

▶ Blood Bank
▶ Buffy Coat
▶ Pooled Platelets
▶ Thrombocytopenia

References

Heddle N, Arnold D, Boye D et al (2008) Comparing the efficacy and safety of pheresis and whole blood-derived platelet transfusions: a systematic review. Transfusion 48:1447–1458
Schrezenmeter H, Walther-Wenke G, Muller TH et al (2007) Bacterial contamination of platelet concentrates: results of a prospective multicenter study comparing pooled whole blood-derived platelets and apheresis platelets. Transfusion 47:644–652
Thiele T, Heddle N, Greinacher A (2013) Donor exposures in recipients of pooled platelet concentrates. N Engl J Med 368:487–489

Vamvakas E (2009) Relative safety of pooled whole blood-derived versus single-donor (apheresis) platelets in the United States: a systematic review of disparate risks. Transfusion 49:2743–2758

Vassallo R, Murphy S (2006) A critical comparison of platelet preparation methods. Curr Opin Hematol 13:323–330

APRV

▶ Neurotrauma and Brain Death, Ventilatory Management

aPTT

▶ Partial Thromboplastin Time

ARDS, Complication of Trauma

Claudia C. dos Santos[1] and Dun Yuan Zhou[2]
[1]Interdepartmental Division of Critical Care, St. Michael's Hospital/University of Toronto, The Keenan Research Centre of the Li Ka Shing Knowledge Institute, Toronto, ON, Canada
[2]Interdepartmental Division of Critical Care, Institute of Medical Sciences, University of Toronto, Toronto, ON, Canada

Synonyms

Acute lung injury; Acute respiratory distress syndrome; Adult respiratory distress syndrome

Definition

Acute respiratory distress syndrome (ARDS) is a well-known complication of major trauma, occurring in 8–82 % of selected patient populations (Hudson et al. 1995). Susceptible subgroups include patients with pulmonary contusions, severe trauma (Injury Severity Score, >25), head injury, marked base deficit, significant blood transfusion requirement, and notable orthopedic injuries such as long-bone and pelvic fractures associated with fat embolus.

Histologically, ALI/ARDS in humans is characterized by diffuse alveolar damage (DAD). Traditionally, the etiology of DAD has been thought to be secondary to a severe acute inflammatory response in the lungs and neutrophilic alveolitis. In practice, ARDS is the clinical expression of a group of diverse processes that produce widespread alveolar damage. Injury to the alveolar capillary barrier leads to exudation of fluid, cells, and proteinaceous contents across the membrane, leading to enough alveolar edema to cause refractory hypoxemia and the cardinal physiological manifestation of the syndrome as defined by the American/ European Consensus Conference in 1994: acute onset of hypoxemia, associated with bilateral infiltrates on chest X-ray (CXR) in the absence of left ventricular failure. In 2011, the Berlin definition aimed to better link consensus definition activities with empirical research (ARDS Definition Task Force et al. 2012). It eliminated acute lung injury (ALI) as a distinct category and classified ARDS by severity based on degree of hypoxemia: mild (200 mmHg $< PaO_2/FIO_2 \leq$ 300 mmHg), moderate (100 mmHg $< PaO_2/FIO_2 \leq$ 200 mmHg), and severe ($PaO_2/FIO_2 \leq$ 100 mmHg) and four ancillary variables for severe ARDS: radiographic severity, respiratory system compliance ($\leq$40 mL/cm H_2O), positive end-expiratory pressure ($\geq$10 cm H_2O), and corrected expired volume per minute ($\geq$10 L/min).

The draft Berlin definition was empirically evaluated using patient-level meta-analysis of 4,188 patients with ARDS from 4 multicenter clinical data sets and 269 patients with ARDS from 3 single-center data sets containing detailed physiologic information (Thille et al. 2013). The four ancillary variables did not contribute to the predictive validity of severe ARDS for mortality and were removed from the definition. Using the Berlin definition, stages of mild, moderate, and severe ARDS were associated with increased mortality (24–30 %; 29–34 %; and 42–48 %, respectively; $P <$ .001) and

increased median duration of mechanical ventilation in survivors (5 days; interquartile [IQR],
2–11; 7 days; IQR, 4–14; and 9 days; IQR, 5–17,
respectively; $p < .001$).

It has been noted that trauma patients may still
have better outcomes than septic patients that
develop ARDS, strongly suggesting that the
etiology of the syndrome may be different despite
given identical manifestations.

Preexisting Condition

ARDS in the Context of Trauma

Initial studies documented that the development
of ARDS in trauma patients resulted in
a significant increase in morbidity, an increased
use of hospital resources, and up to a 4.3-fold
increase in mortality More recent studies
matching patients with similar severity of injury
scores with and without ARDS however have
shown that although the development of ARDS
is associated with increased morbidity, hospital
and ICU length of stay, and costs, it does not
seem to increase the overall mortality in critically
ill trauma patients. Findings from various studies
suggest that the mortality may be explained by
injury severity alone and not by the presence of
ARDS. It has also become apparent that the
mortality from trauma-related ARDS is lower
than that associated with ARDS from other
causes (Hudson et al. 1995). Recent studies
have highlighted the possibility that the type of
lung injury that occurs in the setting of trauma
may in fact differ pathologically from the acute
lung injury (ALI) associated with sepsis, the most
common cause of ARDS. This short entry will
focus on the development of trauma-related
ARDS, how it may differ from sepsis-induced
ARDS, and the implications for treatment.

The pathogenic mechanisms responsible
for the development of ARDS in the context
of trauma have recently gained much attention.
Although the role of preexisting conditions
in mediating susceptibility to ARDS is controversial, specific mechanisms of lung injury,
including genetic susceptibility, should be
highlighted.

How Does Trauma Lead to ARDS?

Given the similarities between posttraumatic systemic inflammatory response syndrome (SIRS)
and the host response to overwhelming sepsis, it
was initially proposed that SIRS develops after
trauma as a result of bacterial translocation from
the bowel to the blood (likely due to hypotension,
leading to poor perfusion of the bowel, possible
subclinical ischemia, loss of bowel wall integrity,
and translocation of bacteria from the lumen to
the circulation; Moore et al. 1996). This hypothesis has been somewhat discredited and more
recent theories posit that the innate immune system and its pattern-recognition receptors are the
main components of the common molecular pathway, leading to SIRS in both infectious and non-
infectious settings (Iwasaki and Medzhitov
2010). Invading pathogens and danger signals
(generated by tissue injury) are recognized by
pathogen and danger-associated molecular
patterns (PAMP and DAMP). These may either
sit on the membrane surface such as Toll-like
receptors (TLRs) or inside the cytoplasm like
Nod-like receptors (NLRs). PAMPs and
DAMPs initiate similar innate immune responses
even in the absence of microbial infection
(Mollen et al. 2006). Recent work has
demonstrated that some DAMPs – including
high-mobility group protein B1 (HMGB1) and
S100 proteins (family of low molecular weight
proteins characterized by their calcium-binding
abilities) – are rapidly released into the blood of
severely injured patients. In keeping with this
hypothesis, elevated levels of HMGB1 in the
blood have been linked to the development of
organ failure after trauma.

Recently, Zhang and colleagues elegantly demonstrated how molecular motifs conserved between
bacteria and mitochondria may explain some of the
similarities in the innate immune responses to
external (infectious) and internal (damage) danger
signals. In the case of severe tissue injury, as that
resulting from trauma, mitochondrial DNA may
gain access to the circulating blood, probably secondary to the tissue necrosis caused by the extensive force of the injury. Mitochondrial DNA or
even mitochondrial DAMPs, such as formyl peptide, attract neutrophils. Neutrophil activation by

these DAMPs may represent the initial response of the innate immune system – triggering a systemic inflammatory response to injury. This hypothesis is supported by evidence that neutrophils are activated through formyl peptide receptor-1 on their surface, which promote a neutrophil-mediated inflammatory response through release of the immune mediators metalloproteinase-8 (MMP-8) and interleukin-8 (IL-8), and phosphorylation of several mitogen-activated protein (MAP) kinase enzymes. Most importantly, injection of mitochondrial DAMPs into rats causes acute lung injury (Zhang et al. 2010). Cumulatively, this data supports the existence of unique pathways that may be responsible for the development of ARDS in trauma patients. The significance of these findings lies in its importance for diagnosis, prognosis, and treatment.

Is There Evidence That Trauma-Associated ARDS May Be Differentiated from Other Forms of ARDS? An important implication of identifying unique biological mechanisms of injury is that this may enable the differentiation of ARDS from different etiologies.

Recent studies evaluating biomarkers in patients with ALI/ARDS have identified a number of markers that are predictive of clinical outcomes; these studies have also provided insight into the underlying pathogenetic mechanisms of ALI/ARDS (Calfee et al. 2007). Biomarkers that are specific to inflammation, endothelial activation and injury, lung epithelial injury, and disordered coagulation and fibrinolysis have all been previously shown to help differentiate patients with ALI/ARDS. In a recent study, Calfee and colleagues compared a panel of eight biomarkers in patients with traumatic ALI/ARDS to patients with nontraumatic ALI/ARDS. They found significant differences in six of the eight biomarkers that were evaluated. This study, however, did not examine the role that biomarkers might play in the diagnosis of ALI/ARDS. In a retrospective nested case control study of 192 patients admitted to a university trauma intensive care unit (ICU), the same authors compared biomarkers from plasma cells collected from 107 patients with ALI to

85 patients without ALI. Results showed that patients with ALI had higher severity of illness scores, more days of mechanical ventilation, longer hospital stays, and higher mortality versus controls. Seven biomarkers (RAGE, PCPIII, BNP, ANG2, IL10, TNF-α, and IL8) had a high diagnostic accuracy, as reflected by the area under the receiver operating characteristic curve of 0.86 (95 % CI 0.82–0.92) in differentiating ALI from controls.

In separate studies, circulating leukotriene B4 (LTB4) identified respiratory complications after trauma. The cutoff to predict pulmonary complications was calculated at 109.6 pg/mL (72 % specificity, 67 % sensitivity), about twice the levels detected in the group of trauma patients that did not develop pulmonary complications. LTB4 was not influenced by overall or chest injury severity, age, gender, or massive transfusion. Patients with pulmonary complications received mechanical ventilation for a significantly longer period of time, and had prolonged intensive care unit and overall hospital stay, suggesting this may be a relatively interesting biomarker that can be used to at least predict likelihood of development of pulmonary complications after major trauma.

Genetic Susceptibility to the Development of ALI
Results from animal studies clearly show that not all ARDS is "created equal." Different genetic molecular mechanisms of injury may be invoked by different insults, and these result in gene expression profiles that characterize injury-specific molecular phenotypes. Injury-specific profiles are the result of differential gene expression, indicating that genes may play an important role in the susceptibility and development of ARDS. There is rapidly growing interest in the potential role of genetic factors in patients who develop ARDS. Single nucleotide polymorphisms (SNPs) are the most commonly studied variations. Genetic studies of ALI/ARDS have largely centered on candidate genes that play a role in the response to external stimuli, because these genes are assumed to have key roles in the ALI/ARDS immune response (Gao and Barnes 2009). Several studies have

reported associations between SNPs and clinical outcomes in patients with trauma-induced ALI susceptibility. In response to a number of stressors including oxidative stress, NF-E2 related factor-2 (NRF-2) dissociates from the cytoplasmic inhibitor, Kelchlike ECH-associated protein (Keap1), and translocates to the nucleus where it binds to the antioxidant response elements (ARE) and upregulates the transcription of protective detoxifying enzymes. Studies have sequenced the NRF2 gene in ethnically diverse subjects, and identified three novel, potentially functional promoter SNPs at positions -617 (C/A),-651 (G/A), and -653 (A/G). The authors used a luciferase construct to detect the different binding affinities of SNPs of NRF2, and the -617 (C/A) mutation showed significantly decreased binding affinity ($p < 0.001$) relative to the wild type. In a nested case-control study, patients with the -617 A SNP had a significantly higher risk for developing ALI after major trauma.

The results of several candidate-gene studies have been summarized in a recent review (Gao and Barnes 2009), and the accompanying editorial provided important additional insights. Another likely contributing factor to the development and severity of lung injury is the virulence of the infecting organism, be it bacterial, viral, fungal, or parasitic. Some studies have shown experimentally that the virulence capacity of *Pseudomonas aeruginosa* is a major determinant of the severity of lung injury. An alternative approach to tradition genetic analysis of individual SNPs is to apply genome-wide association screening (screens the genome in a relatively unsupervised fashion without a priori knowledge of potential SNPs of interest) of patients who either have ARDS or are at risk of developing ARDS. Christie et al. conducted the first investigation to use the genome-wide association (GWA) approach to identify putative risk variants for ALI (Christie et al. 2008). Using a gradated informed target discovery approach, the authors narrowed the number of candidate small nucleotide polymorphisms (SNPs) that they validated using expression quantitative trait loci (eQTL) analyses in stimulated

B-lymphoblastoid cell lines (B-LCL). Using this advanced genetic approach, the group identified a polymorphism in the gene protein tyrosine phosphatase, receptor type, f polypeptide (PTPRF), interacting protein (liprin), alpha 1 (PPFIA1) as significantly associated with the development of ALI in trauma patients ($P = 0.0021$). The PPFIA1 genes encode liprin alpha, a protein involved in cell adhesion, integrin expression, and cell-matrix interactions. This study supports the feasibility of future multicenter GWA investigations of ALI risk, and identifies PPFIA1 as a potential functional candidate ALI risk gene for future research.

The clinical implication is that unlike other forms of ALI/ARDS – we know exactly when the risk of ALI/ARDS begins. This will allow patients to be screened for their genetic susceptibility and for therapies to be instituted preventively rather than retrospectively.

Special Topics in Trauma-Induced ARDS

Lung Contusions

Lung contusion (LC) is common in patients with thoracic trauma and is a leading risk factor for ALI/ARDS development. After blunt chest trauma, pulmonary contusion is a common result that leads to physiologic consequences of alveolar hemorrhage and pulmonary parenchymal destruction, which take place within hours of injury. After pulmonary contusion, acute pathologic changes are associated with important physiologic alterations in hemodynamics. Due to severe vasoconstriction after injury, computed tomography (CT) has been able to show increased pulmonary vascular resistance and shunt fraction. Macrophage chemo-attractant protein (MCP)-1/CC chemokine ligand (CCL)-2 is produced by a number of cells in response to inflammatory stimuli, such as IL-1b, -4, -6, and -10, transforming growth factor-b, secondary to tissue injury. The management of pulmonary contusion is primarily supportive. Optimization of oxygenation and ventilation are the key factors to monitor. Fluid management and control of chest wall pain are critical in the treatment of LC patients. In cases of severe injury, intensive monitoring is also essential for ensuring adequate organ perfusion and oxygenation. Aggressive attempts to alleviate discomfort and restore unhindered pulmonary mechanics are mandatory; otherwise, hypoventilation, atelectasis, and subsequent respiratory deterioration could take place. Also, high frequency oscillatory ventilation and extracorporeal membrane oxygenation have been gaining more acceptance in LC treatment (see entries on "▶ Chest Wall Injury" and "▶ Blast Lung Injury").

Fat Embolus

Fat embolism syndrome (FES) includes hypoxia, deteriorating mental status, and petechiae, tachycardia, fever, anemia, and thrombocytopenia. FES occurs in approximately 47–100 % of patients with long-bone fractures. Within the first 12–72 h after injury, there is an asymptomatic interval with development of pulmonary, neurologic, and dermatologic changes. Currently, there are two theories explaining FES causes. The mechanical theory suggests the release of mechanical emboli from fractures or soft tissue injury into the venous system, which are then transported to the lungs. The biochemical theory proposes that FES is a process where inflammatory reactants, including lipoprotein lipase, cause the release of fatty acids, thus altering the fat transport mechanisms of the plasma. This hemostatic change results in fat droplet aggregation with systemic sequestration in the microvasculature, which is highly inflammatory. The current treatment to FES is largely supportive. Through mechanical ventilation, oxygen therapy aims to maintain the PaO_2 and adequate hydration in the patient (see entries on "▶ Fat Embolism Syndrome" and "▶ Femoral Shaft Fractures").

Transfusion-Related Acute Lung Injury (TRALI)

Transfusion-related acute lung injury (TRALI) is the most severe complication in transfusion medicine, and represents a significant risk for ALI/ARDS in trauma patients who require major transfusions at the time of resuscitation. Transfusion can lead to both immune and nonimmune-mediated TRALI. The immune-mediated TRALI mechanisms are widely accepted and proven in both preclinical and clinical studies. Cells that contain blood products in the beginning stages of nonimmune TRALI have been studied in preclinical and clinical studies. One postulate suggests that pro-inflammatory mediators in the plasma layer of blood products are responsible for the initiation of nonimmune-mediated TRALI. Lysophosphatidylcholines, sCD40L and neutral lipids, which accumulate in the plasma layer during the storage of cell-containing blood products, play a role in the onset of nonimmune-mediated TRALI. Another common hypothesis suggests that the aged erythrocyte or platelet itself is responsible for the onset of nonimmune-mediated TRALI. The loss of Duffy expression on the aged erythrocyte results in a reduction in erythrocyte chemokine scavenging and may result in the onset of TRALI in the presence of an inflammatory condition. Common strategies to prevent TRALI include the exclusion of female plasma donors and the pooling of plasma products. Strategies to prevent immune-mediated TRALI include exclusion of HLA or HNA positive donors, exclusion of donors at risk of being HLA or HNA positive, testing donors for HLA or HNA antibodies, and multiple plasma pooling. To prevent nonimmune-mediated TRALI, transfusing fresh blood only has been the most widely suggested. These strategies have already been implemented in some countries, resulting in a reduction of the incidence of TRALI. Challenges are ahead as preventive strategies reduced but not eliminated onset of TRALI, and still no therapy for this potentially life-treating syndrome exists (see entries on "▶ Blood Therapy in Trauma Anesthesia," "▶ Leukoreduced Red Blood Cells," "▶ Massive Transfusion," "▶ Red Blood Cell Transfusion in Trauma ICU," "▶ Plasma Transfusion in Trauma," and "▶ Platelet Transfusion in Trauma").

Massive Aspiration

Acute aspiration pneumonitits is a well-established complication among trauma patients. Approximately one third of patients with aspiration pneumonitis develop a more severe, protracted hypoxemia course associated with ALI/ARDS. The two most common consequences resulting from aspiration of gastric or oropharyngeal content are chemical pneumonitis and bacterial aspiration pneumonia. Animal studies have confirmed that a combination of acid and particulate matter aspirate results in severe, progressive lung injury compared with the individual gastric components of acid or particulate matter individually. In terms of two-hit gastric aspirates, attention has been focused on a combination of acid plus small non-acidified gastric particles. Data on leukocyte influx and cytokine/chemokine production demonstrate an over-exuberant pro-inflammatory response after the instillation of combination of acid and particulate matter. Once aspiration has taken place, the patient should be positioned so that further inhalation of particulate contents is substantially reduced. Additionally, patients may require intubation to facilitate future bronchoscopy. Other measures to prevent recurrent aspiration should be taken. Furthermore, a vast majority of intensivists prescribe antibiotics in patients with suspected aspiration events in which bacteria colonizing the stomach could be aspirated by the patient through the oropharynx (see entries on "▶ Lung Injury," and "▶ Hypoxemia, Severe").

Application

Treatment for Trauma-Associated ARDS

A large number of pharmacologic therapies have been evaluated in Phase II and Phase III clinical trials for the treatment of ALI/ARDS. These treatments include glucocorticoids, surfactants, inhaled nitric oxide, antioxidants, protease inhibitors, and a variety of other anti-inflammatory treatments. Unfortunately, to date, none of these pharmacologic treatments have proven to be effective, although some of them may be effective in a subgroup of patients with specific causes of lung injury that might make them more responsive than others. Identification of the mortality-reducing effect of lung-protective ventilation using low tidal volumes and pressure limitation is one of the biggest advances in the application of mechanical ventilation. Despite the lack of a specific pharmacologic treatment, lung-protective ventilation has reduced the mortality

of ALI from 40 % in 2000 to 25 % in 2006. Moreover, the use of a fluid-conservative strategy after patients with ARDS are no longer in shock has reduced the duration of mechanical ventilation (see entries on "▶ Mechanical Ventilation, Conventional," "▶ Mechanical Ventilation, High-Frequency Oscillation," "▶ Mechanical Ventilation, Permissive Hypercapnia").

A systematic review and meta-analysis of all publications (between 1966 and 2012) has specifically addressed the question as to the benefit of using neuromuscular-blocking agents (NMBA) as an adjunct to the ventilator management of ARDS patients. The authors found that patients treated with NMBA showed less mortality (risk ratio, 0.71 [95 % CI, 0.55–0.90]; number needed to treat, 1–7), more ventilator-free days at day 28 ($p = 0.020$), higher PaO_2 to FiO_2 ratios ($p = 0.004$), and less barotraumas ($p = 0.030$). The incidence of critical illness neuromyopathy was similar ($p = 0.540$). How this knowledge can be applied to trauma patients at risk or with documented evidence of ARDS remains to be determined by large randomized controlled trials.

In contrast to patients with established ARDS, ventilator practices in patients at risk for ALI/ARDS are unclear. Established ARDS may often be refractory to treatment. As discussed above, the best clinical trials of protective mechanical ventilation have demonstrated modest treatment effects, and mortality remains high. Early ventilatory intervention in patients at risk of developing ARDS may be exploited to block progression to ARDS. Conceptually, the primary goal of protective ventilation strategies in at-risk populations, such as trauma patients, would be to avoid the development of ventilator induced lung injury (VILI) by applying ventilation strategies that maintain alveolar stability and reduces pulmonary edema formation. Studies of VILI in subjects without ALI demonstrate inconsistent results. Retrospective clinical studies, however, suggest that the use of large tidal volumes (VT) favors the development of lung injury in these patients. Side effects associated with the use of lower VT in patients with ALI seem to be minimal. Assuming that this will be the case in patients without ALI/ARDS too, the prevailing thought among critical care intensivists is that the use of lower VT should be considered in all mechanically ventilated patients, whether they have ALI or not. Prospective studies should be performed to evaluate optimal ventilator management strategies for patients without ALI, and these are currently underway.

In terms of future strategies that may come to play an important role in the management of trauma-induced ARDS, a growing number of studies have demonstrated compelling data on the beneficial effects of mesenchymal stem or stromal cells (MSCs). Both systemic and intrapulmonary administration of bone-marrow-derived MSCs have been shown to improve mortality, alveolar fluid clearance, and attenuate inflammation – despite minimal, if any, lung MSC engraftment. The mechanisms of MSC actions on inflammatory and immune cells are not well understood but likely involve both secretion of soluble mediators as well as cell–cell contact. In a rat "fixed volume" model of mild hemorrhagic shock, MSC administration inhibits systemic levels of inflammatory cytokines and chemokines in the serum of treated animals. In vivo MSCs also inhibit pulmonary endothelial permeability and lung edema, with concurrent preservation of the vascular endothelial barrier proteins. Therefore, these data suggest that MSCs, acting directly and through soluble factors, are potent stabilizers of the vascular endothelium and inflammation. These data are the first to demonstrate the therapeutic potential of MSCs in hemorrhagic shock-induced lung injury.

An important area of treatment that is not explored in this manuscript is the use of extracorporeal ventilation for trauma patients at risk or with established ARDS. This is a very active area of research and probably represents a potential strategy for the future (please see entry on "▸ Extracorporeal Membrane Oxygenation").

Conclusions

The primary goal of this entry was twofold: Firstly, to provide an updated review of important issues in the field of trauma-induced ARDS. Secondly, to highlight the importance of understanding individual mechanisms of injury to the development of future therapeutics; especially as it pertains to the management of trauma patients at risk for developing ARDS/ALI.

Acknowledgements Funding Sources: This work is supported by the Canadian Institutes of Health Research (Grant # MOP-106545), the Ontario Thoracic Society (Grants OTS2010/2011/2012), the Physicians Services Incorporate (Grant # PSI 09–21) and the Early Research Award from the Ministry of Research and Innovation of Ontario (Grant ERA/MRI 2011), Canada.

Cross-References

▸ Acute Abdominal Compartment Syndrome in Trauma
▸ Acute Coagulopathy of Trauma
▸ Acute Respiratory Distress Syndrome (ARDS), General
▸ Adrenal Insufficiency in Trauma and Sepsis
▸ Blast Lung Injury
▸ Blood Therapy in Trauma Anesthesia
▸ Chest Wall Injury
▸ Coagulopathy in Trauma: Underlying Mechanisms
▸ Cryoprecipitate Transfusion in Trauma
▸ Extracorporeal Membrane Oxygenation
▸ Fat Embolism Syndrome
▸ Femoral Shaft Fractures
▸ Hypoxemia, Severe
▸ Leukoreduced Red Blood Cells
▸ Lung Injury
▸ Massive Transfusion
▸ Mechanical Ventilation, Conventional
▸ Mechanical Ventilation, High-Frequency Oscillation
▸ Mechanical Ventilation, Permissive Hypercapnia
▸ Multiorgan System Failure (MOF)
▸ Open Abdomen
▸ Plasma Transfusion in Trauma
▸ Platelet Transfusion in Trauma
▸ Pulmonary Hypertension
▸ Red Blood Cell Transfusion in Trauma ICU
▸ Sepsis, General mechanism of
▸ Sepsis, Treatment of

► Shock
► Systemic Inflammatory Response Syndrome
► Ventilator-Associated Pneumonia
► Ventilatory Management of Trauma Patients

References

ARDS Definition Task Force, Ranieri VM, Rubenfeld GD, Thompson BT, Ferguson ND, Caldwell E, Fan E, Camporota L, Slutsky AS (2012) Acute respiratory distress syndrome: the Berlin definition. JAMA 307(23):2526–2533

Calfee CS, Eisner MD, Ware LB et al (2007) Trauma-associated lung injury differs clinically and biologically from acute lung injury due to other clinical disorders. Crit Care Med 35(10):2243–2250

Christie JD, Ma SF, Aplenc R et al (2008) Variation in the myosin light chain kinase gene is associated with development of acute lung injury after major trauma. Crit Care Med 36(10):2794–2800

Gao L, Barnes KC (2009) Recent advances in genetic predisposition to clinical acute lung injury. Am J Physiol Lung Cell Mol Physiol 296(5):L713–L725

Hudson LD, Milberg JA, Anardi D, Maunder RJ (1995) Clinical risks for development of the acute respiratory distress syndrome. Am J Respir Crit Care Med 151(2 Pt 1):293–301

Iwasaki A, Medzhitov R (2010) Regulation of adaptive immunity by the innate immune system. Science 327(5963):291–295

Mollen KP, Anand RJ, Tsung A, Prince JM, Levy RM, Billiar TR (2006) Emerging paradigm: toll-like receptor 4-sentinel for the detection of tissue damage. Shock 26(5):430–437

Moore FA, Sauaia A, Moore EE, Haenel JB, Burch JM, Lezotte DC (1996) Postinjury multiple organ failure: a bimodal phenomenon. J Trauma 40(4):501–510; discussion 510–512

Thille AW, Esteban A, Fernández-Segoviano P, Rodriguez JM, Aramburu JA, Peñuelas O, Cortés-Puch I, Cardinal-Fernández P, Lorente JA, Frutos-Vivar F (2013) Comparison of the Berlin definition for acute respiratory distress syndrome with autopsy. Am J Respir Crit Care Med 187(7):761–767

Zhang Q, Raoof M, Chen Y et al (2010) Circulating mitochondrial DAMPs cause inflammatory responses to injury. Nature 464(7285):104–107

Recommended Reading

Acute Respiratory Distress Syndrome Network (2000) Ventilation with lower tidal volumes as compared with traditional tidal volumes for acute lung injury and the acute respiratory distress syndrome. N Engl J Med 342(18):1301–1308

Angus DC (2012) The acute respiratory distress syndrome: what's in a name. JAMA 307(23):2542–2544

Atkinson JL (1997) Acute lung injury in isolated traumatic brain injury. Neurosurgery 41(5):1214–1216

Auner B, Geiger EV, Henrich D, Lehnert M, Marzi I, Relja B (2012) Circulating leukotriene B4 identifies respiratory complications after trauma. Mediators Inflamm 2012:536156

Cepkova M, Matthay MA (2006) Pharmacotherapy of acute lung injury and the acute respiratory distress syndrome. J Intensive Care Med 21(3):119–143

Funk DJ, Lujan E, Moretti EW et al (2008) A brief report: the use of high-frequency oscillatory ventilation for severe pulmonary contusion. J Trauma 65(2):390–395

Hiss J, Kahana T, Kugel C (1996) Beaten to death: why do they die. J Trauma 40(1):27–30

Hod EA, Zhang N, Sokol SA et al (2010) Transfusion of red blood cells after prolonged storage produces harmful effects that are mediated by iron and inflammation. Blood 115(21):4284–4292

Holland MC, Mackersie RC, Morabito D et al (2003) The development of acute lung injury is associated with worse neurologic outcome in patients with severe traumatic brain injury. J Trauma 55(1):106–111

Kelher MR, Masuno T, Moore EE et al (2009) Plasma from stored packed red blood cells and MHC class I antibodies causes acute lung injury in a 2-event in vivo rat model. Blood 113(9):2079–2087

Lucas G, Win N, Calvert A et al (2012) Reducing the incidence of TRALI in the UK: the results of screening for donor leucocyte antibodies and the development of national guidelines. Vox Sang 103(1):10–17

Madershahian N, Wittwer T, Strauch J et al (2007) Application of ECMO in multitrauma patients with ARDS as rescue therapy. J Card Surg 22(3):180–184

Matthay MA (2008) Treatment of acute lung injury: clinical and experimental studies. Proc Am Thorac Soc 5(3):297–299

Miller PR, Croce MA, Bee TK et al (2001) ARDS after pulmonary contusion: accurate measurement of contusion volume identifies high-risk patients. J Trauma 51(2):223–228; discussion 229–230

Miller PR, Croce MA, Kilgo PD, Scott J, Fabian TC (2002) Acute respiratory distress syndrome in blunt trauma: identification of independent risk factors. Am Surg 68(10):845–850; discussion 850–851

Mudd KL, Hunt A, Matherly RC et al (2000) Analysis of pulmonary fat embolism in blunt force fatalities. J Trauma 48(4):711–715

Navarrete-Navarro P, Rodriguez A, Reynolds N et al (2001) Acute respiratory distress syndrome among trauma patients: trends in ICU mortality, risk factors, complications and resource utilization. Intensive Care Med 27(7):1133–1140

Neto AS, Pereira VG, Esposito DC, Damasceno MC, Schultz MJ (2012) Neuromuscular blocking agents in patients with acute respiratory distress syndrome: a summary of the current evidence from three randomized controlled trials. Ann Intensive Care 2(1):33

Salim A, Martin M, Constantinou C et al (2006) Acute respiratory distress syndrome in the trauma intensive care unit: morbid but not mortal. Arch Surg 141(7):655–658

Schreiter D, Reske A, Stichert B et al (2004) Alveolar recruitment in combination with sufficient positive end-expiratory pressure increases oxygenation and lung aeration in patients with severe chest trauma. Crit Care Med 32(4):968–975

Schultz MJ, Haitsma JJ, Slutsky AS, Gajic O (2007) What tidal volumes should be used in patients without acute lung injury. Anesthesiology 106(6):1226–1231

Treggiari MM, Hudson LD, Martin DP, Weiss NS, Caldwell E, Rubenfeld G (2004) Effect of acute lung injury and acute respiratory distress syndrome on outcome in critically ill trauma patients. Crit Care Med 32(2):327–331

Villar J, Flores C, Perez-Mendez L et al (2008) Angiotensin-converting enzyme insertion/deletion polymorphism is not associated with susceptibility and outcome in sepsis and acute respiratory distress syndrome. Intensive Care Med 34(3):488–495

Wheeler AP, Bernard GR, Thompson BT et al (2006) Pulmonary-artery versus central venous catheter to guide treatment of acute lung injury. N Engl J Med 354(21):2213–2224

Wiedemann HP, Wheeler AP, Bernard GR et al (2006) Comparison of two fluid-management strategies in acute lung injury. N Engl J Med 354(24):2564–2575

ARF

▶ Acute Kidney Injury

Arginine Vasopressin

▶ DDAVP

Arterial Desaturation

▶ Hypoxemia, Severe

Arterial Tourniquet

▶ Tourniquet

Artificial Limb

▶ Prosthetics

Artillery

▶ Mortars

Aseptic Necrosis

▶ Avascular Necrosis of the Femoral Head

ASIA Score

▶ Examination, Neurological

Aspergillus

▶ Fungal Infections

Aspiration

▶ Trauma-Related Dysphagia

Assault

▶ Interpersonal Violence

Assistive Device

▶ Adaptive Equipment

Associations

▶ Trauma Associations

Astragalus

▶ Talus Fractures

Asystole

▶ Cardiopulmonary Resuscitation in Adult Trauma

ATC

▶ Acute Coagulopathy of Trauma

Atelectasis

Ariful Alam[1] and Khanjan H. Nagarsheth[2]
[1]Department of General Surgery, Staten Island University Hospital, Staten Island, NY, USA
[2]R Adams Cowley Shock Trauma Center, University of Maryland School of Medicine, Baltimore, MD, USA

Synonyms

Cicatrization atelectasis; Fleischner lines; Lung collapse; Nonobstructive atelectasis; Obstructive atelectasis; Platelike atelectasis; Postoperative atelectasis

Definition

Atelectasis is the loss of lung volume due to collapse of alveoli resulting in reduced or absent gas exchange (Duggan and Kavanagh 2005). It may occur in either an acute or a chronic setting. Acute atelectasis is primarily notable for airlessness, whereas chronic atelectasis is often characterized by a combination of airlessness, infection along with bronchiectasis, and fibrosis (Woodring and Reed 1996). Atelectasis can be classified according to the pathophysiologic mechanism, the location, or the volume of lung involved.

Preexisting Condition

Both blunt and penetrating chest trauma can cause atelectasis. Other causes include mucus in the airways after surgery, cystic fibrosis, inhaled foreign objects, and severe asthma. Acute atelectasis may occur in premature neonates as a result of surfactant deficiency, which leads to infant respiratory distress syndrome (Woodring and Reed 1996). Three mechanisms have been proposed to explain the development of atelectasis. These include compression of lung tissue, absorption of alveolar air, and impairment of surfactant function (Duggan and Kavanagh 2005).

Compression Atelectasis

Compression atelectasis occurs as a result of alveolar collapse due to the reduction in the transmural pressure that distends the alveolus. This occurs due to an increase in pleural pressure, with the greatest extent in the dependent lung regions, compressing the adjacent lung tissue (Duggan and Kavanagh 2005). It is usually associated with accumulation of fluid, blood, or air within the pleural cavity, which mechanically collapses the adjacent lung. Compression atelectasis is often a result of pleural effusions, caused by congestive heart failure (Woodring and Reed 1996). Leakage of air into the pleural cavity as well as spontaneous pneumothorax can also lead to compression atelectasis. Basal atelectasis can result from an elevated hemidiaphragm. This is commonly seen in bedridden patients and in patients with ascites and spinal cord injury, during and after surgery (Woodring and Reed 1996). Cineradiography can also be used to demonstrate a cephalad shift of the diaphragm during anesthesia and spontaneous breathing. This diaphragmatic shift does not progress after muscle relaxation and results in reduced functional residual capacity (Duggan and Kavanagh 2005).

Injury to the chest from both blunt and penetrating injury results in pulmonary contusions which lead to edema and blood collection in alveolar spaces. This causes compression atelectasis and involves alveoli in one or more regions of the injured lungs. In these circumstances, the degree of collapse among alveoli tends to be quite consistent and complete. Patients with chest trauma with an Injury Severity Score of 15 or above 40–60 % will require mechanical ventilation, and there is an observed mortality rate of 10–25 % (Woodring and Reed 1996).

Resorption Atelectasis

Resorption atelectasis, also known as gas atelectasis, can occur by one of two mechanisms: gas trapped in alveoli distal to an obstruction or disparity in the rate of oxygen uptake versus oxygen delivery in the distal alveoli. In the first scenario, when there is a complete obstruction in the airways, a pocket of trapped gas is created in the distal lung unit. Perfusion of the alveoli persists while further gas inflow is prevented and this gas pocket eventually collapses (Woodring and Reed 1996). Under this condition, the rate of gas absorption from an unventilated part of the lung increases with a rise in the fraction of inspired oxygen (FiO_2) (Duggan and Kavanagh 2005). This type of atelectasis is commonly associated with aspirated foreign body, mucus plugging, mass effect from tumors, lymphadenopathy, aortic aneurysm, cardiomegaly, or incorrect positioning of an endotracheal tube (Woodring and Reed 1996).

The second mechanism proposed to explain resorption atelectasis occurs when there is a disparity in oxygen delivery and uptake. Lung zones that have a low ventilation to perfusion ratio (V/Q) have a lower partial pressure of alveolar oxygen during inspiration. When the FiO_2 is increased, partial pressure of alveolar oxygen increases. This leads to increased rate of oxygen uptake by the blood. The rate of uptake may be greater than the rate of inspired flow of gas, leading to progressive reduction of the lung unit (Duggan and Kavanagh 2005).

Adhesive Atelectasis

The normal alveolar surface is covered by pulmonary surfactant, which reduces pulmonary surface tension, stabilizes alveoli, and prevents alveolar collapse. In conditions causing loss or impairment of surfactant, the alveoli become susceptible to collapse and become atelectatic (Duggan and Kavanagh 2005). Conditions that predispose to adhesive type of atelectasis include anesthesia, acute respiratory distress syndrome, smoke inhalation, uremia, or prolonged shallow breathing (Woodring and Reed 1996).

Relaxation Atelectasis

Relaxation atelectasis occurs when there is a disruption of contact between the parietal and visceral pleurae. Under normal circumstances, the lungs remain in close proximity to the chest wall due the negative pressure in the pleural space. Pleural effusion, pneumothorax, or a large emphysematous bulla can cause the separation between the visceral and parietal pleurae. Due to the loss of the negative pressure, the physiologic elastic recoil of normal lung parenchyma retracts the normal lung and may lead to atelectasis (Woodring and Reed 1996).

Cicatricial Atelectasis

Cicatrization results from loss of lung volume due to severe parenchymal scarring. This is commonly seen in granulomatous diseases such as sarcoidosis, tuberculosis, radiation pneumonia, and necrotizing pneumonia (Woodring and Reed 1996).

Application

Presentation

Atelectasis is associated with the development of several pathophysiologic effects, which include decreased lung compliance, impairment of oxygenation, increased pulmonary vascular resistance, and development of lung injury

(Duggan and Kavanagh 2005). The patient may present with cough, chest pain, difficulty breathing, and cyanosis as a late sign. They may also have decreased oxygen saturation, increased heart rate, and low-grade fever (Woodring and Reed 1996). Late-stage findings may include a shift of the mediastinum with subsequent tracheal deviation and heart displacement towards the atelectatic lung. There is often drooping of shoulder with crowding of ribs (Woodring and Reed 1996).

Detection of Atelectasis

Conventional chest radiography is usually used to confirm the diagnosis of suspected atelectasis. Lobar or segmental atelectasis is classically seen as opacification of the lobe or segment. The most direct and reliable sign on radiograph is displacement of the lung fissures. Other signs include a rise of the hemidiaphragm and mediastinal shift near the point of volume loss. There is compensatory hyperinflation of the remaining aerated segment in the affected lobe evidenced by increased radiolucency, and the collapsed portion of the lung is often triangular in at least one projection. In the case of absorption atelectasis, the features are similar to consolidation with the presence of air bronchograms. Furthermore, the "silhouette" sign, which is the loss of normal borders between thoracic structures, allows identification of the lobe or segment of the lung that is affected (Proto and Tocino 1980).

Computed tomography is emerging as a preferred alternative to CXR because of the widespread availability, resolution, high signal/noise ratio for lung tissue, and speed. CT allows measurement of whole and regional lung volumes and distribution of aerated lung segments. Atelectasis on a CT scan is defined as pixels with attenuation values of -100 to $+100$ Hounsfield units (Duggan and Kavanagh 2005).

Prevention or Reversal

The definitive treatment of atelectasis depends on the underlying etiology. Treatment of acute atelectasis, including postoperative lung collapse, requires removal of the underlying cause. The management of atelectasis depends on whether the lungs are injured or uninjured. Progressive pulmonary atelectasis may occur with constant ventilation without periodic hyperinflation. Recruitment maneuvers using three successive inflations with a pressure of 20 cm H_2O, 30 cm H_2O, and 40 cm H_2O for 10 s, 15 s, and 15 s, respectively, have been described. Tusman reported that high initial pressures are needed to overcome collapsed lungs and that PEEP of 5 cm H_2O or above is required to prevent the newly recruited alveoli from collapsing. This is in the healthy lungs, without any evidence of barotrauma or pulmonary complications. It is important to note that the use of large tidal volumes, high peak airway pressure, and end-expiratory alveolar collapse with cyclic reopening can be detrimental and worsen lung injuries (Duggan and Kavanagh 2005).

Reversing or preventing atelectasis is possible in many patients in the perioperative period by use of techniques or devices that either encourage or force patients to inspire deeply. The goal of these means is to produce and sustain a large increase in transpulmonary pressure, resulting in distension of the lung and reexpansion of collapsed lung units. Commonly used techniques include intermittent positive-pressure breathing, deep-breathing exercises, incentive spirometry, and chest physiotherapy (Pryor 1999; McCool and Rosen 2006). Studies suggest that all regimens are equally effective in reducing the frequency of postoperative pulmonary complications. Judicious use of perioperative analgesia is an essential adjunct. Patient-controlled analgesia, epidural pumps, subcutaneous infusion pumps, as well as lidocaine patches over the affected area all play an important part in permitting patients to breathe deeply, cough forcefully, and participate in chest physiotherapy maneuvers (Ingalls et al. 2010; Karmakar and Ho 2003).

When a mechanically obstructed bronchus is suggested but coughing or suctioning is not successful, flexible bronchoscopy should be performed. Some patients may require repeat bronchoscopy if atelectasis recurs. Patients with poor pain control and those who are chronic smokers may need this repeat procedure (Kreider and Lipson 2003). Therapy with a broad-spectrum antibiotic is started and modified appropriately if a specific pathogen is isolated from bronchial lavage secretions. Although *N*-acetylcysteine aerosols commonly are administered in an effort to promote clearance of tenacious secretions, their efficacy has not been documented. In addition, *N*-acetylcysteine may cause acute bronchoconstriction (Schindler 2005).

Cross-References

► Chest Wall Injury
► Lung Injury
► Oxygen-Carrying Capacity
► Ventilator-Associated Pneumonia
► Ventilatory Management of Trauma Patients

References

Duggan M, Kavanagh BP (2005) Pulmonary atelectasis: a pathogenic perioperative entity. Anesthesiology 102:838–854
Ingalls NK, Horton ZA, Bettendorf M et al (2010) Randomized, double-blind, placebo-controlled trial using lidocaine patch 5 % in traumatic rib fractures. J Am Coll Surg 210:205–209
Karmakar MK, Ho AMH (2003) Acute pain management of patients with multiple fractured ribs. J Trauma 54:615–625
Kreider ME, Lipson DA (2003) Bronchoscopy for atelectasis in the ICU: a case report and review of the literature. Chest 124:344–350
McCool FD, Rosen MJ (2006) Nonpharmacologic airway clearance therapies: ACCP evidence-based clinical practice guidelines. Chest 129(1 Suppl):250S–259S
Proto AV, Tocino I (1980) Radiographic manifestations of lobar collapse. Semin Roentgenol 15(2):117–173
Pryor JA (1999) Physiotherapy for airway clearance in adults. Eur Respir J 14(6):1418–1424
Schindler MB (2005) Treatment of atelectasis: where is the evidence? Crit Care 9(4):341–342
Woodring JH, Reed JC (1996) Types and mechanisms of pulmonary atelectasis. J Thorac Imaging 11:92–108

Atelectrauma

► Barotrauma

Atlanto-Axial Dislocation

► Dislocation, Atlas or Axis

Atlas Fracture

► Fracture, Atlas (C1)

ATLS

► Neurotrauma, Pre-hospital Evaluation and Care

Atrial Fibrillation

► Supraventricular Arrhythmia Management

Atrial Flutter

► Supraventricular Arrhythmia Management

Atrial Tachycardia

► Supraventricular Arrhythmia Management

Atrioventricular Nodal Reentry Tachycardia

► Supraventricular Arrhythmia Management

Atrioventricular Reciprocating Tachycardia

► Supraventricular Arrhythmia Management

Attending Physician

▶ Postgraduate Education

Attest

▶ Credentialing

ATV Injuries

Alison Wilson
Department of Surgery, West Virginia
University, Morgantown, WV, USA

Synonyms

All-terrain vehicle; Four wheeler; Quad;
Quad bike

Definition

An ATV is a motorized vehicle with wide, low-
pressure tires, a seat, and handlebars designed to
be straddled by the rider. It is designed to handle
rugged, off-road terrain (Fig. 1). The weight of
the vehicle ranges from 600 to greater than
1,000 lbs. Engine sizes range from 49 to
1,000 cc and speed can approach 80 mph. ATVs

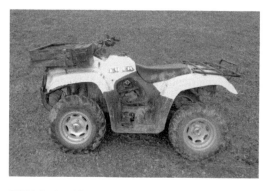

ATV Injuries, Fig. 1 All-Terrain Vehicle (ATV)

are used in a variety of work settings including
farming, ranching, and industrial work. However,
the most common utilization is for recreational
activities. The three-wheeled ATV appeared in
the 1970s, but after an alarming number of injuries and deaths, it was removed from the market
in 1988. The four-wheeled ATV is more stable
than the earlier version, but there remain concerns about the injuries due to these machines.

Application

ATVs are primarily designed for one rider and
require active rider participation to adequately
steer it. To balance the vehicle during a turn, the
rider must actively shift weight away from the
turn. This characteristic contributes to the rate of
rollover accidents when the rider is not able to
provide adequate counter weight, such as when
there is also a passenger or the driver is too small
for the vehicle. This is also why children are at
substantial risk especially when they operate an
adult-sized ATV. ATVs are produced in a variety
of sizes to better match the size of the operator;
however, it is not uncommon that the issue of size
is overlooked.

It is estimated that as of 2010 there were
10.8 million ATVs in use (http://www.atvsafety.
gov/stats.html. Accessed 15 Sep 2013). From the
1990s to 2000s, ATV sales increased 316 %
(Axelband et al. 2007). As the number of ATVs
in the community has increased, so has the
number of ATV-related injuries. The Consumer
Product Safety Commission (CPSC) reported in
2010 that there were 590 confirmed deaths due to
ATV crashes, of which 82 were children under
age 16. The CPSC estimates that the actual
number of ATV-related deaths for 2010 was
726. 115,000 emergency department visits were
recorded in 2010 due to injury after ATV
accidents. 28,300 visits (25 %) were pediatric
patients (http://www.atvsafety.gov/stats.html;
accessed 15 Sep 2013). There has been concern
over the increasing numbers of injuries and
deaths due to ATV injuries. Table 1 illustrates
the trends in injuries and fatalities for both adult
and pediatric patients. Annually, May through

ATV Injuries, Table 1 Trends in injuries and fatalities for adult and pediatric patients

Total deaths		Pediatric deaths	Total ED visits	Pediatric ED visits
2010	590	82	115,000	28,300
2000	447	123	92,200	32,000
1990	235	81	59,500	22,400

Data adapted from http://www.atvsafety.gov/stats.html

ATV Injuries, Table 2 Distribution of injuries by body region in 2011

	Number of injuries	% of total injuries
Head and neck	30,300	28 %
Upper extremity	31,300	29 %
Torso	23,400	22 %
Lower extremity	20,900	20 %
Other	1,500	1 %

Data adapted from http://www.cpsc.gov

September yield the greatest number of both adult and pediatric ATV-related deaths. These injuries predominantly happen in rural environments. Of reported fatalities, 53 % occurred on a roadway, while only 12 % occurred on a farm or pasture and 9 % occurred in forest area (http://www.cpsc.gov/Safety-Education/Safety-Education-Centers/ATV-Safety; accessed 15 Sep 2013). States with the greatest number of deaths due to ATVs are California and Texas. However, West Virginia continues to have the greatest number of fatalities on a per capita basis, and this number appears to be rising. The number of ATV-related fatalities in WV increased from .72 per 100,000 population in 2004 to 1.32 per 100,000 in 2006. The highest death rate is among age 10–17 years and occurs in the southern counties of the state. These counties also have the highest rate of poverty and are the farthest from a trauma center (Center for Disease Control 2008). West Virginia is followed by Kentucky, Tennessee, and North Carolina in per capita ATV-related fatalities. Risk factors for a fatal head injury include lack of a helmet and being a passenger. 95 % of the fatal injuries occurred in riders not wearing helmets (Helmkamp 2003).

Injury patterns can vary depending on the circumstances of the ATV use. Extremity fractures account for approximately half of the total number of injuries, with open extremity fractures being common (Helmkamp et al. 2008). Open elbow fractures are of significant concern in the pediatric population (Kirkpatrick et al. 2007). Facial fractures and spine fractures are also common injuries. Table 2 depicts the anatomic injury distribution as reported by the CPSC for 2011. Severe traumatic brain injury is the most common injury leading to death. Head and neck injuries account for approximately 28 % of the total injuries.

Injury populations due to ATV crashes can vary distinctly. In general, ATVs are designed for an active operator without a passenger, but the actual use and subsequent injury populations expand beyond this group. This is reflected by the trauma registries of injured patients. At one West Virginia Level 1 trauma center, the age range for ATV-related injuries spanned from 2 months of age to 88 years. Geriatric ATV operators tend to be more often using the ATV for occupational use. These vehicles are very useful on farms and ranches where rugged terrain unable to be crossed by a car is common. It is estimated that geriatric ATV riders now comprise 7–9 % of all ATV injury hospitalizations. These accidents tend to be of lower speed and often involve a rollover of the ATV. Helmet use among geriatric patients is low. Recovery from injuries in these patients can be complicated by medical comorbidities, limited physiologic reserves, and pre-injury medications, particularly anticoagulants. Age greater than 60 was an independent predictor of mortality. Patients over age 60 also had a statistically higher Injury Severity Score (12.9 vs. 10.3, $p < 0.001$), longer hospital length of stay (8.3 vs. 4.8 days, $p < 0.001$), and greater number of ICU days (3.1 vs. 1.3 days, $p < 0.001$). Age older than 60 was associated with increased risk of mortality (OR 6.96; 95 % CI 3.75–12.92) (Deladisma et al. 2008).

Pediatric injuries and subsequent mortalities continue to be of concern. Though there are smaller-sized ATVs, children are frequently involved in accidents with adult-sized ATVs. The large size and weight of these machines makes crash injuries and traumatic asphyxia of particular concern in this population. Small-statured children in particular may have difficulty steering appropriately given the need to actively shift weight toward the outside while turning. This makes rollover accidents more likely with a child. Younger children may not have the cognitive development to be able to understand the complexities of steering and balance particularly in uneven terrain (Shah et al. 2012). Children are more likely to be passengers. A passenger on an ATV designed for one person will also cause potential weight shifts that may negatively affect steering. There is evidence that ATV dealers do review the safety recommendations and state legislation, but almost half the ATVs are purchased secondhand. The annualized injury rate is approximately double for boys compared to girls. For children, approximately 70 % of hospitalizations are less than 4 days; however, 10 % had a length of stay greater than 10 days. Also of concern is that the severity of injury as reflected by ISS appears to be increasing (Killingsworth et al. 2005).

An increasing trend is the number of accidents occurring on the roadways. Roadway fatalities increased over twice the rate of off-road fatalities. Roadway crashes were more likely to involve collisions with another vehicle and have multiple fatalities. In fact, ATV crashes that resulted in multiple fatalities were three times greater on roadways as compared to off roadway accidents (Denning et al. 2013a). Roadway crashes are more likely to involve young males and involve alcohol. One in three on road crashes involves collision with another vehicle. This type of collision is 10 times more likely to occur on roadways than off and more likely to result in severe traumatic brain injury (Denning et al. 2013b). Other contributing factors for roadways to pose more danger include structural aspects of the ATV. The wheels are intended for off-road use and do not have the traction interface for paved surfaces. Roadway turns are also more acutely angled than the turn radius that the ATV can usually accommodate. These factors, with the higher center of gravity and high speed of the larger engines, contribute to crashes.

From 2000 to 2004, estimated hospital charges were $1.1 billion with an average charge per patient being approximately $19,000. Intracranial injuries resulted in a longer hospital LOS and hospital cost (Helmkamp et al. 2008). In a pediatric study over a 2-year period total hospital charges were estimated at $74 million (Killingsworth et al. 2005), so the economic impact is significant. Overall, injuries secondary to ATV crashes are increasing, in part due to the increasing popularity of the vehicle. Legislative efforts have been initiated but often are difficult to enforce. Continued education and outreach to high-risk populations, especially young males in rural areas, are warranted.

Cross-References

► Ankle Fractures
► Chest Wall Injury
► Compartment Syndrome, Acute
► Crush Injuries
► Distal Femur Fractures
► Distal Humerus Fractures
► Distal Radius Fractures
► Examination, Neurological
► Femoral Shaft Fractures
► Fracture, Extension Injury
► Fracture, Flexion Injury
► Neurotrauma, Introduction
► Neurotrauma, Pediatric Considerations
► Open Fractures
► Pediatric Airway Management
► Pediatric Femur Fractures
► Pediatric Fractures about the Elbow
► Pediatric Fractures About the Hip
► Tibial Fractures
► Trauma Centers
► Traumatic Brain Injury, Emergency Department Care
► Traumatic Brain Injury, Severe: Medical and Surgical Management

References

Axelband J, Stromski C, McQuay N, Heller M (2007) Are all terrain vehicle injuries becoming more severe? Accid Anal Prev 39:213–215

Center for Disease Control (2008) All terrain vehicle fatalities- West Virginia 1999–2006. Morb Mortal Wkly Rep 57:312–315

Deladisma A, Parker W, Medeiros R, Hawkins M (2008) All-terrain vehicle trauma in the elderly: an analysis of a national database. Am Surgeon 74:767–769

Denning G, Harland K, Ellis D, Jennissen C (2013a) More fatal all-terrain vehicle crashes occur on the roadway than off: increased risk-taking characterises roadway fatalities. Inj Prev 19:250–256

Denning G, Jennissen C, Harland K, Ellis D, Buresh C (2013b) All-Terrain Vehicles (ATVs) on the road: a serious traffic safety and public health concern. Traffic Inj Prev 14:78–85

Helmkamp JC (2003) ATV related deaths in West Virginia: 1990–2003. WV Med J 99:224–227

Helmkamp J, Furbee P, Coben J, Tadros A (2008) All-terrain vehicle related hospitalizations in the United States, 2000–2004. Am J Prev Med 34:39–45

Killingsworth J, Tilford J, Parker J, Graham J, Dick R, Aitken M (2005) National hospitalization impact of pediatric all-terrain vehicle injuries. Pediatrics 115:316–321

Kirkpatrick R, Puffinbarger W, Sullivan A (2007) All-terrain vehicle injuries in children. J Ped Ortho 27:725–728

Shah S, McKenna C, Miller M, Shultz B, Upperman J, Gaines B (2012) Safety factors related to all-terrain vehicle injuries in children. J Trauma Acute Care Surg 73:S273–S276

Authorize

▶ Credentialing

Auto Versus Ped

▶ Pedestrian Struck

Auto Versus Pedestrian

▶ Pedestrian Struck

Autoerotic Strangulation

▶ Strangulation and Hanging

Autologous Donation

Bryan A. Cotton[1] and Laura A. McElroy[2]
[1]Department of Surgery, Division of Acute Care Surgery, Trauma and Critical Care, University of Texas Health Science Center at Houston, The University of Texas Medical School at Houston, Houston, TX, USA
[2]Department of Anesthesiology, Critical Care Medicine, University of Rochester Medical Center, Rochester, NY, USA

Synonyms

Acute normovolemic hemodilution; Homologous donation; Intraoperative cell salvage

Definition

Autologous donation is a method of utilizing a patient's own blood to reduce the number of allogenic blood products needed and the inherent risks associated with their use. Autologous blood donation can be done preoperatively and stored for elective use or intraoperatively using different methods. Indications for autologous donation include large expected blood losses, continued bleeding, and patients that have rare blood types or antibodies or who refuse allogenic blood products (Ashworth and Klein 2010).

Acute normovolemic hemodilution can be utilized in patients with an adequate preoperative hematocrit and expected blood losses near one liter. One to three units of blood are drawn off, anticoagulated, and stored in the operating room for up to eight hours for subsequent transfusion. After the blood is drawn, the volume is replaced with either crystalloid or colloid, producing a temporary hemodilution. This practice has limited application in elective cases but may be associated with increased risk of myocardial ischemia in susceptible patients (Cushing and Ness 2013).

Intraoperative cell salvage (ICS) is an attractive choice for rapidly exsanguinating patients. The process requires a skilled transfusionist and involves collecting blood from the surgical field using a dual-lumen anticoagulating suctioning device, followed by filtration and temporary storage. When an adequate amount of blood has been collected, it is then washed and centrifuged and passed through a semipermeable membrane to recover red blood cells for transfusion. Processing removes free plasma hemoglobin, plasma, white blood cells, platelets, and heparin. Newer devices can separate collected autologous whole blood and separate them into components much like apheresis blood donation, giving red blood cells, platelet-poor liquid plasma, and platelet-rich plasma gels (Waters 2013). Leukocyte reduction filters may also be utilized. Caution must be used, and ICS should be interrupted when the surgical field is contaminated with topical hemostatic agents, antibiotic-laden irrigation, and gross spillage of bowel contents or uterine breach in pregnant females. ICS should be avoided in cases of known bacteremia.

Trauma patients present a complex interplay of pathology and often have contaminated wounds, concomitant gastrointestinal injury, massive inflammatory response, and cytokine release leading to disseminated intravascular coagulopathy (DIC) at the time of surgery. The effects of transfusing blood collected from this environment are being actively studied and are currently unknown, though early studies raise questions about postoperative infection and coagulation problems in these populations (Bhangu 2013; Konig et al. 2013). Meticulous washing of isolated red blood cells may ameliorate some of the detrimental effects (Gruber et al. 2013).

Autologous blood salvage systems can be connected to a variety of devices already utilized in trauma, from thoracostomy drainage systems (first used in 1931) to intra-abdominal suction catheters. There is a paucity of data, but recent studies have looked at the safety and effects of collecting and transfusing autologous blood during trauma surgery and have found that ICS decreases the amount of autologous blood transfused with no difference in morbidity or mortality (Bowley et al. 2006; Brown et al. 2010).

In special social circumstances, such as managing hemorrhagic shock in patients that refuse allogenic blood transfusion, ICS and even use of existing stored preoperative autologous blood donations may be helpful (Gohel et al. 2011).

Cross-References

▶ Disseminated Intravascular Coagulation

References

Ashworth A, Klein AA (2010) Cell salvage as part of a blood conservation strategy in anesthesia. Br J Anesth 105(4):401–416

Bhangu A, Nepogodiev D, Doughty H et al (2013) Intraoperative cell salvage in combat support hospital: a prospective proof of concept study. Transfusion 53:805–810

Bowley D, Barker P, Boffard K (2006) Intraoperative blood salvage in penetrating abdominal trauma: a randomized, controlled trial. World J Surg 30:1074–1080

Brown C, Foulkrod KH, Sadler H et al (2010) Autologous blood transfusion during emergency trauma operations. Arch Surg 145:690–694

Cushing M, Ness P (2013) Principles of red blood cell transfusion. Hematology: basic principles and practice, 6th edn. Elsevier, Philadelphia, pp 1642–1652

Gohel MS, Bulbulia RA, Poskitt KR et al (2011) Avoiding blood transfusion in surgical patients (including Jehovah's Witnesses). Ann R Coll Surg Engl 93:429–431

Gruber M, Breu A, Frauendorf M et al (2013) Washing of banked blood by three different blood salvage devices. Transfusion 53:1001–1009

Konig G, Yazer MH, Waters JH (2013) The effect of salvaged blood on coagulation function as measured by thromboelastography. Transfusion 53:1235–1239

Waters JH (2013) Intraoperative blood recovery. ASAIO J 59:11–17

Autonomy

Jacqueline J. L. Chin
Centre for Biomedical Ethics, Yong Loo Lin
School of Medicine, National University of
Singapore, Singapore, Singapore

Synonyms

Right to decide; Self-determination

Definition

The autonomy of an individual is his or her capacity to think and act in accordance with self-endorsed reasons and motives free from distorting or manipulative forces. Individual autonomy is a central value in biomedical ethics and underpins the ethical and legal requirements of consent, information disclosure, truth-telling, and confidentiality in biomedicine. Autonomy as self-determination is distinct from freedom, which is the ability to act without constraints, whether internal or external. Thus, even constraints upon a person's actions are present or cannot be removed, so that one is not free to act, the autonomy of the individual could remain a matter to be respected, encouraged to certain degrees, and protected in different ways.

Autonomy is a characteristic that could be applied *globally*, and thus, certain beings may be deemed to have autonomy because of their capacity for reason and reflection (e.g., human beings rather than lower animals) or certain persons may be deemed to have autonomy (mentally competent individuals) and not others (e.g., legal minors, patients in PVS or coma, patients with dementia). Or autonomy could be applied *piecemeal* to aspects of decision making, such as to immediate decisions, preferences, wishes, or general values of an individual.

Background

Patients in the Emergency Department

How the autonomy of patients should be protected in a health emergency is a complex question. Patients presenting at the emergency department may be in a critical condition such as trauma, myocardial infarction, and drug overdose and whose survival depends on immediate supportive treatment. Or, they could be seriously ill with rapidly deteriorating functions that could be arrested or reversed by appropriate treatment measures. Many patients in EDs have compromised mental status or regressive behavior due to alcohol or drug-induced intoxication, head trauma, pain, shock, anxiety, or psychiatric conditions. Some may be verbally and physically abusive, requiring stabilization or even restraint. Emergency medicine characteristically demands rapid intervention and, at times, aggressive measures under circumstances when key information is sketchy or simply unavailable (Sanders 2008).

While many patients in the ED may be mentally and decisionally compromised (as legal minors or PVS patients might be) such that their immediate choices are of uncertain reliability, their general preferences, wishes, and values may be known to close friends and relatives who may be at hand to serve as proxy decision makers or collaborators in the decision-making process or through advance directives. However, the availability of knowledgeable proxies or advance directives and their interpretation is not usually assured in the ED. Since present consent to treatment or refusal of treatment carries such an uncertain status with regard to the patient's authentic values, various proposals have been put forward for the protection of patient autonomy in emergency situations.

Paternalism in Emergency Medicine

It used to be assumed in emergency medicine that, while patient consent is an important ethical requirement that underpins patient autonomy, under emergency conditions, it is sufficient that consent be implied (Ramsey 1970, p. 5). Emergency care cannot take into account the idiosyncratic wishes of desperately ill persons. The capacity of emergency room patients to think clearly and the ability of medical professionals to make decisions that accord with the wishes of uniquely individual patients under conditions of limited access to good information in such situations warrant acting in accordance with standards that rational and reflective persons could accept (Tait and Winslow 1977). Emergency care on this account aimed at providing swift intervention and management of patients that emergency medical teams judged to be necessary for preserving life and preventing serious compromise to the patient's health condition. The assumptions behind this practice were the life-preserving aims of medicine, the idea that in a medical emergency patients want physicians and others with experience and expertise in dealing with similar situations to make decisions for them, and that these aims are important enough for most reasonable patients to be willing to take the risk of injury or compromise in quality of life as a result of aggressive management. These assumptions justified medical paternalism on the part of emergency teams (Mattox and Engelhardt 1998).

Limits to Medical Paternalism During Emergencies

In emergency situations involving serious risks to public health, law and ethics support the position that the requirement of consent may be waived. In a pandemic outbreak, for example, quarantine measures may be enforced even against the will of patients. Under such circumstances, the principle of necessity prevails over the principle of liberty. However, such paternalistic actions must be justified by demonstration of sound reasoning and proportionality of the autonomy-limiting interventions. Thus, quarantine measures are normally not recommended until their efficacy has been properly assessed and until public hygiene messages are deemed to be insufficient for addressing the spread of infection. Similarly, the case for more discerning judgement and proportionate action may be applied to patients presenting in the ED, and the assumptions in favor of aggressive intervention and presumed consent by patients have to be subject to careful scrutiny.

The Assumption of Urgency

In an emergency, it may be felt that evaluation and treatment decisions have to be taken within a highly limited time frame (the "golden hour"). However, blanket assumptions of urgency in the emergency situation are unhelpful for medical decision making and may further exacerbate the difficulties of making care decisions in circumstances where the information available is likely to be incomplete, inconclusive, or even incorrect. In situations where surgery is a consideration, for example, urgent surgical conditions such as drainage of subdural hematoma, arresting blood loss or establishment of an airway could represent less than 1 % of the emergency surgery case load (Mattox and Engelhardt 1998, p. 79). Most other surgical decision making in emergency cases is not significantly time constrained and observatory treatment is routine, allowing for better information to emerge for clarifying risks and treatment options.

The Assumption of Aggressive Treatment Pressure

The "vitalist" assumption that all life-preserving measures should be aggressively pursued comes under challenge in the light of considerations of cost, unlikely success, marginal life-prolonging benefit, and quality of life. If treatment is deemed futile or inappropriate, then emergency teams have no obligation to provide it. Ways of classifying emergency patients for aiding decisions on whether to go for cure or comfort care have been proposed (Mattox and Engelhardt 1998). Decision-making guidelines may be drawn up for various categories of emergency patients including those for whom survival of a particular treatment is unprecedented, those who would survive but with likely severe neurological deficits or survive with severe disabilities, or those whose survival chances are low but there is good quality of life among survivors (American College of Emergency Physicians 2004).

Challenges of Informed Consent

Having a patient's informed consent to treatment gives medical teams the right to treat patients. Under emergency conditions, information provided needs to be at a level that is enough for a patient to understand what the medical team intends to do and to authorize them to do it. Fully informed consent may be too difficult, impractical, or unduly burdensome on emergency patients. Hence, quick consent, surrogate consent, or collaborative models of decision making to ascertain a patient's capacity to make specific decisions are common compromises. Again, in the context of a medical emergency, assessment of a patient's capacity to choose or refuse treatment would at times be feasible only at the level of ascertaining whether the patient understands intellectually the intervention to be chosen or refused and what is at stake, appreciates the context of the choice intellectually and affectively, and grasps the causal connections between choosing or refusing particular interventions and their outcomes. This level of understanding may diverge from that of the medical team and the nonemergency patient.

Advance Directives

There is increasing interest in the advance directive or living will as a means of understanding the considered wishes of a patient in a range of anticipated circumstances. These are intended as authoritative instructions even for emergency settings. However, the practical obstacles to their implementation are serious and numerous. Surrogates and medical personnel are often unaware of the existence of any advance directive that the patient might have made. Interpreting the directive is often difficult because some features of the current situation might not have been anticipated and could be seen as relevant exceptions to the circumstances envisaged by the patient. For example, the validity of a DNAR order for "the next episode of respiratory failure" may be called into question if the situation is readily reversed by establishment of an airway and a new significant feature has entered the situation, such as the unexpected diagnosis of terminal illness in a spouse, for instance. There is also evidence of

physician reluctance to implement advance directives due to unwillingness to take on the responsibility of interpreting them in an emergency, especially when trust between doctors, patients and their families have yet to be established (Emanuel et al. 1991).

The Role of the Physician

Within the many constraints of the emergency situation, the responsibility to guide and make decisions that respect the autonomy of the patient rests squarely with physicians. Respect for patient autonomy does not absolve physicians of their critical role in aiding patients, families, and the whole medical team in coming to terms with tough responsibilities accepted under the conditions of human finitude. They have obligations to implement good emergency care and protect the best interests of patients often in the face of emotive interventions by families or against the pressures exerted by law enforcement agencies in some cases.

Application

Refusal of treatment in a medical emergency follows a pattern of practice where the greater the health costs to the patient who refuses treatment, the greater will be the burden on patients to establish their competence or to have left good, clear advance directives that anticipated the current circumstances. Thus, the concern to protect the best interests of patients warrants overriding refusals of lifesaving measures and interventions to prevent grave health risks if a patient's decision-making capacity has not been convincingly established, due to the high cost of the refusal (Sanders 2008, p. 471).

Families are often called upon to be surrogate decision makers in a medical emergency, but the notion that the family possesses decision-making authority over its individual members is a contested one and not well established in most legal jurisdictions. Increasingly, legislative frameworks are providing for involvement of surrogates that take account of traditional family structures. Surrogates are assumed to be good informants on the patient's view of his or her best interests, although this has been repeatedly shown to be false. Family members and surrogates very commonly come to conclusions that are completely different from previously established wishes of a patient. It is also common to find families disagreeing with medical team's judgement of the patient's best interest. Thus, surrogate decision making has not been shown to be a reliable means of preserving patient autonomy. In most Anglo-European countries within the developed world, it is expected of medical teams that patients be asked about the extent to which they would want family to be involved in treatment and care decisions.

In truly emergent conditions where threats to life and limb are imminent, treatment is sometimes undertaken with justification without seeking the patient's consent, such as when capacity is severely compromised (e.g., with patients with trauma, hypotension, or under narcotic influence). The bare semblance of consent or "quick consent" (a grunt or feeble nod) to a quick request to insert a catheter in the bladder or a tube into the chest may suffice. Medical teams have a continuing obligation to then engage the patient and surrogates in gaining understanding of the evolving circumstances and treatment options as time allows.

Cross-References

▶ Evaluating a Patient's Decision-Making Capacity
▶ Informed Consent in Trauma

References

American College of Emergency Physicians (2004) Code of ethics for emergency medicine. Ann Emerg Med 43:686–694
Emanuel LL, Barry MJ, Stoeckle JD, Ettelson LM, Emanuel EJ (1991) Advance directives for medical care – a case for greater use. N Engl J Med 324:889–895
Mattox KL, Engelhardt HT (1998) Emergency patients. In: McCollough LB, Jones JW, Brody BA (eds) Surgical ethics. Oxford University Press, New York, pp 78–96
Ramsey P (1970) The patient as person. Yale University Press, New Haven
Sanders AB (2008) Emergency and trauma medicine ethics. In: Singer PA, Viens AM (eds) The Cambridge textbook of bioethics. Cambridge University Press, New York, pp 469–474
Tait K, Winslow G (1977) Beyond consent-the ethics of decision-making in emergency medicine. West J Med 126:156–159

Autoped

▶ Pedestrian Struck

Auto-PEEP

Stephen E. Lapinsky
Interdepartmental Division of Critical Care, University of Toronto, Toronto, ON, Canada

Synonyms

Dynamic hyperinflation; Intrinsic PEEP; Occult PEEP

Definition

Auto-PEEP is the positive end-expiratory pressure caused by the progressive accumulation of air (air trapping), due to incomplete expiration prior to the initiation of the next breath. This occurs when expiration is limited by airway narrowing or obstruction, or when expiratory time is limited. Total end-expiratory pressure is the sum of the auto-PEEP and the extrinsically applied PEEP, in the mechanically ventilated patient.

Preexisting Condition

Pathophysiology

Inability to fully exhale a tidal volume before the next breath may be caused by increased minute ventilation (i.e., increased tidal volume or respiratory rate) or due to obstruction to exhalation (i.e., airway obstruction or extrinsic resistance), and usually a combination of both.

Elevated minute ventilation: A large tidal volume requires a longer expiratory time to exhale, and increased respiratory rate will shorten the expiratory time. These effects will be aggravated in the patient with airflow limitation. Elevated minute ventilation may occur with a high-set mechanical ventilation, with increased drive to breathe (e.g., acidosis, pneumonia) or may be unrecognized due to rapid manual bag ventilation.

Obstruction to exhalation: This may occur due to airway narrowing (bronchospasm, secretions, airway collapse) or to obstruction to the exhalation circuit, e.g., narrowed endotracheal tube, extrinsic PEEP, or ventilator dyssynchrony.

Identification

Auto-PEEP should be considered in any patient with obstructive airway disease (chronic obstructive pulmonary disease, asthma) receiving mechanical ventilation or any mechanically ventilated patient presenting with potential sequelae of auto-PEEP such as hypotension, pulseless electrical activity, or ventilator dyssynchrony. Identification is relatively simple, but quantification of auto-PEEP is more complex.

Clinical: The patient who continues to exhale (visually, by palpation, or by auscultation of breath sounds) at the time of onset of the next breath likely has a degree of auto-PEEP. However, clinical examination may not be reliable in confidently excluding the presence of auto-PEEP (Kress et al. 1999).

Ventilator graphics: Auto-PEEP can be diagnosed by viewing the flow-time tracing on the ventilator. In the normal situation, expiratory flow gradually approaches the zero level prior to onset of the next breath. In the presence of auto-PEEP, expiratory flow is still present when the upstroke of the next breath occurs (see Fig. 1).

Methods to quantify the degree of auto-PEEP require a patient without spontaneous respiratory efforts, e.g., heavily sedated or paralyzed. By using an end-expiratory breath hold, the end-expiratory pressure in the respiratory system can be measured from the ventilator. Any applied PEEP should be subtracted from the value generated. Another method involves simultaneous measurement of airflow and airway and esophageal pressures (using an esophageal balloon) (Laghi and Goyal 2012). During the respiratory cycle, the negative esophageal pressure (representing pleural pressure) at which expiratory flow ceases correlates with the level of auto-PEEP. Many current ventilators automate one or both of these measurement techniques. The accuracy of measured auto-PEEP is often in question, and all these measurements are affected by active expiratory efforts. The end-inspiratory plateau pressure may be more informative, in terms of the clinical effects and hazards produced by auto-PEEP (Marini 2011).

The presence of spontaneous respiratory effort should be recognized, as this can significantly affect the assessment and quantification of auto-PEEP. Furthermore, the concept of hidden or occult auto-PEEP needs to be appreciated – the presence of widespread airway closure in severe obstructive airway disease may block the continuity between alveoli and the proximal airway where pressure is measured, making the presence of auto-PEEP unrecognized (Stewart and Slutsky 1996).

Application

Clinical Effects

The clinical effects of auto-PEEP are influenced by the compliance of the lungs and chest wall. Auto-PEEP effects on the lungs are also not homogeneous and are influenced by local airway disease, secretions, and positional and gravitational influences.

Hemodynamic effects: Elevated intrathoracic pressure results in a decrease in venous return and reduces cardiac output. In addition, the dynamic hyperinflation also increases pulmonary vascular resistance and therefore right ventricular afterload. The hemodynamic effects are particularly pronounced in the patient who is volume depleted. Hypotension results, which may be

Auto-PEEP,

Fig. 1 Flow-time tracings, demonstrating auto-PEEP. *Panel A* shows expiratory flow returning to zero prior to next breath, while *panel B* shows subsequent breath beginning while expiratory flow continues (*arrow*) implying the presence of auto-PEEP

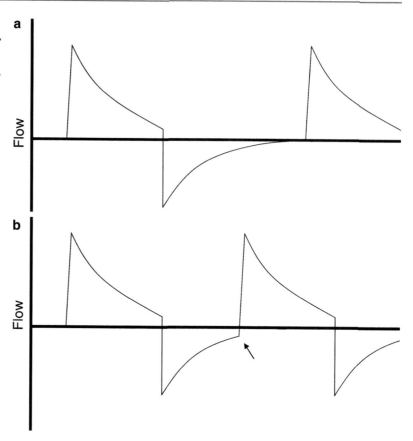

severe, and pulseless electrical activity (PEA) cardiac arrests have been reported (Rogers et al. 1991; Lapinsky and Leung 1996).

Respiratory effects: Alveolar distension may result in barotrauma, manifesting as pneumothorax or pneumomediastinum, which can exacerbate the hemodynamic effects. Compression of the alveolar capillary bed by alveoli under pressure can shunt blood to less well-ventilated areas, causing hypoxemia. In the spontaneously breathing patient, auto-PEEP increases the work of breathing (or work of triggering the ventilator). The respiratory musculature must generate a negative pressure equivalent to the auto-PEEP to the reverse exhalation, before the negative intrathoracic pressure required to initiate the breath becomes effective. Furthermore, the lungs and chest wall are less complaint at high lung volumes. Auto-PEEP may result in patient-ventilator dyssynchrony (i.e., inability to trigger the ventilator) or respiratory muscle fatigue.

Unrecognized auto-PEEP in the mechanically ventilated patient may produce a relatively low respiratory rate due to a proportion of patient efforts being unable to trigger the ventilator. This can be detected clinically by comparing patient efforts (visually or by palpation) with ventilator-assisted breaths and may be corrected when minute ventilation is reduced. A clinical scenario suggestive of intolerance of ventilator weaning may be a manifestation of this effect. An increase in respiratory frequency occurs as ventilator pressure-support level (and therefore minute ventilation) is weaned, due to reduced ineffective triggering of the ventilator (Thille et al. 2008).

Differential Diagnosis

Pneumothorax is a complication of auto-PEEP, but pneumothorax may produce many similar clinical features, i.e., increased intrathoracic pressure and hypotension. In the patient with pneumothorax who does not improve following chest tube drainage, the possibility of associated auto-PEEP should be considered. High levels of extrinsically applied PEEP may produce a similar clinical picture to auto-PEEP.

Management

In the ventilated patient with significant hemodynamic compromise due to auto-PEEP, a rapid solution is to disconnect the ventilator briefly, exposing the airway to room pressure. This will allow the dynamic hyperinflation to "deflate" with resolution of the hypotension within a few heart beats. The ventilator can then be reset to a lower minute ventilation while the patient is reconnected. Fluid resuscitation will also be beneficial in this situation.

Definitive correction of auto-PEEP requires an identification of the cause. Correction of any extrinsic obstruction to the ventilator circuit is essential. Treatment with bronchodilators or steroids may be beneficial in the patient where obstructive airway disease is playing a significant role. Minute ventilation should be reduced, either by decreasing tidal volume, pressure-support level, or respiratory rate or by sedating or paralyzing the spontaneously breathing patient. Reduced ventilation may cause carbon dioxide levels to rise, and a strategy of permissive hypercapnia may be appropriate and lifesaving.

In the spontaneously breathing ventilated patient with auto-PEEP and ventilator dyssynchrony, applying extrinsic PEEP may help to reduce the need for a large negative intrathoracic pressure to trigger the ventilator and improve synchrony and work of breathing. Applied PEEP will generally not increase plateau pressure, if administered in a pressure less than the auto-PEEP level, in patients on volume-cycled ventilation. In the patient on pressure-cycled ventilation, the applied PEEP will increase peak pressure, if driving pressure is maintained. Extrinsically applied PEEP may be beneficial in the patient with expiratory airflow limitation, by opening airways and redistributing PEEP from the most severely air-trapped zones, potentially reducing total PEEP. Applied PEEP should always be significantly less than the auto-PEEP level; otherwise, overall intrathoracic pressure levels may be raised (Marini 2011).

Cross-References

▶ Mechanical Ventilation, Conventional
▶ Mechanical Ventilation, High-Frequency Oscillation
▶ Mechanical Ventilation, Permissive Hypercapnia

References

Kress JP, O'Connor MF, Schmidt GA (1999) Clinical examination reliably detects intrinsic positive end-expiratory pressure in critically ill, mechanically ventilated patients. Am J Respir Crit Care Med 159:290

Laghi F, Goyal A (2012) Auto-PEEP in respiratory failure. Minerva Anestesiol 78(2):201–221

Lapinsky SE, Leung RS (1996) Auto-PEEP and electromechanical dissociation. N Engl J Med 335(9):674

Marini JJ (2011) Dynamic hyperinflation and auto-positive end-expiratory pressure: lessons learned over 30 years. Am J Respir Crit Care Med 184(7):756–762

Rogers PL, Schlichtig R, Miro A, Pinsky M (1991) Auto-PEEP during CPR. An "occult" cause of electromechanical dissociation? Chest 99(2):492–493

Stewart TE, Slutsky AS (1996) Occult, occult auto-PEEP in status asthmaticus. Crit Care Med 24(3):379–380

Thille AW, Cabello B, Galia F, Lyazidi A, Brochard L (2008) Reduction of patient-ventilator asynchrony by reducing tidal volume during pressure-support ventilation. Intensive Care Med 34:1477–1486

Avascular Necrosis (AVN)

▶ Pediatric Fractures About the Hip

Avascular Necrosis of the Femoral Head

Ariful Alam[1] and Khanjan H. Nagarsheth[2]
[1]Department of General Surgery, Staten Island University Hospital, Staten Island, NY, USA
[2]R Adams Cowley Shock Trauma Center, University of Maryland School of Medicine, Baltimore, MD, USA

Synonyms

Aseptic necrosis; AVN; Bone infarction; Ischemic bone necrosis; Osteonecrosis

Definition

Avascular necrosis (AVN) is a pathologic process with various etiologies, the most common of which are trauma and injury. By definition, avascular necrosis of the femoral head is death of bone and marrow cells due to compromise of the blood supply, leading to mechanical failure of the joint. The process is usually progressive, resulting in destruction of the joint within a few months to two years in the majority of patients (Kaushik et al. 2012).

Preexisting Conditions

Anatomy of the Femoral Head

An understanding of the vasculature of the femoral head is necessary to understand the progressive nature of AVN. The main blood supply to the femoral head arises from the medial femoral circumflex artery (MFCA). Branches of MFCA enter the capsule of hip joint near its distal insertion and course proximally along the femoral neck towards the head. The MCFA arises from the posteromedial aspect of the deep femoral artery and less commonly from the common femoral artery. Of the branches of the MCFA, the posterior superior retinacular vessels give rise to the lateral epiphyseal vessels (LEVs), which are the principal sources of blood flow to the femoral head. The LEVs enter the femoral head within a 1-cm-wide zone between the cartilage of the femoral head and the cortical bone of the femoral neck. The LEVs supply the lateral and central thirds of the femoral head. The artery of the ligamentum teres supplies the medial third of the femoral head, when patent (Karatoprak and Karaca 2012).

Etiology and Pathophysiology

Avascular necrosis of the femoral head can be associated with a variety of traumatic and atraumatic factors. It can be a result of a combination of multiple factors which include genetic predisposition, metabolic factors, vascular disease, and mechanical stresses (Kaushik et al. 2012).

Trauma is one of the most common causes of AVN and can occur within 8 h after a traumatic disruption of the blood supply. Fracture in the subcapital region is often accompanied by interruption of the blood supply to the head of the femur resulting in ischemia and eventual necrosis. In addition, intracapsular hematoma can increase intracapsular pressure and cause blockage of blood flow to the vessels within the joint capsule (Kaushik et al. 2012).

Corticosteroids have been associated to the development of osteonecrosis in numerous retrospective studies, with incidence ranging from 27 % to 31 % (Shigemura et al. 2011). Several mechanisms have been suggested, one of which involves alterations in circulating lipids resulting in microemboli in the arteries. Another possible mechanism suggests an increase in the size of bone marrow fat cells that cause an obstruction of the venous flow. Yet another possibility is that corticosteroids cause change in venous endothelium leading to stasis, increased intraosseous pressure, and necrosis (Sen 2009).

Excessive alcohol use may cause fat emboli, adipocyte hypertrophy, venous stasis, and increased cortisol levels, which can lead to osteonecrosis. Systemic lupus erythematosus has been associated with avascular necrosis in 3–30 % of patients (Fukushima et al. 2010). The greatest risk is in patients who use corticosteroids. Osteonecrosis is also seen in patients with

Avascular Necrosis of the Femoral Head, Table 1 Classification systems for avascular necrosis of the femoral head

Stage	Ficat/Arlet	Steinberg/U Penn	ARCO[a]	Treatment options
I	Normal radiographs	Normal radiographs	Normal radiographs	Core – decompression possible, free vascularized fibula grafting
II	Subchondral cyst formation and sclerosis	Femoral head lucency/ sclerosis	Demarcating sclerosis in femoral head, no collapse	Free vascularized fibula grafting
III	Femoral head flattening, subchondral collapse, "crescent sign"	Subchondral collapse without femoral head flattening, "crescent sign"	Femoral head collapse, "crescent sign," no joint space narrowing	Free vascularized fibula grafting. Success depends on degree of changes
IIIA			Collapse < 3 mm	Increasing risk of failure of preventative surgery
IIIB			Collapse > 3 mm	Increasing risk of failure of preventative surgery
IV	Osteoarthritic space narrowing, degenerative changes	Subchondral collapse, femoral head flattening, normal joint space	Osteoarthritic degenerative changes	Total hip replacement, free vascularized fibula grafting
V		Femoral head flattening with joint space narrowing, acetabular changes, or both		Hip replacement required
VI		Advanced degenerative changes, secondary osteoarthritis		Total hip replacement

[a]ARCO: Association Research Circulation Osseous

sickle cell hemoglobinopathies, Gaucher disease, radiation therapy, and type II collagen mutation. There are also two types of osteonecrosis limited to children and adolescents. These include Legg-Calve-Perthes disease and slipped capital femoral epiphysis (Kaushik et al. 2012).

Application

Presentation
Patients presenting with medial thigh or groin pain with limitation of hip motion, particularly hip abduction and internal rotation, should raise suspicion for AVN. Symptoms are usually slow onset and may be unilateral or bilateral. They are aggravated by weight bearing and alleviated by rest. The pain may be present in the buttocks, knees, or anterior and lateral thigh. It is important to remember that early stages of the disease may be asymptomatic. Diagnosis and management of the disease are based upon plain radiographic classification (Karatoprak and Karaca 2012).

Multiple classification systems exist for classifying AVN of the femoral head (Table 1).

Nonoperative Management
Nonoperative management of avascular necrosis of the femoral head includes restricted weight bearing, pharmacological agents, and external, biophysical modalities. Reduced weight bearing was recommended on the expectation that it would prevent femoral head collapse during healing. However, numerous studies have failed to demonstrate the effectiveness of this treatment modality (Sen 2009).

Pharmacological agents such as lipid-lowering drugs, anticoagulants, vasodilators, and bisphosphonates have been suggested as therapies, due to their effects on physiologic risk factors. Pulsed electromagnetic field stimulation has been used on the premise that it affects local inflammation and contributes to the repair of the osteonecrotic head by neovascularization and new bone formation. Hyperbaric oxygen has also been used because it is thought to induce angiogenesis, reduce edema, and improve oxygenation. It should be noted that although various nonoperative methods are available to manage asymptomatic patients or those in early stages of the disease, most authors agree that advanced stages of the disease should be treated operatively (Sen 2009).

Operative Management

Operative management of avascular necrosis of the femoral head can be divided into either joint-preserving procedures or arthroplasty. Joint-preserving techniques have good outcomes if performed at earlier stages of the disease or prior to femoral head collapse. In the event that the femoral head has already collapsed, arthroplasty is the preferred technique (Karatoprak and Karaca 2012).

Joint-sparing techniques include core decompression, vascularized fibular grafting, nonvascularized bone grafting, and rotational osteotomies. Core decompression involves the removal of one or more necrotic cores in order to stimulate repair and is performed as a prophylactic measure in earlier stage of the disease. The procedure may be performed with cancellous bone autograft or structural allograft for stabilization and to augment the repair. Core decompression can be further supplemented by bone morphogenetic proteins, electromagnetic stimulation, or demineralized bone matrix, which has been suggested to improve the healing process (Karatoprak and Karaca 2012).

Vascularized fibular grafts have been used as a supplement to core decompression for more advanced disease. This can delay the progression of disease both before and after femoral head collapse. They provide structural support and promote callus formation and remodeling. Nonvascularized bone grafting provides subchondral and joint cartilage support by replacing necrotic tissue with a cortical or cancellous bone graft. Although there is no consensus regarding the use of this technique, it is usually recommended for patients with depression of the femoral head of less than 2 mm. Osteotomies can be performed in attempt to move necrotic bone away from the primary weight bearing areas in the hip joint.

However, osteotomies make subsequent arthroplasty more challenging, and unfortunately, these procedures are associated with a higher risk of nonunion. Although the aforementioned techniques may delay arthroplasty, ultimately, total hip replacement is the definitive repair for avascular necrosis of the femoral head (Kaushik et al. 2012).

Conclusion

Avascular necrosis of the femoral head is a problem seen after trauma that can result in serious morbidity for the victim. This is a result of interruption in the blood supply to the femoral head, which is usually supplied by an end artery. This injury is classified based on a number of different systems, and treatment is based on its classification. Prompt diagnosis and treatment are necessary to prevent any undue complications and the need for further surgeries and possible total joint replacement.

Cross-References

▶ Amputation

References

Fukushima W, Fujioka M, Kubo T et al (2010) Nationwide epidemiologic survey of idiopathic osteonecrosis of the femoral head. Clin Orthop Relat Res 468:2715

Karatoprak O, Karaca S (2012) Surgical management of avascular necrosis of the femoral head: an update. Orthop Res Rev 4:97–102

Kaushik AP, Das A, Cui Q (2012) Osteonecrosis of the femoral head: an update in 2012. World J Orthop 3(5):49–57

Sen RK (2009) Management of avascular necrosis of femoral head at pre-collapse stage. Indian J Orthop 43(1):6–16

Shigemura T, Nakamura J, Kishida S et al (2011) Incidence of osteonecrosis associated with corticosteroid therapy among different underlying diseases: prospective MRI study. Rheumatology 50:2023

AVN

▶ Avascular Necrosis of the Femoral Head

Awareness and Trauma Anesthesia

Nina Singh-Radcliff
Department of Anesthesiology,
AtlantiCare Regional Medical Center,
Pomona, NJ, USA
Galloway Township, NJ, USA

Synonyms

Recall; Unintentional Consciousness; Unintentional Intraoperative Awareness

Definition

Awareness during anesthesia implies that during a period of intended general anesthesia, the brain is aroused by stimuli that are stored in memory for future explicit recall. It has an estimated incidence between 0.007 % and 0.91 % (Domino et al. 2000; Ghoneim et al. 2009; Sebel et al. 2004). Thus, with over 20 million general anesthetics performed yearly in the United States, the occurrence can be striking. Consequently, in 2004, the Joint Commission issued an alert stating that anesthesia awareness is an "under-recognized and undertreated" problem in health-care organizations. The incidence in trauma patients is even more alarming and has been shown to range from 11 % to 43 % in various studies (Bogetz and Katz 1984; Moerman et al. 1993; Dave and Winikoff 2012). However, ethical considerations have limited intervention-based studies that support recommendations to prevent awareness under anesthesia or treat patients who have experienced it. The current body of evidence is mostly comprised of retrospective studies and data analysis that identify risk factors and associations or have limited interventions.

When discussing and describing awareness, there are several important terms that require defining (ASA Practice Advisory 2006; Ghoneim et al. 2009; Moerman et al. 1993; Dave and Winikoff 2012):

- Consciousness describes a state in which a patient is able to process information from his or her surroundings.
- Unconsciousness results from the interruption in cortical communication and loss of integration that is needed to process information from one's surroundings.
- General anesthesia is a drug-induced state that produces unconsciousness.
- Perceptions while under anesthesia are most commonly auditory (sounds, conversations) and feelings of fear, helplessness, pain, anxiety, and paralysis. Less commonly, they include visual perception, memory of intubation, and feeling the operation without pain.
- Memories are often described as explicit or implicit. Explicit memory, or recall, is the conscious recollection of stored memories, whereas implicit memory describes changes in performance or behavior that are produced by previous experiences but without any conscious recollection of those experiences
- Amnesia is the absence of recall. Patients may follow commands as they are emerging from anesthesia or during "wake-up" testing (e.g., spinal surgery to test the integrity of nerves), but not have conscious recall (explicit memory).
- "Awake paralysis" is a term used to describe errors in the administration of neuromuscular blocking agent resulting in paralysis of the unanesthetized or incompletely anesthetized patient.

Preexisting Condition

Risk Factors

Retrospective studies and closed claims analysis have identified the following risk factors for awareness under anesthesia (Bischoff and Rundshagen 2011; Domino et al. 2000; Ghoneim et al. 2009):

- Patient related: Impaired cardiovascular function and reserve, chronic pain conditions, obesity, and children

- Intervention related: Emergency surgery, procedures performed at night, Cesarean sections, and cardiac surgery
- Drug related: Administration of muscle relaxants, total intravenous anesthesia, and nitrous oxide

Trauma patients may have several of the above-mentioned risk factors including impaired cardiovascular reserve, emergency status, and requiring surgery at night.

Morbidity

The impact of anesthesia awareness is not inconsequential. Studies have shown that postoperative sequelae can range from 33 % to 69 % and may persist for varying durations. They include (Bischoff and Rundshagen 2011; Ghoneim et al. 2009; Moerman et al. 1993; Dave and Winikoff 2012):

- Sleep disturbances, including nightmares.
- Daytime anxiety and panic attacks.
- Post-traumatic stress disorder (PTSD). Patients that experience the inability to move or feelings such as helplessness have a significant increase in PTSD. Studies have shown that 10–25 % of patients who experience PTSD will not recover and will require treatment.
- Avoidance of future medical care including any future anesthetic exposure.

Application

Clinical Signs and Symptoms

Clinical signs and symptoms of perception have been described as surrogate markers and often occur *after* awareness has taken place. Sweating, lacrimation, and movement may be seen (Bischoff and Rundshagen 2011). Vital sign changes include tachycardia and hypertension, and in spontaneously breathing subjects, increases in the respiratory rate and volume can be indicative of inadequate anesthesia and awareness. However, the administration of beta-blockers or calcium channel blockers, medications with sympatholytic effects, or muscle

relaxation can mask these findings. A review of the American Society of Anesthesiologist's Closed Claims Database showed that increased blood pressure was noted in only 15 % of cases, increased heart rate in only 7 % of cases, and movement in only 2 % of cases (ASA Practice Advisory 2006; Domino et al. 2000).

Volatile Anesthetics

Inhaled volatile agents are frequently utilized to maintain unconsciousness, amnesia, and immobility. The main hemodynamic implication of contemporary inhalational agents (desflurane, isoflurane, and sevoflurane) is a decrease in the systemic vascular resistance (SVR); decreases in cardiac contractility occur to a smaller extent. Halothane, which is less commonly used, significantly decreases cardiac contractility and hence cardiac output (CO), in addition to decreasing the SVR. Since blood pressure (BP) is the product of the SVR and CO (BP = SVR × CO), decreases in either parameter can affect perfusion of vital organs. These cardiovascular effects from volatile agents are more profound in patients with advanced age, increased vascular tone, decreased cardiac function/reserve, coadministration of medications affecting the SVR and/or CO, coadministration of intravenous anesthetics (e.g., propofol), and hypovolemia.

The term minimum alveolar concentration (MAC) describes the alveolar concentration of a volatile agent, at 1 atm, that is required to produce immobility in 50 % of patients at skin incision. MAC awake, or MAC awareness, is the term used to describe the concentration at which there is no response to verbal or tactile stimulation in 50 % of patients and is estimated at approximately 0.4 MAC. MAC values have limitations and cannot ensure that a patient will not have awareness. They do not reflect an individual's response and, by definition, 50 % of patients will move or respond to verbal or tactile stimulation.

Intravenous Anesthetics

Intravenous anesthetics can be used to induce or maintain general anesthesia as well as serve as an adjunct to provide a "balanced" anesthetic.

Depending on their hemodynamic profile, these agents may be utilized to offset the deleterious hemodynamic effects of volatile agents and allow a decrease in MAC values. In the unstable patient, intravenous agents may be the only agent that is tolerated.

Propofol is a hypnotic agent that is commonly utilized to induce general anesthesia or as a component of total intravenous anesthesia. It can result in profound decreases in the systemic BP from vasodilation of arterial and venous systems as well as myocardial depression. It demonstrates a dose-dependent reduction in preload, afterload, and contractility, with a consequent decrease in the mean arterial pressure (MAP, up to 40 %) and cardiac output. Additionally, it blocks the arterial baroreceptor response to hypotension and reflex tachycardia. Its effects are more pronounced in elderly patients, states of hypovolemia, and with rapid administration. Consequently, its pharmacodynamic profile often precludes its use, or requires dose reduction, for induction in the trauma patient.

Etomidate is a hypnotic agent that is often preferred for induction of anesthesia in the hemodynamically unstable patient. It does not release histamine and has a unique lack of effect on the sympathetic nervous system and baroreceptor function. Consequently, it has been shown to maintain cardiac contractility, central venous pressure, systemic vascular resistance, heart rate, and stroke volume to a greater extent than propofol. Mild decreases in the MAP can occur from decreased SVR (hypovolemic states may see a drop in the blood pressure).

Ketamine is a phencyclidine derivative that can be utilized for induction of anesthesia; it has one-tenth the potency but maintains many of its psychomimetic effects. In vitro, it is a cardiac depressant. In vivo, administration often results in centrally mediated sympathetic stimulation as well as inhibits reuptake of norepinephrine with resultant increases in mean arterial pressure, heart rate, cardiac output, and systemic vascular resistance (coadministration of benzodiazepines, opioids, and inhaled anesthetics may blunt this effect). However, if catecholamine stores are depleted, as can be seen in the trauma patient, ketamine has a direct depressant effect on the myocardium.

Scopolamine is a nonselective muscarinic antagonist that can cross the blood–brain barrier and produce amnesia with minimal hemodynamic consequences. Its use as a pharmacological model of "cholinergic amnesia" became very popular after the cholinergic hypothesis of geriatric memory dysfunction was postulated. This hypothesis assumes that the age-related decline in cognitive function is predominantly related to the decrease of the integrity of cholinergic neurotransmission. In the trauma patient, intravenous administration of 5–10 mcg/kg (onset time ~20 min) may be given to decrease the incidence of awareness (Mashour et al. 2011; Dave and Winikoff 2012). It is also available for subcutaneous and transdermal patch administration. However, it does not reliably produce amnesia.

In addition to providing anxiolysis and treating seizure activity, benzodiazepines are capable of producing anterograde amnesia by impairing acquisition processes and disrupting the ability to build new associations between events. Midazolam, at large doses (0.3 mg/kg), may also be used as a sole intravenous induction agent. However, it has a slower onset of action and longer duration than propofol, etomidate, and ketamine. Additionally, it is not void of cardiovascular effects; however, they are typically less pronounced than propofol and volatile agents. Benzodiazepine administration can decrease the MAC of volatile agents necessary to prevent awareness. In the setting of hemodynamic embarrassment, it may be the only agent that a patient can tolerate.

Monitors

At this time, cost-effective monitors that can detect the level of consciousness during general anesthesia and prevent awareness with high reliability do not exist. However, these monitors have been shown to potentially be effective and may play an important role in the trauma patient. Most current monitors aim to assess brain electrical activity rather than physiological responses.

The raw electroencephalogram (EEG) is a reflection of cortical brain activity that requires knowledge of the differing waveforms to gain an understanding of anesthetic depth. The complexity of the EEG, however, can mislead even sophisticated quantitative monitors and can lead to erroneous clinical decisions. Classically, the patient requires a full "montage" of electrodes that cover the entire scalp to capture the whole spectrum of EEG activity that is generated (e.g., assessment of seizure activity, during carotid endarterectomy, and clipping of cerebral aneurysms). To assess anesthetic depth, monitoring three or four electrodes (positive, negative, and reference) placed on the forehead close to the hairline will obtain an EEG sufficient to assess the depth of anesthesia. The frontal aspect is more resistant to pharmacologic sleep than posterior aspects, thereby bestowing a margin of safety. Voltage fluctuations that arise from dendritic synapses are sensed by the electrodes, and the sum is reflected in each EEG electrode. The EEG pattern consists of waves of differing frequencies over time. The awake state is demonstrated by low amplitude (or voltage) and high frequency. With increasing anesthetic depth, the amplitude increases and the frequency decreases; there is a loss of fast alpha activity and an increase in beta activity. With further increasing sedation, beta activity will slow, and spindle (theta) activity will appear. Eventually, alpha and beta activity disappears, and theta activity will appear. Even deeper levels of general anesthesia will cause an isoelectric EEG that is interrupted by "bursts," and is referred to as burst suppression. Further deepening of anesthesia will further increase the length spent suppressed and reduce the number of "bursts." Eventually, isoelectricity will prevail without "bursts" (Nadjat-Haiem 2012) (Table 1).

The EEG is influenced not only by the medications administered but also by a myriad of factors in the patient's physiology and underlying pathology. Additionally, the electrodes will also pick up signals generated by other unwanted current sources, such as facial, eye, and heart muscles, and electrical sources. The anesthetist must be aware of these noise generators when making clinical decisions.

Modern monitors, such as the Bispectral Index® (BIS) and Spectral Entropy® (M-entropy), attempt to quantify this raw EEG, yielding an easy-to-interpret number. The BIS monitor provides a single, unitless value based on the weighted sum of electroencephalographic subparameters to indicate the depth of anesthesia. BIS values range from 0 to 100, with higher values suggesting awakeness. Values within 40–60 have been generally accepted to have a low probability of awareness under anesthesia. However, retrospective studies have shown that awareness can occur outside these ranges. Furthermore, BIS values are affected by hypoperfusion and cerebral ischemia and may lead to false positives (O'Connor et al. 2001).

Preventative Measures

Basic preventative measures that can be performed to decrease the likelihood of intraoperative awareness include conducting a preoperative checklist of the anesthesia machine and equipment to ensure that the intended anesthetic drugs and dosages will be delivered (Bischoff and Rundshagen 2011). These procedures should be extended to include proper functioning of intravenous access, infusion pumps, and their connections. Modulation of operating room behavior should also be performed, as patients tend to remember auditory perceptions. The use of electrical function monitors may be useful, in addition to delivering a balanced general anesthetic and assessing clinical signs and symptoms frequently.

Providing a balanced general anesthetic that ensures adequate end-organ perfusion and amnesia is a challenging task in trauma. Several measures that help prevent awareness are often not applicable in trauma patients. These include taking the time to obtain a thorough medical history, reviewing the patient's medical records, or discussing potential risk factors. Additionally, administering between 0.8 and 1.0 MAC of volatile anesthetic, nitrous oxide (potential to expand airspaces), or more than a "sleep dose" of induction agent prior to tracheal intubation is usually not a viable option in trauma anesthesia. The cardiodepressant effects of

Awareness and Trauma Anesthesia, Table 1 Summary of electroencephalogram (EEG) frequencies at different states of anesthesia

Depth of anesthesia	EEG frequency	EEG waveform	EEG morphology	Bispectral Index (BIS)
Awake	Fast, low amplitude	Mostly alpha, some beta		High 90s
Sedation	Slow, increased amplitude	Alpha decreases, beta increases		80s to low 90s
General anesthesia	Increased slowing, prominent slow waves	Mostly theta		40–60
Burst suppression	Varying suppression, with bursts			0–teens

A

volatile agents are the main limiting factor in achieving adequate MAC values and, hence, amnesia in the trauma patient. In the setting of hemodynamic instability, the administration of anesthetic agents can lead to end-organ damage or hemodynamic decompensation and collapse, thereby warranting dose reduction. Additionally, MAC values may be increased with chronic alcoholism or use of sympathetic agents (acute cocaine and amphetamine intoxication), conditions that may be present in the trauma patient and potentially increase the risk of awareness. Conversely, certain physiological derangements and factors that may be coexistent in the trauma patient have been shown to reduce MAC values: hypothermia (decreases 50 % for every 10 °C decrease), hypotension (MAP < 40 mmHg), hyponatremia, metabolic acidosis, anemia (Hct <10 %), hypercarbia ($paCO_2$ >95 mmHg), hypoxia (paO_2 >38 mmHg), and pregnancy (after ~8 weeks). Therefore, assessment of anesthetic depth during trauma anesthesia requires taking into consideration all of these physiologic, pharmacologic, and intraoperative considerations, continuous monitoring of clinical signs of awareness, and use of adjunct monitors if available.

Postoperative Assessment and Management

Awareness under general anesthesia for the trauma patient should be identified, managed, and, if appropriate, referred for further support (ASA Practice Advisory 2006; Bogetz and Katz 1984; Ghoneim et al. 2009). Postoperative follow-up of all trauma patients may be performed with the modified Brice Questionnaire. This four-question list provides a quick and easy way to assess for the occurrence of awareness under anesthesia:

- What was the last thing you remembered before going to sleep?
- What was the last thing you remembered on waking?
- Do you remember anything between going to sleep and waking?
- While you were sleeping during the operation, did you dream?

Studies have shown that explicit memories may not be detected in the immediate postoperative period or hospital stay, however.

In patients in whom awareness has occurred, a discussion should take place to obtain a detailed account of the patient's experience. This should be appropriately documented. Additionally, an occurrence report regarding the event should be completed for the purpose of quality management. The patient should be informed of the Anesthesia Awareness Registry and encouraged to join the registry by calling (206) 616–2669 and request a paper enrollment packet. Apologizing to the patient and offering counseling or psychological support to the patient should also take place (ASA Practice Advisory 2006; Bogetz and Katz 1984; Ghoneim et al. 2009).

Cross-References

- ▶ Benzodiazepines
- ▶ Drug Abuse and Trauma Anesthesia
- ▶ General Anesthesia for Major Trauma
- ▶ Hemodynamic Management in Trauma Anesthesia
- ▶ Pharmacologic Strategies in Adult Trauma Anesthesia

References

American Society of Anesthesiologists Task Force on Intraoperative Awareness (2006) Practice advisory for intraoperative awareness and brain function monitoring. A report by the American Society of Anesthesiologists Task Force on intraoperative awareness. Anesthesiology 104:847–864

Bischoff P, Rundshagen I (2011) Awareness under general anesthesia. Deutsches Arztebl Int 108(1–2):1–7

Bogetz MS, Katz JA (1984) Recall of surgery for major trauma. Anesthesiology 61:6–9

Dave ND, Winikoff S (2012) Awareness under anesthesia. In: Singh-Radcliff N (ed) The 5 minute anesthesia consult, 1st edn. Lippincott, Philadelphia, PA, pp 110–111

Domino KB, Posner KL, Caplan RA, Cheney FW (2000) Awareness during anesthesia. Anesthesiology 90:1053–1061

Ghoneim MM, Block RI, Haffarnan M, Mathews MJ (2009) Awareness during anesthesia: risk factors, causes and sequelae: a review of reported cases in the literature. Intl Anesth Res Soc 108:2

Mashour GA, Orser BA, Avidan MS (2011) Intraoperative awareness from neurobiology to clinical practice. Anesthesiology 114:5

Moerman N, Bonke B, Oosting J (1993) Awareness and recall during general anesthesia. Anesthesiology 79:454–464

Nadjat-Haiem C (2012) Electroencephalogram (EEG). In: Singh-Radcliff N (ed) The 5 minute anesthesia consult, 1st edn. Lippincott, Philadelphia, PA, pp 356–357

O'Connor MF, Daves SM, Tung A, Cook RI, Thisted R, Apfelbaum J (2001) BIS monitoring to prevent awareness during general anesthesia. Anesthesiology 94:520–522

Sebel PS, Bowdle TA, Ghoneim MM, Rampil IJ, Padilla RE, Gan TJ, Domino KB (2004) The incidence of awareness during anesthesia: a multicenter United States study. Anesth Analg 99:833–839

A

B

Bacterial Pneumonia

▶ Empyema

Bag-Mask Ventilation

▶ Airway Management in Trauma, Nonsurgical

Ballistic Trauma

▶ Gunshot Wounds to the Extremity

Ballistic Vest

▶ Body Armor

Ballistics

Craig D. Silverton[1] and Paul Dougherty[2]
[1]Department of Orthopedic Surgery,
Henry Ford Hospital, Detroit, MI, USA
[2]Department of Orthopedic Surgery,
University of Michigan, Ann Arbor, MI, USA

Synonyms

Ammunition; Cavitation; Firearms; Projectiles; Weapons

Definition

Ballistics is the science of a projectile traveling a path and ultimately hitting a target. Once the projectile hits the intended target, this creates another area of science termed wounding or terminal ballistics.

While the bullet or projectile is in the barrel of the weapon, this is termed internal ballistics.

© Springer-Verlag Berlin Heidelberg 2015
P.J. Papadakos, M.L. Gestring (eds.), *Encyclopedia of Trauma Care*,
DOI 10.1007/978-3-642-29613-0

After leaving the barrel and prior to hitting the target, this path of the bullet is termed external ballistics. These three areas are combined to define the study of ballistics.

Internal Ballistics

There are two important variables in studying internal ballistics: the size of the bullet and the barrel velocity. Handguns typically shoot a lower-velocity bullet as compared to a rifle. Handgun chambers are able to handle less pressure as compared to rifles. Rifling of the barrel in both handguns and rifles assists in stabilizing the bullet as it moves down the barrel. Barrel length also is different and contributes to the velocity and accuracy of a weapon. A typical handgun may have a 4- or 6-in. barrel as compared to a rifle with a 22-in. barrel. Once a bullet exits the barrel, no further propulsion is provided by the gunpowder and the bullet will begin the gradually lose velocity.

A typical 9-mm bullet is classified according to the weight of the bullet (125 grain, 147 grain, etc.). The amount and type of powder will determine the exit muzzle velocity. This can vary from 1,100 to 1,300 ft per second (fps). Compare this to a 30-06 rifle with a 168 grain bullet traveling at 2,800 fps. The common M16 military rifle uses a 62 grain bullet with an exit velocity of 3,200 fps. The cartridge in a rifle bullet is able to handle more powder than a handgun. Although different velocities can be achieved with varying powder types and bullet weights, the goal remains the same, accuracy and reliability while maintaining maximum wounding potential.

External Ballistics

Once the bullet exits the barrel, whether a handgun or a rifle, it begins to lose its velocity for several reasons. There is no longer the "push" from the propellant, the air creates a certain amount of drag on the projectile, and some degree of yaw takes effect. Yaw is the amount of deflection seen off a straight line to the target. This rocking back and forth motion has been termed tumbling in the past. The bullet moves very little (1–3°) off the intended course, and there is nothing to suggest it will actually tumble in the air until it hits the target. Once it enters the soft tissue (wounding ballistics), tumbling plays a major role in wounding.

Terminal/Wounding Ballistics

Once the bullet strikes the intended target, a cascade of events transpires. The bullet initially penetrates clothing and enters the skin, muscle, and soft tissue envelope where damage begins to take place. Many have termed this the release of the kinetic energy to the target; however this terminology can be misleading (Fackler 1988; 1996). A faster bullet (62 grain, 3,200 fps M16) may enter and exit a target with minimal soft tissue damage. Conversely, a slower moving bullet (200 grain, 800 fps 45 caliber pistol) may impart significant damage and not exit the target (Swan and Swan 1991). A speed of 160 fps is required to enter the skin and soft tissue (Belkin 1978). Thus the wounding potential of various calibers is difficult to classify since as much has to do with where the bullet strikes anatomically. Any bone that is hit generally will fracture and or become a secondary missile causing additional damage. A rifle bullet striking a bone will generally do significantly more damage as compared to a pistol bullet.

After entering the soft tissues, the bullet may yaw and tumble as well as fragment. This again varies on the size, shape, and velocity of the bullet. A typical handgun bullet (low velocity) will not exhibit this disorderly conduct as compared to a rifle bullet (high velocity) that may fragment as much as 50 % and tumble 180° before exciting the target.

Tumbling, fragmenting, and rotating all contribute to the soft tissue injury present. Softer tip bullets and hollow point bullets are designed to expand once entering their target to enhance the wounding potential by creating a larger cross-sectional diameter. Expansion of bullets reliably occurs above 1,200 fps so this limits certain handgun calibers.

As the bullet traverses the soft tissue envelope, two cavities are created. The permanent cavity is the area of crush and necrosis and a reliable indicator of wounding capacity. Larger diameter bullets create a larger permanent cavity. The temporary cavity is the area that surrounds the permanent cavity as the soft tissues are expanded outward or stretched. This temporary cavity is variable but is usually significantly larger with high-velocity (>2,000 fps) rifles as compared to low-velocity (<1,000 fps) handgun calibers. Most handgun calibers only create a minimal if any temporary cavity thus their wounding potential is limited by the size of the permanent cavity (Peters and Sebourn 1996).

The temporary cavity may damage solid structures such as the kidney or liver that is nonelastic. Muscle however is able to absorb the temporary cavity since it is highly elastic. Other empty hollow organs, blood vessels, and skin are good energy absorbers and are not confined by hard structures. The brain however is not able to absorb this temporary cavity and is surrounded by the hardened bony structure making most ballistic wounds to the head lethal.

Tumbling and fragmentation is generally seen with high-velocity bullets and creates significant soft tissue damage. The bullet will yaw and tumble, creating a larger permanent cavity, and fragmentation of the bullet creates additional permanent cavities in the soft tissue envelope. This fragmentation is one of the major differences in the wounding potential of high-velocity versus low-velocity missile wounds.

Treatment

Debridement of necrotic and nonviable tissue is the mainstay of treatment of any ballistic wound. The permanent cavity creates this wound channel, and depending on the extent of the wound, a more or less aggressive treatment protocol is necessary. The temporary cavity is not debrided as this tissue is generally stretched and is still viable. Overaggressive debridement is not recommended and causes more morbidity without any benefit. All wounds should be left open.

Cross-References

▶ Cavitation
▶ Debridement
▶ Explosion
▶ Fragment Injury
▶ High-Velocity
▶ Mortars
▶ Spalling

References

Belkin M (1978) Wound ballistics. Prog Sur 16:7–2
Fackler ML (1988) Wound ballistics. A review of common misconceptions. JAMA 259:2730–2736
Fackler ML (1996) Gunshot wound review. Ann Emerg Med 28:194–203
Peters CE, Sebourn CL (1996) Wound ballistics of unstable projectiles. Part II: temporary cavity formation and tissue damage. J Trauma 40:S16–S21
Swan KG, Swan RC (1991) Principles of ballistics applicable to the treatment of gunshot wounds. Surg Clinics North Am 71:221–239

Balloon Occlusion

▶ Adjuncts to Damage Control Laparotomy: Endovascular Therapies

Barefoot Doctor (China)

▶ Physician Assistant

Barker Vacuum Pack

▶ Open Abdomen, Vacuum Dressing

Barotrauma

Stephanie Lueckel
Department of Trauma Surgery and Critical Care,
Rhode Island Hospital and Warren Alpert
Medical School, Providence, RI, USA

Synonyms

Atelectrauma; Biotrauma; Volutrauma

Definition

Barotrauma refers to the damage sustained by viscera due to any severe changes in pressure. Pressure changes usually cause injury where there is an interface between fluid-filled and gas-filled structures, for example, the lungs. A simple example of this is decompression illness suffered by some scuba divers. The changes in pressure are usually well tolerated by the body but occasionally a diver ascends too quickly. This pressurizes the gas forcing it into the bloodstream as bubbles, barotrauma. Blast injuries can also result in barotrauma to the lungs, gastrointestinal tract, and ears. In trauma and critical care, mechanical ventilation is the focus of most barotrauma and will be the focus of this entry.

Lung injuries due to mechanical ventilation were initially referred to as "gross barotrauma." It was thought that the barotrauma was a direct result of excessive pressure forced into the lungs by the ventilator (Kumar et al. 1973). The excessive pressure resulted in pneumothoraces mainly but could also cause pneumomediastinum, pneumoperitoneum, subcutaneous emphysema, and gas emboli.

However, as interest grew in the etiology of lung injury, Dreyfuss (et al.) studied the effect of forced *volume* delivery to the lungs. Using a rat model, he showed that the rats subjected to increased tidal volumes had more permeability edema as compared to the rats with smaller tidal volumes (Dreyfuss et al. 1988). Volutrauma, rather than barotrauma, became the term used to define ventilator-associated lung injury.

The relationship between barotrauma and volutrauma is further defined with the terms *stress* and *strain*. *Stress* is the continuous internal distribution of the counterforce (per unit of area) that balances and reacts to an external load. Counterforce refers to the positive pressure delivered by the ventilator. Barotrauma represents *stress*. *Strain* refers to the deformation of the size or shape of the alveolar structures. Volutrauma represents strain. The relationship is represented by the formula:

$$\text{stress} = K^*\text{strain}.$$

K is specific elastance (Chiumello et al. 2008).

Barotrauma and volutrauma are not independent risk factors for the development of ventilator-associated lung injury, but rather demonstrate a linear-type relationship, further expanding the definition of "gross barotrauma."

Pathophysiology

The lung parenchyma is made of two key components: the fibrous skeleton and the alveolar epithelial cells. The fibrous skeleton consists of both elastic and collagen fibers. These fibers absorb the majority of the force delivered by the ventilator. These fibers stretch and unfold in order to accommodate the pressure and volume of air that is forced into the alveoli structure. Once collagen has been unfolded to accommodate total lung capacity, further stress can cause rupture. Unlike the collagen and elastin fibers, the alveolar epithelial cells don't absorb the force of the ventilator. However, mechanoreceptors in the cell sense a change in the fiber system. Mechanoreceptors then cause a release of cytokines initiating an inflammatory response (Gattinoni et al. 2010). This phenomenon is referred to as biotrauma.

Alterations in surface tension also contribute to the damaging effects of mechanical ventilation. When surfactant is lacking, surface tension is unopposed. More pressure is required to open the collapsed alveoli, and the already open alveoli must incur more stress. This is what is known as atelectrauma. All of these factors contribute to "gross barotrauma."

Preexisting Conditions

Gross barotrauma is most commonly seen in patients receiving mechanical ventilation for acute lung injury or acute respiratory distress syndrome (ALI/ARDS). The simplest explanation is that an already injured lung has an increased risk for further injury (Anzueto et al. 2004). ALI/ARDS disrupts the balance of surface tension and surfactant creating areas of the lung susceptible to severe collapse, atelectrauma (Gattinoni et al. 2010). Additionally, there are areas of the lungs that become overdistended to compensate for the collapsed areas.

Other factors that increase the likelihood of gross barotrauma are blood product transfusions, acidemia, previously diagnosed restrictive lung disease, as well as genetic variations (Gajic et al. 2004; Arcaroli et al. 2008).

Application

Understanding the histopathology and pathophysiology allows for physicians to develop ways to interrupt these mechanisms. A significant amount of literature exists, suggesting ways to reduce barotrauma, volutrauma, and lung collapse, labeled lung protective strategies. The National Institute of Health strongly showed that smaller tidal volumes (6 mL/kg) were associated with lower mortality when compared to patients who received higher tidal volumes (12 mL/kg) (ARDSNET, 2000). Other suggestions for the prevention of lung injury include maintaining a plateau pressure below 28–30 (Terragni et al. 2007). Applied positive end-expiratory pressure (PEEP) helps to prevent atelectasis or collapse of the alveoli.

Cross-References

▶ Mechanical Ventilation, Conventional
▶ Mechanical Ventilation, High-Frequency Oscillation
▶ Mechanical Ventilation, Noninvasive
▶ Mechanical Ventilation, Permissive Hypercapnia
▶ Mechanical Ventilation, Weaning

References

Anzueto A, Frutos-Vivar F, Esteban A, Alia I et al (2004) Incidence, risk factors and outcome of barotrauma in mechanically ventilated patients. Intensive Care Med 30(4):612–619

Arcaroli J, Sankoff J, Liu N et al (2008) Association between urokinase haplotypes and outcome from infection-associated acute lung injury. Intensive Care Med 34:300

ARDSNET (2000) Ventilation with lower tidal volumes as compared with traditional tidal volumes for acute lung injury and the acute respiratory distress syndrome. N Engl J Med 342:1301–1308

Chiumello D, Carlesso E, Cadringher P et al (2008) Lung stress and strain during mechanical ventilation for acute respiratory distress syndrome. Am J Respir Crit Care Med 178:346–355

Dreyfuss D, Soler P, Basset G et al (1988) High inflation pressure pulmonary edema: respective effects of high airway pressure, high tidal volume, and positive end-expiratory pressure. Am Rev Respir Dis 137:1159–1164

Gajic O, Dara S, Mendez JL et al (2004) Ventilator-associated lung injury in patients without acute lung injury at the onset of mechanical ventilation. Crit Care Med 32:1817

Gattinoni L, Protti A, Caironi P, Carlesso E (2010) Ventilator-induced lung injury: the anatomical and physiological framework. Crit Care Med 38:539–549

Kumar et al (1973) Pulmonary barotrauma during mechanical ventilation. Crit Care Med 1(4):181–186

Terragni PP, Rosboch G, Tealdi A et al (2007) Tidal hyperinflation during low tidal volume ventilation in acute respiratory distress syndrome. Am J Respir Crit Care Med 175:160–166

Recommended Reading
Pelosi P, Negrini D (2008) Extracellular matrix and mechanical ventilation in healthy lungs: back to baro/volutrauma? Curr Opin Crit Care 14:16–21

Schnapp LM, Chin DP, Szaflarski N, Matthay MA (1995) Frequency and importance of barotrauma in 100 patients with acute lung injury. Crit Care Med 23(2):272–278

Barton Fracture

▶ Distal Radius Fractures

Basic Cardiac Life Support (BCLS)

▶ Life Support Training

Basic Life Support

▶ Cardiopulmonary Resuscitation in Adult Trauma
▶ Cardiopulmonary Resuscitation in Pediatric Trauma

Battlefield Trauma Care

▶ Tactical Combat Casualty Care

Beak Fracture

▶ Calcaneus Fractures

Bed Sore

▶ Pressure Ulcers
▶ Pressure Ulcer, Complication of Care in ICU

Behind Armor Blunt Trauma (BABT)

▶ Body Armor

Benzodiazepines

▶ Sedation and Analgesia

Bicolumn Humerus Fracture

▶ Distal Humerus Fractures

Bicycle Accidents

▶ Bicycle-Related Injuries

Bicycle Crashes

▶ Bicycle-Related Injuries

Bicycle Helmets

▶ Bicycle-Related Injuries

Bicycle Safety

▶ Bicycle-Related Injuries

Bicycle-Related Injuries

Jeanne Mueller
Department of Surgery, Trauma, Loyola
University Medical Center, Maywood, IL, USA

Synonyms

Bicycle accidents; Bicycle crashes; Bicycle helmets; Bicycle safety; Bike helmets; Bike safety; Cycling safety; Head injuries; TBI; Traumatic brain injury

Definition

Bicycle riding is an increasingly popular form of recreation and transportation for adults and children. Resultant injuries cause significant morbidity and mortality. Yearly, crashes involving cyclists cause approximately 900 deaths, 23,000 hospital admissions, 580,000 emergency room visits, and 1.2 million visits to physician offices and clinics in the USA (Rivara 1996). Statistically, more injuries occur in males and are associated with riding at high speeds. The most common injuries are soft tissue and musculoskeletal trauma. Head injuries are responsible for the majority of fatalities and long-term disabilities (Thompson 2001).

Injury prevention interventions have proven to be successful in preventing the occurrence or decreasing the severity of injury through the development and enforcement of safety rules and protective gear (Cheng 2000). Utilization of protective helmets decreases the risk of head injury in all ages (Rivara 1996). They also provide substantial protection against lacerations and fractures to the upper and midface.

Common Injuries

Head injuries occur in 22–47 % of injured bicyclists, often as a result of being struck by a motor vehicle, and are responsible for 60 % of all bicycle-related mortalities (Thompson 2001). It is also the leading cause of long-term disability in an injured bicyclist (Puranic 1998). A large range of severity can occur and can be delineated by head injury, brain injury, and severe brain injury. Head injury can be defined as any and all injuries to the forehead, scalp, ears, skull, and brain, including superficial lacerations, abrasions, and bruises on the scalp, forehead, and ears as well as skull fractures, concussion, cerebral contusions, and all intracranial hemorrhages (subarachnoid, subdural, epidural, and intracerebral). A brain injury includes a diagnosis of concussion or more serious intracranial injury excluding skull fractures without accompanying brain injury. Finally, a severe brain injury indicates an intracranial injury or hemorrhage, including all cerebral lacerations/contusions, and subarachnoid, subdural, and extradural hemorrhages (Rivara 1996). Facial and ocular injuries can include fractures, contusions, dental fractures, or corneal foreign bodies (Thompson 2001).

Musculoskeletal injuries are a common occurrence in bicycle trauma. Fractures are most common in the hand, wrist, forearm, or shoulder due to the rider attempting to brace themselves from impact on an outstretched arm. Separation or dislocation of the shoulder can also occur from impact (Starling 2003). Strains, fractures, and dislocations are readily identified by deformity, swelling, pain, bruising, or lack of function (Thompson 2001). Follow-up imaging may be necessary to dictate further management.

Chest trauma while biking can involve high speeds, falls from height, and impact with hard and/or sharp objects. Impacts involving these significant mechanisms of injury can result in serious damage to the chest, which may not be readily identifiable because the damage is internal (Shotz, International Mountain Biking Association, 2010). Blunt injuries are those that are caused by impact with an object that is typically not sharp and does not penetrate the skin. Penetrating injuries are usually caused by a sharp or narrow object that break the skin and enter the chest cavity. Rapid assessment should include palpation and observing the chest for deformities. There may be contusions, abrasions, punctures, lacerations, swelling, or crepitus, a grinding sensation or noise when broken bones rub together (Shotz, International Mountain Biking Association, unk). Assess respiratory effort and for equal chest rise bilaterally as well as for pain. Injuries that may occur include rib fractures, flail chest, traumatic asphyxia, pulmonary contusion, pericardial tamponade, commotio cordis, pneumothorax, open pneumothorax, tension pneumothorax, hemothorax, and hemopneumothorax (Shotz, International Mountain Biking Association, unk).

Abdominal trauma can be a result of blunt injury or penetration from landing on upturned handlebars. This type of injury generally occurs when a child loses control of the bicycle and begins to fall, the front wheel rotated into a plane perpendicular to the body. The child then lands on the end of the handlebar resulting in serious truncal injury (Winston 1998). Impact with handlebars has been documented as producing traumatic abdominal wall hernia; renal, intestinal, liver, splenic, and pancreatic injuries; abdominal wall rupture; transection of the common bile duct; traumatic arterial occlusion; groin injuries; and even death (Winston 1998). To complicate matters, underlying organ injuries are often occult, as external bruising is infrequent and signs and symptoms may not manifest for hours after time of injury.

Genitourinary trauma exhibits symptoms that are nonspecific and may be masked by or attributed to other injuries (Rivara 1996). Gross hematuria and inability to void can be indicators of bladder or urethral trauma. The degree of hematuria is not directly correlated to the severity of injury. Bladder injuries are best classified as intraperitoneal and extraperitoneal. Extraperitoneal injuries are almost always associated with pelvic fractures, specifically pubic ramus fractures. Blunt trauma, such as a straddle injury from the crossbar of a bicycle, is responsible for 60 % of urethral injuries (Dandan 2011). Vulvar, penile, and scrotal contusions and hematomas can also occur with a straddle injury (Cheng 2000). Other injuries often take priority over injuries of the GU system and can interfere with a timely urologic assessment. Coordinated efforts between services caring for the patient are vital to ensure comprehensive care.

Skin and soft tissue injuries can be significant. Simple abrasions, contusions, and lacerations will require local care, while a "road rash" can involve partial or full-thickness injuries (Thompson 2001). Deeper injuries may require bedside or surgical debridement. Prevention of infection becomes a priority as the wounds can be dirty or embedded with soil or debris. Spoke injuries can often be seen in the toes and feet in children. They often cause significant damage to the soft tissues, which can lead to amputation (Starling 2003). These injuries can be prevented by utilizing spoke shields and wearing proper footwear.

Injury prevention initiatives aim at educating riders and parents of riders in safe operation of bicycles. Helmet use is the single most effective way to reduce bicycle-related fatalities. Statistically, younger children are more likely to wear a helmet over older riders. A child who rides with companions wearing helmets or adults in general are more likely to wear a helmet

themselves. Helmet use can be credited with reducing the risk of head injury by at least 45 %, brain injury by 33 %, facial injury by 27 %, and fatal injury by 29 % (Thompson 1989). In addition to encouraging helmet use, safety education is an important component of injury reduction strategies. Intersections pose substantial risk for cyclist due to cars turning in multiple configurations, and children are frequently injured due to unsafe crossing patterns. Safety education programs that have shown the most promise utilize active learning and feedback in a brief intervention. By using role playing and problem solving to reinforce safety behaviors, educators can positively impact riders.

Cross-References

▶ Acetabulum Fractures
▶ Ankle Fractures
▶ Bladder Rupture (Intra/Extraperitoneal)
▶ Chest Wall Injury
▶ Concussion
▶ Debridement
▶ Delayed Diagnosis/Missed Injury
▶ Distal Humerus Fractures
▶ Distal Radius Fractures
▶ Femoral Shaft Fractures
▶ Head Injury
▶ Intracranial Hemorrhage
▶ Lung Injury
▶ Pelvis Fractures
▶ Pneumothorax
▶ Pneumothorax, Tension
▶ Proximal Femoral Fractures
▶ Subarachnoid Hemorrhage
▶ Subdural Hematoma
▶ Tibial Fractures
▶ Traumatic Brain Injury, Mild (mTBI)

References

Cheng RL (2000) Sports injuries: an important cause of morbidity in urban youth. Pediatrics 105(3):e32
Dandan I (2011) Medscape reference drugs, diseases, and procedures.   http://emedicine.medscape.com/article/ 828251-overview. Retrieved 3 June 2013

Puranic SL (1998) Profile of pediatric bicycle injuries. South Med J 91:1003–1007

Rivara FP (1996) Circumstances and severity of bicycle injuries. http://www.smf.org/docs/articles/report.html. Retrieved 3 June 2013

Shotz S (2010) International Mountain Biking Association. http://www.imba.com/resources/nmbp/assessment-and-treatment-chest-injuries-part-1. Retrieved June 2013

Shotz S (unk) International Mountain Biking Association. Assessment and treatment of chest injuries: part 2. http://www.imba.com/resources/nmbp/assessment-and-treatment-chest-injuries-part-2. Retrieved 3 June 2013

Starling CC (2003) Hughston clinic. http://www.hughston.com/a-15-3-1.aspx. Retrieved 3 June 2013

Thompson RR (1989) A case control study of the effectiveness of bicycle safety helmets. N Engl J Med 320:1361–1367

Thompson MR (2001) Bicycle-related injuries. Am Fam Physician 63:2007–2014, 2017–2018

Winston FS (1998) Hidden spears: handlebars as injury hazards to children. Pediatrics 102:596–601

Bike Helmets

▶ Bicycle-Related Injuries

Bike Safety

▶ Bicycle-Related Injuries

Bioethics

▶ Brain Death, Ethical Concerns
▶ Ethical Issues in Trauma Anesthesia

Biomedical Ethics

▶ Ethical Issues in Trauma Anesthesia

Biotrauma

▶ Barotrauma

Bladder Accident

▶ Bladder Incontinence

Bladder Incontinence

Douglas Fetkenhour
Department of Physical Medicine and Rehabilitation, University of Rochester School of Medicine, Rochester, NY, USA

Synonyms

Bladder accident; Wetting oneself

Definition

Inability to empty the bladder in a controlled fashion resulting in involuntary leakage of urine.

Bladder incontinence following trauma may be the result of injury to the nervous system (SCI, TBI), peripheral nerve injury, or from the basic inability to mobilize adequately. Minimizing incontinence is crucial from the perspective of protecting the perineal skin and upper genitourinary system as well as the psychosocial impact of incontinence.

The neurogenic bladder will be characterized by the type of nerve injury. Upper motor neuron (UMN) injuries as seen in TBI and SCI will cause a hyperreflexic or spastic bladder that has a low maximum storage volume. There may also be contraction of the urinary sphincter during detrusor contraction, or dysergia, that results in incomplete emptying. A peripheral nerve or lower motor neuron (LMN) injury from pelvic trauma might result in an areflexic or flaccid bladder. In this case, the bladder will not void normally, but once volumes exceed the storage capacity of the bladder, the intravesicular pressure will rise rapidly and result in uncontrolled emptying of the bladder. Both UMN and LMN lesions can cause uncontrolled emptying and, therefore, urinary incontinence.

Management of the bladder requires an understanding of the pattern of filling and emptying. "Bladder scans" or ultrasound quantification of bladder volume prior to and following a void is very helpful in characterizing function. A void of 200 cc and a post-void residual (PVR) of 200 cc suggest dyssynergia between the detrusor and sphincter muscle contraction. Patients typically have enough warning time in this situation to maintain continence. A void of 200 cc with negligible PVR volumes suggests a spastic bladder. This may lead to significant urinary urgency resulting in incontinence. Anticholinergic medications like oxybutinin and tolterodine will diminish detrusor muscle contraction and allow the bladder to fill to more normal volumes (400–500 cc) before voiding. A patient who has not voided 8–10 h might have a bladder volume of 1,100 cc. This suggests a flaccid bladder. Ultimately the bladder will exceed the compliance of the bladder wall's transitional epithelium and cause an abrupt rise in intravesicular pressure. This results in "overflow" voiding which rarely occurs in a continent fashion. Of significant importance with the flaccid bladder is the risk of urinary reflux, hydronephrosis, and subsequent structural kidney injury that can occur in a high-pressure bladder. Planned evacuation of bladder is required to avoid overflow voiding and urinary reflux. This is typically accomplished with intermittent catheterization. A straight catheter is passed through the urethra and into the bladder on a timed basis. The interval of catheterization should be based on the volume of the bladder and not time elapsed. The filtration rate of the kidneys and therefore the filling demand on the bladder vary based on fluid intake and body position. If the bladder is catheterized every 6 h, midday volumes may be very low and night time volumes very high secondary to position-related fluid shifts within the body. The bladder should be catheterized when it contains 400–500 cc. Determining this is based on trial and error, but by wearing compression stockings to minimize dependent edema,

hydrating during the day, and taking only sips after dinner, fairly regular intervals for catheterizing can be achieved.

Timed toileting is an important concept in maximizing continence irrespective of the cause for incontinence. Regular, frequent transfers to the toilet or commode (as often as every 2 h) can "catch" the emptying of the bladder. There may be no emptying at some attempts, but in repeating this process over a 48-h period, a pattern will likely emerge when the bladder empties based on the activities of the patient. As an understanding of the intervals between voids is attained, the frequency of regular transfers to the toilet can be changed to match the pattern of the patient.

Cross-References

▶ Rehabilitation Nursing

Recommended Reading

Corocos J, Schick E (2008) Textbook of neurogenic bladder, 2nd edn. CRC Press

Bladder Rupture (Intra/Extraperitoneal)

Rona Altaras
Division of Acute Surgery/Trauma/Surgical Critical Care, Lawnwood Regional Medical Center, Fort Pierce, FL, USA

Synonyms

Intra/extraperitoneal bladder injury

Definition

The bladder is an extraperitoneal muscular urine reservoir located anatomically in the pelvic space behind the pubic symphysis. The proximity to bony structures of the pelvis predisposes this organ to injury. Most injuries are seen at the dome of the bladder, which is its weakest part.

Most bladder ruptures are caused by blunt trauma; penetrating trauma is less common. In motor vehicle collisions, the injury can occur either by direct blow of the steering wheel or by the classic lap belt mechanism.

Gross hematuria is the classic sign of bladder rupture and is present in 90 % of the cases. Rest of the patients will have microhematuria. An important fact is that 85 % of bladder ruptures are the result of pelvic fractures, but that only 10 % of pelvic fractures are associated with bladder injuries. Clinically, most of the patients will present with lower abdominal pain and tenderness associated with inability to void and signs of trauma in the lower pelvic trauma like perineal or suprapubic ecchymosis.

Diagnosis

The diagnosis can easily be established with a CT cystogram utilizing about 400 cm^3 of contrast. CT cystogram is equivalent to contrast cystogram to detect bladder injuries and can be performed as an integral part of the trauma screen (Quagliano et al. 2006). Of note is that the excretion phase of abdominal CT scanning has a high rate of false-negative results and is not adequate to diagnose most bladder ruptures. The sunburst pattern of contrast extravasation is typical of extraperitoneal injury. The intraperitoneal bladder rupture will demonstrate contrast in the peritoneal cavity.

Management

Injuries are divided in intra- or extraperitoneal type, according to their anatomical location. This differentiation matters due to different treatment modalities. The treatment of contusions, which are injuries causing hematuria without contrast leak, is nonoperative, with a large bore bladder catheter. The treatment of extraperitoneal injuries in most of cases is also accomplished with a large bore (18–20 French) bladder catheter. The catheter is removed after

about 14 days, and the healing of the injury is confirmed with a cystogram study. The exception to the nonoperative management of extraperitoneal injuries occurs with involvement of the neck of the bladder containing the anatomically important sphincter. Also, in cases of surgical interventions for orthopedic or abdominal explorations, the bladder should be repaired during the same session.

The treatment of intraperitoneal injuries is surgical on a routine basis. Postoperatively, a bladder catheter is left indwelling for about 2 weeks. And a cystogram should be obtained prior to catheter removal to confirm the healing.

Surgical technique: The bladder is approached through a lower midline incision. It is prudent to palpate the bladder through the laceration in order to exclude other injuries. The edges are debrided to healthy tissue and the laceration is then closed in two layers of absorbable suture. In cases of extraperitoneal ruptures with pelvic hematoma, it is beneficial to avoid severe bleeding by entering the hematoma. To achieve this, the bladder is approached via a cephaladly placed anterior cystotomy. The laceration is then closed after adequate inspection of the bladder intravesically again with absorbable suture (Coburn 2012).

Complications: Urinoma, neurogenic bladder, sexual dysfunction, fistulas to rectum or vagina, and urinary incontinence are the most complications of the bladder rupture.

Cross-References

▶ Bladder Incontinence
▶ Urinoma

References

Coburn M (2012) Genitourinary trauma. In: Mattox KL, Moore EE, Feliciano DV (eds) Trauma, 7th edn. Mc Graw Hill, New York

Quagliano P, Delair S et al (2006) Diagnosis of blunt bladder injury: a prospective ccoperative study of computed tomography cystography and conventional retrograde cystography. J Trauma 61(2):410–422

Blast

Sara J. Aberle
Department of Emergency Medicine, Mayo
School of Graduate Medical Education – Mayo
Clinic, Rochester, MN, USA

Synonyms

Blast injury; Blast wave; Bomb; Explosion

Definition

There are two categories of explosives, high-order explosives (HE) and low-order explosives (LE), which can either be commercially produced such as in military munitions or "improvised explosive devices" (IEDs). "IED" encompasses many types of explosives, to include Molotov cocktails, pipe, and fertilizer bombs, with many being used extensively through recent military conflicts and terrorist attacks (CDC 2006; Wightman and Gladish 2001).

HEs result in a blast wave as a result of a rapid chemical conversion of a solid or liquid into highly pressurized gas. As the pressure from the explosion moves spherically outward from an explosive source, it causes a supersonic blast wave that is greater than the atmospheric pressure, referred to as "overpressure" (Wightman and Gladish 2001). Examples of HE substances include the following: plastic explosives, ammonium nitrate fuel oil ("ANFO"), and triacetone triperoxide (TAPT). LEs are subsonic and are those such as black powder or petroleum-based devices, like "Molotov cocktails" (CDC 2006; Wightman and Gladish 2001).

The biologic effects from a blast on a body depend on a number of factors, such as device type, overpressure magnitude, open or enclosed detonation site, and distance from the blast. There are several different mechanisms of body tissue injury from blasts. Most of these mechanisms occur at the interface of body tissues of different densities and include spalling, shearing, or tearing forces and implosion. "Irreversible work" is a fourth mechanism being studied, in which the tensile strength of a tissue is surpassed (CDC 2006; Wightman and Gladish 2001).

The injuries associated with blasts are categorized into four general groups:

Primary Blast Injury – Injuries that are caused by the blast wave itself, usually at the interface of tissues of different densities. The organs primarily affected in this category are the air-filled structures, such as the ear, lungs, or hollow viscous organs of the gastrointestinal system (Yeh and Schecter 2012; Mackenzie and Tunnicliffe 2011).

Secondary Blast Injury – Injuries that occur as a result of projectile fragmentation, either from an explosive device itself or from debris that is picked up with the blast wave. This type of injury has become more common with the increased use of IEDs, which may be designed with various types of projectiles (nails, nuts, ball bearings, etc.) built into the device, and has been described as being similar to gunshot wounds (Navarro et al. 2012; Ramasamy et al. 2008).

Tertiary Blast Injury – Injuries that come as a result of the blast wave hurling the victim against another object. This can result in both penetrating and blunt injury depending on the object(s) the patient contacts. Normal trauma management concepts apply, to include following spinal precautions.

Quaternary Blast Injury – Those injuries that are not encompassed within the three preceding categories. This includes injuries associated with inhalation, burns, carbon monoxide, crush injuries, and psychiatric illness.

Cross-References

▶ Ballistics
▶ Barotrauma
▶ Body Armor
▶ Cardiopulmonary Resuscitation in Adult Trauma

▶ Cardiopulmonary Resuscitation in Pediatric Trauma
▶ Compressible Hemorrhage
▶ Damage Control Resuscitation, Military Trauma
▶ Damage Control Surgery
▶ Explosion
▶ Extremity Injury
▶ Fluid, Electrolytes, and Nutrition in Trauma Patients
▶ IED (Improvised Explosive Device)
▶ Military Trauma, Anesthesia for
▶ Noncompressible Hemorrhage
▶ Shock Management in Trauma
▶ Spalling
▶ Tactical Combat Casualty Care

References

CDC (2006) Bombings: injury patterns and care. Blast curriculum: one-hour module. http://www.bt.cdc.gov/masscasualties/bombings_injurycare.asp. Accessed 28 July 2013

Mackenzie IM, Tunnicliffe B (2011) Blast Injuries to the lung: epidemiology and management. Philos Trans R Soc Lond B Biol Sci 366(1562):295–299

Navarro SR, Abadía de Barbará AH, Gutierrez OC, Bartolome CE, Lam DM, Gilsanz RF (2012) Gunshot and improvised explosive casualties: a report from the Spanish Role 2 medical facility in Herat, Afghanistan. Mil Med 177(3):326–332

Ramasamy A, Harrisson SE, Clasper JC, Stewart MP (2008) Injuries from roadside improvised explosive devices. J Trauma 65(4):910–914

Wightman JM, Gladish SL (2001) Explosions and blast injuries. Ann Emerg Med 37:664–678

Yeh D, Schecter WP (2012) Primary blast injuries – an updated concise review. World J Surg 36(5):966–972

Blast Chest Wall Trauma

▶ Chest Wall Injury

Blast Injury

▶ Blast

Blast Lung

▶ Blast Lung Injury

B

Blast Lung Injury

Sara J. Aberle
Department of Emergency Medicine, Mayo School of Graduate Medical Education-Mayo Clinic, Rochester, MN, USA

Synonyms

Blast lung; BLI; Primary blast injury

Definition

Blast lung injury (BLI) is a major cause of blast-related on-scene and in-hospital morbidity and mortality. High-order explosives result in a blast wave, as rapid chemical conversion of a solid or liquid into highly pressurized gases occurs. As the pressure moves spherically outward from the explosive source, it causes a supersonic wave that is greater than the atmospheric pressure, referred to as "overpressure" (CDC 2006; Wightman and Gladish 2001). Injuries occur as a result of this wave, secondary to shearing, spalling, and related mechanisms, as energy is transferred between tissue density interfaces (Wightman and Gladish 2001). The organs primarily affected in primary blast injury are the air-filled structures, such as the ear, lungs, and gastrointestinal tract (Yeh and Schecter 2012).

In the lungs, these mechanisms could result in tearing of the lung tissues and cause subsequent pulmonary edema, contusions, and hemorrhage (CDC 2006; Wightman and Gladish 2001). Lung injury has the potential to start occurring at around 30 pounds per square inch (PSI) of pressure, with a 50 % incidence of lung injury reported at 75 PSI. Tympanic membrane (TM) rupture can occur as low as 5 PSI, and therefore while a patient with ruptured TMs may indeed have BLI, they do not necessarily coexist (Kizer 2000).

The clinical presentation of blast lung injury may include shortness of breath, chest tightness or pain, tachypnea, hypoxia, hemoptysis, and subsequent respiratory failure. When severe lung injury is present, the patient tends to clinically decline fairly rapidly, and many blast lung injuries do result in near-immediate death (CDC 2006). Assessment consists of assessing vital signs and obtaining a chest X-ray or even CT scan of the chest. The patient have unilateral involvement if one side is facing the blast, and the blast occurs in an open space, with an increased risk of bilateral lung involvement if closer to the blast or in an enclosed space at the time of the blast. Imaging may show the characteristic "butterfly" or "batwing" appearance. The diagnosis of BLI is sometimes complicated by other injuries, such as a pneumothorax or hemothorax, which may also be identified on imaging (CDC 2006; Wightman and Gladish 2001).

Treatment of BLIs is comprised of providing supplemental oxygen and positive-pressure ventilation and performing intubation and mechanical ventilation if needed. Because the cause of lung injury following a blast can come as a result of the blast but could also be linked to fluid resuscitation or blood product transfusion (Mackenzie and Tunnicliffe 2011), these resuscitative efforts must be performed judiciously in blast-injured patient. Those patients who are at risk of having a BLI should have an X-ray and be considered for arterial blood gas (ABG) evaluation. Should a patient be vitally stable, asymptomatic, and both the chest X-ray and ABG be within normal limits, the patient should be observed for 4–6 h prior to discharge to monitor for potentially delayed presentation of BLI (CDC 2006).

Cross-References

▶ Acute Respiratory Distress Syndrome (ARDS), General
▶ Airway Trauma, Management of
▶ ARDS, Complication of Trauma
▶ Barotrauma
▶ Blast
▶ Body Armor
▶ Cardiopulmonary Resuscitation in Adult Trauma
▶ Cardiopulmonary Resuscitation in Pediatric Trauma
▶ Explosion
▶ Hypoxemia, Severe
▶ IED (Improvised Explosive Device)
▶ Imaging of Aortic and Thoracic Injuries
▶ Lung Injury
▶ Massive Transfusion and Complications
▶ Pneumothorax
▶ Pneumothorax, Tension
▶ Pulmonary Trauma, Anesthetic Management for
▶ Spalling
▶ Ventilatory Management of Trauma Patients

References

CDC (2006) Bombings: injury patterns and care. Blast curriculum: one-hour module. http://www.bt.cdc.gov/masscasualties/bombings_injurycare.asp. Accessed 28 July 2013

Kizer KW (2000) Dysbarism. In: Tintinalli JE, Kelen GD, Stapyczynski JS (eds) Emergency medicine: a comprehensive study guide, 5th edn. McGraw-Hill, New York, p 1276

Mackenzie IM, Tunnicliffe B (2011) Blast injuries to the lung: epidemiology and management. Philos Trans R Soc Lond B Biol Sci 366(1562):295–299

Wightman JM, Gladish SL (2001) Explosions and blast injuries. Ann Emerg Med 37:664–678

Yeh D, Schecter WP (2012) Primary blast injuries – an updated concise review. World J Surg 36(5):966–972

Blast TBI

▶ Neurotrauma, Military Considerations

Blast Wave

▶ Blast

Bleeding Diathesis

▶ Coagulopathy

Bleeding Disorder

▶ Coagulopathy

BLI

▶ Blast Lung Injury

Blood Administration

▶ Blood Therapy in Trauma Anesthesia

Blood Bank

Bryan A. Cotton[1,2] and Laura A. McElroy[2]
[1]Department of Surgery, Division of Acute Care Surgery, Trauma and Critical Care, University of Texas Health Science Center at Houston, The University of Texas Medical School at Houston, Houston, TX, USA
[2]Department of Anesthesiology, Critical Care Medicine, University of Rochester Medical Center, Rochester, NY, USA

Synonyms

Blood donor center; Blood mobile

Definition

A blood bank, historically, referred to hospital laboratory that was responsible for preserving and storing donated blood. Though first appearing in 1932 in Leningrad and 1937 in Chicago, the first civilian blood banks were built on advances in understanding transfusion biochemistry and development of preservation and storage technology in the previous three decades (Nathoo et al. 2009).

Attempts at blood transfusions are recorded as early as the seventeenth century, after William Harvey described the circulation of blood. In 1900, Karl Landsteiner discovered the blood group antigens A, B, and C (later O) and helped study the Rh blood group. Seven years later, blood typing and cross-matching reduced the morbidity associated with transfusion, making it a viable treatment modality for anemia (Sturgis 1941).

Blood storage was feasible only after the discovery of sodium citrate anticoagulation and citrate-glucose solutions just prior to the second decade of the past century, which permitted donated blood to be stored for several days, ending direct vein-to-vein transfusions. Mobile blood units were placed in the battle-field during the Spanish Civil War, brought by the Canadian Norman Bethune in 1936. Plasma was utilized extensively by the British military during the Second World War and saw the creation of blood depots, sterile blood product packaging, and massive donation of plasma organized by the American Red Cross (Learoyd 2006).

As our understanding of the biochemistry of transfusion medicine grew, and transfusions became tools for civilian medicine after the experience in the battlefield, the American Association of Blood Banks (AABB) was founded and provided a foundation for common goals among blood banks, including public education regarding donation.

Currently, blood banks exist either in hospitals or as stand-alone units. Many countries have federal government oversight of the standards and practices of blood bank safety and reliability. Blood banks typically organize and promote donation from the public, process whole blood and aphaeresis donations, characterize blood type and antibodies for each unit, screen donors and products for potential blood borne diseases, store and distribute products, and follow adverse events (Shaz and Hillyer 2010).

Trauma surgeons, a group responsible for the use of large volumes of blood products in a very time-sensitive manner, are recommended to become familiar with local blood banks and the transfusion medicine specialists who administer them. In a series of recent studies, improved communication, ordering flow, and emphasis on the shared goals of patient safety have improved outcomes in critically injured patients (Alter and Klein 2008). Roughly 10–15 % of all injured patients seen in level I trauma centers that require blood transfusion, and we see a large increase in patient mortality as the number of units of blood products infused increases (Como et al. 2004).

Cross-References

- ▶ Antibody Screen
- ▶ Blood Group Antibodies
- ▶ Blood Type
- ▶ Blood Typing
- ▶ Citrate-Dextrose Solutions
- ▶ Crossmatch
- ▶ Cryoprecipitate Transfusion in Trauma
- ▶ FP24
- ▶ Leukoreduced Red Blood Cells
- ▶ Plasma
- ▶ Pooled Platelets
- ▶ Plasma Transfusion in Trauma
- ▶ Red Blood Cell Transfusion in Trauma ICU
- ▶ Rhesus Factor
- ▶ Thrombocytopenia
- ▶ Universal Donor

References

Alter HJ, Klein HG (2008) The hazards of blood transfusion in historical perspective. Blood 112(7):2617–2626

Como J, Dutton R, Scalea T et al (2004) Blood transfusion rates in the care of acute trauma. Transfusion 44:809–813

Learoyd P (2006) A short history of blood transfusion. NBS- Scientific & Technical Training vol 042, pp 1–17

Nathoo N, Lautzenheiser K, Barnet G et al (2009) The first direct human blood transfusion: the forgotten legacy of George W. Crile. Op Neurosurg 64:20–27

Shaz B, Hillyer C (2010) Transfusion medicine as a profession: evolution over the past 50 years. Transfusion 50:2536–2541

Sturgis C (1941) The history of blood transfusion. In: 43rd annual meeting of MLA, 30 May 1941

Blood Clot

- ▶ Venous Thromboembolism (VTE)

Blood Component Administration

- ▶ Blood Therapy in Trauma Anesthesia

Blood Component Resuscitation

- ▶ Blood Therapy in Trauma Anesthesia

Blood Component Therapy

- ▶ Blood Therapy in Trauma Anesthesia

Blood Component Transfusion

- ▶ Blood Therapy in Trauma Anesthesia

Blood Donor Center

- ▶ Blood Bank

Blood Group

- ▶ Blood Type

Blood Group Antibodies

Bryan A. Cotton[1,2] and Laura A. McElroy[2]
[1]Department of Surgery, Division of Acute Care
Surgery, Trauma and Critical Care, University of
Texas Health Science Center at Houston, The
University of Texas Medical School at Houston,
Houston, TX, USA
[2]Department of Anesthesiology, Critical Care
Medicine, University of Rochester Medical
Center, Rochester, NY, USA

Synonyms

Anti-A antibody; Anti-B antibody; Anti-Rh
antibody

Definition

The discovery in 1900 by Karl Landsteiner of
blood group antigens and their associated antibodies heralded the beginning of safe, predictable
transfusions in medicine. The ABO blood groups
are determined by the antigen expressed on erythrocytes and are inherited codominantly. The "I"
alleles can be of the A type ($I^{A}i$ or $I^{A}I^{A}$), B type ($I^{B}i$
or $I^{B}I^{B}$), null type (ii, phenotypically O type), or
the codominant AB type ($I^{A}I^{B}$). Individuals then
develop IgM and IgG antibodies based on this
genotype, with A types having anti-B antibodies,
B types having anti-A antibodies, O types having
both anti-A and anti-B antibodies, and AB types
having neither. These antibodies develop by
4 months of age and are capable of activating the
complement system leading to serious, but thank-
fully rare, hemolytic transfusion reactions. These
antibodies determine what donor blood can be
safely transfused. AB-type recipients can receive
blood from any ABO donor type, while O-type
recipients can only receive O-type red blood cells.

Subsequent to the initial ABO erythrocyte antigen discovery has followed the elucidation of
many weaker variants of the A and B antigens,
notably including the A1 and A2 subtypes. However, these are not clinically significant and play
little role in common transfusion medicine. Antibodies to the A1 subtype seem to be incapable of
activating the complement cascade. All in all,
there are over 300 blood group antigens that can
potentially play clinically significant roles in
human blood transfusion, with the ABO being by
far the most immunogenic. The second most
important group of antigens are of the Rhesus
(Rh) class, currently understood to be a complex
array of over 49 Rh antigens controlled by the
expression of two genes. The Rh D, C, and
e antigens are the most important of these antigens
phenotypically, though clinically we speak of the
global Rh-positive and Rh-negative types. Antibodies to the Rh, D, C, e antigens are primarily of
the IgG variety and do not activate complement,
but can lead to extravascular acute hemolytic
transfusion reactions and cause hemolytic disease
of the newborn in Rh-incompatible pregnant
mothers (Westhoff 2007).

"Naturally occurring" antibodies are not
a result of RBC exposure, but instead occur
after exposure to microbes encountered routinely
in the digestive tract or other mucosal surfaces.
These are the most common antibodies found in
non-transfused children and men. They are
primarily IgM and are referred to collectively as
cold agglutinins. In general, they have little
clinical importance in transfusion reactions, as
they are in low titers, rarely detectable in dilutions greater than 1:10. In patients with cold
agglutinin disease, these titers can exceed $1:10^{5}$.
These antibodies can become clinically relevant
in transfusion below 37 °C, when these IgM
pentamers react with polysaccharides on the surface of red cells, principally the i and I antigens,
causing them to adhere together in clumps. While
this reaction is reversible when the temperature
increases above 37 °C, the attachment of IgM to
the red blood cell allows for the adherence and
activation of complement. Red cells have cell
surface inhibitors to complement that allow
them to survive the initial lysis by the complement system, but through this attachment, the
complement fragments C3b and C4b are left
behind on the cell surface, leaving the red cell
vulnerable to phagocytic engulfment and destruction (Westhoff et al. 2012).

The most common causes of immunization against blood group antigens are transfusion, pregnancy, transplantation, or sharing of needles. Individuals who have had multiple allogenic blood transfusions or exposures, such as those with sickle cell disease or autoimmune hemolytic anemias, are likely to develop antibodies to more uncommon antigens including Kell, Duffy, and Kidd, leading to difficulty crossmatching allogenic blood products and extended delays in beginning transfusions (Schwartz 2011).

Cross-References

▶ Antibody Screen
▶ Blood Bank
▶ Blood Type
▶ Crossmatch
▶ Rhesus Factor

References

Schwartz R (2011) Autoimmune and intravascular hemolytic anemias, Chap 163. In: Goldman's Cecil medicine, 24th edn. Elsevier, Philadelphia, pp 1045–1052
Westhoff C (2007) The structure and function of the Rh antigen complex. Semin Hematol 44(1):42–50
Westhoff CM, Storry JR, Shaz B (2012) Human blood group antigens and antibodies, Chap 111. In: Hematology: basic principles and practice, 6th edn. Elsevier, Philadelphia, pp 1628–1641

Blood Loss

▶ Hemorrhage

Blood Mobile

▶ Blood Bank

Blood Poisoning

▶ Sepsis, Treatment of

Blood Product Administration

▶ Blood Therapy in Trauma Anesthesia

Blood Product Transfusion

▶ Blood Therapy in Trauma Anesthesia

Blood Resuscitation

▶ Blood Therapy in Trauma Anesthesia

Blood Therapy in Trauma Anesthesia

Lejla Music-Aplenc[1] and Mirsad Dupanovic[2]
[1]Children's Mercy Hospital, University of Missouri, Kansas City, MO, USA
[2]Department of Anesthesiology, Kansas University Medical Center, The University of Kansas Hospital, Kansas City, KS, USA

Synonyms

Blood administration; Blood component administration; Blood component resuscitation; Blood component therapy; Blood component transfusion; Blood product administration; Blood product transfusion; Blood resuscitation; Blood transfusion; Hemostatic resuscitation; Massive transfusion; Transfusion; Transfusion therapy

Definition

Blood therapy in trauma anesthesia represents administration of either specific blood components or fresh whole blood (FWB) with the goal of supporting oxygen delivery and/or process of coagulation. Controlling the hemorrhage and increasing the circulating volume directly or indirectly support maintenance of circulation. Initial blood therapy in trauma often involves administration of group O uncrossmatched red blood cells (RBCs), fresh frozen plasma (FFP), and platelets. Group-specific blood components or FWB may be administered if there was enough time to perform type and cross testing in the blood bank. In case of life-threatening injuries, blood therapy is initially guided by the patient's clinical status. However, subsequent therapy is usually guided by a series of hematologic and coagulation tests.

Preexisting Condition

The decision about urgent/emergent administration of blood in trauma usually occurs in an acute setting during life-threatening hemorrhage in the emergency room and/or in the operating room. Sometimes this may occur in the intensive care unit if the patient has bypassed the operating room in need of obtaining adequate vascular access and hemodynamic stabilization. A multidisciplinary clinical team is usually involved in assessment and resuscitation from the time of patient's arrival to the emergency room onward. However, blood component administration in trauma may also be elective in patients that have survived acute trauma; they are recovering and need supportive blood therapy. Since such elective administration of blood is not much different from any other elective blood transfusion, the focus of this entry will be blood therapy in acute hemorrhage.

Historical Prospective

Historically, separation of whole blood into RBCs, plasma, and platelets was started because of better preservation of each component under special storage conditions and more flexibility with administration of blood components than with administration of whole blood. In general, administration of a specific blood component to a patient that is either anemic, coagulopathic, and/or thrombocytopenic represents a goal-oriented therapy and more rational blood utilization. However, it still remains questionable what represents the best blood transfusion strategy for an acutely hemorrhaging patient that is rapidly losing whole blood.

Over a period of 30 years, the American College of Surgeons Committee on Trauma has provided a foundation of care for injured patients by publishing the Advanced Trauma Life Support (ATLS) and teaching the ATLS course. The basic premise is that injured patients should receive two large-bore peripheral intravenous (IV) lines and ongoing crystalloid solutions as soon as possible (ATLS 2008). In case of hypotension, rapid administration of 1–2 L of crystalloids (20 mL/kg for pediatric patients) is recommended. Subsequently, 3-for-1 blood replacement should follow (3 mL of crystalloids for 1 mL of blood lost). Subsequently, excessive crystalloid administration may have significant dilutional effect and can worsen coagulopathy of acute trauma, resulting in even more difficulty controlling the hemorrhage and potential for iatrogenic injury. In case of unacceptably poor perfusion, surgical control of the ongoing hemorrhage and RBC administration are necessary. In the past, administration of FFP and platelets was usually guided by laboratory testing and often delayed: FFP to be given when PT and PTT were prolonged more than 1.5 times the normal value and platelets usually administered when the count was less than 50,000. However subsequently, the delay in obtaining the results of laboratory testing and ongoing hemorrhage worsen the coagulopathy even more. Thus, in order to achieve a timely hemostatic resuscitation, this practice is being replaced by early transfusion of RBCs, FFP, and platelets in the balanced 1:1:1 ratio.

Justification for institution of such transfusion practice is not only clinical. A simple laboratory experiment of diluting plasma and measuring prothrombin time (PT) demonstrated that PT exceeds 1.5 times the normal value when 40 % of plasma was mixed with 60 % of normal saline. On the other hand, when a whole blood unit of 500 mL, with a hematocrit (Hct) of 40–50 %, platelet count of 250,000, and coagulation factor activity of 100 %, is separated into three blood components (RBCs, FFP, and platelets) and leukoreduced, it will lose approximately 15 mL of RBCs, 20 mL of plasma, and 20–50 % of platelets. Additionally, the red cell component is diluted with 110 mL of additive solution. When these three components are transfused in a 1:1:1 ratio, the combined volume of 645 mL has Hct of 29 %, coagulation factor activity of 65 %, and platelet count of 90,000 (Mintz 2011). However, rapid infusion of large volumes of RBCs that have been stored for more than 2 weeks may not provide expected degree of resuscitation because of formation of microaggregates and metabolic changes that occur over time. Thus, in a massively bleeding patient, requiring large amounts of blood components may be desirable to provide the best functioning RBCs (1–2 weeks old). Since approximately 90 % of RBC and only 60 % of platelets actually circulate, balanced blood resuscitation approach results in final Hct of about 26 %, INR of 1.4, and platelet count of 55,000/mL. Attempts to increase the concentration of one component result in dilution of the other two components. This illustrates the limits of hemostatic resuscitation (Mintz 2011).

Application

New Developments

Three major discoveries have changed the traditional resuscitation practice of massively bleeding trauma patients over the past decade:

1. Understanding that early treatment of coagulopathy in acute trauma is a major resuscitation issue
2. Awareness that many of the severely injured arrive to the trauma center already coagulopathic
3. Knowledge that massive crystalloid resuscitation may worsen coagulopathy and lead to intracranial, abdominal, and limb compartment syndromes in acutely injured

These discoveries prompted a recommendation for an early start of a balanced (1:1) transfusion of RBCs and FFP in case of a massive hemorrhage (Stansbury et al. 2009).

Massive Transfusion

Massive transfusion is commonly defined as administration of 20 PRBC units within 24 h. However, administration of more than 4 PRBC units within 1 h with ongoing need for blood transfusion or loss of more than 150 mL of blood per minute with hemodynamic instability are more practical definitions of massive transfusion (ASA 2011). Loss of one blood volume within 24 h is considered massive transfusion in pediatric patients. Exchange transfusion of an infant is also considered massive transfusion.

Massive Transfusion Protocol (MTP)

The MTP represents activation of a procedure that ensures emergent delivery of predefined balanced ratio of blood components to the site of resuscitation of a massively bleeding patient (usually to the emergency room, operating room, or intensive care unit). Every hospital may have its own version of an MTP. The protocol is usually activated by a resuscitation team in the emergency room; basic patient information is provided to the blood bank. Clinical criteria, laboratory criteria, or both are used to make the decision about the MTP activation. Once the MTP is activated, the blood bank ensures rapid and timely availability of a series of balanced blood component packs (ASA 2011).

There are many advantages to using an MTP:

1. MTP ensures expeditious delivery of a balanced ratio of blood products.
2. It may prevent or reverse coagulopathy of acute trauma.
3. It may prevent complications of excessive crystalloid infusion.
4. MTP improves coordination between different departments.
5. Potentially, it improves trauma resuscitation outcomes (Riskin et al. 2009).

Blood Crossmatch

Implementation of the MTP is essential in resuscitation of acutely hemorrhaging trauma patient. Blood bank must release group O RBCs during severe trauma emergencies before patient's blood specimen arrives. When the specimen is received and the patient's ABO/Rh type is determined, the group-specific blood products can begin to be released. Antibody screen is performed as well. If the antibody screen results are negative, then the blood bank proceeds with an abbreviated crossmatch (electronic or immediate spin). An abbreviated cross-match is used to ensure ABO compatibility. If the antibody screen results are positive, then the blood bank needs to determine the type of the antibody and start providing RBC units that do not have matching antigens on their surface. Administration of such PRBC units can result in hemolytic transfusion reaction. Performing all these tests can cause a lot of pressure on the blood bank staff in order to try to identify the antibody as soon as possible and provide appropriate blood products. Some facilities stop crossmatching RBCs as soon as the patient has received ten RBC units in less than 24 h. Such practice is justified by assumption that the circulating blood has been so much diluted with transfused products that pre-existing antibodies have also been diluted.

If during the resuscitation the rhesus (Rh)-negative patient received Rh-positive blood, it may be difficult to determine the patient's true Rh type during the blood bank testing. If there is any question about patient's true Rh type and especially if the patent is a female, the blood bank should provide Rh-negative RBCs due to the concerns of possible Rh alloimmunization. If the resources are limited or the patient already used a significant portion of the blood bank inventory, the switch from providing Rh-negative to Rh-positive units may be inevitable. Under such circumstances, WinRho (RhIG) infusion to prevent Rh alloimmunization may be considered especially in young women (Roback et al. 1999).

The experience regarding the use of FWB in trauma patients is limited to the military experience and comes from Combat Support Hospital in Baghdad (Perkins et al. 2011). Treatment facilities across Iraq and Afghanistan have administered more than 8,000 FWB transfusions to more than 1,000 patients. Many retrospective studies came out of this military experience and demonstrated satisfactory or superior outcomes in patients who received FWB; however, the evidence from large prospective randomized trials is still missing. Despite that this military experience led to a fresh new way of looking into the balanced resuscitation with a fixed RBC to FFP ratio.

Acute Complications of Massive Blood Transfusion

It is not always possible to easily distinguish complications of massive blood transfusion (MBT) from deterioration in clinical condition of an acutely hemorrhaging anesthetized patient. If suspected these complications should be considered in the context of patient's medical history, the injuries being treated, the course of surgery and ongoing blood loss, type of anesthetic being administered, as well as possible vital organ dysfunction.

1. Acid-base and electrolyte abnormalities – Acidosis is primarily metabolic and a consequence of hypoperfusion and anaerobic metabolism. Successful restoration of adequate tissue perfusion will be the best contribution to normalization of metabolic acidosis. Otherwise, with sustained hypoperfusion and continuous production of lactate, administration of sodium bicarbonate and calcium gluconate may be necessary. Citrate (anticoagulant in the RBC units) binds calcium and can cause a dramatic decrease in serum calcium level. However, administration of sodium bicarbonate should be sensible because metabolic alkalosis may ensue post-operatively subsequent to administration of large amounts of sodium bicarbonate, successful resuscitation, and lactate metabolism. Hyperkalemia and hypokalemia may be secondary consequences of acidosis or alkalosis, respectively. These fluctuations are particularly important to consider in children and renal failure patients. Hypernatremia may be a consequence of administration of a large load of sodium citrate during an MBT as well as administration of sodium bicarbonate.

2. Hypothermia is usually caused by multiple environmental factors in the field, skin exposure during the patient assessment in

a cold location, and by administration of cold fluid and blood products. Hypothermia results in worsening of metabolic acidosis, increased intracellular potassium release, and hyperkalemia as well as shift of the oxygen dissociation curve to the left with decreased tissue oxygen delivery and worsened acidosis. Additionally, impaired coagulation, decreased drug metabolism, reduced cardiac output, and increased incidence of cardiac arrhythmias are also consequences of hypothermia.

3. Coagulopathy may be rapidly developing in trauma and is often associated with metabolic acidosis and hypothermia (the lethal triad). The etiology of coagulopathy in trauma is complex. Coagulation factor dilution using large amounts of crystalloids and RBCs may initiate or contribute to the vicious cycle. Preexisting administration of anticoagulants or antiplatelet agents and insufficient hemostatic resuscitation may also be critical. Hypothermia will further contribute to coagulopathy. Traumatic brain injury may also be associated with coagulopathy.

4. Hemolytic transfusion reaction can develop due to error in transfusion and administration of a wrong ABO blood group unit of RBCs. Such transfusion may result in renal failure, disseminated intravascular coagulation, and circulatory collapse. Strict compliance with patient identification procedures is mandatory despite of time pressure to transfuse as soon as possible.

5. Transfusion-related acute lung injury (TRALI) is the leading cause of the transfusion-related fatalities reported to the FDA. It is a consequence of the presence of leukoagglutinins in the donor plasma that forms complexes with HLA or HNA antigens leading to neutrophil activation, sequestration in the lungs, endothelial damage, and pulmonary edema.

Jehovah's Witness Patient, Trauma, and Blood Management

Jehovah's Witnesses may refuse blood therapy despite the possibility of exsanguinations and death. Initial assessment should include identification and documentation of such religious beliefs. If possible a discussion with the patient should occur and the provider should plan accordingly. Ethical issues like competence, capacity, and care of minors are very important in trauma care of Jehovah's Witnesses. If such patient cannot make important decisions about his/her health, significant ethical controversies may be faced by the medical staff.

Hemoglobin-based oxygen carriers are still being investigated and are not available for commercial use. Thus, management strategy of Jehovah's Witness patients comprises blood conservation, maximizing oxygen delivery, minimizing oxygen demand, and stimulation of erythropoiesis (Kulvatunyou and Heard 2004).

1. Blood conservation – Intraoperative considerations include rapid control of hemorrhage with a single intervention if possible, autologous transfusion with a cell salvage device, reducing the frequency of blood testing, and using smaller size sample tubes to reduce iatrogenic blood loss.

2. Maximizing oxygen delivery – Crystalloids are administered to increase intravascular volume and maintain tissue perfusion. Administration of colloids allows use of smaller volumes of fluid. However, Jehovah's Witness patients may refuse administration of albumin while there may be concerns about adverse effects of hetastarch on coagulation in a trauma patient. Hypertonic saline solutions should be considered in view of potential benefit in counterbalancing inflammatory response and decreasing hemodilution. The use of 100 % inspiratory oxygen may maximize oxygen delivery to the tissues.

3. Minimizing oxygen demand may be accomplished by using neuromuscular blockade and mechanical ventilation in order to decrease the work of breathing.

4. Stimulation of erythropoiesis by administration of iron, folic acid, vitamin B12, and erythropoietin takes time and is not effective in acute trauma.

Pediatric Considerations

Trauma is frequent in childhood and is the leading cause of death in teenagers. Unlike adults, children sustain higher rate of blunt trauma versus penetrating trauma, and variations of coagulation factors with age may influence their bleeding tendencies. Trauma in pediatric patients may encompass complex surgeries, MBT, and use of ECMO or cardiopulmonary bypass. Neonates who receive exchange transfusion also qualify as massive transfusion recipients.

Recent studies have shown that coagulopathy of acute trauma is as prevalent in the pediatric as it is in adult population. In addition, pediatric patients who present with coagulopathy of acute trauma have significantly worse outcomes compared with patients who were not coagulopathic. Prolongation of PT is the most common coagulation abnormality, and children with highest degree of PT prolongation had the highest mortality rates (Hendrickson 2012a).

The prevalence of coagulopathy in pediatric trauma and the evidence of improved outcomes with balanced transfusion ratios in adults led to development of MTPs in many pediatric institutions. In addition to fixed and balanced ratio of blood products, pediatric MTP takes into consideration patient's size reflected in weight-based blood product packages. Pediatric MTP allows for rapid provision of balanced blood products to the trauma victim. Larger studies are needed to determine whether MTP will improve clinical outcomes in pediatric trauma patients (Hendrickson 2012b).

Cross-References

- ▶ Adjuncts to Transfusion: Antifibrinolytics
- ▶ Adjuncts to Transfusion: Fibrinogen Concentrate
- ▶ Adjuncts to Transfusion: Prothrombin Complex Concentrate
- ▶ Adjuncts to Transfusion: Recombinant Factor VIIa, Factor XIII, and Calcium
- ▶ Aminocaproic Acid
- ▶ Anticoagulation/Antiplatelet Agents and Trauma
- ▶ Apheresis Platelets
- ▶ Blood Group Antibodies
- ▶ Blood Type
- ▶ Coagulopathy
- ▶ Cryoprecipitate Transfusion in Trauma
- ▶ Electrolyte and Acid-Base Abnormalities
- ▶ Exsanguination Transfusion
- ▶ Factor I Concentrate
- ▶ Factor VIIa
- ▶ Fibrinogen (Test)
- ▶ FP24
- ▶ Hypothermia, Trauma, and Anesthetic Management
- ▶ Massive Transfusion
- ▶ Massive Transfusion Protocols in Trauma
- ▶ Packed Red Blood Cells
- ▶ Plasma Transfusion in Trauma
- ▶ Platelets
- ▶ Pooled Platelets
- ▶ Red Blood Cell Transfusion in Trauma ICU
- ▶ Tranexamic Acid
- ▶ Transfusion Strategy in Trauma: What Is the Evidence?
- ▶ Transfusion Thresholds
- ▶ Whole Blood

References

American College of Surgeons Committee on Trauma (2008) ATLS® student course manual. American College of Surgeons Committee on Trauma, Chicago

American Society of Anesthesiologists (ASA) Committee on Blood Management (2011) Massive transfusion protocol for hemorrhagic shock. http://www.asahq.org/for-members/about-asa/asa-committees/committee-on-blood-management.aspx. Accessed 21 Jan 2012

Hendrickson JE et al (2012a) Coagulopathy is prevalent and associated with adverse outcomes in transfused pediatric trauma patients. J Pediatr 160(2):204–209

Hendrickson JE et al (2012b) Implementation of pediatric trauma massive transfusion protocol: one institution's experience. Transfusion 52(6):1228–1236

Kulvatunyou N, Heard SO (2004) Care of injured Jehovah's Witness patient: case report and review of the literature. J Clin Anesth 16:548–553

Mintz PD (2011) Transfusion therapy: clinical principles and practice, 3rd edn. AABB Press, Bethesda

Perkins JG et al (2011) Comparison of platelet transfusion as fresh whole blood vs. apheresis platelets for massively transfused combat trauma patients. Transfusion 51(2):242–252

Riskin DJ et al (2009) Massive transfusion protocols: the role of aggressive resuscitation vs. product ratio in mortality reduction. J Am Coll Surg 209(2):198–205

Roback J et al. (ed) (1999) Technical manual, 17th edn. AABB Press, Bethesda, Maryland

Stansbury LG et al (2009) Controversy in trauma resuscitation: do ratios of plasma to red blood cells matter. Transfus Med Rev 23(4):255–265

Blood Thinners

▶ Anticoagulation/Antiplatelet Agents and Trauma

Blood Transfusion

▶ Blood Therapy in Trauma Anesthesia

Blood Type

Harvey G. Hawes[1], Laura A. McElroy[2] and Bryan A. Cotton[1]
[1]Department of Surgery, Division of Acute Care Surgery, Trauma and Critical Care, University of Texas Health Science Center at Houston, The University of Texas Medical School at Houston, Houston, TX, USA
[2]Department of Anesthesiology, Critical Care Medicine, University of Rochester Medical Center, Rochester, NY, USA

Synonyms

Blood group

Definition

A person's blood type or blood group is determined by the expression of erythrocyte surface antigens, of which there are over 30 clinically used types. The most important blood group antigens are the ABO and Rhesus (Rh) types. These blood group antigens are transmitted by various genetic mechanisms; the ABO antigens are an example of codominant transmission (Miller 2009). Individuals with specific blood group antigens also then have a complementary set of blood group antibodies, many of which are able to activate the complement system and thus lead to significant, if not fatal, hemolytic transfusion reactions or hemolytic disease of newborns (Ahsan and Noether 2011).

The blood type of an individual patient is then a composite phenotype of as many blood group antigens the clinician cares to measure. In standard clinical practice, the ABO and Rh types are determined for each patient donating or receiving blood products and for pregnant mothers and newborns. In persons with a strong history of blood transfusion or blood exposure, such as those with sickle cell anemia or posttransplantation, it may be necessary to test for more rare antigens like Kidd, Duffy, or Kell to minimize transfusion reactions (Westhoff 2004).

There are geographic differences in the relative frequency of each blood type, with blood type A being more common in Europe and aboriginal populations in Australia and North America and type B being more prevalent in northern India, Asia, and parts of Russia. Some of these differences are likely due to selection pressures, as type O individuals are more susceptible to the bubonic plague and type A people are more vulnerable to the smallpox virus than those of the other blood groups. The areas of the world where type B is predominant have had epidemics of both of these diseases. The most striking example of selection bias in blood groups is the Duffy antigen. This blood type contains a receptor that facilitates the entry of some malarial parasites into the red blood cell. Therefore, in populations with endemic malaria, having Duffy-negative blood would confer a significant survival and thus reproductive advantage. The significance or functionality of most blood types is not known, including the ABO system. Some statistical correlations have been established, for example, people with type A blood have about a 20 % increased risk of stomach cancer versus those with type O blood, whereas type O people are more likely to develop ulcers than those with type A (Klein 2005). These associations are unlikely to be driven by natural selection, as they usually occur past the reproductive years.

Determination of a patient's blood type consists of agglutination reactions and maybe all that is required prior to blood transfusion in emergency situations (as the risk of severe transfusion reaction would be less than the risk of death from hemorrhagic shock). More commonly, a further crossmatch, in which serum from a potential recipient is mixed with donor blood, is performed to assess the specific compatibility of each unit of blood (Goodnough 2011).

Cross-References

- ▶ Antibody Screen
- ▶ Blood Group Antibodies
- ▶ Blood Typing
- ▶ Crossmatch
- ▶ Rhesus Factor

References

Ahsan S, Noether J (2011) Hematology. The Harriet Lane handbook, 19th edn. Chap 14. Mosby, St/Louis, MO

Goodnough LT (2011) Transfusion medicine. Goldman's Cecil medicine, 24th edn. Saunders, Philadelphia, PA, pp 1154–1158, Chap 180

Klein HG (2005) Why do people have different blood types? Sci Am. http://www.scientificamerican.com/article/why-do-people-have-differ/. Accessed 24 Mar 2014

Miller R (2009) Transfusion therapy. Miller's anesthesia, 7th edn. Chap 55. Churchill/Livingstone, London, pp 1739–1766

Westhoff CM (2004) Review: the Kell, Duffy, and Kidd blood group systems. Immunohematology 20:37–49

Blood Typing

Bryan A. Cotton[1] and Laura A. McElroy[2]
[1]Department of Surgery, Division of Acute Care Surgery, Trauma and Critical Care, University of Texas Health Science Center at Houston, The University of Texas Medical School at Houston, Houston, TX, USA
[2]Department of Anesthesiology, Critical Care Medicine, University of Rochester Medical Center, Rochester, NY, USA

Synonyms

Type-specific blood; Uncrossmatched Blood

Definition

Blood typing is the first step used to characterize the array of erythrocyte antigens present in a blood sample. The discovery of the ABO and Rh blood antigens by Dr. Karl Landsteiner in the early 1900s began effective research leading to today's relatively safe and effective transfusion science. The ABO and Rh antigen systems are by far the most immunogenic and thus the first and most important compatibilities to document, although more than 20 known blood group systems are known. A patient or donation's blood type is determined by indirect Coombs test whereby a small sample of red cells is separately mixed with both anti-A and anti-B sera. Antihuman antibodies are then added to the mixture. If the patient's red cells express A or B antigens on their surfaces, the tagged red cells with agglutinate reveal the patient's ABO blood type. The same test is performed on the sample's serum and with the D antigen, determining Rh status. An antibody screen is then performed by mixing commercially prepared RBCs expressing clinically significant antigens with patient serum and watching for agglutination. These are antibodies present in low incidence in the general population (1–2 %). These tests are performed on donor blood before it is made available for transfusion. When performed urgently for the recipient, testing for type specificity takes between 5–15 minutes (Emery 2014).

Type-specific blood is donor blood that is compatible with the recipient's determined ABO and Rh blood types. When combined with a negative antibody screen, the transfused blood product has a less than 1 % chance of resulting in a clinically significant nonhemolytic transfusion reaction. Because of its excellent safety profile, type-specific blood should be considered for transfusion in patients during exigent circumstances including massive hemorrhage and trauma (Gongal 2005).

Cross-References

- ▶ Antibody Screen
- ▶ Blood Bank
- ▶ Blood Group Antibodies
- ▶ Blood Type
- ▶ Crossmatch
- ▶ Rhesus Factor
- ▶ Universal Donor

References

Emery M (2014) Blood and blood components. Mars: Rosen's emergency medicine- concepts and clinical practice, 8th edn. Edinburgh, UK, Mosby/Elsevier pp 75–77, Chap 7
Gongal R (2005) How safe is transfusion of uncrossmatched blood? Kathmandu Univ Med J 3(9):76–78

Blood Volume

Bryan A. Cotton[1] and Laura A. McElroy[2]
[1]Department of Surgery, Division of Acute Care Surgery, Trauma and Critical Care, University of Texas Health Science Center at Houston, The University of Texas Medical School at Houston, Houston, TX, USA
[2]Department of Anesthesiology, Critical Care Medicine, University of Rochester Medical Center, Rochester, NY, USA

Synonyms

Total blood volume

Definition

The blood volume, or the total volume of blood cells and plasma in the circulatory system, is often estimated, but rarely measured directly. Red blood cell (RBC) volume (RCV) and plasma volume (PV) are the primary components of total blood volume (TV), with the remaining contribution of white blood cells making up less than 0.1 % of TV. The hematocrit measures the proportions of RCV and PV (Feldschuh and Katz 2007).

Estimations of blood volume have been historically based on body weight, ideal or actual, and body surface area. Until quite recently, direct measurement of blood TV in patients was quite laborious and fraught with inaccuracies (Jacob et al. 2007). First attempts involved injection of a dye or, later, a radiotracer with subsequent serial measurement of blood levels; the indicator dilution method equation $C_1V_1 = C_2V_2$, where C_1 is the concentration of known injected tracer of volume V_1 and C_2 then is the measured concentration of the tracer in the unknown volume V_2 (Ertl et al. 2007).

The most elaborate test involved two radiotracers, one to label the RBCs and another to label the PV component. This test involved multiple blood draws and injections over the course of 5 h, and the results could be confounded by user error at each of the steps. There exists now an automated, validated rapid device that uses a combination of ^{131}I-radiotracer to measure PV and to measure hematocrit (Hct) to derive the RCV using the equation (Manzone et al. 2007)

$$TV = PV/(1 - Hct)$$

The euvolemic state is regulated by a complex interplay of cardiovascular, renal, and endocrine physiology, including the renin-angiotensin system, antidiuretic hormone, and baroreceptors (Riley et al. 2010). Hypovolemia secondary to hemorrhage, when significant enough to lead to hypoperfusion of organs, is termed hemorrhagic shock. Hypervolemia, or blood volume overload in otherwise healthy trauma patients, is often iatrogenic.

Cross-References

▶ Exsanguination Transfusion
▶ Hemorrhage

References

Ertl A, Diedrich A, Satish R (2007) Techniques used for the determination of blood volume. Am J Med Sci 334:32–36

Feldschuh J, Katz S (2007) The importance of correct norms in blood volume measurement. Am J Med Sci 334:41–46

Jacob M, Conzen P, Finsterer U (2007) Technical and physiological background of plasma volume measurement with indocyanine green: a clarification of misunderstandings. J Appl Physiol 102:1235–1242

Manzone T, Dam HQ, Soltis D et al (2007) Volume analysis: a new technique and new clinical interest reinvigorate a classic study. J Nucl Med Technol 35:55–63

Riley A, Arakawa Y, Worley S et al (2010) Circulating blood volumes: a review of measurement techniques and a meta-analysis in children. ASAIO J 56:260–264

Blunt Aortic Injury (BAI)

▶ Thoracic Vascular Injuries

Blunt Cardiac Injury

▶ Cardiac Injuries

Blunt Cardiac Injury: Cardiac Contusion

▶ Cardiac and Aortic Trauma, Anesthesia for

Blunt Carotid Vertebral Injuries

▶ Neurotrauma, Complications: Blunt Cerebrovascular Injuries

Blunt Chest Trauma

▶ Airbag Injuries

Blunt Chest Wall Trauma

▶ Chest Wall Injury

Blunt Craniocervical Arterial Injuries

▶ Neurotrauma, Complications: Blunt Cerebrovascular Injuries

Blunt Ocular Injury

▶ Eye Trauma, Anesthesia for

Body Armor

Charles A. Frosolone
Medical Department, USS Nimitz CVN-68, Everett, WA, USA

Synonyms

Ballistic vest; Behind armor blunt trauma (BABT); Bullet proof vest; Bullet-resistant vest; Combat helmet; Flak jacket, protective body armor; Personal armor system for ground troops (PASGT)

Definition

Body armor is a protective outer wear clothing usually a type of vest and helmet that is used to prevent injury from being inflicted to an individual by a weapon of direct contact or projectiles used against them.

Preexisting Condition

Anticipation of and/or potential for blunt or penetrating trauma and the need to protect an individual from injury by it.

Body Armor

Different types of body armor, to include helmets, have been utilized throughout history to protect personnel from harm by blows, slashing, stabbing, and projectiles both fragments and bullets. The body armor has been made of materials of increasing protection, from leather to bronze, to iron, to steel, and to synthetic fibers and ceramics, and has increased in sophistication. Each change in material and sophistication has been to increase levels of protection and to minimally degrade performance.

In US military rudimentary body armor was first used in American Civil War 1861–1865 consisting of two plates of steel inserted into a vest. In WW1 individual isolated efforts by combatants were done to develop armor that would protect from low-velocity weapons and fragments. But no body armor was issued to troops. The first usage of the term "flak jacket" refers to the armor originally developed during WW2 for Royal Air Force bomber crews to protect against shrapnel from antiaircraft fire. "Flak" is an abbreviation of the German "Fliegerabwehrkanone" (antiaircraft gun). These flak jackets went on to further development by the USA. Malcolm Grow studied wounds sustained by aircrews and noted that 70 % were from low-velocity fragments and that light body armor and steel helmets would protect against these injuries. Flak jackets consisting of manganese steel plates sewn into ballistic nylon and steel helmets became standard issue on bombers and with many US Navy personnel for protection against low-velocity fragments, but offered no real protection against bullets (ballistic protection).

Body armor was used by US troops in Korea and Vietnam. They were an upgrade from the "flak jacket" of WW 2 made with ballistic nylon layers and with additions of fiberglass plates. This generation of body armor could stop low-velocity fragments and pistol rounds, but was not protective against standard combat rifle rounds. In Vietnam ceramic plates were added to this armor and issued to crews of attack aircraft. The US helmet through Vietnam and into the 1980s was still the "steel pot" from WW2 which offered no substantial protection from high-velocity fragments or any kind of bullets.

The US National Institute of Justice (NIJ) in 1970 began a program to develop effective body armor against most pistol bullets. They also developed rating standards for body armor taking into account the threat level that the armor will protect against. These levels are from II (9 mm pistol rounds) to III (standard military rifle round) through IV (offering protection against .30 caliber armor-piercing rounds). There are subsets of each threat level rating. These levels of protection are now industry standards to rate body armor effectiveness. However the military standards do not require their vests to be NIJ certified, though they do offer protection equivalent to NIJ standards (Hanlon and Gillich 2012).

In the 1970s DuPont introduced kevlar, a synthetic fiber that was woven into a fabric and layered and when used as a vest could offer ballistic protection and be flexible, somewhat comfortable and concealable. Vests made of multiple kevlar fabric layers became widely used in the law enforcement community and are credited with saving many lives, but offer protection against threat level II only. Kevlar vests of the PASGT (personal armor system for ground troops) were issued to US forces, but offered only NIJ level II protection. They did not protect against large fragments or high-velocity rounds that were able to cause severe blunt trauma "behind armor blunt trauma" (BABT).

The "Ranger Armor" began to be issued in the 1990s, and this ultimately incorporated front and rear ceramic ballistic armor plates with flexible kevlar vest panels offering protection against military rifle rounds. The ceramic plates, small arms protective inserts (SAPIs), were made of aluminum oxide decreasing BABT, but covering only a 10 in. by 12 in. area of the chest and back. This body armor was heavy and demonstrated age old problem with body armor of the tradeoffs between protection and mobility.

Body armor in US forces has now evolved to armor with front, back, and side improved SAPI plates (ESAPI enhanced small arms protective inserts made of boron carbide or silicon carbide ceramics) capable of stopping armor-piercing rounds NIJ level IV and soft kevlar panels (capable of stopping 9 mm pistol rounds) that offer improved neck, groin, axillary, and upper arm area coverage. There is a liner behind the ceramic plates to trap fragments from either the projectile or the plate. The US Army fields the Improved Outer Tactical Vest, and the US Marine Corps (USMC) the Modular Tactical Vest. These are the current body armors used in Iraq and Afghanistan. Their mechanism of protection is to absorb and to dissipate the kinetic energy of the projectile by local shattering of the plate and blunting of the bullet. The energy of impact is dispersed into a larger area and decreases the chance of a fatal injury to the wearer. They are of considerable weight (over 30 lb) and add to potential heat stress and exhaustion and decreased mobility. They do have a number of features to decrease the burden and discomfort of wearing them, plus release features for quick removal of the armor. They are designed to take the weight of the vest off the shoulders and move it to the lower torso. The vests have a mesh liner to increase airflow inside the armor and a lower back pad to defeat the injuries caused by projectile impacts to lower back and kidney areas (Fig. 1).

Helmets were some of the oldest forms of protective equipment for soldiers dating back to over 4,000 years ago. They were made of leather, brass, bronze, iron, and later steel. They protected against blows, slash or stabs to the head, and projectiles such as arrows. With the introduction of firearms, the use of helmets for other than ceremonial or decorative use pretty much disappeared. However in WW1 with the increased use of artillery, functional military helmet use returned to the battlefield. Different countries produced various designs made of steel designed to protect against blunt trauma to head or low-velocity fragments or shrapnel. They offered little protection against high-velocity fragments or bullets. The US "doughboy" or Brodie helmet from WW1 evolved to the "steel

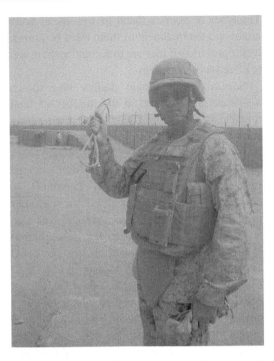

Body Armor, Fig. 1 US marine corps medical personnel with modular tactical vest and lightweight helmet

pot" or M1 helmet of WW2 that continued to be in frontline use until the late 1980s. The M1 offered little to no protection against bullets. The successor to the M1 was the PASGT helmet made of multiple layers of kevlar and resins and is rated at threat level IIIA (pistol bullets including magnums), plus it has increased fragment protection and larger area of coverage over the M1. In the USMC this helmet has been replaced by the lightweight helmet, and in the US Army the Modular Integrated Communications Helmet and Advanced Combat Helmet. These newer helmets offer increased protection and comfort.

Application

No doubt that body armor protects against fragment and bullets injury as evidenced by decreased rates of truncal injury in Iraq and Afghanistan. What is important for providers of medical care to realize is that wearing of the most technologically up-to-date body armor does not eliminate injury from fragments or bullets.

The types of injuries found in wearers of body armor and the treatment of them must be known by the providers if they are to recognize them and to effectively treat them.

Several epidemiologic studies have shown a substantial reduction in the number of fatal thoracic and abdominal injuries incurred during conflict situations in combatants wearing modern body armor. In Iraq and Afghanistan, only 5–7 % of reported injuries were thoracic, the lowest for American military personnel in modem warfare (Owens et al. 2008). A greater proportion of head and neck wounds was also noted in comparison with earlier non-armored conflicts both areas not sufficiently protected by armor. In both Iraq and Afghanistan the *died of wound* rate (DOW) is lower than any earlier conflicts and body armor contributed to this. It is unclear just how much body armor contributed to this improvement as there were many other changes in protection, evacuation, and field and hospital treatment of casualties that were initiated in this conflict.

Injuries noted in wearers of body armor fall into basically two categories. First category is injuries sustained in areas of the body where the body armor does not cover around the armor trauma (AAT). Second category is injuries sustained in areas covered by the armor or behind armor blunt trauma (BABT) where the projectile impacts the body armor and does not penetrate, but causes injury none the less.

First category AAT are treated just like any injury to that particular body area armor or not. Most commonly injured areas are head, neck, axilla, groin, and shoulder areas and of course the extremities. The current body armor has been improved to have kevlar pads to afford some protections to these areas, but projectiles can still get through these "chinks in the armor." Experienced snipers can take advantage of these weaknesses in protection and concentrate fire there causing significant and often fatal injuries. Injuries to the subclavian-axillary arteries, femoral-iliac arteries, carotids, and distal extremity arteries are quite common in AAT injuries. Surgeons tasked with care of combat victims must be facile with proximal vascular control

and exposures for these arteries, not commonly needed in civilian trauma settings. The main target area in civilian penetrating trauma is the trunk, which is covered by armor in combat. Pre-deployment training and practice should be done if one is not familiar with these key exposures. In a forward surgical setting, reestablishing flow to the injured arteries can be obtained by temporary shunting, or vessels may be temporarily or permanently ligated. Surgeons need to know which vessels and in what circumstances they can be safely ligated.

Second category of injuries noted in wearers of body armor is BABT. BABT is defined as the nonpenetrating injury resulting from a ballistic impact on body armor and has two mechanisms causing injury. Deformation of the armor caused by the projectile striking, but not penetrating the armor, can cause injury to the structures directly under the area of armor struck. The other mechanism is similar to primary blast injury with energy transfer causing injury or dysfunction at a distance from the area struck.

The increase in available energy of bullets and the desire of armor designers to minimize the weight and bulk of personal armor systems has increased the risk of BABT in military and security forces personnel. With the lighter flexible armor development, projectiles are stopped from entering the body by allowing deformation inward of the body armor dissipating of the projectile's energy (Bass and Salzar 2006). This injury potential is appreciated and forms a part of how the NIJ determines levels of protection for body armor: the 44-mm standard. Using the NIJ levels of protection, assuming the armor is not penetrated which constitutes vest failure, the measure of performance is based solely on a 44-mm static measurement of the deformation depth backface signature (BFS) created in a clay model. Derived from ballistic impacts on armor in animals, a 44-mm limit was determined as the maximum allowable BFS depth in the clay for a vest to meet ballistic resistance standards and be rated as acceptable for field use. Bass et al. state that the introduction of modern high impact strength, deformable materials into helmets, and body armor for this ballistic impact protection has increased the potential for significant backface deformation under ballistic impact. For most helmet and body armor systems, there is limited space available for this backface deformation. Even if there is no penetration, there is a substantial risk of producing severe head or thorax injury due to large deformations in the protective body armor striking the underlying structures. Possible injuries include bruising and hematoma in underlying skin; hematomas; fractures of underlying bone; lung contusions; blunt cardiac trauma; blunt injury to the liver, spleen, or kidney; rupture of bowel or bladder; or spinal cord or peripheral nerve injury. In animal studies high-velocity BABT of the spine generates high pressure and acceleration of the spine inducing various degrees of paralysis and cerebral dysfunction (Zhang 2011).

The second type of BABT mechanism is characterized by a stress wave that coupled into the body transforms at the point of impact through the armor and clothing into the body at the velocity of sound in the respective media. This mechanism results in injury even remote from the point of impact. This mechanism of injury is very similar to primary blast injury. It can result in primary blast-like effects to the cardiopulmonary system and central nervous system. There are noted behavioral disturbances and EEG changes (Drobin and Gryth 2007). The triad of apnea, bradycardia, and hypotension, noted in primary blast injury, has also been seen in animal studies of BABT. Lung contusions with hemoptysis and a sudden drop in blood pressure may occur. There is an initial apneic period, which has been shown to be a reflex reaction, which is an important factor for hypoxia after BABT. The brain dysfunction following BABT may be due to the hypoxic brain injury caused by this apnea.

Besides AAT and BABT, there are other injuries that can occur from projectile striking, but not penetrating the armor. When a helmet is struck by a projectile even if not penetrating the helmet, the transfer of kinetic energy to the head can cause injury (Komuński et al. 2009). This injury is other than the BABT from helmet deformation striking the underlying head. Head trauma is caused by acceleration/deceleration of the cranium, and with the stresses on the neck, cervical spine trauma can result.

Because of the additional weight burden when wearing body armor and the additional layers of protective clothing, besides impairing physical performance, there are other effects on the wearers. There is a considerable proportion of military personnel reporting noncombat injuries, the majority of which are musculoskeletal such as joint and back disorders. It has been hypothesized that the wearing of modern body armor can alter soldier's movement patterns, increase joint stress, and potentially increase their risk of suffering musculoskeletal injuries. Thermal stresses occur, though were felt unlikely to lead to either exertional heat illness or impaired cognitive function. There is increased oxygen consumption doing certain tasks in armor vs. unarmored. What part that decreased performance caused by wearing body armor may increase potential for injury is not known.

In the current conflicts, Lehman et al. noted a disproportionate number of low lumbar burst fractures among injured wearing body armor with approximately 50 % sustaining neurologic injury (Lehman 2011). The rigidity of current body armor possibly lowers the level of fracture from the usual thoracolumbar junction (T12–L2) where the stiff thoracic spine meets the lumbar spine to the low lumbar area (L3–L5) resulting in burst fractures.

Meralgia paresthetica has been observed in wearers of body armor; it is felt due to the pressure from the armor onto the lateral femoral cutaneous nerve (Fargo and Konitzer 2007 Jun).

Prevention of some injuries and decrease in related stresses can be improved by constant redesign of feature of today's body armor. Effective protection against BABT might be obtained by changing the ESAPIs from ceramic materials to other materials. Backing the armor with a trauma attenuating backing was shown to decrease pulmonary injury in animal models. Decreasing weight of body armor while maintaining protection will help in lessening performance degradation while decreasing chronic musculoskeletal injuries, thermal stress, and oxygen consumption. Improvements in suspension and increased flexibility of armor might lessen incidence of low lumbar fractures and meralgia paresthetica.

Prevention of AAT is to increase coverage of the areas where projectiles can cause injury, without degrading performance. In the latest generation of body armor, the kevlar pads for the neck, groin, and axillary areas have given protection against pistol rounds and lower-velocity fragments. Research and development has improved protection against BABT. Swedish researchers have investigated backing of armor with trauma attenuating backing (TAB). They showed decreased pulmonary injury by use of TAB (Sonden et al. 2009), but this TAB had no effect on brain injuries. Effective protection has been achieved for lungs exposed to short duration external blast waves by the placement of stress wave decouplers to the thoracoabdominal wall in a pig model, thus modifying the energy coupled into the body. A combination of two densities of glass-reinforced plastic plate and Plastazote foam (GRP/PZ) effectively eliminated pulmonary injury (Cripps and Cooper 1996 Mar). Progress is in designing new types of armor that decrease weight, offer improved or equivalent protection (yet are comfortable and nonrestrictive), cause less performance degradation, and decrease chronic musculoskeletal injuries, thermal stress, and oxygen consumption. Modifications of weight bearing of armor could be done to avoid meralgia paresthetica.

Diagnosis

A thorough history and physical exam and indicated laboratories and radiologic studies should establish the diagnosis. Being aware of the potential injuries caused by BABT is also paramount. Some injuries caused by BABT may evidence themselves in a delayed fashion such as pulmonary contusion, blunt enteric injury, and neurologic injury. Being aware of these possibilities, admission overnight may be indicated in victims with suspected BABT injuries, and serial examination is used to diagnose these delayed presentations.

Treatment

Treatment follows established guidelines for blunt and penetrating trauma. Respiratory arrest in BABT is treated with immediate ventilation until adequate spontaneous respirations return, and role 1 providers should be aware of this need for immediate ventilation.

Cross-References

► Ballistics
► Blast Lung Injury
► Firearm-Related Injuries
► High-Velocity

References

Bass CR, Salzar RS (2006) Injury risk in behind armor blunt thoracic trauma. Int J Occup Saf Ergon 12(4):429–442

Cripps NP, Cooper GJ (1996) The influence of personal blast protection on the distribution and severity of primary blast gut injury. J Trauma 40(Suppl 3): S206–S211

Drobin D, Gryth D (2007) Electroencephalogram, circulation, and lung function after high-velocity behind armor blunt trauma. J Trauma 63(2):405–413

Fargo MV, Konitzer LN (2007) Meralgia paresthetica due to body armor wear in US soldiers serving in Iraq: a case report and review of the literature. Mil Med 172(2):663–665

Hanlon E, Gillich P (2012) Origin of the 44-mm behind-armor blunt trauma standard. Mil Med 177: 333–339

Komuński P, Kubiak T, Łandwijt M, Romek R (2009) Energy transmission from bullet impact onto head or neck through structures of the protective ballistic helmet – tests and evaluation. Techniczne Wyroby Włókiennicze (Technical Textiles J) 4:18–22

Lehman RA, Paik H (2012) Low lumbar burst fractures: a unique fracture mechanism sustained in our current overseas conflicts. Spine J 12(9):784–790

Owens BD, Kragh JF, Wenke JC, Macaitisj BS, Wade CE, Holcomb JB (2008) Combat wounds in operation Iraqi freedom and operation enduring freedom. J Trauma 64:295–299

Sonden A, Rocksen D, Riddez L (2009) Trauma attenuating backing improves protection against behind armor blunt trauma. J Trauma 67(6):1191–1199

Zhang B, Huang Y (2011) Neurologica, functional and biomechanical characteristics after high-velocity behind armor blunt trauma of the spine. J Trauma 71(6):1680–1688

Body Heat Loss

▶ Hypothermia, Trauma, and Anesthetic Management

Body Temperature

▶ Monitoring of Trauma Patients During Anesthesia

Bogota Bag

Jamie J. Coleman
Department of Surgery, Indiana University School of Medicine, Indianapolis, IN, USA

Synonyms

Silo dressing; Temporary silo

Definition

A Bogota bag is a method of containment for the open abdomen, also known as a temporary abdominal closure. This technique was first described in Bogota, Colombia, in 1984 and utilizes a large piece of nonadherent material to contain intra-abdominal contents (Wyrzykowski and Feliciano 2013). Many types of materials have been used to create these temporary silos and include large sterile IV bags, silastic sheeting, parachute silk, PTFE, and X-ray cassette covers (Wyrzykowski and Feliciano 2013; Luchette et al. 2007; Demetriades and Salim 2014). The nonadherent material is then sutured to either the skin or fascial edges. The skin is typically preferred as not to potentially damage the fascia and inhibit future fascial closure. Advantages to this technique are its low cost, nonadherence to the bowel, ease of removal, and low incidence of postoperative abdominal

compartment syndrome (Luchette et al. 2007; Demetriades and Salim 2014). In addition, some materials allow for visual inspection of the bowel at the bedside for patients in whom the presence of bowel ischemia is suspected. This technique, however, does not allow for effective fluid removal from the abdomen or prevent retraction of the fascial edges, making future fascial potentially more difficult. Although this technique is still used, it has been replaced at many centers in the United States by negative pressure dressings (Demetriades and Salim 2014).

Cross-References

▶ Abdominal Compartment Syndrome
▶ Damage Control Resuscitation
▶ Methods of Containment of the Open Abdomen, Overview
▶ Open Abdomen, Temporary Abdominal Closure

References

Demetriades D, Salim A (2014) Management of the open abdomen. Surg Clin N Am 94:131–153
Luchette FA, Poulakidas SJ, Esposito TJ (2007) The open abdomen: management from initial laparotomy to definitive closure. In: Britt LD, Trunkey DD, Feliciano DV (eds) Acute care surgery: principles and practice. Springer, New York, pp 176–186
Wyrzykowski AD, Feliciano DV (2013) Trauma damage control. In: Mattox KL, Moore EE, Feliciano DV (eds) Trauma, 7th edn. McGraw-Hill, New York, pp 725–746

Bomb

▶ Blast
▶ Explosion
▶ Mortars

Bone Healing

▶ Principles of Internal Fixation of Fractures

Bone Infarction

▶ Avascular Necrosis of the Femoral Head

Booby Trap

▶ IED (Improvised Explosive Device)

Bowel Accident

▶ Bowel Incontinence

Bowel Active Agents in the ICU

Melissa A. Reger[1], Staci A. Anderson[1] and
Mary M. Wolfe[2]
[1]Department of Pharmacy, Community Regional
Medical Center, Fresno, CA, USA
[2]Department of Surgery, Community Regional
Medical Center, Fresno, CA, USA

Synonyms

Bowel regimens; Cathartics; Constipation;
Evacuants; Laxation; Laxatives; Purgatives

Definition

Constipation is a common problem in patients
with traumatic injuries. Currently there is no
approved definition of acute constipation, but
chronic constipation is described as lack of a
bowel movement for three consecutive days
(Locke et al. 2000). Using this definition, the
frequency of constipation has been found to be
as high as 83 % in the critically ill patient
(Mostafa et al. 2003). Constipation can also
describe difficulty in initiation or passage of
stool, passage of firm or small volume stool, or
the feeling of incomplete evacuation (Pasricha
2008). Unfortunately, proper bowel care is often
overlooked in the intensive care unit and considered a lower priority. Side effects of constipation
include abdominal distension, pain, nausea,
vomiting, anorexia, dehydration, confusion,
overflow fecal incontinence, restlessness,
obstruction, and stercoral perforation (Dorman
et al. 2004). It has also been implicated in
prolonged mechanical ventilation and delayed
start of enteral nutrition (Patanwala et al. 2006;
Mostafa et al. 2003).

Preexisting Condition

Fluid content is the primary determinant of stool
volume and consistency and reflects a balance
between luminal input and output (Pasricha
2008). Alterations in secretion, absorption,
and/or motility along the length of the bowel
can lead to excess fluid removal and constipation.
There are many potential causes for constipation
in the trauma patient including medications,
dehydration, underlying bowel condition, lack
of fiber in diet, immobility, pain, inability to act
or respond to the urge to defecate, hormonal
disturbances, neurogenic disorders, and lack of
privacy (Dorman et al. 2004; Pasricha 2008).
Medications that are commonly associated with
constipation include opiates, anticholinergics,
and others (Table 1) (Cassagnol et al. 2010). As
the population ages, there may be an increase
in the prevalence of constipation, primarily
due to decreased mobility, comorbid medical
conditions, and polypharmacy.

Application

Treatment of constipation should involve
a multidisciplinary team approach including the
physician, nurse, and pharmacist. There are
numerous non-pharmacologic methods of treatment including hydration, physical activity,
enemas, and elimination of offending medications. Another non-pharmacologic remedy for
constipation includes prune juice, which can be

Bowel Active Agents in the ICU, Table 1 Medications associated with constipation

Medication class	Example agents
Opiates	Morphine, hydrocodone, fentanyl, hydromorphone, oxycodone
Anticholinergics	Tolterodine, scopolamine, benztropine, atropine
Antispasmodics	Oxybutynin, hyoscyamine, cyclobenzaprine, baclofen
Tricyclic antidepressants	Amitriptyline, doxepin, desipramine, nortriptyline
Antiparkinsonians	Carbidopa, entacapone, trihexyphenidyl, amantadine, pramipexole
Calcium channel blockers	Verapamil, diltiazem
Diuretics	Furosemide, torsemide, hydrochlorothiazide, metolazone, triamterene
Anticonvulsants	Phenobarbital, phenytoin, carbamazepine, levetiracetam, pregabalin
Vinca alkaloids	Vinblastine, vincristine, vinorelbine
Antihistamines	Diphenhydramine, promethazine, famotidine
Antacids	Calcium carbonate, aluminum hydroxide
Iron supplements	Ferrous sulfate, ferrous gluconate, polysaccharide-iron complex
Antidiarrheals	Loperamide, bismuth, diphenoxylate/atropine, opium tincture

given orally or added to tube feedings. Prune juice acts as a natural laxative because of its high content of sorbitol, a nondigestible sugar that occurs naturally.

The ideal pharmacologic intervention consists of the combination of a stool softener and a motility agent. A stool softener without a motility agent causes "all mush and no push." A retrospective analysis of critically ill patients found that the use of a stimulant or osmotic laxative was associated with the occurrence of a bowel movement, while prokinetic agents (metoclopramide, erythromycin) were not (Patanwala et al. 2006). Rarely, patients may require additional interventions based on their disease states. For example, patients with quadriplegia or paraplegia who have an upper motor neuron cord lesion generally have reflex bowel activity and may require digital rectal stimulation to produce a bowel movement. This is achieved by placing a gloved finger into the rectum and slowly rotating, while maintaining contact with the anterior portion of the rectal wall (Steins et al. 1997). In addition, manual digital pressure applied to the abdomen or manual disimpaction may be necessary to assist with bowel evacuation. Because stimulation of the vagus nerve may occur, this should be used with caution in patients with cardiac disorders and recent bowel or genitourinary surgery.

Medications for Constipation

Numerous drug products are available to help relieve constipation in the ICU patient (Table 2). Bulk-forming agents, such as psyllium and methylcellulose, can assist with constipation and have very few side effects. Bulk-forming agents absorb water in the intestine to form a viscous liquid which promotes peristalsis and reduces transit time. They also soften the stool (Cassagnol et al. 2010). Caution must be taken when administering these to patients with poor intake of liquids as the constipation could worsen if not given with at least 8 oz of water. Since these agents thicken when mixed with water, caution should be taken when administering through a feeding tube as clogging of the tube may occur.

Osmotic agents, such as lactulose, sorbitol, and magnesium hydroxide, exert their action by osmotically drawing water into the bowel and stimulating peristalsis. Saline laxatives, which can contain magnesium or phosphate, should be used with caution in patients with renal impairment, cardiac disease, and preexisting electrolyte abnormalities or in patients on diuretic therapy as electrolyte abnormalities may occur (Pasricha 2008). Effects of these agents may not be seen for 24–48 h after administration, generally with higher doses producing faster results. Polyethylene glycol is a newer agent that produces similar effects to other osmotically active agents but with fewer side effects and improved compliance.

Stool softeners such as docusate and mineral oil are necessary in bowel care to limit the pain associated with bowel movements. Docusate is an anionic surfactant that lowers the surface tension

Bowel Active Agents in the ICU, Table 2 Medications to relieve constipation

Medications	Usual dosage	Expected time to laxation
Bulk-forming laxatives		
Psyllium	2.5–30 g divided 1–4x daily	12–72 h
Methylcellulose	2–20 g divided 1–4x daily	24–72 h
Polycarbophil	1.25–20 g divided 1–4x daily	24–72 h
Wheat dextran	1.3–9 g divided 1–4x daily	24–72 h
Osmotic agents		
Magnesium hydroxide	2.4–9.6 g (30–120 mL) divided 1–4x daily	0.5–6 h
Magnesium citrate	150–300 mL once daily	1–3 h
Sodium phosphate	15–45 mL once daily	3–6 h
Lactulose	10–40 g (15–60 mL) divided 1–4x daily	24–48 h
Polyethylene glycol	17–34 g divided 1–2x daily	24–96 h
Stool softener		
Docusate	200–500 mg/day divided 2x daily	12–72 h
Mineral oil	15–45 mL once daily	6–8 h
Stimulants		
Bisacodyl (PO)	10–40 mg divided 1–4x daily	6–10 h
Senna	8.6–51.6 mg (1–6 tabs) divided 1–3x daily	6–8 h
Enema/suppository		
Phosphate enema	118 mL once daily	2–5 min
Mineral oil enema	118 mL once daily	2–15 min
Bisacodyl suppository	1 suppository 1–4x daily	15–60 min
Glycerin suppository	1 suppository 1–2x daily	15–30 min

of the stool, similar to the action of soap, and allows for softening of the stool. Docusate alone for treatment of constipation has proven to be an ineffective method (Cassagnol et al. 2010). Mineral oil is a nonabsorbable oil that softens the stool. However, this can lead to malabsorption of fat-soluble vitamins, leakage of oil past the anal sphincter, and pneumonitis if aspirated, and thus its regular use is limited (Pasricha 2008).

Stimulant laxatives have a direct effect on the enterocytes and GI smooth muscle to stimulate intestinal motility. Bisacodyl is available as an oral or rectal preparation for use by adults and children over the age of 6. Suppositories generally produce a more rapid effect (within 30–60 min) when compared to the oral route (6 h) (Pasricha 2008). The oral preparation is an enteric-coated tablet, so manipulation (crushing) of the tablet is not advised. Senna is another commonly used stimulant agent. It is derived from the plant *Cassia acutifolia* and is considered an herbal preparation, which makes standardized dosing difficult. It is usually administered orally and produces an effect within 6 h. Due to the stimulating effect of both of these agents, common side effects include abdominal pain and cramping.

Enemas and suppositories generally provide fast and localized effects. Bowel distention alone, by any means, can produce a bowel movement in most patients. This can be facilitated by anything from normal saline to commercially available preparations. Caution should be used with all of these agents and attention paid to their contents. For example, repeated use of tap water enemas can lead to hyponatremia due to an increase in free water or too many sodium phosphate enemas may put a patient at risk for hypernatremia and hyperphosphatemia. Another type of enema is the return-flow enema, also called a Harris flush. In this procedure, a bag filled with a small amount of fluid (usually warm tap water) is elevated above the patient's hips, and the fluid is instilled into the colon through a tube. The bag is then lowered, allowing the solution to run back into the bag. This process is repeated several times, stimulating peristalsis and allowing the patient to expel flatus and stool. Glycerin suppositories act as a colonic lubricant and usually produce a bowel movement in less than an hour (Pasricha 2008). This preparation has very few side effects, except for some local irritation, and is arguably the drug of choice for pediatric trauma patients. As previously mentioned, bisacodyl suppositories are very effective at rapidly producing a bowel movement, by both local irritation and digital stimulation during administration. However, when considering use of enemas and suppositories, care must be taken in those patients with distal bowel injury and/or recent anastomosis.

Prevention of constipation is an exciting new area of research. It would be ideal to limit the adverse effects of medications such as opioids on the bowel. Enteral naloxone, a pure opiate antagonist, has been studied to treat opiate-induced constipation. Enteral administration has the theoretical benefit of little to no systemic exposure due to extensive first-pass metabolism in the liver. However, opiate withdrawal symptoms have still been reported with its use (Foss 2001). Methylnaltrexone is an antagonist of the mu-opioid receptor with limited ability to cross the blood–brain barrier. Therefore, it functions in the periphery and does not affect opiate analgesia efficacy or induce withdrawal symptoms. Methylnaltrexone has been shown to decrease oral-cecal transit times in both acute and chronic opioid administration (Foss 2001). Subcutaneous administration and medication cost limit its usefulness. Alvimopan, another peripherally acting mu-opioid receptor antagonist, has been shown to accelerate gastrointestinal recovery in patients undergoing laparotomy for bowel resection. However, in studies of alvimopan for opiate-induced bowel dysfunction in patients with chronic non-cancer pain, there was a higher incidence of myocardial infarction in alvimopan-treated patients. This led to the implementation of a risk evaluation and mitigation strategy by the FDA and restriction of the medication to patients undergoing bowel resection (Kraft et al. 2010). For this reason, alvimopan cannot be recommended for the prevention of opiate-induced constipation in the trauma patient.

Agents that are not beneficial include erythromycin due to its action on the stomach and small intestine that are mediated through motilin receptors that do not extend into the colon. The effects of metoclopramide are confined largely to the upper gastrointestinal tract. It has no clinically significant effects on the motility of the colon, and its ability to improve transit in motility disorders is limited (Pasricha 2008).

Conclusions and Recommendations

Prevention is the best medicine, and it is no different when it comes to constipation. Treatment recommendations consist of an initial assessment of the patients' medication regimen and removal of unnecessary medications that can predispose patients to constipation. Pharmacologic therapy is most beneficial when it is started early and includes a combination of a stool softener (docusate) twice daily with the addition of a stimulant agent (senna or bisacodyl) at bedtime. Bisacodyl has the advantage of a suppository formulation that is especially useful after surgery, whereas senna is better tolerated via feeding tube administration. If constipation remains a problem, other agents can be added (polyethylene glycol, saline laxatives) until the goal of a bowel movement is attained. Once the sweet smell of success has been achieved, the regimen should be tapered down to limit the occurrence of diarrhea due to these agents, as this can lead to other needless tests and procedures.

Cross-References

- ▶ Acute Pain Management in Trauma
- ▶ Bowel Incontinence
- ▶ Fluid, Electrolytes, and Nutrition in Trauma Patients
- ▶ Geriatric Trauma
- ▶ ICU Management
- ▶ Nutritional Support
- ▶ Pain
- ▶ Sedation and Analgesia
- ▶ Sedation, Analgesia, Neuromuscular Blockade in the ICU

References

Cassagnol M, Saad M, Ahmed E, Ezzo D (2010) Review of current chronic constipation guidelines. US Pharm 35:74–85

Dorman BP, Hill C, McGrath M et al (2004) Bowel management in the intensive care unit. Intensive Crit Care Nurs 20:320–329

Foss JF (2001) A review of the potential role of methylnaltrexone in opioid bowel dysfunction. Am J Surg 182:19S–26S

Kraft M, MacLaren R, Du W, Owens G (2010) Alvimopan (Entereg) for the management of postoperative ileus in patients undergoing bowel resection. P T 35:44–49

Locke GR 3rd, Pemberton JH, Phillips SF (2000) American Gastroenterological Association medical position statement: guidelines of constipation. Gastroenterology 119:1761–1766

Mostafa SM, Bhandari S, Ritchie G et al (2003) Constipation and its implications in the critically ill patient. Br J Anaesth 91:815–819

Pasricha PJ (2008) Goodman and Gilman's manual of pharmacology and therapeutics. In: Treatment of disorders of bowel motility and water flux; antiemetics; agents used in biliary and pancreatic disease, 11th edn. The McGraw-Hill Companies, San Francisco, pp 633–652, Chap 37

Patanwala AE, Abarca J, Huckleberry Y, Erstad BL (2006) Pharmacologic management of constipation in the critically ill patient. Pharmacotherapy 26:896–902

Steins SA, Bergman SB, Goetz LL (1997) Neurogenic bowel dysfunction after spinal cord injury: clinical evaluation and rehabilitative management. Arch Phys Med Rehabil 78:S86–S102

Bowel Incontinence

Douglas Fetkenhour
Department of Physical Medicine and Rehabilitation, University of Rochester School of Medicine, Rochester, NY, USA

Synonyms

Bowel accident; Soiling oneself

Definition

Inability to evacuate stool in a controlled fashion resulting in involuntary excretion of stool.

Bowel incontinence following trauma may be the result of injury to the nervous system (SCI, TBI), peripheral nerve injury, or from the basic inability to mobilize adequately.

Neurogenic Bowel

Nerve injury can impair the normal sensation of a full rectum and ability to store and release stool. An effective bowel program can provide control and predictability over evacuation of the bowels. Components of a successful bowel program include consistency, motility, and evacuation.

The desirable consistency of stool is soft enough to move through the large bowel and formed enough to be stored in the rectum without leakage. The motility and transit time of stool should be consistent to allow a predictable timing of evacuation. Immobility, narcotics, and iron supplementation can make the stool too hard and decrease motility. Antibiotics can make the stool too soft and increase motility.

Utilization of a stimulus to trigger the evacuation of the rectum in an appropriate setting (i.e., toilet or commode) is a major determinant of continence.

Medications recommended by the physiatrist help to control consistency, motility, and evacuation.

Medications for consistency
Docusate – mild softener
Lactulose – moderate softener
Magnesium citrate – potent softener
Fiber (metamucil) – adds bulk
Medications for motility
Senna – mild
Milk of magnesia – moderate
Doculax – potent
Medications/techniques for evacuation
Suppository – routine
Digital stimulation (finger inserted into the rectum)
Enema – rescue therapy

A typical bowel regimen should include a mild softener twice daily, a stimulant once daily (8–12 h prior to evacuation), and a suppository or digital stimulation once daily (can be morning or night based on patient preference). Based on the trauma patient's diet and other medications, bowel medications will be adjusted to optimize consistency and motility.

Physical and occupational therapy to improve bed mobility, transfers, and personal hygiene are implemented irrespective of the etiology of the incontinent episodes.

The goal of a successful bowel program is COT and CIB: Control Over Timing (of evacuation) and Clean In Between (bowel movements).

Cross-References

▶ Rehabilitation Nursing

Recommended Reading

Neurogenic Continence, Part 3. Bowel management strategies in congrave. Br J Nurs, 10; 17(15): 962–968.www.now.aapmr.org/cns/complications/Pages/Neurogenic-Bowel.aspx

Bowel Regimens

▶ Bowel Active Agents in the ICU

Brace

▶ Orthotics

Brain Death

Nahit Çakar and Evren Şentürk
Istanbul Medical Faculty Anesthesiology and Intensive Care, Istanbul, Turkey

Synonyms

Coma depasse; Irreversible apneic coma; Irreversible coma

Introduction

> Life is pleasant. Death is peaceful. It's the transition that's troublesome.
> Isaac Asimov

Brain death is the irreversible loss of all brain function including that of respiratory drive after a direct or an indirect injury to the brain concerning the cerebrum, cerebellum, and mid brain.

Before developments in medicine, especially in the area of intensive care, death was determined according to cardiac and respiratory criteria. This was the case for all primary diagnoses including severely comatose patients with brain injuries. In this group of patients who did not have any reversible brain function including respiratory drive, it was possible to prolong death when death was determined by cardiorespiratory criteria. This caused medical societies to search for new definitions of death in these cases. The new found definition of "brain death" led to some humanitarian benefits:

(a) Patient relatives are released of unnecessary hopes.
(b) Organs of brain death donors can be used for transplantation.
(c) Intensive care unit facilities are used more properly for patients who have chances of survival.

History

Intensive care units began to save lives with positive-pressure ventilation and prevent mortality after the Copenhagen polio epidemic in 1952–1953 (Machado et al. 2007). Patients who had severe devastating neurologic compromise could be sustained by artificial ventilation in intensive care units (Wertheimer et al. 1959). In 1959, Mollaret and Goulon coined the phrase "Le Coma De'passe" meaning a clinical state beyond coma who were apneic and had no brainstem reflexes in deep coma and polyuria (Mollaret and Goulon 1959). Those days, it was a challenge to find a definition that is easy to understand and simple for brain death. Brain death criteria were first defined in 1968 by the "Harvard criteria" (Beecher and Harvard Ad Hoc Committee 1968). According to Harvard Ad Hoc Committee "An organ, brain or other that no longer function and has no possibility of functioning again is for all practical purposes dead" (Beecher 2007). Then in 1971, two neurosurgeons described brain death as "point of no return" (Mohandas and Chou 1971); these criteria were based on a clinical basis and no confirmatory tests were mandatory.

Definition

> We don't know life: how can we know death?
> Confucius.

Brain death defines a clinical situation after a severe direct or an indirect injury to the brain. This is an irreversible loss of the whole brain function above the medulla spinalis which includes unconsciousness with a Glasgow Coma Score of 3, fixed dilated pupils, absence of all cranial nerve functions, and the absence of a spontaneous respiratory drive.

Preexisting Condition

Pathophysiology

Following a direct or an indirect injury of the brain, intracranial pressure increases to a level which interrupts blood flow to the brain. Following the cessation of blood flow to the brain, within 3–5 days, the brain is liquefied which was described as a "respirator brain" by Walker et al. (1975). Microscopic examination shows autolysis and aseptic necrosis. According to Ujihira et al. (1993), neuropathological findings are brain edema, congestion, herniation, and various subarachnoid hemorrhages. Histologically, the neurons' cytoplasm was pale and ghost-like. In the white matter, myelin staining was pale, and nuclei of the glial cells were shrunken and piknotic. Autolysis of the cerebellar granular layer and the pituitary gland was evident in all cases. There was not any reactive astrocytosis or infiltration of the cells in or around necrotic tissue.

Application

Diagnosis of Brain Death

For the diagnosis of brain death, the patient should have a history or findings of direct or indirect insult to the brain which result in a structural brain damage and a deep coma. The patient should also be apneic under controlled mechanical ventilation. An unresponsive coma caused by alcohol, sedative or depressant drug overdose, metabolic or endocrine disorders, electrolyte disturbances, hypothermia, and neuromuscular blocker drugs can be potentially reversible and cannot be classified as brain death. In the absence of these reversible causes, a neurologic examination of a brain death case should lack all evidence of responsiveness to painful stimulus. Eye opening or eye movement to noxious stimuli should be absent. Painful stimuli can be made by nail bed pressure and supraorbital pressure or jaw thrust maneuver. No grimacing or facial muscle movement must be seen.

In the presence of coma as defined above with Glasgow Coma Scale point 3, and absence of brainstem reflexes which includes light, corneal, occulocephalic, occulovestibular, pharyngeal, tracheal reflexes, and a positive apnea test (detailed information about the absence of brain reflexes and the apnea test is given below) shows brain death. In most of the cases, deep tendon reflexes are absent however in some cases spinal reflexes and myoclonus may persist and can be misunderstood both by family members and medical personal.

Several centers usually perform two neurologic examinations within a 12–24-h period, but one should be sufficient to pronounce brain death. One absolute requirement is that the physicians involved with declaration of brain death should have no conflict of interest with organ donation.

Absence of Brainstem Reflexes

[This part is modified from American Academy of Neurology Evidence-based guideline update (Wijdicks et al. 2010).]

- Absence of pupillary response to bright light has to be demonstrated. Both pupils should be fixed in diameter and pupil size is irrelevant although most will be dilated. Constricted pupils raise the possibility of drug intoxication.
- Absence of occulocephalic reflex is determined by observing no movement of the eyes during the head movement to vertical, right, and left positions. Before this test, cervical spine injury should be excluded.
- Absence of occulovestibular reflex is tested by irrigating each ear with ice water (caloric testing) after the patency of the external auditory canal is confirmed. The head is elevated to 30°. Each external auditory canal is irrigated (1 ear at a time) with approximately 50 mL of ice water. Movement of the eyes should be absent during 1 min of observation. Both sides are tested, with an interval of several minutes.
- Absence of corneal reflex is tested by touching the cornea with a cotton swab, or squirts of water. There should be no eyelid movement.
- Absence of facial muscle movement to a noxious stimulus should be determined by pressing the condyles at the level of the temporomandibular joints, and/or a pressure at the supraorbital ridge is performed. There should be no grimacing or facial muscle movement.
- Absence of the pharyngeal or gag reflex is tested with the stimulation of the posterior pharynx with a tongue blade or suction device. The tracheal reflex is most reliably tested by examining the cough response to tracheal suctioning. The catheter should be inserted into the trachea and advanced to the level of the carina followed by 1 or 2 suctioning passes.

Apnea Test

Apnea is defined as absence of spontaneous breathing effort. Documentation of an increase in $PaCO_2$ above normal levels without breathing effort is a positive apnea test (Nakagawa et al. 2011). Before the test, the patient must be normotensive, normothermic, euvolemic, eucapnic ($PaCO_2$ 35–45 mmHg), and not hypoxic.

Procedure:
- Preoxygenation with 100 % oxygen at least 10 min, target PaO_2 is above 200 mmHg to avoid hypoxia.
- Obtain a sample of arterial blood gas for a baseline PaO_2, $PaCO_2$, pH, bicarbonate, and base excess values.
- Disconnect the patient from the ventilator.
- Give oxygen through the endotracheal tube by placing a catheter close to the level of the carina and deliver 100 % O_2 at 6 L/min.
- Observe respiratory movements at least for 8–10 min.
- Stop the procedure if systolic blood pressure decreases to <90 mmHg or pulse oximetry saturation value is below 85 % for 30 s. In this case, apnea test can be repeated with a T-piece or CPAP 10 cm H_2O, and 100 % O_2. Take a sample of arterial blood gas when no respiratory drive is observed.

Apnea test is positive when respiratory movements are absent and $PaCO_2$ is above 60 mmHg (or 20 mmHg increase over a baseline $PaCO_2$).

Ancillary Tests

Brain death is diagnosed clinically. However, ancillary tests are needed when the clinical criteria cannot be applied (cranial nerves cannot be adequately tested and cardiorespiratory criteria that precludes testing for apnea) reliably or if there are confounding factors (possible drug or metabolic effect on coma and cervical vertebra or cord injury is present) and no clear cause of coma exists.

These tests can be divided into two categories: cerebral electrical function (EEG, SSEPs, BAERs) and cerebral blood flow (four vessel cerebral angiography, nuclear brain blood flow tests, transcranial Doppler, MR angiography, and CT angiography). Cerebral blood flow tests provide acceptable data for the declaration of brain death. Cerebral blood flow tests are not influenced by drugs, metabolic disorders, or hypothermia but can be affected from systemic blood pressure. On the other hand, electrical brain function tests are vulnerable to barbiturate overdose or deep anesthesia, conditions that are completely reversible (false positive).

The ideal ancillary test must have no false positives or false negatives and should not be affected by sedatives or metabolic disturbances. An ideal ancillary test should be declarative, available, easily applied, reliable, and safe.

Brain Death in Children

According to the Society of Critical Care Medicine; the Section on Critical Care and Section on Neurology of the American Academy of Pediatrics; the Child Neurology Society task force recommendations (Nakagawa et al. 2011), two examinations with each examination separated by an observation period are required (Wijdicks et al. 2010). Examinations should be performed by different attending physicians. Apnea testing may be performed by the same physician. An observation period of 24 h for term newborns (37 weeks of gestational age) to 30 days of age and 12 h for infants and children (>30 days to 18 years) is recommended. Assessment of neurologic function after cardiopulmonary resuscitation or other severe acute brain injuries should be deferred for >24 h if there are concerns or inconstancy in the examination.

Documentation

The time of brain death must be documented in the medical record. Time of death is the time when an apnea test is confirmed. In patients with an aborted apnea test, the time of death is when the ancillary test have been officially performed (Section "Cross-References").

Cross-References

▶ Brain Death, Ethical Concerns
▶ Examination, Neurological
▶ Organ Donor Management
▶ Neurotrauma, Death by Neurological Criteria
▶ Neurotrauma and Brain Death, Ventilatory Management

References

Beecher HK (2007) A definition of irreversible coma. Int Anesthesiol Clin 45(4):113–119

Beecher HK, Harvard Ad Hoc Committee (1968) A definition of irreversible coma: report of the ad hoc committee of the Harvard Medical School to examine the definition of brain death. JAMA 205: 337–340

Machado C, Kerein J, Ferrer Y et al (2007) The concept of brain death did not evolve to benefit organ transplants. J Med Ethics 33:197–200

Mohandas A, Chou SN (1971) Brain death – a clinical and pathological study. J Neurosurg 35:211–218

Mollaret P, Goulon M (1959) Le coma de'passe'. Rev Neurol (Paris) 101:3–15

Nakagawa TA, Ashwal S, Mathur M, Mysore MR, Bruce D, Conway EE Jr, Duthie SE, Hamrick S, Harrison R, Kline AM, Lebovitz DJ, Madden MA, Montgomery VL, Perlman JM, Rollins N, Shemie SD, Vohra A, Williams-Phillips JA (2011) Guidelines for the determination of brain death in infants and children: An update of the 1987 Task Force recommendations. Society of Critical Care Medicine; the Section on Critical Care and Section on Neurology of the American Academy of Pediatrics; the Child Neurology Society. Crit Care Med 39(9): 2139–2155

Ujihira N, Hashizume Y, Takahashi A (1993) A clinico-neuropathological study on braindeath. Nagoya J Med Sci 56:89–99

Walker AE, Diamond EL, Moseley J (1975) The neuropathological findings in irreversible coma: a critique of the "respirator brain". J Neuropathol Exp Neurol 34:295

Wertheimer P, Jouvet M, Descotes J (1959) Diagnosis of death of the nervous system in comas with respiratory arrest treated by artificial respiration. Presse Med 67:87–88

Wijdicks EF, Varelas PN, Gronseth GS, Greer DM (2010) American Academy of Neurology: Evidence-based guideline update: determining brain death in adults: report of the Quality Standards Subcommittee of the American Academy of Neurology. Neurology 74(23):1911–1918

Brain Death, Ethical Concerns

Abhijit Lele[1] and Gary Gronseth[2]
[1]Department of Anesthesiology, Neurology and Neurosurgery, University of Kansas Medical Center, Kansas City, KS, USA
[2]Department of Neurology, University of Kansas Medical Center, Kansas City, KS, USA

Synonyms

Bioethics; Brain death; Brainstem death; Death; End-of-life issues; Ethics; Medical ethics; Organ donation

Definition, Background

Brief History of Brain Death
Ever since technological revolution occurred about a century ago during the polio epidemics, man has been able to prolong life with artificial support, namely, mechanical ventilation.

The first European country to adopt brain death as a legal definition of death was Finland in 1971.

An ad hoc committee at the Harvard Medical School published a pivotal 1968 report to define irreversible coma.

In the USA, the 1981 President's commission outlined the essential elements that serve as the foundation of the modern criterion of brain death: Cessation of whole brain function including.

1. Unresponsive coma
2. The absence of brain stem reflexes
3. Apnea

The commission also outlined requirements for the irreversibility of the brain function cessation:

1. The cause is established.
2. The possibility of recovery is excluded by ensuring that the cessation of function persists for a period of time.
3. Confounding conditions such as hypothermia are absent.

The commission's report was the catalyst that led to the Uniform Declaration of Death act in the USA that defined death as either:

1. The irreversible cessation of circulatory and respiratory function or
2. The irreversible cessation of all functions of the entire brain

Other countries have adopted somewhat different standards. For example, in the UK, the Royal College of Physicians in 1976 and 1977 rejected the whole brain death criterion and adopted notion of irreversible brain stem dysfunction as an indicator of death.

Application

Ethical Problems in the Determination of Death
The ethical problems commonly encountered in the declaration of brain death can be highlighted by considering seven common brain death myths encountered in practice. These myths can be organized by the four fundamental bioethical principles: Autonomy, Non-maleficence, Beneficence, and Justice.

Autonomy Myth: "Death is a Choice"
Although all four bioethical principles are considered equally important, the principle of autonomy very often dominates medical decisions. With rare exception, patient (or family acting as patient surrogates) values and preferences drive medical decisions.

The preeminence of patient autonomy sometimes inappropriately spills over into the brain death scenario. Physicians at times feel obligated to ask a family member (acting as the patient's surrogates) for permission to declare a patient brain dead. The declaration of brain death becomes confused with a decision to withdraw care – too entirely different situations.

Although keeping family members informed of a patient's condition is crucial, burdening them with this decision is inappropriate. It would be similar to asking a family member's permission to declare someone dead after a cardiac arrest. Death is not a choice.

Indeed, even the terminology we use to describe brain death confuses the issue and can stir some controversies. It is often confusing to practitioners as well as to family members, when they are told that their loved ones are meeting criteria for "brain death," when vital signs often seem to be normal with or without use of vasopressors or inotropes. Since "brain-dead" patients show traditional signs of life as warm, moist skin, a pulse, and breathing, it is not surprising that many people think that "brain death" is a separate type of death that occurs before "real death." This is often confounded when medical providers repeat that "life support" as being removed in such patients (Capron 2001).

Being sensitive to family and explaining the differences between the above terminologies may alleviate some concerns regarding sensitivity in such a difficult situation.

Autonomy Myth: "Physicians Define Death"

Physicians do not define death. Through consensus, the law, and religious beliefs, societies select the vital functions that must irreversibly cease to consider someone dead. Physicians define and execute the medical procedures necessary to determine if someone meets these societal definitions. Societies define death.

Whether someone is dead is dependent on the societal context. Although there is widespread acceptance of the concept of irreversible cessation of whole brain function as a definition of death, the acceptance is not universal.

Because they do not define death, physicians must be aware of the societal and religious context in which they are practicing. Variations in the acceptance of brain death as a concept are outlined below.

Jewish Law:

- There still exists opposition in the Jewish Law regarding the halachic acceptability of brain death criteria.

- The principle of *ain dochin nefesh mipnei nefesh* – that one life may not set aside to ensure another life – applies with full force even where the life to be terminated is of short duration and seems to lack the meaning or purpose and even when the potential recipient has excellent chances for full recovery and long life.

- If on the other hand if the donor is dead, the harvesting of organs to save another life becomes a *mitzvah* of the highest order.

- New York is the only state that requires medical personnel to make a reasonable effort to notify family members before a determination of brain death and to make "reasonable accommodations" for the patient's religious beliefs.

Buddhist:

- In 2006, the family of a Buddhist man in Boston who had been declared legally brain-dead argues that, because his heart was still beating, his spirit and consciousness still lingered and that removing him from life support would be akin to killing him.

- In Tibetan Buddhism, a person has multiple levels of consciousness, which may not correspond with brain activity

Christians:

- Christians who ardently support the traditional circulatory-respiratory definition of death tend to be fundamentalists or evangelicals.

- Most main stream Protestant groups in the United States accept brain death as a valid criterion for death, as does the Roman Catholic Church, albeit some controversy.

Islamic law:

- In 1986, the Academy of Islamic Jurisprudence, a group of legal experts convened by the Organization of the Islamic Conference, issued an opinion stating that a person should be considered legally dead when either "complete cessation of the heart or respiration occurs" or "complete cessation of all functions of the brain occurs."

Hinduism:

- Because artificial life support prolongs life after brain death, it is not viewed favorably. Most Hindus believe that prolonging life after a person's time for death has come interferes with the karma of that person, and does not allow the soul to move back into cycle of incarnation. When the choice is made to discontinue life support, the timing is very important down to the minute. Priests may be consulted to determine the best time to release the soul.
- Organ donation rates are among the lowest in India (2 %) compared to 40 % in the United States.
- In India, four doctors are required to declare brain death, and the criteria used are similar to the ones in the United Kingdom (that of brain stem death) (The Transplantation of Human Organ Act, 1994).

Non-Maleficence Myth: "Physicians Know how to Determine if a Patient is Dead by Brain Criteria"

The foundation of non-maleficence is medical competence. However, most physicians are not familiar with the criteria for determining brain death. There are worrisome knowledge gaps even among physicians likely to be called upon to make a brain death declaration such as intensivists, neurosurgeons, and neurologists.

In a survey of US hospitals, Greer et al. (2008) found even though, there was 100 % compliance in clinical examination with respect to the AAN guidelines in terms of establishing coma and absence of pupillary reflexes, there was less than 50 % compliance in demonstrating no spontaneous respirations, or absence of pain in cranium, or absent jaw jerk The same survey found that preclinical testing compliance with the American Academy of Neurology guidelines was less than 100 %.

- 89 % compliance in demonstrating absence of hypothermia
- 81 % compliance in demonstrating absence of sedatives

- 72 % compliance in demonstrating the electrolyte disturbances were absent
- 71 % compliance that shock was absent
- 63 % compliance that established cause was found
- 55 % compliance was sedatives or paralytics were absent
- 45 % compliance that acid-based disorders were absent
- 42 % compliance that endocrine disorders were absent

Non-Maleficence Myth: "Cessation of Whole Body Function is Sufficient for the Declaration"

Every patient who is considered for brain death testing must meet three basic criteria of irreversibility:

1. Cause is established.
2. Sufficient duration of observation.
3. Absence of confounding conditions.

The diagnosis of brain death requires the physician to exclude any reversible cause leading to an eyes closed, unresponsive state. If the cause is not easily established, then a battery of tests must be carried out to distinguish patients with this condition from other brain-injured individuals for whom recovery of (at least some) brain function remains possible.

The second important consideration must be made for sufficient observation of patients to rule out transient unresponsive state.

Most importantly, absence of confounding variables (e.g., hypothermia or drug intoxication) must be established prior to consideration for brain death.

Beneficence Myth: "Ancillary Tests are Sufficient to Declare Brain Death"

It is the duty of the physician to care for the patient. In the setting of possible brain death, it is the attending physician's responsibility to make the brain death determination. All too often, physicians will try to shift this burden from a skilled examination to an ancillary test.

Brain death is a clinical decision to be made by the attending physician. The concept of brain death and the process of declaration is based on systematic neurological examination focusing on irreversibility of brain dysfunction, in the absence of confounding factors. The determination of irreversibility is a clinical decision, based on available history, evidence of injury on neuroimaging, and absence of brainstem reflexes, including the documentation of apnea despite subjecting the brainstem to hypercarbia.

Ancillary tests are appropriately used in situations where the clinical examination is compromised: for example, in situations where elicitation and interpretation of brainstem reflexes is difficult as in the presence of severe facial injuries obviating documentation of pupillary or corneal reflexes, upper cervical spine injury preventing motor responses, and in clinical conditions that retain carbon dioxide, thus making interpretation of apnea test difficult. These tests are best reserved for the above conditions.

Even if confounding variables may be present, i.e., pentobarbitone coma, physicians may be tempted to use ancillary tests in lieu of clinical criteria; however, many physicians may rather choose to observe patients, until those confounding variables are corrected.

Interestingly, the most common ancillary testing that was performed included:

- EEG (84 %)
- Conventional angiography (74 %)
- Radionuclide scintigraphy (66 %)
- Trans cranial Doppler (42 %)
- Somatosensory-evoked potentials (SSEP) (24 %)
- Magnetic resonance angiography (9 %)
- CT angiography (6 %)
- CT perfusion (3 %)
- Atropine challenge (3 %)
- Mean arterial pressure = intracranial pressure for 30 min (3 %)

Contrary to popular belief, none of the ancillary tests, i.e., cerebral angiography, EEG, and nuclear medicine testing, to demonstrate cessation of cerebral blood flow have been validated as accurate as ancillary tests. We primarily rely on case reports for information about the validity of these tests.

Demonstration of Cessation of Cerebral Blood Flow as a Precise Indicator of Brain Death: (Wijdicks 2010)

- There may be two distinct patterns of bran death. The most common pattern is characterized by increased intracranial pressure (ICP) above the mean arterial pressure (MAP), resulting in no net cerebral blood flow.
- The second pattern is where the ICP does not exceed MAP, but there is an inherent pathology that affects brain tissue on a cellular level to the extent that brain death occurs (Bader et al. 2003; Palmer and Bader 2005).

Role of EEG as Ancillary Test in Declaration of Brain Death:

- EEG was one of the first confirmatory tests that was proposed for brain death declaration. However, isoelectric EEG can be associated with retained cerebral blood flow, and thus, these patients would seem brain dead on one laboratory test but not on another.

Role of Transcranial Doppler in Declaration of Brain Death:

- Transcranial Doppler (TCD) ultrasound has emerged as a noninvasive method in the declaration of brain death. Ten percent of patients do not possess adequate insonation windows to perform TCDs; thus, presence of a baseline is paramount.
- There have been studies demonstrating no flow pattern in middle cerebral artery segments, but indicating flow in basilar arteries.
- Retrospective data showed that TCD confirmed brain death in 57 % of patients, while it was inconclusive in 43 % patients with no flow signals seen on first examination in 8 % and waveform patterns in remaining patients (35 %) being inconsistent with standard brain death criteria for cerebral circulatory arrest (Sharma et al. 2011).
- Recent meta-analysis of TCD data demonstrated a sensitivity of 89 % and a specificity of 99 %. The study found two false-positive

results, in which brain stem function showed brain death shortly thereafter (Monteiro et al. 2006).

Role of Computed Angiography (CTA) in Declaration of Brain Death:

- Greer et al. describe a case in which computed angiography (CTA) was performed to evaluate for cerebral circulatory arrest, later proved wrong by Transcranial Doppler.

Beneficence Myth: "It is Okay to Rely on the Organ Donor Team to Confirm Brain Death"

Clinicians sometimes inappropriately defer decisions regarding brain death to the organ procurement team (OPT). The OPT is a tempting resource because of their familiarity with the concepts and procedures for determining death. This temptation must be resisted. The OPT has an inherent conflict of interest. The duty of the attending physician is to their patient whereas the duty of the OPT is to the patients needing organ transplants. The attending physician must make the determination of brain death completely independent of the OPT.

Brain death and organ donation although intuitively seem related are in fact two separate topics that deserve equal attention. As per federal guidelines, any patient admitted to a hospital with a Glasgow Coma Score of less than equal to 5 must be notified to the local transplant network for possible eligibility for organ donation. This process as it should proceed in parallel with the ICU care of these patients, until either the primary team declares patient's brain death or the family decides to stop continuation of technological support ("withdrawal of care").

Often, treating physicians confuse the two entities: withdrawal of technological support or brain death declaration and at times relies on the organ donor team to declare brain death. This practice should not be encouraged, as brain death declaration is a process that any physician who is intimately familiar with end-of-life issues should be also familiar with, and may be able to guide families in that regard. The organ donation teams' involvement and interaction with the primary treatment team must never cloud any clinical decision that the family may have taken, unless it is a request by the family per se to ask about eligibility regarding organ donation, especially if their loved ones were in fact organ recipients. In this case, it is best to refer them to the organ donation team, once the clinical decision has been made to declare brain death or the family decides to discontinue technological support, in which case donation after cardiac death may happen. The authors have been involved in situations where formal brain death declaration has not been performed, only to the requested by the organ donation team to perform an apnea test, and declare, due to family wishes.

Justice Myth: "The Concept of Death by Brain Criteria was Developed Because of Organ Donation Demands"

Organs suitable for transplant are clearly scarce. Given this and the tragic circumstances that invariably accompany a brain death determination, it seems just to try to salvage some good from the situation.

It is often expressed that concept of death by brain death criteria was developed because of organ donation demands. Physicians often may seem burdened to declare patient's brain death due to institutional, regional, and national pressure to provide organs to patients on the transplant list. Indeed Troug RD (2007) raises significant issues relating to the flourishing organ transplant industry and its demands on declaration of brain death. He cites that in 1968, the Ad Hoc Committee at Harvard claimed that brain death criteria were needed to clarify definition of death as the now obsolete criteria would lead to controversy in obtaining organs for transplantation.

In fact, upon careful review of the history of organ transplantation and the history of brain death declaration processes, it is obvious that brain death concept and organ transplantation arose separately and advanced in parallel, and only began to process together in the late 1960s. It may be impossible to deny that the final successes of transplants were indeed improved by the development and refinement of the concept of brain death (Machado et al. 2007).

Family understanding about brain death is an important factor that contributes to the decision to donate organs after declaration. In a survey conducted by Siminoff et.al (2007), following factors were involved against organ donation:

- Family perception that the patient would not want to donate (51 %).
- Family stamina or emotional turmoil (44 %), that accompany donation especially in younger patients.
- Disfigurement concerns (43 %).
- Mistrust of the health care system (25 %). This was thought to be due to lack of adequate emotional support that the treating physicians provided the families in making decisions regarding organ donation.
- Family determination (incorrectly) that the patient was ineligible (19 %).
- Family disagreed over donated decision (14 %).
- Termination of mechanical support (12 %).

Summary

Brain death is a clinical diagnosis. Physician intimately knowledgeable with the process must be cognizant of social, cultural, and religious practices, and rely on best available clinical evidence during declaration.

Cross-References

▶ Brain Death
▶ Withdrawal of Life-Support

References

Bader MK, Littlejohns LR, March K (2003) Brain tissue oxygen monitoring in severe brain injury, II. Implications for critical care teams and case study. Crit Care Nurse 23(4):29–38
Capron AM (2001) Brain death–well settled yet still unresolved. N Engl J Med 344(16):1244–1246
Greer DM, Varelas PN, Haque S, Wijdicks EF (2008) Variability of brain death determination guidelines in leading US neurologic institutions. Neurology 70(4):284–289
Machado C, Kerein J, Ferrer Y, Portela L, de la C Garica M, Manero JM (2007) The concept of brain death did not evolve to benefit organ transplants. J Med Ethics 33(4):197–200
Monteiro LM, Bollen CW, van Huffelen AC, Ackerstaff RG, Jansen NJ, van Vught AJ (2006) Transcranial Doppler ultrasonography to confirm brain death: a meta-analysis. Intensive Care Med 32(12):1937–1944
Palmer S, Bader MK (2005) Brain tissue oxygenation in brain death. Neurocrit Care 2(1):17–22
Sharma D, Souter MJ, Moore AE, Lam AM (2011) Clinical experience with transcranial Doppler ultrasonography as a confirmatory test for brain death: a retrospective analysis. Neurocrit Care 14(3):370–376
Siminoff L, Mercer MB, Graham G, Burant C (2007) The reasons families donate organs for transplantation: implications for policy and practice. J Trauma 62(4):969–978
Truog RD (2007) Brain death – too flawed to endure, too ingrained to abandon. J Law Med Ethics J Am Soc Law Med Ethics 35(2):273–281
Wijdicks EF (2010) The case against confirmatory tests for determining brain death in adults. Neurology 75(1):77–83

Brain Edema

▶ Traumatic Brain Injury, Anesthesia for

Brain Injury

▶ Traumatic Brain Injury, Mild (mTBI)
▶ Traumatic Brain Injury, Anesthesia for
▶ Neurotrauma, Prognosis and Outcome Predictions
▶ Neurotrauma, Multimodal Neuromonitoring

Brain Tissue Oxygen Tension

▶ Traumatic Brain Injury, Intensive Care Unit Management

Brain-Dead Donor

▶ Organ Donor Management

Brainstem Death

▶ Brain Death, Ethical Concerns

Breathing Passage

▶ Airway Anatomy

Broken Ankle

▶ Ankle Fractures

Brown-Séquard Hemiplegia

▶ Brown-Séquard Syndrome

Brown-Séquard Paralysis

▶ Brown-Séquard Syndrome

Brown-Séquard Syndrome

MariaLisa Itzoe and Daniel M. Sciubba
Department of Neurosurgery, The Johns
Hopkins University School of Medicine,
Baltimore, MD, USA

Synonyms

Brown-Séquard hemiplegia; Brown-Séquard paralysis

Definition

Brown Séquard Syndrome (BSS), sometimes referred to as Brown-Séquard hemiplegia or paralysis, was first observed in 1849 by Mauritian physiologist and neurologist Brown-Séquard (Brown-Sequard 1850). The syndrome is characterized by a functional lateral hemisection of the spinal cord. The most common cause of BSS is trauma involving a penetrating mechanism, for example, a stab or gunshot wound (Musker and Musker 2011). In addition, blunt trauma, pressure contusion, motor vehicle accidents, or severe falls that cause unilateral facet fracture and dislocation may also lead to the development of BSS.

Neurologically, these patients present with loss of motor function (hemiparaplegia) and sensation on the ipsilateral side of the hemisection. Interruption of the lateral corticospinal tracts may lead patients to present with ispilateral spastic paralysis below the level of lesion as well as Babinski's sign. Damage to the posterior column results in ipsilateral loss of tactile discrimination, vibration sense, and proprioception. Nerve fibers of the spinothalamic tract (pain and temperature sensation) crossover within the spinal cord from the periphery; thus, contralateral loss of such sensation usually occurs two to three segments below location of injury.

Overall prognosis for BSS is better than any other spinal cord injury. For example, patients with cervical BSS achieve higher functional improvement by time of discharge compared with patients with CCS (McKinley et al. 2007). In general, treatment focuses on addressing the underlying cause of the syndrome, which may involve first administering to other injuries if any are present. Recovery of function tends to be progressive: motion is regained in the ipsilateral proximal extensor muscles before the ipsilateral distal flexor muscles, and pain/temperature sensation is regained in the ipsilateral extremities before the contralateral extremities (Little and Halar 1985). Voluntary motor strength and functional gate are usually regained within 6 months post injury. Up to 90 % of patients regain some degree of ambulation by the end of their recovery (Little and Halar 1985).

References

Brown-Sequard C-E (1850) De La Transmission Croisee Des Impressions Sensitives Par La Moelle Epiniere. Comptes rendus de la Societe de biologie 2:33–44

Little JW, Halar E (1985) Temporal course of motor recovery after Brown-Sequard spinal cord injuries. Paraplegia 23(1):39–46

McKinley W, Santos K, Meade M, Brooke K (2007) Incidence and outcomes of spinal cord injury clinical syndromes. J Spinal Cord Med 30(3):215–224

Musker P, Musker G (2011) Pneumocephalus and Brown-Sequard syndrome caused by a stab wound to the back. Emerg Med Australas 23(2):217–219

bTBI

▶ Neurotrauma, Military Considerations

Buffy Coat

Harvey G. Hawes[1], Bryan A. Cotton[1] and Laura A. McElroy[2]
[1]Department of Surgery, Division of Acute Care Surgery, Trauma and Critical Care, University of Texas Health Science Center at Houston, The University of Texas Medical School at Houston, Houston, TX, USA
[2]Department of Anesthesiology, Critical Care Medicine, University of Rochester Medical Center, Rochester, NY, USA

Definition

The buffy coat refers to a layer of platelets and white blood cells (WBCs) that is found between the heavier red blood cell (RBC) layer and the lighter plasma layer after centrifuging whole blood at high speed. The term "buff," the yellow-brown color of undyed leather, refers to the color of the buffy coat. This layer was initially removed to improve RBC storage. In the 1970s, European countries began removing the buffy coat layer to reduce WBC contamination that was leading to febrile transfusion reactions. While North American blood banks use a platelet-rich plasma method to separate component blood products, Canada and much of Europe use the buffy coat method as their primary method of platelet product preparation. All of these methods produce high-quality platelets with roughly equivalent yields (Hogman et al. 2010).

During the buffy coat production of platelet concentrates, whole blood first undergoes a "hard spin," after which the heavy layer of RBC concentrate is removed to be processed into packed red blood cells. The middle buffy coat layer is then siphoned off the lighter platelet-poor plasma and subjected to a slower "soft spin." This second spin leaves two layers, a top discard layer and a heavier layer of platelet concentrate. Due to the relatively low platelet counts when run in a single process, pools of 4–5 buffy coats are made and mixed with male donor plasma prior to the final "soft spin." There are many variations on the buffy coat method including the addition of additives at various stages to improve product purity and storage and separation of layers at reduced temperatures to improve platelet yield (Lozano et al. 2000). The buffy coat method has been heavily automated, and when followed by leukocyte reduction, it can decrease WBC levels below 1×10^6 per unit (Ito and Shinomiva 2001).

Cross-References

▶ Apheresis platelets
▶ Blood Bank
▶ Blood Group Antibodies
▶ Blood Therapy in Trauma Anesthesia

References

Hogman CF, Berseus O, Eriksson L et al (2010) International forum: Europe. Buffy-coat-derived platelet concentrates: Swedish experience. Clin Lab 56: 263–279

Ito Y, Shinomiva K (2001) A new continuous-flow cell separation method based on cell density: principle, apparatus, and preliminary application to separation of human buffy coat. J Clin Apher 16:186–191

Lozano M, Escolar G, Mazzara R et al (2000) Effects of the addition of second messenger effectors to platelet concentrates separated from whole blood donations and stored at 4 degrees C or −80 degrees C. Transfusion 40:527–534

Building Collapse

▶ Crush Syndrome

Bullet Proof Vest

▶ Body Armor

Bullet Wound

▶ Firearm-Related Injuries
▶ Gunshot Wounds to the Extremity

Bullet-Resistant Vest

▶ Body Armor

Burn

▶ Flame Burns

Burn and Plastics Trauma Fellowship

▶ Academic Programs in Trauma Care

Burn Anesthesia

Anthony L. Kovac
Kasumi Arakawa Professor of Anesthesiology,
Department of Anesthesiology, University of
Kansas Medical Center, Kansas City, KS, USA

Synonyms

Heat injury; Inhalation injury; Thermal injury

Definition

Burn injury most commonly affects the skin, mucous membranes of the airway, and lungs of the respiratory system. The depth of injury depends on the type of energy (heat, electricity, chemicals, radiation, cold), intensity, and length of time that the energy was applied. In most severe cases, deeper structures like tendons, muscles, joints, or bones may be injured.

Preexisting Condition

Burn Classification

Annually approximately two million people in the USA suffer major thermal injury ($\approx$0.5 % mortality) caused by radiation, chemicals, electricity, or heat. Burn wounds are classified as 1st, 2nd, 3rd, or 4th degree according to depth of injury. First degree (major sunburn with pain and erythema) involves only top epithelial layer. Second degree (pain and vesicles) includes epithelium and part of dermis. Third degree (no pain, destruction of nerve endings) involves entire skin thickness and tough eschar. Fourth degree has destruction of muscle and fascia. Burn size is measured as percent (%) of total body surface area (TBSA). "Rule of nines" is used. For adults, head and upper limbs equal 9 % TBSA, anterior and posterior trunk and lower limbs 18 %, and perineum 1 %. For children <12 years, due to a child's disproportionately larger head and smaller lower extremities

Burn Anesthesia,
Fig. 1 Rule of nines for
adult and child

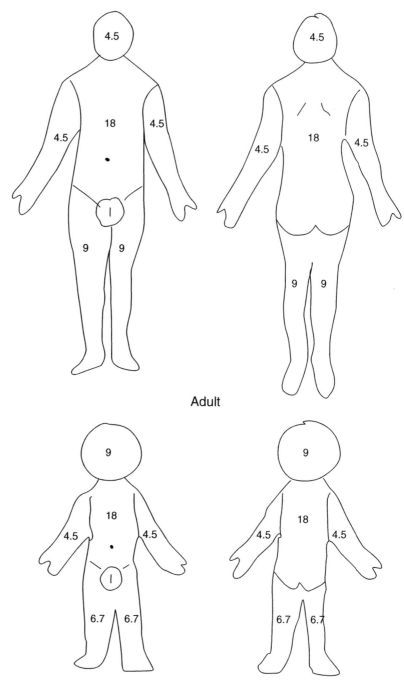

Adult

Child

compared to adults, "modified rule of nines" is
more accurate (Capan et al. 1991; Lovich-
Sapola 2008; Wikipedia, the free encyclopedia
2012) (Fig. 1).

Morbidity and Mortality

Criteria for burn center admission include
(1) 2nd degree $\geq$ 25 % TBSA, (2) 3rd
degree $\geq$ 10 % TBSA, (3) smoke inhalation injury,

(4) electrical burn, (5) children, and (6) age > 60 years. Baux's formula estimates that % mortality for elderly patients is equal to the sum of patient's age plus % TBSA burn. Inhalation injury adds 20–60 % increased mortality to burn of any size in any age group. Patients >80 years old with inhalation injury have high mortality. Young patients have an overall mortality $\approx$30–40 % with burns complicated by inhalation injury. Other mortality factors are (1) coexisting disease, (2) concomitant injuries, (3) location of burn, and (4) physical environment (closed space). Three phases of recovery are (1) resuscitation, 1st 24–48 h; (2) hypermetabolic, 2 days to 2 months; and (3) reconstruction, 2 months to 2 years or until wound heals (Capan et al. 1991; Lovich-Sapola 2008).

Skin Effects

Burn injury patients lose heat. Increased metabolism is needed to generate heat. Burn injury increases metabolic rate 1 week after injury. Edema from fluid resuscitation, hypoproteinemia, and an inelastic eschar (circumferential burns) may compromise neurovascular function (extremities, digits) and restrict chest wall respiration. An escharotomy may be needed to release compression and constriction and restore neurovascular function. Patients with electrical injuries often require a fasciotomy and deep compartment decompression release. Infection is a constant possibility (Capan et al. 1991; Lovich-Sapola 2008).

Cardiovascular Effects

Burn shock occurs immediately following extensive burn injury. Cardiac output initially decreases due to fluid redistribution caused by translocation of intravascular fluids and tissue edema. Within hours, protein and electrolyte loss occurs into the extravascular space. Prostaglandins, oxygen (O_2) radicals, myocardial depressant factor, and leukotrienes are released, causing increased capillary permeability. Plasma volume falls, causing hypovolemia and hemoconcentration. Systemic vascular resistance increases.

Fluid shifts and tissue edema occur in the 1st 8–12 h and may continue for 24 h. Tissue edema

Burn Anesthesia, Table 1 Parkland formula example

4.0 mL crystalloid/kg/% burn/24 h
70 kg female with 50 % TBSA burn
4 ml $\times$ 70 kg $\times$ 50 % TBSA burn = 4 $\times$ 70 $\times$ 50 = 14,000 ml crystalloid in 1st 24 h
7,000 ml crystalloid in 1st 8 h
3,500 ml crystalloid during 2nd $^+$8 h
3,500 ml crystalloid during 3rd 8 h

is related to the amount of TBSA burned. With large superficial, deep partial-thickness, and full-thickness burns, increased fluid requirements require large fluid administration to replace blood volume lost. Various formulas such as the Parkland formula (Table 1) have been used to calculate the fluids needed during the 1st 24 h following injury. The type of fluid used appears to be less important than accurately calculating blood volume replacement. It is important to monitor mental status, heart rate (HR), blood pressure (BP), O_2 saturation (SpO_2), urine output (UO), weight, and skin turgor. One should evaluate arterial blood gas, CBC, electrolytes, BUN, creatinine, CVP, pulmonary artery catheter depending on patient coexisting diseases, and physical status.

An early goal of surgery is to debride to a bleeding viable dermal layer with skin grafting the ultimate goal. Early debridement is often profuse resulting in a large and difficult to estimate intraoperative blood loss. Phenylephrine-soaked gauze pads on burn wounds can reduce blood loss, but a falsely elevated BP may result. Vasopressor support of BP may be necessary. Unstable vital signs may require postponement of surgery. Preoperatively, the patients' hematocrit should be $\geq$25 %, and blood components should be available. Intraoperatively, if the patient is unstable in regard to HR, BP, urine output, and/or SpO_2, a "stop and talk" time should occur between anesthesia and surgery to discuss whether to proceed or stop surgery (Capan et al. 1991; Lovich-Sapola 2008).

Airway and Inhalation Injury

Oxygen consumption and carbon dioxide (CO_2) production are increased in burn patients with inhalation injury. Decreases in O_2 delivery can be due to (1) airway obstruction, (2) inhalation injury, (3) pulmonary disease, (4) infection, and (5) sepsis. Airway obstruction can occur rapidly due to edema and swelling. One should assume inhalation injury with face and neck burns, singed nasal hair, bronchorrhea, soot-tinged sputum, dysphagia, hoarseness, upper airway obstruction, wheezing, rales, unconsciousness, stupor, coughing spells, hypoxia, or burns that occur in a confined space. While facial burns suggest inhalation injury, patients with inhalation injury may not have facial burns. Wheezing, rales, and carbon-tinged sputum may occur 24–48 h post-injury. Of patients who suffer major burns, ≈30 % may have coexisting inhalation injury.

Before extensive edema develops, airway management in suspected inhalation injury is best achieved by prophylactic intubation and humidified 100 % O_2. Inhalation injury patients should initially be given 100 % oxygen. As pulmonary edema is possible, extreme fluid care must be used to prevent overhydration. Avoid steroids which have no benefit in inhalation injury patients. Following inhalation injury, upper airway injury is more common than lower airway injury. Upper airway efficiently dissipates heat, and reflex glottic closure occurs. Lower airway injury below vocal cords occurs with (1) steam inhalation (heat capacity 4,000 times that of air), (2) superheated soot, and (3) other products of combustion: aldehydes, oxides of sulfur and nitrogen, hydrogen cyanide, hydrochloric acid, or sulfuric acid. Clinical manifestations are (1) mucosal edema; (2) impaired ciliary function; (3) ineffective surfactant; (4) small airway collapse; (5) bronchoconstriction; (6) increased capillary permeability; (7) necrotizing bronchiolitis; (8) intra-alveolar hemorrhage; (9) pneumonia and ARDS; and (10) pulmonary fibrosis. Initially, extent of injury is not predictive of severity of oxygenation or degree and duration of needed ventilation. Airway and lung pathology can be assessed with fiber-optic bronchoscopy, pulmonary function tests, and lung scans (Capan et al. 1991; Lovich-Sapola 2008; Herndon et al. 1987).

Carbon Monoxide

Carbon monoxide (CO) is colorless, odorless, tasteless, and nonirritating. It has a hemoglobin (Hb) affinity 210 times that of O_2. With CO toxicity, oxyhemoglobin (O_2Hb) saturation is reduced even if there is normal arterial O_2 content. O_2Hb concentration is reduced to 50 % of normal by prolonged inhalation of air containing 0.1 volume % CO. Carboxyhemoglobin (COHb) shifts the O_2Hb dissociation curve to the left. Thus, Hb is more tightly bound to O_2, decreasing O_2 delivery. Standard pulse oximeters estimate arterial O_2Hb saturation by measuring light absorbance at two wavelengths, 660 and 940 nm. With COHb, SpO_2 monitoring with a standard pulse oximeter is inaccurate, as standard oximeters cannot differentiate between more than two types of Hb (reduced vs nonreduced). With COHb poisoning, SpO_2 via pulse oximeter is normal; the SpO_2 measured is the sum of COHb and O_2. A CO-oximeter is needed to correctly measure COHb levels, measuring light absorbance at six or more wavelengths and concentrations of 4Hb types: (1) reduced Hb, (2) O_2Hb, (3) methemoglobin (MetHb), and (4) COHb. Many heavy cigarette smokers have 10–20 % COHb levels, causing an accelerated effect of CO poisoning during smoke inhalation. A cherry-red skin color is observed with COHb levels >40 %. A majority of inhalation injury deaths are due to CO poisoning. The elimination half-time of CO in a patient breathing room air (21 % O_2) is ≈4 h. A 100 % O_2 decreases this to 30–60 min. All closed-space fire patients should be intubated and given 100 % O_2 until COHb level is <20 %. Patients with CO coma due to hypoxic brain edema should be immediately treated with (1) hyperbaric oxygen therapy, (2) hyperventilation, and (3) osmotherapy. Pregnant patients with COHb levels >20 %, neurologic signs, and/or fetal distress should receive hyperbaric O_2 therapy (Capan et al. 1991; Lovich-Sapola 2008; Herndon et al. 1987).

Cyanide (CN)

When burned, many synthetic materials release CN. Following inhalation, blood CN may reach levels >0.2 mg/L (toxic) and >1 mg/L (lethal).

Patients with COHb >15 % have elevated blood CN levels. Metabolic acidosis indicates possible CN toxicity. O_2 and thiosulfate or hydroxocobalamin (vitamin B_{12}) are treatments of choice. Avoid amyl nitrate and sodium nitrate, as they form MetHb, shifting the O_2 dissociation curve more to the left than COHb (Capan et al. 1991; Lovich-Sapola 2008; Herndon et al. 1987).

Kidney Effects
Renal failure has a high mortality. Oliguria <0.5 ml/kg/h in 1st 24 h is often due to inadequate fluid resuscitation. Hypoxemia, hypovolemia, decreased cardiac output, myoglobinuria, and/or hemoglobinuria can cause renal failure. A urine output (UO) of 0.5–1.0 ml/kg/h suggests adequate fluid replacement and kidney perfusion, unless the patient has received hypertonic saline solution and/or is hyperglycemic. If the UO is inadequate (<0.5 ml/kg/h) despite adequate cardiac filling pressures, osmotic or loop diuretics or low-dose dopamine (1–3 µg/kg/min) may be helpful. If cardiac output is low, hemodynamic support may improve renal perfusion. If Hb or myoglobin is in the urine, urine alkalinization is needed to prevent their deposition in the kidney. After resuscitation phase, a decrease in UO may indicate sepsis (Capan et al. 1991; Lovich-Sapola 2008; Langley and Sim 2002).

Liver Effects
Elevated bilirubin and liver enzymes can occur. Liver injury increases patient mortality. In the resuscitation phase, hypoperfusion, hypoxemia, and hypovolemia adversely affect liver metabolism. Early liver injury can occur without clinical signs of shock. Elevated liver enzymes occurs within 24 h. In the hypermetabolic phase, liver blood flow, gluconeogenesis, and protein catabolism increase. Later, sepsis can decrease glucose synthesis. Acute hypoglycemia may indicate sepsis and/or acute liver failure (Capan et al. 1991; Lovich-Sapola 2008; Langley and Sim 2002).

Gastrointestinal (GI) Effects
Adynamic ileus often develops within 24 h and resolves in 2–3 days. Stress ("Curling") ulcers may occur and correlates with % TBSA burn. Gastritis and duodenitis can occur within 12 h, and ulceration within 72 h. To keep gastric pH >7.0 and decrease GI bleeding, antacids, H_2 blockers, and frequent enteral feedings are methods of therapy (Capan et al. 1991; Lovich-Sapola 2008; Langley and Sim 2002).

Hematologic Effects
During the 1st days postburn, plasma volume decreases cause increased Hct and blood viscosity. Red blood cell half-life decrease; hematopoiesis is suppressed. Factors V and VIII and fibrin split products increase. Increased platelet adhesiveness and aggregation occur. By 2nd week, platelet increases. Disseminated intravascular coagulopathy (DIC) can occur (Capan et al. 1991; Lovich-Sapola 2008; Langley and Sim 2002).

Central Nervous System (CNS) Effects
Hypoxia, electrolyte imbalances, sepsis, and neurotoxic effects of smoke and products of combustion can cause early CNS dysfunction. Burn encephalopathy syndrome presents as lethargy, disorientation, delirium, seizures, or coma. Electrical injury can cause direct nerve injury (Capan et al. 1991; Lovich-Sapola 2008; Langley and Sim 2002).

Endocrine, Metabolic, and Nutritional Effects
Burn injury increases metabolism. Increased caloric requirements (2,500 kcal/m^2 TBSA) are needed for wound healing. A 50 % TBSA burn increases basal metabolic rate to 70 % due to increases in (1) epinephrine, (2) norepinephrine, (3) glucagon, (4) cortisol, (5) renin, (6) antidiuretic hormone, (7) O_2 consumption, (8) CO_2 production, (9) minute ventilation, (10) free fatty acids, (11) glycogen, and (12) gluconeogenesis. Catabolism and protein loss occur (negative nitrogen balance). Relative insulin resistance occurs, associated with glucose intolerance, hypocalcemia, hypermagnesemia, hypophosphatemia, hyperpyrexia, and alterations in fluid and electrolyte balance. In severe burn patients, major heat loss is due to large evaporative water loss. Heat conservation methods

include (1) warming patient's room to >27 °C (77° F); (2) warming skin prep and irrigation solutions, IV fluids, and blood products; (3) use of a radiant heater and warming blanket; (4) covering body parts not part of surgical field; (5) limiting operative exposure time; and (6) ventilation with heated, humidified gases at low fresh gas flows (Capan et al. 1991; Lovich-Sapola 2008; Langley and Sim 2002).

Immunologic Effects

Burn patients have immunosuppression with cellular (T cells) depressed more than humoral (B cells). Wound infection and sepsis are possible. Meticulous attention to sterile technique is required (Capan et al. 1991; Lovich-Sapola 2008; Langley and Sim 2002).

Application

Pediatric Considerations

The smaller airway opening of pediatric patients predisposes to airway obstruction. Neck hyperextension can obstruct the airway. A right main stem intubation may more easily occur in children compared to adults. Compared to adults, in children younger than 8 years old, the subglottic area is more narrow. A ½ decrease in the tracheal radius (r) can increase airway resistance (R) by 16 times (r^4). Poiseuille's equation: Resistance, R is proportional to $1/r^4 (R = 8 \mu LQ/r^4)$.

For fluid resuscitation, the "rule of nines" in children underestimates the TBSA of the head and overestimates the TBSA of the extremities. In children, fluid losses are proportionally greater than adults with similar burn injuries. Hyperglycemia should be monitored the first 24 h postburn. Similar to adults, reliable indicators of resuscitation are mental status, vital signs, pulse pressure, urine output, body temperature, color of the distal extremities, and capillary refill (Capan et al. 1991; Langley and Sim 2002; Lovich-Sapola 2008).

Pharmacologic Effects

Changes in fluid compartments, cardiac output, renal and liver perfusion, and metabolism and decreases in albumin can alter pharmacodynamics and pharmacokinetics of drugs. Changes in free/protein-bound fraction can occur, with a resulting altered drug response. During resuscitation phase, generalized hypoperfusion results in delayed drug absorption with decreased concentration and bioavailability. High or repeated IV doses can cause toxic effects. During the initial phase, small, repeated IV dosing is safer and more effective. During the hypermetabolic phase, increased renal and liver blood flow results in rapid drug metabolism and excretion. Volume of distribution is affected by changes in protein binding and extracellular fluid volume. Increased protein binding causes a decrease in volume of distribution and elimination of glomerular-filtered drugs. Decreased protein binding increases elimination. Adjust antibiotic dosing if renal failure is present. Drug loss through burn wounds increases drug requirements. During hypermetabolic phase, antacids and H_2-receptor blockers should be increased in dosing frequency. It is best to titrate all drugs to their desired effect.

Anesthesia induction depends on the patient's cardiac status. Ketamine is useful if patients are hypovolemic, as it increases HR and myocardial O_2 supply and demand. Optimize volume status. If the blood volume is decreased or catecholamines are depleted, hypotension can occur. Ketamine (1) allows spontaneous ventilation, (2) maintains BP, (3) provides analgesia and amnesia, and (4) preserves gag reflex, but does not fully protect patients from regurgitation and aspiration. Standard NPO criteria should be followed. Use glycopyrrolate to dry secretions. Premedicate with a benzodiazepine (midazolam) to reduce hallucinations. Pentothal or propofol also can be safely used, titrating to effect.

Succinylcholine (Sch) can produce life-threatening hyperkalemia with potassium release from muscle membranes. It is related to dose, time since injury, and TBSA burn. Increased Sch response most likely occurs after 1 day. Hyperkalemia can develop within minutes and results from muscle denervation. Extrajunctional acetylcholine (Ach) receptors increase throughout muscle membranes, causing hypersensitivity to depolarizing and resistance to nondepolarizing muscle relaxants. Sch is best avoided because the period of hyperkalemic response is unclear. Some believe Sch can safely be used up to 8–24 h after burn injury and then again after 8–24 months or until all burned areas have healed. For treatment of hyperkalemia, calcium, sodium bicarbonate, hyperventilation, CPR, glucose, and insulin may be necessary. Precurarization with a nondepolarizing muscle relaxant does not appear to prevent hyperkalemic response.

Burn patients' resistance to nondepolarizing drugs is possibly due to an increase in Ach receptors or altered receptor affinity. This resistance (1) develops with burns >25–30 % TBSA, (2) is rarely seen in <10 % TBSA, (3) is observed <1st week, (4) peaks at 5–6 weeks, and (5) is attenuated at 3 months postinjury. Volume of distribution, wound drug transfer, and increased plasma protein binding have minimal effect on nondepolarizing relaxant requirements. Burn patients require 2–5 times the normal nondepolarizing dose for relaxation. A twitch monitor is useful to determine dosing and redosing. Normal doses of reversal agents (neostigmine) are required (Langley and Sim 2002; Gronert and Theye 1975; Martyn 1986).

Anesthesia for Burn Dressing Changes

Etomidate is not recommended due to adrenal suppression. Fentanyl, ketamine, and remifentanil plus propofol or dexmedetomidine infusions have been used (Langley and Sim 2002; Martyn 1986).

Inhalation Anesthetics

All inhaled agents can be safely used with no single "best" technique. Isoflurane, sevoflurane, and desflurane cause minimal cardiac depression and do not sensitize the myocardium to arrhythmias caused by exogenous catecholamines (Langley and Sim 2002; Martyn 1986).

Monitoring

Electrocardiograph (ECG), BP (cuff, arterial line), and HR monitoring must be adapted to each patient, with electrodes and SpO_2 often placed at nonstandard sites. Sterile needle ECG electrodes instead of pads increase electrical shock risk. IV lines placed through burned skin areas increase infection risk. Invasive central IV lines should be placed through nonburned skin and securely sutured.

Summary

More than other types of trauma, burn injury changes normal homeostasis. Multiple changes must be recognized and adapted. Wound debridement 1 day postburn has different physiologic changes than reconstructive surgery at 1 month or 1 year. Increased opioids are required for pain control. Burn patients deserve our empathy. Anything anesthesia providers can do to decrease burn patients' suffering will be remembered and appreciated by these patients.

Cross-References

▶ Acute Pain Management in Trauma
▶ Airway Assessment
▶ Airway Trauma, Management of
▶ Blast Lung Injury
▶ Chemical Burns
▶ Electrical Burns
▶ Escharotomy
▶ Firework Injuries
▶ Flame Burns
▶ Fluid, Electrolytes, and Nutrition in Trauma Patients
▶ Hypothermia, Trauma, and Anesthetic Management
▶ Scald Burns

References

Capan LM, Miller SM, Turndorf H (eds) (1991) Trauma: anesthesia and intensive care. JB Lippincott Co, Philadelphia, PA, pp 629–648
Gronert GA, Theye RA (1975) Pathophysiology of hyperkalemia induced by succinylcholine. Anesthesiology 43:89–94
Herndon DN, Langner F, Thompson P et al (1987) Pulmonary injury in burned patients. Surg Clin North Am 67:31

Lovich-Sapola J (2008) Anesthesia for burns. In: Smith CE (ed) Trauma anesthesia. Cambridge University Press, Cambridge, pp 322–342

Langley K, Sim K (2002) Anaesthesia for patients with burn injuries. Curr Anaesth Crit Care 13:70–75

Martyn JAJ (1986) Clinical pharmacology and drug therapy in the burned patient. Anesthesiology 65:67

Wikipedia, the free encyclopedia (2012) Total body surface area. http://en.wikipedia.org/wiki/Total_body_surface_area. Accessed 5 Oct 2012

Burn Resuscitation Formula

▶ Rule of Tens

Burning

▶ Pain

Burns Due to Exposure to Cleaning Agents or Petroleum Products

▶ Chemical Burns

Bylaws (Institution)

Martin Morales
Physician Assistant Services, North Shore – LIJ Health System, Great Neck, NY, USA

Synonyms

Constitution; Covenant

Definition

Bylaws are the legally binding rules that govern the behavior of an organization and its members.

Preexisting Condition

Bylaws

Bylaws are the necessary tools of governance of an organization. They are the written rules that control the internal affairs of an organization. They state the mission, goals, and vision of the organization and lay the ground rules for how these are to be accomplished. The structure of the organization is described along with the individual duties and responsibilities of its members.

Bylaws are founded upon basic principles an organization holds to and wishes to project to the community. It states the standards which the organization will uphold and directs its members in their behavior. Bylaws are not meant to micromanage an organization. The bylaws give a general direction to the organization and establish committees to then write the rules/regulation and policies/procedures that will effectuate the goals of the organization.

There is a close relationship between the law and bylaws. The bylaws may exceed the requirements of the law but cannot be used in such a way that it undermines state or federal laws. In most situations, bylaws will be considered invalid in court if they are contradictory to the state/federal law. This is why legal counsel and review is critical in establishing or amending the bylaws. In most states bylaws are filed by nonprofit organizations with the State Attorney General's office in the state where the organization is registered or incorporated. It cannot be overstated that the bylaws are usually considered a legally binding document. There are some that dispute this, but the American Medical Association has a policy that the "by-laws are a contract between the Medical Staff and the Hospital" (Gassiot 2007, p. 96). Bylaws cannot be revised unilaterally. There must be agreement between the Medical Board and the governing body. Intentional violations of the bylaws can lead to prosecution or dissolution of the organization.

Importance of Bylaws

The bylaws define the goals and function of the organization. They keep the organization from deviating from legal requirements, help to resolve internal disputes, and keep the organization on track to accomplish its goals. They help the organization in deciding what to do in difficult situations. They may also indemnify members from legal jeopardy and protect the constitutional rights of the individual.

While much of what is contained in bylaws seems to be onerous and at times irrelevant, it behooves all organizations in our litigious-prone society to have bylaws. Unfortunately, too often we look at bylaws after the litigation process has commenced.

Once established the organization is held to the standards described in the bylaws by the legal system. This can come to haunt the organization if bylaws are written and not adhered to. The bylaws not only set the standards by decree of the governing body, but the governing body is responsible to make sure the standards are adhered to and provides for methods of resolving conflicts when adherence is violated.

Application

Structure of the Bylaws

The bylaws describe who will be members of the organization and their term of office and provide for succession. It describes and gives power to committees to pursue and accomplish the mission of the organization.

The bylaws define the following:

Purpose of the organization

This occurs as a stated mission, vision, and specific goals.

Titles and function of the officers

All positions of the governing body are defined such as chair, president, or CEO. It defines how they are elected and describes a table of succession so that a sudden or prolonged vacancy would not adversely impact the organization.

Requirements for membership

The requirements should speak to academic and professional credentials. It should describe the category of membership such as nonvoting member, adjunct or honorary, or emeritus status. It describes the roles of the members and their authority as well as their ability to vote in elections or other official business.

Terms of office

This should describe the length of the term as well as how many times one can be elected and if there is to be a hiatus before being reelected.

Frequency of meetings

This should address the requirement for a certain number of meetings and the amount of meetings that need to be attended to maintain membership. It provides for emergency meetings to deal with sudden potentially catastrophic events.

Elections

This will address the election process and the quorum needed for election results to be official.

Process for voting

Issues brought before the board should be in a timely manner so as to give its members time for serious consideration. The percentage or number of votes is described and whether this should be by open or secret ballot or whether absentee/electronic ballots are to be considered admissible.

Review, revision, and amendment of the bylaws

Describes how often the bylaws are to be reviewed. The Joint Commission mandates that bylaws be reviewed periodically to assure that they are compatible with current legislation and practice. The process for submission of items to be reviewed and who can introduce new amendments should be so stated.

Conflict resolution

Describes modalities for conflict resolution including "rules of order" and the legal process as it affects the functioning of the organization.

Corrective action

Describes the process of summary suspensions and methods of appropriate notification.

Appeal of corrective actions

Describes who in the membership has rights of appeal and appropriate timelines for notification and granting such appeals. It describes who will be at the review hearings and whether legal counsel will be permitted.

Rules of conduct in meetings

Describes whether "Robert's Rules of Order," the prerogative of the chair, or other guidelines for conducting the meeting in a professional, efficient, and courteous manner are utilized.

Quorum for conducting official business

Describes the number of members necessary to be physically present or by electronic communication to conduct official business. The quorum may be variable for different types of business and must be so stated.

Indemnification of members

States that the members will not be held accountable individually for conduct of the group as a whole.

Compensation to the members

States what if any monetary compensation or otherwise may be due to the members.

It may stipulate the direction any compensation should take.

Conflict of interest

The members will report any conflict of interest circumstances they may be involved in.

Most organizations will require members to sign a declaration regarding potential or actual conflict of interest annually.

Annual reports

The governing body may require monthly, quarterly, or annual reports of the activities of any committees. This may describe who will do the reporting, frequency, and by what means. The governing body may require "hard copies" or electronic documents and may stipulate the time the report should be issued in relation to meetings.

The Medical Model

The hospital's governing board is legally and morally responsible for the quality of medical care a patient receives while hospitalized (The Joint Commission Standard MS01.01.01).

The Joint Commission standards require that the governing body and the organized medical staff work collaboratively, clearly defining their roles, responsibilities, and accountabilities.

The bylaws delineate these rights and responsibilities and the relationships between the leaders of the organized medical staff, its members, and the governing body (The Joint Commission (JCAHO) MS10 2005).

The governing board may control the quality of the medical staff and does so by choosing the leadership for the Medical Board and granting them authority to form committees including the "Medical Staff Credentialing Committee." It is the Credentials Committee that recommends to the Medical Board who should be granted privileges to practice in the hospital.

Ultimate approval is made by the governing body upon recommendation of the Medical Board.

Development of the Bylaws

Most organizations follow a generally accepted format for the bylaws that are considered to have been tested in the courts. This is not unlike the components of corporate bylaws. The components of the bylaws are governed by requirements from the Joint Commission on the Accreditation of Hospitals (JCAHO), the Center for Medicaid and Medicare (CMS), and the National Commission on Quality Assurance (NCQA) (Gassiot et al. 2007, p. 97). Legal counsel is sought to help develop and review the bylaws for compatibility with state and federal laws.

The medical staff bylaws describe how often the committees shall meet, the place, and who shall attend.

It describes the categories of membership and their rights to vote.

Provisions for nonphysician and allied health professional practice are defined.

The quorum is established to pass rules, regulations, or policies and provides for emergency meetings to deal with pressing issues. The use of electronic communication and voting is also described. With rapid changes in development of how all healthcare business is conducted and changes in legislation that govern healthcare, a process for periodic review and changes in the bylaws must be included.

The Joint Commission in M.S. 3.6 states that "when necessary the Medical staff By-Law and rules and regulations are revised to reflect the hospital's current practices with respect to medical staff organization and function" (JCAHO Comprehensive Accreditation Manual 2011). The organization should not wait for the imminent survey to take place before reviewing its rules. The stated policy and practice must be congruent at the time of the survey (Lang et al. 1995). The need for changes in the bylaws should not be sparked by reviews and surveys but by the need for the organization to reflect changes in the landscape of healthcare delivery. With the currently changing paradigm, this is most important.

Establishment of Committees

The board shall appoint such committees and give a "charge" to those committees with guidelines and a commitment to report back to the board.

These may include (North Shore LIJ Health System Medical Staff Bylaws 2012):

Ambulatory Health Services Committee
Bylaws Committee
Cancer Committee
Credentials Committee
Critical Care Committee
Environment and Infection Control Committee
Graduate Medical Education Committee
Health Sciences Library and Informatics Committee

Institutional Review Board Committee
Medical Ethics Committee
Medical Records Committee
Medical Staff Health Committee
Nominating Committee
Nutrition Committee
Performance Improvement Coordinating Group (PICG)
Perioperative Committee
Pharmacy and Therapeutics Committee
Radiation Safety Committee
Surgical Audit Committee
Transfusion Committee

Other committees so deemed necessary to carry out the goals of the governing body, the Medical Board, and the organized medical staff.

Bylaws are a critical component of any organization. They are the reference point for maintaining the standards and direction of the organization. Bylaws must be congruent with practice.

In any test of the legal process, all will look first at the bylaws. Any weakness in the wording or implementation may have severe negative impact on the hospital's case. The time for development of bylaws is at the inception of the organization, and a periodic review is absolutely essential. There will always be conflicts that require resolution, and the bylaws become the essential governing document that helps to resolve these conflicts.

The governing body must appoint reliable members that are vested in the interest of patient care and furthering the goals of the organization. While very difficult, the members need to find the time to review agendas, attend meetings, and make meaningful contributions to the process. Traditional processes of conducting "ritualistic" meetings and of rubber-stamping issues without serious consideration can be detrimental to the overall mission of the hospital. It can potentially have adverse effects on patient care and place the hospital in financial and legal jeopardy. This above all reflects the need for comprehensive, up-to-date, and relevant bylaws.

Cross-References

▶ Activity Restrictions
▶ Advanced Practice Provider Care Delivery
  Models

References

Gassiot CA, Searcy V, Giles CW (2007) The medical staff
  handbook: fundamentals and beyond. Jones and
  Bartlett Publishers, Sudbury
Lang DA, Kadielski M, Liset JR (1995) Managing medi-
  cal staff change through by-laws and other strategies.
  American Hospital Publishing Inc., Chicago

The Joint Commission on Accreditation of Healthcare
  Organizations (JCAHO) (2005) Manual for hospitals.
  WWW.JCAHO.ORG. Accessed 28 Sept 2012
The Joint Commission (JCAHO) (2011) Comprehensive
  accreditation manual

Bywaters' Syndrome

▶ Crush Syndrome
▶ Crush Syndrome, Anesthetic Management for

C1 Fracture

▶ Fracture, Atlas (C1)

C2 Fracture

▶ Fracture, Axis (C2)

Cachexia

▶ Lean Body Mass Wasting

Calcaneus Fractures

John P. Ketz
University of Rochester, Strong Memorial
Hospital, Rochester, NY, USA

Synonyms

Beak fracture; Fracture of the os calcis; Hindfoot injury; Subtalar arthrodesis; Subtalar fracture

Definition

Calcaneal fractures are one of the most challenging injuries to treat in the lower extremity. It is the most common tarsal bone fracture and accounts for 1–2 % of all fractures (Sanders 2000). The calcaneus composes the inferior part of the subtalar joint which is an important joint for hindfoot and ankle biomechanics. Approximately, two-thirds of all injuries involve articular surface. These injuries generally occur as a result of axial loads, commonly through falls from height or because of axial loads encountered in motor vehicle collisions. There is a large predominance in young males and also as a result of work-related injuries. There is a long recovery period as patients are typically impaired long term. Initially, results of treatment were met with poor results and significant complications. Despite advances in surgical treatment strategies and implants, there is still continued morbidity associated with these injuries.

Anatomy

The calcaneus bone plays an important role in the foot. It is the largest bone and has several articular surfaces (Fig. 1). The bone itself has a thin outer cortical shell with abundant cancellous bone throughout. The posterior facet makes up the inferior portion of the subtalar joint which is responsible for hindfoot inversion and eversion. The middle facet, located medially, supports the talar head. The anterior process extends laterally and maintains the length of the lateral column of the foot. Its distal extension has a joint surface that articulates with the cuboid.

© Springer-Verlag Berlin Heidelberg 2015
P.J. Papadakos, M.L. Gestring (eds.), *Encyclopedia of Trauma Care*,
DOI 10.1007/978-3-642-29613-0

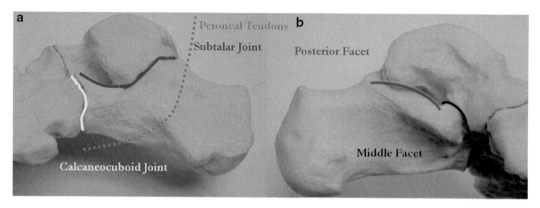

Calcaneus Fractures, Fig. 1 The lateral (*left*) and medial (*right*) aspects of the calcaneus are shown. The posterior facet makes up the inferior portion of the subtalar joint. The peroneal tendons are separated by the peroneal tubercle (**a**) and the strong medial ligaments of the hindfoot attach to the sustentaculum (**b**)

The calcaneus also has several vital soft tissue attachments. The sustentaculum tali is a process located on the medial aspect of the bone. It has strong ligamentous attachments including divisions of the deltoid ligament, including the spring ligament. The lateral wall of the calcaneus includes a small bony prominence, the peroneal tubercle, which separates the peroneal tendons as they course distally. The Achilles tendon inserts into the posterior tuberosity of the calcaneus, creating a strong lever arm for the gastrosoleus complex. There is a dense collection of adipose tissue inferior to the posterior tuberosity which comprises the heel pad. The heel pad houses a rich supply of septa and nerve endings. It functions as a shock absorber during heel strike.

Mechanism

Calcaneal fractures typically occur as a result of high-energy injury. This can occur from a fall from height or through motor vehicle accidents. In both instances, there is a large axial force that is transmitted through the heel pad and foot. Depending on the direction of the force and the foot position at the time of impact, there are several different fracture patterns that can occur. Also, the magnitude of the force can impact the extent of comminution that is seen.

Associated injuries are common in the presence of calcaneal fractures. Lumbar spine fractures can occur in 10–50 % of patients. Associated ipsilateral or contralateral lower extremity fractures occur in 25 % of cases. Open injuries, which are a surgical emergency, are seen in 5–10 % of all calcaneal fractures (Sanders 2000). In the polytrauma patient, closed calcaneal fractures may be initially missed, due to more serious injuries. However, a low suspicion of injury should prompt radiographic evaluation, as foot injuries are a major cause of permanent disability.

Clinical Evaluation

Calcaneus fractures have a wide variety of presentations, and the severity of fracture displacement often dictates the amount of soft tissue injury that is present. Higher-energy patterns create a large amount of swelling as well as visible deformities of the extremity. In evaluating the trauma patient, suspicion of injury should warrant radiologic evaluation. Lower-energy injuries may only have a small amount of swelling and ecchymosis but, if missed, can produce long-term disability. The clinical exam typically used is the calcaneal "squeeze test." The hand is cupped around the heel and gentle pressure is applied. If the patient has pain with this maneuver, further imaging workup is needed.

Particular attention should be paid to the soft tissue envelope. With any severe swelling

Calcaneus Fractures, Fig. 2 Figure (**a**) shows a lateral radiograph of a joint depression injury where the posterior facet (*) is separate from the posterior tuberosity. In Figure (**b**), the posterior facet is contiguous with the posterior tuberosity

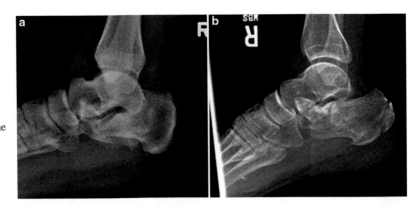

fracture blisters can appear. This is due to separation of the dermal-epidermal layers. These blisters can either contain clear serous fluid or serosanguinous fluid. The latter denotes a deeper injury and longer time period before the skin becomes healthy. The treatment of skin blistering is controversial and surgeon dependent. As the soft tissues improve, the foot will begin to show "skin wrinkles." This denotes that the skin is ready for surgical treatment, if indicated. The foot should be immobilized in a well-padded splint that extends to the proximal leg and extends to the foot.

The foot has relatively little soft tissue overlying the osseous structures. There are four main compartments in the lower extremity: the lateral, medial, central, and interosseous. Significant swelling and hemorrhage can create a compartment syndrome due to the limited space surrounding the calcaneus. Compartment syndrome of the foot creates significant pain that is not alleviated with elevation and immobilization. The treatment and diagnosis of foot compartment syndrome remains controversial because of limited studies. The long-term sequelae of foot compartment syndrome include rigid claw toes, weakness, neuritis, and loss of function.

Open fractures can occur in 10–17 % of all intra-articular calcaneal fractures (Heier et al. 2003). This denotes a high-energy injury with significant soft tissue implications and greater fracture deformity and comminution. These injuries have increased complications including wound issues, deep infections, osteomyelitis, and progression to amputation. The typical location for the open wound is plantar medial but can occur anywhere given the direction and force of impaction. The treatment for open injuries of the calcaneus is the same as any other lower extremity fracture. It includes antibiotics, tetanus, a clean dressing, and initial immobilization. Prompt operative irrigation and debridement is paramount to decrease the aforementioned complications.

Imaging

The complete initial radiographic evaluation of the calcaneus should include a lateral and anteroposterior (AP) view of the foot and an axial (Harris) view of the heel. A mortise view of the ankle should also be included. A lateral radiograph of the foot is the best for identifying most calcaneal fractures. This view offers many of the anatomical landmarks of the calcaneus, the Bohler's angle and angle of Gissane. It also shows articular injury and incongruity of the posterior facet and helps distinguish between a tongue-type injury and a joint depression injury (Fig. 2). If the calcaneus fracture is well visualized on the lateral radiograph, no further plain radiographs are needed as a computed tomography (CT) scan is the preferred method to evaluate the fracture and its articular injury.

The AP view of the foot shows involvement of the calcaneocuboid joint, lateral wall, and the anterior process of the calcaneus. The axial or Harris view (Fig. 3) shows the position of the tuberosity with relation to the posterior facet, typically impacted and in varus as well as lateral wall expansion. The mortise of the ankle identifies any posterior facet involvement. If there is abutment of the posterior facet on the fibula, it

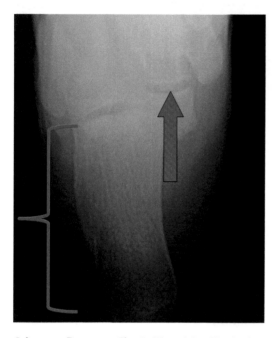

Calcaneus Fractures, Fig. 3 The axial or Harris view depicts the lateral wall (*bracket*) and the sustentaculum and middle facet (*arrow*)

may denote a fracture dislocation. Also, fibular avulsion fractures may denote associated soft tissue injuries such as a peroneal dislocation.

CT scans are the most beneficial imaging study because they reveal the exact location and size of the fragments. Typically images are needed using 1–2 mm cuts in the axial, sagittal, and semicoronal planes. The semi coronal plane is obtained by using images perpendicular to the posterior facet, which is different than the true coronal plane of the calcaneus (Fig. 4). As with imaging each plane of imaging offers different information about the fracture. The axial plane identifies the posterior tuberosity and its relation to the axis of the body (varus or valgus), lateral wall expansion, as well as the anterior process and involvement of the calcaneocuboid joint. The sagittal plane images offer information of the loss of height and length of the bone, the anterior process, and the delineation between a joint depression and tongue-type pattern. The semicoronal plane is the best to visualize the number and displacement of the articular fragments.

The Broden view is a plain radiograph image that is taken in neutral flexion with the leg internally rotated 30–40° (Fig. 5). The X-ray beam is centered over the fibula, and sequential images

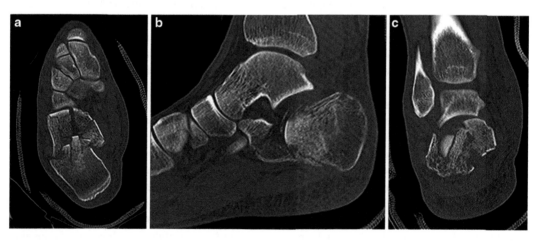

Calcaneus Fractures, Fig. 4 (**a**) The axial image of the CT scan shows injury to the calcaneocuboid joint and varus angulation with shortening of the posterior tuberosity. (**b**) Sagittal images showing the posterior facet fragment is impacted and rotated inferiorly with respect to the undersurface of the talus. (**c**) Semicoronal image showing a three-part fracture of the posterior facet (Sanders IIIAB) with displacement of the middle and lateral articular fragments

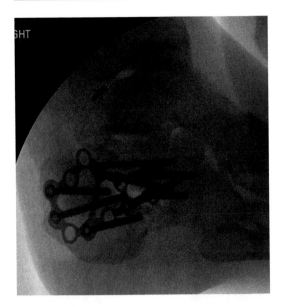

Calcaneus Fractures, Fig. 5 The Broden view is used intraoperatively to confirm anatomic reduction of the posterior facet to restore its congruency with the undersurface of the talus

are taken with the beam angled at 10°, 20°, 30°, and 40°. These views offer complete visualization of the posterior facet. Specialized views such as the Broden view are not needed for initial diagnosis, although they are important during operative fixation and postoperative monitoring for the development of arthrosis. Magnetic resonance imaging (MRI) is not typically used for these injuries and offers no advantage over CT scan.

Classification

Two main classifications exist for calcaneal fractures. The first is the Essex-Lopresti classification that separates calcaneal fractures into two types, tongue type and joint depression, based on plain radiographs. The tongue-type fracture is a pattern that has the entire posterior facet fragment intact with the posterior tuberosity. In the joint depression pattern, the articular surface is a separate fragment. This classification is beneficial in that it helps the surgeon determine the method of treatment, but it did not correlate with clinical outcomes.

The most commonly used classification used currently is the Sanders classification which was based on the semicoronal imaging from computed tomography. The basis of the classification was to determine the number and location of the fragments. This classification is more useful because it determines surgical treatment and prognosis. It, however, only includes intra-articular fractures of the calcaneus. Other patterns such as an intra-articular tongue, calcaneal fracture dislocation, anterior process, and posterior tuberosity fractures are not included in the classification.

Treatment

Historically calcaneal fractures were treated conservatively. This led to poor clinical results and patient dysfunction. Early attempts at operative fixation were also met with poor results, and it was not until the 1970s that operative treatment became more prominent for the treatment of calcaneal fractures. This was due to improvements in operative care and the availability of intraoperative fluoroscopy. As operative treatment has become more popular, newer techniques have emerged in an aim to improve outcomes and decrease complications.

Conservative treatment should be reserved for truly nondisplaced fractures. Displaced fractures typically have yielded poor results due to the rapid rate of subtalar arthrosis and the effect on the ankle joint (Buckley and Tough 2004). Although delayed fusion of the subtalar joint is possible, the treatment of a calcaneal malunion is technically difficult and also carries high rates of complications. Studies have shown improved outcomes in patients who had operative fixation followed with later arthrodesis compared to patients who underwent correction of malunion with arthrodesis (Radnay et al. 2009). Patient-specific comorbidities are also a concern. Patients with uncontrolled diabetes, peripheral vascular disease, noncompliant patients, peripheral neuropathy, or nonambulators are probably best treated with conservative care. Smoking is considered a relative contraindication, as there is a higher complication rate and poorer outcomes.

The goal of operative treatment is to restore the anatomy of the bone and anatomically restore the articular surface. There are four main surgical techniques that can be used for operative management of calcaneal fractures: percutaneous, open reduction internal fixation (ORIF), primary fusion, and external fixation.

Percutaneous Fixation

Percutaneous techniques are best suited for simple fracture patterns or for patients with significant deformity that are poor candidates to perform formal open incisions. The classic fracture pattern that is amenable to percutaneous techniques is the simple tongue-type fracture. This fracture pattern can be manipulated by K-wires, Shanz pins, and periosteal elevators using fluoroscopic imaging. Once the fracture is reduced, percutaneous screws can be placed across the fracture for stability using small incisions. This technique should be performed within 7 days of the injury date (Fig. 6). As the calcaneus begins to heal, there is significant scarring and partial healing that make percutaneous manipulation of the fragments difficult. This technique has limitations in reducing articular incongruity and should not routinely be used for complex fracture patterns. Some authors have described

Calcaneus Fractures, Fig. 6 An open calcaneal fracture that was treated with initial irrigation and debridement with external fixation. Note the displaced posterior facet fragment cannot be reduced with ligamentotaxis alone. Percutaneous techniques were used to reduce this fragment with continued use of the external fixation

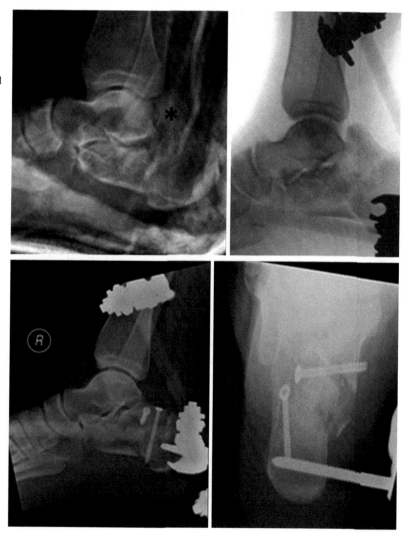

Calcaneus Fractures, Fig. 7 (**a**) Extensile lateral exposure of the calcaneus which allows for plate fixation. (**b**) Broden view following ORIF with anatomical alignment of the subtalar joint. (**c**) Lateral fluoroscopic image showing appropriate plate placement and reduction of the calcaneocuboid joint. (**d**) Axial fluoroscopic view showing restoration of the normal valgus alignment and appropriate screw length

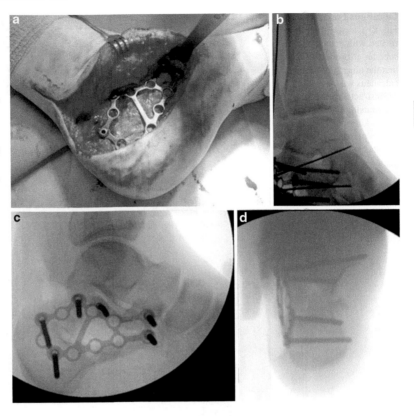

percutaneous reduction techniques with arthroscopically aided joint reduction (Rammelt et al. 2010).

Operative Fixation

Classical operative fixation of calcaneal fractures is done using an extensile lateral incision popularized by Palmer (Fig. 7). Prior to surgical stabilization the skin should be inspected and should have the presence of skin wrinkles and healing of any skin blisters, typically 14–28 days. This requires that the patient be placed in the lateral decubitus position with the affected leg closer to the surgeon and flexed at the knee. The nonaffected leg should be extended away from the operative leg. A tourniquet is used for the procedure and is placed high on the thigh. Prior to the start of the case, fluoroscopic imaging should be obtained to make sure a lateral ankle, axial, and Broden view can be obtained easily during the case.

The incision is based between the posterior edge of the fibula and lateral aspect of the Achilles tendon. It is carried distally to the junction of the glabrous skin and carried distally over the anterior process. Proximally, the sural neurovascular structures are at risk and distally the peroneal tendons and cutaneous branches of the sural nerve are at risk. A large subperiosteal flap is created and K-wires are placed into the fibula, talar neck, and cuboid and used for retraction purposes. A large 5.0 mm Shanz pin is placed into the posterior tuberosity and used to maneuver the posterior tuberosity and open the subtalar joint. The fracture is then reassembled using a variety of different techniques with the goal of anatomic articular reduction, restoration of the angle of Gissane and Bohler's angle, and the natural hindfoot alignment (5 deg. of valgus). Following fixation final fluoroscopic images should be obtained, and the wound should be meticulously closed in layered fashion. The use of a drain is typically performed to avoid large hematomas under the skin flap which can cause necrosis.

Calcaneus Fractures,
Fig. 8 Calcaneal fracture
treated with primary
subtalar arthrodesis. Note
that the alignment of the
calcaneus was
reconstructed prior to
fusion using plate fixation
with additional 7.3 mm lag
screws placed across the
subtalar joint for
compression

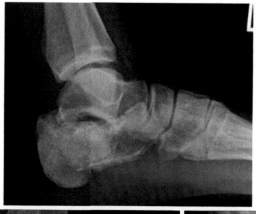

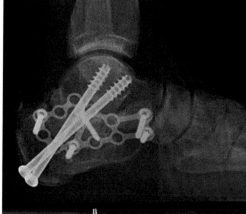

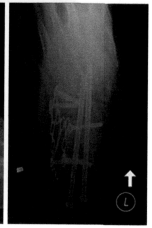

More recently the use of a sinus tarsi surgical approach has been described (Kikuchi et al. 2013). This goal of this technique is to minimize the wound complications seen with the classic extensile lateral incision by using a small incision that allows for direct visualization and reduction of the articular surface. The remainder of the calcaneal anatomy is reduced using percutaneous techniques as mentioned above. For this reason, if the sinus tarsi technique it to be used, it should be performed within 7 days of the injury.

Primary Arthrodesis

Primary arthrodesis had been described for calcaneal fractures as early as 1912 due to the poor outcomes and rapid progression of arthrosis seen with calcaneal fractures (Fig. 8). It still remains a viable option for treatment of fractures in which the articular surface is not able to be reconstructed. It offers the advantage of having

one surgery and one recovery period, particularly because subtalar arthrosis is common following calcaneal ORIF. However, this technique relies on reconstruction of the calcaneal anatomy prior to proceeding with arthrodesis. Fusing the joint in a malreduced position will create a painful, stiff hindfoot that will yield poor outcomes. Studies have suggested that this technique is particularly useful in Sanders type IV fractures and some Sanders type III fractures.

External Fixation

This technique is rarely used for definitive treatment in calcaneal fractures but can be of use in selected cases. Injuries with severe soft tissue problems may benefit from external fixation because it can stabilize the fracture, while allowing for local wound care and treatment. It may be beneficial to patients who are not good surgical candidates who have severe deformity.

This technique can reduce the anatomical length and valgus hindfoot alignment. This is done with placement of fixator pins, medial into the tibia, medial talar neck, and first metatarsal. Using sequential distraction along the triangular fixator pattern, the length, height, and hindfoot alignment can be reduced. However, since the posterior facet fragments are not connected to the tuberosity in joint depression injuries, reduction of the articular surface is not possible with external fixation alone.

Special Considerations

Calcaneal "beak" fractures can occur. This fracture involves the superior aspect of the posterior tuberosity of the calcaneus (Fig. 9). This injury commonly occurs in elderly patients with poor bone quality. The mechanism involves a forceful contraction of the gastrosoleus complex resulting in fracture. This is a true surgical emergency as the posterior skin is at risk for necrosis. Typically percutaneous techniques are used for surgical

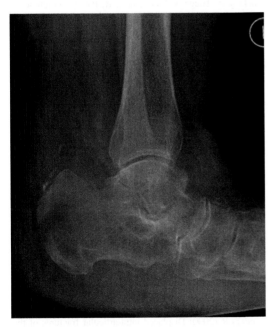

Calcaneus Fractures, Fig. 9 A lateral radiograph showing a calcaneal beak fracture that shows osteopenic bone with proximal displacement due to the strong forces of the gastrosoleus complex

stabilization, as the soft tissue envelope is already compromised. Due to poor bone quality and strong forces from the gastrosoleus complex, there is a relatively high failure rate of fixation with these injuries.

Anterior process fractures are uncommon and are typically treated conservatively. The mechanism of these injuries is due to forceful plantar flexion and inversion. These are commonly missed initially, due to lack of imaging. Operative consideration could be given to large (>1 cm) fragments or ones that are significantly displaced. Surgical excision is also an option for comminuted, displaced fractures.

Sustentacular fractures occur from a direct blow on an inverted foot. These produce medial swelling and ecchymosis. Most are comminuted and nondisplaced which are best treated with conservative care. Injuries that have a large fragment, have significant displacement (>2 mm), or have loss of medial ligament stability benefit from operative stabilization.

Posterior tuberosity fractures are almost exclusively treated conservatively. Plain imaging and CT scans should be used to be certain there is no intra-articular involvement. If there is not associated joint injury, earlier weight bearing can be started in a fracture boot or cast, typically 4 weeks, because the calcaneus is a fast healing bone due to the abundance of cancellous bone. If there is significant shortening or loss of hindfoot alignment, consideration may be given to operative treatment.

Outcomes

Historically, conservative treatment for these fractures produced poor functional outcomes. Initial surgical techniques also were met with a high incidence of complications with limited improvement in outcomes. As time has evolved improved surgical techniques have improved results from operative treatment. However, calcaneal fractures continue to pose issues for the treating orthopedic surgeon due to high complication rates and continued pain and dysfunction. Several recent studies have advocated for operative

C

treatment in patients with displaced intra-articular fractures. One meta-analysis by Buckley et al. showed improved outcomes in females, younger patients, patients with sedentary jobs, higher Bohler's angle, and those not involved in worker's compensation claims. Another study also showed improved outcomes for elderly population compared to conservative treatment (Herscovici et al. 2005). Calcaneal fractures typically occur in young males in their working prime (90 %) and represent a huge economic implication as studies show up to a 3-year complete impairment and partial impairment in work for up to 5 years. In the polytrauma patient, if they survive the initial critical period, foot injuries compromise the majority of the permanent disability (Tornetta et al. 2013).

Postoperative Complications

The majority of complications are due to wound dehiscence which can occur in 2–25 % of cases (Buckley and Tough 2004). The majority of these can be treated with local wound care, but some may require repeat surgeries and soft tissue coverage and can even progress to amputation. Risk factors for wound problems include smoking, diabetes, noncompliance with weight bearing, open fractures, and high body mass index (BMI). Deep infection and osteomyelitis occurs in 0–4 % of closed fractures and up to 19 % in open injuries.

Subtalar arthritis is a typical complication, and there is a high incidence of radiographic changes. Studies have shown that there is a 3.5–7 % conversion to subtalar joint arthrodesis by 2 years. Other studies have shown that there is a 2–5.5 times higher rate of subtalar fusion for nonoperatively treated fractures (Buckley et al. 2002). Repair of calcaneal malunions requires expertise with this problem as reconstructive procedures are often performed in association with arthrodesis.

Soft tissue complications are also prevalent with calcaneal fractures. Typical associated injuries can involve peroneals tendonitis or residual peroneal tendon dislocation associated with the initial fracture. Post-injury neuritis is common and can affect the heel pad, sural, and other nerves supplying the foot. Iatrogenic injury to the sural neurovascular structures has been documented.

Cross-References

► Ankle Fractures
► Compartment Syndrome of the Leg
► Complex Regional Pain Syndrome and Trauma
► Falls from Height
► Midfoot Fractures
► Open Fractures
► Orthopedic Trauma, Anesthesia for
► Talus Fractures
► Trauma Patient Evaluation

References

Buckley RE, Tough S (2004) Displaced intra-articular calcaneal fractures. J Am Acad Orthop Surg 12(3): 172–178

Buckley R, Tough S, McCormack R, Pate G, Leighton R, Petrie D, Galpin R (2002) Operative compared with nonoperative treatment of displaced intra-articular calcaneal fractures: a prospective, randomized, controlled multicenter trial. J Bone Joint Surg Am 84-A(10):1733–1744

Heier KA, Infante AF, Walling AK, Sanders RW (2003) Open fractures of the calcaneus: soft-tissue injury determines outcome. J Bone Joint Surg Am 85-A(12):2276–2282

Herscovici D Jr, Widmaier J, Scaduto JM, Sanders RW, Walling A (2005) Operative treatment of calcaneal fractures in elderly patients. J Bone Joint Surg Am 87(6):1260–1264

Kikuchi C, Charlton TP, Thordarson DB (2013) Limited sinus tarsi approach for intra-articular calcaneus fractures. Foot Ankle Int 34(12):1689–1694

Radnay CS, Clare MP, Sanders RW (2009) Subtalar fusion after displaced intra-articular calcaneal fractures: does initial operative treatment matter? J Bone Joint Surg Am 91(3):541–546

Rammelt S, Amlang M, Barthel S, Gavlik JM, Zwipp H (2010) Percutaneous treatment of less severe intraarticular calcaneal fractures. Clin Orthop Relat Res 468(4):983–990

Sanders R (2000) Displaced intra-articular fractures of the calcaneus. J Bone Joint Surg Am 82(2):225–250, Review

Tornetta P 3rd, Qadir R, Sanders R (2013) Pain dominates summed scores for hindfoot and ankle trauma. J Orthop Trauma 27(8):477–482

Calcium

▶ Adjuncts to Transfusion: Recombinant Factor VIIa, Factor XIII, and Calcium

Calf Hypertension

▶ Compartment Syndrome, Acute

911 Call Center

▶ Prehospital Emergency Preparedness

Canadian C-Spine

▶ Clearance, Cervical Spine

Candida

▶ Fungal Infections

Cannon

▶ Mortars

Capitellar Fractures

▶ Pediatric Fractures About the Elbow

Capsular Decompression

▶ Pediatric Fractures About the Hip

Car Accident

▶ Motor Vehicle Crash Injury

Car Crash

▶ Motor Vehicle Crash Injury

Cardiac and Aortic Trauma, Anesthesia for

James Osorio
Department of Anesthesiology, New York Presbyterian Hospital Weill Cornell Medical College, New York, NY, USA

Synonyms

Agitation of the heart; Aortic dissection: aortic tear; Blunt cardiac injury: cardiac contusion; Cardiac concussion; Commotio cordis; Penetrating cardiac injury: cardiac injury from piercing force

Definition

Cardiac and major vessel trauma is caused by force, either blunt or penetrating, to the heart and/or great vessels that results in abnormal function of the heart and circulatory system.

Preexisting Condition

Following a blunt or penetrating force to the heart and great vessels, alterations in function of the heart and circulatory system can range from no interruption in circulation or cardiac function to life-threatening conditions resulting in organ malperfusion or shock.

Blunt cardiac trauma:

1. *Cardiac contusion* that can result in the development of acute impairment of ventricular function and ECG changes ranging from ST abnormalities, QT interval prolongation, and different degrees of AV block to supraventricular and ventricular arrhythmias.
2. Free-wall myocardial rupture with *cardiac tamponade* or fatal bleeding.
3. *Septal rupture* with acute left to right intracardiac shunt placing a substantial strain on right ventricular function and subsequent low cardiac output.
4. *Acute valvular insufficiency* of the aortic or mitral valve and less commonly tricuspid valve. A condition least well tolerated when acutely developed is acute aortic insufficiency, leading to frequently *acute pulmonary edema* and decreased forward flow and cardiac output.
5. *Coronary injury* that can present with acute ischemia, hemopericardium, and cardiac tamponade or as fistulae.

Blunt major vessel trauma:

1. Blunt aortic dissection which commonly occurs just distally of the takeoff of the left subclavian artery. This segment, isthmus, is anchored by the ligamentum arteriosum and supported by the left mainstem bronchus making more immobile and susceptible to forces of traction and tear (dissection). Distal extension of the tear (Stanford type B dissection) can compromise blood supply to the abdominal mesentery with the development of mesenteric ischemia and to the spinal cord resulting in paraplegia or renal blood flow, causing acute renal failure. If the dissection affects the thoracic aorta proximal to the takeoff of the left subclavian artery towards the heart (Stanford type A dissection), this can cause acute cerebral ischemia, cardiac ischemia, acute aortic insufficiency, and cardiac tamponade.
2. Blunt trauma can result in the aorta being completely transected with fatal exsanguination at the scene.

Penetrating trauma (cardiac and major vessel) can lead to:

1. Hemopericardium and cardiac tamponade caused by injuries from sharp objects
2. Hypovolemia as a result of rapid and significant blood loss in patients that sustain a gunshot wound to the chest with a large defect

Penetrating aortic injuries are often rapidly fatal. Therefore, prompt thoracotomy with proximal control of the aorta is essential (Baum 2000; Salehian et al. 2003).

Application

The goal of the preoperative anesthetic assessment is to identify the nature of injuries that will require surgical intervention and that will impact anesthetic management.

Preoperative assessment starts with a directed history and information obtained from the ATLS (advanced trauma life support) primary and secondary survey. For the anesthesiologist, a focused physical examination is needed to help identify facial, head, and neck injuries in planning airway management. Careful attention is needed to identify clinical signs of *cardiac tamponade*, which includes Beck's triad ((1) fall in arterial blood pressure, (2) jugular venous distention, and (3) distant muffled heart sounds), pulsus paradoxus (inspiratory decrease in SBP greater than 10 mmHg), and Kussmaul's sign (rise in JVP jugular venous pressure during inspiration indicative of limited right ventricular filling). Signs of a *tension pneumothorax are* sought by auscultation and chest radiograph. Unrecognized tension pneumothorax and/or cardiac tamponade can precipitate life-threatening hypotension and acute cardiogenic shock further pronounced with induction of general anesthesia. The mechanisms responsible for precipitating an acute decompensated state post induction of general anesthesia are negative effects of positive pressure ventilation on venous return in an already compromised ventricular filling from hypovolemia as well as pharmacological effects of anesthetic induction and inhalation agents on the heart and sympathetic nervous system. Chest radiograph can also confirm the diagnosis of a *pleural effusion*, which in the case of acute trauma is likely to be hemothorax. ECG can provide clues to acute ischemic changes secondary to coronary circulation disruption as well as rhythm disturbances from ischemia or blunt injury. A CT scan provides comprehensive information about thoracic and intra-abdominal injuries. In this early post-trauma period of assessment and management, the surgical decisions are guided by identifying life-threatening injuries that require immediate surgical intervention with the best conditions for surgical control and maintenance of stable hemodynamics, managed either in the emergency room or operating room. The decision to commit the patient for a diagnostic exam commonly requiring a trip to the CT scan often out of the ER (emergency room) or vicinity of the OR (operating room) will depend on the recognition and management of immediate life-threatening injuries.

TTE and TEE (ultrasonography) provide rapid, valuable bedside preoperative and intraoperative information. Preoperative and intraoperative TEE can offer a comprehensive assessment of cardiac injuries and function as well as serve as an intraoperative monitor for assessing volume status, cardiac function, and response to therapy (Mollod and Felner 1996). Preoperative TTE is a rapid, focused bedside diagnostic evaluation performed in a systematic fashion that includes the FAST, FATE, and RUSH protocol (Price et al. 2008).

The FAST (focused assessment with sonography in trauma patients) exam is a protocol that enables a rapid bedside assessment for presence of blood in the:

1. Pericardial sac (see Fig. 1).
2. Intraperitoneal space (Morison's pouch, subphrenic space, and pelvis)

The FATE (focused assessed transthoracic echocardiography) (Scalea et al. 1999) exam is a protocol designed for the evaluation of critically ill patients. In the setting of trauma, the skilled sonographer (cardiologist/

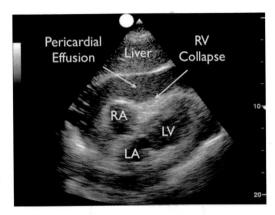

Cardiac and Aortic Trauma, Anesthesia for, Fig. 1 FAST exam. Step 1. Evaluation for presence of blood in the pericardial sac; *also* rapid ultrasound in shock (RUSH) step 1. Evaluation of the pump (*Subcostal/subxiphoid four-chamber view: cardiac tamponade*)

anesthesiologist or intensivist/surgeon) can obtain an essential rapid bedside evaluation of the heart:

1. Assessment of cardiac chamber size and myocardial function (global and regional)
2. Evaluation of valvular function (presence of valvular regurgitation)
3. Presence of intrapericardial fluid (cardiac tamponade)
4. Intracavitary pathology (intracardiac shunts ASD and VSD, ruptured papillary muscles, and intracardiac masses) (see Figs. 1 and 2)

The RUSH (rapid ultrasound in shock) (Perera et al. 2010) protocol provides valuable, rapid preoperative differentiation between cardiogenic and hypovolemic shock secondary to an acute aortic dissection. The examination includes assessment of the following:

1. *Pump* (heart) – which is the essence of the FATE exam described above
2. *Tank* (volume status) – by assessing echo signs of hypovolemia such as parasternal mid-papillary short-axis view and subxiphoid 2D or M-mode image of IVC collapsibility (sniff test)
3. *Pipes* (blood vessels) – systematic examination of the aorta with assessment for an acute dissection (see Figs. 3 and 4)

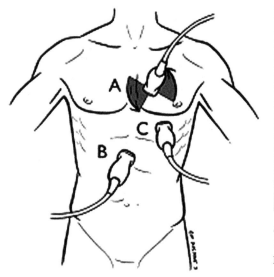

A) Parasternal Views
    Long / Short Axies
B) Subxiphoid View
C) Apical View

Cardiac and Aortic Trauma, Anesthesia for,
Fig. 2 Illustration of probe position on the chest for
image acquisition (*Standard transthoracic echo-TTE*
windows)

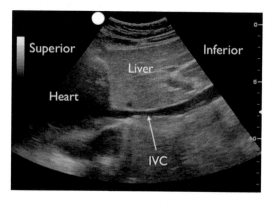

Cardiac and Aortic Trauma, Anesthesia for,
Fig. 3 *Subcostal/subxiphoid view 2D image* probe
rotated about 90° cursor facing towards the patients head
until image acquisition. Evaluation of the tank (inferior
vena cava (IVC) "sniff test"): low cardiac filling pressures

Intraoperative Course

Pericardial tamponade and tension pneumothorax are treated by the surgeon upon recognition,
prior to induction of general anesthesia with

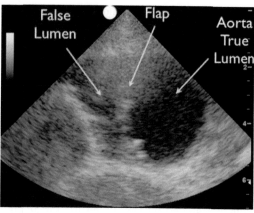

Cardiac and Aortic Trauma, Anesthesia for,
Fig. 4 *Short-axis view of the aorta.* Evaluation of the
pipes: aortic dissection

local anesthesia. If the surgeon requires general
anesthesia in patients with cardiac tamponade
secondary to difficult anatomy or patients'
noncompliance, the patient must be prepped and
draped with the surgeon prepared to expeditiously access the pericardial sac and relieve the
tamponade, control bleeding with the anesthesia
team prepared to replace lost blood volume.
Induction is performed with hemodynamic goals
in mind (fast, full, and tight).

Induction of General Anesthesia

Endotracheal intubation of trauma patients with
cardiac injuries is achieved with a rapid sequence
intubation and cervical spine controlled with
manual in-line traction, when cervical spine is
not cleared. Difficult airway when recognized
secondary to head and neck trauma or due to
patient's anatomy is addressed by the principles
of the difficult airway algorithm.

The goal of anesthetic management in trauma
patients is to avoid myocardial depressants and
agents with potent vasodilatory properties. For
patients with suspected hypovolemia and hemodynamic instability, the following agents are
recommended: (1) ketamine (1–2.5 mg/kg IV)
and (2) succinylcholine (1.5 mg/kg IV). Maintenance is achieved with inhalation agents and narcotics (Yao 2008; Round and Mellor 2006). For
patients with thoracic aortic dissections, the anesthesiologist needs to be prepared to control

sudden increases in heart rate and blood pressure to prevent free aortic rupture.

Intraoperative Access and Monitors

In addition to routine monitoring (ECG, pulse oximetry, end-tidal CO_2, temperature, and urine output measurements – foley or suprapubic catheter), it is essential to have good intravenous access with at least two large-bore IVs for resuscitation, an arterial line for close blood pressure monitoring and frequent arterial blood draws, and a prepared rapid volume infuser with a capacity of infusion rate of 1 l/min. A 9 French cordis central line has advantages for central venous pressure monitoring, administration of drips, and fluid resuscitation. If cardiac function is compromised, placement of a pulmonary artery catheter is justified for intra- and postoperative management. In the absence of contraindication, such as esophageal injury, use of intraoperative TEE (transesophageal echocardiography) will provide real-time assessment of cardiac function and cardiac volume status, impart a comprehensive assessment of life-threatening cardiac injuries, and help guide management.

Intraoperative Challenges

Intraoperative challenges include ventilation, hypothermia, ongoing surgical bleeding, coagulopathy, and cardiac arrhythmias. Lung-protective ARDS network ventilation strategy recommends the use of 4–6 ml/kg tidal volumes. If the clinical situation dictates, institution of one-lung independent ventilation (OL-ILV) to avoid contamination of normal lung alveoli and trial of other ventilator modes may be necessary (e.g., pressure control ventilation). ECMO is an option for temporary replacement for lungs where there is a catastrophic failure to provide oxygenation and ventilation, and all conventional efforts have failed, as well as full cardiopulmonary bypass may be necessary for repair of cardiac injuries. It is important to actively warm trauma patients as hypothermia develops rapidly. Available means include rushed air warmer, warming pads, and warm gastric lavage. Of note, use a fluid warmer for all fluids, except platelets. Intraoperative bleeding secondary to

coagulopathy is managed based on clinical assessment and with information obtained from the standard coagulation laboratory (PT/aPTT, platelet count, hemoglodin and fibrinogen level) as well as, when available, information obtained by either thromboelastometry and thromboelastography. Massive transfusion protocol should be activated to limit delays in the availability of blood products. Patients should be continuously monitored for rhythm disturbances. Close attention to ECG changes will provide clues to acute ischemic changes from coronary circulation disruption, rhythm disturbances secondary to ischemia, and cardiac contusion (i.e., supra and ventricular tachyarrhythmias/bradydysrhythmias and heart block).

Special Cases

Specific anesthetic requirements are dictated by the surgical procedure. Traditional open surgical approach for the repair of blunt aortic injury (BAI) distal to the isthmus is through a left thoracotomy, requiring single-lung ventilation, preferably right intra-arterial blood pressure monitoring for possible high position of cross clamp, rapid fluid infuser, aortic cross clamp, and partial heparinization (100 units/kg). Common surgical technique is the "clamp and sew" method. For an anticipated longer clamp time (La/Fa – left atrial to femoral artery), partial left heart bypass technique can be used. This surgical technique can involve rapid and significant blood loss with a relatively high complication rates and mortality.

Alternative surgical technique for BAI is an endovascular repair. The TEVAR approach eliminates the need for a thoracotomy, single-lung ventilation, and aortic cross clamp (Singh and Baum 2011; Hoffer 2008). Anesthetic management includes preferable right intra-arterial blood pressure monitoring and large-bore vascular access for rapid volume expansion. Placement of central venous access for monitoring right atrial pressure and administration of vasoactive drug therapy to control the circulation is justified, as well as ensuring immediate availability of packed red blood cells. During stent deployment and balloon expansion, the anesthesiologist should be prepared to transiently decrease the blood pressure to avoid proximal hypertension. When performing electroencephalograph (EEG), inhaled anesthetic concentrations should be maintained at half minimum anesthetic concentration (MAC). This surgical approach is associated with less bleeding, rate of early complications, and mortality compared to the open approach.

Cross-References

▶ Cardiac Injuries
▶ Heart-Lung Interactions
▶ Hemodynamic Management in Trauma Anesthesia
▶ Massive Transfusion Protocols in Trauma
▶ Thoracic Vascular Injuries
▶ Transesophageal Echocardiography (TEE)

References

Baum VC (2000) Review article-the patient with cardiac trauma. J Cardiothorac Vasc Anesth 14(1):71–81
Hoffer EK (2008) Endovascular intervention in thoracic arterial trauma. Injury 39(11):1257–1274
Mollod M, Felner JM (1996) Transesophageal echocardiography in the evaluation of cardiothoracic trauma. Am Heart J 132(4):841–849
Perera P et al (2010) The RUSH EXAM: rapid ultrasound in shock in the evaluation of critically ill. Emerg Med Clin North Am 28:29–56
Price S et al (2008) Echocardiography practice, training and accreditation in the intensive care: document for the World Interactive Network Focused on Critical Ultrasound (WINFOCUS). Cardiovasc Ultrasound 6:49
Round JA, Mellor AJ (2006) Anaesthetic and critical care management of thoracic injuries. J R Army Med Corps 156(3):139–149
Salehian O, Teoh K, Mulji A (2003) Blunt and penetrating cardiac trauma: a review. Can J Cardiol 19(9):1054–1059
Scalea TM et al (1999) Focused Assessment with Sonography for Trauma (FAST): results from an international consensus conference. J Trauma 46(3):466–472
Singh KE, Baum VC (2011) The anesthetic management of cardiovascular trauma. Curr Opin Anesthesiol 24:98–103
Yao F-SF (2008) Yao & Artusio's anesthesiology – problem oriented patient management, 6th edn. Lippincott Williams & Wilkins, Philadelphia

Cardiac Concussion

▶ Cardiac and Aortic Trauma, Anesthesia for

Cardiac Contusion

▶ Cardiac Injuries

Cardiac Defibrillation

▶ Cardiopulmonary Resuscitation in Pediatric Trauma

Cardiac Injuries

Franklin Wright[1] and Fred A. Luchette[2]
[1]Division of Trauma, Surgical Critical Care and Burns, Department of Surgery, Stritch School of Medicine, Loyola University Medical Center, Maywood, IL, USA
[2]Department of Surgery, Stritch School of Medicine, Loyola University Medical Center, Maywood, IL, USA

Synonyms

Blunt cardiac injury; Cardiac contusion; Cardiac laceration; Cardiac rupture; Traumatic wounding of the heart

Definition

Cardiac injury may involve damage to pericardial tissue, myocardium, septum, valves, papillary muscles, or coronary arteries. Blunt or penetrating trauma may place the patient at risk for a life-threatening cardiac injury, requiring careful but timely diagnostic workup and therapeutic intervention.

Preexisting Condition

Many trauma patients with cardiac injury present with no relevant preexisting conditions. However, the elderly, those with known heart disease, or previously undiagnosed atherosclerosis or structural disease may suffer either penetrating or blunt cardiac injury which may complicate management. Cardiogenic shock may need to be treated in addition to hemorrhagic shock.

Application

Incidence

Blunt cardiac trauma is frequently associated with significant chest pathology and may be difficult to diagnose clinically. Estimated rates vary from 16 % to 76 %, depending on whether clinical or autopsy reviews are conducted. Pathology in blunt cardiac injury (BCI) may range along a spectrum from mild cardiac contusion to cardiac rupture. Right-sided pathology is much more common, although multiple-chamber injury has been found in 50 % of patients suffering BCI (Karalis et al. 1994).

Penetrating cardiac injuries are rare, estimated at 0.1 % of all trauma admissions. However, it should be noted that prehospital mortality from these injuries is 90 %. Improved prehospital care in the last few decades appears to have made no difference in mortality from these lethal injuries. In fact, well-developed prehospital systems appear to lead to worse hospital outcomes, presumably by allowing attempted resuscitation of patients with profound physiologic derangement. Despite the relatively small profile of the heart in relation to total body volume, cardiac injuries account for up to 25 % of mortalities of patients who suffer any form of penetrating trauma. Relative frequencies of shooting versus stabbing injuries in the civilian world depend on local access to firearms. In the USA, firearm injuries occur at nearly a twofold rate compared to stabbings. Penetrating injuries may also occur secondary to impalement, fractures of the ribs or sternum, or iatrogenic misadventures.

History

Surgical intervention on cardiac injuries was not successfully attempted until the late 1890s. Operative pericardial drainage procedures were reported as early as 1801 by the Spanish surgeon Francisco Romero. However, reticence remained widespread among the surgical community that the heart could tolerate suture repair, despite successful animal studies in the 1880s–1890s. Theodor Billroth was (perhaps falsely) quoted as stating "Any surgeon who should attempt to suture a wound of the heart should lose the respect of his colleagues." However, following unsuccessful attempts by Axel Cappelen of Norway in 1895 and Guido Farina of Italy in 1896, Ludwig Rehn of Germany successfully repaired a right ventricular injury in 1896. This patient, a 22-year-old male named William Justus, had been stabbed in the heart 2 days prior to operation, suffering a 1.5 cm laceration of the right ventricle, repaired with three silk sutures. Seven other successful repairs were reported within the subsequent 3 years. Rehn himself later described a 124-patient series with a rather remarkable 60 % mortality rate. The need for surgeons to address life-threatening penetrating cardiac injuries thus gave birth to the field of cardiac surgery.

Anatomy

The precordium refers to the body surface overlying the heart. The technical boundaries extend from the 3rd to 6th intercostal spaces just lateral to the right of the sternal border and on the left side from the 2nd intercostal space 2 cm lateral to the sternal border to the 5th intercostal space in the midclavicular line. Functionally, the "cardiac box" is considered the high-risk region for penetrating trauma to the heart. The "box" extends between the midclavicular lines from the clavicles to the costal margins. Clearly, projectile injuries may still produce cardiac injury with entrance wounds outside of this region.

In BCI, direct sternal blow or compression against the underlying heart may lead directly to damage to the right ventricle, rupture at the atrial appendage, or acute elevation of the intracavitary pressure from the chest or abdominal trauma may cause rupture of the right-sided heart chambers or valves. Blunt forces to the thorax may result in the following injuries that are listed in decreasing frequency: cardiac contusion, cardiac rupture, valvular or septal damage, coronary arterial injury, or pericardial injury.

Given the orientation of the heart in situ and relative size of the chambers, the right ventricle is at highest risk for injury from an anterior penetrating wound, while the left atrium is at least risk. Analysis of injury patterns supports this bias. In combined reviews of 3401 penetrating cardiac wounds, rates of injury are as follows: right ventricular injury 43 %, left ventricular injury 34 %, right atrial injury 18 %, and left atrial injury 5 %. Multiple-chamber injury occurred 18 % of the time and coronary injury of less than 5 %.

Pathophysiology

Cardiac wounds present unique physiologic challenges. Cardiac tamponade especially provides distinctive physiologic derangement. The pericardium, a fibrous and inelastic sac, lacks compliance to respond to acute bleeding. Thus, intrapericardial pressure climbs rapidly, resulting in failure of venous inflow to the heart. Decreased right and left ventricular stroke volume stimulates the adrenergic response leading to tachycardia and increased cardiac contractility. As intrapericardial pressure rises, end-diastolic pressure must rise to prevent cardiac chamber collapse and loss of filling. This leads to pulsus paradoxus, as the normal respiratory variation in arterial pressure increases while pulse pressure decreases. As intracardiac and intrapleural pressures equalize, cardiac arrest ensues.

Of note, the degree of hemorrhage possible from cardiac wounds that are not contained by the pericardium clearly overshadows bleeding from anywhere else in the body other than at the root of the great vessels. Despite the profound physiologic derangements found with cardiac tamponade, it may actually allow a brief time frame for repair by temporarily controlling life-threatening exsanguination. Retrospective analyses have suggested that cardiac tamponade may indeed provide a paradoxical survival advantage in penetrating trauma (Tyburski et al. 2000). However, these studies include a preponderance of stab wounds rather than gunshot victims, suggesting that survival in fact may be due to the degree of damage to cardiac tissue and subsequent volume of hemorrhage more than a protective tamponade effect.

Cardiac tamponade and exsanguination combine to present immediate and profound threats to life. In both of these situations, resuscitation provides limited benefit compared to emergent operative intervention. Studies consistently demonstrate that for the hemodynamically unstable patient or the patient who presents in cardiac arrest, shorter prehospital time leads to improved outcomes.

While less common, there are a variety of rare other injuries that may occur with penetrating wounds associated with significant morbidity and mortality. Injuries to coronary arteries, valves, papillary muscles, or myocardial tissue damage can result in cardiac ventricular dysfunction or arrhythmias. Projectiles may lead to a foreign body embolism resulting in acute vascular occlusion in major organs. Intracardiac shunt due to a septal injury may produce a hemodynamically significant left to right shunt with left heart failure.

Similarly, BCI may lead to heart failure due to complex arrhythmias or atrial or ventricular septal rupture leading to intracardiac shunts. Valvular leaflet injury or papillary muscle rupture can result in ventricular regurgitation. Mitral and aortic valvular incompetence tend to be symptomatic in the first few days after injury, while pulmonary or tricuspid injury may not manifest for years following the traumatic injury. Coronary artery injury following blunt trauma may involve dissection, spasm, or occlusion resulting in an acute myocardial syndrome.

Late complications include endocarditis, suppurative pericarditis, ventricular aneurysms, and coronary-cameral fistulae (fistula between the coronary artery and a cardiac chamber). Undiagnosed and drained hemopericardium may result in constrictive pericarditis months to years after injury.

Diagnostic Modalities: Noninvasive

Physical examination findings in patients with penetrating cardiac injury can be quite variable, ranging from no derangements in hemodynamics to full cardiac arrest. While classically discussions of pericardial tamponade include Beck's triad (hypotension, elevated jugular venous pressure, and muffled heart sounds), it is in fact observed in a minority of patients. Pulsus paradoxus (exaggerated decrease in systolic pressure during inspiration) may be present but can be difficult to appreciate in the hectic trauma bay. In general, nonspecific indicators of shock, including hypotension, tachycardia, tachypnea, agitation, and decreased temperature of extremities, may be the primary markers of cardiac injury. Therefore, it is critical to have a high index of suspicion for these injuries, especially in any penetrating wounds to the thorax or upper abdomen.

Findings on physical examination of a cardiac injury after BCI are likewise generally nonspecific. Nonspecific chest pain is the most common symptom. This patient complaint may be difficult to interpret, however, given a high concurrent rate of associated injuries due to high-energy impact to the thorax. Suspicion for blunt cardiac injury should be high with the following: dyspnea, flail chest, sternal fractures, and chest wall ecchymoses (Schultz and Trunkey 2004).

All patients with any suspicion of blunt cardiac injury should have a 12-lead electrocardiogram (ECG) in the trauma bay. Unfortunately, no specific ECG finding is seen reliably in blunt cardiac injury. In fact, the leading dysrhythmia noted in patients with BCI is sinus tachycardia. An initial ECG with normal sinus rhythm has been shown to correlate with a very low risk of complications, leading to recommendations that young patients without hemodynamic instability require no further diagnostic workup (Illig et al. 1991).

Cardiac enzyme monitoring remains a controversial topic in BCI. Creatine phosphokinase (CPK) and CK-MB were historically used as diagnostic tests for BCI; however, numerous studies have found poor sensitivity for these laboratory studies. The results from studies of more specific biomarkers such as cardiac troponin I (cTnI) and troponin T (cTnT) have been mixed. Some investigations suggest that patients with mild ECG abnormalities who have a normal cTnI at 4–6 h have a low risk of complications from BCI (Collins et al. 2001). Other authors have suggested no role for measurement of cTnI in the evaluation of BCI (Biffl et al. 1994) or have found that cTnI is not related to cardiac injury but is simply a marker of overall stress and injury suggesting mortality benefit with beta-blockade (Martin et al. 2005). Insufficient evidence exists to support the use of cTnI as a diagnostic test for BCI, especially in patients with significant dysrhythmias after major trauma.

Radiologic diagnostic options include chest radiograph, ultrasound, echocardiogram, multidetector CT, and MRI. Chest radiography is inadequate for evaluation of a cardiac injury, although it may diagnose concomitant injuries such as a pneumothorax, pneumopericardium, hemothorax, retained foreign bodies, or mediastinal hematoma. Any of these diagnoses should lead the clinician to have a high index of suspicion for an associated cardiac injury. Of note, the cardiac silhouette is rarely enlarged following acute traumatic injury of the heart, so plain radiography is not reliable for evaluation. Ultrasound may be rapidly employed, is minimally invasive, is readily available in the trauma bay, and is widely used to diagnose traumatic hemopericardium. The FAST (focused abdominal sonogram for trauma) provides excellent positive and negative predictive values despite being somewhat operator dependent. Echocardiography may assess valvular dysfunction, septal injury, wall motion, and cardiac tamponade/effusion. More sensitive than the FAST, echocardiography may detect as little as 25 mL of hemopericardium. Unfortunately, the sensitivity of transthoracic echocardiography may be significantly limited by body habitus, tubes, and dressings. In contrast, transesophageal echocardiography (TEE) has improved sensitivity, but is invasive, requires specially trained operators and sedation, and can be technically complicated by associated cervical spine, esophageal, or facial

C

trauma. In acute penetrating cardiac trauma, there are limited if any indications for TEE. With the exception of cardiac tamponade, FAST has not been found to be a useful screening tool for blunt cardiac injury but may be useful in evaluating the patient with unexplained hypotension, dysrhythmias, or evidence of cardiac failure (Karalis et al. 1994).

Both multidetector CT and MRI generally require placing patients at risk for rapid decompensation in areas with limited ability to closely monitor the patient and poor resources to acutely intervene should the patient's clinical status deteriorate. Patients with any evidence of hemodynamic instability, signs of pericardial fluid on FAST and undrained or rapidly draining hemothorax, or indicators of shock should not travel to the radiologic suite. While blunt cardiac injury may lead to injury patterns detectable on CT/MRI, in "hemodynamically stable" patients with penetrating wounds, these imaging modalities may be most useful to rule out other occult intrathoracic injuries (contained great vessel injury/ pseudoaneurysm, trachea injury, esophageal injury, etc) rather than to assess for a penetrating cardiac wound.

Diagnostic Modalities: Invasive

Historically, patients presenting with presumed penetrating cardiac injuries, not in extremis, underwent subxiphoid pericardial window (SPW) as a diagnostic procedure to evaluate for pericardial blood. SPW involves anesthesia, surgical division of the linea alba, detachment of the xiphisternal attachments, and sharp division of the pericardium. Management with the finding of blood in the pericardium classically mandated further operative exploration. The use of bedside ultrasound in the trauma bay has largely supplanted SPW as the gold standard for ascertaining the need for operative intervention. Again, fluid in the pericardium immediately following penetrating trauma must be presumed to be blood. Of note, FAST false negatives may occur if the pericardial injury allows drainage into the mediastinum or hemithorax. Residual hemothorax or high-volume thoracostomy tube

drainage suggests the need for SPW to further evaluate for an undiagnosed cardiac injury.

Controversial management of hemopericardium has been proposed by a few trauma centers seeing a high volume of patients with penetrating chest wounds. These centers have questioned the dogma that the diagnosis of hemopericardium mandates operative intervention beyond a SPW in a hemodynamically stable patient. The Ryder Trauma Center reported that 38 % of patients with hemopericardium following blunt or penetrating injury did not have any injury that required repair, suggesting a high rate of nontherapeutic median sternotomies. Similarly, a study from Cook County Hospital described that 25 % of sternotomies were nontherapeutic even after limiting the analysis to sternotomies performed after there was evidence of ongoing bleeding at the time of SPW. Use of SPW as a therapeutic maneuver in patients without active bleeding despite blood in the pericardium has also been advocated by the University of Cape Town in South Africa. In a prospective study, they found that 71 % of hemodynamically stable patients with penetrating chest wounds underwent a nontherapeutic sternotomy and therefore advocated SPW and drainage alone (Navsaria and Nicol 2005). One criticism of these studies is the small numbers of patients in each. However, for hemodynamically stable patients, these data suggest a potential if unproven role for drainage rather than sternotomy in select patients with penetrating cardiac injury.

Pericardiocentesis does not have a role in the management of penetrating thoracic trauma, with few exceptions. Despite medical literature suggesting that pericardial blood does not clot, in practical experience, this is not the case. Percutaneous drainage of hemopericardium with a catheter is not adequate since the catheter promotes clot formation. From a diagnostic standpoint, FAST is more accurate (significantly higher sensitivity and specificity) and is without complications. Therapeutic management should be definitive as will be discussed in the following section. At best, pericardiocentesis should be considered a temporizing maneuver in a patient sustaining cardiac arrest or hemodynamic insta-bility when there is no surgical capability available.

Surgical Approaches

The operative approach will depend, in part, upon patient presentation. Patients who present in extremis generally require an emergency depart-ment thoracotomy (EDT), also referred to as resuscitative thoracotomy. Patients with evidence of cardiac tamponade or severe hemorrhage who can tolerate being transported to the operating room (which varies by institution) will benefit from having a median sternotomy due to the lower morbidity compared to an anterolateral thoracotomy. Patients with combined thoracoabdominal injuries in whom the predom-inant source of hemodynamic instability is unclear may require SPW in the OR to evaluate for a cardiac injury before exploratory laparot-omy and potential median sternotomy. If during laparotomy the patient remains hemodynami-cally unstable, the pericardium can be easily assessed transperitoneally by creating a transdiaphragmatic pericardiotomy. Hemody-namically stable patients on presentation with high-risk injuries suggesting the possibility of cardiac injury should first be evaluated with FAST examination plus either echocardiography or potentially CT angiography. As mentioned previously, patients with hemopericardium on FAST require at the minimum SPW with drain-age and generally a median sternotomy to address the source of the bleeding. Leaving patients with undrained hemopericardium risks both sudden and profound clinical deterioration as well as post-traumatic constrictive pericarditis.

Patients who present with suspicion of pene-trating cardiac injury and shock or in cardiac arrest may be salvaged with an EDT. Following, or ideally concurrent during intubation, the trauma surgeon should perform a left anterolateral thoracotomy in the 4th or 5th inter-costal space. Deviating somewhat from the advanced trauma life support (ATLS) that focuses on large bore intravenous lines and aggressive fluid bolus, this subset of patients requires immediate release of cardiac tamponade and/or control of hemorrhage. Resuscitation plays a less critical role than in other trauma scenarios. While left thoracotomy or extension into the so-called "clamshell" thoracotomy does not provide optimal exposure of the heart and great vessels, they allow for release of tamponade, temporary control of most major sources of cardiac hemorrhage, and if needed cross clamping of the descending aorta at the diaphragm.

Selecting patients who benefit from an EDT remains a controversial topic. Overall, survival following EDT for penetrating trauma is 11 % in merged data sets. However, the survival rate in patients with a penetrating cardiac injury is sig-nificantly higher at 31 %. The American College of Surgeons Committee on Trauma guidelines emphasize that patients with penetrating cardiac wounds have the best chance of survival with hospital discharge when the patient arrives after "a short scene and transport time with witnessed or objectively measured physiologic parameters (signs of life)." This does not address hard criteria for futility of EDT. The Denver Health group in collaboration with the Western Trauma Associa-tion prospectively analyzed resuscitative thora-cotomies and found survival benefit for those patients who had undergone less than 15 min of CPR without return of vital signs. Trauma patients arriving without cardiac activity should not undergo resuscitative efforts with the excep-tion of those patients with a pericardial tamponade from a penetrating wound (Moore et al. 2011). These data support previous studies concluding the patients with penetrating injuries who arrest shortly before arrival to or in the emergency department may respond to resuscita-tive thoracostomy without neurologic sequelae (Powell et al. 2004). Most experts would argue that patients presenting with profound hypoten-sion (systolic blood pressures in the 60–70 mmHg range) require emergent resuscita-tive thoracotomy in the trauma bay as well.

During resuscitative thoracotomy for cardiac injury, the primary goal is to open the pericar-dium to relieve potential tamponade and to tem-porarily control massive hemorrhage. Pericardial clot may not be immediately visualized;

therefore, the pericardium should be rapidly opened in all patients. A knick in the pericardium is made with a scalpel anterior to the left phrenic nerve and then opened longitudinally with scissors or bluntly with a fingertip to avoid damage to the phrenic nerve. As the heart is delivered from the pericardial sac and inspected for penetrating wounds, both anteriorly and posteriorly, fingertip pressure on injured areas should be applied. Insertion of a Foley catheter into gaping wounds with inflation of the balloon and gentle traction has been described to occlude the wound; however, this risks expanding the hole with any increase in tension. Atrial wounds may be occluded with a Satinsky clamp to allow a more controlled repair. Ventricular wounds may be sutured with a 2–0 or 3–0 nonabsorbable suture such as a nylon or polypropylene; given the thinner wall of the right ventricle, Teflon pledgets may be helpful. Atrial wounds may be closed in a running fashion, while ventricular wounds are generally closed with an interrupted horizontal mattress, figure of eight, or simple sutures. The use of standard 6 mm skin staplers has also been described to temporarily control bleeding from cardiac injuries in 93 % of patients. Wounds in direct proximity to major coronary vessels should be repaired using a horizontal mattress placed underneath the vessels. Additionally, if broader access is required in the emergency department, the left anterolateral thoracotomy may be extended into the right chest by crossing the sternum and creating a bilateral anterior thoracotomy ("clamshell" incision). The sternum may be divided with trauma shears, a Lebsche knife, or a Gigli saw. Note that if the patient recovers vital signs, both internal mammary arteries will result in significant hemorrhage and should be quickly ligated before transporting the patient to the operating room for further exploration and resuscitation.

Median sternotomy provides excellent exposure for most cardiac injuries. Of note, patients with penetrating cardiac injury stable enough for exploration in the OR are compensated due to excessive catecholamine levels and sympathetic activity. Anesthetic induction at the beginning of the operative procedure frequently results in cardiovascular collapse and even arrest. Positive end expiratory pressure and mechanical ventilation may also impair venous return to the heart, worsening the hemodynamic status of previously relatively stable patients with cardiac tamponade. It is therefore recommended that the patient be prepped and draped with the surgeon immediately ready to enter the chest prior to induction of anesthesia. Ideally, the SPW is performed using local anesthesia to relieve the tamponade prior to induction. Additionally, it should be noted that opening the pericardium may release massive exsanguination, and, if at all possible, cardiopulmonary bypass should be available. Intraoperative transesophageal echocardiography should also be available to identify otherwise occult traumatic injuries.

Blunt cardiac injuries, especially atrial or ventricular rupture, may require emergent surgical treatment as discussed above. Septal, valvular, or coronary arterial injury may necessitate consultation with a cardiac surgeon or interventional cardiologist for management of complex cardiac wounds. Coronary arterial injuries, whether from blunt or penetrating mechanisms, may rarely be managed by direct repair of the vessel but more commonly require bypass grafting.

Following repair of cardiac wounds, patients should be followed up with echocardiography to evaluate for pericarditis, valvular or septal damage, or development of aneurysms. Traumatic BCI with myocardial damage has been shown to generally resolve within 1 year without significant functional sequelae.

Conclusion

Penetrating cardiac injuries are highly lethal injuries, requiring the clinician to have a high index of suspicion and aggressive and timely interventions to prevent significant morbidity and mortality. Widespread use of FAST in the trauma bay may greatly aid early diagnosis and treatment, although subxiphoid pericardial window still may play an important diagnostic role, and some would argue potentially therapeutic role. In patients maintaining cardiac output in the trauma bay, median sternotomy allows for optimal management of cardiac injuries. However, emergency department thoracotomy in this patient population still offers a reasonable chance of survival for patients presenting in extremis. Despite the high incidence of prehospital death, in patients who are hemodynamically unstable after cardiac injury enough to require an EDT, penetrating cardiac wounds offer the best chance of survival. Ventricular stab wounds, in particular, may be rapidly controlled and produce favorable outcomes if treated expeditiously.

Blunt cardiac injury following major trauma may be difficult to diagnose, but screening should begin with ECG. Evidence of major chest trauma, including chest pain, flail chest, sternal fracture, or chest wall ecchymoses should prompt screening and further workup. Cardiac enzyme testing has a limited role in the evaluation and diagnosis. At most, they may allow for exclusion of a BCI and avoid further testing in lower-risk patients. Additional imaging with computed tomography and echocardiogram leading to the diagnosis of an intracavitary injury may require the assistance of a cardiac surgeon for management.

Cross-References

▶ ABCDE of Trauma Care
▶ Cardiac and Aortic Trauma, Anesthesia for
▶ Cardiopulmonary Resuscitation in Adult Trauma
▶ Firearm-Related Injuries
▶ Imaging of Aortic and Thoracic Injuries
▶ Motor Vehicle Crash Injury
▶ Trauma Emergency Department Management

References

Biffl W, Moore F, Moore E et al (1994) Cardiac enzymes are irrelevant in the patient with suspected myocardial contusion. Am J Surg 168:523–528

Collins J, Cole F, Weireter L et al (2001) The usefulness of serum troponin levels in evaluating cardiac injury. Am Surg 67:821–826

Illig K, Swierzewski M, Feliciano D, Morton J (1991) A rational screening and treatment strategy based on the electrocardiogram alone for suspected cardiac contusion. Am J Surg 162:537–543

Karalis D, Victor M, Davis G et al (1994) The role of echocardiography in blunt chest trauma: a transthoracic and transesophageal echocardiographic study. J Trauma 36:53–58

Martin M, Mullenix P, Rhee P et al (2005) Troponin increases in the critically injured patient: mechanical trauma or physiologic stress? J Trauma 59:1086–1091

Moore E, Knudson M, Burlew C et al (2011) Defining the limits of resuscitative emergency department thoracotomy: a contemporary western trauma association perspective. J Trauma 70:334–339

Navsaria P, Nicol A (2005) Haemopericardium in stable patients after penetrating injury: is subxiphoid pericardial window and drainage enough? Injury 36:745–750

Powell D, Moore E, Cothren C et al (2004) Is emergency department resuscitative thoracotomy futile care for the critically injured patient requiring prehospital cardiopulmonary resuscitation. J Am Coll Surg 199:211–215

Schultz J, Trunkey D (2004) Blunt cardiac injury. Crit Care Clin 20:57–70

Tyburski J, Astra L, Wilson R et al (2000) Factors affecting prognosis with penetrating wounds of the heart. J Trauma 48:587–590

Recommended Reading

Asensio J, Wall M Jr, Minei J et al (2001) Working group sub-committee on outcomes, American College of Surgeons-Committee on Trauma. Practice management guidelines for emergency department thoracotomy. J Am Coll Surg 193:303–309

Bottcher VA-M (2011) Suturing of penetrating wounds to the heart in the nineteenth century: the beginnings of heart surgery. Ann Thorac Surg 92:1926–1931

Cook C, Gleason T (2009) Great vessel and cardiac trauma. Surg Clin N Am 89:797–820

Kang N, Hsee L, Rizoli S, Alison P (2009) Penetrating cardiac injury: overcoming the limits set by nature. Inj Int J Care Inj 40:929–27

Pretre R, Chilcott M (1997) Blunt trauma to the heart and great vessels. N Engl J Med 336:626–632

Rozycki G, Feliciano D, Ochsner M et al (1999) The role of ultrasound in patients with possible penetrating cardiac wounds: a prospective multicenter study. J Trauma 46:543–551

Thorson C, Namias N, Van Haren R et al (2012) Does hemopericardium after chest trauma mandate sternotomy? J Trauma Acute Care Surg 72:1518–1525

Cardiac Laceration

▶ Cardiac Injuries

Cardiac Rupture

► Cardiac Injuries

Cardiopulmonary Interactions

► Heart-Lung Interactions

Cardiopulmonary Resuscitation

► Cardiopulmonary Resuscitation in Adult Trauma

Cardiopulmonary Resuscitation (CPR)

► Life Support Training

Cardiopulmonary Resuscitation in Adult Trauma

John Nachtigal
Department of Anesthesiology, University of Kansas Medical Center, Kansas City, KS, USA

Synonyms

Advanced cardiac life support (ACLS); Asystole; Basic life support; Cardiopulmonary resuscitation; Defibrillation; Out-of-hospital cardiac arrest; Pulseless electrical activity; Return of spontaneous circulation; Traumatic cardiopulmonary arrest; Ventricular fibrillation

Definition

Cardiac arrest is the cessation of cardiac mechanical activity, confirmed by the absence of signs of circulation. The arrest may be traumatic or nontraumatic and precipitated by a variety of causes including acute myocardial infarction, hypovolemia, hypoxia, diminished cardiac output, and hypothermia. Cardiopulmonary resuscitation (CPR) is a series of lifesaving actions that improve the chance of survival following cardiac arrest. CPR includes an attempt to restore spontaneous circulation (ROSC) by chest compressions or defibrillation, with or without ventilation.

Preexisting Condition

Traumatic injury is the leading cause of death among adults under 44 years of age, and up to 34 % of deaths in trauma victims occur before hospital arrival (Tobin and Varon 2012). Traumatic cardiopulmonary arrest (TCPA) may be due to a number of different causes, including hypoxia, hypovolemia due to hemorrhage, decreased cardiac output due to pneumothorax or pericardial tamponade, hypothermia, or in more rare cases, commotio cordis (sudden ventricular fibrillation after blunt chest trauma). Compared to cardiac arrests of a presumed cardiac etiology, patients with TCPA tend to be younger, are more likely to be male, and are less likely to have a shockable rhythm of ventricular fibrillation (VF) or ventricular tachycardia (VT) (Pickens et al. 2005).

There may be numerous presentations in TCPA victims: the injury may be due to either blunt or penetrating trauma; the initial rhythm may be asystole, pulseless electrical activity (PEA), or some other nonperfusing rhythm; the cardiac arrest may be present in the field or may occur in the hospital; and they may present after already having basic or advanced cardiac life support (BLS or ACLS) performed. In some cases a cardiac cause such as an acute myocardial infarction may have precipitated their trauma. Regardless of the cause, victims of TCPA have been found to have very low survival rates of only 0–2.6 %, with poor outcomes for many survivors (Mollberg et al. 2011).

Application

In general, BLS and ACLS for the adult trauma patient are fundamentally the same as for the patient with primary, nontraumatic cardiac arrest (Vanden Hoek et al. 2010). The focus is on support of the airway, breathing, and circulation. In 2010 the American Heart Association (AHA) issued their latest Guidelines for CPR and Emergency Cardiovascular Care. The fundamental tenets of early recognition and activation, early CPR, early defibrillation, and early access to emergency medical care have not changed. Similarly, the emphasis on ensuring CPR is of high quality: compressions with adequate depth and rate, allowance of full chest recoil, minimizing interruptions in compressions, and avoiding excessive ventilation are continued. The universal compression-ventilation ratio for lone rescuers of 30:2 and the defibrillation sequence of one shock followed by immediate CPR remain and are intended to minimize interruptions in chest compressions.

The most significant modification in the 2010 Guidelines is the change in the BLS sequence of steps from A-B-C (airway, breathing, circulation or chest compressions) to C-A-B (chest compressions, airway, breathing). This change was instituted because the vast majority of cardiac arrests occur in adults and the highest survival rates are in those patients with a witnessed arrest and either VF or pulseless VT as the presenting rhythm (Travers et al. 2010). In these patients the most important initial components of CPR are chest compressions and early defibrillation. Note, however, that the Guidelines do retain flexibility for healthcare providers to tailor the rescue sequence to the most likely cause of arrest. For example, in a presumed drowning or other likely asphyxial arrest, providing conventional CPR, including rescue breathing, would be the initial priority.

With respect to BLS, the algorithm has been simplified. The "look, listen, feel" mantra has been removed. Instead, the Guidelines stress immediate activation of the emergency response system and immediately starting chest compressions for any unresponsive adult victim with either no breathing or no normal breathing (i.e., agonal breaths or gasping). Chest compressions should be initiated before giving rescue breaths (C-A-B rather than A-B-C) to shorten the delay to first compression. Additionally, the recommended depth of chest compressions has increased from 1.5 to 2 in. to a recommended depth of at least 2 in.. The importance of pulse checks by healthcare providers is also de-emphasized in the new Guidelines, as chest compressions in patients subsequently found to not be in cardiac arrest rarely lead to significant injury.

ACLS algorithms have also been modified. The first major change is a new Class I recommendation for use of quantitative waveform capnography for confirmation and monitoring of endotracheal tube placement, rather than simple carbon dioxide detection. The routine use of cricoid pressure during airway management of patients in cardiac arrest is also no longer recommended. With respect to management of symptomatic arrhythmias, adenosine may now be considered for the diagnosis and treatment of stable undifferentiated wide-complex tachycardias, so long as the rhythm is regular and the QRS waveform monomorphic. For symptomatic or unstable bradycardias, when atropine is ineffective IV infusion of chronotropic agents is now recommended as an alternative to external pacing. Atropine is also no longer recommended for routine use in the management of PEA and asystole due to the low likelihood of therapeutic benefit. Instead, epinephrine continues to be recommended as the first-line agent, with or without a dose of vasopressin (Neumar et al. 2010).

Lastly, the Guidelines contain a new Early Post-Cardiac Arrest Treatment Algorithm, recognizing that ACLS does not end when ROSC is achieved. Recommendations include implementation of a comprehensive, multidisciplinary system of care and goal-oriented management, with the objective of optimizing cardiopulmonary function and vital organ perfusion after ROSC. Key objectives in the pathway include temperature control via therapeutic hypothermia to optimize neurological recovery and anticipation, treatment, and prevention of multiple organ dysfunction. Therapeutic hypothermia in particular warrants further exploration. While its benefits in the nontraumatic setting are widely accepted, its potential benefits in trauma patients, while promising, must be weighed against risks such as dysrhythmias, coagulopathy, and acidosis, particularly given that the combination of hypothermia, coagulopathy, and acidosis constitutes the "lethal triad" of trauma (Tuma et al. 2011).

Unlike in primary cardiac arrest, CPR in the pulseless trauma patient has frequently been considered futile, with survival rates of only 0–2.6 % reported. The most important factor contributing to an increased chance of survival is the presence of a shockable rhythm (either VF or pulseless VT) on the initial EKG. In these situations the chance of survival increases significantly. Unfortunately, a shockable rhythm is present in as little as 1.6 % of TCPA. Asystole (75.4 %) and PEA (13.4 %) are much more likely. Penetrating injuries have also previously been associated with an improved chance of survival, due to more localized or isolated organ injury and the potential benefit of resuscitative thoracotomy (Deasy et al. 2012).

This low probability of survival, as well as concerns over neurological and quality of life outcomes, led the National Association of EMS Physicians (NAEMSP) and the American College of Surgeons Committee on Trauma (ACSCOT) to produce Guidelines regarding the withholding or termination of resuscitation for prehospital TCPA. These Guidelines attempt to identify which TCPA patients are more likely to survive so that unrecoverable patients can be triaged as do not resuscitate (DNR) in the field, thus allowing resources to be focused more appropriately. However, TCPA is associated with several reversible causes that if promptly corrected could be lifesaving. Additionally, there are several modifications to BLS and ACLS in the trauma setting that must be considered.

During BLS, when trauma involves the head and neck or multisystem trauma is present, the cervical spine must be stabilized. A jaw thrust should be used instead of a head tilt-chin lift to establish a patent airway. If breathing is inadequate and the patient's face is bloody, ventilation should be provided with a bag-mask device while maintaining cervical spine stabilization. After initiation of BLS, if bag-mask ventilation is inadequate, an advanced airway should be inserted, again while maintaining cervical spine stabilization. If endotracheal intubation is not possible, a cricothyrotomy should be considered (*See* ► *Airway Trauma, Management of*).

A unilateral decrease in breath sounds during positive-pressure ventilation should prompt consideration of a pneumothorax, hemothorax, or diaphragmatic rupture. Chest decompression via needle thoracostomy or resuscitative thoracotomy may be lifesaving. A resuscitative thoracotomy may also be indicated for the treatment of pericardial tamponade, primarily seen in victims of penetrating trauma to the chest. In many European trauma systems such thoracotomies are often performed in the field by physicians, and studies focused on trauma outcomes in these settings often show decreased mortality compared to American studies, where thoracotomies are generally performed only after trauma victims are transported to the emergency department.

When the airway, oxygenation and ventilation are adequate, circulation should be evaluated and supported. Treatment of the PEA frequently seen in TCPA victims requires identification and treatment of reversible causes such as severe hypovolemia, hypothermia, tamponade, acid–base abnormalities, or tension pneumothorax. Ventricular fibrillation and pulseless ventricular tachycardia are treated using the ACLS algorithms, focusing on CPR and defibrillation. Severe hypovolemia should be treated with transfusion of appropriate blood components and volume resuscitation (*See* ► *Blood Component Transfusion*). Additionally, ongoing hemorrhage should be controlled when possible, as resuscitation from cardiac arrest will likely be ineffective in the setting of uncorrected severe hypovolemia (*See* ► *Massive Transfusion*).

The Guidelines for withholding or terminating resuscitation for victims of TCPA, developed jointly by the National Association of EMS Physicians and the American College of Surgeons Committee on Trauma, should also be consulted (Millin et al. 2013). These Guidelines were published in 2003 due to numerous studies reporting the abysmal survival rates in TCPA patients. Due to both ongoing debate over the original Guidelines and the development of new evidence, the Guidelines and position statements were revised in 2013. They attempt to identify patients who are unlikely to survive and minimize the risks of futile resuscitation to the victims, families, and healthcare providers and minimize consumption of healthcare resources, both personnel (prehospital, ED, surgical, and ICU) and medical products (blood, medications, and equipment). The Guidelines (Table 1) provide evaluation criteria which can be utilized to identify patients who are unlikely to survive TCPA. These criteria include blunt trauma patients who are found apneic, pulseless, and without organized ECG activity; penetrating trauma patients found apneic, pulseless, and without other signs of life; victims with injuries obviously incompatible with life, such as decapitation; victims with evidence of significant time lapse since TCPA occurred, such as rigor mortis; patients with prolonged resuscitation efforts of greater than 15 min without ROSC; and other criteria.

Some newer studies suggest use of cardiac ultrasound in the trauma bay as an adjunct to the Focused Assessment with Sonography for Trauma (FAST) exam, as patients without cardiac motion on ultrasound have an exceedingly low chance of survival (Cureton et al. 2012). Further study is needed in this area. Additionally, EMS and hospital protocols for termination of resuscitative efforts should be instituted to ensure that resources are allocated to appropriate victims and that risks to healthcare providers, patients, and families are minimized whenever possible.

Cardiopulmonary Resuscitation in Adult Trauma, Table 1 NAEMSP/ACSCOT Guidelines for withholding or termination of resuscitation in prehospital traumatic cardiopulmonary arrest[1]

1. It is appropriate to withhold resuscitative efforts for certain trauma patients for whom death is the predictable outcome
2. Resuscitative efforts should be withheld for trauma patients with injuries that are incompatible with life, such as decapitation or hemicorporectomy
3. Resuscitative efforts should be withheld for patients of either blunt or penetrating trauma when there is evidence of prolonged cardiac arrest, including rigor mortis or dependent lividity
4. Resuscitative efforts may be withheld for a blunt trauma patient who, on the arrival of EMS personnel, is found to be pulseless and apneic and without organized ECG activity
5. Resuscitative efforts may be withheld for a penetrating trauma patient who, on the arrival of EMS personnel, is found to be pulseless and apneic and there are no other signs of life, including spontaneous movement, ECG activity, and papillary response
6. When the mechanism of injury does not correlate with the clinical condition, suggesting a nontraumatic cause of cardiac arrest, standard resuscitative measures should be followed
7. A principle focus of EMS treatment of trauma patients is efficient evacuation to definitive care, where major blood loss can be corrected. Resuscitative efforts should not prolong on-scene time
8. EMS systems should have protocols that allow EMS providers to terminate resuscitative efforts for certain adult patients in traumatic cardiopulmonary arrest
9. TOR may be considered when there are no signs of life and there is no ROSC despite appropriate field EMS treatment that includes minimally interrupted CPR
10. Protocols should require a specific interval of CPR that accompanies other resuscitative interventions. Past guidance has indicated that up to 15 min of CPR should be provided before resuscitative efforts are terminated, but the science in this regard remains unclear
11. TOR protocols should be accompanied by standard procedures to ensure appropriate management of the deceased patient in the field and adequate support services for the patient's family
12. Implementation of TOR protocols mandates active physician oversight
13. TOR protocols should include any locally specific clinical, environmental, or population-based situations for which the protocol is not applicable. TOR may be impractical after transport has been initiated
14. Further research is appropriate to determine the optimal duration of CPR before terminating resuscitative efforts

[1]J Trauma Acute Care Surg 75:461

Cross-References

► Airway Trauma, Management of
► Blood Component Transfusion
► Massive Transfusion

References

Cureton EL, Yeung LY, Kwan RO, Miraflor EJ, Sadjadi J,
  Price DD, Victorino GP (2012) The heart of the matter:
  utility of ultrasound of cardiac activity during trau-
  matic arrest. J Trauma Acute Care Surg 73:102–110
Deasy C, Bray J, Smith K et al (2012 Apr) Traumatic out-
  of-hospital cardiac arrests in Melbourne Australia.
  Resuscitation 83(4):465–470
Millin MG, Galvagno SM, Khandker SR, Malki A, Bulger
  EM (2013) For the Standards and Clinical
  Practice Committee of the NAEMSP and the Subcom-
  mittee on Emergency Services-Prehospital of the
  ACSCOT. Withholding and termination of resuscita-
  tion of adult cardiopulmonary arrest secondary to
  trauma: Resource document to the joint NAEMSP-
  ACSCOT position statements. J Trauma Acute Care
  Surg 75(3):459–467
Mollberg NM, Wise SR, Berman K et al (2011) The
  consequences of noncompliance with guidelines for
  withholding or terminating resuscitation in traumatic
  cardiac arrest patients. J Trauma 71:997–1002
Neumar RW, Otto CW, Link MS et al (2010) Part 8: adult
  advanced cardiovascular life support: 2010 American
  Heart Association Guidelines for Cardiopulmonary
  Resuscitation and Emergency Cardiovascular Care.
  Circulation 122:S729–S767
Pickens JJ, Copass MK, Bulger EM (2005) Trauma
  patients receiving CPR: predictors of survival.
  J Trauma 58:951–958
Tobin JM, Varon AJ (2012) Update in trauma anesthesi-
  ology: perioperative resuscitation management.
  Anesth Analg 115:1326–1333
Travers AH, Rea TD, Bobrow BJ, Edelson DP, Berg RA,
  Sayre MR, Berg MD, Chameides L, O'Connor RE,
  Swor RA (2010) Part 4: CPR overview: 2010
  American Heart Association Guidelines for Cardiopul-
  monary Resuscitation and Emergency Cardiovascular
  Care. Circulation 122(Suppl 3):S676–S684
Tuma MA, Stansbury LG, Stein DM et al (2011) Induced
  hypothermia after cardiac arrest in trauma patients:
  a case series. J Trauma 71:1524–1527
Vanden Hoek TL, Morrison LJ, Shuster M, Donnino M,
  Sinz E, Lavonas EJ, Jeejeebhoy FM,
  Gabrielli A (2010) Part 12: cardiac arrest in special
  situations: 2010 American Heart Association guide-
  lines for cardiopulmonary resuscitation and emergency cardiovascular care. Circulation 122(suppl 3):
  S829–S861

Cardiopulmonary Resuscitation in Pediatric Trauma

Mirsad Dupanovic[1] and
Svjetlana Tisma-Dupanovic[2]
[1]Department of Anesthesiology, Kansas
University Medical Center, The University of
Kansas Hospital, Kansas City, KS, USA
[2]Department of Cardiology, Children's Mercy
Hospital, University of Missouri, Kansas City,
MO, USA

Synonyms

Basic life support; Cardiac defibrillation; External
chest compressions; Open-chest cardiopulmonary
resuscitation; Pediatric advanced life support

Definition

Cardiac arrest represents cessation of spontaneous mechanical activity of the heart with
resulting absence of circulation. In general, etiology is either cardiac or respiratory. However, in
pediatric trauma etiology of cardiac arrest is typically either circulatory or respiratory. If not
treated severe hypotension or hypoxemia lead to
significant physiologic derangements with consequent bradycardia and asystole. Unrespon-
siveness, apnea, and the inability to palpate the
central pulse are symptoms and signs of
a cardiopulmonary arrest.

Cardiopulmonary resuscitation (CPR)
includes series of lifesaving procedures that if
initiated promptly and properly may undo effects
of cessation of cardiac mechanical activity,
absence of blood circulation, and arrested
ventilation. Quick and deliberate actions are
required in order to improve chance of victim's
survival and to minimize the risk of secondary
injury. Thus, call for help must be sent immediately and external chest compressions of adequate depth and frequency started. The major
goal of CPR is restoring spontaneous circulation
(ROSC) represented by perfusing heart rhythm

for more than 20 min in the absence of chest compressions (Donoghue et al. 2005). Success of the CPR depends on multiple factors of which timely delivery of high-quality chest compressions and efficient teamwork are the most important. Providing oxygenation and ventilation and reversing underlying pathologic cardiac rhythm are also essential factors in obtaining rapid ROSC and improving chances for victim's survival following cardiopulmonary arrest. Because of physiological differences between children and adults, American Heart Association has created the CPR guidelines specifically adapted to children. Those guidelines have been published in the pediatric advanced life support (PALS, Kleinman et al. 2010). A separate consensus on neonatal CPR is in existence as well (Perlman et al. 2010).

Preexisting Condition

Injuries are the leading cause of death in children in the United States. Two largest groups of injured are teenagers and children aged 1–4, usually involved in motor vehicle collisions and a variety of other accidents, respectively. In general, the tallest peak of trauma-related deaths occurs within minutes of injury as a result of abrupt apnea and/or exsanguination that rapidly results in cardiac arrest and death (ATLS 2008). In those that survive until medical teams arrive, cardiopulmonary arrest is either caused by compromised oxygenation/ventilation or is a consequence of major external or internal hemorrhage and hypovolemic shock. A progressive respiratory failure that culminates in cardiac arrest is called asphyxial arrest. Primary cessation of cardiac mechanical activity due to ventricular fibrillation (VF) or pulseless ventricular tachycardia (VT) is a less common cause of cardiopulmonary arrest in children than in adults because of lower incidence of primary cardiac disease in pediatric population. Approximately 5–15 % of pediatric inhospital and out-of-hospital cardiac arrests have VF or pulseless VT as the initial cardiac rhythm (Kleinman et al. 2010).

Pediatric out-of-hospital cardiopulmonary arrest is a rare event that has very poor outcome. Survival to discharge of children who suffered an out-of-hospital cardiopulmonary arrest is low at approximately 6 % compared to 27 % survival from an inhospital cardiopulmonary arrest (Kleinman et al. 2010). The primary cause of such low survival rate in an out-of-hospital cardiopulmonary arrest situation is frequent absence of witnesses capable of initiation of resuscitation, hesitation to start the CPR, lack of necessary medical resources, and limited time frame for reversal of severe physiologic derangements. Thus, there is significantly greater likelihood of survival in children whose cardiac arrest was witnessed versus non-witnessed cardiac arrest. A large meta-analysis reported 13.1 % survival when cardiac arrests were witnessed compared to 4.4 % survival with non-witnessed cardiac arrests (Donoghue et al. 2005). The same study reported 9.4 % survival in those who received bystander CPR versus 4.7 % in those who did not. However, ROSC and survival are not guaranteed for maintenance of a full neurological capacity of cardiac arrest victims. The above study reported intact neurologic survival in 4 % of patients who suffered a cardiopulmonary arrest (Donoghue et al. 2005).

Trauma-associated cardiopulmonary arrest in children represents 22 % of all pediatric out-of-hospital arrests (Crewdson et al. 2007). It may be associated with blunt trauma (traffic accidents, falls, assaults, being struck by falling objects, air crushes), penetrating trauma (most commonly stab wounds and rarely firearm injuries), burns, electrocution, systemic hypothermia, drowning (submersion injury), and hanging. Consequences of child abuse may be a combination of some of the pathologic factors listed. Children with penetrating trauma have the highest morbidity, while those with asphyxial cardiopulmonary arrest have the highest survival rate. Major hemorrhage associated with shock resulting in hypovolemic cardiac arrest is unlikely to respond to CPR measures without a prompt surgical hemostasis and administration of fluid and blood products to support the circulation. Sufficient tissue oxygen delivery depends not only on pulmonary ventilation and satisfactory cardiac output but also on adequate blood oxygen content, which is mainly determined by hemoglobin concentration and oxyhemoglobin saturation. Thus, common errors in pediatric trauma CPR include not only failure to start delivering chest compressions and open the airway but also failure to recognize and treat internal bleeding and provide appropriate volume resuscitation. Multiple organs are closely situated in a small body of a child, and thus, multiple-organ injury is a frequent consequence of a blunt trauma. Thoracic injury should be suspected in all thoraco-abdominal trauma cases (Kleinman et al. 2010). Tension pneumothorax and hemothorax may be consequences of thoraco-abdominal trauma and are usually successfully treated by a qualified surgical team. However, if these two entities are unrecognized, compression of great vessels may result in obstructive shock and cardiac arrest.

Paradoxically, cardiac arrest in pediatric trauma may be a consequence of resuscitation. Acute hyperkalemia associated with rapid transfusion of red blood cells (RBCs) containing high potassium level is the major culprit. RBCs with a longer shelf life and irradiated blood usually contain higher potassium level. Use of central venous line rather than a peripheral IV line for RBC transfusion will contribute to increased RBC destruction and greater leak of potassium (Lee and Heitmiller 2014). Low cardiac output state slows intracellular distribution of potassium and contributes to a higher serum potassium level. Acidosis and hyperglycemia that are frequently associated with hemorrhagic shock contribute to increased serum potassium levels, while hypothermia and hypocalcemia increase the risk of potassium-associated cardiac toxicity (Smith et al. 2007). In addition, small circulating blood volume and immature renal function may place children at additional risk of hyperkalemia when compared to adults. Survival rate is very low.

Abnormal cardiac rhythms, as initial causes of cardiac arrest, are similar between pediatric trauma population and general pediatric out-of-hospital cardiac arrest population: asystole (75 % vs. 78 %), pulseless electrical activity (PEA, 6.7 % vs. 12.8 %), VF/pulseless VT (5 % vs. 8.1 %), and bradycardia (1 % vs. none). Please note that there were 13.4 % of patients with unknown (not recorded) rhythm in the trauma cardiac arrest group in this meta-analysis (Donoghue et al. 2005).

Application

Cardiac arrest associated with trauma usually occurs in the out-of-hospital setting. However, irrespective of the setting, quick recognition of the arrest and prompt activation of the emergency response system are crucial measures in mobilizing multiple capable responders, gathering necessary medical resources, and ultimately increasing chances of victim's survival.

Basic Life Support

Regardless of the etiology or setting of a pediatric traumatic cardiac arrest, effective CPR starts with immediate delivery of high-quality chest compressions by a first responder. The ABC resuscitation sequence (airway, breathing, chest compressions) has been changed to the CAB sequence (chest compressions, airway, breathing) in the 2010 BLS Guidelines (Kleinman et al. 2010). The main impetus for this change was avoiding delay in chest compression delivery, restoring blood circulation, and tissue oxygenation. It takes less time to place hands on the victim's chest and start compressing than to do any meaningful airway management procedure. This is especially important in cases of arrest of primary cardiac etiology and in the out-of-hospital setting. Minimum chest compression rate should be 100/min, compression depth should be at least 1/3 of the thoracic anteroposterior diameter, and full chest recoil should follow each compression. Simultaneous delivery of chest compressions and ventilation by a single rescuer is impossible. Thus, the recommended compression to ventilation ratio in non-intubated children (mouth-to-mouth, mouth-to-mask, or bag-mask ventilation) is 30:2 for a lone rescuer and 15:2 for two rescuers. The aim of this recommendation is to provide the most beneficial balance between blood circulation and lung ventilation under specific circumstances.

Prompt pulmonary delivery of oxygen in case of asphyxial cardiopulmonary arrest along with other CPR measures often reverses causative physiologic derangements, allowing ROSC and potentially a good recovery (Crewdson et al. 2007). Pulmonary ventilation may be as important as chest compressions for the success of the CPR following an asphyxial arrest, frequent in pediatric population. Bag-mask ventilation using 100 % oxygen can be a very effective CPR method in children because delivery of chest compressions does not have to be interrupted for placement of an artificial airway. However, the rescuer should possess the skills in maintaining the airway open and delivering positive pressure ventilation with minimal cervical spine extension. Newborns, infants, and young children have disproportionately larger head compared to the rest of the body, and their optimal positioning for mask ventilation and tracheal intubation requires elevating the torso by placing appropriately sized towel roll under the shoulders. This maneuver helps avoid undesirable cervical flexion. Victims should not be routinely hyperventilated. A brief hyperventilation may be used only as a temporizing measure if signs of impending brain herniation like dilatation of one or both pupils with decreased response to light, bradycardia, and hypertension are present (Kleinman et al. 2010).

Advanced Life Support

In general, delivery of chest compressions should not be interrupted to perform tracheal intubation. However, healthcare providers may adapt the CPR sequence in order to provide the most benefit to the victim. Thus, in the case of an asphyxial arrest, if highly skilled personnel consider tracheal intubation an indispensable resuscitation measure, endotracheal tube (ETT) placement may be performed as soon as feasible. Use of cuffed ETTs is associated with increased likelihood of correct ETT size selection, lowered re-intubation rate, and decreased risk of pulmonary aspiration with a comparable frequency of

other complications (Kleinman et al. 2010). Decreased time spent on intubation leads to minimized interruption in delivery of chest compressions. Visualization of ETT passage through the glottis, presence of bilateral breath sounds, absence of auscultatory signs of gastric insufflation, and presence of exhaled end-tidal CO_2 are confirmatory signs of tracheal intubation. Absence of end-tidal CO_2 following ETT placement is most commonly either a consequence of the ETT misplacement or severely reduced cardiac output resulting in very low pulmonary blood flow. If end-tidal CO_2 is not detectable, a differential diagnosis between esophageal intubation and a low flow state has to be made using laryngoscopy. Some other causes of altered colorimetric end-tidal CO_2 reading are detector contamination with gastric contents or acidic drugs (e.g., epinephrine), a large glottic leak, severe airway obstruction (e.g., status asthmaticus, massive aspiration), pulmonary edema, or injections of epinephrine just preceding the end-tidal CO_2 test resulting in low pulmonary blood flow (Kleinman et al. 2010). Use of continuous capnography during the CPR is not only important for confirmation of tracheal intubation but also for monitoring the effectiveness of chest compressions and detecting the ETT dislocation. Quantitative waveform capnography is recommended. However, it needs to be remembered that in extremely low flow states, capnography may be falsely negative and visualization of the ETT and lung auscultation may be the only confirmatory method available. In addition, bronchial intubation cannot be excluded with the capnography.

Following successful tracheal intubation, chest compressions and ventilation proceed simultaneously with the approximate ratio of 10:1 in older children and lower ratios in infants and neonates (Table 1). Regardless of the ventilation strategy used, high peak airway pressures should be avoided in order to minimize the risk of unnecessary increases of intrathoracic pressures, which in turn reduce venous return, diminish cardiac output, decrease cardiac and cerebral blood flow, and diminish the likelihood of ROSC. In addition, excessive ventilation in

Cardiopulmonary Resuscitation in Pediatric Trauma, Table 1 Recommended compression to ventilation ratios in pediatric cardiopulmonary resuscitation

	Compression to ventilation ratios					
	Children		Infants		Neonates	
	Non-intubated	Intubated	Non-intubated	Intubated	Non-intubated	Intubated
Single rescuer	30:2		30:2		30:2[b]	
					3:1[c]	
Two rescuers	15:2		15:2		15:2[b]	
					3:1[c]	
		10–5:1[a]		5:1		3:1

[a]Younger intubated children require increased rate of ventilation relative to chest compressions
[b]Arrest of cardiac etiology
[c]Arrest of respiratory etiology

a non-intubated victim may lead to gastric inflation, increased risk of regurgitation, pulmonary aspiration, and further ventilatory compromise. Cricoid pressure may be used in patients that are considered at high risk for pulmonary aspiration during mask ventilation or tracheal intubation unless cricoid pressure interferes with effective ventilation or distorts the airway during intubation, respectively. In apneic intubated children with a perfusing rhythm, respiratory rate may be increased above 10/min up to 20/min depending on the age (the younger the child, the higher the respiratory rate). There are a few airway management options in case that tracheal intubation was unsuccessful. Resuming to bag-mask ventilation with or without an oropharyngeal airway or nasopharyngeal airway in place is the fastest way of delivering oxygen and eliminating CO_2. If bag-mask ventilation is inadequate, a supraglottic airway, of which laryngeal mask airway has been studied the most, may be placed and pulmonary ventilation resumed.

Cardiopulmonary arrest in pediatric trauma is less frequently caused by "shockable" rhythms (pulseless ventricular tachycardia and ventricular fibrillation) than "non-shockable" rhythms (asystole and pulseless electrical activity). During delivery of chest compressions, after cardiac rhythm monitor is attached, "shockable" versus "non-shockable" rhythm is documented and a 2 J/kg shock vs. epinephrine bolus delivered, respectively. Delivery of chest compressions then continues, and if the rhythm remains "shockable" and there is no ROSC, another 4 J/kg shock

should be delivered. Chest compressions and epinephrine administration in appropriate sequence follow those steps (Table 2). If after another 2 min of high-quality chest compressions cardiac rhythm still remains "shockable," delivery of another ≥4 J/kg shock is followed by amiodarone administration. Continued chest compressions and treatment of reversible causes of cardiac arrest follow those steps. Drug administration occurs during chest compressions that may be only briefly interrupted for tracheal intubation, rhythm check, and shock delivery. In case that "non-shockable" rhythm at any time becomes "shockable," a 4 J/kg shock should be delivered and resuscitation continued as described for a "shockable" rhythm. On the other hand, if the "non-shockable" rhythm continues, sequential administration of CPR and epinephrine continues until there is ROSC or termination of CPR efforts. Intravenous drug administration is a preferred method of drug delivery during CPR. However, any ATLS drug, IV fluids, and blood products can be safely and effectively administered by intraosseous route as well. On the other hand, endotracheal drug administration is limited to lidocaine, epinephrine, atropine, and naloxone ("LEAN"). However, doses of these drugs should be tripled, and for epinephrine, the dose is increased tenfold.

Emergency treatment of bradycardia is needed if despite effective ventilation with oxygen heart rate of less than 60/min is associated with hemodynamic compromise. Epinephrine is the first drug of choice. Atropine is the treatment choice

Cardiopulmonary Resuscitation in Pediatric Trauma, Table 2 Selected ATLS medications

Drug	IV/IO dose	Endotracheal dose	Indication
Epinephrine[a]	10 mcg/kg bolus (1:10,000 solution)	100 mcg/kg (1:1,000 solution)	Cardiac arrest of any type (every 3–5 min)
Amiodarone	5 mg/kg bolus; may repeat X3 (max. single dose 300 mg)	N/A	"Shockable" cardiac arrest
Atropine	20 mcg/kg (max. single dose 0.5 mg)	40–60 mcg/kg	Bradycardia
Magnesium sulfate	25–50 mg/kg (max dose 2 g)	N/A	Torsades de Pointes
Calcium chloride	20 mcg/kg (max single dose 2 g)	N/A	Hypocalcemia
Sodium bicarbonate	1 mEq/kg per dose	N/A	Metabolic acidosis
Glucose	0.5–1 g/kg	N/A	Supportive care

[a]Maximum for a single epinephrine dose is 1 mg IV

of bradycardia with high vagal tone or primary AV block. Polymorphic ventricular tachycardia (torsades de pointes) is treated with rapid infusion of magnesium sulfate.

The child's weight is the most accurate method to calculate drug doses. However, if that information is not available, a body length tape with pre-calculated doses is the best next method for estimating drug doses.

Newborns and Infants

Heart rate assessed by auscultation of the precordium is the primary vital sign in newborn resuscitation. In case of respiratory distress and heart rate below 100/min, respiratory support is necessary. It requires ensuring of adequate ventilation and oxygenation. Recommended inflation pressures are 20–25 cm H_2O and 30 cm H_2O in preterm and term infants, respectively. Use of bag-mask ventilation, endotracheal intubation, and the laryngeal mask airway is a preferred ventilatory method. In addition to clinical signs, use of exhaled CO detectors is the most reliable method in confirming proper tracheal tube placement. If heart rate falls below 60/min, chest compressions are coordinated with positive pressure ventilation (Table 1). Two thumb encircling method centered over the lower third of the sternum and compressing 1/3 of the anterior-posterior diameter of the chest is recommended for the delivery of chest compressions in the newborn. If despite adequate ventilation and

chest compressions heart rate remains below 60/min, epinephrine administration should be started (Table 2). In case of known or suspected hemorrhage, volume replacement should start (crystalloids, blood products). Therapeutic hypothermia may be considered for newborns and infants with evolving hypoxic-ischemic encephalopathy. Intravenous glucose administration should be considered in order to avoid hypoglycemia.

The rate and route of RBC administration are very important factors in pathogenesis and prophylaxis of transfusion-associated hyperkalemic cardiac arrest. Anticipation of a need for massive transfusion leading to an early blood transfusion at a slower rate is a recommended preventive measure. It has also been recommended that the rate of RBC transfusion does not exceed 0.5 mL/kg/min (Lee and Heitmiller 2014). Administering PRBCs through a large caliber peripheral IV will decrease RBC destruction and lower potassium leak compared to RBC administration through central venous line. In addition, blood bank processing measures to decrease potassium content in stored red blood cells may be performed depending on the availability of time.

Cross-References

▶ ABCDE of Trauma Care
▶ Airway Management in Trauma, Nonsurgical
▶ Airway Management in Trauma, tracheostomy

▶ Airway Trauma, Management of
▶ Cardiac and Aortic Trauma, Anesthesia for
▶ Cardiopulmonary Resuscitation in Adult Trauma
▶ Hypothermia, Trauma, and Anesthetic Management
▶ Pediatric Trauma, Assessment, and Anesthetic Management
▶ Pneumothorax
▶ Shock
▶ Vascular access in trauma patients

References

American College of Surgeons Committee on Trauma (2008) Advanced Trauma Life Support® for Doctors (ATLS®) student course manual, 8th edn. American College of Surgeons Committee on Trauma, Chicago

Crewdson K, Lockey D, Davies G (2007) Outcome from paediatric cardiac arrest associated with trauma. Resuscitation 75:29–34

Donoghue AJ, Nadkarni V, Berg RA et al (2005) Out—of hospital pediatric cardiac arrest: epidemiologic review and assessment of current knowledge. Ann Emerg Med 46:512–522

Kleinman ME, Chameides L, Schexnayder SM et al (2010) Part 14: Pediatric advanced life support: American Heart Association guidelines for cardiopulmonary resuscitation and emergency cardiovascular care. Circulation 122(Suppl 3):S876–S908

Lee AC, Heitmiller ES (2014) Preventing pediatric transfusion-associated incidents of hyperkalemic cardiac arrest. Anesth Patient Saf Found Newsl 29:1 and 6. http://issuu.com/enews/docs/spring2014?e=1607375/8073163. Accessed 25 June 2014

Perlman JM, Wyllie J, Kattwinkel J et al (2010) Neonatal resuscitation: international consensus on cardiopulmonary resuscitation and emergency cardiovascular care science with treatment recommendations part 11. Circulation 22(Suppl 2):S516–S538

Smith HM, Farrow SJ, Ackerman JD et al (2007) Cardiac arrests associated with hyperkalemia during red blood cell transfusion: a case series. Anesth Analg 106:1062–1069

Cardiovascular Monitoring

▶ Hemodynamic Monitoring

Cardiovascular System Management in Trauma Anesthesia

▶ Hemodynamic Management in Trauma Anesthesia

Case Fatality Rate (CFR)

Mary Ann Spott[1] and Donald H. Jenkins[2,3]
[1]U.S. Army Institute of Surgical Research, JBSA Fort Sam Houston, TX, USA
[2]Department of Surgery, Division of Trauma, Critical Care and Emergency General Surgery, Saint Marys Hospital, Rochester, MN, USA
[3]Mayo Clinic, Rochester, MN, USA

Synonyms

Died of wounds; Killed in action

Definition

Case fatality rate (CFR) refers to the fraction of an exposed group who died of their wound. This includes all those wounded in action (sum of three subgroups: (1) Died of Wounds, vide infra, (2) casualties admitted to a military treatment facility and subsequently survived/evacuated, and (3) casualties who returned to duty (RTD) within 72 h suffering minor wounds) and all those who die (at any level), expressed as a percentage. This confers the risk that if injured in combat, the percent likelihood of death. This definition is distinctly different than the other, more commonly known terms such as Died of Wounds (DOW) or Killed in Action (KIA) both of which refer to death due to combat injury at a particular location in the combat zone. KIA occur on the battlefield, while DOW occur after the casualty arrives for medical treatment at a military medical treatment facility. Neither is inclusive as the CFR and does not capture all those who die related to combat injury; only

CFR is inclusive of all combat-related deaths and is deemed to be a more appropriate tool for comparison purposes (Holcomb et al. 2006).

Of historical note, CFR for US forces in World War II was over 22 % (meaning, if injured, the likelihood of dying in WWII was 1 in 4 to 1 in 5), dropped to approximately 16 % in Vietnam, and is less than 10 % for US troops in the current conflict in Iraq and Afghanistan. The reasons for this decline are myriad, but a combination of better body armor, better armored vehicles, better field care (tourniquets, hemostatic adjuncts, etc.), and rapid evacuation to Forward Surgical Teams are all important factors to consider (Holcomb et al. 2006).

Cross-References

▶ Joint Trauma Registry

References

Holcomb JB, Stansbury LG, Champion HR, Wade C, Bellamy RF (2006) Understanding combat casualty care statistics. J Trauma 60(2):397–401

CASEVAC

Frank K. Butler
Department of the Army, Committee on Tactical Combat Casualty Care, U.S. Army Institute of Surgical Research, Fort Sam Houston, TX, USA
Department of the Army, Prehospital Trauma Care, Joint Trauma System, U.S. Army Institute of Surgical Research, Fort Sam Houston, TX, USA

Synonyms

Casualty evacuation

Frank K. Butler has retired.

Definition

The term Casualty Evacuation (CASEVAC) is used to describe the movement of casualties from the point of wounding to a medical treatment facility using transportation assets that are not designated Medical Evacuation (MEDEVAC) assets (Butler et al. 2010). MEDEVAC is defined later in this section. CASEVAC platforms are generally armed tactical assets that bear no Red Cross markings. CASEVAC and MEDEVAC are often collectively referred to as TACEVAC, which is an abbreviation for Tactical Evacuation. The CASEVAC phase of prehospital care is critical in that this phase represents what may be the first opportunity to bring an advanced medical treatment capability directly to the injured Soldier, Sailor, Airman, or Marine.

Two significant differences will be present in progressing from the Tactical Field Care phase of Tactical Combat Casualty Care (TCCC) to the TACEVAC phase of care. The first is that additional medical personnel may accompany the evacuating asset. The practice in the past for many units in Special Operations was that medical care during CASEVAC was expected to be rendered by the corpsman or medic present on the mission phase of the operation. This was a problem for several reasons: (1) the corpsman or medic may be among the casualties; (2) the corpsman or medic may be dehydrated, hypothermic, or otherwise debilitated; (3) the evacuation platform's medical equipment will need to be prepared prior to the extraction mission; and (4) there may be multiple casualties, which make it difficult for a single corpsman, medic, or pararescueman to care for them all simultaneously (Butler et al. 1996).

TACEVAC capabilities are not standardized in the Afghanistan area of operations at present. Some platforms are staffed with EMT-B trained flight medics, while others have paramedic-level providers and others (the UK Medical Emergency Response Team or MERT) have a physician on the aircraft as well as a larger team (Mabry 2011).

The 2011 memo from the Defense Health Board (Dickey et al. 2011) makes recommendations regarding a number of the key aspects of TACEVAC care, to include response time, size of the evacuation platform, number and types of providers recommended, availability of blood products for resuscitation from hemorrhagic shock, pre-deployment training experience required to ensure optimized care, supervision of medical providers in TACEVAC platforms, and considerations for evacuation from a hostile landing zone.

Cross-References

▶ Damage Control Resuscitation
▶ Damage Control Resuscitation, Military Trauma
▶ Fluid, Electrolytes, and Nutrition in Trauma Patients
▶ FP24
▶ Hemodynamic Monitoring
▶ Hemorrhage
▶ Hemostatic Adjunct
▶ Hypothermia
▶ IED (Improvised Explosive Device)
▶ Intraosseous Device
▶ Monitoring of Trauma Patients During Anesthesia
▶ Noncompressible Hemorrhage
▶ Packed Red Blood Cells
▶ Plasma Transfusion in Trauma
▶ Pneumothorax, Tension
▶ Rule of Tens
▶ Shock
▶ Shock Management in Trauma
▶ TACEVAC
▶ Tactical Combat Casualty Care
▶ TBI
▶ Tourniquet
▶ Tranexamic Acid
▶ Whole Blood

References

Butler FK, Giebner SD, McSwain N, Salomone J, Pons P (eds) (2010) Prehospital trauma life support manual, 7th edn. Military Version, Mosby JEMS, Elsevier, St. Louis, MO
Butler FK, Hagmann J, Butler EG (1996) Tactical combat casualty care in special operations. Mil Med 161:1
Dickey N, Jenkins D, Butler F (2011) Tactical evacuation care improvements within the Department of Defense. Defense Health Board Memo, 8 Aug 2011
Mabry R (2011) OEF MEDEVAC and enroute care director after-action report, 7 Feb 2011

Casualty and Resource Alignment

▶ Rationing Hospital Resources During Mass Casualty Disasters
▶ Triage: Ethics in the Field

Casualty Evacuation

▶ CASEVAC

Catastrophe Intervention – Interference – Involvement

▶ Crisis Intervention

Cathartics

▶ Bowel Active Agents in the ICU

Catheter Associated Urinary Tract Infection

Dima Danovich[1] and Khanjan H. Nagarsheth[2]
[1]Department of General Surgery, Staten Island University Hospital, Staten Island, NY, USA
[2]R Adams Cowley Shock Trauma Center, University of Maryland School of Medicine, Baltimore, MD, USA

Synonyms

Pyelonephritis; Urinary retention; Urinary tract infection; UTI

Definition

An infection of the urinary tract in a patient who has had an indwelling urinary catheter for a minimum two days or has had a catheter recently removed that was present for 2 days.

Preexisting Condition

Of the 1.7 million healthcare-associated infections that occur annually in the USA, urinary tract infection (UTI) is by far the most common. These infections account for up to 32 %, or 900,000 patients infected (Klevens et al. 2007). Of these infections, approximately 80 % are associated with indwelling urinary catheters (Conway et al. 2012). These are referred to as catheter-associated urinary tract infections (CAUTI).

Application

Diagnosis

According to the Infectious Disease Society of America (ISDA), the following are required for diagnosis of a CAUTI:

1. Presence of an indwelling urinary catheter for more than 2 calendar days with either fever or suprapubic/costovertebral tenderness and a positive urine culture with less than two species of microorganisms. This continues to apply even if the catheter was removed in the last 24 h and there is no other likely cause.
2. Presence of an indwelling catheter for more than 2 calendar days with fever, suprapubic tenderness, and a positive dipstick for nitrite and leukocyte esterase, or pyuria, or positive urine gram stain. This also continues to apply even if the catheter was removed within the last 24 h (Hooton et al. 2010).

Microbiology

In the hospital environment, the spectrum of pathogens that cause UTI is slightly different from those in the community. The most prevalent, just as in community acquired infections, is

E. coli, making up 47 % of infections. The next most common pathogens are *Enterococcus spp.* (13 %), *Klebsiella spp.* (11 %), and *Pseudomonas aeruginosa* (8 %). Together, they make up almost 80 % of hospital-acquired UTI causes. The remaining 20 % are a variety of other species with very low incidences (Gordon and Jones 2003).

Causes and Prevention

Inappropriate use and extended length of urinary catheterization are the most frequent causes of CAUTI. Therefore, optimizing the use and monitoring of catheterization make these infections highly preventable and can significantly decrease the incidence and morbidity associated with them (Gould et al. 2010). Recent studies have found that a single episode of catheter-associated asymptomatic bacteria and a single episode of CAUTI cost an addition of $589 and $676, respectively. If CAUTI leads to bacteremia, this adds an additional cost of $2836 (Tambyah et al. 2002).

The National Institute of Health has approved guidelines concerning the appropriate indications for using an indwelling urinary catheter. Patients who require a urinary catheter include those with urinary retention, those who need close monitoring or intake and output and perioperatively in those who are undergoing long procedures. Other indications include use to assist in healing of perineal or sacral wounds in incontinent patients, but these are special circumstances where alternatives, such as condom catheters in males, should also be considered (Conway et al. 2012).

Even when urinary catheters are used for appropriate indications, best practice dictates expedient removal, when possible. Intraoperative catheters should be used only as necessary instead of routinely and discontinued within 24 h of the end time of operation.

When inserting a catheter, the smallest diameter possible should be used to avoid trauma to the urethra, which can serve as an entry point for infection. Sterile equipment and aseptic technique should be employed upon insertion, and only personnel trained in aseptic technique should participate in catheter insertion. Antiseptic lubricants have shown to be unnecessary for insertion, but the use of antiseptic agents versus sterile water to clean the urethral meatus prior to insertion remains a question that has yet to be answered. Lastly, catheters should be secured after insertion to prevent movement and trauma to the urethra from traction (Gould et al. 2010).

When maintaining a catheter, it is recommended to use a sterile drainage system and most guidelines recommend using a preconnected system with sealed junctions. If the drainage system becomes inadvertently disconnected, the entire apparatus, including the indwelling catheter, must be removed and replaced with a new one using aseptic technique. The drainage bag must be kept below the level of the bladder to prevent backflow, and routine irrigation, without indication, should be avoided (Conway et al. 2012).

Due to the preventable nature of CAUTI, many hospitals in the USA have put in place systems of quality assurance and close monitoring of catheter insertion and maintenance. These systems include urinary catheter removal prompts or reminders, nurse-initiated catheter discontinuation protocols, bedside ultrasound monitoring, and intermittent catheterization. With these methods in place, an annual decrease in CAUTI rates has been observed nationwide. There has been a 6 % decrease in CAUTI from 2009 to 2010, and some states report an even more substantial decrease, such as Michigan with a 25 % decrease (Saint et al. 2013).

Treatment

Two of the most pressing questions when it comes to treatment of CAUTI include duration of therapy and the use of prophylactic antibiotics immediately after catheter removal. In terms of duration, it has been shown that the appropriate course of antibiotics is somewhere between 3 and 10 days, depending on how long the catheter had been in place. More research needs to be done in the area of prophylaxis as no definitive evidence exists. What evidence does support is changing of a long-term catheter prior to beginning treatment for a CAUTI, as this will remove a possible nidus for infection (Traunter 2010).

Cross-References

▶ Acute Kidney Injury
▶ Bladder Incontinence
▶ Catheter-Related Infections
▶ Sepsis, General Mechanism of
▶ Sepsis, Treatment of
▶ Urinoma

References

Conway LJ, Pogorzelska M, Larson E, Stone PW (2012) Adoption of policies to prevent catheter-associated urinary tract infections in United States intensive care units. Am J Infect Control 40:705–710

Gordon KA, Jones RN (2003) SENTRY participant groups (Europe, Latin America, North America). Susceptibility patterns of orally administered antimicrobials among urinary tract infection pathogens from hospitalized patients in North America: comparison report to Europe and Latin America. Results from the SENTRY Antimicrobial Surveillance Program (2000). Diagn Microbiol Infect Dis 45:295–301

Gould CV, Umscheid CA, Agarwal RK, Kuntz G, Pegues DA (2010) Guideline for prevention of catheter-associated urinary tract infections 2009. Infect Control Hosp Epidemiol 31(4):319–326

Hooton TM, Bradley SF, Cardenas DD et al (2010) Diagnosis, prevention, and treatment of catheter-associated urinary tract infections in adults: 2009 international clinical practice guidelines from the infectious disease society of America. Clin Infect Dis 50:625–663

Klevens RM, Edward JR et al (2007) Estimating health care-associated infections and deaths in U.S. hospitals, 2002. Public Health Rep 122:160–166

Saint S, Greene MT, Kowalski CP, Watson SR, Hofer TP, Krein SL (2013) Preventing catheter associated urinary tract infection in the United States: a national comparative study. JAMA Intern Med 173:874–879

Tambyah PA, Knasinski V, Maki DG (2002) The direct costs of nosocomial catheter-associated urinary tract infection in the era of managed care. Infect Control Hosp Epidemiol 23:27–31

Traunter BW (2010) Management of catheter-associated urinary tract infection (CAUTI). Curr Opin Infect Dis 23(1):76–82

Catheter-Related Blood Stream Infection (CRBSI)

▶ Catheter-Related Infections
▶ Central Line Associated Blood Stream Infection

Catheter-Related Infections

Shannon Goddard
Sunnybrook Health Sciences Centre,
University of Toronto, Toronto, ON, Canada

Synonyms

Catheter-related blood stream infection (CRBSI); Central line infection; Central venous catheter infections; Line infections

Definition

Catheter-related bloodstream infection (CRBSI) refers to an infection caused by an intravascular catheter with positive blood cultures (either bacteria or fungi). *Catheter colonization* refers to culture growth of an organism from a segment of the catheter without bloodstream infection. *Exit site infection* refers to growth of an organism around the site of skin entry of a catheter and may or may not be associated with clinical evidence of infection. A *tunnel infection* is an infection at least 2 cm from the skin site and may occur with bloodstream infection. A *pocket infection* is a local infection with a collection of infected fluid in the soft tissue around the catheter (Mermel et al. 2001).

Preexisting Condition

In the ICU, patients may have venous or arterial catheters. Venous catheters include multi-lumen catheters, dual-lumen dialysis catheters, and introducer sheaths, which may be used as conduits for pulmonary artery catheters or pacemakers or alone as resuscitation lines. These catheters function for infusions of medications, fluids and blood products, and most can be used to transduce pressures. Arterial catheters are largely used for monitoring in the ICU, although may be used occasionally as access ports for interventional procedures, such as embolizations.

Occasionally, these lines are tunneled, where the catheter skin entry site is remote from the entry site to the vessel. Tunneled lines are uncommonly placed in the ICU, although patients may come to the ICU with them.

Infections associated with vascular catheters in the intensive care unit (ICU) are common. However, with the introduction of clinical evidence and best practice guidelines around introduction and maintenance, rates have recently declined (Daniels and Frei 2012). Although any bacterial or fungal organism can cause a CRBSI, certain organisms are more common. Skin flora are the most common; they include coagulase-negative staphylococci, *S. aureus*, gram-negative bacilli, and enterococci (Pittet et al. 1994). *Candida albicans* is the most common fungal infection. The specific gram-negative species generally depend on hospital-specific colonization profiles and patient length of stay.

Catheter infections are significant; they are associated with increased mortality, increased hospital length of stay, and increased cost. Although any organism can cause serious infection, *S. aureus* and candida infections are the most virulent; they are the most likely to lead to metastatic seeding (e.g., endocarditis, endophthalmitis) and are associated with the highest mortality.

Application

Diagnosis of Catheter-Related Infections

The diagnosis of a CRBSI is based on microbiologic testing; clinical findings alone (e.g., fever) are nonspecific. Cultures should be drawn from both the catheter and from a peripheral site; a negative catheter culture helps to exclude a catheter infection. Quantitative cultures are preferred to qualitative cultures in the diagnosis of a CRBSI because of increased specificity but are not available at all hospitals. The details of microbiologic techniques are beyond the scope of this chapter; clinicians should familiarize themselves with techniques at their hospitals and seek microbiologic or infectious disease consultation when uncertainty exists.

Specific infections may require further investigation, beyond establishing bacteremia or fungemia. For example, when a diagnosis is made of an *S. aureus* infection, the clinician should rule out infective endocarditis with transesophageal echocardiography. Similarly, candida infections should be investigated with echocardiography and an ophthalmic examination, because of the potential for endophthalmitis.

Management

Management of any CRBSI generally focuses on two key principles; catheter removal and appropriate antimicrobial therapy. In addition, "complicated" infections require consideration of additional management. A complicated infection is one involving an abscess, a remote focus (e.g., endocarditis, ophthalmitis, splenic or liver abscess, osteomyelitis), or septic thrombosis. Complicated infections may require surgical management, image guided or other drainage, and usually require prolonged antibiotic therapy.

Line removal is the cornerstone of therapy for all organisms, except coagulase-negative staphylococcus, in which case the line can usually be salvaged with appropriate antimicrobial therapy. For all other established infections, or when infection is highly suspected in a patient who is systemically unwell or unstable, the line should be promptly removed and replaced if still necessary. Line change over a guidewire is not recommended when treating infection.

Empiric therapy before the organism is known should always include coverage for *S. aureus* infection, because of high morbidity and mortality associated with this pathogen. The clinician should also consider common organisms in his/her own unit when making a decision about empiric antimicrobial coverage. If *S. aureus* methicillin-resistance is common in the unit, the clinician should include vancomycin in empiric coverage. Although candida infections are also quite virulent, empiric therapy without microbiologic evidence is not usually recommended because of low prevalence.

Specific antibiotics of choice, dose, and duration of therapy depend on the infecting organism, the resistance profile, and on patient characteristics (e.g., organ failure, allergies). Common organisms and sample treatment regimes are shown in Table 1. Management of an immunocompromised patient (e.g., neutropenia) may require consultation by an infectious diseases specialist or a medical microbiologist.

Prevention of Catheter-Related Infections

Prevention of CRBSI is the most effective strategy to reduce morbidity. Detailed guidelines exist to guide clinicians on the insertion and maintenance of intravascular catheters; key interventions will be reviewed in detail in this section (O'Grady et al. 2011). Prevention can be highly effective; in a large prospective cohort study of 108 intensive care units in Michigan, Pronovost et al. showed that implementation of five key evidence-based maneuvers led to a significant reduction in catheter-related infections (Pronovost et al. 2006). Furthermore, recent data indicate a significant decreased in CRBSI in the United States coincident with guidelines on insertion and maintenance (Daniels and Frei 2012).

Insertion of the Catheter

In Pronovost et al.'s study, a bundle of insertion techniques included handwashing prior to insertion, skin preparation with chlorhexidine, full barrier precautions, avoidance of the femoral site, and prompt removal of unnecessary catheters (Pronovost et al. 2006). These techniques should be closely followed, although avoidance of the femoral site of insertion may not always be possible. The operator should choose the most appropriate line site for the patient, taking into account expertise, patient-specific risk of complications, and indication for the line. For example, in a patient on with high ventilation requirements, one might choose not to use the subclavian site because of pneumothorax risk. In one randomized trial, the subclavian site had a lower risk of infections than the femoral site (19.8 % vs. 4.5 %, $p < 0.001$), when both were inserted using maximal barrier precautions (Merrer et al. 2001). In a large cohort study, the femoral site was inferior to all other sites, although the result was not statistically

Catheter-Related Infections, Table 1 Antimicrobial regimens by organism

Infecting organism	Pharmacologic regimen	Duration of therapy (for usual infections)[a]
S. aureus, uncomplicated[b]	Empiric therapy with vancomycin until sensitivity established.	14 days after CVC removal
	Synthetic penicillin (e.g., cloxacillin) preferred if sensitive organism. First-generation cephalosporin also acceptable. If MRSA, vancomycin is the agent of choice	
S. aureus, complicated	Same as above	4–8 weeks, depending on complication and source control. Consultation with infectious disease specialist recommended
Coagulase-negative staphylococcus	Vancomycin as empiric therapy and for most isolates. If sensitive, change to synthetic penicillin	7 days
Gram-negative bacilli	Empiric therapy as dictated by local resistance profiles should include an agent with activity against pseudomonas	14 days
Candida spp.	Fluconazole or an echinocandin (e.g., caspofungin)	14 days after last positive blood culture

[a]For infections with unusual characteristics (e.g., persistent or recurrent bacteremia, metastatic foci, unusual organisms), consideration should be given to infectious disease or medical microbiology consultation
[b]Uncomplicated S. aureus infectious are those with a negative transesophageal echocardiogram and no other identified or suspected metastatic focus of infection

significant (Goetz et al. 1998). If a clinician must insert a line that does not follow adherence to this protocol (e.g., during a resuscitation), the line should be changed as soon as possible.

Other evidence also supports the use of a catheter with the minimum required number or lumens (Clark-Christoff et al. 1992). One randomized trial in patients on total parenteral nutrition supports this practice; otherwise, evidence is largely observational and may be confounded by severity of illness (Early et al. 1990; Yeung et al. 1988). Although it may seem self-evident, it should be specifically stated that the clinician should only insert a central venous catheter when it is truly indicated and should remove it promptly when it is no longer necessary. Central catheters should not be used when peripheral intravenous catheters would be adequate, because of higher risk of infectious complications.

Catheter Maintenance

The catheter insertion site should be dressed with either a transparent cling dressing or with sterile gauze. A Cochrane review found a higher risk of infection with transparent dressings (Webster et al. 2011), but the quality of studies was very low and current recommendations support either practice (O'Grady et al. 2011). Dressings should be changed either every 7 days (transparent dressings) or every 2 days (gauze dressings) and the site examined at every change (O'Grady et al. 2011). Catheters should not be changed prophylactically or for fever, but should be changed if infection is suspected or confirmed. Prophylactic topical or systemic antibiotics are not recommended.

In summary, catheter-related infections are common, although incidence is decreasing in the United States. Prevention should be the focus of efforts to reduce morbidity from catheter-related infections, both at the time of insertion and while the catheter is in place. When these precautions are taken, infection rates decrease significantly. Management should focus on catheter removal and appropriate antimicrobial therapy. Treatment of complicated infections or infections in immunocompromised patients should involve specialty consultation with infectious diseases or medical microbiology.

Cross-References

▶ Antibiotic Therapy
▶ Central Line Associated Blood Stream Infection
▶ Fungal Infections
▶ Infection Control

References

Clark-Christoff N, Watters VA, Sparks W, Snyder P, Grant JP (1992) Use of triple-lumen subclavian catheters for administration of total parenteral nutrition. JPEN J Parenter Enteral Nutr 16(5):403–407

Daniels KR, Frei CR (2012) The United States' progress toward eliminating catheter-related bloodstream infections: Incidence, mortality, and hospital length of stay from 1996 to 2008. Am J Infect Control 41:118–121

Early TF, Gregory RT, Wheeler JR, Snyder SO Jr, Gayle RG (1990) Increased infection rate in double-lumen versus single-lumen Hickman catheters in cancer patients. South Med J 83(1):34–36

Goetz AM, Wagener MM, Miller JM, Muder RR (1998) Risk of infection due to central venous catheters: effect of site of placement and catheter type. Infect Control Hosp Epidemiol 19(11):842–845

Mermel LA, Farr BM, Sherertz RJ, Raad II, O'Grady N, Harris JS, Craven DE, Infectious Diseases Society of A, American College of Critical Care M, Society for Healthcare Epidemiology of A (2001) Guidelines for the management of intravascular catheter-related infections. Clin Infect Dis 32(9):1249–1272

Merrer J, De Jonghe B, Golliot F, Lefrant JY, Raffy B, Barre E, Rigaud JP, Casciani D, Misset B, Bosquet C et al. (2001) Complications of femoral and subclavian venous catheterization in critically ill patients: a randomized controlled trial. JAMA 286(6):700–707

O'Grady NP, Alexander M, Burns LA, Dellinger EP, Garland J, Heard SO, Lipsett PA, Masur H, Mermel LA, Pearson ML et al. (2011) Guidelines for the prevention of intravascular catheter-related infections. Am J Infect Control 39(4 Suppl 1):S1–S34

Pittet D, Tarara D, Wenzel RP (1994) Nosocomial bloodstream infection in critically ill patients. Excess length of stay, extra costs, and attributable mortality. JAMA 271(20):1598–1601

Pronovost P, Needham D, Berenholtz S, Sinopoli D, Chu H, Cosgrove S, Sexton B, Hyzy R, Welsh R, Roth G et al. (2006) An intervention to decrease catheter-related bloodstream infections in the ICU [Erratum appears in N Engl J Med. 2007 Jun 21;356(25):2660]. New Engl J Med 355(26):2725–2732

Webster J, Gillies D, O'Riordan E, Sherriff KL, Rickard CM (2011) Cochrane Database Syst Rev (11). Art No.: 10.1002/14651858.CD003827.pub2.

Yeung C, May J, Hughes R (1988) Infection rate for single lumen v triple lumen subclavian catheters. Infect Control Hosp Epidemiol 9(4):154–158

Cave-In Syndrome

▶ Crush Syndrome

Cavitation

Craig D. Silverton[1] and Paul Dougherty[2]
[1]Department of Orthopedic Surgery, Henry Ford Hospital, Detroit, MI, USA
[2]Department of Orthopedic Surgery, University of Michigan, Ann Arbor, MI, USA

Synonyms

High powered; High velocity; Muzzle velocity; Permanent cavity; Tumble; Yaw

Definition

During the nineteenth century, wound ballistics investigators noticed that sometimes remote effects, away from a bullets path, occurred in tissue. Investigators developed methodology to study wound ballistics and found that the remote effects were due to the effects of what we called temporary cavity.

Originally derived from the marine industry, cavitation describes the inefficient air (bubbling) that develops around a low-pressure area surrounding the propeller. This cavitation prevents the propeller from capturing the consistency of the water, and although the propeller increases in revolutions, the boat will slow in speed.

Woodruff, in 1898, adopted this term in describing the effects of temporary cavity that he saw in tissue.

In the field of wound ballistics, there are three potential mechanisms of injury: the permanent cavity and the temporary cavity. There is also a pressure wave or shock wave that is antecedent to the bullet in the tissue.

The temporary cavity is a stretching of the soft tissues surrounding the permanent cavity. This happens very quickly (5–10 mil/s). The size of this area of stretching is related to several factors: speed of the projectile, yaw, as well as fragmentation. Typically, low-velocity bullets (<1,000 fps, i.e., handguns) have a small temporary cavity, whereas high-velocity bullets (>2,500 fps, i.e., military and hunting rifles) have a larger temporary cavity. Velocity however is not the sole determinant of the size of the temporary cavity. Vintage military rifles with lower velocities (<1,500 fps) can have devastating temporary and permanent cavities. In the case of most high-velocity bullets, the temporary cavity may be up to 10 times the size of the permanent cavity. Some describe this temporary cavity as a "splash" similar to a diver entering the water. The damage imparted by the temporary cavity is related to the location of nonelastic structures (Fackler 1984). The lungs, muscles, and other "stretchable" soft tissues may have minimal if any injury from the temporary cavity, whereas solid nonelastic structures like the liver, kidneys, and spleen may have devastating consequences. Most nerves and blood vessels may not be permanently injured by the stretch of this temporary cavity. Although bone is nonelastic, the temporary cavity rarely is the cause of a long-bone fracture. These fractures associated with bullet wounds are usually the result of the permanent cavity and are in the direct path of the bullet or projectile (Fig. 1).

In discussing the various wound channels produced by handguns and rifles, the bullet composition is a key factor to understand. Vintage military bullets were soft lead and slow by today's standards and produced large wound channels. The Hague Convention of

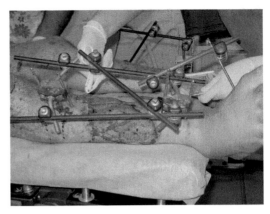

Cavitation, Fig. 1 Use of external fixation allows fracture stabilization while allowing treatment of soft tissue wounds

1899 and subsequently the Geneva Convention forbade the use of expanding deformable bullets in wartime. Therefore, the bullet composition in modern military weapons consists of a copper-jacketed cover over the lead or steel core. This theoretically prevents the "mushrooming" seen with vintage military non-jacketed lead bullets. However, once the jacketed bullets fragment in the soft tissue as seen with the M16 and 7.62 military rifles, the consequences of the permanent and temporary cavities are impressive (Fackler and Dougherty 1991). Hunting rifles are not subject to this declaration and thus civilian high-velocity wounds may impart a slightly different wounding channel based on bullet composition. A non-jacketed lead bullet however is limited to <2,000 ft/s due to the heat generated and the possibility of the lead melting.

Cross-References

▶ Ballistics
▶ Debridement
▶ Explosion
▶ Fragment Injury
▶ High-Velocity
▶ Mortars
▶ Spalling

References

Fackler ML (1984) Bullet fragmentation: a major cause of tissue disruption. J Trauma 24(1):35–39

Fackler ML, Dougherty PJ (1991) Theodor Kocher and the Scientific Foundation of Wound Ballistics. Surg Gynecol Obstet 172:153–160

Celiac Artery Injury

▶ Abdominal Major Vascular Injury, Anesthesia for

Centenarian Trauma

▶ Elderly Trauma, Anesthetic Considerations for

Central Catheters

▶ Monitoring of Trauma Patients During Anesthesia

Central Cord Syndrome

MariaLisa Itzoe and Daniel M. Sciubba
Department of Neurosurgery, The Johns Hopkins University School of Medicine, Baltimore, MD, USA

Definition

First described by Schneider in 1954, central cord syndrome (CCS) is the most common type of incomplete spinal cord injury (Schneider et al. 1954). It usually occurs when individuals suffering from long-term degeneration of the cervical spine, associated with changes in vertebral bodies and intervertebral disks (cervical spondylosis),

sustain a hyperextension injury. Nearly 50% of patients with CCS also suffer from congenital or degenerative spinal stenosis (Aarabi et al. 2008), which can lead to fracture dislocation and compression fractures. While such pathophysiology is most commonly seen in older patients who sustain falls, CCS can affect people of any age (Schneider et al. 1954). In younger patients, CCS is generally a result of sports-related trauma (Hayes and Kakulas 1997). MRI and pathophysiological studies suggest that CCS is primarily a white matter injury with relative preservation of gray matter as the central part of the spinal cord is a vascular watershed zone, making this area more susceptible to edematous injury. Intramedullary hemorrhage can also occur (Quencer et al. 1992). CCS may be caused by bleeding into the central part of the cord, disk compression, bone fragment or syrinx formation.

CCS is typically associated with symmetrical bilateral injury and it affects upper extremities more severely than lower extremities (Nowak et al. 2009). While motor function is greatly compromised, the effect of injury on sensory function is variable among patients and sensation may be retained in some cases (Lenehan et al. 2009). Sacral sensation is usually preserved. More than half of patients affected by CCS demonstrate spontaneous recovery from motor weakness over time; however, in more extreme cases, lack of manual dexterity, neuropathic pain, spasticity, bladder dysfunction, and imbalance of gait can significantly diminish a patient's quality of life and functional independence (Aarabi et al. 2008). The outcomes related to central cord syndrome vary. Evidence suggests that surgical decompression in select patients improves neurologic outcomes, although there is a debate in the literature on the indications for surgery (Fong and Eismont 2007; Bosch et al. 1971; Bose et al. 1984; Chen et al. 1997).

Cross-References

▶ Fractures

References

Aarabi B, Koltz M, Ibrahimi D (2008) Hyperextension cervical spine injuries and traumatic central cord syndrome. Neurosurg Focus 25(5):E9

Bosch A, Stauffer ES, Nickel VL (1971) Incomplete traumatic quadriplegia. A ten-year review. JAMA 216(3):473–478

Bose B, Northrup BE, Osterholm JL, Cotler JM, DiTunno JF (1984) Reanalysis of central cervical cord injury management. Neurosurgery 15(3):367–372

Chen TY, Lee ST, Lui TN, Wong CW, Yeh YS, Tzaan WC, Hung SY (1997) Efficacy of surgical treatment in traumatic central cord syndrome. Surg Neurol 48(5):435–440 discussion 441

Fong W, Eismont FJ (2007) Controversies in the treatment of central cord injuries. Semin Spine Surg 19:260–271

Hayes KC, Kakulas BA (1997) Neuropathology of human spinal cord injury sustained in sports-related activities. J Neurotrauma 14(4):235–248

Lenehan B, Street J, O'Toole P, Siddiqui A, Poynton A (2009) Central cord syndrome in Ireland: the effect of age on clinical outcome. Eur Spine J 18(10):1458–1463

Nowak DD, Lee JK, Gelb DE, Poelstra KA, Ludwig SC (2009) Central cord syndrome. J Am Acad Orthop Surg 17(12):756–765

Quencer RM, Bunge RP, Egnor M, Green BA, Puckett W, Naidich TP, Post MJ, Norenberg M (1992) Acute traumatic central cord syndrome: MRI-pathological correlations. Neuroradiology 34(2):85–94

Schneider RC, Cherry G, Pantek H (1954) The syndrome of acute central cervical spinal cord injury; with special reference to the mechanisms involved in hyperextension injuries of cervical spine. J Neurosurg 11(6):546–577

Central Line Associated Blood Stream Infection

Lindsay O'Meara[1] and Khanjan H. Nagarsheth[2]
[1]Shock Trauma Center, University of Maryland Medical Center, Baltimore, MD, USA
[2]R Adams Cowley Shock Trauma Center, University of Maryland School of Medicine, Baltimore, MD, USA

Synonyms

Catheter-related blood stream infection (CRBSI); Central line infection; Central venous catheter infection

Definition

The Center for Disease and Control and Prevention (CDC) recognizes that central line associated blood stream infection (CLABSI) is an increasing problem within the healthcare system. Approximately 1/3 of all bloodstream infections reported in the United States each year are due to catheter-related blood stream infections (CRBSIs) within the intensive care unit (ICU). Many institutions have made attempts to improve patient outcomes and reduce healthcare costs related to CLABSI. It was found that the average CRBSI increased a patient's length of hospitalization by 12 days and cost approximately $18,000 (Jeong et al. 2013). CLABSIs are defined by the CDC as a primary blood stream infection (BSI) in patients who have had a central venous catheter placed 48 h prior to developing a BSI and is not bloodstream related to another source of infection, whereas a CRBSI is confirmed when synchronous bloodstream and central venous catheter tip cultures demonstrate the same colonization of identified organisms (O'Connor et al. 2013).

Preexisting Condition

Many trauma patients sustain serious injuries and require immediate, life-saving resuscitation. Unstable trauma patients also often require the use of vasoactives to help assist with hemodynamic stability. In order to help facilitate resuscitation, emergent central venous catheters and arterial catheters are placed in potentially a clean, as opposed to sterile environment. The most likely emergent site for central venous catheter (CVC) placement is the femoral vein, which has been shown to have the highest incidence of CLABSI (O'Connor et al. 2013). The site at which the catheter is placed influences the risk of developing a CLABSI. The density of body flora plays a significant role in the development of a CVC infection. Obese patients were found to have an even higher incidence of femoral related CLABSI as compared to those with a normal body mass index (Center for Disease and Control, 2011).

Critically ill trauma patients often have prolonged ICU stays and require the need for long-term CVC access with multiple lumens. The duration that a CVC is left in place has been shown to correlate with the development of a blood stream infection. Studies have shown that the average length from the time of catheter insertion to the development of a BSI was approximately 11 days (Jeong et al. 2013). CRBSI were shown to be more prevalent with 3 or 4 lm as compared to 2 lm. Central venous catheters with just 2 lm were found to have an infection rate similar to that of a tunneled line, which was found to have the lowest incidence of CRBSI (O'Connor et al. 2013). Severe trauma patients often require operative intervention such as an exploratory laparotomy, which in itself has not shown to increase the risk of developing a CLABSI. However, a retrospective cohort study performed by Lissauer and colleagues demonstrated that patients requiring reopening of a recent laparotomy had a statistically significant development of a CLABSI compared to those who did not require further operative intervention past their initial surgical procedure (Lissauer et al. 2011).

Application

In an effort to help reduce CLABSI and improve outcomes, the CDC developed guidelines for the prevention of intravascular catheter-related infections (Center for Disease and Control, 2011). These guidelines were developed for healthcare personnel who are responsible for inserting CVC as well as for those who are responsible for infection control in the hospital, outpatient, and home health settings. The guidelines to help reduce CLABSI are based on 5 strategies: education and training for those who insert and maintain CVCs, using maximal sterile barrier precautions, using chlorhexidine skin preparation with alcohol for antisepsis, avoiding routine replacement of CVC to avoid infections, and using antiseptic-/antibiotic-impregnated short-term CVC and chlorhexidine-impregnated sponge dressings if the rate of infection is not

decreasing despite strict adherence to the other strategies listed (Center for Disease and Control 2011). If femoral venous catheters are placed, even under strict adherence to the CDC guidelines, the line should be changed as soon as possible to either a subclavian or internal jugular vein site. Once the CVC is no longer indicated, it should be removed as soon as possible.

Conclusion

The severity of injuries found in trauma patients places them at an increased risk for developing a CLABSI. Independent factors that have been shown to increase the risk of CLABSI include poor patient hygiene, leading to development of dense body flora, emergent central venous access, and to an extent the severity of the illness that can determine the length that a catheter may need to stay in place (O'Connor et al. 2013). It is important that healthcare providers adhere to the CDC guidelines to help reduce the risk of CLABSI and improve outcomes and reduce cost.

Cross-References

▶ Catheter-Related Infections

References

Grady NP, Alexander M, Burns LA, Dellinger EP et al. Centers for Disease control and prevention. 2011 Guidelines for the prevention of intravacular Catheter-Related infections. 1 April 2011. Available at http://www.cdc.gov/hicpac/BSI/BSI-guidelines-2011.html. Accessed 1 march 2013

Jeong I, Park S, Lee J, et al (2013) Effect of central line bundle on central line-assoicated bloodstream infections in intensive care units. Am J Infect Control 41(8):1–7

Lissauer M, Leekha S, Preas M et al (2011) Risk factors for central line-associated bloodstream infections in the era of best practice. J Trauma 72(5):1174–1180

O'Connor A, Hanly A, Francis E et al (2013) Catheter associated blood stream infections in patients receiving parenteral nutrition: a prospective study of 850 patients. J Clin Med Res 5(1):18–21

Central Line Infection

▶ Catheter-Related Infections
▶ Central Line Associated Blood Stream Infection

Central Pain

▶ Phantom Limb Pain

Central Venous Catheter Infection

▶ Central Line Associated Blood Stream Infection

Central Venous Catheter Infections

▶ Catheter-Related Infections

Cerebral Blood Flow

▶ Neurotrauma, Pharmacological Considerations

Cerebral Concussion

▶ Traumatic Brain Injury, Concussion

Cerebral Contusion

▶ Neurotrauma, Anesthesia Management
▶ Traumatic Brain Injury, Intensive Care Unit Management

Cerebral Hemorrhage

▶ Neurotrauma, Anesthesia Management

Cerebral Perfusion Pressure

▶ Traumatic Brain Injury, Intensive Care Unit Management

Cerebral Salt Wasting

Ani Aydin[1] and Khanjan H. Nagarsheth[2]
[1]Shock Trauma Center, University of Maryland Medical Center, Baltimore, MD, USA
[2]R Adams Cowley Shock Trauma Center, University of Maryland School of Medicine, Baltimore, MD, USA

Synonyms

Salt wasting nephropathy

Definition

Cerebral salt wasting (CSW) was first described by Peters et al. in 1950 as a cerebral condition that leads to the inability of the kidneys to conserve salt (Peters et al. 1950). With the newly described syndrome of inappropriate antidiuretic hormone (SIADH) in 1957, CSW was clumped with this new condition (Uygun et al. 1996). While CSW is often misdiagnosed as SIADH, many argue that it is a separate clinical entity and requires a different treatment regimen (Palmer 2003; Yee et al. 2010).

Preexisting Condition

To better understand this syndrome, we will begin with a review of the causes of hyponatremia. Causes of low plasma sodium concentration, or hyponatremia, can be differentiated first by the plasma osmolality, followed by the plasma volume status (Adrogue and Madias 2000). Hypertonic hyponatremia is due to an excess of osmotically active agents in the plasma, such as glucose, which draw water out of cells, thereby diluting the serum plasma concentration (Adrogue and Madias 2000). Pseudohyponatremia, or normo-osmolar hyponatremia, is due to an elevation in proteins or lipids in the plasma, which leads to a relative decrease in the water and therefore solute concentration of the plasma; the absolute sodium concentration in plasma is, however, normal (Adrogue and Madias 2000).

The causes of hypotonic hyponatremia can be further differentiated based on the patient's plasma volume status (Adrogue and Madias 2000). Hypervolemic hypotonic hyponatremia is due to conditions such as congestive heart failure, in which the patient can be total body volume overloaded, with relative intravascular volume depletion (Adrogue and Madias 2000). Euvolemic hypotonic hyponatremia is due to conditions such as hypothyroidism, secondary adrenal failure, low salt diet, polydipsia, and SIADH (Adrogue and Madias 2000).

Application

Hypovolemic hypotonic hyponatremia can be due to extra-renal causes such as hemorrhage (Adrogue and Madias 2000). In addition, renally mediated causes such as diuretic use, primary adrenal failure, and cerebral salt wasting are possible (Adrogue and Madias 2000).

Many authors over the last 50 years have argued that the condition known as CSW, or salt wasting nephropathy, is not a distinct entity; rather, it is a result of inappropriate treatment of SIADH (Harrigan 2001). More specifically, it occurs during saline solution infusion treatment of SIADH (Ellison and Berl 2007). If the incorrect concentration of the sodium chloride solution is chosen, the salt content in the solution will be appropriate exceeded in a patient with SIADH, drawing excess water into the urine and leading to a relative dehydration (Adrogue and Madias 2000).

However, more recently, some authors have argued that CSW is a distinct entity. Therefore, it is important to understand the similarities and distinctions between CSW and SIADH. Both CSW and SIADH occur in patients with cerebral insults with hypotonic hyponatremia (Yee et al. 2010). Both conditions present with high urine osmolality ($\geq$100 mOsm/kg urine) and high urine sodium ($\geq$40 mEq/L urine) (Palmer 2003). The main distinction between these clinical entities is the patient's volume status (Palmer 2003). While SIADH is found in patients who are euvolemic, CSW occurs in those hypovolemic (Palmer 2003). Therefore, in CSW patients can present with signs of dehydration, hypotension, decreased skin turgor, elevated blood urea nitrogen to creatinine ratio, and elevated hematocrit (Palmer 2003).

There is also some overlap in the conditions that can lead to SIADH and CSW. For example, CSW can be due to many disorders of the central nervous system, such as tumors, trauma (epidural, subdural, subarachnoid), infections (meningitis, encephalitis, poliomyelitis), or following surgery (Uygun et al. 1996). Occasionally, CSW and SIADH can coexist in a patient (Uygun et al. 1996).

While the first-line treatment in SIADH is fluid restriction, the primary treatment in CSW is fluid hydration to correct the hypovolemia (Adrogue and Madias 2000). With correction of the dehydration, the stimulus for antidiuretic hormone, or arginine vasopressin, is suppressed, and the hyponatremia resolves. In contrast, inappropriate fluid hydration in SIADH can lead to additional urinary solute excretion and worsen the existing hyponatremic state (Palmer 2003).

In summary, cerebral salt wasting is a clinical syndrome due to a cerebral insult which results in inappropriate renal salt excretion. This entity shares many features with SIADH, and it is often misdiagnosed as such (Harrigan 2001). While some argue that CSW is not a discrete condition, rather results of inappropriate treatment of SIADH, other authors argue that CSW is a separate syndrome that requires a different treatment regimen (Yee et al. 2010). The primary treatment of CSW is hydration, which resolves the hypovolemia and corrects the hyponatremia (Ellison and Berl 2007).

Cross-References

► Head Injury
► Syndrome of Inappropriate Antidiuresis (SIADH)

References

Adrogue HJ, Madias NE (2000) Hyponatremia. NEJM 342:1581–1589
Ellison DH, Berl T (2007) The syndrome of inappropriate antidiuresis. NEJM 356:2064–2074
Harrigan MR (2001) Cerebral salt wasting syndrome. Crit Care Clin 17:125–138
Palmer BF (2003) Hyponatremia in patients with central nervous system disease: SIADH versus CSW. Trends Endocrinol Metab 14:182–187
Peters JP, Welt LG, Sims EA, Orloff J, Neeham J (1950) A salt-wasting syndrome associated with cerebral disease. Trans Assoc Am Physicians 63:57–64
Uygun MA, Ozkal E, Acar O, Erogun U (1996) Cerebral salt wasting syndrome. Neurosurg Rev 19:193–196
Yee AH, Burns JD, Wijdicks EFM (2010) Cerebral salt wasting: pathophysiology, diagnosis, and treatment. Neurosurg Clin N Am 21:339–352

Cerebrospinal Fluid

► Traumatic Brain Injury, Intensive Care Unit Management

Cerebrospinal Fluid Fistula

► Neurotrauma, Management of Cerebrospinal Fluid Leak

Certify

► Credentialing

Cervical Spine Fractures, Indications for Surgery

Mari L. Groves and Daniel M. Sciubba
Department of Neurosurgery, The Johns Hopkins University School of Medicine, Baltimore, MD, USA

Synonyms

Decompression; Instrumented fusion; Stabilization

Definition

Management of cervical spine fractures should consider the need for stability or decompression, and in some cases both. Even patients with unstable fractures can be managed with a range of fixation from traction and orthosis to surgical fusion. The Surgical Timing in Acute Spinal Cord Injury Study (STASCIS) found in a study of 313 patients with acute cervical SCI, 19.8 % of patients undergoing surgical decompression early (mean 14.2 h after injury) had a $>=2$ grade improvement in neurologic function, as assessed by the American Spinal Injury Association (ASIA) score compared to 8.8 % of patients undergoing late surgery (mean 48.3 h after injury) (Fehlings et al. 2012). Neurologic function was assessed at 6-month follow-up. Surgical decompression also plays a role for patients with incomplete neurologic deficit (La Rosa et al. 2004). Patients are typically stratified into those with complete or incomplete spinal cord lesions. In general, surgery is reserved for those patients with incomplete lesions. Patients with a complete cord injury typically do not have improvement of their symptoms despite decompression. However, surgical stabilization can be indicated to allow better post-injury mobilization and rehabilitation. Any correction of spinal deformity can also help prevent worsening cervical kyphosis. These patients may have pulmonary complications secondary to paraparesis and their underlying injury and so should be medically stabilized prior to proceeding to surgery.

Patients who have incomplete cord injuries with compromise of the spinal canal should be considered for immediate decompression. The modified recommendations of Schneider (Schneider et al. 1973) include decompression of those patients with extrinsic compression who, following maximal possible reduction of subluxation, show progression of neurological signs, complete subarachnoid bloc by Queckenstedt test or radiographically, bone fragments or soft tissue encroachment of the spinal canal causing spinal cord compression, compound fracture or penetrating trauma of the spine, non-reducible fracture dislocations from locked facets causing spinal cord compression. They also recommend surgery for decompression of a vital cervical root or in cases of acute anterior spinal cord syndrome. General contraindications to emergent operation include a complete spinal cord injury that presents greater than 24 h after loss of function, a medically unstable patient, and central cord syndrome. Surgery for central cord syndrome has been debated in the literature, and is discussed in a separate entry.

The technical decision to perform an anterior or posterior decompression and/or fusion depends, in large part, on the mechanism of injury. The instrumentation should ideally counteract the instability and bridge the area of failure while bony fusion occurs. Extensive lesions through all three columns of the spine and disrupting both anterior and posterior elements will sometimes require a combined approach.

Posterior immobilization and fusion is the treatment of choice for most flexion injuries. In the absence of injury to the vertebral body or anterior compression of the spinal cord, posterior fixation will address the compromised area. Typical injuries include unilateral or bilateral locked facets, wedge compression fractures, traumatic subluxation, or posterior ligamentous instability. The most common technique is either an open or closed reduction followed by lateral mass screws and rods at the level above and below the injury site.

Anterior approaches are favored for extension injuries in which the posterior elements are typically intact. These include fractures through the vertebral body with or without compression of the anterior neural elements. This approach may also be used in traumatic subluxation cases. Typically a discectomy is insufficient to decompress the bony elements and a corpectomy is performed to remove the fractured and structurally compromised bone as well as removal of any epidural component. A synthetic cage or bone graft is typically placed and augmented with an anterior plate for stabilization and fusion.

Cross-References

▶ Central Cord Syndrome

References

Fehlings MG, Vaccaro A, Wilson JR, Singh A, Cadotte D, Harrop DW, Aarabi B, Shaffrey C, Dvorak M, Fisher C, Arnold P, Massicotte EM, Lewis S, Rampersaud R (2012) Early versus delayed decompression for traumatic cervical spinal cord injury: results of the surgical timing in acute spinal cord injury study (STASCIS). PLoS One 7(2):e32037
La Rosa G, Conti A, Cardali S, Cacciola F, Tomasello F (2004) Does early decompression improve neurological outcome of spinal cord injured patients? Appraisal of the literature using a meta-analytical approach. Spinal Cord 42(9):503–512
Schneider RC, Crosby EC, Russo RH, Gosch HH (1973) Chapter 32. Traumatic spinal cord syndromes and their management. Clin Neurosurg 20:424–492

Cervical Spine Injury

▶ Spinal Cord Injury, Anesthetic Management for

Chance Fracture

▶ Seatbelt Injuries

Chemical Burns

Mary-Margaret Brandt
St. Joseph Mercy Hospital, Ann Arbor, MI, USA

Synonyms

Acid burns; Alkali burns; Burns due to exposure to cleaning agents or petroleum products; Ingestion or inhalation of chemicals

Definition

Chemical burns can be caused by acids, alkalis also called bases, or petroleum products and organic solvents that come into contact with the skin, eyes, or through ingestion. Both acids and bases can be defined as caustics. These chemicals may cause significant tissue damage on contact. The strength of acids and bases is defined by using the pH scale, which ranges from 1 to 14 and is logarithmic. A strong acid has a pH of 1, and a strong base has a pH of 14. A pH of 7 is neutral. Petroleum products include gasoline, kerosene, and other hydrocarbons. In addition to injury to the body surfaces, petroleum products can be absorbed systemically through the skin, eyes, and mucous membranes, causing pulmonary, cardiovascular, neurologic, renal, and hepatic derangements.

As with thermal injuries, clinical signs and symptoms vary depending on the route of exposure and the duration of contact. Additional information regarding the particular substances involved is important to determine the tissue damage and potential therapeutic interventions. In general, acids and bases should not be neutralized because the chemical reaction will result in heat production and additional injury (Taira et al. 2010). Some exposures, such as cement, a base, may present without immediate pain and should be considered in patients with complaints of slow-onset deep pain occurring after exposure to wet cement. This is described further in the heading "Alkalis/Bases" below.

Preexisting Condition

Additional patient history should include the following: the offending agent; its concentration and physical form; pH; route of exposure; time of exposure, including the time of the event as well as the duration of the exposure to the chemical; volume of exposure, for example, immersion versus splash; possibility of coexisting injury(ies), including fractures or lacerations; and timing and extent of irrigation or any other treatment that occurred prior to this evaluation. For children presenting with chemical burns, in addition to a thorough history as described above, the possibility of neglect and/or abuse must be considered.

Physical Examination

If the exposure was by ingestion, the immediate concern is to protect the patient's airway. If there is evidence of airway compromise (e.g., oropharyngeal edema, hoarseness, stridor, difficulty breathing, or use of accessory muscles) or the presence of oral burns, oral edema, or drooling, prompt establishment of a definitive airway is the first priority (Ramasamy and Gumaste 2003). Orotracheal intubation is the preferred route and should be obtained early in order to secure a patent airway before extensive swelling occurs. Hypoxia is a late finding and may indicate the need for a surgical airway, cricothyrotomy/tracheotomy. Evaluation of the esophagus and alimentary tract is important if there was a significant volume ingested (Howell 1986).

If the skin is the route of exposure, specific physical findings to assess the extent of the injury include the area of skin involved, using the rule of nines to estimate total body surface area. The depth of the injury is also important to assess. This may be difficult to determine initially and may not declare itself for 24–48 h. It is important to remove all of the chemical to stop the burning, before trying to determine the size and depth. Also important to assess is the location of the injury; especially concerning are injuries to the hands, face, feet, joints, or genitalia. As in thermal burns, function needs to be maintained in these areas, as much as possible following an injury. This can best be done with optimal initial care.

The presence of circumferential burns is also of urgent concern. The circumferential injury may cause a constricting band of damaged tissue, compromising underlying living tissue resulting in compartment syndrome or ischemia distal to the circumferential injury. In addition to evaluating the all of the patient's skin, there needs to be a high index of suspicion for eye injuries. Liquid chemicals can splash, and powders can be blown or brushed into the eye. It is important to assess initial visual acuity and to irrigate the eye with copious amounts of balanced salt solution to remove all of the chemical. Some suggest checking the pH of the effluent solution when irrigating acid or alkali injuries, and continuing to irrigate the eye(s) until the pH is neutral.

Application

Chemicals That May Cause Burn Injuries

Many large numbers of industrial and commercial products contain potentially toxic concentrations of acids, bases, or other chemicals that can cause burns (Mozingo et al. 1988). Some of the more common products are listed as follows:

Acids

Sulfuric acid is commonly used in toilet bowl cleaners, drain cleaners, metal cleaners, automobile battery fluid, munitions, and fertilizer manufacturing. Concentrations range from 8 % acid to almost pure acid. The concentrated acid is very viscous and denser than water. It also generates significant heat when diluted. These attributes make sulfuric acid an effective drain cleaner. Concentrated sulfuric acid is hygroscopic; it produces dermal injuries not only by direct chemical injury but by dehydration and thermal injury. Nitric acid is commonly used in engraving, metal refining, electroplating, and fertilizer manufacturing.

Hydrofluoric acid is commonly used in rust removers, tire cleaners, tile cleaners, glass etching, dental work, tanning, semiconductors, refrigerant and fertilizer manufacturing, and petroleum refining. This is actually a weak acid, and, in dilute form, it may not cause immediate burning

or pain on contact. Hydrofluoric acid burns require special consideration (Bertolini 1992). Hydrofluoric acid is used in manufacturing as a cleaning agent. These burns should initially be treated as any other burn, with thorough irrigation. Due to the penetrating power of the fluoride ion, specific neutralization procedures are indicated. Fluoride can be neutralized by either calcium or magnesium (Cox and Osgood 1994). For small superficial burns, topical calcium or magnesium gels can be applied. Deeper burns may require subcutaneous injections of calcium gluconate. Hand burns can be treated with subcutaneous injections of calcium, intra-arterial calcium infusions, or intravenous infusions of magnesium. Keeping the hand warm and adequately treating pain will help to increase local circulation and the body's natural supply of calcium and magnesium. These injuries are potentially very serious and must be treated urgently to preserve full function of the patient's hand.

Hydrochloric acid is commonly used in toilet bowl cleaners, metal cleaners, soldering fluxes, dye manufacturing, metal refining, plumbing applications, swimming pool cleaners, and laboratory chemicals.

Hydrochloric acid is also known as muriatic acid and may be used in pool maintenance. Phosphoric acid is commonly used in metal cleaners, rustproofing, disinfectants, detergents, and fertilizer manufacturing. Acetic acid is commonly used in printing, dyes, rayon and hat manufacturing, disinfectants, and hair wave neutralizers. Vinegar is a dilute acetic acid. Formic acid is commonly used in airplane glue, tanning, and cellulose manufacturing. In nature, it is found in the stings and bites of many insects, especially ants.

Alkalis/Bases

Sodium hydroxide (NaOH) and potassium hydroxide (KOH) are used in drain cleaners, oven cleaners, Clinitest tablets, and denture cleaners. They are extremely corrosive. Clinitest tablets contain 45–50 % sodium hydroxide (NaOH) or potassium hydroxide (KOH). Solid or concentrated NaOH or KOH is denser than water and generates significant heat when diluted. Both the heat generated and the alkalinity contribute to burns. Calcium hydroxide also is known as slaked lime. It is used in mortar, plaster, and cement. It is not as caustic as NaOH, KOH, or calcium oxide. Chlorites are the primary chemicals used as bleaches in the United States. Household bleach is alkaline with a pH of 11–12, but it is dilute enough that it is minimally irritating to the skin. More concentrated, industrial strength chlorites may be more damaging to the skin. Sodium and calcium hypochlorite are common ingredients in household bleach and pool chlorinating solution. Pool chlorinators also contain NaOH and have a pH around 13.5, making them very caustic. Household bleach with its pH between 11 and 12 is much less corrosive. Calcium oxide, also known as lime, is the caustic ingredient in cement. It generates heat when diluted with water and can produce a thermal or caustic burn. In cooler climates the quantity of lime may be increased to allow curing of the cement before it freezes. The exposure may occur in someone working on cement installation, without the person initially being aware. The concentration of lime is proportional to the extent of injury as the concentration of caustic material. Ammonia is used in cleaners and detergents. The dilute form is not highly corrosive. Gaseous anhydrous ammonia is used in a number of industrial applications, particularly in fertilizer manufacturing. It is very hygroscopic (has a high affinity for water). It produces injury by desiccation and heat of dilution in addition to causing a chemical burn. It can cause severe skin burns as well as pulmonary injury. Phosphates commonly are used in many types of household detergents and cleaners. Substances include tribasic potassium phosphate, trisodium phosphate, and sodium tripolyphosphates. Silicates include sodium silicate and sodium metasilicate. They are used to replace phosphates in detergents. Dishwashing detergents are alkaline, primarily due to components such as silicates and carbonates. They are moderately corrosive. Sodium carbonate is also used in detergents. It is moderately alkaline, depending on the concentration.

Other Substances

Lithium hydride is used to absorb carbon dioxide in space technology applications. It vigorously reacts with water to generate hydrogen and lithium hydroxide. It can produce thermal and alkaline burns. Household-grade hydrogen peroxide, 3 % concentration, produces minimal skin irritation. Concentrations of 10 % may cause irritation and blanching of the skin. Concentrations of 35 % or more will cause immediate blistering. Hair coloring agents contain persulfates and concentrated solutions of peroxides. Hair straightening agents may contain concentrated alkali. Chemical burns can result if these are not diluted properly or have a prolonged contact time with the scalp. Potassium dichromate and chromic acid are common industrial chemicals used in tanning, waterproofing fabrics, corrosion inhibition, painting, and printing, and they are also used as an oxidizing agent in chemical reactions. Chromates can result in severe skin burns and subsequent systemic toxicity, including renal failure. Potassium permanganate is a strong oxidizing agent that is used in dilute solutions as a disinfectant or sanitizing agent. In dilute solutions, it is minimally irritating to the skin. In concentrated form or pure crystals, it can cause severe burns, ulcerations, and systemic toxicity.

White phosphorus (Barillo et al. 2004) is poisonous and can spontaneously ignite when it comes in contact with air. For this reason, white phosphorus must be stored under water. This chemical is used as an incendiary in the manufacture of munitions, fireworks, and fertilizer. White phosphorus is spontaneously oxidized in air, giving off a yellow flame and a dense white smoke with a garlic odor. After explosions of munitions or fireworks, small particles of phosphorus can become embedded in the skin and continue to smolder. Elemental lithium, sodium, potassium, and magnesium react violently with water, including water on the skin in an exothermic reaction. If these metals are thought to be on the skin of a patient, do not irrigate with water. The water may increase local heat production extending the depth of the injury. The metallic pieces should be removed manually with forceps and placed in a container of mineral oil.

Conclusion

The care of chemical burns relies upon the same principles as those for thermal injuries, stop the burning, wash the wounds with gentle soap and water after removing the burning agent, and provide supportive care. Information about the chemical involved is important for the initial care and subsequent management.

Cross-References

▶ ABCDE of Trauma Care
▶ Escharotomy
▶ Flame Burns

References

Barillo DJ, Cancio LC, Goodwin CW (2004) Treatment of white phosphorus and other chemical burn injuries at one burn center over a 51-year period. Burns 30(5):448–452

Bertolini JC (1992) Hydrofluoric acid: a review of toxicity. J Emerg Med 10(2):163–168

Cox RD, Osgood KA (1994) Evaluation of intravenous magnesium sulfate for the treatment of hydrofluoric acid burns. J Toxicol Clin Toxicol 32(2):123–136

Howell JM (1986) Alkaline ingestions. Ann Emerg Med 15(7):820–825

Mozingo DW, Smith AA, McManus WF et al (1988) Chemical burns. J Trauma 28(5):642–647

Ramasamy K, Gumaste VV (2003) Corrosive ingestion in adults. J Clin Gastroenterol 37(2):119–124

Taira BR, Singer AJ, Thode HC, Lee C (2010) Burns in the emergency department: a national perspective. J Emerg Med 39(1):1–5

Recommended Reading

Bronstein AC, Spyker DA, Cantilena LR Jr, Green JL, Rumack BH, Dart RC (2012) 2011 Annual report of the American Association of Poison Control Centers' National Poison Data System (NPDS): 29th annual report. Clin Toxicol 50:911–1164

Fulton JA, Hoffman RS (2007) Steroids in second degree caustic burns of the esophagus: a systematic pooled analysis of fifty years of human data: 1956–2006. Clin Toxicol (Phila) 45(4):402–408

Maguina P, Shah-Khan M, An G, Hanumadass M (2007) Chemical scalp burns after hair highlights. J Burn Care Res 28(2):361–363

Mannan A, Ghani S, Clarke A, Butler PE (2007) Cases of chemical assault worldwide: a literature review. Burns 33(2):149–154

Scarlett A, Gee P (2007) Corneal abrasion and alkali burn secondary to automobile air bag inflation. Emerg Med J 24(10):733–734

Spector J, Fernandez WG (2008) Chemical, thermal, and biological ocular exposures. Emerg Med Clin North Am 26(1):125–136, vii

Chemical Element "Ca^{2+}"

▶ Adjuncts to Transfusion: Recombinant Factor VIIa, Factor XIII, and Calcium

Chemical Exposure

▶ Toxicology

Chest Radiograph

▶ Thoracic Vascular Injuries

Chest Wall Injury

Kosar Khwaja[1] and Jalal Alowais[2]
[1]Departments of Surgery and Critical Care Medicine, McGill University Health Centre, Montreal, QC, Canada
[2]Department of Surgery, Al Imam Mohammad Ibn Saud University, Riyadh, Saudi Arabia

Synonyms

Blast chest wall trauma; Blunt chest wall trauma; Penetrating chest wall trauma; Thoracic cage injury

Definition

Thoracic trauma comprise 10–15 % of all traumas and are the causes of death in 25 % of all fatalities due to trauma. Chest wall trauma includes any injury to the chest outside the

Chest Wall Injury, Table 1 High risk for severe chest wall trauma

2 or more rib fractures
Fracture of the 1st or 2nd rib
ISS $> = 16$
Age $> = 60$
Presence of shock
Combination of lung contusion and flail chest

pleural cavity, including the skin, subcutaneous tissue, chest wall muscle, bony cage, and intercostal neurovascular bundle.

Preexisting Condition

Chest wall injury can be secondary to blunt mechanism (70 %) or penetrating mechanism (30 %). The three main types of blunt injury forces are compression, shearing, and blast. Soft tissue and the bony thoracic cage are the locations most commonly affected by blunt mechanism of injury. Chest wall trauma can present in several forms of injuries (rib fracture, flail chest, intercostal bleed, and subcutaneous tissue injury). Most of the fractures of the bony thorax are benign entities and can be followed up without hospitalization, but some trauma limited to the thoracic cage itself may cause profound physiologic alterations, which may be fatal if not promptly treated (Liman et al. 2003).

Table 1 shows factors indicating high risk for severe chest wall trauma.

Application

Several forms of injury can present after blunt chest wall trauma:

1. Rib fractures
2. Flail chest
3. Sternal fracture
4. Intercostal bleed

Rib Fractures
Rib fractures are a common result of compressive blunt mechanism of injury to the thoracic cage.

Most of the fractures are located anteriorly, however, when frontal and lateral impaction is applied, this may result in multiple anterior and posterior rib fracture points (Pettiford et al. 2007a). Fractured ribs may have minor consequences like minimal pain or may lead to serious events, such as lacerations to the pleura, lungs, or abdominal organ. Upper rib fracture may be an indicator of brachial plexus or vascular injuries.

Fractures are more easily detected with chest-computed tomography (CT), but still chest X-ray plays a major role in chest wall trauma. The management of a simple rib fracture is mainly directed toward controlling patient pain and to rule out associated injury.

Pain Management
The presence of three or more rib fractures after a motor vehicle crash (MVC) has been associated with an increase in mortality, hospital stay, and number of days in the intensive care unit (ICU) (Wu et al. 1999). The pain associated with rib fracture is variable in severity. This pain can be severe enough to adversely affect respiration, which may lead to serious consequences like pneumonia and respiratory failure. Pain management must be a priority when managing rib fractures as adequate analgesia has shown improvement in pulmonary function and potentially decreases patient morbidity (Wu et al. 1999).

Route of Administration
Analgesia could be provided using systemic opioids or regional analgesic techniques such as intercostal nerve block or epidural analgesia. Based on current evidence it is difficult to recommend a single method that can be safely and effectively used for analgesia in all circumstances in patients with multiple fractured ribs. By understanding the strengths and weaknesses of each analgesic technique, the clinician can weigh the risks and benefits and individualize pain management based on the clinical setting and the extent of trauma. In general, regional blocks tend to be more effective than systemic opioids and produce less systemic side effects especially in the presence of three or more rib fractures (Karmakar and Ho 2003). Epidural pain

control is the cornerstone of acute management and has been shown to improve pulmonary mechanics and reduce pneumonia rates and ventilator days (Nirula and Mayberry 2010).

Fixation of Fracture

Historically, the fixation or "healing" of ribs was promoted by using various techniques such as the use of sandbags, external strapping, or positioning the patient in a lateral position. These maneuvers were often ineffective and involved significant bed rest and immobilization. The concept of internal fixation of flail chest and rib fractures was initially described in 1950 (Nirula and Mayberry 2010). This practice lost popularity as regional analgesic techniques and positive pressure ventilation provided an alternative method to manage flail chest. However, recently there has been a renewed interest in internal fixation of rib fractures with small series suggesting a decrease in length of ventilation and positive long term effects on pain control and functional outcome. More studies are needed to better understand the indications, methods, and timing of internal fixation of rib fractures.

Indication of Fixation

Potential indications for rib fixation are summarized in Tables 2 and 3.

Method of Fixation

Body ribs are classified as membranous bone with thin cortex (1–2 mm), and usually do not tolerate high stress; membranous bone therefore does not hold screws as strong as cortical bone. Many techniques for rib fixation have been described, yet at the present moment none have shown clear superiority over the others. Below are some examples of internal fixation techniques.

Anterior Plates with Cerclage Wire Cerclaging the rib with a permanent material can potentially impinge the intercostal nerve and lead to chronic pain.

Anterior Plating with Bicortical Screws Locking screw designs are a relatively recent

Chest Wall Injury, Table 2 Potential indications and inclusion criteria for rib fracture repair (Nirula et al. 2008)

1. Flail chest
Inclusion criteria
(a) Failure to wean from ventilator
(b) Paradoxical movement visualized during weaning
(c) No significant pulmonary contusion
(d) No significant brain injury
2. Reduction of pain and disability
Inclusion criteria
(a) Painful, movable rib fractures
(b) Failure of narcotics or epidural pain catheter
(c) Fracture movement exacerbates pain
(d) Minimal associated injuries (AIS B 2)
3. Chest wall deformity/defect
Inclusion criteria
(a) Chest wall crush injury with collapse of the structure of the chest wall and loss of thoracic volume
(b) Severely displaced, multiple rib fractures, or tissue defect that may result in permanent deformity or pulmonary hernia
(c) Severely displaced fractures are significantly impeding lung expansion or rib fractures are impaling the lung
(d) Patient is expected to survive any other injuries
4. Symptomatic rib fracture nonunion
Inclusion criteria
(a) CT scan evidence of fracture nonunion (2 months after injury)
(b) Patient reports persistent, symptomatic fracture movement
5. Thoracotomy for other indications (i.e., "on the way out")

Chest Wall Injury, Table 3 Current status of potential indications for operative rib fracture fixation (Nirula and Mayberry 2010)

1. Flail chest	Supported in select patients but expert opinion divided
2. Reduction of acute pain and disability	Unproven and controversial
3. Open chest defect	Supported by case series and expert opinion
4. Pulmonary herniation	Supported by case series and expert opinion
5. Nonunion	Supported by case series but expert opinion divided
6. Thoracotomy for other indications	That is, "on the way out," supported by case series but expert opinion divided

innovation where threads in the screw head "lock" to threads in the plate hole that may improve fixation in softer bone.

Intramedullary Fixation This technique carries a risk of wire dislodgement and is technically demanding. Internal wire fixation has also been criticized because it does not provide rotational stability.

Judet Strut The Judet strut is a bendable metal plate that grasps the rib with tongs both superiorly and inferiorly without transfixing screws. This type of fixation still can injure the neurovascular bundle below the rib and chronic pain may persist.

RibLoc™ In a simulation of an unstable rib fracture with a small bony gap, RibLoc™ fixation was superior in durability to anterior plate fixation, despite its reduced length. The RibLoc™ may facilitate the application of a much less invasive rib fracture fixation than the anterior plate technique.

Absorbable Plates Absorbable plates have practical and theoretical advantages over titanium plates. First, they do not need to be removed, as may be the case in the minority of metal plates. Additionally, because metal plates are much stiffer than the bone, "stress-shielding" of the plated bone is possible. "Stress-shielding" occurs because the plated bone is protected from normal stress and therefore does not heal as nonplated bone. Animal models support the concept that fractures heal faster and stronger with absorbable plates as compared with metal (Vu et al. 2008).

Timing of Fixation

Controversy exists regarding the optimal timing of rib fixation. Authors have suggested that delays that were made to stabilize the patient, treat associated injuries, and plan orthopedic reconstruction did not adversely affect patient outcome (Reynolds et al. 1995). Pulmonary complications may be related to the severity of injury rather than to the timing of fracture fixation. However recently, proponents of rib fixation suggest that early fixation can improve the chances of having a successful outcome. More studies are needed to clarify the ideal timing of fixation.

Rib Fracture in the Elderly

Elderly trauma patients with rib fractures should receive special attention. A low threshold to admit these patients to hospital is preferable, even in cases of isolated thoracic injury with multiple rib fractures. It was clear that old patient (65 years and above) who sustains rib fractures would have twice the mortality and thoracic morbidity of younger patients with similar injuries. For each additional rib fracture in the elderly, mortality increases by 19 % and the risk of pneumonia by 27 % (Bergeron et al. 2003).

Flail Chest

Double fractures of three or more adjacent ribs or contiguous combined rib and sternal or costochondral fractures can produce a focal area of chest wall instability, in a form of paradoxical movement of a "flail" segment during the respiratory cycle. Flail chest injury is an uncommon entity with mortality rate exceeding 10% and is dependent on patient age, presence of shock, and severity of associated injuries. The combination of flail chest and pulmonary contusion is associated with a mortality rate more than double that of either injury alone (Collins 2000). Pain management is the cornerstone in dealing with these cases and may contribute in return to normal respiration. Early intubation and mechanical ventilation is mandatory for the patient with refractory respiratory failure or the presence of other severe injury.

Ventilation Support

The initial management of flail chest is focusing on maintaining adequate ventilation. The positive pressure ventilation was first successfully used to manage flail chest in mid-1950.

Fixation

The aim of operative chest wall stabilization in patients with flail chest and respiratory insufficiency is to reduce ventilator time and avoid ventilator associated complications. In patients with flail chest and respiratory insufficiency without pulmonary contusion, operative chest wall stabilization permits early extubation. Patients with pulmonary contusion may not benefit from chest wall stabilization. Surgical stabilization is associated with a faster ventilator wean, shorter ICU time, less hospital cost, and recovery of pulmonary function in a select group of patients with flail chest (Pettiford et al. 2007b). The surgical management of flail chest has traditionally been reserved for the following indications:

1. Patients with flail chest who require thoracotomy for other intrathoracic injury
2. Those who are unable to be successfully weaned from mechanical ventilatory assistance
3. Severe chest wall instability
4. Persistent pain secondary to fracture malunion
5. Persistent or progressive loss of pulmonary function

Unilateral Versus Bilateral Flail Chest

Unilateral flail chest has better outcome than the bilateral one. In comparisons to unilateral flail chest, mortality and morbidity increased by the presence of bilateral flail chest. Early intubation and fixation should be considered in these cases, as bilateral flail chest is considered as a predictive factor for outcome (Borman et al. 2006).

Sternal Fracture

Incidence and Diagnosis

Sternum fracture is observed in 4 % of traffic accident victims and 3–8 % of blunt thoracic trauma. It was noticed that the death rates in traffic accidents have decreased in Europe due to the widespread use of seat belts, but at the same time the rate of sternal fractures has increased for the same reason (Budd 1985). It is reported that the risk for sternal fracture increased with old age trauma victims and for front seat victims during the crash. Sternal fractures are diagnosed clinically by presence of sternal tenderness, deformity, crepitation, and swelling of the sternum. The radiological images required for definitive diagnosis are lateral chest X-ray, or CT scan. As a new modality in diagnosing the sternal fracture, US shows good sensitivity and specificity in detecting the fracture. US is operator dependent and should be considered in patients with symptoms suggesting sternal fractures whose radiographs remain indeterminate (You et al. 2010). Many times sternal fractures are discovered from the CT chest done as part of a Trauma workup.

Associated Injury

Displaced sternal fractures have higher chances of associated injury. In the literature, it has been reported that sternal fractures are often accompanied by vertebral fractures, specifically by fractures of the thoracic vertebrae. It was once thought that sternal fractures occurred together with cardiac trauma, but this belief has changed over time (Celik et al. 2009). Traumatic aortic rupture does not occur more commonly in patients with sternal fracture when compared with other patients with blunt chest injuries (STURM et al. 1989).

Management

The fracture is typically in a transversal position. Fractures can be end to end, partially displaced or overriding. Most patients with sternal fracture required pain control medications and pulmonary toilet for symptom control. Some cases may need surgical fixation especially in overriding fracture. Placing a rolled cushion under the patient's back is a simple method for stabilization of overriding fractures in the emergency department.

In general, sternal fractures are not a marker for clinically significant myocardial injury. The management of sternal fracture patients should be directed toward the treatment of associated injuries. Sternal fractures are benign and do not require special treatment nor an expensive workup, and there is no need to admit these patients solely for observation if their initial clinical condition is satisfactory and there are no abnormalities identified by chest radiograph and electrocardiography (Bar et al. 2003).

Intercostal Bleed

Hemothorax secondary to rib fracture can develop as a result of intercostal vascular bleed in 13 % of all rib fracture cases. It is frequently more common with posterior rib fracture than anterior one (McLoughlin et al. 1987). There are many factors suggested as predictors for intercostal bleed associated with rib fracture (severe mechanism of injury, number of ribs fractured, the higher rib involved, severe degree of rib fracture).

Delayed hemothorax after rib fracture is uncommon but can be fatal. It can be delayed as long as 3–4 days post trauma.

Management

Most intercostal bleeds will stop spontaneously. Patients must be resuscitated adequately for the blood loss. The resulting hemothorax is evacuated with chest tube insertion. Patients unstable with ongoing bleeding should undergo thoracotomy for surgical control with ligation of the bleeding intercostal vessel. Patients that are hemodynamically stable with evidence of contrast blush on a CT chest should be considered for angioemoblization to obtain hemostasis.

Cross-References

▶ Blast
▶ Geriatric Trauma
▶ Hemorrhage
▶ Hemorrhagic Shock
▶ Retained Hemothorax

References

Bar I et al (2003) Isolated sternal fracture – a benign condition? Isr Med Assoc J 5(2):105–106

Bergeron E et al (2003) Elderly trauma patients with rib fractures are at greater risk of death and pneumonia. J Trauma Inj Infect Crit Care 54(3):478–485

Borman JB et al (2006) Unilateral flail chest is seldom a lethal injury. Emerg Med J 23(12):903–905

Budd JS (1985) Effect of seat belt legislation on the incidence of sternal fractures seen in the accident department. Br Med J (Clin Res Ed) 291(6498):785

Collins J (2000) Chest wall trauma. J Thorac Imaging 15(2):112–119

Karmakar MK, Ho AM-H (2003) Acute pain management of patients with multiple fractured ribs. J Trauma Inj Infect Crit Care 54(3):615–625

Liman STS et al (2003) Chest injury due to blunt trauma. Eur J Cardiothorac Surg 23(3):374–378

McLoughlin R et al (1987) Haemothorax after rib fracture—incidence, timing and prediction. Ir J Med Sci 156(4):117–119

Nirula R, Mayberry JC (2010) Rib fracture fixation: controversies and technical challenges. Am Surg 76(8):793–802

Nirula R et al (2008) Rib fracture repair: indications, technical issues, and future directions. World J Surg 33(1):14–22

Pettiford BL, Luketich JD, Landreneau RJ (2007a) The management of flail chest. Thorac Surg Clin 17(1):25–33

Pettiford BL, Luketich JD, Landreneau RJ (2007b) The management of flail chest. Thorac Surg Clin 17(1):25–33

Reynolds MA et al (1995) Is the timing of fracture fixation important for the patient with multiple trauma? Ann Surg 222(4):470–478, discussion 478–81

STURM JT et al (1989) Does sternal fracture increase the risk for aortic rupture. Ann Thorac Surg 48(5):697–698

Vu K-C et al (2008) Reduction of rib fractures with a bioresorbable plating system: preliminary observations. J Trauma Inj Infect Crit Care 64(5):1264–1269

Wu CL et al (1999) Thoracic epidural analgesia versus intravenous patient-controlled analgesia for the treatment of rib fracture pain after motor vehicle crash. J Trauma Inj Infect Crit Care 47(3):564–567

You JS et al (2010) Role of sonography in the emergency room to diagnose sternal fractures. J Clin Ultrasound 38(3):135–137

Recommended Reading

Avery EEE, Benson DWD, Morch ETE (1956) Critically crushed chests; a new method of treatment with continuous mechanical hyperventilation to produce alkalotic apnea and internal pneumatic stabilization. J Thorac Surg 32(3):291–311

Bulger EM et al (2000) Rib fractures in the elderly. J Trauma Acute Care Surg 48(6):1040–1047

Celik B et al (2009) Sternum fractures and effects of associated injuries. Thorac Cardiovasc Surg 57(8):468–471

Chiu WCW, D'Amelio LFL, Hammond JSJ (1997) Sternal fractures in blunt chest trauma: a practical algorithm for management. Am J Emerg Med 15(3):252–255

Engel CC et al (2005) Operative chest wall fixation with osteosynthesis plates. J Trauma Inj Infect Crit Care 58(1):181–186

Freedland MM et al (1990) The management of flail chest injury: factors affecting outcome. J Trauma Inj Infect Crit Care 30(12):1460–1468

von Garrel TT et al (2004) The sternal fracture: radiographic analysis of 200 fractures with special reference to concomitant injuries. J Trauma Inj Infect Crit Care 57(4):837–844

Knobloch KK et al (2008) RETRACTED: sternal fractures are frequent among polytraumatised patients following high deceleration velocities in a severe vehicle crash. Injury 39(1):8–8

Ross RMR, Cordoba AA (1986) Delayed life-threatening hemothorax associated with rib fractures. J Trauma Inj Infect Crit Care 26(6):576–578

Roy-Shapirga AA, Levi II, Khoda JJ (1994) Sternal fractures: a red flag or a red herring? J Trauma Inj Infect Crit Care 37(1):59–61

Sales JR et al (2008) Biomechanical testing of a novel, minimally invasive rib fracture plating system. J Trauma Inj Infect Crit Care 64(5):1270–1274

Sırmalı M (2003) A comprehensive analysis of traumatic rib fractures: morbidity, mortality and management. Eur J Cardiothorac Surg 24(1):133–138

Tanaka HH et al (2002) Surgical stabilization of internal pneumatic stabilization? A prospective randomized study of management of severe flail chest patients. J Trauma Inj Infect Crit Care 52(4):727–732

Voggenreiter GG et al (1998) Operative chest wall stabilization in flail chest–outcomes of patients with or without pulmonary contusion. J Am Coll Surg 187(2):130–138

Chest X-Ray (CXR)

▶ Thoracic Vascular Injuries

Child Abuse

▶ Pediatric Trauma, Assessment, and Anesthetic Management

Child Occupant Injuries

Katrina B. Altenhofen
Iowa Department of Public Health-Bureau of EMS, Washington, IA, USA

Synonyms

Child occupant restraints; Child passenger safety

Definition

Injury is the physical damage that results when a human body is suddenly subjected to energy in amounts that exceed the threshold of physiologic tolerance – or else the result of a lack of one or more vital elements, such as oxygen (Baker 1992).

Crash is an event that produces injury and/or property damage, involves a motor vehicle in transport, and occurs on a roadway or when the vehicle is still in motion after running off the roadway (National Highway Traffic Safety Administration 2004). Child occupant injuries occur when a child is unrestrained or improperly restrained or the crash forces of the motor vehicle crash are so severe that they exceed the protection capacity of the safety devise utilized.

Common Indications

Unintentional injuries are the leading cause of death and disability for children and teenagers in the United States. Motor vehicle-related injuries are the leading cause of fatalities among children and young adults.

A statistical projection of traffic fatalities for the first quarter of 2012 shows that an estimated 7,630 people died in motor vehicle traffic crashes; this represents a significant increase of about 13.5 % as compared to the 6,720 fatalities that were projected to have occurred in the first quarter of 2011 (National Highway Traffic Safety Administration 2012).

Parents and caregivers often utilize occupant protection devices such as a child passenger safety seat; however, the correct usage of the device is poor. Compatibility of the child passenger safety device and the vehicle as well as the instructions for use of the device is often complicated, resulting in misuse of the product. Incorrect use of child passenger safety seats is widespread and it is estimated that 82 % of child safety seats are not installed and used correctly. Inappropriately restrained children are nearly three and a half times more likely to be injured in a crash (National Highway Traffic Safety Administration 2004).

Challenges beyond the misuse of the child restraint devices also lie in the fact that vehicle restraint use drops as children get older. Parents and caregivers often feel that infants and young children are more fragile and need more protection, but as the child reaches the age of 4–7, the use of a child passenger safety seat drops, and parents or caregivers believe that the vehicle safety belt system is protection enough despite the poor fit due to the child still being too small for that system.

Currently child passenger safety devices are broken down into four types:

1. Rear-facing car seat: Utilized by a child who birth to at a minimum of 2 years or to the maximum of the child restraint rear-facing seat height and weight limit. It has a harness and in a crash cradles and moves with the child to reduce the stress to the child's neck and spinal cord. There are different types of the rear-facing child safety seats – an infant-only seat which can only be used rear-facing and a convertible and 3-in-1 child safety seat that can be used in a rear-facing or forward-facing position. Typically the convertible and 3-in-1 seats have higher weight limits which allows for longer use.
2. Forward-facing car seat: Utilized by a child who is at a minimum of 1 year and then to the maximum of the child restraint height and weight limit. The restraint has a harness and tether that limits the child's forward movement during a crash.
3. Booster seat: Positions the seat belt so that it fits properly over the stronger parts of the child's body. A child should remain in this type of restraint until the seat belt system of the vehicle fits properly.
4. Vehicle seat belt: Should be positioned to lie across the upper thighs and snug across the shoulder and chest to restrain the child safely in a crash. It should not rest on the abdominal area or across the neck.

The National Highway Traffic Safety Administration has implemented a "four-step" program for parents to assist in providing education on the right child passenger safety seat for the right size of the child. The intent is for the parent or caregiver to select a child passenger safety seat based on the child's age and size and choose a seat that fits in the vehicle and will be used every time. This process looks at four age ranges and matches those with one of the appropriate child passenger safety seat devices.

Sir Isaac Newton's theory of gravitation and motion states that an "object in motion stays in motion at the original speed until acted on by an outside force." Occupant protection devices can help reduce the burden of injury by keeping occupants in the vehicle, contacting the occupant at the strongest parts of the body, spreading crash forces over a larger body surface area, and slowing the body down to minimize crash forces and to protect the brain and spinal cord.

In a motor vehicle crash, three separate collisions are occurring – vehicle collision, human collision, and internal collision. Within the first collision of the vehicle, the vehicle begins to stop as it collides with another object; as the vehicle slows, the point of collision crushes, absorbing some of the crash energy. The second collision happens as the occupant continues to move toward the point of impact at the same speed despite the vehicle beginning to stop upon impact. The occupant will begin to stop once they connect with an outside force that is in the path of motion. As the individual collides with the outside force, the body starts to slow its motion toward impact; however, the body is now the object that absorbs the crash energy. During the internal collision, the occupant's internal organs move toward the point of impact and hit other organs or bones. Injuries can be classified as blunt trauma and either is closed or open.

If an occupant is not utilizing an occupant protection device, there is the potential for the body to go "up and over" or "down and under." In an up and over, there is potential for head, face, and neck injuries upon impact with the windshield and chest and/or abdominal injuries due to impact of the steering wheel. The lower extremities can become injured if entangled in the dashboard, brake or gas pedals, or steering column. With the down and under mechanism of injury, lower extremities could experience crushing injuries, entrapment again of the brake or gas pedals, impalement or crush injuries could also affect the abdominal organs.

When an occupant only uses a lap belt for protection, the upper body is at risk of injury due to no type of restraint device holding the occupant. Injuries to the head, neck, and face could happen if the occupant impacts an object in front of them.

Improperly worn restraints can result in a variety of injuries depending on where the restraint is located on the occupant's body. If the lap belt is too high, then abdominal, thoracic, and lumbar spine injuries could be present. If the lap belt is too loose, the occupant could become ejected from the vehicle.

When an occupant is not in the appropriate position with a properly utilized occupant protection device, there is the added risk of impact with the vehicle's airbag system resulting in injuries to the head, neck, face, and chest.

Different types of vehicle crashes create different risks for the vehicle occupants. The crash can be frontal, side, or rear impact as well as various types of rollovers.

Frontal impact is the most frequent type, happening when the vehicle is moving forward and is stopped suddenly by an object in the front of the vehicle. Common injuries to occupants can be skull or spinal fractures, broken ribs, liver, spleen, or larynx injuries as well as lacerations or bruising to the head and face.

In a side collision, the vehicle is impacted on one side or the other which creates an increase in injury to an occupant sitting on the same side as the impact. There is minimal vehicle space to absorb the crash force between the vehicle and the occupant sitting on the side of the impact. Chest and pelvic injuries as well as skull fractures or lacerations are often experienced in a side impact crash. Depending on the position of the occupant and the safety restraint device, there is also a possibility of liver and spleen injuries.

Rear collisions account for a small number of fatalities; however, several injuries such as cervical fractures and stretching or tearing of the anterior ligaments or tendons could possibly be experienced. These injuries are often due to the vehicle moving forward after impact pushing the occupant's body out from under the head. The occupant's head moves toward the point of impact and often rotates back and then is thrown forward.

In a rollover or vault, there is always a potential for an unrestrained or not properly restrained occupant to be thrown from the vehicle creating potentially life-threatening and/or fatal injuries.

Cross-References

► Abdominal Compartment Syndrome
► Airway Exchange in Trauma Patients
► Airway Management in Trauma, Cricothyrotomy
► Airway Management in Trauma, Nonsurgical
► Airway Management in Trauma, Tracheostomy
► Airway Trauma, Management of
► Brain Death
► Cardiac Injuries
► Cardiopulmonary Resuscitation in Pediatric Trauma
► Chest Wall Injury
► Crush Injuries
► Damage Control Resuscitation
► Delayed Diagnosis/Missed Injury
► Diaphragmatic Injuries
► Head Injury
► Hemorrhage
► Hemorrhagic Shock
► Informed Consent in Trauma
► Massive Transfusion Protocols in Trauma
► Motor Vehicle Crash Injury
► Pediatric Airway Management
► Shock
► TBI
► Thoracic Vascular Injuries
► Trauma Patient Evaluation

References

Baker SP (1992) The injury fact book, 2nd edn. Oxford University Press, New York

National Highway Traffic Safety Administration (2004) Motor vehicle occupant protection fact book. National Highway Traffic Safety Administration, Washington, DC

National Highway Traffic Safety Administration (2012) Traffic safety facts. National Highway Traffic Safety Administration, Washington, DC

Child Occupant Restraints

▶ Child Occupant Injuries

Child Passenger Safety

▶ Child Occupant Injuries

Child Trauma

▶ Pediatric Trauma, Assessment, and Anesthetic Management

Children's Femoral Shaft Fractures

▶ Pediatric Femur Fractures

Children's Femur Fractures

▶ Pediatric Femur Fractures

Choking

▶ Strangulation and Hanging
▶ Trauma-Related Dysphagia

Cholecystitis

▶ Acalculous Cholecystitis

Cicatrization Atelectasis

▶ Atelectasis

Circulatory Shock

▶ Shock

Citrate-Dextrose Solutions

Bryan A. Cotton[1] and Laura A. McElroy[2]
[1]Department of Surgery, Division of Acute Care Surgery, Trauma and Critical Care, University of Texas Health Science Center at Houston, The University of Texas Medical School at Houston, Houston, TX, USA
[2]Department of Anesthesiology, Critical Care Medicine, University of Rochester Medical Center, Rochester, NY, USA

Synonyms

Acid-citrate-dextrose, ACD; Citrate-phosphate-dextrose, CPD

Definition

The current state of liquid storage of blood products is the result of over 100 years of research testing both storage containers and solutions. The ideal storage solution supplies red blood cells (RBCs) with appropriate nutrients such as a sugar energy source and phosphate, prevents clotting, reduces the risk of bacterial contamination, and can be sterilized.

The first major acid-citrate-dextrose (ACD) solution was reported in 1943 by Loutit and Mollison in the frenzy of blood bank research centered around World War II. The original ACD solution had a pH of 5; was made with citric acid, dextrose, and sodium citrate; and stably survived being autoclaved. It was used primarily for glass bottle storage of whole blood and allowed for 72 % RBC survival after 21 days with little hemolysis, which was a vast improvement over the prior trisodium citrate solution, which only preserved 22 % of erythrocytes after 7 days (Loutit and Mollison 1943).

Further research revealed that the addition of phosphate to the anticoagulant solution increased the RBC survival rate, by mitigating the loss of intracellular phosphate concentrations, thus supporting cellular metabolism (Sohmer and Dawson 1979). This new solution, a mixture of citric acid, sodium citrate, monosodium phosphate, and dextrose (CPD), was utilized in the new plastic flexible storage bags and is the basis of RBC storage in North America.

Continued advancements have been made in improving blood storage. Additional additives have been used, the nucleoside adenine being important. In Europe, solutions of phosphate, adenine, glucose, guanosine, saline, and mannitol (PAGGS-M) are used, while alternative solutions based on saline, adenine, glucose, and mannitol (SAG-M) are used and bear the name AS-1 and AS-5 (Cushing and Ness 2009).

Blood products continue to be a limited and precious commodity in trauma resuscitation, and work is ongoing to increase storage times and improve effective yields of transfused stored blood products (Nishino et al. 2009; Wagner et al. 2013).

Cross-References

- ▶ Blood Bank
- ▶ Leukoreduced Red Blood Cells
- ▶ Packed Red Blood Cells

References

Cushing M and Ness P (2009) In Hematology: Basic principles and practice. 6th Edition, Ch 112. Hoffman R et al, Eds. Churchill, Philadelphia, PA.

Loutit JF, Mollison PL (1943) Disodium-citrate-glucose mixture as a blood preservative. Br Med J 2(4327):744–745

Nishino T, Yachie-Kinoshita A, Hirayama A et al (2009) In silico modeling and metabolome analysis of long-stored erythrocytes to improve blood storage methods. J Biotechnol 144:212–223

Sohmer PR, Dawson RB (1979) The significance of 2,3-DPG in red blood cell transfusions. Crit Rev Clin Sci 11(2):107–174

Wagner SJ, Glynn SA, Welniak LA (2013) Research opportunities in optimizing storage of red blood cell products. NHLBI working group conference report. Transfusion. Apr 2013. doi:10.1111/trf.12244

Citrate-Phosphate-Dextrose, CPD

▶ Citrate-Dextrose Solutions

Classification of Traumatic Brain Injury

▶ Traumatic Brain Injury, Emergency Department Care

Clauss Fibrinogen Assay

▶ Fibrinogen (Test)

Clearance, Cervical Spine

Patricia L. Zadnik and Daniel M. Sciubba
Department of Neurosurgery, The Johns Hopkins University School of Medicine, Baltimore, MD, USA

Synonyms

Canadian C-spine; National Emergency X-radiography Utilization Study (NEXUS)

Definition

The Canadian C-spine and the National Emergency X-radiography Utilization Study (NEXUS) define the criteria for clearance of the cervical spine in an adult patient who has sustained blunt injury to the cervical spine (Mower et al. 2001; Stiell et al. 2001, 2003; Holmes et al. 2002; Lowery et al. 2001). Debate has emerged over which criteria provide the greatest specificity and sensitivity; however, both tests have demonstrated an excellent sensitivity (98–100 %) in identifying patients who do not need spinal imaging (Fig. 1) (Stiell et al. 2003; Panacek et al. 2001).

According to the NEXUS low-risk criteria, if the patient is alert and responsive (GCS 15), is not intoxicated, has no palpable pain in the posterior neck, has no distracting injury such as a long bone fracture, and no neurological deficits (sensory or motor), they do not require imaging for clearance of their cervical spine (Mower et al. 2001). They can be safely extricated from any cervical immobilization devices without imaging (Fig. 1).

The Canadian C-Spine criteria dictates that in the absence of risk factors, the mechanism of injury is not "dangerous," the patient is under 65 years old, and there are no paresthesias in the extremities, imaging is not necessary. Specifically, dangerous mechanisms of injury are

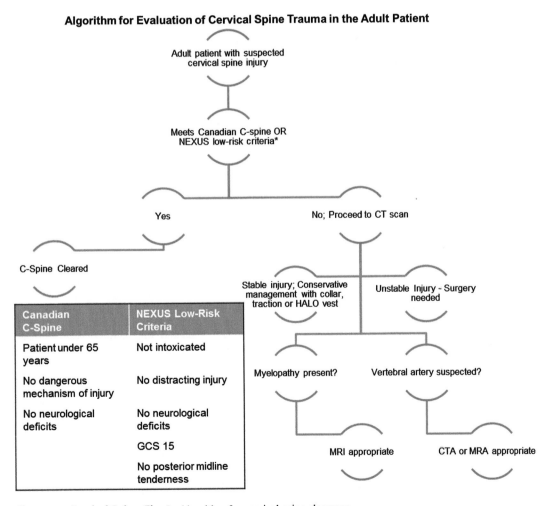

Clearance, Cervical Spine, Fig. 1 Algorithm for cervical spine clearance

defined as a fall from an elevation of greater than 3 ft or 5 stairs, an axial load to the head, motor vehicle accident >60 mph or 100 kph, or with rollover or ejection, or involving a recreational vehicle or bicycle (Fig. 1) (Stiell et al. 2001, 2003).

When a patient fails to meet the exclusion criteria dictated above, a CT scan is the recommended imaging modality. Although adequate three-view plain radiographs (AP, lateral and open mouth odontoid) have been used in the past with good sensitivity and specificity, logistical issues often prevent the acquisition of an adequate series. In the original NEXUS study, up to one-third of patients with cervical spine injury did not have adequate three-view plain films to assess for spinal column injury (Mower et al. 2001). According to the American College of Radiology (ACR) Appropriateness Criteria, a CT scan is the most appropriate first-line imaging for all patients with blunt cervical spine trauma who fail to meet the Canadian C-Spine or NEXUS low-risk criteria, or who have a known rigid spinal disease (ankylosing spondylitis or diffuse idiopathic skeletal hyperostosis) and blunt cervical spine trauma (Daffner and Hackney 2007). If the CT scan does not demonstrate an unstable injury, and the patient does not have myelopathy, the patient's cervical spine can be cleared and immobilization can be removed.

In an obtunded patient with a dangerous mechanism of injury, or if CT scan fails to demonstrate a fracture in a patient with myelopathy, the ACR recommends MRI for assessment for spinal cord injury (Daffner and Hackney 2007). MRI is also appropriate for patients who are unable to be evaluated for greater than 48 h following their traumatic event due to intoxication, sedation for ventilation assistance, or neurologic deficit. In patients with CT scan demonstrating vertebral artery injury, such as the absence of a flow void on CT, a CTA of the head and neck or an MRA of the neck, and a cervical spine and brain MRI is warranted (Daffner and Hackney 2007). If the CT spine demonstrates findings consistent with ligamentous injury, such as dislocated facets or suspended bone fragments, an MRI of the cervical spine should be performed to evaluate the extent of soft tissue damage as well as any compression of the neural elements. Further, if the CT scan is normal, but there is significant clinical evidence of posterior ligamentous injury, such as pain on palpation, or concern for an abnormal neurological exam, MRI should be performed (Daffner and Hackney 2007).

Flexion and extension (FE) radiographs are almost never clinically appropriate in the first-line evaluation of blunt cervical spine trauma as it is contraindicated in patients who have distracting injuries, neurological deficits, or patients who are obtunded and unable to cooperate. FE radiography may be performed at later clinical follow-up, and the ACR recommends FE radiographs for patients with pain but no unstable injury who are returning for evaluation (Daffner and Hackney 2007). FE radiographs are also contraindicated in patients with greater than 3.5 mm of subluxation on any C-spine imaging.

Cross-References

▶ Trauma Patient Evaluation

References

Daffner RH, Hackney DB (2007) ACR appropriateness criteria on suspected spine trauma. J Am Coll Radiol 4(11):762–775

Holmes JF, Mirvis SE, Panacek EA, Hoffman JR, Mower WR, Velmahos GC, NEXUS Group (2002) Variability in computed tomography and magnetic resonance imaging in patients with cervical spine injuries. J Trauma 53(3):524–529 discussion 530

Lowery DW, Wald MM, Browne BJ, Tigges S, Hoffman JR, Mower WR, NEXUS Group (2001) Epidemiology of cervical spine injury victims. Ann Emerg Med 38(1):12–16

Mower MR, Hoffman JR, Pollack CV, Zucker MI, Browne BJ, Wolfson AB, NEXUS Group (2001) Use of plain radiography to screen for cervical spine injuries. Ann Emerg Med 38(1):1–7

Panacek EA, Mower WR, Holmes JF, Hoffman JR, NEXUS Group (2001) Test performance of the individual NEXUS low-risk clinical screening criteria for cervical spine injury. Ann Emerg Med 38(1):22–25

Stiell IG, Wells GA, Vandemheen KL, Clement CM, Lesiuk H, De Maio VJ, Laupacis A, Schull M,

McKnight RD, Verbeek R, Brison R, Cass D, Dreyer J, Eisenhauer MA, Greenberg GH, MacPhail I, Morrison L, Reardon M, Worthington J (2001) The Canadian C-spine rule for radiography in alert and stable trauma patients. JAMA 286(15):1841–1848

Stiell IG, Clement CM, McKnight RD, Brison R, Schull MJ, Rowe BH, Worthington JR, Eisenhauer MA, Cass D, Greenberg G, MacPhail I, Dreyer J, Lee JS, Bandiera G, Reardon M, Holroyd B, Lesiuk H, Wells GA (2003) The Canadian C-spine rule versus the NEXUS low-risk criteria in patients with trauma. N Engl J Med 349(26):2510–2518

Clinical Associate

▶ Physician Assistant

Clinical Ethics

▶ Ethical Issues in Trauma Anesthesia

Clinical Officer (Sub-Saharan Africa)

▶ Physician Assistant

Clinical Trials

▶ Neurotrauma, Emerging Research

Close Friend

▶ Family Preparation for Organ Donation

Closed Head Injury

▶ Neurotrauma, Introduction
▶ Traumatic Brain Injury, Emergency Department Care

Clostridium Tetani Infection

▶ Tetanus

Clothes-Line Injury

▶ Strangulation and Hanging

Clottafact®

▶ Adjuncts to Transfusion: Fibrinogen Concentrate

Clotting Disorder

▶ Coagulopathy

CNS Device Infections

▶ Neurotrauma, Infectious Considerations

CNS Infections

▶ Neurotrauma, Infectious Considerations

Coagulation Disorders

▶ Coagulopathy

Coagulation "Factor IV"

▶ Adjuncts to Transfusion: Recombinant Factor VIIa, Factor XIII, and Calcium

Coagulopathy

Adriana Laser[1] and Khanjan H. Nagarsheth[2]
[1]Department of General Surgery, University of
Maryland Medical Center, Baltimore, MD, USA
[2]R Adams Cowley Shock Trauma Center,
University of Maryland School of Medicine,
Baltimore, MD, USA

Synonyms

Bleeding diathesis; Bleeding disorder; Clotting
disorder; Coagulation disorders; Hypocoaguability

Definition

Prolonged or excessive bleeding due to an
alteration in the body's ability to clot which can
manifest spontaneously, or after trauma or
a surgical procedure.

Preexisting Condition

Victims of trauma can present with underlying
coagulation disorders, so a basic understanding
is important in treating these patients. There are
several types of coagulation disorders that fall
under this umbrella term. The most common
genetic defects are in clotting factors: von
Willebrands disease and the hemophilias A and
B. Von Willebrands is the most common inherited
coagulation disorder and has subtypes for qualitative and quantitative forms. X-linked hemophilia
A (factor VIII deficiency) and B (factor IX deficiency) are present in 1 in 5–10,000 and
20–35,000 male births, respectively. Other more
rare diseases include Bernard-Soulier syndrome,
a defect in von Willebrand receptor glycoprotein
Ib, and Wiskott-Aldrich syndrome, an X-linked
mutation in the WASp protein that leads to
small and dysfunctional platelets. Glanzmann's
thrombasthenia is also very rare and is due
to a defective glycoprotein IIb/IIIa fibrinogen
receptor. Congenital afibrinogenemia as its

name implies is a complete lack of fibrinogen
(Factor I). Unlike its more common Factor V
Leiden mutation leading to thrombophilia, a deficiency in Factor V leads to a coagulopathy. So
does Factor X (prothrombinase) deficiency, with
a prevalence of 1 in 500,000.

Other sources of coagulopathy include
defective or decreased number of circulating
platelets. Iatrogenic sources are seen with
prescribed anticoagulation. Nutritional sources
can include a vitamin K deficiency. Liver failure
consists of decreased coagulation protein synthesis, and an associated coagulopathy. Disseminated Intravascular Coagulation (DIC) leads to
bleeding due to reduced platelets, fibrinogen, and
other factors plus thrombosis by way of intravascular fibrin deposition. Coagulation disorders are
also seen with leukemia, certain snake venoms,
and viral hemorrhagic fevers like Dengue fever.

Application

Complications
A coagulopathic state can lead to bleeding in soft
tissues, cerebral, retinal, joints or hemarthrosis
(which can lead to joint destruction and arthritis),
heavy menses, and epistaxis. Specific populations
have been investigated more thoroughly. The
development of acute coagulopathy of trauma
(ACoT) or acute traumatic coagulopathy (ATC),
usually defined as an elevated PT or INR > 1.6, has
been shown to result in increased mortality (Brohi
et al. 2003). Multiple studies have shown ACoT is
associated with base deficit and tissue loss (Sixta
et al. 2012). Chronically, anemia or infectious risks
from multiple transfusions can result.

Pathophysiology
In ACoT, there is interplay between direct loss
and consumption of coagulation factors (activity
levels <50 %), acidemia, hypothermia, dilution,
and fibrinolysis (Murthi et al. 2011). Initiation of
both anticoagulant and fibrinolytic pathways by
endothelial activation of protein C is involved in
the mechanism of the early coagulopathy associated with shock, and the capacity of the coagulation system is overwhelmed (Hess et al. 2008;

Davenport 2013). Increases in ICU coagulopathic derangements have been attributed to many new anticoagulant and antiplatelet therapies (Levy et al. 2013).

Diagnosis

Workup can be rapid including laboratory tests for a complete blood count (CBC), Bleeding time, partial thromboplastin time (PTT), platelet aggregation test, prothrombin time (PT), fibrinogen, fibrin split products, and reptilase time. Viscoelastic tests on whole blood, TEG (thromboelastogram), and the enhanced ROTEM (thromboelastometry) measure the interaction of coagulation factors, inhibitors, and cellular components during clotting and lysis. The reduction in clot strength can be rapidly diagnosed in an acute situation and is associated with increased transfusions and mortality; using these tests have not yet been proven to increase outcomes and therefore new standard has not been established as of 2013 (Davenport 2013).

Treatment

Treatment regimen depends on factor replacement, platelet and fresh frozen plasma (FFP) transfusion, hemodialysis, prohemostatic pharmacologic agents, or other therapies. By 2008, damage control resuscitation with 1:1 plasma to red blood cells became the national standard in the USA. Platelets have also been shown recently to improve mortality in trauma and shock scenarios (Holcomb et al. 2008). Evidence is forthcoming; however, for example, some trauma literature has posited a shift from empirical therapy with FFP to targeted with coagulation factors. However, there is a noted lack of data on the subject to settle the controversy yet (Grottke 2012).

Cross-References

- ▶ Coagulopathy in Trauma: Underlying Mechanisms
- ▶ Hypocoaguability
- ▶ Platelet Transfusion in Trauma

References

Brohi K, Singh J, Heron M et al (2003) Acute traumatic coagulopathy. J Trauma Inj Infect Crit Care 54:1127–1130

Davenport R (2013) Pathogenesis of acute traumatic coagulopathy. Transfusion 53:23S–27S

Grottke O (2012) Coagulation management. Curr Opin Crit Care 18:641–646

Hess JR, Brohi K, Dutton RP et al (2008) The coagulopathy of trauma: a review of mechanisms. J Trauma 65:748–754

Holcomb JB, Wade CE, Michalek JE et al (2008) Increased plasma and platelet to red blood cell ratios improves outcome in 466 massively transfused civilian trauma patients. Ann Surg 248:447–458

Levy J, Faraoni D, Sniecinski R (2013) Perioperative coagulation management in the intensive care unit. Curr Opin Anaesthesiol 26:65–70

Murthi S, Stansbury LG, Dutton RP et al (2011) Transfusion medicine for trauma patients: an update: the coagulopathy of trauma. Expert Rev Hematol 4:527–537

Sixta SL, Hatch QM, Matijevic N et al (2012) Mechanistic determinants of the acute coagulopathy of trauma (ACoT) in patients requiring emergency surgery. Int J Burns Trauma 2:158–166. Epub 2012 Dec 5

Coagulopathy (ATC)

▶ Coagulopathy in Trauma: Underlying Mechanisms

Coagulopathy in Trauma: Underlying Mechanisms

Barto Nascimento[1] and Sandro Rizoli[2]
[1]Trauma Program, Department of Surgery, Sunnybrook Health Sciences Centre, University of Toronto, Toronto, ON, Canada
[2]Trauma & Acute Care Surgery, Departments of Critical Care & Surgery, St. Michael's Hospital, University of Toronto, Toronto, ON, Canada

Synonyms

Acute coagulopathy of trauma; Acute Traumatic; Coagulopathy (ATC); Consumptive coagulopathy; Dilutional coagulopathy;

Disseminated intravascular coagulation; Early coagulopathy of trauma; Hyperfibrinolysis; Microvascular hemorrhage; Nonsurgical hemorrhage; Trauma-associated Coagulopathy (TAC); Trauma-induced Coagulopathy (TIC)

Definition

Coagulopathy in trauma is a multifactorial phenomenon frequently associated with massive hemorrhage and aggressive clotting factor-deprived fluid resuscitation. Traditionally, trauma-induced coagulopathy was understood as the loss of procoagulant factors accompanying massive hemorrhage; dilution ensuing aggressive crystalloid infusion and red blood cell (RBC) transfusion; and metabolic acidosis and hypothermia associated with hemorrhagic shock. However, evolving evidence suggests the existence of an early intrinsic coagulopathy, not explained by consumption and dilution, which is linked to an imbalance of the complex interplay in procoagulant, anticoagulant, and fibrinolytic pathways, and also associated with platelet and endothelial dysfunction (Frith and Brohi 2012; Hess et al. 2008). The presence of coagulopathy is known to be an independent predictor of multiple organ dysfunction and mortality in trauma.

Preexisting Condition

Imbalance in Procoagulant, Anticoagulant, and Fibrinolytic Pathways

Hemostasis following vascular injury and bleeding is maintained by a dynamic equilibrium involving mainly procoagulant elements (coagulation factors and platelets) and anticoagulant pathways (thrombomodulin and protein C pathways). Recent prehospital and emergency department research documented the presence, based on the standard coagulation assays (PT, INR, aPTT) and thromboelastography/metry (TEG and ROTEM), of an early hemostatic impairment, within the first hour following injury, in bleeding trauma patients (Frith and

Brohi 2012). The activation of protein C (aPC), which induces systemic anticoagulation by cleaving and degrading factor V, is responsible in part for the development of this early trauma coagulopathy. Normally, factor V functions as a cofactor to allow factor Xa to activate thrombin. Thrombin in turn cleaves fibrinogen into fibrin, which polymerizes to constitute the fibrin net that is the clot's main structure. In severely injured patients with hemorrhagic shock, high levels of circulating aPC and critical deficit of factor V have been reported (Rizoli et al. 2011a). Furthermore, hypoperfusion during hemorrhage leads to release of tissue-type plasminogen activator inhibitor-1 (t-PA) from vascular endothelial cells leading to fibrinolysis. Capillary cells contain receptors for thrombomodulin and protein C, which bind thrombin and exponentially stimulate protein C activation. aPC also depletes plasminogen activator inhibitor-1 (PAI-1), major antagonist of t-PA. Although rare, an overwhelming imbalance in these fibrinolytic pathways leading to hyperfibrinolysis may develop and is associated with high mortality in severe trauma. Fibrinogen concentrations are known to be reduced shortly after traumatic injury. Other markers of endothelial glycocalyx degradation have been identified and shown to be correlated with traumatic coagulopathy (Frith and Brohi 2012). Finally, significant differences in platelet function have recently been reported between survivors and non-survivors in trauma. Of note, platelet count is only mildly reduced in the vast majority of trauma patients. However, minor differences in platelet count and function have been associated with worse outcomes following injury.

Tissue destruction following trauma leads to exposure of tissue factor (TF) in the vascular endothelium which binds FVII to initiate normal clot formation. This response is normally limited to the injury site. However, in the presence of systemic hypoperfusion, this mechanism may lead to clinically relevant coagulation changes. The activation of a systemic inflammatory response by hemorrhage induces TF exposure in vascular beds systemically, which in turn leads to generalized activation of coagulation. It remains unclear whether this delocalized coagulation response constitutes the mechanism underlying the disseminated intravascular coagulation (DIC) in trauma. Furthermore, the diagnosis and incidence of DIC is currently an area of scientific debate. As oppose to traditional understanding, a recent study utilizing histopathological examination of organs removed during operation of severely injured patients failed to detect any evidence of DIC (Rizoli et al. 2011b).

Hemodilution, Metabolic Acidosis, and Hypothermia

Loss of clotting factors compounded by their dilution during resuscitation with hypocoagulable fluids are major causes of TIC (Frith and Brohi 2012; Hess et al. 2008). High-volume crystalloid- and/or colloid-based prehospital resuscitation is independently associated with worse emergency department coagulation tests and increased need for blood transfusion. Hypoperfusion due to hemorrhagic shock and excess ionic chloride administration commonly leads to metabolic acidosis. Acidosis impairs the activity of coagulation proteases. The activities of FVII and the complexes tissue factor-FVII and Fxa-Va are markedly reduced at pH levels of 7.0 or below. Hypothermia is also common in trauma and inhibits platelet function and coagulation protease activity. Clinically, relevant changes on platelet function are observed in moderate hypothermia when core temperatures drop below 34 °C. Clotting factor activity is critically affected with more severe hypothermia at temperatures below 32 °C.

Application

Our current understanding that TIC is not only the result of severe hemorrhage, dilution, acidosis, and hypothermia but also due to an early, intrinsic, coagulopathy initiated by shock and amount of tissue destruction has challenged traditional resuscitation strategies utilizing hypocoagulable fluids. A more balanced resuscitation, addressing not only volume loss but also early coagulopathy,

has been proposed (Holcomb 2007). It recommends early activation of a ratio-based transfusion protocols (plasma and platelets at a near 1:1 ratio with RBC) while limiting hypocoagulable fluids. This novel trauma resuscitation also promotes liberal use of fibrinogen and hemostatic drugs, such as tranexamic acid in severely injured bleeding patients. The different strategies currently available for the management of TIC are discussed in subsequent chapters of this section.

Cross-References

- ▶ Acute Coagulopathy of Trauma
- ▶ Coagulopathy
- ▶ Coagulopathy in a Trauma Patient
- ▶ Hypocoaguability
- ▶ International Normalized Ratio
- ▶ Prothrombin Time
- ▶ Thrombocytopenia

References

Frith D, Brohi K (2012) The pathophysiology of trauma-induced coagulopathy. Curr Opin Crit Care 18(6):631–636, 24, Epub ahead of print

Hess JR, Brohi K, Dutton RP et al (2008) The coagulopathy of trauma: a review of mechanisms. J Trauma 65(4):748–754

Holcomb JB (2007) Damage control resuscitation. J Trauma 62(Suppl 6):S36–S37

Rizoli SB, Scarpelini S, Callum J et al (2011a) Clotting factor deficiency in early trauma-associated coagulopathy. J Trauma 71(5 Suppl 1):S427–S434

Rizoli S, Nascimento B Jr, Key N et al (2011b) Disseminated intravascular coagulopathy in the first 24 hours after trauma: the association between ISTH score and anatomopathologic evidence. J Trauma 71(5 Suppl 1):S441–S447

Cognition

▶ Traumatic Brain Injury: Cognitive/Speech-Language Issues

Cognitive Impairment

▶ Cognitive-Linguistic Deficits, Trauma-Related

Cognitive-Communication Disorder

▶ Cognitive-Linguistic Deficits, Trauma-Related

Cognitive-Linguistic Deficits, Trauma-Related

Inga Simning[1] and Douglas Fetkenhour[2]
[1]Department of Speech Pathology, University of Rochester School of Medicine, Rochester, NY, USA
[2]Department of Physical Medicine and Rehabilitation, University of Rochester School of Medicine, Rochester, NY, USA

Synonyms

Cognitive-Communication Disorder; Cognitive impairment

Definition

Disorder of memory, problem-solving, and ability to understand or produce language.

Many patients beginning rehabilitation after significant trauma will have cognitive deficits resulting from a known or unknown traumatic brain injury, side effects of multiple medications, lingering encephalopathy, or baseline deficits. Healthcare providers should be sensitive to patients who have difficulty accurately responding to orientation questions, are tangential or incoherent in conversation, make inappropriate jokes or comments, are easily distracted, do not comprehend the gravity or impact of their injuries, or need alarms, restraints, or supervision for safety. Patients with suspected cognitive

deficits should be referred to an SLP for cognitive-linguistic evaluation. It is especially important to identify and refer these patients because even mild cognitive impairments can significantly impact patient safety after discharge.

Cognitive-Linguistic Evaluation and Treatment

Speech-language pathologists working in acute rehabilitation are trained to evaluate and treat all aspects of cognition. SLPs use a combination of formal and informal tools to assess language, memory, attention, insight, problem-solving, reasoning, judgment, and executive functioning. Treatment involves frequent reorientation, teaching and practicing compensatory strategies, use of assistive devices, and drills to improve specific deficit areas (Brookshire 2007). The SLP will assist with discharge planning by providing information regarding the need for supervision or assistance to ensure patient safety after discharge.

Trauma-Related Speech Deficits

Trauma patients can have speech disorders resulting from intubation trauma, tracheostomy, or poor respiratory support for speech. A patient with a speech disorder can have a hoarse voice, run out of breath when talking, speak too quietly, or be completely aphonic.

Treatment of Trauma-Related Speech Deficits

SLPs treat speech disorders through breathing exercises to increase respiratory support; voicing exercises to improve loudness, pitch, or quality; and education about vocal hygiene to keep the vocal folds healthy.

For the patient who has a tracheostomy and is aphonic, a speaking valve may be the most appropriate way to restore oral communication. A speaking valve is a small, one-way valve that is placed on the end of a tracheostomy tube. The application of a speaking valve will redirect expiratory airflow past the vocal folds and out of the oral cavity (rather than out of the tracheostomy, which is below the level of the vocal folds) allowing the patient to phonate. The speaking valve is ordered by a physician and initially placed by the SLP, usually in conjunction with a respiratory therapist.

Cross-References

▶ Speech-Language Pathologist (SLP)

References

Brookshire RH (2007) Introduction to neurogenic communication disorders, 7th edn. Mosby Elsevier, St. Louis

Colles' Fracture

▶ Distal Radius Fractures

Colon and Rectal Injuries

Joshua A. Marks and Patrick K. Kim
Division of Traumatology, Surgical Critical Care and Emergency Surgery, Department of Surgery, Perelman School of Medicine at the University of Pennsylvania, Philadelphia, PA, USA

Synonyms

Penetrating colon injuries; Perforating injuries of the colon and rectum; Trauma of the large bowel

Definition

Anatomy
The colon extends from the ileocecal valve to the rectosigmoid junction at the level of the sacral promontory. The rectosigmoid junction is marked by the splaying of the three taenia coli and the disappearance of the epiploic appendages.

The colon is both a retro- and intraperitoneal structure tethered to the retroperitoneum along the right and left avascular white lines of Toldt.

The rectum is an intraperitoneal structure for approximately 8 cm from the rectosigmoid junction to the middle traverse fold where the peritoneal reflection ends and then the rectum becomes completely extraperitoneal. Thus, injuries to the lower one-third of the rectum and to the entire posterior wall are considered to be extraperitoneal. The relation of the rectum to the peritoneum defines the management of injuries to the region.

Mechanism of Injury
The majority of injury to the colon is caused by penetrating objects or projectiles either from transabdominal or transgluteal gunshot or stab wounds or iatrogenically during endoscopy or from swallowing or inserting objects rectally. Blunt trauma to the colon is rare, often caused by motor vehicle collisions, and frequently the result of sheer injury from acute increase in intraluminal pressure causing blowout or from avulsion injury to the mesocolon (Cayten et al. 1998; Johnson and Steele 2013; Steele et al. 2011).

AAST Colon Injury Scale (Moore et al. 1996)

Grade[a]	Type of injury	Description of injury	AIS-90
I	Hematoma	Contusion without devascularization	2
	Laceration	Partial thickness, no perforation	2
II	Laceration	<50 % of circumference	3
III	Laceration	≥50 % of circumference without transection	3
IV	Laceration	Transection of the colon	4
V	Laceration	Transection of the colon with segmental tissue loss	4
	Vascular	Devascularized segment	4

AIS abbreviated injury scale
[a]Advance one grade for multiple injuries up to grade III

AAST Rectum Injury Scale (Moore et al. 1996)

Grade[a]	Type of injury	Description of injury	AIS-90
I	Hematoma	Contusion without devascularization	2
	Laceration	Partial thickness	2
II	Laceration	<50 % of circumference	3
III	Laceration	≥50 % of circumference	4
IV	Laceration	Full thickness with extension in the perineum	5
V	Vascular	Devascularized segment	5

AIS abbreviated injury scale
[a]Advance one grade for multiple injuries up to grade III

Preexisting Condition

Historical Perspective

The management of colorectal trauma has evolved over the last number of decades (Cayten et al. 1998; Johnson and Steele 2013; Steele et al. 2011). Once held military dogma regarding mandatory colostomy for all colonic injuries now largely has been abandoned favoring primary repair of colonic injuries, especially in the civilian population, when and where possible (Woodhall and Ochsner 1951; Stone and Fabian 1979). Similarly, for penetrating rectal injury, former recommendations of routine fecal diversion, distal rectal washout, presacral drainage, and rectal repair have been challenged (Lavenson and Cohen 1971).

Diagnosis

Patients with peritoneal signs or who develop peritonitis while following serial abdominal examinations require exploratory laparotomy. On CT imaging, the presence of pneumoperitoneum, extraluminal contrast, and colonic wall thickening and stranding of the mesentery are suggestive signs of colonic injury. Triple contrast CT scanning (oral, intravenous, and rectal) is utilized in some centers to evaluate hemodynamically stable penetrating trauma to the flank and back to aid in identification of injury to the colon. However, the value of oral contrast is debated. In the acute trauma setting, oral and rectal contrast is impractical, but in select stable patients, it may be helpful. Triple contrast helical CT in penetrating trauma has been shown to demonstrate up to a 100 % sensitivity, 96 % specificity, 100 % negative predictive value, and 97 % accuracy in patients evaluated for peritoneal violation, or colonic, major vascular or urinary tract injuries (Johnson and Steele 2013).

Rectal injury is often a result of pelvic fractures or penetrating injury as in a transpelvic gunshot wound. On physical exam, gross blood seen on digital rectal exam should increase suspicion of a rectal injury. It is important to first wipe the perineum clean and assure that the gloved finger is clean of blood prior to insertion into the rectum. If rectal injury is suspected, rigid proctoscopy is indicated even if an exploratory laparotomy is otherwise planned (Cayten et al. 1998). On proctoscopy, hematoma, perforation, and intraluminal blood indicate rectal injury. In select hemodynamically stable patients without peritonitis, laparoscopy is an option to assess for penetration of the peritoneal cavity (Johnson and Steele 2013; Steele et al. 2011).

Application

Control of Contamination

Injuries to the colon are identified as part of a complete trauma laparotomy. Control of major hemorrhage is the first priority, followed by control of gross GI contamination. The intraperitoneal and retroperitoneal aspects of the colon should be inspected. The right and left colon are mobilized along the white lines of Toldt to fully evaluate the retroperitoneal aspect. The avascular gastrocolic ligament is also opened to both evaluate the lesser sac and fully explore the transverse colon to the splenic flexure. In penetrating trauma, the finding of a colon injury should prompt the careful and thorough inspection for another traumatic defect, as most projectiles will cause a through-and-through injury (Cayten et al. 1998; Johnson and Steele 2013; Steele et al. 2011).

Traumatic defects of the colon can be temporarily controlled with a "whipstitch" suture, clamp (Babcock or Allis), umbilical tapes, or bowel staplers. All methods of temporary fecal containment have a risk of threatening additional colon tissue, which should be considered when performing definitive repair.

Injury Location

Until recently, left colon injuries were more likely to be treated by fecal diversion compared to right colon injuries, for which primary repair was more common. Current data suggests that colon injury location per se (ascending/hepatic flexure, transverse, descending/splenic flexure, or sigmoid) does not affect morbidity (i.e., leak or abscess formation) or mortality (Sharpe et al. 2012). Other factors, such as tissue destruction of the wound itself and presence of shock, have greater impact on outcomes. Thus, the treatment of colon injury should take all these factors into account, not simply injury location (Cayten et al. 1998; Johnson and Steele 2013; Steele et al. 2011).

Conversely, management of rectal injury depends on location of the injury in relation to the peritoneal reflection. Proximal intraperitoneal rectal injuries are managed similar to injuries of the colon. Extraperitoneal injuries are treated with proximal fecal diversion, usually via sigmoid loop colostomy, with or without direct repair of the injury (Cayten et al. 1998; Johnson and Steele 2013; Steele et al. 2011). The available data suggest that primary repair of extraperitoneal wounds is unnecessary in the setting of proximal rectal diversion and that the added time, blood loss, and morbidity of the dissection and repair is not worth the potential benefit (Johnson and Steele 2013). In general the extraperitoneal rectum only needs to be mobilized if there is massive adjacent hemorrhage, as in bleeding from the mesorectum; however, this too can be managed frequently with pelvic packing alone (Johnson and Steele 2013).

Primary Repair Versus Resection

The preponderance of the current evidence supports primary closure of all nondestructive colon injuries. Destructive wounds are those involving greater than 50 % circumference of the colonic wall, complete transection of the colon, significant loss of tissue, and devascularized segments of colon (Miller et al. 2002). In the absence of comorbidities (medical conditions that reduce wound healing, including chronic renal failure, congestive heart failure, HIV, cirrhosis, and use of chronic steroids) or significant transfusion requirement (≥ 6 units PRBCs), destructive wounds should be treated with appropriate segmental resection and primary anastomosis (Miller et al. 2002; Demetriades et al. 2001). Patients with destructive wounds and significant comorbidities or preoperative or intraoperative transfusion requirements should undergo diversion either via proximal diverting ostomy or Hartmann's procedure (Miller et al. 2002). If the distal segment (Hartmann's pouch) is long enough, a mucus fistula should be considered. Primary repair of an injury involving more than 50 % of the colonic wall circumference narrows significantly the colon and could result in obstructive symptoms (Miller et al. 2002).

Anastomosis Versus Diversion

Generally, a colostomy is performed only if primary repair cannot safely be done due to patient instability, serious concomitant injury, or significant bowel edema or ischemia (Demetriades et al. 2001). The degree of contamination should probably not affect the decision to divert (Miller et al. 2002). Furthermore, complications from colostomy closure should be considered part of the overall decision to commit a patient to fecal diversion. The decreased morbidity associated with avoiding a colostomy, the disability associated with the time interval from creation to closure of the colostomy, and the charges incurred with colostomy creation and subsequent closure all add support to primary repair of nondestructive colon wounds as the standard of care (Demetriades et al. 2001). Stable patients with destructive penetrating wounds and without significant associated injuries should undergo resection with primary anastomosis (Cayten et al. 1998; Johnson and Steele 2013; Steele et al. 2011). Again, extraperitoneal rectal injuries are treated with proximal fecal diversion, usually via sigmoid loop colostomy (Johnson and Steele 2013; Steele et al. 2011).

Stapled Versus Handsewn

The technique of anastomosis has been studied and evaluated to determine its impact on leak rates. Two Cochrane reviews examining ileocolic and colorectal anastomoses respectively concluded that stapled functional end-to-end ileocolic anastomoses are associated with fewer leaks than handsewn but identified no superiority of one over the other in colorectal anastomoses. Stapled versus handsewn techniques (either single or two layer) have demonstrated no difference in terms of anastomotic leak in the setting of trauma (Demetriades et al. 2002). Either technique can be used and should be dictated by the surgeon's experience, comfort, and preference. If the patient is unstable, a damage control technique should be utilized and anastomosis delayed (Johnson and Steele 2013; Steele et al. 2011).

Open Abdomen/Damage Control

After controlling hemorrhage and contamination, an abbreviated laparotomy may be performed in order to interrupt the trauma lethal triad. The definitive surgical procedure reestablishing gastrointestinal continuity can occur after the patient is warmed, resuscitated, and stabilized. Debate exists over whether a primary anastomosis should be performed at this point or if diversion is more prudent (Miller et al. 2007). Some data suggest that if the first reoperation is within 36 h, then a delayed colonic anastomosis is acceptable; otherwise an ostomy may be best management (Miller et al. 2007; Burlew et al. 2011). Other data advocate that there is a single opportunity to restore colonic continuity following damage control laparotomy and that if fascial closure cannot be achieved on the second operation, then patients should be treated with an ostomy as there may be as high as an eightfold increase in anastomotic leak (Anjaria et al. 2014).

Presacral Drains

Popularized during World War II, the use of presacral drains either via the traditional transperineal or transabdominal routes is controversial due to the potential complications and associated patient discomfort (Johnson and Steele 2013; Steele et al. 2011). If used, proper positioning of the drains adjacent to the injury is necessary to drain the presacral space adequately (Johnson and Steele 2013; Steele et al. 2011). While studies have shown presacral drains to reduce pelvic infection in a series of combat wounds, several retrospective studies have demonstrated no difference with and without presacral drainage in patients who underwent fecal diversion (Ivatury et al. 1991). One small prospective randomized trial concluded that presacral drainage had no role in the reduction of infectious complications (Gonzalez et al. 1998). Overall the available data indicate that the use of presacral drains should be limited, possibly only to lower third (essentially anal canal) injuries, and, when used, should communicate with the injury (Johnson and Steele 2013).

Distal Rectal Washout

The goal of distal rectal washout is to minimize fecal contamination of an open rectal wound, thereby reducing the risk of pelvic sepsis. Ironically, the process of flushing irrigant into the rectum may actually deliver bacteria into tissue planes that would otherwise have been minimally contaminated (Ivatury et al. 1991). Most recent published series have demonstrated no significant advantage to distal washout in civilian trauma. The technique offers no significant protective effect on the prevention of infectious complications (Johnson and Steele 2013).

Colostomy Reversal

Timing of takedown of diverting colostomies is debated. Most injuries heal within 10 days, and, therefore, most colostomies performed for colon and rectal trauma can be closed within 2 weeks if the patient is otherwise stable without evidence of non-healing bowel injury or unresolved wound sepsis (Berne et al. 1998). A barium enema need not be performed to rule out colon cancer or polyps prior to colostomy reversal for trauma patients without risk factors or other indication for screening (Johnson and Steele 2013).

Antibiotics

Numerous studies demonstrate the importance of administering a single preoperative dose of prophylactic broad-spectrum aerobic and anaerobic antibiotic coverage for all penetrating abdominal wounds to reduce the risk of surgical site infection (SSI). The current data clearly show that antibiotics should be continued for no more than 24 h in the presence of hollow viscus injury and that with absent hollow viscus injury, no further administration of antibiotics beyond the preoperative dose is necessary (Goldberg et al. 2012). Furthermore, the damage control laparotomy in and of itself does not warrant the continuation of prophylactic antibiotics for any longer than 24 h. Despite the emergent nature of operative procedures in trauma, adherence to the four Surgical Care Improvement Project (SCIP) antibiotic prophylaxis guidelines ((1.) prophylactic antibiotics given, (2.) antibiotics received within 1 h before incision, (3.) correct antibiotic selection, and (4.) discontinuation of antibiotic within 24 h after surgery) should be maintained in order to effectively reduce the risk of SSI (Smith et al. 2012). Of note, in the hemorrhaging patient, the administered dose of antibiotics may be increased two- or threefold and repeated after transfusion of every 10 units of blood until there is no further blood loss.

Conclusions

Specific surgical procedures should be tailored to the patient based not only on the degree of injury but also on hemodynamic stability and associated injuries. Technical excellence and sound surgical judgment remains paramount in the management of these injuries.

Cross-References

▶ Damage Control Resuscitation
▶ Damage Control Surgery
▶ Imaging of Abdominal and Pelvic Injuries
▶ Open Abdomen
▶ Surgical Site Infections
▶ Trauma Laparotomy

References

Anjaria DJ, Ullmann TM, Lavery R, Livingston DH (2014) Management of colonic injuries in the setting of damage-control laparotomy: one shot to get it right. J Trauma Acute Care Surg 76(3):594–598, discussion 598–600

Berne JD, Velmahos GC, Chan LS, Asensio JA, Demetriades D (1998) The high morbidity of colostomy closure after trauma: further support for the primary repair of colon injuries. Surgery 123(2):157–164

Burlew CC, Moore EE, Cuschieri J, Jurkovich GJ, Codner P, Crowell K et al (2011) Sew it up! A western trauma association multi-institutional study of enteric injury management in the postinjury open abdomen. J Trauma 70(2):273–277

Cayten CG, Fabian TC, Garcia VF, Ivatury RR, Morris Jr, JA (1998) Patient management guidelines for penetrating intraperitoneal colon injuries. East Assoc Surg Trauma

Demetriades D, Murray JA, Chan L, Ordonez C, Bowley D, Nagy KK et al (2001) Penetrating colon injuries requiring resection: diversion or primary anastomosis? an AAST prospective multicenter study. J Trauma 50(5):765–775

Demetriades D, Murray JA, Chan LS, Ordonez C, Bowley D, Nagy KK et al (2002) Handsewn versus stapled anastomosis in penetrating colon injuries requiring resection: a multicenter study. J Trauma 52(1):117–121

Goldberg SR, Anand RJ, Como JJ, Dechert T, Dente C, Luchette FA et al (2012) Prophylactic antibiotic use in penetrating abdominal trauma: an eastern association for the surgery of trauma practice management guideline. J Trauma Acute Care Surg 73(5 Suppl 4): S321–S325

Gonzalez RP, Falimirski ME, Holevar MR (1998) The role of presacral drainage in the management of penetrating rectal injuries. J Trauma 45(4):656–661

Ivatury RR, Licata J, Gunduz Y, Rao P, Stahl WM (1991) Management options in penetrating rectal injuries. Am Surg 57(1):50–55

Johnson EK, Steele SR (2013) Evidence-based management of colorectal trauma. J Gastrointest Surg 17(9):1712–1719

Lavenson GS, Cohen A (1971) Management of rectal injuries. Am J Surg 122(2):226–230

Miller PR, Fabian TC, Croce MA, Magnotti LJ, Elizabeth Pritchard F, Minard G et al (2002) Improving outcomes following penetrating colon wounds: application of a clinical pathway. Ann Surg 235(6):775–781

Miller PR, Chang MC, Hoth JJ, Holmes JH 4, Meredith JW (2007) Colonic resection in the setting of damage control laparotomy: is delayed anastomosis safe? Am Surg 73(6):606–609, discussion 609–10

Moore EE, Cogbill TH, Malangoni MA, Jurkovich GJ, Champion HR (1996) Scaling system for organ specific injuries. Curr Opin Crit Care 2(6):450–462

Sharpe JP, Magnotti LJ, Weinberg JA, Zarzaur BL, Shahan CP, Parks NA et al (2012) Impact of location on outcome after penetrating colon injuries. J Trauma Acute Care Surg 73(6):1428–1432, discussion 1433

Smith BP, Fox N, Fakhro A, LaChant M, Pathak AS, Ross SE et al (2012) "SCIP"ping antibiotic prophylaxis guidelines in trauma: the consequences of noncompliance. J Trauma Acute Care Surg 73(2):452–456, discussion 456

Steele SR, Maykel JA, Johnson EK (2011) Traumatic injury of the colon and rectum: the evidence vs dogma. Dis Colon Rectum 54(9):1184–1201

Stone HH, Fabian TC (1979) Management of perforating colon trauma: randomization between primary closure and exteriorization. Ann Surg 190(4):430–436

Woodhall JP, Ochsner A (1951) The management of perforating injuries of the colon and rectum in civilian practice. Surgery 29(2):305–320

Colon Injury

▶ Gastrointestinal Injury, Anesthesia for

Coma

▶ Traumatic Brain Injury, Severe: Medical and Surgical Management

Coma Depasse

▶ Brain Death

Comatose

▶ Traumatic Brain Injury, Severe: Medical and Surgical Management

Combat Disorder

▶ Post Traumatic Stress Disorder

Combat Fatigue

▶ Post Traumatic Stress Disorder

Combat Helmet

▶ Body Armor

Combat Neurosis

▶ Post Traumatic Stress Disorder

Comfort, Neuromuscular Blockade

▶ Sedation, Analgesia, Neuromuscular Blockade in the ICU

Commotio Cerebri

▶ Traumatic Brain Injury, Concussion

Commotio Cordis

▶ Cardiac and Aortic Trauma, Anesthesia for

Communication – Interaction, Discussion, Information Transfer, Comforting

▶ End-of-Life Care Communication in Trauma Patients

Compartment Release, Aponeurotomy

► Fasciotomy

Compartment Syndrome

Philip N. Collis and Craig S. Roberts
Department of Orthopaedic Surgery, University
of Louisville School of Medicine, Louisville,
KY, USA

Synonyms

Fasciotomy; Foot; Gluteal; Lumbar paraspinal;
Pelvic; Thigh

Definition

Although compartment syndrome has been most
commonly described in the calf and the forearm,
there is an increased recognition of compartment
syndrome occurring in other less common
regions of the body (thigh, foot, gluteal, lumbar
paraspinal, and pelvic). Compartment syndrome
is commonly attributed to an elevated interstitial
pressure confined within an osteofascial compartment that surpasses the capillary perfusion
pressures and causes decreased perfusion to muscles and nerves. Although the classic clinical
findings seen in compartment syndrome
include disproportionate pain, paresthesias, pain
with passive stretch, pallor, paralysis, and
pulselessness, compartment pressure measurements can be made to assist in diagnosis, and
a delta P (ΔP = diastolic blood
pressure – compartment pressure) is calculated.
A $\Delta P < 30$ is commonly referenced as an indicator of compartment syndrome (Roberts et al.
2011). We will discuss the less commonly seen
compartment syndromes: lumbar paraspinal, gluteal, pelvic, thigh, and foot.

Thigh

Upper leg three compartments: anterior, posterior, medial.

Etiology

Compartment syndrome of the thigh is most commonly seen as a result of direct trauma associated
with femur fractures. Atraumatic causes of thigh
compartment syndrome include external compression of the thigh for a prolonged period of
time. Associated risk factors include vascular
injury, coagulopathy, and systemic hypotension
(Ojike, 2010a, *Injury*).

Diagnosis

Consideration of patient risk factors and high
clinical suspicion are helpful in the early diagnosis of thigh compartment syndrome. Common
clinical exam findings include pain out of proportion and a tense, uncompressible thigh. Elevated
compartment pressures have a limited role, but
can assist in the determination of compartment
syndrome. Laboratory findings such as elevated
creatinine kinase should also be taken into
consideration (Ojike, 2010a, *Injury*).

Treatment

In addition to aggressive resuscitation, patients
with thigh compartment syndrome warrant timely
decompressive fasciotomies of the three compartments of the thigh (anterior, posterior, and medial
compartments). The anterior and posterior compartments are primarily accessed through a direct
lateral incision along the thigh. Release of the
anterior and posterior compartments through
a single lateral incision usually results in decompression of the medial compartment as well. If
there is any doubt as to whether or not the medial
compartment is released, a second incision can be
made medially to release the adductor, or medial,
compartment (Ojike, 2010a, *Injury*).

Foot

Muscles of the foot are separated into nine
compartments.

Etiology

Crush injuries to the foot are among the most common causes for foot compartment syndrome, along with calcaneal fractures, Lisfranc injuries, metatarsal fractures, and phalangeal fractures. There have also been reports of foot compartment syndrome in patients with associated lower leg fractures outside the foot (Ojike, 2010b, *Acta*).

Diagnosis

Diagnosis of compartment syndrome is by clinical exam, high index of suspicion, and associated elevated compartment pressures. Delayed or missed diagnosis can lead to muscle necrosis and the development of claw toes (Ojike, 2010b, *Acta*).

Treatment

There are nine described compartments within the foot (four interosseous compartments, as well as the lateral, medial, superficial, calcaneal, and adductor compartments). Decompression of the osteofascial compartments of the foot has been performed with one to four incisions. A three-incision approach has been advocated, consisting of two dorsal incisions and one medial incision. Delayed primary closure or skin grafting is commonly required to expedite healing of the incisions (Ojike, 2010b, *Acta*).

Gluteal

Buttock region, including the gluteus maximus, gluteus medius, and gluteus minimus muscles and tensor fascia lata.

Etiology

Causes of gluteal compartment syndrome include direct trauma, prolonged period of immobilization, vascular injury, epidural analgesia, and infection (Henson et al. 2009).

Diagnosis

Diagnosis of gluteal compartment syndrome relies primarily on history and clinical findings common to compartment syndrome of other regions and compartment pressure measurements.

Although no standardized pressure threshold is absolutely diagnostic, a measurement greater than 30 mmHg is thought to be suggestive of gluteal compartment syndrome (Henson et al. 2009).

Treatment

There are three myofascial compartments within the gluteal region: gluteus maximus, the gluteus medius and minimus, and tensor fascia lata. Decompressive fasciotomy should be performed in acute compartment syndrome. The most commonly described technique is through the posterior or Southern approach similar to that used in total hip arthroplasty while ensuring release of the three major myofascial compartments. The necessity for exploration and release of the sciatic nerve at the time of fasciotomy is controversial (Henson et al. 2009).

Lumbar Paraspinal

Lower back including the iliocostalis, longissimus, multifidus muscles.

Etiology

Causes of lumbar paraspinal compartment syndrome can be classified as acute versus chronic and traumatic versus atraumatic. The most common causes are downhill skiing, surfboarding, and weight lifting, followed by aortic bypass surgery and gastric bypass surgery (Nathan et al. 2012).

Diagnosis

Common clinical symptoms and findings include extreme pain with localized loss of sensation, localized tenderness, board-like rigidity of the paraspinal region, and decreased abdominal sounds. Chronic exertional symptoms are relieved with extension and worsened with flexion and exertion. Magnetic resonance imaging (MRI) may play an added role in diagnosis of lumbar compartment syndrome. Other investigational studies which can assist in diagnosis are elevated creatinine phosphokinase (CPK) levels, serum glutamic oxaloacetic transaminase (SGOT) levels, urine myoglobinuria, and intracompartmental pressure measurements (Nathan et al. 2012).

Treatment

Initial treatment should consist of aggressive fluid resuscitation, pain control, urine alkalization, and bed rest in order to prevent rhabdomyolysis and acute renal failure. Fasciotomies have an important role in the treatment of acute lumbar paraspinal compartment syndrome and involve decompression of the paraspinal muscles within the lumbodorsal fascia (Nathan et al. 2012).

Pelvic

Retroperitoneal space, including the iliopsoas and intrapelvic muscles.

Etiology

Pelvic compartment syndrome is rare. The most common cause is direct pelvic trauma resulting in hematoma and increased pressures in the retroperitoneal space. Atraumatic pelvic compartment syndrome is associated with infection and drug and alcohol abuse leading to prolonged compression-type injury. It has also been associated with hip arthroscopy in cases with higher-than-usual fluid requirements. Injury to intrapelvic vessels can also cause pelvic compartment syndrome from bleeding and hematoma, with compromise of neuromuscular perfusion and compression of the ureters (Ojike et al. 2012).

Diagnosis

Diagnosis of pelvic compartment syndrome can be difficult. History of trauma and/or coagulopathies is a risk factor, as well as unstable pelvic fracture and hematoma formation as depicted on CT scan. Burning pain, pelvic tenderness, swelling in the buttocks, palpable lower abdominal mass, lower extremity weakness, and decreased urinary output are clinical findings associated with pelvic compartment syndrome (Ojike et al. 2012).

Treatment

Decompression of pelvic compartment syndrome is performed by decompression of the retroperitoneum. Skin incisions are usually made parallel with and centered over the iliac crests, similar to the anterior approach to the sacroiliac joints. Upon entry into the iliac fossa, the retroperitoneal hematoma can be evaluated. In addition, a Pfannenstiel incision can be made in order to enter the space of Retzius if additional decompression and evacuation of a hematoma is needed. The ureters are usually decompressed by evacuation of the hematoma. Visualization and decompression of the ureters or nephrostomy tubes have also been recommended, but are controversial.

Conclusion

Compartment syndrome is recognized in less common areas of the body: lumbar paraspinal muscles, gluteal region, pelvic, thigh, and foot. Each of these compartment syndromes has special clinical features. Despite increased appreciation for these rarer types of compartment syndrome, their diagnosis and management remain challenging problems.

Cross-References

▶ Compartment Syndrome of the Forearm
▶ Compartment Syndrome of the Leg
▶ Compartment Syndrome, Acute
▶ Compartment Syndrome: Complication of Care in ICU
▶ Orthopedic Trauma, Anesthesia for

References

Henson JT, Roberts CS, Giannoudis PV (2009) Gluteal compartment syndrome. Acta Orthop Belg 75:147–152
Nathan ST, Roberts CS, Deliberato D (2012) Lumbar paraspinal compartment syndrome. Int Orthop 36:1221–1227

Ojike NI, Roberts CS, Giannoudis PV (2010a) Compartment syndrome of the thigh: a systematic review. Injury 41:133–136

Ojike NI, Roberts CS, Giannoudis PV (2010b) Foot compartment syndrome: a systematic review of the literature. Acta Orthop Belg 75:573–580

Ojike NI, Roberts CS, Giannoudis PV (2012) Pelvic compartment syndrome: a systematic review. Acta Orthop Belg 78:6–10

Roberts CS, Gorczyca JT, Ring D, Pugh KJ (2011) Diagnosis and treatment of less common compartment syndromes of the upper and lower extremities: current evidence and best practices. In: Egol KA, Tornetta P (eds) AOS instructional course lectures, vol 60. AAOS, Rosemont, pp 43–50, Chapter 5

Compartment Syndrome of the Forearm

Xuan Luo[1] and Phil Blazar[2]
[1]Harvard Combined Orthopedic Residency Program, Massachusetts General Hospital, Boston, MA, USA
[2]Department of Orthopedics, Brigham and Women's Hospital, Boston, MA, USA

Synonyms

Acute Compartment Syndrome; Compartmental syndrome

Definition

Compartment syndrome occurs when pressures within an enclosed compartment, usually muscles within a fascial envelope, become elevated to the point that tissue perfusion is compromised, resulting in cell ischemia and if untreated eventual muscle necrosis.

Compartment syndrome can happen in any enclosed space in the body, most commonly seen in the fascial compartments of the leg, however it can occur in the abdomen, chest, head, and in the focus of this chapter, in the upper extremity as well. Compartment syndrome is a true surgical emergency, with devastating results if not diagnosed and treated promptly. Diagnosis of compartment syndrome however, is fraught with misconceptions and pitfalls, namely the confusion between physical exam findings descriptive of acute arterial occlusion with those of compartment syndrome.

History

Though compartment syndrome occurs most frequently in the lower extremity, one of its earliest descriptions was in the upper extremity. In 1881 Richard Von Volkman described an irreversible flexor contracture in patients he hypothesized had splints or bandages placed too tightly, leading to decreased blood flow and thus muscle death leading to contracture (Twaddle and Amendola 2009).

Though this early description was surprisingly accurate, up until the 1960s the pathology of compartment syndrome was not well understood. Prior to that time, many physicians believed that muscle ischemia during compartment syndrome was caused by injury, spasm, or constriction of a major artery. This false belief was further confirmed by operative attempts to address a presumed damaged artery resulting in resolution of compartment syndrome, likely due to the fasciotomy performed during surgical exposure of the arterial system rather than any arterial repair (McQueen 2010). The false belief that arterial flow is compromised in compartment syndrome perpetuates false idioms that persist today.

Pathophysiology

To have compartment syndrome, there are two necessary components. There must be an enclosed compartment and there must be an insult to the tissues within that compartment. At the heart of compartment syndrome is a positive feedback loop, involving muscle ischemia and perfusion.

The cycle starts with the initial insult that causes either direct increase of pressure within a fascial compartment, such as hemorrhage or direct fluid infiltration; or local tissue damage which then also leads to edema and increased local pressures. When pressure in the compartment increases tissue perfusion decreases and then ceases. As the muscle becomes ischemic an inflammatory response results that involves free calcium accumulation, myolysis, and release of toxic intracellular chemicals. Cellular death and inflammation leads to further capillary leak and increase of interstitial fluid and further elevated pressures. This in turn causes further cell death, which then causes yet more capillary leak and elevated pressures. Thus once pressures in a compartment exceeds the threshold beyond which tissue perfusion is compromised, the process is self-perpetuating. It is typically impossible to undo the initial insult; however it is possible to remove the only other necessary component of compartment syndrome, the enclosed compartment itself. Surgical fasciotomy of the compartment and thus opening of the enclosed space is the only reliable treatment for compartment syndrome (Twaddle and Amendola 2009).

As the process of compartment syndrome becomes intractable only after a of the rising intramuscular pressure reaches a threshold information about this threshold pressure is of great clinical interest. There is however, debate as to pressure level should be used. The absolute number of arteriolar pressure in the normal body is close to 30 mmHg. Thus many have advocated for clinical use of 30 mmHg within a muscular compartment as indicative of compartment syndrome. This is based on the hypothesis that beyond 30 mmHg of interstitial pressure, that the surrounding tissues will force these small vessels closed. This 30 mmHg can be thought of as a "closing pressure." Others have countered that the concept of closing pressure is flawed, because in animal studies; the small vessels are never seen to actually close even with high interstitial pressures. . It is likely that ischemia in compartment syndrome is due to the concept of a decreased perfusion gradient rather than vessel closure. I It is the loss of pressure differential that slows blood flow to the point of inadequacy for tissue perfusion. This critical factor appears to be a pressure difference of less than 20–30 mmHg between the diastolic blood pressure and the compartment pressure (ΔP) (McQueen 2010).

Compartment syndrome progresses through six stages. In the acute incipient stage, pressures remain below the critical threshold values and true (i.e. irreversible) compartment syndrome has not set in. At this point removal of the insult may still reverse the process, as the syndrome has not reached its positive feedback cycle stage. As pressures rise, the acute established stage begins and the positive feedback loop of compartment syndrome begins. Tissues become ischemic, however this stage precedes muscle necrosis and permanent damage is avoided if emergent fasciotomy is performed. Muscle tissues likely remains viable for 4–6 h during this period. With a time interval beyond 8 h however, muscle necrosis occurs and the damage is no longer reversible with fasciotomy. Continued neglect of compartment syndrome results in late established compartment syndrome, in which prolonged elevation of pressures results in cell death. Over weeks to months the dead muscle will be replaced with fibrous tissue, which contracts, resulting in the characteristic flexion contractures described by Volkman (Leversedge et al. 2011).

Diagnosis

As missed compartment syndrome is such a devastating and irreversible injury, diagnosis and treatment emergently prior to tissue infarction is paramount.

The most important point for diagnosing compartment syndrome is having a high index of suspicion, especially in the setting of high-risk insults. Recognition of causes of compartment syndrome is invaluable to the diagnosis, and will be covered later in the chapter.

Many clinicians are taught the six P's of compartment syndrome being pain, parathesia, pallor, pressure, paralysis, and pulselessness. The constellation of these findings is more consistent with acute arterial occlusion than with acute compartment syndrome. In compartment syndrome, often only one P, perhaps two of these clinical findings are present. Surgical intervention is indicated/mandatory prior to the development of all six "p"s.

The most common and earliest finding in compartment syndrome is pain. While all patients with injury have some degree of pain, the pain of compartment syndrome is increasing and disproportionate to the expected pain of the particular injury. Many clinicians find that pain on passive stretch, and tenderness with palpation of the affected compartment to add diagnostic value; however some studies have shown these findings are no more sensitive or specific than pain alone. Often times the affected compartments will feel firm or distinctly hard to the touch, however some of the compartments may be to deep to be felt manually, and palpation of compartments has poor inter-observer reliability. With severe swelling the skin may be stretched taut with shiny and hard surface, however this may be confounded by superficial swelling without compartment syndrome. Parathesias involving the cutaneous distribution of the nerves which run within the affected compartment is another sign, which indicates thatthe nerve is ischemic. However, by the time sensory changes have occurred, permanent damage is likely to have already occurred. Paralysis is a late sign and usually a finding of a late compartment syndrome. Pulses are almost never absent (McQueen 2010).

Compartment syndrome is first and foremost a clinical diagnosis. If a patient has the mechanism and symptoms consistent with compartment syndrome, no further studies are needed prior to surgical fasciotomy. However many times diagnosis is not nearly as straight forward. Many patients have issues that confound interpretation of levels of pain including patients with a history of illicit drug use, distracting injuries, nerve/spinal injuries, cerebral injury, or sedation/intubation In these scenarios, assessment for compartment syndrome may require compartment pressure measurements (McQueen 2010).

Compartment measurements can be done with any needle linked to a pressure transducer, though many clinicians use an off the shelf compartment measurement device. Measurements should be performed as close to the area of insult as possible, as a difference in as little as 4 cm distance results in significant changes in pressure measurements within a compartment (Leversedge et al. 2011).

Causes of Upper Extremity Compartment Syndrome

As previously mentioned, one of the greatest tools for diagnosis is having a high index of suspicion with recognition of high-risk causes of compartment syndrome. Though compartment syndrome can occur in anyone, it occurs often in younger males, who have tighter compartments at baseline and more muscle mass.

The most common cause of upper extremity compartment syndrome is fracture with or without dislocation. Particularly high-risk fractures include high energy distal radius fractures, both bone forearm fractures, carpometacarpal dislocations, and supracondylar humerus fractures in children. Any high-energy trauma with a crush component is also at high risk for compartment syndrome, even in the absence of fracture or dislocation. Patients with prolonged pressure over the upper extremity due to intoxication or immobilization are at risk (McQueen 2010).

Tight bandages, casts or splints are a common contributor to compartment syndrome. Volume resuscitation with infiltration into the upper extremity is another described iatrogenic cause of compartment syndrome. Patients with bleeding disorders, innate or due to anticoagulants are at higher risk for significant hemorrhage leading to compartment syndrome with and sometimes without trauma. Restoration of arterial flow after arterial injury or reconstruction has been reported up to 21% of cases. "Reperfusion" compartment syndrome is caused by free radical release, inflammation and swelling after reperfusion. This may not become clinically abnormal for several hours after restoration of arterial inflow. Frequently after upper extremity reperfusion the distal compartments are released prophylactically to avoid the need for urgent return to the OR in the immediate post operative period (McQueen 2010).

Further causes of compartment syndrome include electrical injury or burn, after which constriction of circumferential burned skin acts like

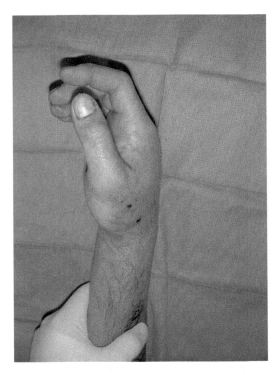

Compartment Syndrome of the Forearm, Fig. 1 Snake bite to hand (Personal image (Phil Blazar))

a tight fascia causing tissue ischemia. Other rarer described causes include venomous snakebites and severe soft tissue infections (Fig. 1) (Leversedge et al. 2011).

Application

Treatment of compartment syndrome can start with preventing iatrogenic causes of compartment syndrome. Bandages and dressings should not be placed too tightly and in cases with a moderate risk of compartment syndrome a low threshold to remove (or avoid) circumferential dressing should clinical symptoms warrant. Limbs should be placed at heart level. Elevation of the affected limb seems intuitive; however this can reduce mean arterial pressure and thus decrease ΔP, so elevation should be avoided (Leversedge et al. 2011).

Once compartment syndrome sets in however, the only treatment is emergent fasciotomy.

Anatomy of Compartments and Surgical Releases

Both compartment measurements for diagnosis and fasciotomy involve knowledge of the anatomy of the upper extremity. Each segment of the upper extremity, the arm, forearm, and hand, has its own unique sets of compartments. The focus of this chapter is on the forearm as compartment syndrome of the forearm is much more common; however the arm and hand will be briefly mentioned

In the forearm, traditionally three or four compartments are described, depending on the source.

The muscles of the volar forearm compartment can be subdivided into superficial and deep. In the superficial compartment, one finds the flexor digitorum superficialis, pronator teres, palmaris longus, flexor carpi radialis and ulnaris. In the deep volar compartment, one finds the flexor digitorum profundus, flexor pollicis longus, and pronator quadratus. The median nerve, anterior interosseous branch of the median nerve, and the ulnar nerve innervate and traverse this compartment (Leversedge et al. 2011).

The dorsal forearm can also be divided into superficial and deep subdivisions.

The superficial muscle layer includes the extensor digitorum communis, extensor digitorum minimus, and extensor carpi ulnaris. The deep muscles include the extensor indicis proprius, extensor pollicis longus, supinator, extensor pollicis brevis, and abductor pollicis longus. These muscles are innervated by the posterior interosseous nerve which traverses this compartment (Leversedge et al. 2011).

The final forearm compartment is the "mobile wad", compromising the extensor carpi radialis longus and brevis and the brachioradialis, all innervated by the radial nerve. This compartment also contains the radial sensory nerve (Leversedge et al. 2011).

The forearm is frequently released by a combination of volar and dorsal incisions, although a number of approaches have been described. The volar aspect is often opened through a traditional Henry approach centered around the FCR tendon distally and carried

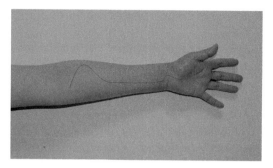

Compartment Syndrome of the Forearm,
Fig. 2 Image of volar incision for compartment release
(Personal images (Xuan Luo))

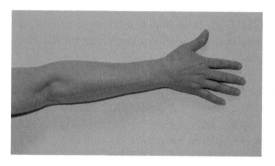

Compartment Syndrome of the Forearm,
Fig. 3 Image of dorsal incision for compartment release
(Personal images (Xuan Luo))

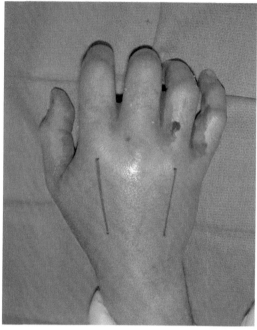

Compartment Syndrome of the Forearm,
Fig. 4 Location of hand fasciotomy Incision (Personal
image (Phil Blazar))

proximally. The carpal tunnel is commonly
opened as well to fully release the forearm
(Fig. 2). The dorsal incision is usually 3–4 cm
distal to lateral epicondyle and extended towards
Listers' tubercle (Fig. 3) (Twaddle and
Amendola 2009).

In the arm there are three compartments, the
anterior posterior and deltoid. The anterior and
posterior compartments are divided by the
humerus in the middle, and the lateral and medial
intermuscular septum on either side. The anterior
compartment of the arm includes the biceps,
brachialis, coracobrachialis muscles. These are
innervated by the musculocutaneous nerve.
Within this compartment are the radial, median,
ulnar nerves, and the medial and lateral
antebrachial cutaneous nerves. The posterior
compartment of the arm includes the three
heads of the triceps muscle, innervated by the
radial nerve. In addition the ulnar nerve,

posterior antebrachial cutaneous nerve, and
nerve to anconeus are located in this compartment. The deltoid compartment predictably
includes the deltoid muscle, innervated by the
axillary nerve. Decompression of the arm can be
carried out with either separate anterior or
posterior incisions or a single lateral incision
to reach both anterior and posterior
(Leversedge et al. 2011).

The hand is classically described as having 10
compartments, most of which include only one
muscle. The muscles involved include the four
dorsal interosseus, three volar interosseus, adductor pollicis; the thenar muscles including flexor
pollicis brevis, opponens pollicis, and abductor
pollicis brevis; and hypothenar muscles comprising of the flexor digiti minimi, opponens minimi,
and abductor digiti minimi. No true compartments exist in the fingers, however severe swelling can cause compromised digital perfusion. All
of the interosseous compartments can be opened
with two incisions between index and long and
ring and small fingers (Fig. 4). The thenar compartment can be released along the radial margin

of the thenar eminence. Likewise the hypothenar can be released through an ulnar border incision. The adductor can be released with a dorsal incision over first webspace (Gulgonen and Ozer 2011).

The majority of the time after compartment release, the incisions are left open to allow for further swelling and closure is performed on a delayed basis. In the forearm and arm this frequently is done with a skin graft, however, the smaller incisions of the hand are typically left to heal by secondary intention.

Summary

Compartment syndrome is a surgical emergency. The process is driven by a positive feedback loop of increased pressures causing ischemia, which in turn causes swelling which keads to even higher pressures. Diagnosis is made by clinical exam, and pain is the most common finding. When exam is unobtainable or equivocal, compartment pressures measurements with a delta P of less than 20–30 mmHg are suggestive of compartment syndrome. With onset of true compartment syndrome, the only treatment is emergent surgical fasciotomy. Untreated compartment syndrome results in muscle necrosis and contractures, often rendering the limb functionless. Fasciotomy of the forearm requires release of the deep and superficial volar compartments, along with the extensor and mobile wad compartment.

Cross-References

- ▶ Abdominal Compartment Syndrome as a Complication of Care
- ▶ Compartment Syndrome of the Leg
- ▶ Compartment Syndrome, Acute
- ▶ Compartment Syndrome: Complication of Care in ICU
- ▶ Compartment Syndrome
- ▶ Crush Injuries
- ▶ Crush Syndrome

References

Gulgonen A, Ozer K (2011) Compartment syndrome. In: Wolfe SW, Hotchkiss RN, Pederson WC, Kozin SH (eds) Green's operative hand surgery. Churchill Livingstone, London, pp 1929–1948
Leversedge FJ, Moore TJ, Peterson BC, Seiler JG III (2011) Compartment syndrome of the upper extremity. J Hand Surg 36(3):544–559
McQueen M (2010) Acute Compartment syndrome. In: Bucholz RW, Heckman JD, Tornetta P (eds) Rockwood and Green's fractures in adults. Lippincott Williams & Wilkins, Philadelphia, pp 689–705
Twaddle B, Amendola A (2009) Compartment syndromes. In: Browner B, Levine A, Jupiter J, Trafton P, Krettek C (eds) Skeletal trauma, 4th edn. Saunders, Philadelphia, chapter 13

Compartment Syndrome of the Leg

John T. Gorczyca
Division of Orthopaedic Trauma, Department of Orthopedic Surgery, University of Rochester School of Medicine, Rochester, NY, USA

Synonyms

Fracture complications; Ischemic contracture; Swelling; Traumatic injuries

Definition

Compartment syndrome is a condition in which the tissue pressure within in a body compartment exceeds the threshold necessary to maintain capillary perfusion. If left untreated, compartment syndrome progresses to ischemia and eventual necrosis of the tissues within the compartment. Compartment syndrome occurs most commonly in one or more of the four compartments of the leg. When not detected and treated early, compartment syndrome in the leg will result in significant functional loss.

Preexisting Conditions

The majority of leg compartment syndromes are caused by trauma. Establishing the diagnosis in

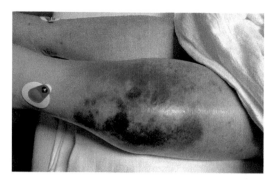

Compartment Syndrome of the Leg, Fig. 1 Photo depicts compartment syndrome of leg which occurred after a minor injury in an anticoagulated patient. The *left leg* has significant swelling and ecchymosis, and the compartments are firm.

cases of trauma can be challenging because it is difficult to distinguish the symptoms of compartment syndrome from the symptoms of the fracture/trauma. A tight or constrictive cast or dressing may contribute to compartment syndrome by elevating the local tissue pressure, thereby reducing the perfusion of the tissue.

Another cause of compartment syndrome is pharmaceutical anticoagulation, which is becoming increasingly more common as the number of patients treated with anticoagulation for thromboembolism or atrial fibrillation increases. The anticoagulated patient is at a higher risk for compartment syndrome from bleeding within the compartments, even with a relatively minor injury (Fig. 1).

Application

Pain is the most common symptom in alert patients with compartment syndrome. This pain may be difficult to treat with analgesics and thus may seem to be out of proportion to the injury. It must be emphasized; however, that with significant trauma, it may be impossible for the physician to distinguish between pain from an injury and pain from a compartment syndrome.

The leg with compartment syndrome often feels swollen and tense. Pressure applied to the leg will cause pain. Passive stretching of the muscles in the compartment will produce pain

in the area of the muscle belly. Paralysis occurs late in the course of compartment syndrome.

Sensory nerves which pass through the compartment may have paresthesias or sensory loss, although this may result from the trauma itself, and the absence of sensory changes does not rule out compartment syndrome. Likewise, the patient may have palpable pulses and good capillary refill distal to a compartment syndrome. Thus, the clinical findings in a patient with compartment syndrome are sometimes inconsistent, which further complicates establishing the diagnosis.

Other factors may complicate establishing the diagnosis. For instance, the patient may be unable to comply with physical examination due to head injury, sedation, spinal cord injury, or peripheral nerve injury. If these patients have a swollen, firm extremity, the examining physician will have a difficult time ruling out compartment syndrome without measuring compartment pressures. Similarly, patients with significant trauma to the leg may have unbearable pain, paresis, and pain with passive stretch due to the traumatic injury alone. Establishing whether or not that patient has a compartment syndrome that requires emergent fasciotomy is best done by measuring compartment pressures.

Some patients may develop compartment syndrome due to the constrictive effect of a cast. If the patient has symptoms of compartment syndrome, the physician should bivalve the cast, then split the cast padding, and position the extremity at the level of the heart with the ankle in neutral position or slight plantar flexion. Often, within 15 min, the release of the constriction will result in improvement of the symptoms as tissue perfusion improves. If there is no improvement, then pressure measurement or fasciotomy is indicated. Compartment syndrome can also be caused by excessive wrapping of soft dressings, such as an overstretched ace wrap, on the leg. The dressing should be loosened, and the patient evaluated briefly for improvement before further intervention is performed.

Traction which is applied to a fractured leg will cause a rise in the compartment pressures. For this reason, prolonged or excessive traction on a leg with a tibial fracture should be avoided, especially if the patient is anesthetized or neurologically impaired and cannot participate in clinical evaluation (Tornetta and French 1997). Likewise, dorsiflexion of the ankle is associated with a rise in pressure of the posterior compartment of the leg. Neutral position or a slightly plantar-flexed position of the ankle is more desirable.

Intraoperative use of a well-leg holder or use of the lithotomy position has been associated with compartment syndrome, probably due to external pressure on compartments, hip and knee flexion that impairs arterial flow, and sedation or anesthesia that interferes with patient feedback.

Compartment Pressure Measurements

In most patients, the diagnosis of compartment syndrome can be established or ruled out based on physical examination findings alone. When the diagnosis is unclear, then measurement of compartment pressures should be performed to clarify the clinical situation. Common clinical scenarios in which compartment pressure measurement will help clarify the diagnosis are (1) an obtunded, anesthetized, or sedated patient with a swollen leg; (2) nerve injury in a patient with a swollen or injured leg; (3) unclear clinical examination; and (4) prolonged hypotension with extremity injury. In patients with progressive exacerbation of symptoms but with pressure measurements that do not indicate compartment syndrome at that time, an indwelling catheter may be placed to provide ongoing monitoring of compartment pressures.

The perfusion of tissue within a compartment is related to both the arterial pressure and the compartment pressure. For that reason, both arterial and intracompartmental pressures should be measured in order to establish the diagnosis of compartment syndrome. When the difference between the patient's diastolic pressure and the compartment pressure (i.e., ΔP) is less than 30 mmHg, it is probable that tissue perfusion is inadequate and thus emergent fasciotomy should be performed. There is some discrepancy about when tissue perfusion becomes impaired in compartment syndrome. Perfusion studies of

non-traumatized canine legs have shown that muscle will tolerate a ΔP as low as 20 mmHg (Bernot et al. 1996). After a period of ischemia, however, a ΔP of 40 mmHg may be insufficient to maintain muscle perfusion (Matava et al. 1994). Thus, using $\Delta P < 30$ mmHg as an indication for fasciotomy appears to be a safe threshold in the traumatized leg and has solid clinical support in humans with compartment syndrome of the leg (McQueen et al. 2013).

One should be cautious in diagnosing compartment syndrome in intraoperative patients because they may have transient diastolic hypotension due to the anesthesia. Thus, intraoperative patients with normal or high-normal compartment pressures with diastolic hypotension may have $\Delta P < 30$ mmHg at that time. It should be understood that most often the diastolic hypotension will be corrected when the anesthesia wears off and that fasciotomy should not be performed unless clinical exam justifies it. The patient's preoperative diastolic pressure is a good predictor of the patient's diastolic pressure in the recovery room and should be included in the consideration of whether or not to perform fasciotomy.

Compartment syndrome can occur in any or all of the four compartments in the leg, so measurements should be taken in all of them. It is recommended that compartment pressure measurements be made within 5 cm of the fracture, as the pressure will be highest in that area and will be closer to normal at larger distance. Only a small amount of fluid (enough to clear the tip of the needle of tissue) should be injected through the needle/catheter, and the monitor should be given time to completely equilibrate before determining the pressure.

Treatment of Compartment Syndrome of the Calf

When the diagnosis of compartment syndrome is confirmed, surgical release of the compartments should be performed emergently. In most cases, all four compartments should be released. Four-compartment fasciotomy of the leg is most easily performed through two skin incisions: a longitudinal medial incision located

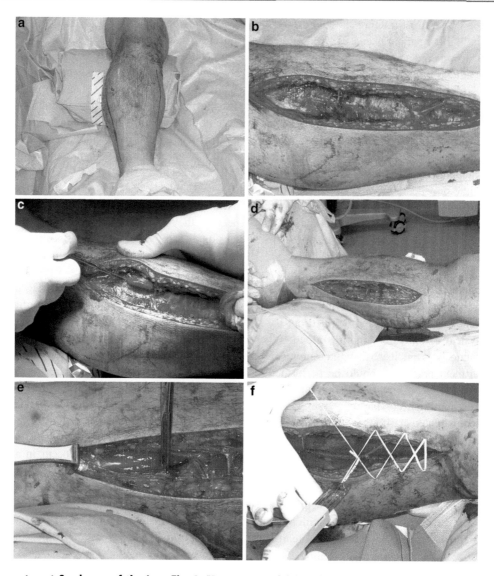

Compartment Syndrome of the Leg, Fig. 2 Young man with compartment syndrome involving all four compartments of *right leg* after gunshot wound. Anteroposterior view (**a**) shows markings for dual incision technique. Closeup views of lateral incision demonstrate perforating vessels at fascial interval (**b**) which should be preserved if possible and bulging of anterior compartments musculature upon release of the fascia (**c**). The superficial medial incision reveals swollen posterior compartments (**d**). After release of the readily identifiable superficial posterior compartment fascia, the deep posterior compartment fascia is best identified *distally* and is shown partially incised (**e**). After evacuating any hematoma and irrigating the tissue, gentle tension is placed on the skin using vessel loops which are stapled to the skin in a crisscross fashion (**f**)

approximately 1 cm posterior to the medial edge of the tibia for the superficial posterior and the deep posterior compartments and a longitudinal anterior-lateral incision located approximately two cm anterior to the fibula for the anterior and lateral compartments (Fig. 2). Alternatively, all four compartments may be released through a single lateral incision located over the fibula which leaves the fibula intact (Maheshwari et al. 2008), but this is a more technically demanding approach.

If compartment syndrome of the calf is associated with a tibia fracture, then the fracture should be reduced and stabilized to facilitate soft-tissue monitoring and management. Depending on the fracture type and the character of the soft tissues, bony stabilization can be achieved by intramedullary nailing, open reduction and internal fixation, or external fixation.

The tissues should be covered with moist or occlusive dressings to prevent desiccation. Use of crisscrossed elastic bands or vessel loops to gently pull the skin edges together will prevent skin retraction and facilitate secondary wound closure. Vacuum-assisted wound closure can be used to reduce postoperative edema, thereby improving the surgeon's ability to perform delayed primary wound closure. The patient should return to the operating room in 2–3 days for irrigation and debridement and closure. If skin closure is not possible after the second or third debridement, then skin grafting should be considered.

Outcomes of Compartment Syndrome

There is limited data on functional outcomes of compartment syndrome of the calf. In a retrospective study of 44 patients with 66 cases of acute compartment syndrome, Sheriden and Matsen reported an indisputable relationship between delayed fasciotomy and worse functional results (Sheriden and Matsen 1976). In the patients treated with fasciotomy within 12 h of symptom onset, 68 % had normal function and 4.5 % had complication. In the patients treated with fasciotomy more than 12 h after symptom onset, only 8 % had normal function, and 54 % had complications, including infection, amputation, renal failure, and death.

Heemskerk and Kitslaar analyzed the outcomes of 40 patients with compartment syndrome of the lower leg treated by fasciotomy (Heemskerk and Kitslaar 2003). They did not analyze the timing of surgery. Their outcomes included 15 % mortality, 25 % amputation, and 15 % nerve injury rates. Only 45 % had a good functional result. In multivariate analysis, younger (<50 years old) patients did better.

Fitzgerald et al. evaluated 60 patients with compartment syndrome over 8 years and noted that most suffered long-term sequelae including altered sensation (77 %), dry scaly skin (40 %), pruritus (33 %), swollen limbs (15 %), wound pain (10 %), and recurrent ulceration (8 %) (Fitzgerald et al. 2000).

Giannoudis et al. evaluated 39 compartment syndrome patients at 12 months and noted worse self-reported overall quality of health in patients with skin grafts and in patients with delayed closure/coverage of fasciotomy wounds (Giannoudis et al. 2002).

Tremblay et al. reported "secondary extremity compartment syndrome" in 10 patients out of 11,996 (0.1 %) trauma patients in 6 years (Tremblay et al. 2002). The unique features of this syndrome are that it occurs in *non-traumatized extremities* of *hemodynamically unstable* patients with systemic inflammatory response syndrome. The compartment syndromes probably resulted from reperfusion of extremities that had been ischemic after administration of vasopressors during prolonged resuscitation efforts. In their experience, each patient had an average of 3.1 extremities involved, and the mortality rate was 70 %. They recommended checking compartment pressures in patients with severe diffuse edema after resuscitation for injury.

Finkelstein and Hunter, however, reported on five patients with fasciotomy performed >35 h after compartment syndrome (Finkelstein et al. 1996). Several of these patients were transferred to their trauma center on a delayed basis after significant trauma and hemodynamic instability. One patient died from multisystem failure and the remaining four patients had amputation, three of which were performed for infection. This study concluded that the benefits of fasciotomy should be reconsidered if considerable delay is present. Olson and Glasgow also weighed in on the topic of whether or not fasciotomy on a significantly delayed basis would be of benefit: they stated that if compartment syndrome has been present for greater than 8 h in a patient with intact cognitive and neurologic function, and the patient is unable to contract muscles within the compartment, that irreversible necrosis had already occurred and it was too late to perform fasciotomy (Olson and Glasgow 2006).

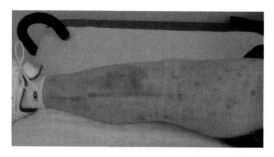

Compartment Syndrome of the Leg, Fig. 3 Photo shows leg 8 years after compartment syndrome treated surgically. The muscle function is excellent, but the patient has dysesthesias in the region of the incisions

Thus, the limited data on functional outcomes identifies problems with muscle strength, functional loss, and skin symptoms after compartment syndrome. These problems are more common in older patients and can occur even when fasciotomy is performed early. While it is clear that surgical fasciotomy has therapeutic benefit, it may contribute to some of the morbidity and disability in patients after compartment syndrome (Fig. 3). There is weak (level IV–V) evidence showing high morbidity and mortality rates with late fasciotomy.

Cross-References

▶ Coagulopathy
▶ Compartment Syndrome
▶ Crush Syndrome
▶ Delayed Diagnosis/Missed Injury
▶ Tibial Fractures

References

Bernot M, Gupta R, Dobrasz J, Chance B, Heppenstall RB, Sapega A (1996) The effect of antecedent ischemia on the tolerance of skeletal muscle to increased interstitial pressure. J Orthop Trauma 10:555–559
Finkelstein JA, Hunter GA, Hu RW (1996) Lower limb compartment syndrome: course after delayed fasciotomy. J Trauma 40:342–344
Fitzgerald AM, Gaston P, Wilson Y, Quaba A, McQueen MM (2000) Long-term sequelae of fasciotomy wounds. Br J Plast Surg 53:690–693
Giannoudis PV, Nicolopoulos C, Dinopoulos H, Ng A, Adedapo S, Kind P (2002) The impact of lower leg compartment syndrome on health related quality of life. Injury 33:117–121
Heemskerk J, Kitslaar P (2003) Acute compartment syndrome of the lower leg: retrospective study on prevalence, technique, and outcome of fasciotomies. World J Surg 27:744–747
Maheshwari R, Taitsman LA, Barei DP (2008) Single-incision fasciotomy for compartment syndrome of the leg in patients with diaphyseal tibial fractures. J Orthop Trauma 22:723–730
Matava MJ, Whitesides TE Jr, Seiler JG III, Hewan-Lowe K, Hutton WC (1994) Determination of the compartment pressure threshold of muscle ischemia in a canine model. J Trauma 37:50–58
McQueen MM, Duckworth AD, Aitken SA, Court-Brown CM (2013) The estimated sensitivity and specificity of compartment pressure monitoring for acute compartment syndrome. J Bone Joint Surg Am 95:673–677
Olson SA, Glasgow RR (2006) Acute compartment syndrome in lower extremity musculoskeletal trauma. J Am Acad Orthop Surg 13:436–444
Sheriden GW, Matsen FA 3rd (1976) Fasciotomy in the treatment of the acute compartment syndrome. J Bone Joint Surg 58:112–115
Tornetta P III, French BG (1997) Compartment pressures during nonreamed tibial nailing without traction. J Orthop Trauma 11:24–27
Tremblay LN, Feliciano DV, Rozycki GS (2002) Secondary compartment syndrome. J Trauma 53:833–837

Compartment Syndrome, Acute

David S. Morris
Division of Trauma, Critical Care, and General Surgery, Mayo Clinic, Rochester, MN, USA

Synonyms

Calf hypertension; Compartment syndrome; Volkmann ischemia

Definition

Acute compartment syndrome refers to the clinical entity that is marked by increased pressure within an anatomic compartment of finite volume. The syndrome occurs when the perfusion pressure to the tissues within the compartment is lower than the pressure of the compartment itself. The increased pressure within the compartment is most often due to tissue edema following injury or reperfusion, particularly in the setting of hypotension or shock.

The most commonly observed compartment syndromes involve the myofascial compartments of the lower leg (Watson and Lee 2008), but elevated compartment pressures are not infrequently observed in the thigh, the forearm, and the hand. Physiologically, abdominal compartment syndrome, cardiac tamponade, and elevated intracranial pressure are similar specialized types of acute compartment syndrome, with important clinical consequences specific to these anatomic regions.

Risk Factors: Acute compartment syndrome should be suspected in any injury that results in increased edema to the tissues within a myofascial compartment. Certain types of injury may be more prone to compartment syndrome, such as crush injuries, vascular injuries with prolonged limb ischemia and reperfusion, combined arterial and venous injury, and fractures in the extremities, particularly tibial fractures. Bony injury may not be present in some instances, such as in patients who are found down after a prolonged period who develop pressure necrosis in the dependent regions.

Diagnosis: Acute compartment syndrome is a clinical diagnosis. The key to diagnosis is a high degree of suspicion for the syndrome in patients who are at risk. The clinical presentation is severe pain, particularly with passive stretch of the muscles within the compartment. Later signs include paresthesias and signs of critical ischemia, such as mottling or pulse deficits of the affected extremity. These signs are classically described as the 5 Ps of compartment syndrome, namely, pain, pallor, paresthesia, poikilothermia, and pulselessness.

Measurement of the compartment pressures can be performed to assist with the diagnosis. This is performed by transducing the pressure after introducing a sterile needle into the compartment in question after prepping and anesthetizing the skin. Compartment pressures

higher than 30 mmHg are consistent with acute compartment syndrome. Another helpful calculation is termed "delta p" (McQueen and Court-Brown 1996) which is defined as the difference between the diastolic pressure and the compartment pressure, which should be greater than 30 mmHg (ΔP (diastolic BP – compartment pressure) <30 mmHg).

Treatment: Acute compartment syndrome treatment consists of surgically opening the involved compartment(s). This intervention allows the edematous tissues to expand without increasing the intracompartment pressure. Blood flow is restored to the tissues of the compartment as the compartment pressure drops below the perfusion pressure. The resulting surgical wounds are dressed, sometimes with a negative pressure dressing, until the amount of tissue edema decreases sufficiently to allow closure of the wounds. If the wounds cannot be closed, split-thickness skin grafts may be required.

Morbidity: Without adequate compartment release, acute compartment syndrome may result in ischemic loss of muscle or nerve tissue. Rhabdomyolysis may develop with attendant acute kidney injury and potential need for dialysis. The necrotic muscle and nerve is at risk for infection, with bacterial contamination from the injury itself, or secondary hematogenous seeding. Surgical debridement of the infected tissue may be required, resulting in loss of limb function. In some cases, amputation may be the only treatment option.

Cross-References

▶ Compartment Syndrome
▶ Compartment Syndrome of the Forearm
▶ Compartment Syndrome of the Leg

References

McQueen MM, Court-Brown CM (1996) Compartment monitoring in tibial fractures. The pressure threshold for decompression. J Bone Joint Surg Br 78(1):99–104
Watson GA, Lee JC (2008) Compartment syndrome. In: Peitzman AB, Rhodes M, Schwab CW, Yealy DM, Fabian TC (eds) The trauma manual: trauma and acute care surgery, 3rd edn. Lippincott, Williams & Wilkins, Philadelphia/Pennsylvania (Chap 34)

Compartment Syndrome: Complication of Care in ICU

Ashika Jain
Trauma Critical Care, Emergency Ultrasound,
Department of Emergency Medicine, Kings
County Hospital Center, SUNY Downstate
Medical Center, Brooklyn, NY, USA

Synonyms

Abdominal compartment syndrome; Extremity compartment syndrome

Definition

Acute Compartment syndrome occurs when the tissue pressure within a closed muscle compartment exceeds the perfusion pressure and results in muscle and nerve ischemia.

Preexisting Condition

The normal pressure of the abdominal compartment is 0–16 mmHg, this can vary based on body habitus and recent abdominal surgery (Sanchez et al. 2001; Balogh et al. 2004). This pressure can be elevated by many different processes. Abdominal compartment syndrome can develop in intensive care patients within 12 h. Factors leading to elevated compartment pressures include over-fluid resuscitation leading to bowel edema, pancreatitis, blunt, and penetrating trauma. Crush injuries, reperfusion injuries after bowel ischemia.

Normal pressure in the extremity compartments ranges from 0 to 8 mmHg. Extremity compartments are bound by facial planes. Any internal or external event that increases pressure within a compartment can cause compartment syndrome. Thus, increased fluid content or decreased compartment size can lead to the condition (Mubarak and Hargens 1983). Most common etiologies include long bone fractures, comminuted fractures, penetrating vascular injuries, crush injuries, vascular injuries, intravenous/intra-articular drug injections, phlegmasia cerulea dolens, circumferential burns, and compressive dressings and casts are among the many causes (Tiwari et al. 2002).

The sequence of events that leads to compartment syndrome begins when the tissue pressure in a compartment exceeds the venous pressure, thereby obstructing outflow. As metabolic waste builds up, pain ensues as well as decreased peripheral sensation from nerve irritation. As the pressure continues to rise and progresses to exceed arteriolar pressure, lack of oxygenated blood furthering tissue damage, eventually leading to muscle, tissue, and nerve necrosis (Weinmann 2003; Olson and Glasgow 2005; Matsen 1980). As the process continues, renal failure can ensue as well as permanent nerve damage, contractures, and altered mentation.

Application

Acute compartment syndrome requires a high index of suspicion to make the diagnosis. The 5 "p"s of compartment syndrome include pain, pallor, parasthesias, paralysis, and pulselessness, the latter being a very ominous sign of arterial occlusion and ensuring necrosis.

Objective data is paramount to confirm the diagnosis. Intra-abdominal pressure measured via the urinary catheter is the current standard of care monitor for compartment syndrome and has excellent correlation with directly measured intra-abdominal pressure; however, its intermittent nature is its major limitation (Saggi et al. 1998). An 18-Fr standard three-way catheter can be used for continuous pressure monitoring in the intensive care unit for patients suspected of having elevated intra-abdominal pressures. Measurement is performed via the irrigation port of the three-way catheter, in which continuous normal saline perfusion (4 mL/h) is maintained and connected through a two-way stopcock and normal saline filled tubing to a pressure transducer placed in line with the iliac crest at the mid axillary line. The transducer should be zeroed and the measurement recorded on the bedside monitor. Measurements greater than 20 mmHg raise concern to abdominal compartment syndrome and should prompt a discussion with a surgeon to definitive release of the anterior fascia to relieve the increasing pressure (Balogh et al. 2004).

There are commercially available devices to measure extremity pressures. When these are not accessible, an 18-gage needle, an 18-gage spinal, or side port needle can be connected to an arterial line transducer to achieve a pressure reading. There are new devices including those that use spectrography on the market, but are not as widely used. Other supplies needed to perform this procedure including high pressure tubing, pressure transducer with cable, pressure monitor, sterile saline, stopcock, 20-ml syringe. Once an elevated pressure is noted, prompt surgical evaluation should be considered to release the fascia and relieve increasing pressures.

Fasciotomy is the treatment of choice. This involves opening the skin and muscle fascia at key points overlying the involved compartment or compartments. The release of enclosed muscles causes a decrease in compartment pressure, thereby restoring blood flow to the tissues. Indications for fasciotomy are not definite. Some indications include an absolutely pressure greater than 30 mmHg. There is much data to suggest a rise to within 10–30 mmHg of the patient's diastolic blood pressure is a more reliable measure than absolute pressure measurement (Whitesides et al. 1975a, b). Other indications include patients who are normotensive with positive clinical findings, with compartment pressures of greater than 30 mmHg, and whose duration of increased pressure is unknown or thought to be longer than 8 h.

Other indications also include patients who are uncooperative or unconscious, with a compartment pressure of greater than 30 mmHg, and patients with low blood pressure and a compartment pressure of greater than 20 mmHg (Mubarak and Hargens 1983).

Outcomes and prognosis greatly depend on time to diagnosis and time to intervention. Performing fasciotomy within 6 h can preserve tissue viability (Rorabeck and Macnab 1975; Matsen et al. 1980). With late diagnosis, irreversible tissue ischemia can develop in the acute setting; thus, permanent muscle and nerve damage, along with chronic pain, may occur. Volkmann contracture is the residual limb deformity that results over weeks to months following untreated acute compartment syndrome or ischemia from an uncorrected arterial injury. Renal failure or multiple organ failure may occur preoperatively or postoperatively. Most fatalities are due to prolonged intensive care admissions with sepsis and multisystem organ failure.

Cross-References

▶ Abdominal Compartment Syndrome as a Complication of Care
▶ Acute Abdominal Compartment Syndrome in Trauma
▶ Compartment Syndrome
▶ Compartment Syndrome of the Forearm
▶ Compartment Syndrome of the Leg
▶ Compartment Syndrome, Acute
▶ Crush Injuries
▶ Multiorgan System Failure (MOF)

References

Balogh Z, Jones F, D'Amours S et al (2004) Continuous intra-abdominal pressure measurement technique. Am J Surg 188(6):679–684

Matsen FA (1980) Compartmental syndromes. Grune & Stratton, New York

Matsen FA 3rd, Winquist RA, Krugmire RB Jr (1980) Diagnosis and management of compartmental syndromes. J Bone Joint Surg Am 62(2):286–291

Mubarak SJ, Hargens AR (1983) Acute compartment syndromes. Surg Clin North Am 63(3):539–565

Olson SA, Glasgow RR (2005) Acute compartment syndrome in lower extremity musculoskeletal trauma. J Am Acad Orthop Surg 13(7):436–444

Rorabeck CH, Macnab I (1975) The pathophysiology of the anterior tibial compartmental syndrome. Clin Orthop Relat Res 1:52–57

Saggi BH, Sugerman HJ, Ivatury RR, Bloomfield GL (1998) Abdominal compartment syndrome. J Trauma 45:597–609

Sanchez NC, Tenofsky PL, Dort JM et al (2001) What is normal intra-abdominal pressure? Am Surg 67(3):243–248

Tiwari A, Haq AI, Myint F et al (2002) Acute compartment syndromes. Br J Surg 89:397–412

Weinmann M (2003) Compartment syndrome. Emerg Med Serv 32(9):36

Whitesides TE, Haney TC, Morimoto K, Harada H (1975a) Tissue pressure measurements as a determinant for the need of fasciotomy. Clin Orthop Relat Res. Arch Surg 110(11):1311–1313

Whitesides TE Jr, Haney TC, Harada H, Holmes HE, Morimoto K (1975b) A simple method for tissue pressure determination. Arch Surg 110(11):1311–1313

Compartmental Syndrome

▶ Compartment Syndrome of the Forearm

Competence to Consent to Treatment

▶ Evaluating a Patient's Decision-Making Capacity

Competency

Robert Grabenkort
Emory Center for Critical Care, Atlanta, GA, USA

Synonyms

Ability; Accomplishment; Adeptness; Expertise; Mastery; Proficiency; Prowess; Skill

Definition

Competency comes from the Latin word "competentia" meaning to agree with. Later (circa 1790) definitions of the word refer to a "sufficiency to deal with what is at hand"

(Random House 1984). More contemporary meanings include the words "ability" and "knowledge" as important constituents in the understanding of the word. Educational sources add further refinement describing, "a combination of skills, abilities, and knowledge needed to perform a specific task" (Soars 2012). Other texts add that the defined skill must be performed to a previously established standard (Sullivan 1995).

Preexisting Condition

Medical training has traditionally been taught using a predetermined period of educational experiences including lectures in large group settings, intensive written examinations, group laboratory experiences, and clinical clerkships with supervised patient care. At the end of the training period, additional written examinations, usually comprehensive in design, are taken, and upon successful completion, the practitioner was assumed to be "competent" to deliver good patient care.

Over the past decade, however, program directors and educators have reexamined the concept of determining competency in the trainee and new graduate. Because of the increasing ease and speed with which new data and facts are available, the trainees must be educated to adapt to an ever-changing medical environment in order to provide best practice care for their patients. Therefore, new methods of instruction using competency-based training are needed to assure up-to-date practice methods for the graduate.

Application

Applying a competency-based approach to the education of medical trainees changes the focus from an objective-driven, time-based program to a program that is focused on mastery of specific competencies, promoting knowledge and performance of designated skills and their assessment. This approach makes the trainee the primary object of the educational track, thus shifting away from the traditional faculty-centered program.

The two most significant concerns when developing a competency are the specific identification of the desired skill and the establishment of an ongoing process for evaluation during training (Sherwin 2011). When designing these integral pieces, the following steps are useful (adapted from Sullivan 1995):

- Identification of specific masteries or "entrustable professional activities," acquiring the integration of skills needed for day-to-day practice (Sherwin 2011).
- Identification of conditions under which these skills must be demonstrated.
- Development of criteria and standards to which these tasks must be performed. During training these are most easily followed using checklists distributed at the beginning of the training period.
- Development and deployment of references and learning tools for self-guided learning which are foundational to the specific objectives and skill sets to be achieved.
- Development of a course outline and syllabus which present an overview of the program and its objectives.

Didactic resources may be obtained from a variety of sources. Web-based professional programs for the advancement of knowledge in a particular discipline are widely available from specific society websites such as the Society of Critical Care Medicine, American Thoracic Society, American Society of Anesthesiologists, and American Academy of Pediatrics. Pertinent textbooks can be reviewed and made available. Traditional, preexisting institutional lectures can be used to reinforce objectives. Clinical simulation laboratories can be used to emulate patient clinical scenarios and family encounters in a "risk-free" environment while also providing periodic assessment as training advances.

Another important element of competency-based education is the experienced clinical mentor. Mentors should clearly convey the previously determined expectations and objectives of the particular portion of training to the trainee. While training, the mentor can provide real-time feedback to the trainee as well as assurance that goals are met. They represent an interactive mode of learning by reinforcing analytic thought, relevant problem solving, and self-evaluations of decisions made (Rogers 2005). The goal of the mentor is to progress the trainee as efficiently as possible, initially providing intense watch care but withdrawing slowly as the expectations of learning are met, allowing more autonomy.

The learning process itself must be imbedded with assessment tools so that each step provides the trainee with guidance and support toward the goals set and the mentor's standard of practice. As an integral part of this process, the trainee must assume an active role in the learning process. Educational methods shift away from traditional large group settings and intensive examinations to small group seminars involving discussions and clinically interactive experiences to impart and support knowledge. The goal of assessment is to assure mastery of defined competencies.

In addition to establishing clearly defined competencies, assessment of the trainee throughout the educational course is critical and must be a high priority set in advance. The goal of frequent evaluation is to measure the skill level and progression of mastery of the competencies. The tools for these evaluations should be crafted to grade not only knowledge but also performance of specific, well-defined tasks. These should measure the impact of training on improved patient care and assess the ability of the provider to be a self-directed, reflective thinker (Sherwin 2011). Adeptness is the sole determinant of progress.

Assessment methods for competency should be varied. This process is dictated by the necessity for multiple data points for trends in progress or failure to advance. Traditional written exams are only one form that may be used but should be given prior to the beginning of training, at the midpoint, and as one part of the final evaluation. Self-evaluation provides a useful insight into the trainee's confidence level. Taken at the beginning of the training and in the final days, the trainee can express his/her confidence in performing the key competencies using a printed form containing the self-check categories of "uncomfortable performing," "comfortable performing with assistance," or "comfortable performing independently."

As previously mentioned a well-advised team of seasoned clinical mentors can provide not only real-time feedback but also a progressive vision of direction of training. Written records using checklists comprised of expected proficiencies will provide a clear progress record. These lists should contain the initials of the mentors written under the appropriate performance column entitled "performed with supervision" or "performed independently."

Evaluation of the educational process must also be performed. Trainees should be asked for their assessment of each phase of training particularly in the early stages of the formation of the program. This data may be used to adjust the program to best achieve the goals of the program and to customize the training to assure the competency of the students.

The following are practical applications of using clinical competency-based education:

Example 1

In 1999 the Accreditation Council for Graduate Education (ACGME) introduced six domains of clinical competency. These domains included patient care, medical knowledge, professionalism, practice-based learning and improvement, and systems-based practice. The key element of these objectives was the measurement and reporting of educational milestones. In 2009 the ACGME began restructuring the accreditation process to be based on educational outcomes using these categories (Nasca 2012).

Example 2

An example of competency-based medical training is the Competency-Based Training Intensive Care Europe (CoBaTrICE) initiative, which has established an educational pathway for training in critical care medicine.

CoBaTrICE defines 12 domains of competency which include resuscitation, diagnosis, disease management, therapeutic intervention, practical procedures, perioperative care, comfort and recovery, end-of-life issues, pediatric care, transport, patient safety, and professionalism. Under each domain are specific competencies, which are required to be performed under observation and evaluated as the doctor progresses. A separate section contains a "work-based toolbox" which provides 10 "tools" for the documentation of the evaluation process. These tools vary in scope from written exams to different forms of oral interaction including one-on-one sessions and suggestions for successful bedside teaching (www.cobatrice.org).

In conclusion, competency is an entity that involves knowledge and performance of a specific skill accomplished according to a previously set standard. Achieving clinical competency involves a multilayered training program requiring observation, mentoring, and frequent evaluation.

References

Competency Based Training Intensive Care Europe (CoBaTrICE) (2006). www.cobatrice.org. Accessed 1 Sept 2012

Nasca TJ et al (2012) The next GME accreditation system-rational and benefits. N Eng J Med 366:1051–1056. www.nejm.org. Accessed 26 Mar 2012

Random House (1984) Random House college dictionary. Revised edn, p 274

Rogers PL (2005) Textbook of critical care medicine, 5th edn, vol 265, pp 2261–2268, Lippincott, Williams, and Wilkins

Sherwin J (2011) Competency-based medical education takes shape. www.aamc.org/newsroom/reporter/april11/184286/competency_based_medical_education.html. Accessed 12 Sept 2012

Soars L (2012) A disruptive look at competency-based education. www.americanprogress.org/issues/2012/06/comp_based_education.html. Accessed 12 Aug 2012

Sullivan RS (1995) The competency-based approach to training, paper #1, September 1995. www.rhrc.org/resources/general_fieldtools/toolkit/51b%20CBT.pdf. Accessed 1 Aug 2012

Complex Regional Pain Syndrome and Trauma

Dawood Sayed and Erin Griffeth
The University of Kansas Medical Center,
Department of Anesthesiology and Pain
Medicine, Kansas City, KS, USA

Synonyms

Minor causalgia; Posttraumatic dystrophy; Reflex sympathetic disorder (RSD); Shoulder-hand syndrome; Sudeck atrophy

Definition

CRPS describes an array of painful conditions that are characterized by a continuing (spontaneous and/or evoked) regional pain that is seemingly disproportionate in time or degree to the usual course of any known trauma or other lesion. The pain is regional (not in a specific nerve territory or dermatome) and usually has a distal predominance of abnormal sensory, motor, sudomotor, vasomotor, and/or trophic findings. The syndrome shows variable progression over time. Other causes for the constellation of symptoms that encompass CRPS must be ruled out prior to diagnosing a patient. There is no specific test or pathognomonic clinical feature to diagnosis CRPS. Distinguishing a collection of signs and symptoms from clinical history, physical exam, and specific supporting laboratory findings makes the diagnosis of CRPS.

Preexisting Conditions

Epidemiology and Pathophysiology

Two population-based studies, one in the USA and the other in the Netherlands, yielded quite different data. There were 5.5 cases per 100,000 person/year in the USA and 26.2 cases per 100,000 person/year in the Netherlands. Women are 3–4 times more likely to be affected than men (Stanton-hicks et al. 1995). The incidence also increases with age until 70. The mean age of diagnosis in females is around 53 years (Stanton-hicks et al. 1995). The upper extremity (60 %) is affected more frequently than the lower extremity (40 %) (Harden et al. 2010). The most frequently reported triggering events are fractures (~45 %), sprains (~18 %), and elective surgery (~12 %), with orthopedic surgeries having the highest rate of CRPS postoperatively (Stanton-hicks et al. 1995).

It is believed that an important trigger for the cascade of events leading to CRPS, even in CRPS I, is some form of initial nerve trauma. There are small nociceptive nerve fibers (A delta and C fibers) in the mixed peripheral nerves that sense pain (Harden et al. 1999; Stanton-hicks et al. 1995). Recent studies suggest that perhaps the nerve trauma, albeit nearly negligent, causes a release of proinflammatory cytokines (e.g., tumor necrosis factor-alpha, interleukins, which are also seen in inflammatory conditions such as asthma), which in turn increase the synthesis and release of neuropeptides from C fibers.

The central nervous system has recently been implicated to play a crucial role in the pathophysiology of CRPS; there are not only patterns of autonomic dysfunction but also motor and sensory symptoms that suggest alterations in the CNS.

Diagnosis

The diagnosis of CRPS is based on clinical criteria. A detailed medical history including the initiating trauma, disturbances of sensation, and autonomic and motor dysfunction should be noted. Information about pain characteristics, distribution of pain, and time course of disease development should be obtained. Swelling, skin color changes, atrophy, and motor abnormalities should be a specific focus of the physical exam. A general neurological exam is also necessary. While there is no specific diagnostic test available for CRPS, there are several tests that can be supportive in making the diagnosis. Testing is utilized not only to rule out other etiologies but also to assist in identifying features of CRPS,

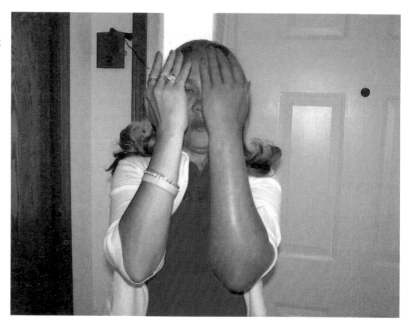

Complex Regional Pain Syndrome and Trauma, Fig. 1 Early stage CRPS 2 after work related injury

such as abnormal sympathetic activity or abnormal limb blood flow, although these are not always present. Commonly employed tests are thermography, sweat testing, three-phase bone scan, electrodiagnostic testing, and sympathetic blocks (Wilson et al. 2005; Harden et al. 2007; Bruehl et al. 2002) (Figs. 1 and 2).

In an effort to increase specificity and reduce over diagnosis of CRPS, the Budapest criteria were developed in 2003 to help guide the accurate identification of this syndrome.

The Budapest clinical diagnostic criteria for CRPS are as follows: (Lau 2004; Bruehl et al. 1999)

1. Continuing pain, which is disproportionate to any inciting event.
2. Must report at least one symptom in three (3) of the four (4) following categories:
   (a) *Sensory*: reports of hyperesthesia and/or allodynia
   (b) *Vasomotor*: reports of temperature asymmetry and/or skin color changes and/or skin color asymmetry
   (c) *Sudomotor/edema*: reports of edema and/or sweating changes and/or sweating asymmetry

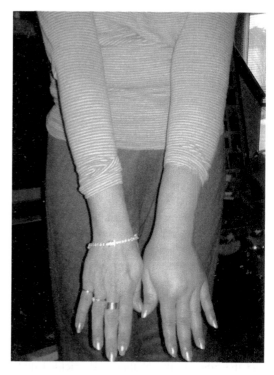

Complex Regional Pain Syndrome and Trauma, Fig. 2 Late stage CRPS 2 in same patient after comprehensive treatment

    (d) *Motor/trophic*: reports of decreased range of motion and/or motor dysfunction (weakness, tremor, dystonia) and/or trophic changes (hair, nail, skin)

3. Must display at least one (1) sign at time of evaluation in two (2) or more of the following categories:

    (a) *Sensory*: evidence of hyperalgesia (to pinprick) and/or allodynia (to light touch and/or deep somatic pressure and/or joint movement)

    (b) *Vasomotor*: evidence of temperature asymmetry and/or skin color changes and/or asymmetry

    (c) *Sudomotor/edema*: evidence of edema and/or sweating changes and/or sweating asymmetry

    (d) *Motor/trophic*: evidence of decreased range of motion and/or motor dysfunction (weakness, tremor, dystonia) and/or trophic changes (hair, nail, skin)

4. There is no other diagnosis that better explains the signs and symptoms.

The research diagnostic criteria for CRPS require that there should be at least one symptom in *all four symptom categories* and *at* least one sign (observed at evaluation) in *two or more sign categories*.

Classification

Three subtypes of CRPS have recently been recognized, as by the Budapest consensus group in 2003. There are two subtypes as defined by the 1994 Orlando Conference: CRPS type I (without distinct major nerve damage, most like the formerly known reflex sympathetic dystrophy, RSD) and CRPS type II (with major nerve damage, most like the formerly term, causalgia). A third subtype with vasomotor signs predominating was also described. Of the three subtypes, the subtype with the briefest pain duration, yet highest levels of motor and trophic signs, as well as possible disuse-related changes (osteopenia) on bone scan, was the third type. Subtype 2 was most suggestive of CRPS type II (causalgia) by testing including EMG (electromyography) and NCV (nerve conduction

velocity) (Wilson et al. 2005; Harden et al. 2007; Bruehl et al. 2002). While the Budapest consensus group did review these subtypes, they considered the data too preliminary to justify including in the formal diagnostic criteria of CRPS. The consensus group also agreed there are problems with the distinctions between the two types of CRPS, I and II. The definition as to what characterizes "major" nerve damage and how it should objectively be defined is vague at best. To clinically define the two types of CRPS is complicated by the fact that the definitive tests for nerve damage (e.g., EMG, NCV) are deemed unnecessarily painful for these patients. Furthermore, the specific therapeutic approach employed is not influenced by the distinction of the two types. The Budapest group retained both subtypes CRPS I and II until further data becomes available regarding the clinical importance of distinction. The group also added another subtype to the formal diagnostic criteria out of recognition that nearly 15 % of those previously diagnosed with CRPS did not meet all criteria of the newly formulated clinical diagnostic considerations for CRPS, but were "not better explained by any other condition." (Wilson et al. 2005).

The three proposed subtypes of CRPS, all three must meet the Budapest diagnostic criteria:

1. CRPS I (old name, RSD).
2. CRPS II (old name, causalgia) has electrodiagnostic or other definitive evidence of a major nerve lesion.
3. CRPS-NOS (not otherwise specified) partially meets CRPS criteria, not better explained by any other condition.

The Budapest consensus group defined general features of the syndrome in their 2004 proposal to the Committee for Classification of Chronic Pain of the IASP as follows: (National Guideline Clearinghouse (NGC) 2011; Reflex Sympathetic Dystrophy Syndrome Association (RSDSA) 2002).

CRPS describes an array of painful conditions that are characterized by a continuing (spontaneous and/or evoked) regional pain that is seemingly disproportionate in time or degree to the usual course of any known trauma or other lesion. The pain is regional (not in a specific nerve territory or dermatome) and usually has a distal predominance of abnormal sensory, motor, sudomotor, vasomotor and/or trophic findings. The syndrome shows variable progression over time.

Application

Treatment

Since complete understanding of the underlying pathophysiology of CRPS is lacking and only a more recent set of objective diagnostic criteria have come about, only a few controlled studies on the therapy for CRPS have been conducted. With this preface, treatment options currently rely on studies for other neuropathic pain syndromes and ideas derived from animal experiments on peripheral nerve lesions.

A multidisciplinary therapeutic approach, beginning immediately and directed toward restoration of full function of the extremity, is the general principle to treatment of CRPS. Treatment should be managed by an experienced pain therapist or provider familiar with the treatment of CRPS. Physical rehabilitation and pain control are the main treatment objectives as pain and limb dysfunction are the major clinical problems. The severity of the pain, and the presence, or absence, of sympathetic dysfunction should guide the selection of pain management modalities. Existing comorbid conditions should be addressed as well: depression, anxiety, sleep disturbance, and generalized physical deconditioning. Treatment guidelines focus on a systematic algorithm with basic principles of motivation, desensitization, and mobilization aided by non-pharmacological, pharmacological, and interventions.

First-line treatment is physical and occupational therapy with the ultimate goal to improve function of the affected extremity (Bonica 1990). Encouragement, education of the disease, and adequate analgesia are essentials for successful implementation and progression of these therapies. These physical modalities include desensitization, isometric exercises, resisted range of motion, and stress loading. Studies demonstrated that these physiotherapies reduced not only pain but also motor impairment, especially if initiated early. The next steps involved are gentle active ROM, stress loading, isotonic strengthening, and general conditional and postural normalization. Final steps involve normalization of use, assessment of any modifications at home and workplace. Failure to progress requires more intensive therapy, including pain relief and psychotherapy. Patients may require weeks to several months to progress through this stage of treatment.

As adequate pain control is essential in the treatment of CRPS, pharmacological strategies are commonly employed. NSAIDs may provide mild to moderate pain relief in CRPS. Although no controlled trials exist for the use of antidepressants in CRPS, they have been studied extensively in other neuropathic pain states. Of these, the norepinephrine and serotonin reuptake inhibitors such as nortriptyline, amitriptyline, and desipramine appear to be the most efficacious. Anticonvulsants such as gabapentin and pregabalin have shown efficacy in postherpetic neuralgia and diabetic peripheral neuropathy and have shown to be effective in CRPS in small studies. Opioids can be very effective in the acute or early phase of CRPS, but its long-term use in chronic cases is controversial.

Interventional treatment modalities can be utilized in cases where first-line therapy has failed or as part of a multimodal approach. Sympathetic nerve blocks with local anesthetics can provide both short-term and long-term pain relief in certain individuals. Stellate ganglion blocks can be performed for upper extremity pain, while lumbar sympathetic blocks are employed for pain in the lower extremities. More invasive treatments for very recalcitrant cases of CRPS include spinal cord stimulation, intrathecal analgesia, and ketamine infusions.

Cross-References

► Acute Pain Management in Trauma
► Pain
► Phantom Limb Pain

References

Bonica JJ (1990) Causalgia and other reflex sympathetic dystrophies. In: Bonica JJ (ed) Management of pain, 2nd edn. Lea and FEibiger, Philadelphia, pp 220–243

Bruehl S, Harden RN, Galer BS, Saltz S, Bertram M, Backonja M, Gayles R, Rudin N, Bhugra MK, Stanton-Hicks M (1999) External validation of IASP diagnostic criteria for complex regional pain syndrome and proposed research diagnostic criteria. Pain 81(1–2):147–154, ISSN:0304–3959, 10.1016/S0304-3959(99)00011-1. (http://www.sciencedirect.com/science/article/pii/S0304395999000111). Accessed 10 Mar 2012

Bruehl S, Harden RN, Galer BS et al (2002) Complex Regional Pain Syndrome: are there distinct subtypes and sequential stages of the syndrome? Pain 95:119–124

Harden RN, Bruehl S, Galer BS, Saltz S, Bertram M, Backonja M, Gayles R, Rudin N, Bhugra MK, Stanton-Hicks M (1999) Complex regional pain syndrome: are the IASP diagnostic criteria valid and sufficiently comprehensive? Pain 83(2):211–219, ISSN:0304–3959, 10.1016/S0304-3959(99)00104-9. http://www.sciencedirect.com/science/article/pii/S030 4395999001049. Accessed 10 Mar 2012

Harden RN, Bruehl S, Stanton-Hicks M, Wilson PR (2007) Proposed new diagnostic criteria for complex regional pain syndrome. Pain Med 8(4):326–331

Harden RN, Bruehl S, Roberto SGM, Perez FB, Marinus J, Maihofner C, Lubenow T, Buvanendran A, Mackey S, Graciosa J, Mogilevski M, Ramsden C, Chont C, Vatine JJ (2010) Validation of proposed diagnostic criteria (the "Budapest Criteria") for Complex Regional Pain Syndrome. Pain 150(2):268–274

Lau FH (2004) Silas Weir Mitchell, MD: the physician who discovered causalgia. J Hand Surg Am 29(2):181. ISSN:0363–5023, 03/2004. doi:10.1016/j.jhsa.2003.08.016

National Guideline Clearinghouse (NGC) (2011) Complex regional pain syndrome: treatment guidelines, 3rd edn. Guideline summary NGC-5233. Agency for Healthcare Research and Quality (AHRQ), Rockville. www.guidelines.gov. Accessed 10 Jan 2011

Reflex Sympathetic Dystrophy Syndrome Association (RSDSA) (2002) Clinical practice guidelines (second edition) for the diagnosis, treatment, and management of reflex sympathetic dystrophy/complex regional pain syndrome (RSD/CRPS). Reflex Sympathetic Dystrophy Syndrome Association (RSDSA), Milford, p 46 [47 references]

Stanton-hicks M, Janig W, Hassenbusch S, Haddox JD, Boas R, Wilson P (1995) Reflex sympathetic dystrophy: changing concepts and taxonomy. Pain 63:127–33

Wilson P, Stanton-Hicks M, Harden RN (eds) (2005) CRPS: current diagnosis and therapy. Progress in pain research and management, vol 32. IASP Press, Seattle

Complications

▶ Damage Control, History of

Compound Fracture

▶ Open Fractures

Compressible Hemorrhage

Frank K. Butler
Department of the Army, Committee on Tactical Combat Casualty Care, U.S. Army Institute of Surgical Research, Fort Sam Houston, TX, USA
Department of the Army, Prehospital Trauma Care, Joint Trauma System, U.S. Army Institute of Surgical Research, Fort Sam Houston, TX, USA

Synonyms

External hemorrhage; Extremity hemorrhage

Definition

Compressible hemorrhage is hemorrhage that can be seen on external examination of a trauma patient and possibly controlled by direct pressure or a tourniquet. Compressible hemorrhage includes extremity hemorrhage and non-extremity external hemorrhage.

The merits of tourniquet use on the battlefield to control extremity hemorrhage have been debated widely and for centuries. Perhaps as a result, exsanguination from extremity hemorrhage was the most common cause of preventable death in combat during the Vietnam War (Maughon 1970). Because of their effectiveness at controlling extremity hemorrhage and the speed with which they can be applied, tourniquets are the best option for temporary control of life-threatening extremity hemorrhage in the tactical environment. Tourniquets have, therefore, been heavily emphasized in Tactical Combat Casualty Care (Butler et al. 1996, 2007, 2010). Studies by Kragh and Lakstein have confirmed the lifesaving benefit and low incidence of complications from prehospital tourniquet use in combat casualties (Kragh et al. 2008, 2009; Lakstein et al. 2003). Although tourniquet use has been discouraged by civilian EMS systems in the past because of concern about ischemic damage to the extremity, limb loss from tourniquet ischemia has not been found to be a problem when tourniquets have been used appropriately during recent combat operations (Kragh et al. 2009).

Compressible hemorrhage also includes non-extremity external bleeding, which may occur from large vessels in the groin, axilla, or neck. Bleeding in these areas may be addressed either with hemostatic agents or with external pressure devices. The TCCC Guidelines now recommend Combat Gauze™ as the hemostatic agent of choice based on testing at the US Army Institute for Surgical Research (USAISR), which found it to be safe and effective at controlling hemorrhage in a lethal swine model of femoral artery bleeding (Kheirabadi et al. 2009, 2010).

Compressible bleeding in the groin may be successfully addressed with a junctional pressure device such as the Combat Ready Clamp if the bleeding site is not anatomically feasible for tourniquet use and Combat Gauze does not control the hemorrhage (Dubick and Kragh 2012).

Cross-References

▶ Corpsman
▶ Damage Control Resuscitation
▶ Damage Control Resuscitation, Military Trauma
▶ Exsanguination Transfusion
▶ Fluid, Electrolytes, and Nutrition in Trauma Patients
▶ FP24
▶ Hemorrhage
▶ Hemostatic Adjunct
▶ Hypothermia

▶ IED (Improvised Explosive Device)
▶ Intraosseous Device
▶ Noncompressible Hemorrhage
▶ Packed Red Blood Cells
▶ Plasma Transfusion in Trauma
▶ Shock
▶ Shock Management in Trauma
▶ TACEVAC
▶ Tactical Combat Casualty Care
▶ Tourniquet
▶ Tranexamic Acid
▶ Whole Blood

References

Butler FK, Giebner SD, McSwain N, Salomone J, Pons P (eds) Prehospital Trauma Life Support Manual. Seventh Edition – Military Version. Mosby JEMS, Elsevier, St. Louis, MO. November 2010.

Butler FK, Hagmann J, Butler EG (1996) Tactical combat casualty care in special operations. Mil Med 161(Suppl):1

Butler FK, Holcomb JB, Giebner SG, McSwain NE, Bagian J (2007) Tactical combat casualty care 2007: evolving concepts and battlefield experience. Mil Med 172(Suppl):1–19

Dubick M, Kragh JF (2012) Evaluation of the combat ready clamp to control bleeding in human cadavers, manikins, swine femoral artery hemorrhage model and swine carcasses. U.S. Army Institute of Surgical Research Technical Report, June 2012

Kheirabadi B, Mace J, Terrazas I et al (2010) Safety evaluation of new hemostatic agents, smectite granules, and kaolin-combat gauze in a vascular injury wound model in swine. J Trauma 68(2):269–278

Kheirabadi BS, Edens JW, Terrazas IB et al (2009) Comparison of new hemostatic granules/powders with currently deployed hemostatic products in a lethal model of extremity arterial hemorrhage in swine. J Trauma 66:316–328

Kragh JF, Walters TJ, Baer DG, Fox CJ, Wade CE, Salinas J, Holcomb JB (2008) Practical use of emergency tourniquets to stop bleeding in major limb trauma. J Trauma 64:S38–S50

Kragh JF Jr, Walters TJ, Baer DG, Fox CJ, Wade CE, Salinas J, Holcomb JB (2009) Survival with emergency tourniquet use to stop bleeding in major limb trauma. Ann Surg 249:1–7

Lakstein D, Blumenfeld A, Sokolov T et al (2003) Tourniquets for hemorrhage control on the battlefield: a four-year accumulated experience. J Trauma 54: S221–S225

Maughon JS An inquiry into the nature of wounds resulting in killed in action in Vietnam. Milit Med. 1970

C

Computed Tomography (CT)

▶ Imaging of Aortic and Thoracic Injuries

Computed Tomography (CT) of Abdominal and Pelvic Injuries

▶ Imaging of Abdominal and Pelvic Injuries

Concentrated Lyophilized Protein

▶ Adjuncts to Transfusion: Fibrinogen Concentrate

Concussion

▶ Traumatic Brain Injury, Mild (mTBI)

Confined Space

▶ Crush Syndrome

Consequences of Damage Control Surgery

▶ Damage Control Surgery: Outcomes of the Open Abdomen

Constipation

▶ Bowel Active Agents in the ICU

Constitution

▶ Bylaws (Institution)

Consumptive Coagulopathy

▶ Coagulopathy in Trauma: Underlying Mechanisms

Continuous Process Improvement

▶ Performance Improvement

Continuous Quality Improvement

▶ Performance Improvement

Contractures

Indraneil Mukherjee[1] and
Khanjan H. Nagarsheth[2]
[1]Department of General Surgery, Staten Island
University Hospital, Staten Island, NY, USA
[2]R Adams Cowley Shock Trauma Center,
University of Maryland School of Medicine,
Baltimore, MD, USA

Synonyms

Flexion contractures; Joint contractures

Definition

Joint contractures are also called flexion contractures. It is defined as a limitation in the passive range of motion of a joint due to fixed shortening of the periarticular soft tissue including the connective tissues, tendons, muscles, and skin. Contraction is a normal process of wound healing, where as a contracture forms when this process becomes pathological.

Preexisting Condition

Immobility is a major cause of joint contractures. Immobility could be a result of trauma, burn, stroke, or prolonged illness. It can also be iatrogenic after immobilization in a cast or a splint. It can also be formed by scarring after burn or surgery or as a reaction to foreign body like breast implant causing capsular contractures. It is also seen in neurological conditions like muscular dystrophy and cerebral palsy. Inflammatory disease like rheumatoid arthritis and other autoimmune diseases also increase the risk of contractures. There is also a lot of variable in genetic and environmental factors in formation of these contractures. Male predilection has been seen in Dupuytren's contracture (palmar fascia), Ledderhose's disease (plantar fascia), and Peyronie's disease (tunica albuginea), whereas adhesive capsulitis is seen more in women.

It has also been seen in the intensive care units. Many studies have shown functionally significant contracture of major joints that persisted till discharge. Some have seen it in one third of patients who stayed in the ICU for only 2 weeks (Clavet 2008). Contractures also cause severe debility to burn victims as well. Polio used to be a common cause of contractures and still is in the endemic part of the world. A severe polio contracture can cause the skin to contract over a joint; shorten the muscles, intermuscular septa, nerves, and vessels; contract the joint capsule; and deform the epiphyses. Correcting them is often impractical and difficult. It is easier to correct contractures in the pediatric population than adults which might need orthopedic procedures like osteotomies or arthrodesis.

Limb-lengthening surgeries can also cause undesirable effects of contractures. In the femur lengthening, both rectus femoris and hamstring muscles can cause contractures, while in tibial lengthening the gastrocnemius and toe flexors cause contractures. This can result in contractures at the knee, ankle, and toes. In the upper extremity biceps and brachioradialis can cause contracture in the arm, while in the forearm, hand flexors cause flexion at the interphalangeal and hyperextension of the metacarpophalangeal joints.

Application

Diagnosis of contractures is done clinically. The assessment of the patient and the contractures is very important in treating them. The cause of the contractures and the extent of the contractures should be assessed. The involvement of the skin, subcutaneous tissues, muscles, tendons, nerves, or joints should be assessed. The range of motion and the power in the muscles around them also need to be assessed. Apart from flexion and extension at various joints, the other ranges of adduction and abduction, as well as varus and valgus deformities, should be noted. All contracted joints usually are associated with nearby joints. Hip contractures can fully or partially be hidden by the spine and the pelvis. Therefore, all joints of the involved extremity should be examined and the ROM be documented.

Imaging is usually not needed to diagnose contractures. X-rays of bones and joints involved may be performed to look for deformities of the joint, presence of active disease, and degree of osteoporosis. MRI can be used as an adjunct to X-ray images.

The treatment of contractures is complex, and multiple modalities need to be involved. We should always understand that the predisposing factors persist after treatment of contractures; thus, for treatment to be effective, long-term management programs need to be developed; otherwise in many cases contractures persist or redevelop (Farmer 2001).

Medications can be used in its care, but rarely as a sole therapy. Spasmolytic medications like baclofen are used for its antispasmodic properties. Along with it, diazepam and clonidine have side effects depressing the central nervous system and should be sparingly used in patients with traumatic brain injury. Tizanidine, which is relatively less sedative, may be preferred. Dantrolene may also be used as it affects calcium channels in the muscles. Hepatotoxicity should be actively looked for as it is quite common.

Active and passive movements are the best prevention for contractures. In spite of the best intentions of patients and their caregivers, contractures do develop. These active and passive movements do retard their formation and assist in correction too. Active assisted movements are active movements that are aided in their terminal range of motion. Passive movements are done without any voluntary movement by the patient.

Skin traction is a simple kind of traction. It can be used temporarily as a bridge to skeletal tractions or used episodically. It is also used a lot in burn traumas as skin contractures are very debilitating.

Skeletal tractions are usually used in traumatic bone injury. In preventing contractures, they are used in extreme cases, when extensive injuries like burns are involved. Skeletal traction has advantages of being able to take care of the skin as well as assisted movements. The drawback of skeletal tractions is usually related to the pin site infection and osteomyelitis.

Manipulations and serial corrective casting are important adjuncts in managing contractures. These are especially important in joints that were active and where passive movements or traction have failed. These are usually hip contractures of less than 45°, knee contractures of less than 30°, and ankle contractures of less than 20°. Anesthesia might be required and helpful. Technique includes applying a very well-padded cast at a position close to maximal range of movement of the joint. Extreme positioning can cause necrosis of the cartilage. Inadequate padding can cause skin breakdown. During this process, hemorrhage into the joint capsule might happen, causing further arthritis, and in some cases bones and tendons can fracture. The cast must be taken down every couple of weeks, the skin and the joint examined, and a new case placed at the new maximal range of movement.

Splinting is also an option. These splints are used to place a muscle group under tension for long durations which helps prevent contractures

in the connective tissue. In a study by (Steffen 1995), prolonged stretch with the use of splints was equivocal in efficacy in reducing flexion contractures when compared to passive range of motion. Therefore, splinting should be employed only when active and passive movement exercises are not possible or need to be delayed for some duration.

In certain cases like fingers and toes, dynamic splints are preferred over static splints. In these, elastic mechanisms of rubber bands are used to produce elongation of the tissues and tendons through a low-load prolonged-duration stretch. Dynamic splints are also used in treating knee and elbow contractures.

Adjuvants like electrical stimulation, nerve blocks, hydrotherapy, and pressure dressings are also used in various scenarios, by various practitioners with varied goals and results.

Transcutaneous electrical stimulation can be used as an aid to cause muscle contractions. A calculated electrical signal is used to stimulate the underlying muscle to contract, which helps in improving muscle strength and reducing contractures.

In spastic neurological conditions like cerebral palsy, botulinum toxins can be used to reduce muscle contraction and thus contracture formation. Other agents like lidocaine, phenol, and alcohol derivatives have also been used for differentiating fixed contractures from spastic muscle contractions and also to treat them.

Hydrotherapy is used by physiotherapist as a preventive and therapeutic aid. It helps in increasing the active range of motion and prevents muscle weakness.

Pressure dressings with a pressure of 25–30 mmHg applied to the skin helps prevention of hypertrophic scar and contracture. It is continued for as long as 6–12 months.

Surgery offers a good option when nonoperative managements have failed and contractures are debilitating.

Release of skin contractures are the relatively simpler techniques but more commonly used. These skin contractures are usually because of large wounds, resulting from burns and other trauma. It can also result from iatrogenic causes, usually complicated by either infection or malnutrition. It can also happen from radiation and other chemical agents. Z-plasty and other kinds of releases should be made to reduce tension on the skin.

In elective surgeries, incisions perpendicular to the join crease should be avoided. These incisions should be made in a Z shape when possible. If that is difficult, it should be grafted with full-thickness grafts or at least thick split-thickness skin grafts. Some scenarios may need flaps for closure. These should be done before the setting of contractures, because once the contracture has set, fasciocutaneous flaps might be needed.

More significant surgeries like tendon-lengthening procedures are used in more fixed contractures when deeper tissues are also involved.

When the hip joint is involved, the knee should also be considered in the management and surgery as the contractures at the hip and knee are often seen together. It usually needs release of four tendons, the iliotibial band in several places, the iliopsoas, the tendon of the biceps femoris, and the medial hamstrings.

The contractures around the knees are very difficult to operate upon especially when they are more than 90°. If corrected too much, it might stretch the vessels and nerves causing pain, paralysis, or gangrene. After tenotomies described for the hip, they are usually treated by other adjuncts like manipulation and casting, wedging a cast, Russell traction, reversed sling on a Thomas splint, or skeletal traction with pins through the tibia.

At the ankle and feet, the release of the flexor digitorum longus and brevis tendons at the base of each toe corrects toe curling. It can be done alone as well as with the lengthening of the Achilles tendon.

In the upper extremity when the shoulder joint is involved in the contracture, the four shoulder muscles, the pectoralis major, the subscapularis, the latissimus dorsi, and the teres major, are usually released. A Z-plasty of the axillary skin is required for the skin contracture. After the wounds heal, the shoulder should be exercised gently.

Flexion contracture of the elbow commonly has breakdown of the antecubital skin and compression neuropathy of the ulnar nerve. The brachioradialis muscle and biceps tendon are usually completely transected. The brachialis muscle tendon is lengthened. The ulnar nerve is transposed anteriorly.

In the hands and fingers, the normal motion requires bony support, intact articular surfaces between them, unhindered gliding of the tendons, and intact collateral ligaments and volar plate. Compromise of any of them can cause reduced finger joint motion and thus contractures. Nonoperative treatment such as splinting or serial casting is tried before attempting any surgical interventions like external fixators and release of contractures. Even though it can improve extension at the joints, it carries the risk of pin site infection and flexion contracture (Hogan 2006). The wrist contractures are corrected by release of the wrist flexors. An arthrodesis is done sometimes to maintain the hand in a neutral position, thus eliminating the need for a permanent splint.

Cross-References

▶ Orthotics

References

Clavet H, Hébert PC, Fergusson D, Doucette S, Trudel G (2008) Joint contracture following prolonged stay in the intensive care unit. CMAJ 178(6):691–697. doi:10.1503/cmaj.071056

Farmer SE, James M (2001) Contractures in orthopaedic and neurological conditions: a review of causes and treatment. Disabil Rehabil 23(13):549–558

Hogan CJ, Nunley JA (2006) Posttraumatic proximal interphalangeal joint flexion contractures. J Am Acad Orthop Surg 14(9):524–533

Leblebici B, Adam M, Bağiş S, Tarim AM, Noyan T, Akman MN, Haberal MA (2006) Quality of life after burn injury: the impact of joint contracture. J Burn Care Res 27(6):864–868

Steffen TM, Mollinger LA (1995) Low-load, prolonged stretch in the treatment of knee flexion contractures in nursing home residents. Phys Ther 75(10):886–895, discussion 895–7

Contrast-Enhanced Multidetector Computed Tomography (MDCT)

▶ Thoracic Vascular Injuries

Controlled Mechanical Ventilation

▶ Ventilatory Management of Trauma Patients

Conversion of a Dedicated Airway into a Definitive Airway

▶ Airway Exchange in Trauma Patients

Coordination of Trauma Care

▶ Teamwork and Trauma Care

Cord Injury

▶ Neurotrauma, Introduction

Core Temperature

▶ Monitoring of Trauma Patients During Anesthesia

Core Temperature Redistribution

▶ Hypothermia, Trauma, and Anesthetic Management

Corifact™ (Coagulation Factor XIII Made from Pooled Human Plasma)

▶ Adjuncts to Transfusion: Recombinant Factor VIIa, Factor XIII, and Calcium

Coronal Shear Humerus Fracture

▶ Distal Humerus Fractures

Coronoid Fractures

▶ Pediatric Fractures About the Elbow

Corpsman

Frank K. Butler
Department of the Army, Committee on Tactical Combat Casualty Care, U.S. Army Institute of Surgical Research, Fort Sam Houston, TX, USA
Department of the Army, Prehospital Trauma Care, Joint Trauma System, U.S. Army Institute of Surgical Research, Fort Sam Houston, TX, USA

Synonyms

Hospital corpsman

Definition

The term corpsman refers to a Navy enlisted medical provider. Navy corpsmen serve in fixed medical treatment facilities, aboard ships, and in support of U.S. Marine Corps combat operations.

Frank K. Butler has retired.

Basic training for Navy corpsmen includes anatomy and physiology, in-hospital patient care, and the basics of emergency trauma care. Advanced training is situationally dependent and may vary from medical specialty training such as a surgical technician to paramedic training for corpsmen serving with Naval Special Warfare or Marine Corps Special Operations units.

Corpsmen who support Marine Corps combat operations receive additional training at one of the Marine Corps' two Field Medical Training Battalions. Here they learn both how to operate as part of a small combatant unit in the field and how to manage combat trauma using the principles of EMT-Basic and TCCC (Fox 2011).

Historically, corpsmen who serve as operators with Navy SEAL units must pass the rigorous Basic Underwater Demolition/SEAL training course, SEAL Qualification Training, jump school, and the 6-month Special Operations Combat Medic school at Fort Bragg, NC, as well as other specialized training. SEAL corpsmen have now been redesignated as "SEAL Operators." Naval Special Warfare units may also have a variety of other types of corpsmen, to include Diving Medical Technicians, Independent Duty Corpsmen, and nonspecialized corpsmen, in support roles (Butler 2002).

Additionally, corpsmen may be trained to provide independent medical care as an Independent Duty Corpsman (IDC). These training programs are typically a year or longer. IDCs are often the only medical provider on board Navy vessels and must be prepared to manage a wide range of medical and traumatic disorders.

Cross-References

- ▶ Cardiopulmonary Resuscitation in Adult Trauma
- ▶ CASEVAC
- ▶ Compressible Hemorrhage
- ▶ Damage Control Resuscitation
- ▶ Damage Control Resuscitation, Military Trauma
- ▶ Exsanguination Transfusion
- ▶ FP24
- ▶ Hemorrhage

- ▶ Hemostatic Adjunct
- ▶ Hypothermia
- ▶ IED (Improvised Explosive Device)
- ▶ Intraosseous Device
- ▶ Monitoring of Trauma Patients During Anesthesia
- ▶ Noncompressible Hemorrhage
- ▶ Pneumothorax, Tension
- ▶ Shock
- ▶ Shock Management in Trauma
- ▶ Tactical Combat Casualty Care
- ▶ Tourniquet
- ▶ Tranexamic Acid
- ▶ Triage

References

Butler FK (2002) Medical support of special operations. In: Pandolph KB, Burr RE (eds) Textbook of military medicine: harsh environments, vol 2. Office of the Surgeon General, U.S. Army, Falls Church VA

Fox RC (2011) Tactical Combat Casualty Care (TCCC) guidelines and updates. Marine Corps Administrative message 016/11, dated 10 Jan 2011

Corticosteroid Insufficiency

- ▶ Adrenal Insufficiency

COT

- ▶ Acute Coagulopathy of Trauma

Councils

- ▶ Trauma Associations

Court Case

- ▶ Litigation

Covenant

▶ Bylaws (Institution)

Covered Stenting

▶ Adjuncts to Damage Control Laparotomy: Endovascular Therapies

Cranial Doppler

▶ Neurotrauma, Transcranial Doppler Ultrasonography

Credentialing

John E. Mack
Surgical Physician Assistant Service,
Health Quest Medical Practice, PC,
Poughkeepsie, NY, USA

Synonyms

Attest; Authorize; Certify; Privileges; Verification

Definition

Credentialing is a process by which hospitals and health-care organizations obtain, review, and validate a physician's and other health-care providers' ability to practice based on education, training, practice history, licensure, certifications, and other professional qualifications. Based on the examination of information obtained, recommendations and determinations are made by medical staff and governing bodies as to whether an individual is entitled to clinical privileges to practice in a particular organization or setting.

Preexisting Condition

It has been well established by case law that a hospital has a legal obligation to ensure that good medical care is provided to its patients. If the hospital fails to use care in medical staff appointments and privileges, in monitoring clinical practice, or in removing physicians or other health-care providers in extreme cases, the hospital may be held liable (Southwick 1988).

This position has not always been the case nor at the forefront of importance. Prior to the 1970s, hospitals were seen as charitable organizations. They were simply places where physicians practiced medical care. They were protected by common law and essentially thought to have no legal responsibility to the patient for care rendered or any adverse outcomes associated with that care. In two benchmark court cases, Darling v. Charleston Community Memorial Hospital (1965) and Gonzales vs. Nork and Mercy Hospital (1973), the decisions handed down dramatically changed the landscape of accountability and liability. The court decisions emphasized that a hospital has a responsibility and duty to not only know but to evaluate, intervene, and take necessary action when there exists potential risk or harm to a patient from the care being provided by one of its physicians. These, along with other landmark cases, set the stage for the development of the medical staff department, its governing bodies, and the process and procedures for initial and ongoing evaluation and granting of clinical privileges.

Application

The objective of well-defined credentialing policies and procedures is to fulfill a hospital or health-care organization's duty to exercise reasonable care when selecting and granting privileges to its medical staff. Credentialing decisions can impact the overall quality of care rendered, degree of legal risk, allocation of financial resources, marketability, and even long-term sustainability of an organization. It is essential that an objective, well-documented, standard process be followed. This process must define roles and responsibilities, accountability, and areas of authority. The medical staff office, medical executive committee, and governing bodies such as the board of directors must set a clear direction and objective for the credentialing process. The ultimate goal is to credential the highest-quality practitioner, improve marketability, attract customers, ensure financial viability, reduce legal risk, and provide the highest-quality care possible for its patients.

A hospital accomplishes these goals by complying with the standards set by its accrediting body – one example is the Joint Commission on Accreditation of Healthcare Organizations (JCAHO). Additionally, a thorough review of state law, guidelines, and regulations for accreditation standards should be conducted. With these requirements and foundations in mind, credentialing agents must determine whether education and training requirements are met, what additional information must be requested to validate and support an application, who will collect the necessary information, and who will evaluate and make the final determination on an applicant's appointment.

A successful credentialing process is one that is universally applied and covers the following areas: defining membership categories and obligations, granting initial appointments, granting initial clinical privileges, monitoring during provision periods, granting full privileges, and conducting ongoing and periodic evaluation and reappointment based on profession practice evaluations and competency reviews. Typically, the medical staff department and its medical staff services professionals (MSSP) are responsible for initiating, processing, and maintaining the credentials file (Pybus, 2003). They are also responsible for ensuring compliance with the most up-to-date JCAHO standards, state and federal requirements, continuing medical education requirements, and medical staff rules, regulations, and bylaws.

The JCAHO and other accrediting bodies require that a hospital or health-care organization credential all licensed independent practitioners (LIPs). They are defined as podiatrists, dentists and physicians, and some nurse practitioners. These are individuals who provide patient care services without direction or supervision (JCAHO, 2005). All individuals are appointed through a fair and defined process. Many organizations also choose to credential nonphysician providers or those who work under supervision. Often referred to as allied health providers (AHPs), midlevel or complementary providers include nurse practitioners, physician assistants, nurse midwives, psychologists, and counselors (Pybus, 2002). Despite the category, the JCAHO standard MS.5.4.3 requires that minimal core criteria for credentialing include:

- Current licensure
- Relevant education, training, and experience
- Current competence and ability to perform the requested privileges

A key component of the credentialing process is the verification of credentials. This process is known as primary source verification. As of 1988, hospitals and health-care organizations are required by JCAHO to validate credentials such as profession, education, licensure, and postgraduate training with a person or organization that can attest to their validity. The purpose of primary source verification is to reduce the possibility of credential forgery (JCAHO, 2005).

In addition, a typical medical staff services professional or outside commercial verifications organization (CVOs) will conduct the following standard verifications of any applicant:

Standard Verifications Performed
- All history; undergraduate to present day – Competency Evaluation and Public Health Law as well as date verification
- Malpractice history – 10-year look back (all carriers will be queried for claims history requests)
- Primary Source Verification
  - NPDB – National Practitioner Data Bank
  - ECFMG – Educational Commission for Foreign Medical Graduates
  - OPMC – Office of Professional Medical Conduct   https://www.deadiversion.usdoj.

gov/webforms/validateSelect.do Accessed February 2013

- AMA – American Medical Association https://profiles.ama-assn.org/amaprofiles/ Accessed February 2013
- Board certification status (certificates or NCCPA) https://www.certifacts.org/dc/Login.aspx?err=nr http://www.nccpa.net/ Accessed February 2013
- Kroll – background check (state/county criminal, DMV, SS, FACIS) https://www.baionline.net/index.cfm Accessed February 2013
- DEA – Drug Enforcement Administration https://www.deadiversion.usdoj.gov/webforms/validateSelect.do Accessed February 2013
- FSMB – Federation of State Medical Boards https://s1.fsmb.org/docinfo/ Accessed February 2013
- Google
- SanctionCheck – (US Treasury and Blocked Persons, General Services Administration, HHS Office of Inspector General, Medical Inspector General, Office of Professional Medical Conduct) https://app.sanctioncheck.com/Scripts/logon.asp Accessed February 2013
- All applicable state licensure
- Health History
  - Current medical clearance, rubella and rubeola immunity, TB status

Competency Evaluation Performed (Requested of Peers and Affiliation Directors – Ratings: Excellent, Good, Fair, Poor, and Unknown)

- Medical/clinical knowledge
- Professional judgment
- Clinical competence/technical skill
- Practice-based learning and improvement
- Interpersonal and communication skills
- Patient care and management
- System-based practice
- Ethical conduct and professionalism
- Participation in medical affairs
- Cooperativeness and ability to work well with others
- Physician–patient relationship

- Timely completion and quality of medical records
- Ability to speak/understand English

A detailed explanation of the medical staff standards can be found in the JCAHO's Comprehensive Accreditation Manual for Hospitals (CAMH).

Depending on the membership category and specialty, typically, a division chief or department chair will review a fully completed application and make an informed recommendation to the chair of the credentials committee. If approved by the credentials committee, a slate is presented to the Medical Executive Committee (MEC). JCAHO requires that the MEC reviews, approves, and submits to the board of directors or overarching governing body all recommendations for appointment, reappointment, resignation, status changes, and disciplinary action. As the final authority, the board in conjunction with the CEO will make ultimate determination to grant or deny privileges accordingly (Fritz 2003).

The length of the application process is determined by the complexity of an applicant's history, the efficiency and availability of resource of an institution, and the overall credentialing system. It is important to note that the burden for obtained required information and completion of an application for credentialing and privileges is the responsibility of the applicant. No action can be rendered on an applicant's application until all information has been received and verified.

One vital component and often the most difficult in the credentialing process is determining the appropriate clinical privileges that will be granted to an applicant at the conclusion of the credentialing process. Though the terms "credentialing" and "privileging" are often used interchangeably, they in fact are two distinct processes. Commonly known as the delineation of privileges (DOP), the Joint Commission standard MS.4.15 states: "The decision to grant or deny a privilege(s), and/or to renew an existing privilege(s), is an objective, evidence-based process" (JCAHO 2005). According to CMS, the process must include criteria for determining the privileges that may be granted to individual practitioners and a procedure for applying the criteria to individual practitioners (Pybus, 2003).

The process of privileging involves several important components. First, an organization must analyze and determine the services they wish to offer their patients and whether sufficient resources exist to support such initiatives. Second, a determination of minimal educational and training requirement for the practitioner must be established. These are then organized into specific categories and define a scope of practice for a given specialty and practitioner. Lastly, an evaluation of the qualifications of the practitioner against the established criteria will determine if qualifications allow for the granting or denial of requested privileges.

In the past, many hospitals and health-care institutions had used a comprehensive "laundry" list of conditions and procedures. The applicant would simply check the box next to the item they wished to include in their delineation of privileges. Since every item listed must be used in conjunction with defined credentialing criteria, it was often fraught with difficulty to administratively manage. Lists were also very lengthy, were often outdated, required continual maintenance, and lacked specificity for a given specialty.

An alternative and now more widely used approach is the use of defined credentialing criteria for a "core" group of privileges. Each core group is designed specifically for a given specialty or treatment area. It is thought that successful completion of academic training and residency adequately prepares and ensures baseline competency for a core group of privileges (Pybus, 2003). However, keeping in mind that the goal of the credentialing process is to provide the highest quality of care and reduce risk, it cannot be assumed that all applicants are equal in their abilities and must be assured. Therefore, if a hospital feels that an individual applicant is not competent in any area requested, the list must be modified accordingly.

In addition to the core, an applicant can often apply for "specialty" or "noncore" privileges. Again, according to CMS: "Any procedure/task/activity/privilege requested by and recommended for a practitioner beyond the specified list of privileges for their particular category of practitioner would require evidence of additional qualifications and competencies, and be an activity/task/procedure that the hospital can support and is conducted within the hospital. Privileges cannot be granted for tasks/procedures/activities not conducted within the hospital despite the practitioner's ability to perform the requested tasks/procedures/activities" (CMS 2004).

In the case of nonphysician or supervised provider, the DOP approved must be supported by the same scope of practice and privileges of the supervising physician (Pybus, 2002). Privileges should be subject to any licensure requirements or other limitations, exercise independent judgment within the areas of his or her professional competence, and participate in the management of patients under the supervision of a physician who has been granted privileges to provide such care.

According to the JCAHO MS.5.15, privileges granted must be hospital-specific and based on an individual's demonstrated current competency. It further requires that privileges are related to an individual's documented experience in categories of treatment areas or procedures; the results of treatment; and the conclusions drawn from quality assessment and improvement activities when available (JCAHO 2005). Also, any decision related to reappointment must consider criteria that are directly related to quality of care.

For additional guidance and practice-related details, one might refer to organizations such as the Advisory Board. Clinical Privilege White Papers are available in a variety of practice areas and can be used to assist hospitals and credentials committees in developing policies and criteria for credentialing and privileges.

One of the defining principles of credentialing is the adoption of the five Ps: "Our Policy is to follow our Policy. In the absence of a Policy, our Policy is to create a Policy." Despite the intricacies of the process and even the policies which govern, credentialing and privileging have one central focus: the patient. If conducted in an organized, consistent, and fair manner, it reduces potential adverse medical and surgical outcomes, decreases costs, promotes business, and most importantly ensures quality health care.

Cross-References

▶ Advanced Practice Provider Care Delivery Models
▶ Bylaws (Institution)
▶ Interdisciplinary Team
▶ Nurse Practitioners in Trauma Care
▶ Physician Assistant
▶ Postgraduate Education
▶ Trauma Centers

References

Centers for Medicare and Medicaid Services, Centers for Medicare & Medicaid Services (CMS) (2004) Requirements for hospital medical. http://www.cms.gov/Medicare/Provider-Enrollment-and-Certification/SurveyCertificationGenInfo/downloads/SCLetter05-04.pdf
Darling v Charleston Community Memorial Hospital, 33 111, 2nd 326, 211 N. E.2d 253 1965
Fritz AL (2003) The medical executive committee handbook. HCPro, Marblehead
Gonzales v. Nork and Mercy Hospital, No, 228566 Sacramento Co, Super. Ct., Calif 1973
Joint Commission on Accreditation of Hospitals (JCAHO) (2005) Comprehensive accreditation manual for hospitals
Pybus B (2002) A guide to AHP credentialing. HcPro, Marblehead
Pybus B (2003) The comprehensive guide to medical staff credentialing and privileging. HCPro, Marblehead
Southwick AF (1988) The law of hospital and health care administration. Heath Administration Press, Ann Arbor

Recommended Reading
Zusman J (1999) The credentialing desk reference. Opus communications, Marblehead

Cricothyroidotomy

▶ Airway Management in Trauma, Cricothyrotomy

Crisis- Disaster

▶ Crisis Intervention

Crisis Intervention

Maureen Byrne
St. Francis Hospital-The Heart Center, Roslyn, NY, USA

Synonyms

Catastrophe intervention – interference – involvement; Crisis- disaster

Definition

The Chinese translation of the word "crisis" consists of two separate characters, which paradoxically mean danger and opportunity. Crisis intervention is defined as an active but temporary and supportive entry into the life situations of an individual or group during a period of extreme distress (Mitchell 2003).

Preexisting Condition

Crisis-inducing events are increasing in prevalence in our day-to-day routine. The September 11 attacks are notably the most horrific events to reach American soil in recent history. Natural disasters, from Hurricane Katrina to the recent events of Hurricane Sandy, emphasize the fear of nature and the unpredictable impact that nature has on the lives of people and the vulnerable ecosystem. The tragedy of the massacre at Newton Elementary Connecticut School and the recent attack suffered by participants and spectators at the Boston Marathon only contribute to the fear of society, are we really safe? If society is not safe or subject to happenings that are out of their control, how do we manage the repercussions of a crisis?

Dr. Gerald Caplan, a psychiatry professor at Massachusetts General Hospital and Harvard School of Public Health, initially "defined a crisis as occurring when individuals are confronted with problems that cannot be resolved." A crisis is an acute emotional reaction to some powerful stimulus or demand. It is also known as a state of emotional turmoil. A crisis is ignited by a stressful event, trauma, act of terrorism, or a situation that disrupts the balance or normal equilibrium of one's daily activity. This state of flux, instability, and uncertainty triggers emotional turmoil within the victim of the crisis. Familiar coping mechanisms become ineffective and fail to help regain homeostasis in one's life. Whether a crisis is related to a stage in life or an unexpected situation and event, the effects can be staggering (Mitchell 2003).

There are three main characteristics of any crisis:

- The relative balance that usually exists between a person's thinking abilities and emotions is disrupted.
- The usual coping methods fail to work in the face of the critical incident.
- There is evidence of mild-to-severe impairment in the individual or group involved in the critical incident (Mitchell 2003).

At times, a crisis may overpower the emotions and intellect of the entity of the crisis-inducing event, hence the birth of crisis intervention. As a consequence of historical events, crisis intervention has gained acceptance and validity in the treatment of victims of a traumatic event. Literature review and historical event analysis identify the initial origin of crisis intervention to World War I. The World War II era constructed a future framework for crisis intervention. It is reported that World War II soldiers who received immediate intervention near front lines and who were presented with suggestions for positive outcomes were more likely to recover and return to combat than those without such intervention (Mitchell 2003).

Dr. Erich Lindemann and Dr. Caplan, two community psychiatrists, are considered to be the forefathers of crisis intervention. The horrific event of a Boston Night Club fire, Coconut Grove, in 1943, resulted in the tragic death of 493 victims. It was this event that led Dr. Lindemann to his theory on crisis intervention. Crisis intervention is often dependent on the variables of society. Development and advancement in communications, particularly the phone, led to the inception of suicide hotlines in the 1950s. In 1963, under the Presidential leadership of John F. Kennedy, the National Community Mental Health Act was passed by Congress. This act supported community outreach programs to provided crisis intervention as a preventive attention to crisis-inducing events. The conceptual foundation for this congressional initiative was by the work of Dr. Caplan (Mitchell 2003).

Application

The goal of crisis intervention is to help the victim adapt to the traumatic event and foster positive coping skills. The individual who first engages in this process may not always be an educated and trained psychotherapist. Often the first contact is with a first responder, police personnel, or emergency room physician and or nurse. Hence, the multidimensional role of the emergency responder to identify characteristics of crisis is paramount. Identifying symptoms such as fear, anger, isolation, and loneness promptly will aid the recovery of the victim. Rapid assessment and intervention is essential. Early crisis intervention is the first stepping stone to the road to recovery for the prey of a traumatic event. It does not replace the professional benefit of a psychotherapist but serves as a bridge to the next level. The effectiveness of coping mechanisms is based on the initial incident and past experiences of the affected individual. The emergency responder must quickly assess the crisis event. If danger is imminent, prompt action is invaluable to secure safety of the situation. Identifying the needs of the victim whether it be first aid, medication, warmth, or shelter will aid in the triage process of crisis intervention. Recognizing intrinsic factors, such as emotional stability, state of present physical and mental health, and sense of self, needs to be explored to aid in the application of the process of crisis intervention. External resources, such as community assistance, personal income and financial stability, family support system, and if a death occurred due to the traumatic event, also play a role in crisis intervention.

Post September 11, Dr. A. Roberts developed the ACT Model for crisis intervention. This three-part model framework begins with assessment/appraisal of medical needs, connecting to support groups, and traumatic stress reduction. Emergency response personnel are educated to identify and intervene judiciously to aid the victim of a crisis (Roberts 2002). Roberts and Ottens (2005) also identified seven critical stages through which clients typically pass on the road to crisis stabilization, resolution, and mastery (Roberts and Ottens 2005). The stages are:

1. Plan and conduct a thorough biopsychosocial and lethality/imminent danger assessment.
2. Make psychological contact and rapidly establish the collaborative relationship.
3. Identify the major problems, including crisis precipitants.
4. Encourage an exploration of feelings and emotions.
5. Generate and explore alternatives and new coping strategies.
6. Restore functioning through implementation of an action plan.
7. Plan follow-up and booster sessions.

Cross-References

▶ Damage Control Surgery
▶ Damage Control, History of
▶ Disaster Preparedness
▶ Emergency Medical Services (EMS)
▶ Post Traumatic Stress Disorder
▶ Prehospital Emergency Preparedness

References

Mitchell J (2003) Major misconceptions in crisis interventions. Int J Emerg Ment Health 5(4):185–197
Roberts A (2002) Assessment, crisis intervention, and trauma treatment: the integrative ACT intervention model. Brief Treat Crisis Interv 2(1):2–21
Roberts A, Ottens A (2005) The seven-stage crisis intervention model: a road map to goal attainment, problem solving, and crisis resolution. Brief Treat Interv 5(4):330–339

Recommended Reading

Dass-Brailsford P (2007) A practical approach to trauma empowering interventions. Sage, Thousand Oak
Mitchell J (1999) Essential factors for effective psychological response to disasters and other crisis. Int J Emerg Ment Health 1:51–58
Mitchell J (2011) Collateral damage in disaster workers. Int J Emerg Ment Health 13(2):121–125

Crisis Standards of Care

▶ Disaster Management

Critical Care

▶ ICU Management
▶ Spinal Cord Injury, Intensive Care Unit (Hospital) Management

Critical Care Air Transport Team (CCATT)

Donald H. Jenkins
Department of Surgery, Division of Trauma, Critical Care and Emergency General Surgery, Saint Marys Hospital, Rochester, MN, USA

Synonyms

Air transport; Flight medic; Flight nurse; Tactical evacuation

Definition

The concept of moving a critically injured/ill service member through the echelons of care and advancing that care en route was developed by Maj. Gen. (Dr.) P. K. Carlton and Col. Chris Farmer at the 59th Medical Wing (Wilford Hall Medical Center), Lackland Air Force Base,

Texas, in a pilot program initiated in May 1994 (Wiki link 2013; Fang 2008).

The mission of CCATT is to operate an intensive care unit in an aircraft cabin during a flight which adds critical care capability to the US Air Force Aeromedical Evacuation System and allows for rapid evacuation of stabilized patients to definitive care at a higher echelon. CCATT patients have received initial stabilization and even surgery in the combat zone but are still critically ill, and they require evacuation from a less capable to a more capable hospital outside of the combat zone (see echelons/roles of care definition section). This allows smaller surgical units with fewer personnel in the combat zone with rapid evacuation of casualties.

One CCATT cares for up to three critically ill patients. By June 1996, the CCATT was formally approved and adopted into the USAF Aeromedical Evacuation System.

While the CCATT is designed to support combat casualties being evacuated from the combat zone, CCATTs have operated in other settings as well such as military operations other than war, pullout of US troops from Somalia, Khobar Towers bombing (Dhahran, Saudi Arabia), non-combatant evacuation from US Embassy in Liberia, special operations support, and peacetime movement of critically ill beneficiaries of military healthcare system. CCATT was extensively employed during Hurricane Katrina, evacuating civilian patients from coastal hospitals in the Southern USA to other US hospitals out of the hurricane evacuation zone (Grathwohl et al. 2008).

The CCATT is a three-member team consisting of the following: a critical care physician (intensivist, pulmonologist, anesthesiologist, general surgeon, emergency medicine physician), a critical care nurse, and a respiratory therapist. CCATT supplies and equipment are designed to supplement what the Aeromedical Evacuation System already carries, fit into four backpacks, can be hand-carried and floor-loaded onto an aircraft, and are lightweight, portable, and battery operated. This equipment includes ventilator, cardiac/physiologic monitor, three-channel computerized intravenous infusion pump, and a handheld point-of-care laboratory testing device.

The CCATT also carries advanced medications needed to provide ICU-level care as well as procedure kits needed to manage patient complications and perform lifesaving interventions (endotracheal intubation, chest tube insertion, etc.). Team members get initial training in aircraft safety procedures, air evacuation principles, as well as extensive hands-on equipment training in a real-world environment. Refresher training is also available just prior to deployment to update CCATT members on the latest equipment and medical treatment algorithms (Lairet et al. 2013).

Cross-References

- ► CASEVAC
- ► Damage Control Surgery
- ► Joint Trauma System (JTS)
- ► Mass Casualty
- ► MEDEVAC
- ► TACEVAC

References

Fang R Experience with long range enroute care. RTO-MP-HFM-157 NATO publication 2008. http://en.wikipedia.org/wiki/Critical_Care_Air_Transport_Team. Accessed 9 Sept 2013

Grathwohl KW, Venticinque SG, Blackbourne LH, Jenkins DH (2008) The evolution of military trauma and critical care medicine: applications for civilian medical care systems. Crit Care Med 36(7 Suppl): S253–S254. doi:10.1097/CCM.0b013e31817e325a. PMID:18594249

Lairet J, King J, Vojta L, Beninati W (2013) Short-term outcomes of US Air Force Critical Care Air Transport Team (CCATT) patients evacuated from a combat setting. Mil Med 17(4):486–490. doi:10.3109/10903127.2013.811564

Critical Care Management

► Trauma Intensive Care Management

Critical Care Support

► Life Support Training

Critical Illness Myopathy and/or Neuropathy

▶ ICU Acquired Weakness

Critical Illness Neuromyopathy

▶ ICU Acquired Weakness

Critical Illness-Related Corticosteroid Insufficiency

▶ Adrenal Insufficiency in Trauma and Sepsis

Crossmatch

Bryan A. Cotton[1,2] and Laura A. McElroy[2]
[1]Department of Surgery, Division of Acute Care Surgery, Trauma and Critical Care, University of Texas Health Science Center at Houston, The University of Texas Medical School at Houston, Houston, TX, USA
[2]Department of Anesthesiology, Critical Care Medicine, University of Rochester Medical Center, Rochester, NY, USA

Definition

Prior to the safe transfusion of blood products, a type and screen must be performed to identify the recipient's ABO and Rh D blood types and to evaluate the recipient's blood for other less common, but clinically significant, antibodies that most commonly form after pregnancy or prior transfusion. Though in theory the type and screen alone will eliminate over 99 % of transfusion reactions, a further test called a crossmatch is then done to maximize compatibility between the recipient and donor blood product.

Blood crossmatching, in the strict sense, involves mixing a sample of the recipient's serum with the actual RBCs to be transfused to test if the recipient has preformed antibodies to the donor erythrocyte antigens. The complete test takes 40–60 min and contains three phases. The first phase takes place at room temperature, and agglutination of the sample within 5–10 min signifies major incompatibility, such as ABO mismatch or the presence of antibodies of the Lewis, NM, or P systems. The next phase occurs if phase one is negative and involves further incubation of the mixture at body temperature (37 °C) after the addition of salt solution or albumin. The second phase tests primarily for Rh antibodies, but can also detect incomplete antibodies (Dean 2005). Completion of this phase takes from 20 to 45 min. If phase two is negative, antihuman globulin (also known as Coombs reagent) is added for the third phase. These antihuman antibodies attach to antibodies on affected RBCs, leading to agglutination. This phase detects incomplete antibodies in several blood group systems, including Kidd, Duffy, and Kell (Miller 2009). While all three phases constitute a complete crossmatch, they are not all routinely required. If a patient's type and screen and clinical history indicate no evidence of or risk factors for alloantibodies, the likelihood of antibodies leading to a positive phase 2 or 3 test result is minimal and is often unnecessary (Lee et al. 2007). Criteria guiding decisions on who needs extended crossmatching are developed by national and regional organizations evaluating transfusion research and formalized for every institution and blood bank (Working Party 2004).

An electronic crossmatch is a computer-generated assessment of donor and recipient compatibility. To be used, both parties must have fully characterized blood typing and no detectible atypical antibodies. This computer-assisted crossmatch allows blood products to be released rapidly, and its use is restricted to patients with known hematologic history and testing. Neonates and patients with significant antibodies cannot safely be included in the electronic crossmatch system (Aslan 2006).

Cross-References

▶ Antibody Screen
▶ Blood Bank
▶ Blood Group Antibodies
▶ Blood Type
▶ Blood Typing
▶ Rhesus Factor

References

Aslan O (2006) Electronic crossmatching. Transfus Med Rev 20(1):75–79

Dean L (2005) Blood groups and red cell antigens [Internet]. National Center for Biotechnology Information (US), Bethesda, Chap 3, Blood transfusions and the immune system. Available from: http://www.ncbi.nlm.nih.gov/books/NBK2265/

Lee E, Redman M, Burgess G et al (2007) Do patients with autoantibodies or clinically significant autoantibodies require and indirect antiglobulin test crossmatch? Transfusion 47:1290–1295

Miller RD (2009) Transfusion therapy, Chap 55. In: Miller's anesthesia, 7th edn. Churchill Livingstone, Maryland Heights, pp 1742–1745

Working Party of the British Committee for Standards in Haematology Blood Transfusion Task Force (2004) Guidelines for compatibility procedures in blood transfusion laboratories. Transfus Med 14:59–73

Crush Injuries

Dane Scantling[1] and Steven R. Allen[2]
[1]Philadelphia College of Osteopathic Medicine, Philadelphia, PA, USA
[2]Department of Traumatology, Surgical Critical Care and Emergency Surgery, Hospital of the University of Pennsylvania, Philadelphia, PA, USA

Synonyms

Crush syndrome; Extremity injury; Prolonged extrication; Reperfusion syndrome; Traumatic rhabdomyolysis

Epidemiology

Crush injury is relatively uncommon in first world nations, and only 1 in 100,000 Americans will experience a crush injury annually that results in myocyte damage (Pinto and White-Guthro 2012). Twenty percent of natural disaster survivors and 40 % of structural collapse survivors have been estimated to have incurred a crush injury (Better and Stein 1990). Internationally, war, terrorism, and industrial accidents contribute substantially to the overall burden of disease. In developed nations and civilian populations, crush injuries are most commonly found in structural collapses following natural disasters such as hurricanes, earthquakes, landslides and tsunamis, as well as motor vehicle crashes or industrial accidents Fig. 1.

Structural collapse is a common cause of crush injury and has many causes Fig. 2.

Crush injury may also be caused by any condition in which an individual remains stationary for extended periods of time. This may occur in conditions of debility, drug use or iatrogenically in health care settings such as lengthy anesthesia times with inadequate padding. Injury patterns overall are predictable. Three quarters of crush injuries affect the lower extremities, 10 % affect the upper extremities, and 9 % affect the trunk (Pinto and White-Guthro 2012).

The occurrence of crush syndrome, a potentially deadly systemic manifestation of crush injury involving metabolic derangements, organ dysfunction, and local tissue damage, has similarly been studied.

In the case of earthquakes causing major structural damage, crush syndrome is estimated to occur in 2–15 % of patients (CDC 2013). Half will experience renal failure and up to 50 % will require a fasciotomy (CDC 2013). The magnitude of complications can be anticipated and is related to the amount of compressive force applied and the length of time the damage was incurred (Jagodzinski et al. 2010).

Anatomy of Injury

Crush injury occurs when one experiences a compressive force, most commonly to the extremities

Crush Injuries,
Fig. 1 (**a**) This photograph
shows the rescue effort
following a recent
industrial accident and
building collapse in
Philadelphia, PA, which
injured 13 people and killed
six civilians (Photo credit:
Ashley Hahn, Eyes on the
Street/PlanPhilly). (**b**) This
image shows multiple
collapsed homes in the
wake of a tornado in
Monson, MA (Photo credit:
FIREGROUND360).
(**c**) A natural gas explosion
has leveled a business in
Springfield, MA (Photo
credit: FIREGROUND360)

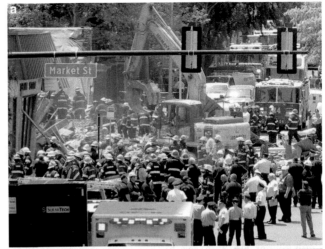

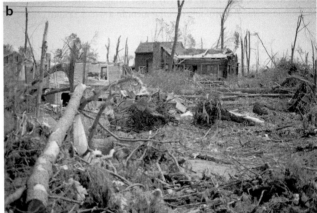

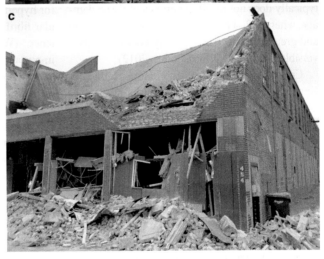

and occasionally to the torso, which causes
injury to the muscle, nerves or both (CDC
2013). Compression of tissue leads to direct
damage as well as a loss of circulation, ischemia
and further myolysis (Pinto and White-Guthro
2012).

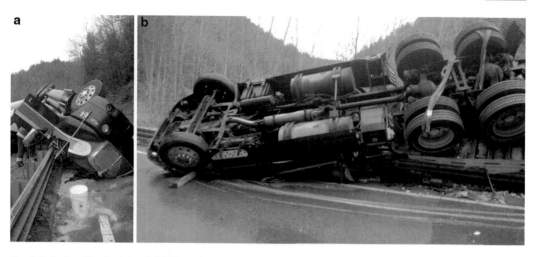

Crush Injuries, Fig. 2 (**a**) and (**b**) These images show emergency personnel conducting a vehicle rescue where the individual suffered a prolonged entrapment in a wreck (Photo credits: FIREGROUND360)

Direct complications of the initial injury should not be overlooked. These include hemorrhage, potential infection and subsequent sepsis as well as the potential for asphyxiation in the setting of a crush into to the torso.

Severity of the injury and the likelihood of complications are related to the force applied, the amount of tissue involved, and the duration of the crush injury (Jagodzinski et al. 2010). Compressive force inducing ischemia lasting less than 2 h typically does not result in permanent tissue damage, whereas 2–4 h may induce reversible damage and greater than 6 h is typically considered irreversible (Pinto and White-Guthro 2012).

Crush injury's most common, clinically significant complication is crush syndrome, a systemic manifestation of a localized injury induced by traumatic rhabdomyolysis (Jagodzinski et al. 2010). Crush syndrome occurs when the compressive force is relieved and metabolic by-products of myocyte injury and death enter the systemic circulation (Smith and Greaves 2003). In fact, most damage to myocytes is believed to occur after the release of compressive forces (Jagodzinski et al. 2010). Cellular contents released include electrolytes, urate, phosphate and most importantly myoglobin, an oxygen binding substance and phosphate from damaged muscle tissue (Jagodzinski et al. 2010). In the acidic conditions found in crush syndrome, these three substances are released from solution, become tubular casts, and directly obstruct kidney function (Jagodzinski et al. 2010) Fig. 3.

Systemic manifestations include electrolyte abnormalities such as hyperkalemia, metabolic acidosis, cardiac arrhythmias, acute renal failure, and death (CDC 2013). While the ECG findings of hyperkalemia are classically described as peaked T waves, a loss of P waves, and widened QRS complexes, it is worth noting that ECG sensitivity for hyperkalemia is low and asystole and ventricular fibrillation may be the first signs of its existence (Weisberg and Dellinger 2008). More important are potassium's physical effects on the heart which include depolarization of cellular membranes, a shortened action potential, and a reduced electrical conduction in the ventricles (Weisberg and Dellinger 2008). All of these aspects may rapidly lead to cardiac arrest, and severity is tied to both the total amount of extracellular potassium and the speed at which the increase occurred (Weisberg and Dellinger 2008).

Another common complication of crush injury is compartment syndrome, a condition in which increasingly edematous muscle, enclosed by a fascial envelope, results in ischemia of that compressed tissue (Smith and Greaves 2003). This may result in permanent muscle or nerve damage and lead to limb loss if the fascia is not adequately released with fasciotomies Figs. 4 and 5.

Crush Injuries,
Fig. 3 This graphic shows
the evolution of untreated
crush syndrome (Photo
credit: Dr. Samir Mehta)

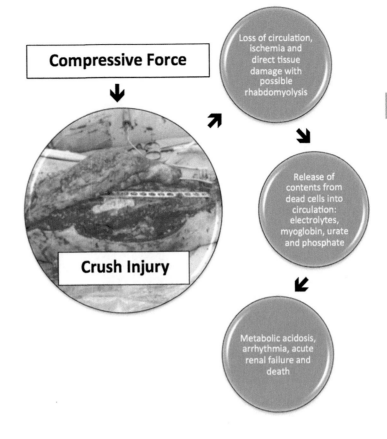

Crush Injuries,
Fig. 4 This image shows
substantial pallor, a late
finding, of a limb with
compartment syndrome
(Photo credit: Dr. Samir
Mehta)

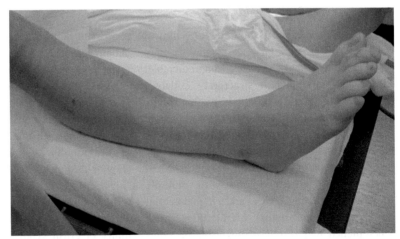

Clinical Impact

Trauma Triage Significance

Although uncommon in the United States, crush injury may have profound consequences. These complications and the expansive list of potential causes require caregivers to have a high level of clinical suspicion. Over-triage is an acceptable outcome in an attempt to identify the condition. All patients suspected to have sustained a crush injury should be transferred to a designated trauma center emergently by prehospital personnel.

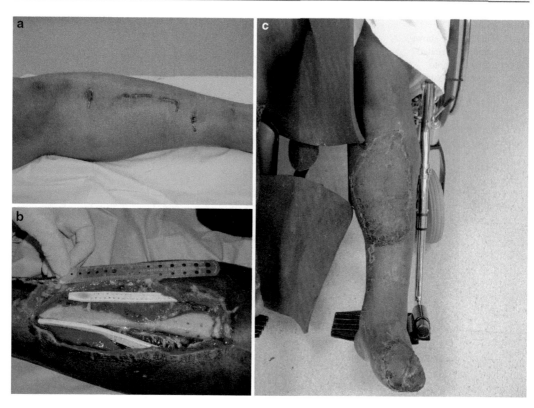

Crush Injuries, Fig. 5 (**a**, **b** and **c**) This image sequence shows a presenting crush injury, resultant fasciotomy, and end result in the same patient (Photo credits: Dr. Samir Mehta)

Mechanism of injury should guide clinical suspicion of crush injury as symptoms may be variable and prove unpredictable. Prolonged entrapment, structural collapse, altered mental status, and immobility that results in long periods of stasis are important indicators that crush injury and crush syndrome may be present.

Mechanisms that lead to crush injuries often result in multisystem trauma with multiple additional distracting injuries and a high potential for altered mental status. Alert patients with a heightened fear response may have no complaints even with significant injury and may not exhibit abnormal vital signs upon presentation. Many of the complications of crush injury may also take substantial time to become clinically apparent.

Crush syndrome may not proceed until compressive force is relieved, and patients in the process of being freed from lengthy entrapment should be monitored carefully, an important consideration for prehospital personnel.

As direct arterial injury from crush injury is unlikely, peripheral pulses are often unaffected even if compartment syndrome is rapidly evolving. Limbs frequently do exhibit uneven numbness, bruising, and discoloration (Jagodzinski et al. 2010).

Clinical Care/Care Caveats

Treatment of patients suspected of having a crush injury or crush syndrome should be performed initially in a similar manner to other traumas. Advanced cardiac life support, prehospital trauma life support, and advanced trauma life support protocols should be followed as appropriate based on resources and personnel available.

All patients suspected to develop crush syndrome should, at a minimum, be monitored for blood pressure, heart rate and rhythm, respiratory rate, and oxygen saturation. Urine output and lactic acid are also vital gauges of a patient's condition. Serum potassium and calcium should be assessed three to four times daily for several days following admission. The short half-life of myoglobin released by damaged muscle allows comparison of urine and serum levels to track the progression of the patient's clinical course. Creatine kinase allows a longer-term snapshot of muscle breakdown, and levels correlate well with the likelihood of renal complications (Jagodzinski et al. 2010). A rising creatine kinase level should be considered indicative of rhabdomyolysis and the need for emergent fasciotomy, or revision of existing fasciotomies should be considered. Ongoing blood gas monitoring is helpful to determine the progression of metabolic acidosis.

Hyperkalemia, as mentioned, is a rapidly fatal complication of crush syndrome and must be quickly corrected. In the prehospital setting, copious isotonic intravenous fluids should be administered, if possible, prior to the release of the crushed tissue (CDC 2013). If this is not possible, a tourniquet may be applied to an affected limb prior to removing compressive forces (CDC 2013). Selective beta 2 agonists such as albuterol or terbutaline and alkalinizing agents like sodium bicarbonate can be used to shift potassium intracellularly. Alkalinization may also aid in preventing crystal deposition into the kidneys (Weisberg and Dellinger 2008). Calcium gluconate can be given to stabilize the cardiac membrane (Shingarev and Allon 2010). Additional therapies reserved for emergency in-hospital treatment include administration of insulin (with glucose to maintain blood sugar levels), which will more rapidly reduce extracellular potassium levels in a manner similar to beta agonists and alkalinizing agents (Weisberg and Dellinger 2008). Ultimately, dialysis is the most definitive treatment for removing potassium from the body and should be accomplished with continual ECG monitoring (Weisberg and Dellinger 2008). It provides additional benefit in the setting of rhabdomyolysis (Shingarev and Allon 2010).

Cross-References

▶ ABCDE of Trauma Care
▶ Compartment Syndrome
▶ Crush Syndrome
▶ Extremity Injury
▶ Mass Casualty Incident
▶ Motor Vehicle Crash Injury

References

Better OS, Stein JH (1990) Early management of shock and prophylaxis of acute renal failure in traumatic rhabdomyolysis. N Engl J Med 322: 825–829

Centers for Disease Control and Prevention (2013) Blast injuries: crush injuries & crush syndrome. Retrieved from http://emergency.cdc.gov/masscasualties/blastinjury-crush.asp. Accessed 22 July 2013

Jagodzinski NA, Weerasinghe C, Porter K (2010a) Crush injuries and crush syndrome – a review. Part 1: the systemic injury. Trauma 12: 69–88

Jagodzinski NA, Weerasinghe C, Porter K (2010b) Crush injuries and crush syndrome – a review. Part 2: the local injury. Trauma 12: 133–148

Pinto S, White-Guthro M (2012) Evidence-based care sheet: crush injury and crush syndrome. Cinahl Information Systems

Shingarev R, Allon M (2010) A physiologic-based approach to the treatment of acute hyperkalemia. Am J Kidney Dis 56(3): 578–584

Smith J, Greaves I (2003) Crush injury and crush syndrome: a review. J Trauma 54(5): S226–S230

Weisberg LS, Dellinger RP (2008) Management of severe hyperkalemia. Crit Care Med 36(12): 3247–3251

Crush Syndrome

Charles A. Frosolone
Medical Department, USS Nimitz CVN-68, Everett, WA, USA

Synonyms

Building collapse; Bywaters' syndrome; Cave-in syndrome; Confined space; Crush injuries; Earthquake; Trapped in vehicle; Traumatic rhabdomyolysis with acute renal failure

Definition

Crush syndrome is traumatic rhabdomyolysis caused by entrapment usually of an extremity under rubble, in a vehicle, or other mechanism that results in acute renal failure and ultimately if untreated death.

The syndrome was first noted in pre-WW1 earthquake/tsunami in Sicily and again in WW1 German medical literature. Bywaters appreciated it in WW2 victims of the 1941 London Blitz noting the classic signs and symptoms resulting in rhabdomyolysis, renal failure, and ultimately death (Bywaters and Beall 1941). He went on to conduct animal studies on prevention of the resulting renal failure caused by the crush syndrome rhabdomyolysis and put these principles into practice during the Vengeance weapon blitz later in the war. His animal studies and treatment still are applicable today in treatment of crush syndrome victims. Coupled with today's therapies for renal failure, if available and applied in an appropriate time, the death rate from crush syndrome treated early and appropriately is negligible.

Preexisting Condition

Crush syndrome is fundamentally based on three criteria (Gonzales 2005): (1) trapped extremity with involvement of muscle mass, (2) prolonged compression (greater than 2 ½–4 h of unrelenting pressure), and (3) compromised local circulation. After release from entrapment and reperfusion of the muscle mass/extremity, there is muscle damage and death (rhabdomyolysis) occurring in the now untrapped muscle mass that if untreated results in renal failure and ultimately death. Not due to entrapment, there are other causes of rhabdomyolysis important to the military provider caused by strenuous prolonged exertion that is seen in elite military units and military recruits in hot, humid training conditions combined with dehydration and downhill marching. Treatment for this exertional rhabdomyolysis or other causes of rhabdomyolysis follows the guidelines below.

The pressure and ischemia from entrapment are more damaging to the muscle than ischemia alone and result in a sarcolemmic leak. This allows Na+, Ca+, and water to enter causing destruction of the muscle tissue by activation of autolytic enzymes and loss of mitochondrial integrity, release of nephrotoxic metabolites (myoglobin and purines) and intracellular ions (potassium, phosphate), and edema of the muscle. When the ischemic limb is released from pressure and reperfused, the toxic metabolites and ions are released into the circulation. The resulting edema can cause significant third spacing of fluid (up to 10 l per limb) resulting in hypovolemic shock and acidosis. These factors contribute to cardiac depression and acute kidney injury (AKI). This renal failure untreated will result in death usually by cardiac arrest from elevated potassium. Medical problems other than renal failure can occur to include sepsis, acute respiratory distress syndrome, disseminated intravascular coagulation, hemorrhage, cardiac arrhythmias, other electrolyte disturbances, pulmonary problems from inhaled dust, and psychological trauma.

Crush syndrome can occur in "epidemics" from entrapment of victims in earthquakes, landslides, mine collapses, terrorist bombings, etc. After major earthquakes, crush syndrome, which results in AKI, is the second most frequent cause of mortality after direct trauma. After the earthquake in Tangshan, China (1976:deathtoll 242,769), 2–5 % of all those injured had crush syndrome. After the Kobe earthquake (1995), this syndrome was observed in 13.8 % of hospitalized patients, and AKI developed in half these patients (Gonzales 2005). The incidence of crush syndrome can rise up to 2–5 % overall in disaster victims, and up to 25 % of hospitalized victims appear to be at risk for AKI. More crush syndrome is noted in areas where buildings are not constructed to earthquake standards and rescue options are limited, and noted less where single-story mud-type buildings predominate or where there are few or no survivors from the building collapse (9–11 attacks). Once AKI occurs, the fatality rate can go as high as 25 %.

Of 200,000 killed and 300,000 injured in Haiti earthquake (2010), only 19 patients with crush syndrome were referred for hemodialysis. Probably this was related to an overwhelming number of severely injured people who died early on (Vanholder et al. 2010), survivors who were pulled from the rubble early by bystanders who were not crushed for long periods, many who could not receive timely medical care, and delayed initiation of dialysis because of complex logistical issues. As contrasted with the L'Aquila, Italy (2009) earthquake where the number of crush syndrome victims not only was low, there were few deaths from crush syndrome even in those requiring dialysis (Vanholder et al. 2009). Many factors may have contributed to these small numbers in L'Aquila, which the most obvious ones are the prompt and effective rescue efforts, the recognition of the syndrome, and transfer of rescued victims quickly to optimal medical care.

Application

Prevention: The best preventive option for decreasing casualties in the event of an earthquake or similar disaster is strict building codes requiring the construction of high-quality buildings and strict safety practices. Also contributing to decreasing the sequelae of crush syndrome are rescue capabilities limiting the time victims that might be trapped, being able to administer to entrapped victims intravenous fluid, and medical infrastructure to respond to those with crush syndrome.

Diagnosis: suspect in victims with a possible entrapment event (Emerg War Surg 2004). Compression >2 h is likely to result in crush syndrome, but this has been seen in as little as 20 min. A thorough examination must be done with attention to extremities, trunk, and buttocks. Typically affected areas of the body include lower extremities (74 %), upper extremities (10 %), and trunk (9 %). The physical findings depend on the duration of entrapment, treatment rendered, and time since the victim's release. Extremities may initially appear normal just after extrication, but soon edema develops and the extremity becomes swollen, cool, and tense. Victims may have severe pain out of proportion

to examination. Anesthesia and paralysis of the extremities can mimic a spinal cord injury with flaccid paralysis; however there will be normal bowel and bladder function. In exam of the trunk and buttocks, there may be severe pain out of proportion to examination and tense compartments. Nausea, vomiting, confusion, and agitation may occur as consequences of disturbed body chemistry.

The urine may appear as hematuria, "port wine urine," and tests positive by dipstick as blood, but has no red blood cells on microscopic. Creatinine phosphokinase is elevated with values usually >100,000 IU/ml. Hemoglobin and hematocrit may be elevated due to hemoconcentration, or normal or low due to hemorrhage from other trauma. Potassium may be elevated, sometimes markedly, averaging 7–8 mmol/L in victims from Haiti earthquake, and many patients' renal functions may already reflect renal failure.

Prehospital treatment: Rapid extrication of crush victims from under the rubble is one of the mainstays of renal disaster rescue and treatment. Beyond rescue, prehospital treatment consists of fluid administration, alkalinization of the urine, and diuresis if indicated. Some casualties who do well while trapped under the rubble may deteriorate and even die immediately after extrication (rescue death). However, early fluid resuscitation within the first 6 h, preferably before the victim is extricated, is essential. Fluid resuscitation to a victim while still entrapped gives a better chance for the victim to remain hemodynamically stable after extrication. Permissive hypotension is unwise! The preferred fluid is isotonic saline, given at a rate of 1–1.5 l per hour (10–15 ml per kilogram of body weight per hour) to a maximum of 6–10 l/day, while the victim is still trapped into a free arm or leg. Use isotonic fluids and avoid solutions containing dextrose, potassium, and lactate. For example, during extrication, administer 1–1.5 l 0.9 % NS/h; consider adding 1 amp bicarbonate and 10 g of mannitol to each liter. Once released from entrapment, patients should be then transferred if possible to a trauma center or medical facility capable of the further care necessary. However, in some disaster situations, like an earthquake, the medical facilities may be destroyed, damaged, or their capabilities degraded by infrastructure damage.

In-hospital treatment: consists of intravenous fluid (IVF) administration, alkalinization of urine, compartment release, rarely amputations, and, if indicated, dialysis. Once in hospital ½ NS without potassium is initiated. Adding 40–50 mEq of sodium bicarbonate to each second or third liter of hypotonic saline (usually a total of 200–300 mEq the first day) will maintain urinary pH above 6.5 and prevent intratubular deposition of myoglobin and uric acid. 50 ml of 20 % mannitol (1–2 g per kilogram per day [total, 120 g], given at a rate of 5 g/h) may be added. The addition of mannitol increases urine output and also decreases compartmental pressures. Once a patient with the crush syndrome has been hospitalized, urinary output should ideally exceed 300 ml per hour. Such a goal may require the intravenous infusion of up to 12 l of fluid per day (4–6 l of which will contain bicarbonate). This should be continued until clinical or biochemical evidence of myoglobinuria disappears (usually by day 3). Fluid treatment needs to be individualized by response and laboratory testing, and, if available, central venous pressure measurements are useful. Electrolyte abnormalities are frequent in patients with crush-related AKI with fatal hyperkalemia being the most important. Victims with elevated potassium should have cardiac monitoring if available. Close monitoring of electrolyte levels is essential, especially potassium, phosphate, and calcium, and if indicated treatment following accepted guidelines should be initiated. Calcium may be low early to rise later in course, so treatment should only be when hypocalcemia is symptomatic or causing ECG changes.

Recognition and treatment of compartment syndrome is important: usually occurring in the lower leg or forearm, but remember to check torso and buttocks as well. Tense compartments, pain out of proportion, paresthesias, and elevated relative compartment pressures are all indicative of compartment syndrome (McQueen et al. 1996). Treatment can consist of mannitol. Betters feels a trial of mannitol before surgery (Betters and Stein 1990), but most commonly surgical compartment release, is done (fasciotomy). It is indicated if the compartment pressures are elevated when compared to the diastolic pressure (differential pressure: diastolic pressure – compartment pressure <30 mmHg). The role of amputation is very limited in the management of crush syndrome. Amputation **may** be necessary for rescue of entrapped casualties (ketamine 2 mg/kg IV for anesthesia and use of proximal tourniquet). Amputation may be considered in casualties with irreversible muscle necrosis/ necrotic extremity. Hyperbaric oxygen may be useful after surgery to improve extremity survival.

If AKI or dangerous levels of serum potassium, acidosis, encephalopathy, or volume overload occur, dialysis may be necessary. Depending on circumstances some form of hemodialysis or peritoneal dialysis might be used. Before return of sufficient renal function, dialysis may be necessary two or three times a day for an average of 13–18 days. Intermittent hemodialysis allows the treatment of several patients per day with a single dialysis machine. Even short hemodialysis sessions (2–3 h daily) will avert life-threatening hyperkalemia. However, implementing this strategy requires significant technical support, experienced personnel, electricity, and water supplies, all of which are often affected by the disaster. Peritoneal dialysis is technically simple, does not require electricity and tap water supplies, and can be initiated rapidly. However, it is difficult to use in patients with abdominal or thoracic trauma, requires substantial quantities of sterilized dialysate, and may cause complications related to the field conditions of the disaster. Recovery of renal function and survival in crush-induced AKI are markedly better than for other causes of AKI.

Prognosis: Appropriate fluid administration and treatment of AKI improve prognosis. The mortality rate for crush syndrome following the earthquake in northern Turkey in 1999 was 15.2 %. However, rates in subsequent quakes have varied, and it is thought that many factors may affect survival, such as less than optimal rescue and transport, infrastructure damage, and availability or not of sophisticated therapeutic options.

When an epidemic occurs, there are large resource demands for crush syndrome victims beyond need for dialysis equipment and expertise, including needs for water, food, and other medical needs caused by the disaster. For example, fluid needs can be 5 l IVF per victim first day times number of victims and continuing need of even more up to IVF 20 l per victim per day, plus blood products, potassium binders, etc. (Sever et al. 2006). Stockpiling equipment to be used in emergencies should be considered in earthquake-prone regions and forming coalitions between medical suppliers, nongovernmental organizations, and governments that can transport ready staged materials into the area of need.

International organizations exist for response to large-scale epidemics of crush syndrome after earthquakes such as the Renal Disaster Relief Task Force (RDRTF) of the International Society of Nephrology (ISN) (Sever et al. 2009). The disappointing experiences of the Armenian earthquake convinced the ISN to create the RDRTF as a logistic organization to avoid similar problems in future disasters. The RDRTF has responded to earthquakes in Haiti and Italy where they functioned along with NGOs and the US military (USNS Comfort) to improve crush syndrome care and dialysis as needed.

Care by Role (ECHELON)

1) **Prior to extrication**: control of A, B, Cs. IV Fluid administration. Field amputation
1,2) **After rescue**: continued A, B, Cs management and IV fluid administration. Resuscitative surgery if indicated and available. Fasciotomy if indicated or prolonged transport to next role
3,4,5) **Hospital care**: management of accompanying injuries and crush injury. Fasciotomy, muscle debridement, or amputation as indicated. Follow electrolytes and renal function. Dialysis if indicated. Hyperbaric oxygen. Eventual reconstructive surgery. Rehabilitation

Cross-References

▶ Compartment Syndrome, Acute
▶ Crush Injuries
▶ Crush Syndrome, Anesthetic Management for
▶ Dialysis
▶ Fasciotomy

References

Betters OS, Stein JH (1990) Early management of shock and prophylaxis of acute renal failure in traumatic rhabdomyolysis. NEJM 322:825–829
Bywaters EGL, Beall D (1941) Crush injuries with impairment of renal function. BMJ 1:427–432
Emergency War Surgery. Third United States Revision (2004) Chapter 22: Soft tissue injuries. Borden Institute, Washington, DC
Gonzales D (2005) Crush syndrome. Crit Care Med 33(1): S34–S41
McQueen et al (1996) Compartment monitoring in tibial fractures: the pressure threshold for decompression. J Bone Joint Surg [Br] 78:99–104
Sever MS, Vanholder R, Lameire N (2006) Management of crush-related injuries after disasters. N Engl J Med 354:1052–1063
Sever MS, Lameire N, Vanholder R (2009) Renal disaster relief: from theory to practice. Nephrol Dial Transplant 24:1730–1735
Vanholder R, Stuard S, Bonomini M, Sever MS (2009) Renal disaster relief in Europe: the experience at L'Aquila, Italy, in April 2009. Nephrol Dial Transplant 24:3251–3255
Vanholder R, Gibney N, Luyckx VA, Sever MS (2010) Renal disaster relief task force in Haiti earthquake. Lancet 375:1162–1163

Crush Syndrome, Anesthetic Management for

Jean Charchaflieh
Department of Anesthesiology, Yale University School of Medicine, New Haven, CT, USA

Synonyms

Bywaters' syndrome; Traumatic rhabdomyolysis

Definition

Crush injury refers to local tissue injury, mainly skeletal muscles, due to compression by heavy object or explosion injury.

Crush syndrome refers to systemic manifestations of crush injury.

Skeletal muscle compartment syndrome (SMCS) refers to traumatic or ischemic muscle swelling and increased pressure within a muscle compartment (surrounded by intact fascia), which can lead to further muscle ischemia and injury.

Preexisting Condition

By definition, crush syndrome is the traumatic form of rhabdomyolysis. Common scenarios of TR include explosion injuries or entrapment under heavy objects (building collapse, vehicular collision). As mentioned, the earliest descriptions of TR occurred in military settings. TR most commonly (75 %) involves lower extremities because of muscle mass followed by upper extremities (10 %), trunk (10 %), and others, e.g., buttocks (5 %).

Nontraumatic causes of rhabdomyolysis can compound TR. Particularly important causes include seizures or mind-altering drugs such as alcohol since they can contribute to the occurrence of trauma. Similarly, complications of TR can aggravate nontraumatic rhabdomyolysis.

Examples of nontraumatic causes of rhabdomyolysis include:

1. Muscle ischemia
2. Muscle swelling and SMCS
3. Delirium tremens (DTs)
4. Seizures
5. Heat stroke
6. Hypokalemia
7. Hypophosphatemia
8. Hyperosmolar states (hyperglycemia, hypernatremia)
9. Illicit drugs (alcohol, heroin, phencyclidine, cocaine, amphetamine)
10. Prescription drugs (statins, terbutaline, aminophylline, diuretics)
11. Infections (bacterial [clostridium] and viral)

Application

Pathophysiology

Traumatic, as well as ischemic, injury to muscle cells (rhabdomyolysis) produces influx of sodium, calcium, and water and efflux of potassium, myoglobin, phosphate, thromboplastin, creatine, and creatine kinase (CK). The influx of sodium, water, and calcium leads to hypovolemia and relatively mild hypocalcemia. Hyponatremia is usually non-evident due to hypovolemia. The efflux of muscle contents leads to acute hyperkalemia, hyperphosphatemia, hyperuricemia, and metabolic acidosis. Hyperkalemia, worsened by metabolic acidosis, can lead to lethal arrhythmias. Decrease intracellular phosphate can decrease the activity of the energy-dependent sodium-potassium adenosine triphosphatase (Na-K ATPase) enzyme, which leads to further influx of sodium and calcium. Increased intracellular calcium can activate phospholipases and endopeptidases which cause further cell lysis. High levels of thromboplastin can lead to disseminated intravascular coagulation (DIC). High levels of myoglobin and uric acid can lead to deposition of insoluble pigments or crystals in renal tubules leading to acute tubular necrosis (ATN) and acute renal failure (ARF).

Influx of sodium and water leads to muscle cell swelling, which increases the risk of SMCS and further worsening of muscle ischemia and swelling. During the crush and ischemia phase of crush syndrome, products of rhabdomyolysis accumulate within the crushed ischemic area. Once the compression is relived and reperfusion is established, rhabdomyolysis products circulate throughout the body and produce systemic toxic effects. Risk of death due to acute massive release of metabolic products once the crushing pressure has been released from affected area has resulted in the term "smiling death" which refers to sudden death after relieving the pain and agony of compression. This risk has lead to recommendations to emergency medical services (EMS) units to avoid sudden release of compression in cases of compressing injuries of longer than 15 min of duration by applying tourniquets proximal to injured areas and then release the pressure in stages while assessing the patient.

Diagnosis

The trauma component of TR is usually evident. Clinical signs of SMCS may not be evident in early stages, are not sensitive or specific, and can be overshadowed by other overwhelming aspects of crush injury. SMCS produces compression of muscles, nerves, and vessels and leads to signs and symptoms referred to as the 5 Ps of increased compartmental pressure:

1. Pain with either palpation or passive stretch of muscle
2. Paresthesia
3. Palsy
4. Palor
5. Pulselessness

SMCS should be suspected in crush injury, and periodic or continuous measurement of skeletal muscle compartment pressure (SMCP) should be implemented early. Pressures above capillary pressure (25 mmHg) are considered diagnostic of SMCS. Newer diagnostic modalities aim to assess muscle perfusion and include near-infrared spectroscopy, ultrafiltration catheters, and radiofrequency identification implants (Harvey et al. 2012).

Laboratory signs of muscle injury include elevated serum levels of specific enzymes (aldolase), nonspecific enzymes (creatine kinase, lactate dehydrogenase, and glutamic oxaloacetic transaminase), myoglobin, uric acid, creatinine, potassium, and phosphate.

Serum CK is usually markedly elevated in all patients that it is considered a hallmark in diagnosing rhabdomyolysis. Serum myoglobin analysis requires special techniques such as gel electrophoresis, radioimmunoassay, or enzymelinked immunosorbent assay (ELISA).

Hyperuricemia occurs due to release of proteins and purines from injured muscle cells and contributes to the development of metabolic acidosis and AKI.

Elevated serum creatinine occurs both due to hydrolyzation of released creatine from muscle cells as well as AKI. Metabolic acidosis occurs due to dehydration, electrolytes abnormities, and AKI. DIC produces thrombocytopenia; elevation of prothrombin time (PT), partial thromboplastin time (PTT), fibrin degradation products (FDPs), and d-dimers; and decreased levels of fibrinogen and platelets.

Myoglobinuria may be detected using simple urine dipstick, which contains the reactant orthotoluidene, which also reacts with globin in the hemoglobin, or relying on more sensitive, specific, and expensive tests, such as radioimmunoassay, immunodiffusion, immunoelectrophoresis, and hemagglutination. EKG changes occur due to electrolytes abnormalities, particularly hyperkalemia.

Complications

SMCS represents local complications of crush injury. SMCS produces its own rhabdomyolysis that further aggravate TR of the crush injury. Crush syndrome represents systemic complications of crush injury. These complications can be fatal acutely or progressively. Acute complications include:

1. Hypovolemia and hypovolemic shock
2. Metabolic abnormalities leading to fatal arrhythmias (hyperkalemia, hyperphosphatemia, hypocalcaemia, hyperuricemia, and metabolic acidosis)
3. Disseminated intravascular coagulation (DIC)
4. Acute renal failure (ARF)

Late complications consist mainly of hypercalcemia:

1. Water influx into muscle cells can exceed 10 l/day leading to hypovolemia and hypovolemic shock, which can lead to lactic acidosis.
2. Metabolic complications can be severe and fatal. Rapid efflux of large amounts of potassium from muscle cells can result in fatal cardiac arrhythmias. Metabolic acidosis and AKI aggravate hyerkalemia. Injury to muscle

cells impairs mechanism of shifting extracellular potassium into intracellular compartment. Efflux of large amounts of organic phosphate from muscle cells leads to hyperphosphatemia, which may worsen hypocalcemia by decreasing 1,25-dihydroxycholecalciferol production. Hyperphosphatemia in the presence of normocalcemia may produce metastatic calcifications of phosphate-calcium products, which may cause disseminated clotting. Metabolism of large amounts of purines released from damage muscle cells can result in hyperuricemia, which contributes to metabolic acidosis, which in conjunction with hypovolemia and decreased urinary flow increases the risk of uric acid crystals precipitation in renal tubules and the development of ATN. Mechanisms of metabolic acidosis in TR include anion gap acidosis due to the release of large amounts of sulfur-containing proteins from injured muscle cells, lactic acidosis due to hypoperfusion, and uremic acidosis due to AKI. Mechanisms of the early-occurring hypocalcemia include calcium influx into muscle cells, decreased levels of 1,25-dihydroxycholecalciferol, and decreased bone cell responsiveness to parathyroid hormone and AKI. During recovery from TR and AKI, hypercalcemia may occur due to mobilization of calcium deposits from injured muscle cells and recovery of 1,25-dihydroxycholecalciferol levels.

3. DIC can be activated by the release of muscle contents particularly thromboplastin. Laboratory findings are more common than over bleeding or thrombosis.

4. ARF occurs in about 30 % of patients with TR. The combination of myoglobinuria and aciduria seems to be most nephrotoxic. At pH < 5.6, myoglobin is converted to ferrihemate which precipitates in renal tubules and acts as a source of iron-derived free radicals. Hypovolemia, hyperkalemia, and hyperphosphatemia are more predictive than CK levels of the risk of development of ARF. Once established, TR-induced ARF requires hemodialysis in 50–70 % of patients. Small observational series suggest that forced alkaline diuresis may significantly reduce the risk of TR-induced ARF.

Treatment

Treatment of crush syndrome begins in the field and continues throughout hospitalization phases.

By definition, TR patients are trauma patient and should be treated as such. TR patients are likely to have polytrauma and should be treated systemically according to Advanced Trauma Life Support (ATLS) protocols. The primary and secondary surveys of trauma should be performed.

The primary survey consists of the ABCDE components:

A. Airway maintenance with cervical spine protection
B. Breathing and ventilation
C. Circulation with hemorrhage control
D. Disability (neurologic evaluation) using Glasgow Coma Scale
E. Exposure and environmental control to prevent hypothermia

During airway control if a muscle relaxant is to be used, depolarizing muscle relaxants such as succinylcholine should be avoided in order to avoid lethal hyperkalemia. Sources of hyperkalemia under such circumstances include:

1. TR and potassium efflux from muscle cells
2. Metabolic acidosis
3. Respiratory acidosis due to apnea or hypoventilation
4. Succinylcholine-induced basic increase in serum potassium by about 0.5 mEq/L from baseline level
5. Succinylcholine-induced additional massive increase in serum potassium due to TR-induced proliferation in extra-neuromuscular-junction acetylcholine receptors

The combination of these sources of hyperkalemia calls for avoiding its use in TR.

Wound care of severe crush injury may call for amputation as a means of decreasing the risk of progression into crush syndrome when means of treatment of crush syndrome are not readily available.

Crush injuries due to entrapment of longer than 15 min may benefit from staged release of pressure by applying a proximal tourniquet and subsequent staged release of pressure under monitored condition and availability of means of treatments for potential complications.

Open wounds should be treated with surgical debridement as indicated with control of bleeding and application of local and systemic antibiotics and tetanus toxoid as needed. Fasciotomy is the definitive treatment of SMCS. Local hyperbaric oxygen therapy has been advocated as an adjunct therapy to decrease ischemia-reperfusion injury (Strauss 2012).

The mainstay of systemic treatment of crush syndrome is aggressive intravascular volume repletion and correction of hyperkalemia.

Intravascular volume repletion improves most aspects of TR. It corrects hypovolemia, prevents or treats hypovolemic shock, reduces hypoperfusion-induced metabolic acidosis, and ameliorates myoglobinuria-induced ATN and ARF. The correction of metabolic acidosis facilitates the treatment of hyperkalemia and hypotension. Based on an estimated extracellular fluid deficit of 10 l, an initial bolus of 2–3 l of an isotonic crystalloid (normal saline or lactated Ringer's solution) is provided followed by an infusion rate of 300–500 ml/h.

Intravascular volume expansion and maintenance of high urine flow are the mainstay of prevention and treatment of TR-induced AKI. The aim of intravenous hydration is to produce a urinary output of 200–300 ml/h. Early volume expansion is more effective than late. In experimental rhabdomyolysis-induced AKI that resulted in reduction in both renal blood flow (RBF) and glomerular filtration rate (GFR), early (within 6 h) volume expansion resulted in restoration of both RBF and GFR while late (after 12 h) volume expansion resulted in restoring only RBF but not GFR (Reineck et al. 1980).

Sodium bicarbonate can be used as an adjunct to IV hydration to both alkalize the urine (pH 6.5–8) and produce solute diuretic effect. Alkaline urine increases solubility of myoglobin and uric acid, which decreases the risk of cast formation, tubular obstruction, ATN, and ARF. Sodium bicarbonate-induced metabolic alkalosis can be ameliorated with acetazolamide. If volume resuscitation is achieved and urine flow is less than 200 ml/h, mannitol can be used as an adjunct therapy to maintain high urine flow.

The combination of IV fluid hydration and alkalization with sodium bicarbonate and osmotic diuresis with mannitol has been called forced alkaline diuresis and advocated for the prevention of TR-induced AKI.

Support for such therapy is provided by two small observational studies. One study reported 20 patients of crush injury due to entrapment in collapsed building. All 20 patients received aggressive fluid resuscitation in the field, 7 of which had myoglobinuria on arrival to the hospital. All seven patients received treatment with forced alkaline diuresis (IV fluids plus sodium bicarbonate plus mannitol), and none of them developed ARF. The authors attributed the successful outcome to the forced alkaline diuresis therapy (Eneas et al. 1979).

The other study indicates that patient's response to forced alkaline diuresis therapy might determine the outcome of therapy. The authors reported the use of forced alkaline diuresis therapy (IV fluids plus sodium bicarbonate plus mannitol) in 20 oliguric patients with due to nontraumatic rhabdomyolysis. Nine patients had increased urine output, recovered without need for HD, and had no mortality. The other 11 patients remained oliguric, required HD, and had 9 % mortality (Ron et al. 1984).

These small observational studies provide low degree of support for the use of forced alkaline diuresis therapy (IV fluids plus sodium bicarbonate plus mannitol) in TR.

Potential risks of forced alkaline diuresis include alkalemia, electrolyte disturbance, pulmonary edema, muscle edema, SMCS, and precipitation of calcium salts in damaged muscles.

Serum electrolytes and pH should be monitored and treated as needed. Continuous EKG should be used to detect arrhythmia. Severe cases of electrolytes imbalance or acidosis are best treated with hemodialysis (HD).

Correction of metabolic acidosis facilitates the treatment of hyperkalemia.

Treatment of hyperkalemia that relies on intracellular shifting potassium (insulin and adrenergic B-2 agonists) can be attempted with the expectation that it is likely to be less effective due to muscle cell injury. Use of the exchange resins kayexalate (25–50 g with sorbitol 20 % 100 mL PO or PR) may be more effective but slow therapy. Hemodialysis (HD) or other forms of renal replacement therapy (RRT) are most effective in achieving rapid and reliable correction of hyperkalemia.

Hyperuricemia in excess of 20 mg/dl can be treated with allopurinol.

Hyperphosphatemia should be treated with phosphate binders.

Calcium infusion in the presence of hyperphosphatemia should be avoided due to the risk of precipitation of phosphate-calcium compounds and calcium deposits in injured muscle cells.

Prognosis

With appropriate treatment, survival of TR can exceed 90 %. ARF may decrease survival rates to 80 %.

Cross-References

▶ Crush Injuries
▶ Crush Syndrome

References

Bywaters EG, Beall D (1941) Crush injuries with impairment of renal function. Br Med J 1(4185):427–432
Eneas JF, Schoenfeld PY, Humphreys MH (1979) The effect of infusion of mannitol-sodium bicarbonate on the clinical course of myoglobinuria. Arch Intern Med 139(7):801–805
Harvey EJ, Sanders DW, Shuler MS, Lawendy AR, Cole AL, Alqahtani SM, Schmidt AH (2012) What's new in acute compartment syndrome? J Orthop Trauma 26 (12):699–702
Minami S (1923) Über Nierenveränderungen nach Verschüttung. Virchows Arch Patho Anat 245 (1):247–267
Reineck HJ, O'Connor GJ, Lifschitz MD, Stein JH (1980) Sequential studies on the pathophysiology of
glycerol-induced acute renal failure. J Lab Clin Med 96(2):356–362
Ron D, Taitelman U, Michaelson M, Bar-Joseph G, Bursztein S, Better OS (1984) Prevention of acute renal failure in traumatic rhabdomyolysis. Arch Intern Med 144(2):277–280
Strauss MB (2012) The effect of hyperbaric oxygen in crush injuries and skeletal muscle-compartment syndromes. Undersea Hyperb Med 39(4):847–855

Cryoprecipitate (CRYO) Transfusion

▶ Cryoprecipitate Transfusion in Trauma

Cryoprecipitate Transfusion in Trauma

Barto Nascimento[1] and Sandro Rizoli[2]
[1]Trauma Program, Department of Surgery, Sunnybrook Health Sciences Centre, University of Toronto, Toronto, ON, Canada
[2]Trauma & Acute Care Surgery, Departments of Critical Care & Surgery, St. Michael's Hospital, University of Toronto, Toronto, ON, Canada

Synonyms

Cryoprecipitate (CRYO) transfusion; Cryoprecipitated antihemophilic factor transfusion; Damage control resuscitation; Fibrinogen replacement; Hemostatic transfusion strategy; Hyperfibrinolysis management

Definition

CRYO is a diverse blood product considered to be a subproduct of frozen plasma preparations. Frozen plasma is thawed at 1–6 °C for the preparation of CRYO. After thawing, the product is centrifuged at 5,000× g for about 6 min, and then the supernatant is removed. The original bag is left with only 5–15 mL of plasma and the cold insoluble precipitate. This residual material, the cryoprecipitate, is refrozen within 1 h of thawing and stored at -18 °C or colder. Under ideal storage conditions, the final product has a shelf life of 12 months.

Developed in the mid-1960, Pool's cryoprecipitate was originally transfused as the main source of factor VIII for patients with congenital factor VIII deficiency. Its use was subsequently expanded to the treatment of patients with von Willebrand's disease (vWD) and hypofibrinogenemia with some benefit. Currently, CRYO is most commonly indicated for the management of acquired hypofibrinogenemia in patients with hemorrhage (O'Shaughnessy et al. 2004). However, in some European countries, the use of CRYO exclusively for fibrinogen replacement has been recently challenged and increasingly replaced with the use of virally inactivated fibrinogen concentrate (Fenger-Eriksen et al. 2008; Bundesaertzekammer 2009). The latter exhibits a safer profile due to decreased risks of pathogen transmission and immune-mediated complications and has a more standardized concentration of fibrinogen.

CRYO Transfusion Basics

The fibrinogen content of a unit of CRYO may vary widely (range, 120–796 mg), with each unit containing 30–50 % of the original fibrinogen in the source plasma. The content of a standard dose of CRYO is equivalent to the amount of fibrinogen found in an average adult dose of fresh frozen plasma (FFP) (4 units), where each unit of plasma contains 0.5 g of fibrinogen. Factor VIII and von Willebrand factor correspond to approximately 5 % of the total pool of proteins in this concentrate. Other components of CRYO include fibronectin, factor XIII, immunoglobulins (IgG and IgM), albumin, and platelet microparticles.

Due to the small volume of plasma transfused, ABO-compatible CRYO is not required, although this may be significant in patients receiving large volumes of cryoprecipitate relative to their red blood cell mass. The selection of this product for transfusion usually does not require consideration of Rh compatibility. CRYO is a frozen blood product that needs to be thawed and can also be pooled for use. After thawing, CRYO should be used immediately. In case the product is not used without delay, it should be stored at 20–24 °C and used within 4–6 h in most jurisdictions for up to 24 h, by when it expires.

Preexisting Condition

The Role of Fibrinogen in Trauma-Associated Coagulopathy

Fibrinogen is fundamental in the coagulation process and clot stabilization in order to form a firm clot. It is cleaved by thrombin to form fibrin polymers, which are capable of binding factor XIII, with subsequent cross-linkage to produce a robust fibrin network. Furthermore, fibrinogen plays an important role in platelet activation and aggregation by its binding to $\alpha2\beta3$ integrin glycoprotein (GP) IIb/IIIa fibrinogen receptors present on the surfaces of platelets, which are the main substrate for primary hemostasis. However, in trauma-associated coagulopathy, multiple causal factors may directly affect fibrinogen polymeration and metabolism (Fries and Martini 2010).

Dilutional Coagulopathy

Conventional resuscitation strategies utilize crystalloid in order to maintain euvolemia, blood pressure, cardiac output, and thus adequate oxygen delivery to tissues. Aggressive fluid replacement causes dilution, which impairs coagulation and has been associated with worse outcomes in trauma. Despite being affected by direct dilution, fibrinogen metabolism is not directly disturbed by crystalloid use.

Hydroxyethyl starch (HES) is also a solution used as fluid replacement in acute resuscitation in trauma. HES may have several deleterious effects on coagulation and has been associated with increased bleeding tendency. It induces a blockage of the fibrinogen receptor (GIIb/IIIa), interferes with fibrin polymerization, and causes platelet coating, hypocalcemia, and a vWD-like syndrome. HES solutions are routinely used in resuscitation protocols in European countries, but not commonly employed in North America. Gelatin products may also cause dilution and impair fibrinogen polymerization.

Hyperfibrinolysis

Fibrinolysis is a physiologic response to diverse insults such as surgery, trauma, infection, and ischemia in order to preserve hemostasis. Normally, this initial fibrinolytic phase is followed by a suppression phase when antifibrinolytic systems are activated. Tissue and endothelial damage result in the release of tissue plasminogen activator (t-TPA), which causes fibrinolysis through the conversion of plasminogen to plasmin, and its antagonist, plasminogen activator inhibitor type 1 (PAI – 1), which regulates fibrinolysis by inhibiting the formation of plasmin. In trauma, hyperfibrinolysis (increased fibrinolysis) occurs due to the combined effects of both extensive tissue injury and shock (Hess et al. 2008). It is believed that this hyperfibrinolysis develops to limit coagulation to the site of bleeding, but in the context of extensive tissue damage, this regulatory process may be imbalanced (Hess et al. 2008). This exacerbated fibrinolysis is considered to be an important contributor of hemorrhage and coagulopathy. It seems to be associated with the severity of trauma and specific tissue traumas, where the increased release of thromboplastins is present, such as traumatic brain injury and long-bone fractures.

The hemorrhagic tendency in hyperfibrinolysis can be treated with antifibrinolytic drugs such as tranexamic acid and aprotinin. In fact, a recent randomized controlled trial evaluated 20,110 trauma patients at risk of significant hemorrhage who were treated with either 2 g tranexamic acid or placebo and showed reduced mortality rates in favor of the intervention for all-cause inhospital mortality if administered within 3 h of injury (Roberts et al. 2011). The efficacy of antifibrinolytic therapy has also been documented in liver transplant, cardiac, and orthopedic surgery.

Hypothermia

In trauma, hypothermia is defined as core temperature of 34 °C or below. The detrimental effects of hypothermia on coagulation are well documented and include decrease in fibrinogen synthesis, reduction in activity of the complex tissue factor-FVIIa, and inhibition of platelet function (Fries and Martini 2010). Core temperatures below 32 °C are associated with excessive mortality rates in trauma.

Acidosis

In trauma, due to the shock state and excessive infusion of ionic chloride solution during acute resuscitation, acidosis is commonly present. Acidosis adversely affects coagulation by reducing protease activity and depleting fibrinogen levels and platelet counts. Unlike hypothermia, acidosis does not affect fibrinogen synthesis, but increases fibrinogen degradation by almost twofold in animal models of coagulopathy.

Application

Guidelines for CRYO Transfusion

Major guidelines on blood component therapy in Europe and North America suggest transfusion of CRYO when plasma fibrinogen level is <1.0 g/L in the context of bleeding and/or disseminated intravascular coagulation (O'Shaughnessy et al. 2004; Levi et al. 2009). Typically, an adult dose of 8–12 units (one unit per 5–10 kg of body weight) is utilized.

There is limited scientific evidence supporting a fibrinogen cutoff of 1.0 g/L as a trigger for CRYO transfusion. In 1987, Ciavarella et al. reviewed 36 massively transfused patients and observed that microvascular bleeding occurred in four patients whose fibrinogen levels were below 0.5 g/L and only occurred in two out of ten patients with fibrinogen levels 0.5–1.0 g/L of whom both were severely thrombocytopenic. The authors then suggested a threshold of 1.0 g/L as a trigger for CRYO transfusion. However, this "historical" 1.0 g/L threshold has recently been considered inadequate, being associated with excessive blood loss during cardiac surgery and severe postpartum bleeding.

In trauma, a European multidisciplinary Task Force for Advanced Bleeding Care in Trauma (Rossaint et al. 2010), recognizing the key role of fibrinogen in the trauma-associated coagulopathy, recommends the replacement of fibrinogen (by fibrinogen concentrate infusion or CRYO transfusion) for plasma fibrinogen level of less than 1.5–2.0 g/L (Rossaint et al. 2010). These guidelines also suggest increased doses of CRYO (15–20 units in a 70 Kg adult) and the use of thrombelastometric monitoring, as a way to detect functional fibrinogen deficits. A fibrinogen concentrate dose of 3–4 g or 50 mg/Kg of CRYO (15–20 units) for an average weight adult (70 kg) is recommended for fibrinogen <1.5–2.0 g/L. Fibrinogen concentrate is currently licensed for use in congenital bleeding throughout Europe, USA, China, and Japan and for use in acquired bleeding in more than 15 countries worldwide. These recommendations were based on a growing body of evidence on improved outcomes with a more aggressive strategy in replacing fibrinogen in trauma (Hess et al. 2008; Stinger et al. 2008; Fries and Martini 2010).

Recently, the issue of long turnaround time for fibrinogen results during acute resuscitation was addressed in a study by Chandler et al. The authors implemented a series of modifications to stat coagulation testing such that (i) the emergency hemorrhage panel was prioritized and (ii) speed in processing samples was improved at the expense of precision, but to still produce clinically relevant results (shortened centrifugation time [from 8 at 2,000 g to 2 min at 4,440 g instead]; elimination of checks for clots and hemolysis; and extension of fibrinogen calibration curve down to 0.53 mg/dL with repeated test, but results as <0.53 mg/dL released). They were able to reduce their turnaround time from 34 to 13 min.

The impact of CRYO transfusion on plasma fibrinogen levels in massively transfused trauma patients was recently evaluated. In 83 trauma patients who did not receive plasma components 2 h prior to CRYO, a dose of 8.7 ($\pm$1.7) units caused a modest increase in fibrinogen levels of 0.55 ($\pm$0.24) gL^{-1} or 0.06 gL^{-1} per unit.

Evidence for CRYO Transfusion in Trauma

Fibrinogen can be provided through plasma, CRYO, and fibrinogen concentrate. Currently, during the acute resuscitation of a trauma patient, fibrinogen is mostly replaced by plasma transfusion. Although the role of fibrinogen for the management of coagulopathy in massive transfusion has been increasingly recognized, the evidence on the clinical efficacy of plasma or CRYO for the replacement of fibrinogen is limited. A recent retrospective review of 252 combat-related trauma patients requiring massive transfusion demonstrated an association between increased fibrinogen (mainly from plasma and CRYO transfusion) to RBC ratios and improved survival (Stinger et al. 2008). In preparation for a larger multicenter trial which will evaluate the effects of an early administration of CRYO in major traumatic hemorrhage, a feasibility trial is currently under way in the UK (ISRCTN55509212).

In a study of coagulopathic patients undergoing major abdominal surgery with estimated blood loss of more than 200 % of the patients' calculated total volemia, fibrinogen was the first clotting factor to decrease to critical levels. Furthermore, in a porcine model of moderate dilutional coagulopathy, compensatory mechanism of synthesis failed to increase fibrinogen levels to overcome the increased breakdown, suggesting that hypofribrinogenemia cannot be entirely explained by blood loss and dilution. It has been shown that low preoperative levels of fibrinogen are associated with increased postoperative bleeding. In postpartum patients, low levels of fibrinogen had a PPV of 100 % for severe bleeding. Finally, besides the importance of fibrinogen in fibrin formation and platelet function, the replacement of exogenous fibrinogen could theoretically bypass other missing components of the coagulation cascade.

Besides their unproven efficacy, the use of human blood products as a source of fibrinogen has important and practical limitations, such as extended turnaround time for thawing and pooling, and transfusion-related risks. Of note, CRYO is not available in most European countries, but it still widely used in North America and the UK. As an alternative to plasma and CRYO, there is growing interest in the use of fibrinogen concentrate, particularly in Europe. A comprehensive review on fibrinogen concentrates for bleeding trauma patients recently published identified four relevant studies on the topic. None of these studies were randomized controlled trials. The main finding of these studies was that the administration of fibrinogen concentrate sometimes associated with prothrombin complex concentrate might be an alternative hemostatic strategy in trauma patients treated with synthetic colloids during resuscitation, as compared to the traditional plasma strategy. No published studies comparing the efficacy of CRYO with fibrinogen concentration are available to date. As compared to plasma and CRYO transfusion, fibrinogen concentrate does not require thawing, and due to their small volume, the turnaround and administration times are much shorter.

Risks of CRYO Transfusion in Trauma

Although pathogen inactivation treatments can be used for FFP – which can reduce the content of fibrinogen present in the product – these procedures are rarely utilized for FFP and cannot be employed for the CRYO product itself. Therefore, these human blood products carry, although low, risks of infectious disease transmission. Other potential complications of these products, particularly FFP, include transfusion-associated circulatory overload (TACO) and transfusion-related acute lung injury (TRALI). TRALI is the commonest cause of transfusion-related mortality.

Fibrinogen concentrate preparations are routinely subjected to pathogen reduction technologies treatment in their manufacturing process, which minimizes the risk of infectious disease transmission.

Conclusion

Cryoprecipitate transfusion is commonly used when plasma fibrinogen level is <1.0 g/L in the context of bleeding and/or disseminated intravascular coagulation. Although there is growing recognition of the pivotal role of fibrinogen in trauma-associated coagulopathy, the efficacy and safety of CRYO transfusion, as well as its dosage, remain uncertain. Recent evidence suggests the potential role of fibrinogen concentrate

and thromboelastographic monitoring for the management of fibrinogen deficiency in trauma.

Cross-References

- ▶ Adjuncts to Transfusion: Antifibrinolytics
- ▶ Adjuncts to Transfusion: Fibrinogen Concentrate
- ▶ Adjuncts to Transfusion: Prothrombin Complex Concentrate
- ▶ Adjuncts to Transfusion: Recombinant Factor VIIa, Factor XIII, and Calcium
- ▶ Blood Component Transfusion
- ▶ Damage Control Resuscitation
- ▶ Damage Control Resuscitation, Military Trauma
- ▶ Disseminated Intravascular Coagulation
- ▶ Factor I Concentrate
- ▶ Fibrinogen (Test)
- ▶ Massive Transfusion
- ▶ Massive Transfusion Protocols in Trauma
- ▶ Plasma Transfusion in Trauma
- ▶ Transfusion Strategy in Trauma: What Is the Evidence?

References

Bundesaertzekammer/ German Medical Association (2009) Cross-sectional guidelines for therapy with blood components and plasma derivates, 4th edn. German Medical Association. http://www.bundesaert-zekammer.de/page.asp?his=0.6.3288.6716. Accessed 30 Nov 2010

Fenger-Eriksen C, Lindberg-Larsen M, Christensen AQ, Ingerslev J, Sorensen B (2008) Fibrinogen concentrate substitution therapy in patients with massive haemorrhage and low plasma fibrinogen concentrations. Br J Anaesth 101:769–773

Fries D, Martini WZ (2010) Role of fibrinogen in trauma-induced coagulopathy. Br J Anaesth 105:116–121

Hess JR, Brohi K, Dutton RP, Hauser CJ, Holcomb JB, Kluger Y, Mackway-Jones K, Parr MJ, Rizoli SB, Yukioka T, Hoyt DB, Bouillon B (2008) The coagulopathy of trauma: a review of mechanisms. J Trauma 65:748–754

Levi M, Toh CH, Thachil J, Watson HG (2009) Guidelines for the diagnosis and management of disseminated intravascular coagulation. British Committee for Standards in Haematology. Br J Haematol 145:24–33

O'Shaughnessy DF, Atterbury C, Bolton MP, Murphy M, Thomas D, Yates S, Williamson LM (2004) Guidelines for the use of fresh-frozen plasma, cryoprecipitate and cryosupernatant. Br J Haematol 126:11–28

Roberts I, Shakur H, Afolabi A, Brohi K, Coats T, Dewan Y, Gando S, Guyatt G, Hunt BJ, Morales C, Perel P, Prieto-Merino D, Woolley T (2011) The importance of early treatment with tranexamic acid in bleeding trauma patients: an exploratory analysis of the CRASH-2 randomised controlled trial. Lancet 377:1096–1101

Rossaint R, Bouillon B, Cerny V, Coats TJ, Duranteau J, Fernandez-Mondejar E, Hunt BJ, Komadina R, Nardi G, Neugebauer E, Ozier Y, Riddez L, Schultz A, Stahel PF, Vincent JL, Spahn DR (2010) Management of bleeding following major trauma: an updated European guideline. Crit Care 14:R52

Stinger HK, Spinella PC, Perkins JG, Grathwohl KW, Salinas J, Martini WZ, Hess JR, Dubick MA, Simon CD, Beekley AC, Wolf SE, Wade CE, Holcomb JB (2008) The ratio of fibrinogen to red cells transfused affects survival in casualties receiving massive transfusions at an army combat support hospital. J Trauma 64:S79–S85

Cryoprecipitated Antihemophilic Factor Transfusion

▶ Cryoprecipitate Transfusion in Trauma

CSF Leak

▶ Neurotrauma, Management of Cerebrospinal Fluid Leak

CSF Otorrhea

▶ Neurotrauma, Management of Cerebrospinal Fluid Leak

CSF Rhinorrhea

▶ Neurotrauma, Management of Cerebrospinal Fluid Leak

Curling's Ulcer

Ariful Alam[1] and Khanjan H. Nagarsheth[2]
[1]Department of General Surgery, Staten Island University Hospital, Staten Island, NY, USA
[2]R Adams Cowley Shock Trauma Center, University of Maryland School of Medicine, Baltimore, MD, USA

Synonyms

Peptic ulcer; Stress ulcer

Definition

Curling's ulcer is an acute ulceration of the stomach or duodenum (Silen et al. 1981). This entity was first described by Swan in 1823, and then in 1842, Thomas Curling further described this ulcer as the most frequent life-threatening gastrointestinal complication in burn patients (Pruitt et al. 1970). Curling's ulcer is commonly described under the term stress ulcer, since it shares common features of acute ulcers following major surgery, mechanical ventilation, shock, or sepsis and is suggested to have a similar pathophysiologic origin (Silen et al. 1981).

Preexisting Condition

Histology

Stress ulcers commonly develop in the parietal cell mucosa, the duodenum is affected in about 30 % of patients, and sometimes both the stomach and duodenum are involved. Morphologically, Curling's ulcer is characteristically shallow and sharply demarcated; however, individual lesions may be extensive and penetrate all layers of the gastric or duodenal wall. There is often congestion and edema, but little inflammatory reaction noted histologically, and no fibrosis is seen. Hemorrhage is the major clinical problem and occurs in 10 % of patients as a result of extension of the ulcer through the muscularis mucosa with erosion into a mural vessel. Transmural extension may also result in free perforation into the peritoneal cavity, the lesser sac, or the head of the pancreas. Gastroduodenal endoscopy performed early in burn patients has shown acute gastric erosions in the majority of the patients within 72 h of injury. However, the disease frequently remains subclinical and becomes apparent in 20 % of patients. Clinically evident bleeding is usually seen in 3–5 days after injury and massive bleeding generally does not appear until 4–5 days later (Pruitt et al. 1970).

Pathophysiology

Several mechanisms have been proposed regarding the pathophysiology of stress ulcers. Necheles and Olson proposed hyperacidic gastric secretion as a possible cause of stress ulcers. Burn patients who manifest serious bleeding have a higher gastric output. In 1934, Kapsinow suggested that concentration of "burn toxins" in the blood resulted in stasis with rupture of the capillaries underlying the duodenal mucosa with tissue anoxia, necrosis, and ulceration (Hartman 1945). The current accepted mechanism of the ulcer formation is multifactorial. Decreased mucosal resistance occurs due to the effects of ischemia and circulating toxins, followed by decreased mucosal renewal, decreased production of endogenous prostanoids, and thinning of the mucus layer. Decreased blood supply also indicates low level of serum buffers available to neutralize hydrogen ions which diffuse into the weakened mucosa. Thus, the mucosa is more susceptible to acid-pepsin ulceration and lysosomal enzymes. Disruption of the gastric mucosal barrier has been found in about half of the patients with this disease (Stollman and Metz 2004).

Risk Factors

In 1970, Pruitt and colleagues published a study of 323 cases of patients with Curling's ulcers. This study was conducted over a 16-year period and found that Curling's ulcers occurred in 323 patients of 2,772 patients equating to 11.7 %. It was noted that the incidence of Curling's ulcers increased in proportion to the size of the burn area. Sepsis in the patient group was shown to

be an additional stressor predisposing patients with burns to developing Curling's ulcers. In patients with less than 50 % burns, sepsis played a significant part in the development of these ulcers (Pruitt et al. 1970).

Application

Clinical Presentation

Hemorrhage is usually the first manifestation of Curling's ulcer, whereas pain rarely occurs. Physical examination is usually not helpful except for gross or peritonitis or signs of shock.

One of the best historic descriptions of a patient with a Curling's ulcer was by Maes in the *Annals of Surgery* 1929. He described a case of an 11-year-old male with burns to his lower extremities. On admission the patient had a temperature of 96.5 °F and pulse of 90 bpm. The next day, the patient's condition worsened with a temperature of 100.8 °F and a pulse of 160 bpm. The patient had evidence of severe toxemia and emesis, with involuntary voiding and extreme delirium. After initially improving, the patient progressed to have severe abdominal pain. Shortly after the patient developed hematemesis and blood per rectum. The patient continued to deteriorate with a blood pressure drop from 100/64 mmHg to 80/0 mmHg. Blood transfusions were given with some improvement, but then the patient became delirious and died within several hours. Autopsy was performed and the findings included acute splenitis and acute glomerular nephritis. The jejunum and ileum were both distended and the ileum was full of blood. A small purple brown area was discovered at the junction of the 1st and 2nd portions of the duodenum. This was the site of the patient's Curling's ulcer (Maes 1930).

In the Pruitt study, approximately one fourth of patients had no signs or symptoms of ulceration while they were living. Of the 323 patients, gastrointestinal bleeding was the presenting clinical sign in 60 % with 45 % of that group having massive bleeding (Pruitt et al. 1970). Fiddian-Green and colleagues demonstrated that GI bleeding was seen only in patients whose intramucosal pH has fallen below the lower limit of 7.24 (1983).

Prevention

Prevention of ulcer-related bleeding is the most effective strategy for patients. This may be accomplished by preventing gastric ischemia or acid injury (Stollman and Metz 2004). A meta-analysis of clinical trials by Cook and colleagues reported that prophylaxis with antacids, sucralfate, and histamine-2 receptor antagonists (H$_2$RA) reduced the incidence of overt or clinically important bleeding compared to no bleeding. However, they demonstrated that H$_2$RA were significantly better than placebo, antacids, and sucralfate in reducing the incidence of bleeding (Cook et al. 1996). Marinating the gastric pH between 3.5 and 4.5 is a surrogate endpoint and should be the minimum goal of prophylactic therapy. Although the efficacy and utility of proton pump inhibitors (PPIs) have been established for several acid-related GI disorders, they have not been approved as prophylaxis for GI bleeding associated with stress ulcers (Stollman and Metz 2004).

Enteral nutrition has significant advantages over parenteral nutrition. Total enteral nutrition maintains the integrity of the GI tract by preservation of gut mucosa and its immune function, thereby reducing bacterial translocation and the incidence of gut-derived infection. Enteral nutrition also increases splanchnic perfusion with an improvement in gastric oxygen balance. Aggressive, early, intragastric enteral nutrition alone has proven to be adequate ulcer prophylaxis and virtually eliminated Curling's ulcer (Andel et al. 2001).

Treatment

Initial management should consist of gastric lavage with chilled solutions. Varying success has been reported with selective infusion of vasoconstricting agents into the left gastric artery percutaneously. However, laparotomy should be performed to control bleeding if nonoperative management fails. Surgical treatment may consist of vagotomy and pyloroplasty, with ligation of bleeding points, or vagotomy and subtotal gastrectomy (Felig and Carafa 2000).

Cross-References

▶ Burn Anesthesia
▶ Gastritis
▶ Gastrointestinal Bleeding: Indications for Prophylaxis Post-trauma and Treatment

References

Andel H, Rab M, Andel D et al (2001) Impact of early high caloric duodenal feeding on the oxygen balance of the splanchnic region after severe burn injury. Burns 27:389

Cook DJ, Reeve BK, Guyatt GH et al (1996) Stress ulcer prophylaxis in critically ill patients: resolving discordant meta-analyses. JAMA 275:308–314

Felig DM, Carafa CJ (2000) Stress ulcers of the stomach. Gastrointest Endosc 51:596

Fiddian-Green RG, McGough E, Pittenger G, Rothman E (1983) Predictive value of intramural pH and other risk factors for massive bleeding from stress ulceration. Gastroenterology 85:613–620

Hartman FW (1945) Curling's ulcer in experimental burns. Ann Surg 121:54–64

Maes U (1930) Curling's ulcer: duodenal ulcer following superficial burns. Ann Surg 91:527–532

Pruitt BA Jr, Foley FA, Moncrief JA (1970) Curling's ulcer: a clinical-pathology study of 323 cases. Ann Surg 172:523–539

Silen W, Merhav A, Simson JNL (1981) The pathophysiology of stress ulcer disease. World J Surg 5:165–174

Stollman N, Metz DC (2004) Pathophysiology and prophylaxis of stress ulcer in intensive care unit patients. J Crit Care 20:35–45

Cushing's Ulcer

Ariful Alam[1] and Khanjan H. Nagarsheth[2]
[1]Department of General Surgery, Staten Island University Hospital, Staten Island, NY, USA
[2]R Adams Cowley Shock Trauma Center, University of Maryland School of Medicine, Baltimore, MD, USA

Synonyms

Peptic ulcer; Rokitansky-Cushing ulcer

Definition

Cushing's ulcer is an acute ulcer associated with tumors or injuries of central nervous system. It is a complication of neurosurgery, head trauma, and other causes of increased intracranial pressure. The ulcer was first described by Rokitansky who associated the development of peptic ulcers in patients with brain and meningeal lesions (Rokitansky 1846). In 1932, Cushing described 11 cases of cerebral pathology that were found to have upper gastrointestinal tract ulceration at autopsy (Cushing 1932). It is for this reason that ulcer associated with CNS abnormalities is called Rokitansky-Cushing ulcer or more commonly known as Cushing ulcer.

Preexisting Condition

Pathophysiology

Several theories have been proposed regarding the mechanism of Cushing's ulcer formation. Cushing himself suggested several theories. One included a bile-vomiting theory, which suggested formation of hemorrhagic ulceration by a combination of bile and acid in a patient who had postoperative emesis during recovery from the anesthetic. Another theory was the association of gastric erosions with malignant hypertension (Cushing 1932). Rokitansky suggested that ulcer formation was through the mediation of the vagus nerve that when the diencephalon was stimulated, hemorrhagic erosions and perforations in the stomach and duodenum occurred. Cook, Hartman, Sarnoff, and Berenberg have all shown that there is an association between ulceration and acute bulbar poliomyelitis (Wijdicks 2011).

This is due to the involvement of the sympathoadrenal response with angiotensin constricting the gastric vasculature. The result is hypoperfusion with diminished mucous production and compromise of the mucous barrier, thereby exposing the gastric lining to acidic material (Wijdicks 2011).

It is important to distinguish Cushing's ulcer from stress ulcers. Morphologically, these ulcers tend to be deep with full-thickness dissolution of the esophagus, stomach, or duodenum. For this reason, perforations are more common in Cushing's ulcer than they are in stress ulcers. Furthermore, elevated levels of gastrin and pepsin are commonly seen with Cushing's ulcer, a finding not present in stress ulcers (Silen et al. 1981).

Application

Presentation

In his 1932 paper, Cushing described three patients with large cerebellar tumors who had a progressively worsening course. All patients developed clinical signs of a general peritonitis with submucosal hemorrhages and perforations in the cardia of the stomach. The perforations and peritonitis were unexpected as a postoperative complication in all three patients. One of the patients developed a distended abdomen that was tender to palpation. In another patient, there was acute onset of severe epigastric pain along with general abdominal pain and pain radiating to the shoulders. In the last case, there was copious emesis of "brownish black fluid." Schlumberger reported that these ulcers are more common in the stomach than in the duodenum (Wijdicks 2011).

Walsh and colleagues reported that use of high-dose corticosteroids for CVA in an aphasic patient may obscure the symptoms and physical findings of a perforated Cushing's ulcer (1982). It should also be noted that sever traumatic brain injury is a well-recognized risk factor for Cushing's ulcer and has an incidence of around 10 % (Alain and Wang 2008).

Prevention

Prevention and treatment is the same for all critically ill patients and is well documented. Prevention of ulcer-related bleeding is the most effective strategy for patients. This may be accomplished by preventing gastric ischemia or acid injury (Stollman and Metz 2004). A meta-analysis of clinical trials by Cook et al. reported that prophylaxis with antacids, sucralfate, and histamine-2 receptor antagonists (H$_2$RA) reduced the incidence of overt or clinically important bleeding compared to no bleeding. However, Cook et al. demonstrated that H_2RA were significantly better than placebo, antacids, and sucralfate in reducing the incidence of bleeding (1996). It is also important to note that maintaining the pH between 3.5 and 4.5 is a surrogate endpoint and should be the minimum goal of prophylactic therapy. Although the efficacy and utility of proton pump inhibitors (PPIs) have been established for several acid-related GI disorders, they have not been approved as prophylaxis for GI bleeding associated with stress ulcers. Finally, clinical studies have conflicting results in establishing a significant relationship between decreasing gastric acidity with H_2RA and an increase in the rate and severity of nosocomial pneumonia from gastric bacterial overgrowth (Stollman and Metz 2004).

Treatment

Initial management should consist of gastric lavage with chilled solutions. Varying success has been reported with selective infusion of vasoconstricting agents into the left gastric artery percutaneously. However, laparotomy should be performed to control bleeding if nonoperative management fails. Surgical treatment may consist of vagotomy and pyloroplasty, with ligation of bleeding points, or vagotomy and subtotal gastrectomy (Felig and Carafa 2000).

Cross-References

▶ Head Injury
▶ Traumatic Brain Injury, Mild (mTBI)

References

Alain BB, Wang YJ (2008) Cushing's ulcer in traumatic brain injury. Chin J Traumatol 11:114–119
Cook DJ, Reeve BK, Guyatt GH et al (1996) Stress ulcer prophylaxis in critically ill patients: resolving discordant meta-analyses. JAMA 275:308–314
Cushing H (1932) Peptic ulcer and the interbrain. Surg Obst 55:1–34
Felig DM, Carafa CJ (2000) Stress ulcers of the stomach. Gastrointest Endosc 51:596
Rokitansky K (1846) Handbuch Der Pathologischen Anatomie, vol 3. Wien, Braumüller & Seidel, Hamburg, Print
Silen W, Merhav A, Simson JNL (1981) The pathophysiology of stress ulcer disease. World J Surg 5:165–174
Stollman N, Metz DC (2004) Pathophysiology and prophylaxis of stress ulcer in intensive care unit patients. J Crit Care 20:35–45
Walsh TJ, Raine T, Chamberlin WH, Rice CL (1982) Occult duodenal perforation complicating cerebral infarction: new problems in diagnosis of Cushing's ulcer. Am J Gastroenterol 77:608–610
Wijdicks EF (2011) Cushing's ulcer: the eponym and his own. Neurosurgery 68:1695–1698; discussion 1698

Cycling Safety

▶ Bicycle-Related Injuries

D

Dabigatran

▶ Neurotrauma, Anticoagulation Considerations

Daily Rounding

▶ Trauma Floor Management

Damage Control Orthopedics

Colin D. Booth[1] and Bruce H. Ziran[2]
[1]Orthopaedic Surgery Resident, Atlanta Medical Center, Atlanta, GA, USA
[2]Orthopaedic Trauma Surgery, The Hughston Clinic at Gwinnett Medical Center, Lawrenceville, GA, USA

Synonyms

Temporary stabilization

Definition

Damage control orthopedics (DCO) is a treatment strategy that is adaptive in nature and uses temporary stabilization (i.e., splinting, casting, traction, external fixation) of musculoskeletal injuries while for the patient's physiological status improves in order that he may tolerate the physiologically challenging procedures required for definitive fixation of these injuries (Schmidt et al. 2010). The term damage control was originally coined by the United States Navy to describe methods of keeping battle-damaged ships afloat and functioning until a definitive repair could be performed. The term was later adopted and modified to "damage control surgery" by Rotondo et al. as a treatment strategy for near-death patients after penetrating trauma. This strategy involved rapid but nondefinitive control of bleeding to avoid the fatal sequelae of acidosis, hypothermia, and coagulopathy that is commonly seen in patients that are exsanguinating (Rotondo et al. 1993). Trauma patients usually have a combination of injuries, soft tissue and bony, that stresses the body's hemodynamic system as well as the immune system. Further stress to an already unstable patient can adversely affect resuscitation efforts and increase proinflammatory messengers in the body, i.e., cytokines that have been shown to increase postsurgical complications. The goal of DCO is to stabilize fractures through numerous methods without significantly increasing stress upon the patient.

Preexisting Conditions

DCO has become a very useful tool for the trauma team when treating multisystem trauma patients. The adaptive strategy of DCO has

P.J. Papadakos, M.L. Gestring (eds.), *Encyclopedia of Trauma Care*,
DOI 10.1007/978-3-642-29613-0

allowed for early orthopedic intervention without compromising the patient's overall stability. Before DCO became the gold standard of care, multi-trauma patients were commonly treated with early total care of skeletal injuries under the belief that the patient was "only going to get sicker" with any delay of skeletal stabilization. Long operative procedures to achieve definitive bony stabilization regardless of the patient's physiological status were felt to mitigate further damage to surrounding soft tissues and decrease the patient's inflammatory load (Schmidt et al. 2010). Several landmark studies led orthopedists and general surgery traumatologists to advocate for early definitive fixation of long bones and external stabilization of the pelvis. Unbeknownst to practitioners, early major orthopedic procedures sometimes had unexpected consequences, such as adult respiratory distress syndrome, multiple organ failure syndrome, as well as occasional cases of fat embolism syndrome (FES) (Pape et al. 2009). Other early studies, using logistic regression, correctly identified a combination of injuries, with chest injuries and head injuries being the most risky, as major risk factors for such complications when early fixation was attempted (Ziran et al. 1997). Further studies, mostly from European literature, eventually identified subgroups of patients at risk for such complications when too early and aggressive skeletal fixation was performed. Unfortunately, stratification of risk for the individual patient proved more challenging. The patient's serum base deficit and lactate levels are currently the most helpful indicators of a patient's overall clinical state and are used by traumatologists use to help direct orthopedic care.

Current approaches of DCO focus on trying to minimizing the risk of second hit phenomenon by delaying major orthopedic procedures until the optimal physiologic "window," which generally varies being somewhere between 2 and 9 days after initial traumatic insult (Pape et al. 2009). While delay times were lessened, complications and remote organ injury still arose. It was this ultimate back and forth on fixation timing that drove physicians to the creation of DCO which would allow early orthopedic intervention without contributing to further physiological compromise or triggering a greater physiological injury, known as the 2nd hit.

The 2nd hit is a concept of an additive orthopedic impact on the patient after the "1st hit" of the initial trauma. The first insult activates inflammatory mediators causing the patient's immune response to be hyperactive and primed to respond to a future insult. The 2nd hit can trigger a larger and more harmful response to the patient and in some patients could lead to unexpected demise. Premature major orthopedic intervention in an under-resuscitated patient can initiate the 2nd hit through numerous methods such as significant blood loss or further soft-tissue damage. This can result in hypoperfusion, hypoxia, and tissue damage resulting in necrosis, inflammation, and acidosis (Schmidt et al. 2010). Both the 1st and the 2nd hit cause the release of proinflammatory proteins and cytokines which can cause major complications as seen with early orthopedic intervention (Pape et al. 2000).

More recently, the cytokine IL-6, a proinflammatory protein, has been analyzed as a marker to monitor the patient's stress response to treatment. While IL-6 indicates a patient's response to stress, other research has determined numerous biochemical markers of patient status that can be used to steer the physician's treatment algorithm toward DCO. Pape et al. identified significant thresholds of the markers as a serum lactate greater than 2.5 (mmol/L), a base excess greater than 8 (mmol/L), a pH less than 7.24, a temperature less than 35 °C, a surgical duration longer than 90 min, any coagulopathy, and a transfusion of more than 10 units of packed red blood cells (Pape et al. 2005). Despite these parameters, one should always approach each patient as a unique case because these parameters represent complex interactions between physiology and genetics that we do not fully understand.

Applications

After the initial assessment of the trauma patient has been done, it is the job of the trauma team to determine if the patient would benefit from DCO (i.e., the risks of total fracture care outweigh the benefits). Once proper imaging has been obtained and the patient's biochemical markers and clinical findings have been taken into account, the trauma team will be able to decide whether early total care versus DCO would be most appropriate and beneficial. Once the decision to employ DCO has been made, it must be decided whether noninvasive or invasive techniques should be used.

Noninvasive

Noninvasive DCO most often utilizes splints and/or traction to stabilize fractures until the patient can tolerate final stabilization/reconstruction. All fractures amendable to splinting should be splinted as soon as possible. The benefits of splinting over operative stabilization are that there is no need to transport the patient to the operating room (OR), there is minimal blood loss, and there is minimal stress to the patient. The disadvantages are that the soft tissues are not readily assessable after splinting, which makes neurovascular and compartment monitoring difficult. Changing a splint can reintroduce fracture instability. Splinting also immobilizes joints, which can lead to long turn stiffness.

Proper splint technique involves immobilization of the joints above and below the fracture to gain proper rotatory control of the fracture pieces and to remove any lever arm that may displace the fracture further. Sir John Charnley who realized that fracture displacement was dictated more by the surrounding soft tissues and the soft tissues that were still attached to the fracture pieces published the basic splinting technique and the ideals behind it (Charnley 1974). Proper understanding of these soft-tissue attachments will allow for near anatomic reduction as allowed by the fracture pattern.

As a general rule, upper extremity fractures are more amenable to splint stabilization than lower extremity fractures. For some lower extremity fractures, control of the fracture with a splint can be difficult and not appropriate. For middle one third to distal one third tibia, ankle, and foot fractures, splinting is very useful for stabilization, but proximal to the middle tibial

splinting can cause issues. As mentioned before, splinting limits a clinician's access to the soft tissues, so if compartment monitoring needs to be done regularly, like in tibial plateau or proximal tibial fractures which have high propensities toward compartment syndrome, the soft tissues must be left relatively free. A way to stabilize such fractures and have easy access for compartment monitoring is to use a removable knee immobilizer until definitive fixation can be done or compartment monitoring is complete.

In addition to splinting, traction is a very useful tool for lower extremity fractures – especially femoral shaft fractures. A major deforming force of femoral shaft fractures is spasm and contraction of thigh muscles which if not treated properly will result in shortening of the thigh and ultimately a leg length discrepancy. Skeletal traction applied across a fracture uses the remaining soft-tissue attachments to the fracture pieces to counteract the shortening forces of the muscles (i.e., ligamentotaxis). Not only does this restore length and relative stability of the limb, it also relieves pain and helps tamponade bleeding from the bone. Besides femoral fractures, traction is also useful in holding the hip in a reduced position when the patient has suffered an unstable acetabular fracture. This prevents the femoral head from putting pressure on the posterior neurovascular structures of the hip. The major disadvantages of traction are the difficulties in getting the patient out of bed, ongoing discomfort from the fracture, and irritation from transfixion pins.

Noninvasive temporary stabilization of pelvic fractures is slightly different from that of the extremities. Severe pelvic fractures are usually caused by significant trauma which results in active hemorrhage internally into the pelvis. One such fracture can be seen in Fig. 1. The most effective way to reduce these fractures, close the widening of the pelvic girdle, and tamponade any bleeding is to apply a pelvic binder or wrap sheets around the patient's pelvis with the binder or sheets placed at the level of the patient's greater trochanters. Commercially available binders are increasingly used by first responders, but a simple sheet can also be effective. An important point

Damage Control Orthopedics, Fig. 1 The above radiography depicts a vertical shear pelvic fracture. Pubic symphyseal diastasis and displacement of the right sacroiliac joint are hallmarks of the fracture pattern and can lead to mortality if not treated quickly

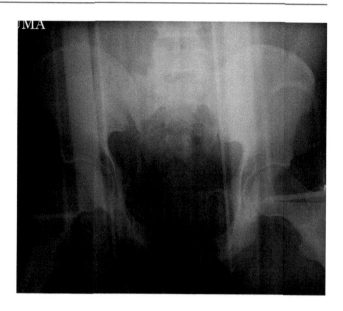

about use of such a damage control device is the attention to the soft-tissue envelope. The binder should be loosened, and the skin should be checked on a regular basis in order that any skin compromise can be detected early. Otherwise, the binder may obstruct visualization of skin lesions from the clinician until they have progressed to an irreversible state. Applying tension of approximately 180 Newtons (N) around the pelvis has been shown to decrease transfusion requirements as well as length of stay and mortality (Hak et al. 2009).

Invasive

In certain circumstances, fractures cannot be appropriately stabilized with splinting or traction. In these cases, brief but operative intervention is usually warranted. As a general rule under DCO algorithms, any operative intervention should have minimal blood loss as well as less than 2 h of operative time (Pape et al. 2009). So selection for operative/invasive intervention is usually reserved for severely, comminuted, open fractures (i.e., Grade 2–3 open fractures). Any open fracture should be treated with intravenous antibiotics and receive an excisional debridement and lavage in the operating room. If this is not possible, the wound should be gently cleansed and then left covered with sterile dressing until

a planned dressing change. Frequent uncovering of the traumatic wound may make it more likely to become contaminated/infected. We recommend the use of plastic saline bottles in which the lid has multiple perforations made by large bore needles as a "squeeze" bottle to provide controlled lavage of wounds. In relatively clean wounds, a provisional cleansing lavage and sterile dressing will suffice until the operating room. In heavily contaminated wounds, a sterile gauze or brush can be use to provide some "macro" debridement of contaminants. While antiseptic solutions such as betadine, alcohol, and chlorhexidine are known to be toxic to living tissues, there comes a point where the contamination burden is so great that the downside risk of tissue toxicity is outweighed by the need for immediate benefit of antisepsis directly into the wound, until formal operative debridement can be performed. The decision for this relies on the judgment of the treating surgeon.

In the operating room, debridement is the key factor for mitigating damage from contamination. Damage control debridement consists of removing as much necrotic or contaminated tissue as possible in a given amount of time. In very sick patients, a thorough debridement is not always possible, and thus supplemental modalities such as antibiotic-impregnated methylmethacrylate beads, antibiotic powder, and negative pressure wound therapy may be useful. Our philosophy is that closure or coverage of the wound should be considered at the time of "definitive" debridement, whether it is the first session or subsequent session, with the state of the wound and soft-tissue envelope being the driving factor.

Once the soft-tissue injury has been addressed, attention is turned to the fracture itself. The main tool used in invasive DCO is the external fixator. The external fixator can be applied quickly without the risks of second hit events as seen with early total care. The external fixator can be applied nearly anywhere, from the battlefield, the emergency room, to the intensive care unit. The main indications for an external fixator are unstable fractures with associated vascular injury, multiply injured patients, segmental bone loss, unstable fractures with soft tissue requiring frequent evaluation and time to evolve prior to fixation, closed unstable extremity fractures, and complex periarticular fractures (Camuso 2006).

The areas that benefit most from external fixators in damage control are the lower extremities: across the ankle, the knee, and the pelvis (Fig. 2). When used to treat an unstable pelvis, an external fixator allows some control of the intrapelvic volume and provides stability to the skeletal structure of the pelvis. The reduced pelvic volume results in a higher intrapelvic pressure which provides some tamponading of blood loss, but most importantly, the stabilized pelvis protects the initial clot that has formed so that ongoing hemorrhage is less likely than in the unstabilized. The initial clot that forms is rich in clotting factor but as crystalloid resuscitation in initiated and blood loss continues, the patient's blood will not contain as many clotting factors and thus may not clot as well, leading to an ongoing cycle of blood loss. Thus, the external fixator plays a significant role in protecting that "initial" clot in the pelvis. This helps with resuscitation and may decrease transfusion requirements. Similarly, the use of an external fixator on the femur can decrease blood loss as well as minimize tissue damage and pain (Fig. 3).

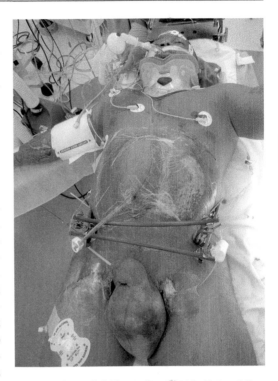

Damage Control Orthopedics, Fig. 2 External fixation of the pelvis is an effective and timely method of stabilizing severe pelvic fractures in trauma patients

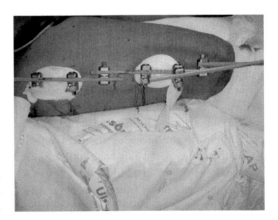

Damage Control Orthopedics, Fig. 3 External fixation of the femur with lateral pins, which avoid medial neurovascular structures

Historically, distal femoral or proximal tibial skeletal traction was used to provide temporary traction for femoral shaft fractures, but as the use of diagnostic CT and MRI scans for multi-trauma patients has become the standard of care, the use

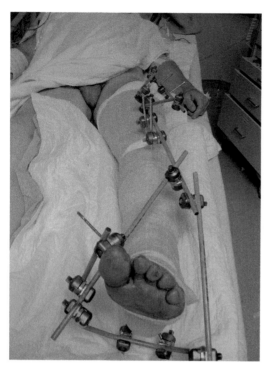

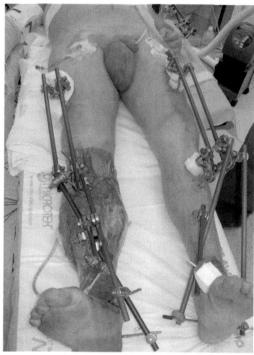

Damage Control Orthopedics, Fig. 4 A version of the "Z" frame construct for the spanning knee external fixator can be seen on the patient's left lower extremity. This construct can be expanded down to span the ankle as shown above

Damage Control Orthopedics, Fig. 5 These patient's bilateral intra-articular knee fractures were stabilized using the cluster clamp method. Both constructs where lengthened to stabilize the ankle joint as well

of skeletal traction has become more problematic with transfers, nursing care, and patient comfort. In such critically ill patients, and with new self-drilling and self-tapping external fixator pins, a four pin external fixation construct can be placed safely in almost any location and provides adequate stability of the long bone until definitive treatment can occur. In addition to their use for femoral shaft and distal femoral fractures, external fixators are commonly used as provisional stabilization for tibial plateau, tibial shaft, and tibial pilon fractures.

The spanning knee frame is one of the most commonly applied fixator constructs and is used for distal femoral or proximal tibial fractures. The two most popular configurations are shown in Figs. 4 and 5. In the "Z" frame, anterolateral pins in the femur and anteromedial pins in the tibia are created to make two "stable bases" which are manipulated, reduced, and connected

with an intercalary bar to create an elongated "Z" shape. The alternative method uses two cluster clamps and long connecting bars. The tibia is best suited for anteromedial pins and bars due to the lack of soft tissues on the anteromedial tibia, which makes pin care easier and results in less irritation. In the ankle, the construct often involves a transfixion pin across the calcaneus with the two ends of the transfixion pin connected to two bars that are attached to pins in the tibial shaft. An alternative ankle construct that avoids use of a calcaneal transfixion pin can sometimes be utilized, mitigates these issues and additionally allows better visualization, and elevates the heel off the bed, while also giving a dorsiflexion moment to the ankle. Using posteriorly placed pins, the construct shown in Figs. 6 and 7 can last a much longer time, has much fewer pin issues, and keeps fixator hardware out of the radiographic view which helps with subsequent evaluations.

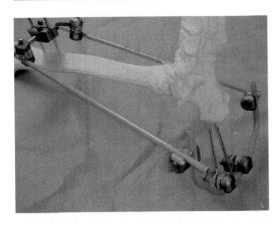

Damage Control Orthopedics, Fig. 6 The saw bones model has an ankle-spanning external fixator using two posterior, calcaneal pins instead of the common single transverse calcaneal pin. As seen, this construct elevates the calcaneus off the bed as well as decrease pin irritation

soft tissues are allowed to settle down as the swelling to decreases which ultimately decreases the patient's infection risk during open reduction and internal fixation procedures. It is the mainstay of damage control orthopedics.

Cross-References

► Damage Control Surgery
► Damage Control, History of

References

Camuso MR (2006) Far-forward fracture stabilization: external fixation versus splinting. J Am Acad Orthop Surg 14:S118–S123

Charnley J (1974) The closed treatment of common fractures, 3rd edn. Churchill Livingstone, New York

Hak DJ, Smith WR, Suzuki T (2009) Management of hemorrhage in life-threatening pelvic fracture. J Am Acad Orthop Surg 17:447–457

Pape HC, Schmidt RE, Rice J, van Griensven M, das Gupta R, Krettek C, Tscherne H (2000) Biochemical changes after trauma and skeletal surgery of the lower extremity: quantification of the operative burden. Crit Care Med 28(10):3441–3448

Pape HC, Giannoudis PV, Krettek C, Trentz O (2005) Timing of fixation of major fractures in blunt polytrauma: role of conventional indicators in clinical decision making. J Orthop Trauma 19:551–562

Pape HC, Tornetta P 3rd, Tarkin I, Tzioupis C, Sabeson V, Olson SA (2009) Timing of fracture fixation in multitrauma patients: the role of early total care and damage control surgery. J Am Acad Orthop Surg 17:541–549

Rotondo MF, Schwab CW, McGonigal MD, Phillips GR 3rd, Frutcherman TM, Kauder DR, Latenser BA, Angood PA (1993) 'Damage control': an approach for improved survival in exsanguinating penetrating abdominal injury. J Trauma 35:375–383

Schmidt AH, Anglen J, Nana AD, Varecka TF (2010) Adult trauma: getting through the night. J Bone Joint Surg Am 92:490–505

Ziran BH, Le T, Zhou H, Fallon W, Wilber JH (1997) The impact of the quantity of skeletal injury on mortality and pulmonary morbidity. J Trauma 43(6):916–921

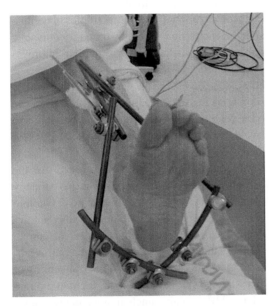

Damage Control Orthopedics, Fig. 7 The two posterior calcaneal pins construct for an ankle-spanning external fixator of the ankle as seen on a patient. Just as with the saw bones model depicted earlier, the posterior calcaneal pins provide many benefits such as heel elevation and decreased pin irritation

We currently use this construct on all-ankle frames, and its cost is commensurate with standard transfixion methods.

In summary, external allows fractures to be held in relative anatomic alignment while the

Damage Control Procedure

► Damage Control, History of

Damage Control Resuscitation

Joseph V. Sakran and Alicia Privette
Department of Surgery, Medical University
of South Carolina, Charleston, SC, USA

Synonyms

Damage control surgery; Lethal triad; Open
abdomen; Open abdomen, intensive care unit
management of a patient with an; Trauma
celiotomy

Definition

Damage control resuscitation (DCR) has revolutionized our approach to managing the unstable
trauma patient. Providing an abbreviated initial
surgical intervention (damage control surgery)
to allow for control of hemorrhage and contamination was the cornerstone of change in
allowing clinicians to focus on the physiologic
insult commonly referred to as the "lethal triad."
Since the landmark article by Rotondo and
Schwab in 1993, the evolution of DCR has
been widespread as we continue to learn how
best to not only improve survival but also
decrease morbidity in this group of critically ill
trauma patients.

Permissive Hypotension

The concept of permissive hypotension in damage control resuscitation refers to the practice of
maintaining a blood pressure that is low enough
to limit exsanguination but still maintains end-
organ perfusion (SBP = 90 mmHg) (Duchesne
et al. 2010). This lower pressure is maintained
until hemorrhage control can be definitively
achieved. This concept is in direct contrast to
traditional resuscitation strategies which have
focused on aggressive fluid resuscitation using
crystalloid/colloid solutions or blood products to
rapidly restore circulating blood volume and
physiologic pressures. Proponents of permissive
hypotension argue that the elevation in blood
pressure produced by aggressive resuscitation
increases bleeding rates and dislodges
established blood clots.

Although the use of permissive hypotension
has gained renewed popularity in the last several
years due to its widespread adoption in combat
settings, the idea has been advocated by physicians since World War I. More recently, Bickell
et al. demonstrated improved survival, fewer
complications, and shorter hospital stays in
patients with penetrating thoracic trauma who
had intravenous fluid resuscitation delayed until
operative intervention (Bickell et al. 1994). The
study had several limitations, including concerns
that it could not be applied to the overall trauma
population as the majority of trauma patients
undergo blunt injury. In addition, several subsequent observational and animal studies of permissive hypotension demonstrated equivalent
outcomes but failed to show similar improvements in mortality (Dutton et al. 2002; Duchesne
et al. 2010). However, more recent data has
supported the use of permissive hypotension in
both penetrating and blunt trauma patients and
has demonstrated decreased coagulopathy and
increased survival rates (Morrison et al. 2011;
Cotton et al. 2011). Cotton et al. found that the
use of a damage control resuscitation strategy
(permissive hypotension, minimizing crystalloid
use) resulted in decreased blood product administration and increased 30-day survival among
trauma patients undergoing damage control laparotomy (Cotton et al. 2011). The applicability of
this strategy in patients with traumatic brain
injury (TBI) remains unclear since many studies
have excluded patients with suspected TBIs.
Although there are currently no definitive guidelines regarding permissive hypotension, the preponderance of available evidence suggests that
initial resuscitation should target a systolic blood
pressure of 90 mmHg until definitive hemorrhage
control can be achieved. However, permissive
hypotension should probably be avoided in
patients with suspected traumatic brain injury
given the known risk of hypotension-induced
secondary brain injury.

Transfusion Ratios

Over the last 10 years, the military's treatment of severely injured combat casualties in Iraq and Afghanistan has resulted in significant advances in resuscitation strategies. Traditionally, early resuscitation efforts consisted of high volumes of crystalloid and PRBCs, and the use of FFP and platelets was often dictated by the presence of laboratory abnormalities. In 2004, US combat hospitals instituted a clinical practice guideline that supported the early use of a 1:1:1 ratio of plasma to RBC to platelets in patients at a high risk for massive transfusion. The 1:1:1 ratio was selected in order to more closely approximate the whole blood lost by the patient. The subsequent analysis of military outcomes demonstrated improved clinical outcomes among patients receiving higher ratios of blood components to packed red blood cells (Borgman et al. 2007; Duchesne et al. 2010). The use of increased transfusion ratios of packed red blood cells to fresh frozen plasma and platelets has since been extrapolated to the civilian trauma center (Holcomb et al. 2008).

Since its widespread adoption in both the military and civilian trauma population, multiple studies have demonstrated decreased mortality rates with the use of higher ratios of FPP and platelets to PRBCs (Duchesne et al. 2010). The exact ratio administered at various trauma centers has varied widely, but the use of a ratio of at least 1:1:2 for FFP/platelets/PRBCs appears to improve patient outcomes significantly (Holcomb and Pati 2013). Most recently, the importance of early administration of balanced blood component therapy was demonstrated by Holcomb et al. using the Prospective Observational Multicenter Major Trauma Transfusion (PROMMTT) Study (Holcomb et al. 2013). The early administration of higher plasma and platelet ratios (1:1:1) within the first 6 h was associated with a three- to fourfold decrease in mortality compared to a lower ratio (1:1:2). Despite the plethora of retrospective and observational data, these studies remain susceptible to survivor bias and have failed to clearly define an ideal transfusion ratio. In order to address these issues,

a prospective randomized trial is currently underway at multiple North American trauma centers. The Pragmatic Randomized Optimal Platelet and Plasma Ratios (PROPPR) trial will compare a 1:1:1 ratio of plasma/platelets/PRBCs with a 1:1:2 ratio among patients that receive PRBCs within 1 h of emergency room arrival and are predicted to require massive transfusion (Holcomb et al. 2013). Study data should be available for analysis in 2014.

Massive Transfusion Protocol

The vast majority of trauma patients (>90 %) do not require blood transfusion during initial resuscitation. However, approximately 3–5 % of civilian trauma patients arrive severely injured and require massive transfusion (administration of ≥10 units of packed red blood cells within a 24 hour period) (Nunez et al. 2010). Several studies have also demonstrated that among these patients, approximately 25 % will arrive at the hospital coagulopathic and are at an increased risk of mortality (Brohi et al. 2008; Nunez et al. 2010). As a result, these patients require early, rapid, and systematic administration of blood products. This delivery system has been streamlined in many institutions by the creation of a massive transfusion protocol. The protocol is activated by the trauma team following clinical patient evaluation and is not based on laboratory values, unless point-of-care testing is available, as this causes unacceptable delays. The protocol is designed so that the blood bank has blood products readily available in predefined ratios that are delivered in large quantities. The ratio of blood components and the amount delivered is determined by individual institutions. For example, an initial container may consist of 10 units of PRBC, 6 units of plasma, and 2 packs of platelets, and this is followed by subsequent containers containing 6 units of PRBCs, 4 units of plasma, and 2 packs of platelets. The delivery of blood products continues until the protocol is discontinued by the trauma team following achievement of hemostasis, completion of operation, or patient death (Nunez et al. 2010).

Indications for Damage Control Principles

The majority of trauma patients will not sustain injuries severe enough to warrant activation of damage control resuscitation. However, uncontrolled hemorrhage remains the leading cause of preventable death among trauma patients and accounts for 30–40 % of trauma-related deaths (Duchesne et al. 2010). For this reason, early and appropriate recognition of patients that will benefit from damage control resuscitation is extremely important. Several studies have attempted to identify clinical factors which correlate with the need for early aggressive resuscitation. A simple four-parameter scoring system using only systolic blood pressure ≤90 on arrival, positive-focused assessment sonography for trauma (FAST), heart rate ≥120 bpm on arrival, and penetrating mechanism was found to be 75 % sensitive and 86 % specific for predicting massive transfusion in the presence of two or more criteria (Nunez et al. 2009). A more recent study by Callcut et al., based on the prospectively collected PROMMTT data, expanded these parameters and examined the predictive ability of systolic blood pressure <90, hemoglobin <11 g/dL, temperature <35.5, INR >1.5, base deficit ≥6, heart rate ≥120 bpm, presence of penetrating trauma, and positive FAST exam. All factors were predictive of massive transfusion except for temperature. If any two triggers were present (not including temperature), the sensitivity for predicting massive transfusion was 85 % (Callcut et al. 2013). Early recognition of these factors can aid in appropriate triage of patients who will benefit from damage control principles.

The diagnosis of coagulopathy can also be an important driver of damage control resuscitation. As mentioned above, INR >1.5 is a marker for the need for massive transfusion. However, the accuracy of laboratory values for PT, PTT, and INR can be affected by the presence of hypothermia, and obtaining results can produce an unacceptable delay in patient care. In order to address the shortcomings of traditional laboratory testing, thromboelastography (TEG) has been developed as a rapid method to assess all portions of the coagulation cascade, including fibrinolytic activity and platelet function. TEG allows clinicians to identify deficiencies in specific phases of clot formation and to tailor resuscitation to those factors (Duchesne et al. 2010). Although the popularity and availability of TEG is growing, there is still little data comparing TEG to standard transfusion ratios, and the exact role of TEG in directing trauma resuscitation remains unclear.

Cross-References

► Abdominal Compartment Syndrome
► Acid-Base Management in Trauma Anesthesia
► Blood Bank
► Blood Therapy in Trauma Anesthesia
► Coagulopathy
► Cryoprecipitate Transfusion in Trauma
► Hypothermia, Trauma, and Anesthetic Management
► Hypothermia
► Massive Transfusion
► Massive Transfusion Protocols in Trauma
► Open Abdomen
► Plasma Transfusion in Trauma
► Resuscitation Goals in Trauma Patients
► Transfusion Strategy in Trauma: What Is the Evidence?
► Trauma Operating Room Management
► Vacuum Dressing

References

Bickell WH, Wall MJ, Pepe PE et al (1994) Immediate versus delayed fluid resuscitation for hypotensive patients with penetrating torso injuries. N Engl J Med 331:1105–1109

Borgman MA, Spinella PC, Perkins JG et al (2007) The ratio of blood products transfused affects mortality n patients receiving massive transfusions at a combat support hospital. J Trauma 63(4):805–813

Brohi K, Singh J, Heron M, Coats T (2008) Acute traumatic coagulopathy. J Trauma 65:986–993

Callcut RA, Cotton BA, Muskat P et al (2013) Defining when to initiate massive transfusion: a validation study of individual massive transfusion riggers in PROMMTT patients. J Trauma Acute Care Surg 74(1):59–68

Cotton, BA, Reddy, N, Hatch QM et al (2011) Damage control resuscitation is associated with a reduction in resuscitation volumes and improvement in survival in 390 damage control laparotomy patients. Ann Surg 254(4):598–605

Duchesne JC, McSwain NE, Cotton BA et al (2010) Damage control resuscitation: the new face of damage control. J Trauma 69(4):976–990

Dutton RP, Mackenzie CF, Scalea TM (2002) Hypotensive resuscitation during active hemorrhage: impact on in-hospital mortality. J Trauma 52(6): 1141–1146

Holcomb JB, Wade CE, Michalek JE et al (2008) Increased plasma and platelet to red blood cell ratios improves outcome in 466 massively transfused civilian trauma patients. Ann Surg 248(3): 447–458

Holcomb JB, Pati S (2013) Optimal trauma resuscitation with plasma as the primary resuscitative fluid: the surgeon's perspective. Hematol Am Soc Hematol Educ Prog 2013:656–659

Holcomb JB, DelJunco DJ, Fox EE et al (2013) The prospective, observational, multicenter, major trauma transfusion (PROMMTT) study: comparative effectiveness of a time-varying treatment with competing risks. JAMA Surg 148(2):127–136

Morrison CA, Carrick MM, Norman MA et al (2011) Hypotensive resuscitation strategy reduces transfusion requirements and severe postoperative coagulopathy in trauma patients with hemorrhagic shock: preliminary results of a randomized controlled trial. J Trauma 70(30):652-663

Nunez TC, Vokresensky IV, Dossett LA et al (2009) Early prediction of massive transfusion in trauma: simple as ABC (assessment of blood consumption)? J Trauma 66(2):346–352

Nunez TC, Young PP, Holcomb JB, Cotton BA (2010) Creation, implementation, and maturation of a massive transfusion protocol for the exsanguinating trauma patient. J Trauma 68(6):1498–1505

Damage Control Resuscitation, Military Trauma

Martin D. Zielinski
Department of Surgery, Mayo Clinic, Rochester, MN, USA

Synonyms

Damage control surgery; Limited crystalloid; Permissive hypotension; Plasma resuscitation

Definition

Damage control resuscitation (DCR) is a treatment paradigm addressing the elements which intensify bleeding in massively hemorrhaging patients. Originally defined by the US Navy to salvage a damaged sinking ship, this concept can be applied to critically ill patients with active hemorrhage and severe physiologic derangements. Specifically, the elements for patient care include damage control surgery, 1:1:1 blood product resuscitation, limited crystalloid use, and permissive hypotension (see the separate definition of "▶ Damage Control Surgery") (Cotton et al. 2011; Duchesne et al. 2010; Neal et al. 2012).

1:1:1 Blood Product Resuscitation: Traditional resuscitation of hemorrhaging patients focused on reversal of lab tests measuring hemoglobin levels and coagulation parameters. There was a paradigm shift during the Middle East conflicts, however, as it was noted that those soldiers who received proactive plasma resuscitation without waiting for the return of blood tests had a significantly improved mortality. In fact, a 1:1 ratio of plasma to red blood cell (RBC) transfusions conferred the greatest survival benefit. Going one step further, recreation of whole blood from its components in the form of 1:1:1 ratios of plasma to RBC to platelet transfusion conferred an even greater mortality benefit in follow-up studies. These articles have come under critique given the strong potential for survivorship bias; nevertheless, 1:1:1 plasma to RBC to platelet resuscitation has become the standard of care in the trauma community.

Limited Crystalloid: Crystalloid has been the traditional fluid for resuscitation of the hemorrhaging patient since the 1950s. Given the inherent differences between crystalloid solutions and blood, however, this dogma has been challenged. In particular, crystalloid solutions are acidotic with supraphysiologic levels of sodium and chloride as well as the documented risk of developing hyperchloremic metabolic acidosis. High ratios of crystalloid to RBC transfusions at 24 h (>1.5 L:1 Unit) have been associated with multiple organ failure, adult respiratory distress syndrome, and abdominal compartment syndrome, but not death. Whether the ratio benefit was due to purposeful limitation of crystalloid resuscitation or a consequence of the greater use of blood product transfusions remains unclear.

Permissive Hypotension: The concept of permissive hypotension revolves around limited use of both blood product and crystalloid resuscitation during the early stages of injury in an effort to allow the patient to be hypotensive until definitive hemorrhage control can be accomplished. This has been shown to reduce blood product requirements and actually limit further bleeding by avoiding pressures which may "pop the clot." The safety analysis of the initial 90 subjects (out of 271) included in the only prospective, randomized, clinical trial to date studying the effects of permissive hypotension compared to standard resuscitation has been published. This preliminary report demonstrated an early postoperative mortality benefit resulting from permissive hypotension; however, there was no benefit at 30 days. Final results from this study are pending (Morrison et al. 2011).

Cross-References

- ▶ Blood Bank
- ▶ Blood Therapy in Trauma Anesthesia
- ▶ Blood Volume
- ▶ Damage Control Resuscitation
- ▶ Damage Control Surgery
- ▶ Massive Transfusion
- ▶ Open Abdomen
- ▶ Packed Red Blood Cells
- ▶ Red Blood Cell Transfusion in Trauma ICU
- ▶ Whole Blood

References

Cotton BA, Reddy N, Hatch QM, LeFebvre E, Wade CE, Kozar RA, Gill BS, Albarado R, McNutt MK, Holcomb JB (2011) Damage control resuscitation is associated with a reduction in resuscitation volumes and improvement in survival in 390 damage control laparotomy patients. Ann Surg 254(4):598–605

Duchesne JC, McSwain NE Jr, Cotton BA, Hunt JP, Dellavolpe J, Lafaro K, Marr AB, Gonzalez EA, Phelan HA, Bilski T, Greiffenstein P, Barbeau JM, Rennie KV, Baker CC, Brohi K, Jenkins DH, Rotondo M (2010) Damage control resuscitation: the new face of damage control. J Trauma 69(4): 976–987

Morrison CA, Carrick MM, Norman MA, Scott BG, Welsh FJ, Tsai P, Liscum KR, Wall MJ Jr, Mattox KL (2011) Hypotensive resuscitation strategy reduces transfusion requirements and severe postoperative coagulopathy in trauma patients with hemorrhagic shock: preliminary results of a randomized controlled trial. J Trauma 70(3):652–663. doi:10.1097/TA.0b013e31820e77ea

Neal MD, Hoffman MK, Cuschieri J, Minei JP, Maier RV, Harbrecht BG, Billiar TR, Peitzman AB, Moore EE, Cohen MJ, Sperry JL (2012) Crystalloid to packed red blood cell transfusion ratio in the massively transfused patient: when a little goes a long way. J Trauma 72(4):892–898

Damage Control Surgery

David S. Morris
Division of Trauma, Critical Care, and General Surgery, Mayo Clinic, Rochester, MN, USA

Synonyms

Abbreviated laparotomy

Definition

Damage control surgery (DCS) is an approach to major trauma which places the emphasis on controlling life-threatening bleeding and controlling contamination. After these issues have been controlled, the operation is terminated and the focus shifts to reversing the "trauma triad of death," namely, acidosis, hypothermia, and coagulopathy, with aggressive resuscitation in the ICU environment (Wyrzykowski and Feliciano 2013). Paramount to the concept of damage control surgery is the idea that lengthy, complex reconstructive procedures, such as bowel anastomosis or vascular reconstruction, are deferred until such time as the patient has had return of normal physiologic parameters. Damage control techniques include ligation or shunting of vascular injuries, leaving the intestine in discontinuity, packing of solid organ injuries, and temporary abdominal closure.

The concept of DCS was first suggested by Stone and colleagues in 1983. The technique was described more formally in several reports from different institutions during the early 1990s. Rotondo et al. (1993) described three separate phases of damage control surgery:

I. Abbreviated laparotomy after control of compelling hemorrhage and major contamination.
II. Aggressive restorative resuscitation in the intensive care unit to reverse hypothermia and coagulopathy.
III. Return to the operating room for definitive repair of injuries and abdominal closure. This phase may actually take several return trips to the operating room to accomplish; indeed, fascial closure may not be possible and split-thickness skin grafting may be required for closure.

A fourth phase has also been described in the patient population that requires skin grafting for abdominal closure wherein the resulting ventral hernia is repaired.

The use of damage control surgery techniques, in conjunction with damage control resuscitation (also termed permissive hypotensive resuscitation) and balanced ratio blood product resuscitation, has resulted in a marked decrease in mortality in the severely injured and exsanguinating trauma patient. In a large review (Shapiro et al. 2000), the salvage rate was found to be approximately 60 %, which is a dramatic improvement over historical rates in this severely injured patient population.

Damage control surgery principles and techniques have been adapted to other clinical scenarios where the patient's physiologic reserve may be minimal or nonexistent, including emergency general surgical problems, thoracic surgery, and orthopedics (Duchesne et al. 2010).

Cross-References

▶ Abdominal Solid Organ Injury, Anesthesia for
▶ Acute Coagulopathy of Trauma
▶ Damage Control Resuscitation
▶ Damage Control Resuscitation, Military Trauma
▶ Military Trauma, Anesthesia for
▶ Open Abdomen
▶ Traumatology

References

Duchesne JC, McSwain NE, Cotton BA, Hunt JP, Dellavolpe J, Lafaro K, Marr AB, Gonzalez EA, Phelan HA, Bilski T, Greiffenstein P, Barbeau JM, Rennie KV, Barker CC, Brohi K, Jenkins DH, Rotondo MF (2010) Damage control resuscitation: the new face of damage control. J Trauma 69(4): 976–990

Rotondo MF, Schwab CW, McGonigal MD et al (1993) "Damage control": an approach for improved survival in exsanguinating penetrating abdominal injury. J Trauma 35(3):375–382; discussion 382–3

Shapiro MB, Jenkins DH, Schwab CW, Rotondo MF (2000) Damage control: collective review. J Trauma 49:969–978

Stone HH, Strom PR (1983) Management of the major coagulopathy with onset during laparotomy. Ann Surg 197(5):532–535

Wyrzykowski AD, Feliciano DV (2013) Chapter 38. Trauma damage control. In: Mattox KL, Moore EE, Feliciano DV (eds) Trauma, 7th edn. McGraw Hill, New York

Damage Control Surgery: Outcomes of the Open Abdomen

Michael Mackowski and Jason W. Smith
Department of Surgery, University of Louisville, Louisville, KY, USA

Synonyms

Abbreviated laparotomy outcomes; Consequences of damage control surgery

Definition

The use of damage control surgery is not without complications. The patient population in which this technique is applied usually has severe hemodynamic, hematologic, and metabolic derangements, and, in the setting of trauma, this technique is often applied to patients with ongoing nonsurgical hemorrhage; therefore, the complication rate following these procedures is not insignificant.

Overview

The use of temporary abdominal closure has become an increasingly common modality for the management of trauma patients and intra-abdominal hypertension. Rotondo et al. reported a complication rate of 36 % in patients surviving damage control for penetrating abdominal injury with a mortality rate of 42 %; most of these deaths occurred early in the hospital stay or during the initial laparotomy (Rotondo et al. 1993). Liao reported an early mortality rate, within the initial 48 h of injury, of 54 % after institution of damage control techniques, with a late mortality of 20 % (Liao et al. 2014; Sutton et al. 2006). The independent predictors on the arrival of late mortality in this patient population were lower temperature, GCS <=8, active cardiopulmonary resuscitation while in emergency department (ED), acidosis, and worsening base deficit. Independent predictors in the same population while in the intensive care unit were higher Apache II score, coagulopathy, need for hemodialysis or ECMO, and increased transfusion requirements. Essentially, patients who present with worse derangements, who suffer early organ failure, or who fail to respond to resuscitation are at increased risk of late mortality.

This self-selecting group of patients is also at risk to significant complications associated with their deranged physiologic state, their injuries, and the procedures required to repair their injuries. Miller and colleagues reported that of the patients who survive to closure of their abdomen, 25 % came to experience complications

(Miller et al. 2005). Complications included intra-abdominal abscess, wound infection, enteric fistula, ventral hernia, or loss of abdominal wall domain. These complications were more likely to be seen in those patients who were unable to achieve primary fascial closure within 8 days time. In treating those patients who fail to achieve primary fascial closure, other management strategies are employed to gain visceral coverage including temporizing closure with mesh, or local wound therapy with eventual split-thickness skin grafting of exposed viscera (Miller et al. 2004). Failure to achieve primary fascial closure in these patients also subjects these patients to increased financial burden, with those patients primarily closed having less than half of the total hospital charges compared with those who underwent a temporizing closure strategy. The goal of the surgical team should be to adequately treat the acutely ill patient and try to achieve early definitive fascial closure, decreasing the overall chances of postoperative complications.

Closure

Temporary Abdominal Closure
While all efforts should be made to achieve early definitive closure in patients and avoid the increased risk of complications, readmissions, and reoperations, temporary abdominal closure is an invaluable option in the management of patients who fail to obtain definitive abdominal closure. Temporary closure in patients who survive to discharge allows for coverage of the abdominal viscera with plan for later definitive fascial closure. The mainstay of the temporary closure technique centers around granulation tissue formation on exposed viscera, allowing for delayed skin grafts over this wound bed. The abdominal contents should be protected from the environment; this can be performed with local wound care with wet-to-dry dressing over a protective nonadherent layer, such as Vaseline impregnated gauze, permanent polypropylene mesh, or absorbable polyglactin mesh. Negative-pressure wound therapy with a VAC may be used

in place of wet-to-dry dressings. Once the underlying tissue has a sufficient granulation bed, split-thickness skin grafting can be performed over the visceral block to achieve wound coverage. Application of this technique may be necessary in the setting of enterocutaneous fistula, fascial retraction, abdominal wall infection or necrosis, or severe visceral edema prohibiting abdominal closure. In the end, temporary closure of the abdomen may be the only option remaining for select patients; however, definitive fascial closure and abdominal wall reconstruction will still be needed in this patient population.

Wound Care

Prior to fascial closure, patients with damage control laparotomies are managed with a large open wound. Temporary closure techniques are used early in the care, negating the need to complicated wound care. During the open phase of damage control surgery, complications, such as fistulas, can arise, creating the need for other more advanced wound care techniques, which have been mentioned earlier. After the fascia has been closed, there is good evidence to support leaving the wound open to heal by secondary intention. Velmahos, in a randomized controlled trial in 2002, found that allowing the wound to heal by secondary intention after colon injury caused a statistically significant decrease in the rate of surgical site infection, from 65 % to 36 % (Velmahos et al. 2002). Further analysis of wound care in the setting of damage control comparing skin closure of any type ("loose" closure and full closure) to open wound management, in a study by Seamon in 2013, demonstrated lower rates of superficial or deep surgical site infection (9.8 % vs. 31 % and 0 % vs. 4.7 %) and lower rates of fascial dehiscence (2.6 % vs. 8.6 %) all with statistical significance (Seamon et al. 2013). Many dressing options exist for the management of the open surgical wound including wet-to-dry dressings to vacuum-assisted closure techniques. Regardless of the dressing used, keeping the skin open and allowing the surgical wound to heal by secondary intention has been shown to decrease the surgical site complication rate in this already complication-burdened patient population.

Complications

Intra-abdominal Infections

Intra-abdominal infections/sepsis is a severe complication of the application of damage control laparotomy. Damage control is often employed in the setting of peritoneal contamination with enteric contents, either succus or stool, and additionally in coagulopathic patients as well. This mixture of bacteria-rich inoculum with blood as a culture medium can set the stage for intra-abdominal infection. A thorough irrigation of the peritoneal cavity is essential, but does not guarantee infection prevention. In the setting of damage control, it can be difficult to determine if infection would preclude definitive primary fascial closure or if delay in closure contributes to increased infection. Surgical site infection more frequently occurred in patients who failed to achieve definitive primary fascial closure. Additionally, the rate of intra-abdominal infection has been examined by DuBose from the AAST Open Abdomen Study Group. The results indicate that abscess/infection occurred overall in 20 % of patients undergoing management with an open abdomen with an increase to 33 % in those patients who fail to achieve primary closure on the first take-back exploration. Additionally the same group failed to identify any management components that helped decrease the risk, including the use of prophylactic antibiotics. In the setting of a colonic injury, statistically significant results have been further verified with rates of intra-abdominal abscess increasing from 17 % of patients not requiring damage control to 31 % of patients being closed at first reoperation to 50 % of patients requiring multiple repeat laparotomies (Dubose et al. 2013). The presence of intra-abdominal infection may also set the stage for further complications including enterocutaneous or enteroatmospheric fistula formation as well. Prior to fascial closure, it is essential that the abdomen is explored and any undrained fluid collections are broken up. Once fascial closure has occurred, the use of radiographic-assisted techniques can be employed to drain any intra-abdominal abscesses or fluid collections with concomitant use of antibiotics to treat the infection.

Enterocutaneous Fistula

Few complications are as dreaded in the damage control surgery patients as the formation of an enterocutaneous fistula. Patients who suffer abdominal trauma requiring open abdomen management have an incidence of enterocutaneous fistula ranging from 4.5 % to 25 %. In a study analyzing the American Association for the Surgery of Trauma (AAST) open abdomen registry over a 2-year enrollment period, 111 patients out of 517 suffered this complication. Patient factors that were associated with fistula were almost twice the number of bowel resections and bowel being left in discontinuity after the initial damage control procedure (Fischer et al. 2009). These patients were not any different on arrival in terms of their laboratory testing or initial intraoperative management. Factors that were identified to be independent predictors of fistula formation were large bowel resection, with an adjusted odds ratio (AOR) of 3.56, total fluid intake at 48 h of between 5 and 10 L, AOR 2.1, and greater number of abdominal re-explorations, AOR 1.1. Further studies have analyzed the location of the injury with respect to fistula formation, and Burlew and colleagues noted that the rate of fistula formation increases as the injury to the bowel progresses more distal within the colon. They noted that patients who had an enteric fistula were associated with having an elevated 12 h heart rate and a higher 12 h base deficit after initial damage control procedure; both of which indicate the presence of an ongoing shock state. Patients who achieved early primary fascial closure were less likely to fistulize with a break point at day 5–7 days with patients closed after this point being four times more likely to develop enteric fistula. It is difficult to discern whether enteric fistula formation precludes definitive primary fascial closure in this patient population, or if the presence of prolonged use of open abdomen management places the patient at risk for the development of enteric fistula. The location of the primary injury along with the presence of ongoing shock has been identified as risk factors for the development of enteric fistula. Patients who develop fistula have complications associated with management of fluid balance, nutrition, wound management difficulties, and challenges with electrolyte management.

Fistula Management

Fistula management in patients with open abdomen should follow the same guidelines as those patients who develop a postoperative enteric fistula. Some factors of fistulas that are favorable, more likely to close spontaneously, include: esophageal, duodenal stump, pancreaticobiliary, and jejunal, all with small defects and long tracts. Unfavorable fistulas, those less likely to close spontaneously, include: gastric, lateral duodenal, ligament of Treitz, ileal, fistulas with adjacent abscesses, fistulas that occur in strictured or diseased bowel, the presence of foreign bodies, or distal obstruction. Additionally, fistulas that have lower output (<200 ml/day) are more likely to close spontaneously compared to those with higher output (>500 ml/day); and higher output fistulas, or fistulas that occur in a malnourished patient population, are associated with a higher patient mortality rate. Early management of enteric fistula requires recognition, stabilization of the patient, control of fistula output, resuscitation, and infection control. In patients who have high-output fistulas, minimizing fistula output with NPO status and parental nutrition may allow for decreased fistula output and correction of electrolyte and nutritional deficiencies. The use of octreotide or somatostatin analogues fails to consistently show any statistically significant decrease in fistula output, time frame to closure, mortality benefit, or spontaneous closure rates (Martineau et al. 1996). Protecting the integrity of the surrounding skin will assist in decreasing local inflammation and infection. This may be a difficult problem in patients who undergo damage control techniques and are unable to achieve primary fascial closure.

All efforts should be made to control the flow of the fistula to allow for granulation and eventual coverage with split-thickness skin grafting, deferring fistula closure to a later date. The use of medical appliances, i.e., catheters and stomal appliances, and fistula management systems all works toward the same purpose, to protect the surrounding tissues from inflammation and infection; enterostomal therapists can be a great resource in the application of these devices. For patients that will be discharged to home or to rehabilitation, ensuring adequate ongoing wound care can be facilitated by trained wound care or enterostomal therapists at the rehabilitation facility and the use of home health nursing for ongoing home care. In some instances a VAC system may be used to assist in protecting the surrounding skin by diverting fistula flow. Definitive management of the enteric fistula is often deferred to a later date; adequate time must be given to correct electrolyte abnormalities and optimize the patient's nutritional status.

After the patient has been stabilized and the fistula tract has matured to the point to allow for intubation, it is appropriate to investigate the patient's GI anatomy to define the anatomic location of the fistula. This is most readily performed with the use of fluoroscopy and water-soluble enteric contrast media given proximally in the GI tract or thru the fistula itself (fistulogram) to help define the anatomic location of the fistula, the characteristics of the fistula tract including length and course, the presence of distal obstruction, and potential communication with an abscess cavity. With optimum control of fistula flow, and nutrition of the patient, favorable enterocutaneous fistulas should spontaneously close within 6 weeks time postoperatively. This delay in the definitive management of fistulas allows those fistulas that will close spontaneously to do so, preventing unnecessary and risky surgical procedures. The mortality of patients who undergo reoperation between the first 10 days postoperatively and week 6 is significantly higher than those repaired later.

Operative Fistula Treatment

When the decision is made to perform resection of the enterocutaneous fistula, careful consideration to surgical incision should be made. Ideally a new incision should be used to avoid entering the abdomen in a location of adhesions to avoid enterotomy; should the old incision be used, then care should be taken to enter cranially or caudally for the same reasons. Once access to the peritoneum is attained, the entirety of the bowel should be explored so that any abscesses or sources of obstruction can be identified and treated. A thorough adhesiolysis should be performed sharply, to avoid unrecognized thermal intestinal injury, and in a controlled manner to reduce the chances of enterotomy formation. Once the fistulous segment of the bowel is isolated, resection should be carried out to non-diseased segments of the bowel. Anastomosis is often performed in an end-to-end or side-to-side manner, should be tension free, and is generally performed in a hand-sewn fashion. Prior to closure all enterotomies or serosal tears should be identified and addressed. Thought should be given to placement of gastrostomy tube for proximal decompression or jejunostomy tube for the delivery of nutrition depending on the location of the resection and to assist in the management of the patient postoperatively. Additionally, the abdomen should be copiously irrigated, and, if possible, omentum should be positioned between the anastomosis and the peritoneal closure. Complete fascial coverage of the abdominal contents is critical in reducing the amount of abdominal inflammation postoperatively and preventing new fistula formation. Patients who suffer from enterocutaneous fistula and loss of abdominal domain secondary to failure to achieve primary fascial closure during their initial hospitalization represent a difficult-to-manage subset of patients and may be best benefited by a multidisciplinary approach, in conjunction with plastic and reconstructive surgery, for the creation of myocutaneous flaps to assist with definitive fascial closure at the time of fistula takedown. After operative fistula closure occurs, all efforts should be made to prevent infection and sepsis, and optimization of patient nutrition should be made to assist with the healing of the postoperative patient.

Nutritional Support

Nutritional deficiencies commonly arise in this patient population and require special attention by the treatment team. Patients treated with open abdominal techniques have significant protein and nitrogen losses. The sources of this nitrogen and protein deficit are twofold; patients with open abdomen had less intake of protein and had higher rates of nitrogen loss including loss of protein from peritoneal fluid effluent, with about 2 g of nitrogen per liter of abdominal fluid. Once bowel continuity is restored, enteral nutrition should be instituted as early as possible even in the presence of open abdominal management. Contraindications to the use of enteral feeding include: ongoing hypovolemic shock state without adequate resuscitation, bowel obstruction, ileus, gastrointestinal hemorrhage, or gastrointestinal ischemia. Caloric needs can be estimated using predictive equations, such as the Harris-Benedict equation or the Ireton-Jones equations. Metabolic cart studies approximating the respiratory quotient (RQ) may also be useful. Early involvement of nutritionist in the intensive care unit can be extremely valuable in performing nutritional assessment in this patient population.

Special consideration should be paid to patients who suffer an enteric fistula complicating their damage control laparotomy, and the nutritional needs in this patient population can differ greatly from the norm. It is first important that once a fistula is identified, efforts should be made to achieve restoration of homeostasis with resuscitation and correction of electrolyte abnormalities, control of sepsis, and control of fistula output. Nutrition should not be initiated until the previously mentioned abnormalities have been treated. The major goal of providing nutrition in this patient population is to prevent malnutrition and the complications associated. Patients with low output fistulas can be approached in a similar manner as those without, with predictive equations to assess the patients caloric needs. Patients who are capable of providing adequate oral intake should be allowed to do so, and caloric supplementation may not be required in these patients. If a patient has a high-output fistula, higher nutritional requirements will be necessary to prevent malnutrition. The sources of malnutrition in these patients are loss of proteins from the GI tract, inadequate PO intake, and accentuated catabolic states due to ongoing sepsis. Patients with higher output fistulas may not be able to meet their dietary needs with oral intake, and supplemental enteric nutrition can be initiated

thru gastric, post-pyloric, jejunal access routes or thru the fistula itself. Supplementation with trace minerals and vitamins should be provided to patients with favorable fistula and may need to be given at twice the daily recommended rates for patients with high-output fistulas.

Parenteral nutrition supplementation may be necessary in patient with enterocutaneous fistula. General indications includes "inability to obtain enteral access, high-output fistulas (>500 ml/ 24 h), GI intolerance with enteral nutrition, and multiple unfavorable factors." Total parenteral nutrition (TPN) should be considered in patients to prevent the complications of malnutrition. Although some studies have attributed increased rates of spontaneous fistula closure to the use of TPN, to date no definitive evidence in the form of prospective randomized trials exists to state that there is increased healing of enterocutaneous fistula with the solo use of parenteral nutrition. Additionally there is a large body of evidence to support that enteral nutrition is superior to parenteral nutrition in an ICU setting with a reduced incidence of infections in patients receiving enteral nutrition. Generally, once a patient is able to tolerate enteral nutrition, it should be initiated with the goal of preventing malnutrition and liberation from parenteral nutrition. In patients with open abdominal management, and those complicated by enterocutaneous fistula, adequate provision of caloric and protein intake is paramount in the nutritional management of these patients and will aid in the successful surgical management should the fistula fail to close spontaneously.

Long-Term Sequelae

Work/Functional Status

Care for the patient who suffers severe abdominal trauma requiring damage control techniques does not end once, and if, the patient undergoes definitive fascial repair These patients are left to recover from a host of other physical and psychological ailments. Readmission to the hospital was a common theme among patients who survived initial injury; 76 % of patients were readmitted in an initial study with a 2-year follow-up period reported by Sutton and colleagues (Sutton et al. 2006). The two most common reasons for readmission in this group of patients were ventral hernia repair and infection, totaling 107 readmissions. This patient group spends a significant amount of time in the hospital after initial discharge with an average length of stay on first readmission of 6 days. This does not include time spent in recovery or physical rehabilitation from initial injury or subsequent readmissions and procedures.

All of the factors mentioned above lead to decreased quality of life. The problem with the assessment of pain post injury is the subjective nature in which pain is perceived and reported. Perhaps the best objective long-term measure of outcomes for patients who underwent damage control laparotomy is return to work after injury, and studies demonstrate that 21–78 % of patients who were managed with an open abdomen were able to return to work. In the patient population analyzed by Sutton, return to work was found to be 81 % by 3 years post injury (Sutton et al. 2006). Timing of closure may be critical to reemployment, with abdominal closure prior to day 7 having a statistically significant higher return to work rate compared to those patients closed after 1 week.

Psychological

Patients who require damage control for abdominal trauma have other long-term complications as well. These patients sustained great deal of emotional and psychological stress from both their initial injury and from the hospital stay with multiple procedures that ensue. Zauzar and colleagues analyzed a group of patients who underwent delayed abdominal wall reconstruction looking at quality of life. Screening patients with Short-Form 36-Item Health Survey, they found that 65 % of patients screened positive for depression and 22.5 % for PTSD. Patients who screened positive for depression or PTSD had a reduced quality of life screening respectively. Quality of life returned to baseline levels in 60 % of patients who had undergone successful abdominal wall reconstruction. The authors

found that quality of life tended to gradually increase in the initial 12–18-month recovery period. A significant aspect to a patient's reported quality of life is the presence of long-term pain (Zarzaur et al. 2011). The presence of pain after abdominal wall reconstruction was observed to occur in 41 % of the patients who underwent abdominal wall reconstruction with patients who underwent late closure (>7 days) being 2.5 times more likely to experience chronic pain post injury. The presence of long-term pain, coupled with the high incidence of psychological comorbidities post trauma, greatly reduced the quality of life in the patient who undergoes abdominal wall reconstruction after suffering polytrauma.

Cost

The cost of damage control laparotomy and subsequent repair is born out over several factors. The injury with the subsequent hospitalization, re-hospitalizations, and surgical procedures places most patients at increased risk of having postoperative pain or suffering from depression or PTSD. This is compounded with increased costs of both initial hospitalization and rehabilitation and decreased earning potential over the months to follow. Quality of life and return to work have both clearly adversely affected this patient population. Knowledge of the emotional, physical, psychological, and monetary costs to the patient should not be underestimated by the treatment team, and multidisciplinary treatment should be instituted early in the management of the patient to help improve the patient's post injury quality of life and hasten return to pre-injury functional status.

Summary

Care for patients requiring damage control laparotomy is complex and requires a dedicated trauma team along with well-trained nursing and other support staff. Patients requiring the use of damage control techniques are exposed to a statistically significantly higher mortality rate and complication rate. Early fascial closure, if possible, is clearly better for the patient, placing them at a lower risk of having complications.

To help facilitate early closure, a multitude of techniques have been described, all centered around maintaining adequate abdominal domain, preventing the formation of intra-abdominal infection and fistulas, and decreasing bowel edema. Some patients may progress to require a planned ventral hernia at their initial operation, and operations have been described to assist in achieving definitive abdominal wall reconstruction in this subgroup as well. Patients requiring the application of these techniques will additionally be subject to a higher cost of care compared to patients who are closed on first operation, and will likely need physical rehabilitation before they are capable of returning to pre-injury functional status. Additionally these severely injured patients suffer from emotional and psychological problems. The treating team should be equipped to expeditiously recognize and treat these other complications that arise in this patient population.

Cross-References

▶ Abdominal Compartment Syndrome
▶ Repair of the Open Abdomen Hernia, Scope of the Problem

References

Dubose JJ, Scalea TM, Holcomb JB, Shrestha B, Okoye O, Inaba K et al (2013) Open abdominal management after damage-control laparotomy for trauma: a prospective observational American Association for the Surgery of Trauma multicenter study. J Trauma Acute Care Surg 74(1):113–120; discussion 1120–2

Fischer PE, Fabian TC, Magnotti LJ, Schroeppel TJ, Bee TK, Maish GO 3rd et al (2009) A ten-year review of enterocutaneous fistulas after laparotomy for trauma. J Trauma 67(5):924–928

Liao LM, Fu CY, Wang SY, Liao CH, Kang SC, Ouyang CH et al (2014) Risk factors for late death of patients with abdominal trauma after damage control laparotomy for hemostasis. World J Emerg Surg 9(1):1

Martineau P, Shwed JA, Denis R (1996) Is octreotide a new hope for enterocutaneous and external pancreatic fistulas closure? Am J Surg 172(4):386–395

Miller PR, Meredith JW, Johnson JC, Chang MC (2004) Prospective evaluation of vacuum-assisted fascial closure after open abdomen: planned ventral hernia rate is substantially reduced. Ann Surg 239(5):608–614; discussion 14–6

Miller RS, Morris JA Jr, Diaz JJ Jr, Herring MB, May AK (2005) Complications after 344 damage-control open celiotomies. J Trauma 59(6):1365–1371; discussion 71–4

Rotondo MF, Schwab CW, McGonigal MD, Phillips GR 3rd, Fruchterman TM, Kauder DR et al (1993) 'Damage control': an approach for improved survival in exsanguinating penetrating abdominal injury. J Trauma 35(3):375–382; discussion 82–3

Seamon MJ, Smith BP, Capano-Wehrle L, Fakhro A, Fox N, Goldberg M et al (2013) Skin closure after trauma laparotomy in high-risk patients: opening opportunities for improvement. J Traumatol Acute Care Surg 74(2):433–439; discussion 9–40

Sutton E, Bochicchio GV, Bochicchio K, Rodriguez ED, Henry S, Joshi M et al (2006) Long term impact of damage control surgery: a preliminary prospective study. J Trauma 61(4):831–834; discussion 5–6

Velmahos GC, Vassiliu P, Demetriades D, Chan LS, Murray J, Salim A et al (2002) Wound management after colon injury: open or closed? A prospective randomized trial. Am Surg 68(9):795–801

Zarzaur BL, DiCocco JM, Shahan CP, Emmett K, Magnotti LJ, Croce MA et al (2011) Quality of life after abdominal wall reconstruction following open abdomen. J Trauma 70(2):285–291

Recommended Reading

Anjaria DJ, Ullmann TM, Lavery R, Livingston DH (2014) Management of colonic injuries in the setting of damage-control laparotomy: one shot to get it right. J Traumatol Acute Care Surg 76(3):594–598; discussion 8–600

Asensio JA, McDuffie L, Petrone P, Roldan G, Forno W, Gambaro E et al (2001) Reliable variables in the exsanguinated patient which indicate damage control and predict outcome. Am J Surg 182(6):743–751

Barker DE, Kaufman HJ, Smith LA, Ciraulo DL, Richart CL, Burns RP (2000) Vacuum pack technique of temporary abdominal closure: a 7-year experience with 112 patients. J Trauma 48(2):201–206; discussion 6–7

Berry SM, Fischer JE (1996) Classification and pathophysiology of enterocutaneous fistulas. Surg Clin North Am 76(5):1009–1018

Bradley MJ, Dubose JJ, Scalea TM, Holcomb JB, Shrestha B, Okoye O et al (2013) Independent predictors of enteric fistula and abdominal sepsis after damage control laparotomy: results from the prospective AAST Open Abdomen registry. JAMA Surg 148(10):947–954

Brenner M, Bochicchio G, Bochicchio K, Ilahi O, Rodriguez E, Henry S et al (2011) Long-term impact of damage control laparotomy: a prospective study. Arch Surg 146(4):395–399

Burlew CC, Moore EE, Cuschieri J, Jurkovich GJ, Codner P, Crowell K et al (2011) Sew it up! A Western Trauma Association multi-institutional study of enteric injury management in the postinjury open abdomen. J Trauma 70(2):273–277

Burlew CC, Moore EE, Biffl WL, Bensard DD, Johnson JL, Barnett CC (2012) One hundred percent fascial approximation can be achieved in the postinjury open abdomen with a sequential closure protocol. J Trauma Acute Care Surg 72(1):235–241

Cheatham ML, Safcsak K, Llerena LE, Morrow CE Jr, Block EF (2004) Long-term physical, mental, and functional consequences of abdominal decompression. J Trauma 56(2):237–241; discussion

Cheatham ML, Safcsak K, Brzezinski SJ, Lube MW (2007) Nitrogen balance, protein loss, and the open abdomen. Crit Care Med 35(1):127–131

Dudrick SJ, Maharaj AR, McKelvey AA (1999) Artificial nutritional support in patients with gastrointestinal fistulas. World J Surg 23(6):570–576

Edmunds LH Jr, Williams GM, Welch CE (1960) External fistulas arising from the gastro-intestinal tract. Ann Surg 152:445–471

Evenson AR, Fischer JE (2006) Current management of enterocutaneous fistula. J Gastrointest Surg 10(3):455–464

Fansler RF, Taheri P, Cullinane C, Sabates B, Flint LM (1995) Polypropylene mesh closure of the complicated abdominal wound. Am J Surg 170(1):15–18

Fantus RJ, Mellett MM, Kirby JP (2006) Use of controlled fascial tension and an adhesion preventing barrier to achieve delayed primary fascial closure in patients managed with an open abdomen. Am J Surg 192(2):243–247

Fazio VW, Coutsoftides T, Steiger E (1983) Factors influencing the outcome of treatment of small bowel cutaneous fistula. World J Surg 7(4):481–488

Fox N, Crutchfield M, LaChant M, Ross SE, Seamon MJ (2013) Early abdominal closure improves long-term outcomes after damage-control laparotomy. J Traumatol Acute Care Surg 75(5):854–858

Foy HM, Nathens AB, Maser B, Mathur S, Jurkovich GJ (2003) Reinforced silicone elastomer sheeting, an improved method of temporary abdominal closure in damage control laparotomy. Am J Surg 185(5):498–501

Gross T, Amsler F (2011) Prevalence and incidence of longer term pain in survivors of polytrauma. Surgery 150(5):985–995

Hadeed JG, Staman GW, Sariol HS, Kumar S, Ross SE (2007) Delayed primary closure in damage control laparotomy: the value of the Wittmann patch. Am Surg 73(1):10–12

Heyland DK, Dhaliwal R, Drover JW, Gramlich L, Dodek P (2003) Canadian critical care clinical practice guidelines C. Canadian clinical practice guidelines for nutrition support in mechanically ventilated, critically ill adult patients. JPEN J Parenter Enteral Nutr 27(5):355–373

Hill GL, Bourchier RG, Witney GB (1988) Surgical and metabolic management of patients with external fistulas of the small intestine associated with Crohn's disease. World J Surg 12(2):191–197

Jamshidi R, Schecter WP (2007) Biological dressings for the management of enteric fistulas in the open abdomen: a preliminary report. Arch Surg 142(8):793–796

Jernigan TW, Fabian TC, Croce MA, Moore N, Pritchard FE, Minard G et al (2003) Staged management of giant abdominal wall defects: acute and long-term results. Ann Surg 238(3):349–355; discussion 55–7

Kirkpatrick AW, Baxter KA, Simons RK, Germann E, Lucas CE, Ledgerwood AM (2003) Intra-abdominal complications after surgical repair of small bowel injuries: an international review. J Trauma 55(3):399–406

Lloyd DA, Gabe SM, Windsor AC (2006) Nutrition and management of enterocutaneous fistula. Br J Surg 93(9):1045–1055

Lynch AC, Delaney CP, Senagore AJ, Connor JT, Remzi FH, Fazio VW (2004) Clinical outcome and factors predictive of recurrence after enterocutaneous fistula surgery. Ann Surg 240(5):825–831

MacFadyen BV Jr, Dudrick SJ, Ruberg RL (1973) Management of gastrointestinal fistulas with parenteral hyperalimentation. Surgery 74(1):100–105

Majercik S, Kinikini M, White T (2012) Enteroatmospheric fistula: from soup to nuts. Nutr Clin Pract 27(4):507–512

Makhdoom ZA, Komar MJ, Still CD (2000) Nutrition and enterocutaneous fistulas. J Clin Gastroenterol 31(3):195–204

Peppas G, Gkegkes ID, Makris MC, Falagas ME (2010) Biological mesh in hernia repair, abdominal wall defects, and reconstruction and treatment of pelvic organ prolapse: a review of the clinical evidence. Am Surg 76(11):1290–1299

Ramirez OM, Ruas E, Dellon AL (1990) "Components separation" method for closure of abdominal-wall defects: an anatomic and clinical study. Plast Reconstr Surg 86(3):519–526

Rasilainen SK, Mentula PJ, Leppaniemi AK (2012) Vacuum and mesh-mediated fascial traction for primary closure of the open abdomen in critically ill surgical patients. Br J Surg 99(12):1725–1732

Rose D, Yarborough MF, Canizaro PC, Lowry SF (1986) One hundred and fourteen fistulas of the gastrointestinal tract treated with total parenteral nutrition. Surg Gynecol Obstet 163(4):345–350

Schnuriger B, Inaba K, Wu T, Eberle BM, Belzberg H, Demetriades D (2011) Crystalloids after primary colon resection and anastomosis at initial trauma laparotomy: excessive volumes are associated with anastomotic leakage. J Trauma 70(3):603–610

Sitges-Serra A, Jaurrieta E, Sitges-Creus A (1982) Management of postoperative enterocutaneous fistulas: the roles of parenteral nutrition and surgery. Br J Surg 69(3):147–150

Smith JW, Garrison RN, Matheson PJ, Franklin GA, Harbrecht BG, Richardson JD (2010) Direct peritoneal resuscitation accelerates primary abdominal wall closure after damage control surgery. J Am Coll Surg 210(5):658–664, 64–7

D

Soeters PB, Ebeid AM, Fischer JE (1979) Review of 404 patients with gastrointestinal fistulas. Impact of parenteral nutrition. Ann Surg 190(2):189–202

Teixeira PG, Inaba K, Dubose J, Salim A, Brown C, Rhee P et al (2009) Enterocutaneous fistula complicating trauma laparotomy: a major resource burden. Am Surg 75(1):30–32

Tsuei BJ, Skinner JC, Bernard AC, Kearney PA, Boulanger BR (2004) The open peritoneal cavity: etiology correlates with the likelihood of fascial closure. Am Surg 70(7):652–656

Vogel TR, Diaz JJ, Miller RS, May AK, Guillamondegui OD, Guy JS et al (2006) The open abdomen in trauma: do infectious complications affect primary abdominal closure? Surg Infect (Larchmt) 7(5):433–441

Damage Control, History of

Joseph V. Sakran and Alicia Privette
Department of Surgery, Medical University of South Carolina, Charleston, SC, USA

Synonyms

Complications; Damage control procedure; History; Outcomes; Open abdomen

Definition

While the concept of damage control surgery is not a new technique, the latter half of the twentieth century has resulted in significant evidence-based medicine identifying the necessary steps surgeons must take to care for such critically ill patients. This has decreased the morbidity and mortality of such patients. Despite the importance of this lifesaving strategy, it is paramount that clinicians are cognizant of the potential complications associated with the implementation of damage control in order to ensure optimal patient care.

Since antiquity, surgeons have utilized the technique of packing to control hemorrhage. This technique has been most commonly described in patients with substantial hepatic trauma. Despite the description of hepatic packing by Pringle in the early twentieth century

(Pringle 1908), the practice of packing during World War II and the Vietnam War was discouraged by the US military. The rebirth of hepatic packing occurred secondary to a number of reports within the civilian sector and perhaps more specifically to the principles described by Lucas and Ledgerwood in a series of patients who underwent packing for major liver injuries (Lucas and Ledgerwood 1976). This concept was repeated by Feliciano et al. (1981), who demonstrated a 90 % survival rate in a small group of patients with massive liver trauma. Several years later, Stone and his colleagues extrapolated this principle to demonstrate the concept of intra-abdominal packing during laparotomy for the exsanguinating, hypothermic, and coagulopathic patient (Stone et al. 1983). This set the stage for the landmark article in 1993 by Rotondo and Schwab where the term "damage control" was introduced into the trauma lexicon (Rotondo et al. 1993). Damage control was originally a term defined by the Navy as "the capacity of a ship to absorb damage and maintain mission integrity" (DOD 1996). The importance of this article is twofold. The first was the concept of an abbreviated operation that allowed for continued resuscitation in the intensive care unit (ICU) with a delayed definitive repair, which was associated with an improved survival. The second was the description of this triphasic approach and specific logistics of how it is accomplished. Since then, the proliferation of damage control surgery (DCS) within the trauma community and beyond has been pervasive. This concept has grown to recently include what is now called damage control resuscitation (DCR), which includes DCS and other basic principles tailored towards reversing the "lethal triad" of coagulopathy, acidosis, and hypothermia.

The Three Phases of Damage Control

Part One: Initial Laparotomy (DCI)

The first phase of damage control has four main objectives: control hemorrhage, control contamination, intra-abdominal packing, and temporary closure device (Rotondo et al. 1993). This is performed with the idea that time is of the essence.

The importance of adequate preparation cannot be overemphasized. It is essential that a multidisciplinary team approach be developed in caring for these critically ill patients. The groundwork for effectively executing damage control surgery is significant and further described by Johnson and colleagues as damage control ground zero (DC0) (Johnson et al. 2001). Trauma centers must ensure that appropriate protocols are in place in order to promptly activate and implement concepts like the massive transfusion protocol (MTP), having immediate access to standardized operating room instruments, and the ability to quickly mobilize experienced surgical assistance. Controlling hemorrhage is the most important step in part one of DCS, and typically this can be initially achieved by methodically packing each of the four abdominal quadrants. More aggressive maneuvers, such as control of aortic inflow, are required when this is not successful. Initial control of vascular injuries is best managed with clamps and/or suture ligation. Shunting of major vessels that are not appropriate be considered appropriate for ligation (i.e., SMA) is a described option (Reilly et al. 1995) and should be considered in order to decrease the length of time spent in the operating room. Solid organ injury (spleen, kidney) is typically best dealt with by resection. When it comes to hepatic injury, the majority of parenchymal injuries can be addressed via suture ligation and/or hepatic packing. At times a number of different temporizing measures can be utilized such as occlusion of hepatic vascular inflow (Pringle maneuver), manual compression, packing, and plugging of through-and-through penetrating wounds. Once control of hemorrhage is established, attention should be turned to controlling contamination from hollow viscus injury. This is not the time to attempt anastomosis, and patients should be left in discontinuity. Techniques such as stapled closure, resection, or primary repair should be employed. At this point it is important to pack the abdomen at both sites of organ injury and at areas where dissection took place. Lap pads can be utilized in this process and have the added benefit of having a radiopaque strip that can be identified when abdominal x-ray is performed prior to definitive reconstruction. Temporary abdominal closure can now be performed. A variety of techniques for temporary abdominal closures exist, ranging from the rarely utilized towel clips, to closing the skin with running suture, to the more commonly applied negative-pressure (vacuum-pack) dressing. There is consensus that closure of the fascia at this stage is not recommended is not recommended due to concern for the development of abdominal compartment syndrome (Hoey and Schwab 2002). Ensuring that the bowel is appropriately protected during dressing placement is critical. By keeping these four objectives in mind, surgeons can systematically address life threatening injuries in a prompt yet elegant manner and achieve the most optimal patient outcomes.

Part Two: ICU Resuscitation (DCII)

The second part of DCS is tailored towards reversing the "lethal triad" (acidosis, coagulopathy, and hypothermia), which many patients in these circumstances develop. Reversal of these physiologic derangements requires a multidisciplinary team with open lines of communication between the ICU nursing staff, intensivist, surgeons, specialty services, blood bank, and other ancillary staff. A number of strategies working in parallel are utilized in the approach to treating these physiologic abnormalities. Invasive monitoring, ventilatory support, and laboratory tests (i.e., serial ABG, lactate) allow for and are essential in the optimization of tissue perfusion. These adjuncts also guide the clinician in their resuscitation efforts as blood volume is restored. Reversal of these physiologic derangements can go hand in hand. For example, providing an optimal ICU room temperature, delivering warm resuscitative crystalloid and/or blood products, and implementing other rewarming techniques (i.e., blankets) allow for not only improvement of hypothermia but can also affect coagulopathy. These patients typically require a significant amount of attention and resources during the first 24 h. As the resuscitation process continues, care is directed toward evaluation of patient injuries to ensure that they are addressed in a timely manner, including early utilization of specialty consultations. Certain circumstances (i.e., hepatic injury) will require further diagnostic and/or therapeutic intervention (i.e., angioembolization). One cannot stress the importance of having these patients supervised by the critical care team during this process in order to ensure that the resuscitation is continued regardless of patient location. As experience with DCS continues to grow, one of the pitfalls that have been described is the development of abdominal compartment syndrome (ACS) can occur secondary to aggressive, yet necessary, resuscitation. Clinicians should remain vigilant for the development of ACS even in the presence of an open abdomen. ACS has been described in patients with temporary closure devices and has subsequently resulted in cardiopulmonary decompensation.

Part Three: Definitive Reconstruction (DCIII)
Depending on the physiologic status of the patient, in the majority of cases, patients can be taken back to the operating room (OR) within 24–48 h. It is essential that patients are optimized prior to returning to the OR with resolution of their acidosis, hypothermia, and coagulopathy. The case should begin with removal of packs and reexploration of the abdomen to identify injuries potentially missed during the first exploration. At this point definitive repair of major vascular injuries or bowel anastomosis is performed. An attempt should be made to close the abdominal fascia at the first take-back in order to reduce the risk of potential morbidities related to an open abdomen. A useful adjunct in determining whether or not fascial closure is appropriate is to determine the change in peak airway pressure (PAP) before and after "temporary" closure. If a difference in PAP >10 is seen, then the abdomen should be left open with application of another negative-pressure (vacuum-pack) dressing (Hoey and Schwab 2002). If the abdominal fascia is closed, the skin is typically left open due to the high rate of surgical site infection associated with skin closure. In such complex wounds, great care must be taken to avoid the presence of retained sponges. An incidence of 1 in 700 has been described after emergent trauma laparotomy (Teixeira et al. 2007). Obtaining an adequate abdominal x-ray intraoperatively prior to fascial closure will allow the surgeon to potentially avoid this complication. Within 1 week, the majority of patients will have successful closure of their fascia. In patients where this is not possible, placement of a Vicryl mesh is recommended given the increased complications associated with an open abdomen as the time interval from initial operation increases (Miller et al. 2005). Within a couple of weeks, granulation through the mesh occurs at which point a split thickness skin graft (STSG) can be performed. These patients usually need at least 9–12 months for the STSG to mature and separate, at which point they can return for definitive reconstruction.

Damage Control Outcomes
When looking at outcomes in DCS, an important concept to remember is that this measure is employed as a lifesaving strategy in critically ill patients. Initial reports have demonstrated that patients who underwent damage control versus a definitive surgery at initial laparotomy have a decreased mortality (Stone et al. 1983;

Damage Control, History of, Table 1 Morbidities in damage control surgery patients

Complications	Prevalence (%)	References
Abscess (intra-abdominal)	0–83	Feliciano et al. 1981; Stone et al. 1983; Rotondo et al. 1993; Moore et al. 1998; Hirshberg et al. 1994; Burch et al. 1992; Barker et al. 2007; Garner et al. 2001; Finlay et al. 2004; Abikhaled et al. 1997; Ekeh et al. 2006
Enteroatmospheric fistula (EAF)	2–25	
Abdominal compartment syndrome (ACS)	10–40	
Dehiscence	9–25	

Rotondo et al. 1993). As the notion of DCS become more widespread, additional data has confirmed this survival advantage. Rotondo and colleagues reviewed 961 patients who had undergone damage control surgery and found an associated overall mortality of 50 % and morbidity of 40 % (Rotondo and Zonies 1997). Understanding the wide variety of complications seen with DCS is critical. Morbidities range from intra-abdominal abscess, dehiscence, enteroatmospheric fistula, to abdominal compartment syndrome (Table 1). The wide variability seen within the literature regarding morbidities is likely secondary to the myriad factors (i.e., length of time open abdomen, type of closure) present within studies, all of which may affect outcomes (Miller et al. 2005).

Cross-References

▶ Abdominal Compartment Syndrome
▶ Acid-Base Management in Trauma Anesthesia
▶ Blood Bank
▶ Blood Therapy in Trauma Anesthesia
▶ Coagulopathy
▶ Hypothermia
▶ Massive Transfusion Protocols in Trauma
▶ Open Abdomen
▶ Trauma Operating Room Management
▶ Vacuum Dressing

References

Abikhaled JA, Granchi TS, Wall MJ, Hirshberg A, Mattox KL (1997) Prolonged abdominal packing for trauma is associated with increased morbidity and mortality. Am Surg 63:1109–1112

Barker DE, Green JM, Maxwell RA, Smith PW, Mejia VA, Dart BW et al (2007) Experience with vacuum-pack temporary abdominal wound closure in 258 trauma and general and vascular surgical patients. J Am Coll Surg 204:784–792

Burch JM, Ortiz VB, Richardson RJ, Martin RR, Mattox KL, Jordan GL Jr (1992) Abbreviated laparotomy and planned reoperation for critically injured patients. Ann Surg 215:476–483

Department of Defense (1996) Surface ship survivability, Naval war publications 3-20.31. Department of Defense, Washington, DC

Ekeh AP, McCarthy MC, Woods RJ, Walusimbi M, Saxe JM, Patterson LA (2006) Delayed closure of ventral abdominal hernias after severe trauma. Am J Surg 191:391–395

Feliciano D, Mattox K, Jordan G (1981) Intra-abdominal packing for control of hepatic hemorrhage: a reappraisal. J Trauma 21:285–290

Finlay IG, Edwards TJ, Lambert AW (2004) Damage control laparotomy. Br J Surg 91:83–85

Garner GB, Ware DN, Cocanour CS, Duke JH, McKinley BA, Kozar RA et al (2001) Vacuum-assisted wound closure provides early fascial reapproximation in trauma patients with open abdomens. Am J Surg 182:630–638

Hirshberg A, Wall MJ Jr, Mattox KL (1994) Planned reoperation for trauma: a 2 year experience with 124 consecutive patients. J Trauma 37:365–369

Hoey BA, Schwab CW (2002) Damage control surgery. Scand J Surg 91(1):92–103

Johnson JW, Gracias VH, Schwab CW, Reilly PM, Kauder DR, Dabrowski GP, Rotondo MF (2001) Evolution in damage control with exsanguinating penetrating abdominal injury. J Trauma 49(6):1166

Lucas C, Ledgerwood A (1976) Prospective evaluation of hemostatic techniques for liver injuries. J Trauma 16:442–451

Miller RS, Morris JA Jr, Diaz JJ Jr, Herring MB, May AK (2005) Complications after 344 damage-control open celiotomies. J Trauma 59(6):1365

Moore EE, Burch JM, Franciose RJ, Offner PJ, Biffl WL (1998) Staged physiologic restoration and damage control surgery. World J Surg 22:1184–1190

Pringle J (1908) Notes on the arrest of hepatic hemorrhage due to trauma. Ann Surg 48:541–549

Reilly P, Rotondo M, Carpenter J, Sherr S, Schwab C (1995) Temporary vascular continuity in damage control: intraluminal shunting for proximal superior mesenteric artery injury. J Trauma 39:757–760

Rotondo MF, Zonies DH (1997) The damage control sequence and underlying logic. Surg Clin North Am 77:761–777

Rotondo MF, Schwab CW, McGonigal MD et al (1993) Damage control: an approach for improved survival in exsanguinating penetrating abdominal injury. J Trauma 35:375–382

Stone HH, Strom PR, Mullins RJ (1983) Management of the major coagulopathy with onset during laparotomy. Ann Surg 197:532–535

Teixeira PG, Inaba K, Salim A, Brown C, Rhee P, Browder T, Belzberg H, Demetriades D (2007) Retained foreign bodies after emergent trauma surgery: incidence after 2526 cavitary explorations. Am Surg 73(10):1031

Databank

▶ Trauma Registry

Database

▸ Trauma Registry

DCBI (Dismounted Complex Blast Injury)

▸ Military Trauma, Anesthesia for

DDAVP

Harvey G. Hawes[1], Bryan A. Cotton[1] and
Laura A. McElroy[2]
[1]Department of Surgery, Division of Acute Care
Surgery, Trauma and Critical Care, University of
Texas Health Science Center at Houston, The
University of Texas Medical School at Houston,
Houston, TX, USA
[2]Department of Anesthesiology, Critical Care
Medicine, University of Rochester Medical
Center, Rochester, NY, USA

Synonyms

Arginine vasopressin; 1-Desamino-8-D-arginine
vasopressin; Desmopressin

Definition

A synthetic analogue of vasopressin, initially utilized as a treatment for inherited bleeding disorders causing a lack of von Willebrand factor
(vWF) and coagulation factor VIII deficiency
hemophilia (Hemophilia A) (Federici and
Mannucci 2007). It is used in the treatment of
bleeding in mild von Willebrand disease or
hemophilia A and also has a role when used
prophylactically and perioperatively for these
patients.

Administration of DDAVP at a standard dose
of 0.3 µg/kg increases megameric vWF release
from endothelium, and factor VIII levels in
humans can augment primary hemostasis when
these factors are deficient. Dosing can be
repeated every 12 h for up to three days, through
tachyphylaxis or depressed response can be seen
as depletion of endogenous vWF occurs
(Schulman 2012). It can be administered in oral,
IV, or intranasally, and all seem to be similarly
efficacious. Adverse events include dilutional
hypernatremia with rare associated seizures and
thromboembolic events, especially coronary
artery thrombosis and myocardial infarction
after coronary artery bypass grafting (Federici
and Mannucci 2007).

DDAVP had been used specifically in high
blood loss surgeries such as CABG and partial
liver resection to mitigate blood loss, though the
data have not been convincing (Sniecinski and
Levy 2011). To support idea that DDAVP does
not alter significantly primary hemostasis in
patients without factor level deficiencies,
DDAVP had no demonstrable role in changing
thromboelastography on blood samples drawn on
normal control patients (Kawasaki et al. 2007).

Desmopressin has also been studied in reversing ADP-mediated antiplatelet effects of
clopidogrel preoperatively in carotid endarterectomy patients. DDAVP as treatment for uremic
syndrome associated bleeding has demonstrated
conflicting results. In patients with chronic uremia,
erythropoietin therapy has largely supplanted the
need for DDAVP (Ranucci et al. 2007).

For injured patients, DDAVP plays a role in
managing head-injured patients with intracranial
hemorrhage on antiplatelet therapy. These patients
have significant mortality and are a challenge to
treat (Sorensen et al. 2012). Though there are no
direct reversal agents for antiplatelet therapies
such as aspirin or the inopyridine clopidogrel and
ticlopidine, DDAVP has been included as therapy
in these patients along with platelet transfusion
(Campbell et al. 2010).

Cross-References

▸ Coagulopathy
▸ Factor I Concentrate

References

Campbell PG, Sen A, Yadia S et al (2010) Emergency reversal of antiplatelet agents in patients presenting with an intracranial hemorrhage: a clinical review. World Neurosurg 74(2–3):279–285. doi:10.1016/j.wneu.2010.05.030

Federici AB, Mannucci PM (2007) Management of inherited von Willebrand disease in 2007. Ann Med 39(5):346–358

Kawasaki J, Katori N, Taketomi T et al (2007) The effects of vasoactive agents, platelet agonists, and anticoagulation on thromboelastography. Acta Anaesthesiol Scand 51:1237–1244

Ranucci M, Nano G, Pazzaglia A et al (2007) Platelet mapping and desmopressin reversal of platelet inhibition during emergency carotid endarterectomy. J Cardiothorac Vasc Anesth 21(6):851–854

Schulman S (2012) Pharmacologic tools to reduce bleeding in surgery. Hematol Am Soc Hematol Educ Progr 12:517–521. doi:10.1182/asheducation-2012.1.517

Sniecinski RM, Levy JH (2011) Bleeding and management of coagulopathy. J Thorac Cardiovasc Surg 142(3):662–667

Sorensen B, Moore G, Hochleitner G et al (2012) Levels of fibrinogen and thromboelastometry fibrin polymerization following treatment with desmopressin (DDAVP). Thromb Res 129(4):e164–e165. doi:10.1016/j.thromres.2012.01.006

D-Dimer

Bryan A. Cotton[1,2] and Laura A. McElroy[2]
[1]Department of Surgery, Division of Acute Care Surgery, Trauma and Critical Care, University of Texas Health Science Center at Houston, The University of Texas Medical School at Houston, Houston, TX, USA
[2]Department of Anesthesiology, Critical Care Medicine, University of Rochester Medical Center, Rochester, NY, USA

Synonyms

XDP

Definition

D-dimers are small polypeptide products resulting from the fibrinolytic action of plasmin on fibrin. D-dimers were measured initially as an attempt to distinguish between fibrin and fibrinogen degradation products. During clot formation, fibrinogen is first converted to fibrin by the action of thrombin. This thrombin molecule then remains bound to fibrin and activates clotting factor XIII to XIIIa. The activated factor XIIIa then acts to cross-link fibrin fibrils. It is at this stage that activated plasmin binds and can lyse fibrin to its constituent parts, including D-dimers and fibrin degradation products (FDP) (Palareti 1993).

Strictly speaking, D-dimers consist of two polypeptide fibrin D subunits covalently linked to an E fragment (Gaffney 1975) that are the result of complete degradation of fibrin from a stable clot. Current generation assays measure D-dimer antigens, which could be high molecular weight soluble fibrin fragments that have either not entered a stable fibrin clot or are released before complete terminal fibrin degradation has occurred. Each manufacturer's assay system measures different epitopes, and standardization between each assay has been a subject of some controversy (Dempfle et al. 2001).

In practice, evaluation of the significance of D-dimer levels is placed in the context of assessment of the patient's clinical picture in addition to other investigations to diagnose venous thrombotic events such as deep venous thrombosis and pulmonary embolus. Fibrin degradation products also play a role in the diagnosis disseminated intravascular coagulopathy (DIC). Trauma, recent surgery, and other inciting inflammatory events can elevate D-dimer levels (Bates 2012), and examinations into the role of a thrombolytic phenotype of DIC early in severely injured patients have begun to include markedly elevated D-dimer levels as part of the diagnostic criteria (Sawamura et al. 2009).

Cross-References

▶ Disseminated Intravascular Coagulation
▶ Fibrinogen Split Products (Test)
▶ Pulmonary Embolus
▶ Venous Thromboembolism (VTE)

References

Bates SM (2012) D-Dimer assays in diagnosis and management of thrombotic and bleeding disorders. Semin Thromb Hemost 38(7):673–682. doi:10.1055/s-0032-1326782

Dempfle CE, Zips S, Ergul H et al (2001) The fibrin assay comparison trial (FACT): correlation of soluble fibrin assays with D-dimer. Thromb Haemost 86:1204–1209

Gaffney PJ (1975) Distinction between fibrinogen and fibrin degradation products in plasma. Clin Chim Acta 65(1):109–115

Palareti G (1993) Fibrinogen/fibrin degradation products: pathophysiology and clinical application. Fibrinolysis 7(1):60–61

Sawamura A, Hayakawa M, Gando S et al (2009) Disseminated intravascular coagulation with a fibrinolytic phenotype at an early phase of trauma predicts mortality. Thromb Res 124(5):608–613. doi:10.1016/j.thromres.2009.06.034

Deafferentation Pain

▶ Phantom Limb Pain

Death

▶ Brain Death, Ethical Concerns

Debridement

Charles A. Frosolone
Medical Department, USS Nimitz CVN-68, Everett, WA, USA

Synonyms

Excision of devitalized tissue; Wound excision; Wound incision and exploration

Definition

Debridement comes from the French *debrider*, meaning to unbridle. It came into use when an incision was made through investing fascia of a battlefield wound that unbridled, or released, the underlying expanding tissue. In the pre-Napoleonic era, some principles of debridement were developed and practiced but were largely forgotten in later conflicts. In the American Civil War, most wounds were not explored (97 %) with many deaths resulting from infection. After Lister's 1867 discovery of antiseptics, instead of debridement, antiseptics were used as treatment of gunshot-type extremity wounds. Due to the devastating wounds caused by the new weapons in WW1, the basic principles of debridement were developed by Belgian surgeon Antoine Depage and others. He showed that antiseptics should be an adjunct to wound care and that wounds needed to have foreign bodies and necrotic tissues removed (Helling and Daon 1998). These principles are still practiced today in care of battlefield wounds.

The goal in debridement is to save lives, preserve function, minimize morbidity, and prevent infections. The tissues devitalized by the high explosives form a culture medium for the bacteria introduced with the shell fragments, debris, or pieces of clothing, and they must be removed surgically (Emergency War Surgery 2004).

Timing: usually best within 6 h or as soon as possible.

Priority of treatment: antibiotics, life saving, limb saving by restoring perfusion/compartment release, and then debridement of soft tissues.

Technique: longitudinal incisions in the extremities allow for extension of the incision and more thorough visualization of the wound. Skin and subcutaneous tissues should, as a rule, not be extensively debrided, excising usually only a few mm of necrotic skin. Damaged or contaminated fat should be widely removed. Underlying fascia should be opened longitudinally to expose the full extent of the wound beneath and shredded fascia areas excised, performing full fasciotomy as indicated. Accurate assessment of muscle viability can be initially difficult, with obviously necrotic and contaminated muscle removed, and marginal muscle reexamined at a later surgery. To assess muscle viability the four Cs can be used: color, consistency, circulation, and contractility. Most reliable are circulation (bleeding) and consistency. Remove bone fragments that are not connected to soft tissues, avascular, necrotic, and less than thumbnail in size. Leave most nerves and tendons alone. Irrigate, not under high pressure, until wound is clean. Avoid packing as it inhibits drainage. Immobilize fractures: External fixation is best. No primary closure of extremity wounds. Do another look and debridement at about 24–72 h to maximize ultimate tissue salvage and extremity length. To spare resources the International Committee of Red Cross uses more aggressive initial debridement with no second look unless infection signs occur and delayed primary closure at 4–5 days (Gray 1994). Soft tissue coverage or closure if possible done at 5–6 days is optimum. Vacuum wound closure is very useful when available for closure. With multiple small superficial "peppering" by fragments with no evidence of underlying significant injuries, cleansing of the wounds and antibiotics is usually all that is necessary.

Cross-References

- ▶ Delayed Wound Closure
- ▶ Fragment Injury
- ▶ Negative Pressure Dressing

References

Emergency War Surgery. Third United States Revision (2004) Chapter 22: soft tissue injuries. Borden Institute, Washington, DC

Gray R (1994) War wounds, basic surgical management. International Committee of the Red Cross publication, Geneva

Helling TS, Daon E (1998) In flanders fields: the great war, Antoine Depage, and the resurgence of debridement. Ann Surg 228(2):173–181

Decision Making in Trauma Patients

- ▶ Informed Consent in Trauma

Decompression

- ▶ Cervical Spine Fractures, Indications for Surgery

Decubitus Ulcer

- ▶ Pressure Ulcer, Complication of Care in ICU

Decubitus Ulcer (Misnomer)

- ▶ Pressure Ulcers

Deep Vein Thrombosis

- ▶ DVT, as a Complication
- ▶ Neurotrauma, Anticoagulation Considerations
- ▶ Thromboembolic Disease

Deep Vein Thrombosis (DVT)

- ▶ Venous Thromboembolism Prophylaxis and Treatment Following Trauma

Deep Venous Thrombosis

- ▶ DVT, as a Complication

Deep Venous Thrombosis (DVT)

- ▶ Venous Thromboembolism Prophylaxis in the Intensive Care Unit

Defibrillation

▶ Cardiopulmonary Resuscitation in Adult Trauma

Definitive Airway

▶ Airway Management in Trauma, Nonsurgical

Delayed Diagnosis/Missed Injury

Jason Moore
Department of Surgery, Lawnwood Regional Medical Center, Fort Pierce, FL, USA

Synonyms

Misdiagnosis; Untreated injury

Definition

Despite the many advances in medical technology and the development of guidelines for the appropriate diagnosis and treatment of medical conditions, there are still patients who unfortunately do not receive the proper treatment. There is no other patient who has more potential to suffer from this problem than the acutely ill trauma patient with multiple injuries. Although not frequently life-threatening, these missed injuries may result in significant long-term disability. Furthermore, a missed injury may stand out as the most memorable event in a patient's course, overshadowing the heroic efforts of the trauma surgeon and trauma team. In addition to proving embarrassing to the surgeon and institution, missed injuries are a common reason for litigation (Biffl et al. 2003). The missed injury may lead to a delay in diagnosis which can significantly add to the morbidity of the initial insult and may result in permanent disability or even mortality.

Furthermore, missed injuries may contribute to greater length of stay in the hospital and increased patient costs (Stawicki and Lindsey 2009).

For the purposes of this discussion, the definition of delay in diagnosis is when an injury is identified sometime after the initial diagnostic phase of resuscitation, but before the injury presents itself as a clinical problem. A missed injury occurs when the injury is not diagnosed in a timely fashion but is later discovered after it causes clinical symptoms. The common ideology that is understood from these two definitions is that the injury would normally have been detected in an awake, alert patient who had the appropriate clinical investigation and diagnostic studies performed (Stawicki and Lindsey 2009). We will review common reasons associated with missed injuries and emphasize the steps that members of the trauma team can take to minimize delays in diagnosis.

Preexisting Condition

There are many possible reasons why missed injuries and delays in diagnosis occur. The etiology of "missed injury" is multifactorial and involves the interplay of the key elements of patient, provider, and environment (Stawicki and Lindsey 2009). Throughout the literature, the two broad categories of missed injuries are avoidable and unavoidable. In general, the factors most commonly implicated in unavoidable types of missed injuries include altered level of consciousness because of brain injury, intoxication, or sedation, hemodynamic or respiratory compromise, delayed assessment, distracting injuries, multiple injuries, presence of traumatic or pharmacologic paralysis, and delayed presentation (Stawicki and Lindsey 2009). Any of these may require immediate operative intervention or transfer to the ICU before the completion of the secondary survey. The most commonly cited factors for potentially avoidable missed injuries are inadequate initial or post-admission clinical exam (over 50 % of cases), trauma team inexperience, overall urgency of the clinical situation, and numerous factors related to radiologic workup (appropriate test not ordered, testing delayed, technically inadequate study, radiologist level of experience, or misinterpretation) (Stawicki and Lindsey 2009).

Application

Overall, the most commonly missed injuries are fractures. By region, the extremity injuries are mostly fractures, and thorax injuries are aortic rupture, rib fractures, pneumothorax, and hemothorax. Abdominal injuries include solid organ, intestinal, and diaphragm injuries. Missed skull and facial fractures are routinely reported, as well as spine and pelvic fractures (Smith et al. 2008). According to the literature focusing on missed injuries, the three most common anatomic regions are extremities (52 %), thorax (15 %), and abdomen (13 %), with head and spine injuries not far behind (Stawicki and Lindsey 2009). Of note, only a relatively small number of missed injuries required procedural interventions, while most were treated nonoperatively. In two studies, 11 % and 12 % of patients with missed injuries were clinically significant, and 14 % and 50 % of these injuries, respectively, were associated with mortality (Stawicki and Lindsey 2009). Other reported rates of missed injuries vary from 2 % to 50 %. These missed injuries are more common in those in motor vehicle crashes, those with higher injury severity scores, and those with a greater number of injuries (Smith et al. 2008).

The American College of Surgeons Advanced Trauma Life Support (ATLS) course provides a framework for the systematic evaluation of the injured patient and is considered the gold standard (Smith et al. 2008). The primary survey is designed to recognize and treat immediately life-threatening problems within minutes of arrival. The secondary survey is described as a head-to-toe examination, including "tubes and fingers in every orifice," and is intended to diagnose all injuries before formulating a definitive management strategy (Biffl et al. 2003). Unfortunately, it is widely recognized that not every injury is identified at the time of presentation due to factors mentioned above which may especially interfere with completing the secondary survey. This will lead to missed injuries of the unavoidable and avoidable types.

We can strive to improve both types; however, limited improvement is to be expected in unavoidable types of missed injury as we have little control in how patients present. This leaves room for improvement in the avoidable types when the trauma team matures and a higher index of clinical suspicion arises while assessing patients with an altered level of consciousness, hemodynamic or respiratory compromise, distracting and/or multiple injuries, and presence of paralysis. Improvements in radiologic studies are to be expected as well.

Finally, the use of a tertiary survey has been found to decrease the number of missed injuries in many institutions and trauma centers. It consists of a complete head-to-toe examination with additional radiographic or other investigation as necessary on all patients admitted to the trauma service within 24 h of admission and after all contributing sources of examination difficulty have resolved (Smith et al. 2008). ATLS emphasizes frequent reevaluations; however, the tertiary survey prompts the trauma team to do another complete exam on all patients in a timely fashion, which can yield new findings.

It is ideal that all trauma centers strive to decrease the incidence of missed injuries and delays in diagnosis. We must be cognizant of the fact that our ever-changing health-care system may not have the resources needed to reduce these events. Trauma team members must be more aware of missed injuries and eliminate pathways that lead to their persistent appearance. The tertiary survey is fast, practices good patient care, and should be performed in a timely fashion in all trauma patients. Notably, it may detect new injuries and potentially decrease harmful outcomes for patients and increase good outcomes for physicians.

Cross-References

▶ Diaphragmatic Injuries
▶ Head Injury
▶ Motor Vehicle Crash Injury

► Pelvis Fractures
► Pneumothorax
► Retained Hemothorax
► Sedation and Analgesia
► Teamwork and Trauma Care
► Thoracic Vascular Injuries

References

Biffl WL, Harrington DT, Cioffi WG (2003) Implementation of a tertiary survey decreases missed injuries. J Trauma 54:38–44
Smith RS, Nold RJ, Dort JM (2008) Common errors in trauma care. In: Asensio JA, Trunkey DD (eds) Current therapy of trauma and surgical critical care, 1st edn. Mosby/Elsevier, Philadelphia, pp 583–588
Stawicki SP, Lindsey DE (2009) Trauma corner – missed traumatic injuries: a synopsis. OPUS 12 Sci 3(2):35–43

Delayed Primary Closure

► Delayed Wound Closure

Delayed Splenic Rupture

Khanjan H. Nagarsheth
R Adams Cowley Shock Trauma Center,
University of Maryland School of Medicine,
Baltimore, MD, USA

Synonyms

Latent period of Baudet

Definition

Delayed splenic rupture (DSR) is a scene of blunt splenic injury in the form of significant hemorrhage from a ruptured spleen more than 48 h after injury. The 48-h time interval is also known as the latent period; it is named after Baudet who first described this entity in 1907 (Baudet 1907).

Preexisting Condition

The spleen is the most frequently injured organ after blunt trauma. The reported incidence of DSR spans a wide range from 0.3 % to 24 % when looking through the literature (Peitzman and Richardson 2010). The true significance of this entity lies in the mortality rates. It has been noted that the mortality rate from DSR is 5–15 %, whereas the mortality for an acute splenic rupture is in the realm of 1 % (Cogbill et al. 1989). In recent years, the incidence has decreased, possibly due to the use of multi-detector computed tomography (MDCT) to make the diagnosis of splenic injury and a more sophisticated method of treating splenic injuries, such as nonoperative management (NOM) with splenic artery embolization (SAE).

There are several large reviews of the literature that look at the true incidence of DSR. A large review looking at 306 cases of DSR in the literature found that 80 % of patients with DSR ruptured within 14 days of their injury and 95 % of patients with DSR ruptured within 21 days of their injury (Sizer et al. 1966). Another such review was performed by Gamblin et al. This group found the mean day of rupture was day 13 post injury (range 2–30 days). In this series, they found one death and one patient management with NOM, everyone else received a splenectomy (Gamblin et al. 2005).

Application

The majority of reported cases of DSR are based on clinical suspicions and did not have an initial MDCT scan to verify that they were truly delayed ruptures. With this in mind, many experts believe an initial CT scan needs to be performed to show the presence of a splenic injury if a diagnosis of DSR is to be made later.

There have been several theories proposed as to why DSR is seen. Some of these theories revolve around the protocol that was used to obtain the initial CT images. For example, if the images are obtained too early after the trauma, some injuries like subcapsular hemorrhages may not be seen (Kluger et al. 1994). Another theory involves the timing and quantity of intravenous contrast material given during these scans. Scans performed before the peak arterial contrast bolus peak result in images with a very heterogeneous appearing spleen and images obtained after the peak yield images that are suboptimal as injuries may be missed due to the phenomenon known as "fill-in," where contrast will obscure the injuries (Gamblin et al. 2005).

These studies and findings have raised the question of whether a repeated CT scan is necessary in patients with splenic injury, who have been deemed candidates for NOM. Typically, patients who exhibit signs of hemodynamic instability have a significant drop in their hemoglobin levels or have worsened abdominal tenderness and will get a repeat CT scan looking for DSR. It has been recommended that all patients who sustained blunt splenic injury should undergo repeat CT scan to identify arterial pseudoaneurysm formation or worsening injury (Weinberg et al. 2007). In general, DSR should be kept in the differential diagnosis for patients who recently sustained blunt splenic injury and have the aforementioned signs.

Patients in whom DSR is identified usually managed with splenectomy. Several studies reviewing DSR found that simple splenectomy was the preferred method of treatment in the majority of patients (Farhat et al. 1992). The use of NOM and SAE in the setting of DSR has been advocated because of a high rate of success in preserving the spleen and avoiding the immunologic and physical morbidities associated with splenectomy (Liu 2012). This group found a success rate of 83 % for NOM of DSR and a splenic salvage rate of 80 % in those treated with SAE. This group feels that NOM and SAE are not superior to surgical therapy. Instead NOM and SAE for DSR should be used in conjunction with surgical splenectomy when necessary.

Delayed splenic rupture after blunt splenic injury is an entity that has been described in the literature but is still seen relatively infrequently in clinical practice. When patients do have DSR, it can be anywhere from post-injury day two to thirty, so a high clinical suspicion should be kept in patients who have a recent history of blunt abdominal injury and worsening hemodynamics or physical exam. Imaging should be obtained if possible, in the form of a CT scan. The mainstay of treatment has been surgical splenectomy, but more recently, NOM and SAE have been gaining more importance for their role in the treatment of DSR.

Cross-References

▶ Thoracic Vascular Injuries

References

Baudet R (1907) Ruptures de la rate. Med Practique 3:565

Cogbill TH, Moore EE, Jurkovich GJ et al (1989) Nonoperative management of blunt splenic trauma: a multicenter experience. J Trauma 29(10):1312–1317

Farhat GA, Abdu RA, Vanek VW (1992) Delayed splenic rupture: real or imaginary? Am Surg 58:340–345

Gamblin TC, Wall CE Jr, Royer GM, Dalton ML, Ashley DW (2005) Delayed splenic rupture: case reports and review of the literature. J Trauma 59:1231–1234

Kluger Y, Paul DB, Raves JJ, Fonda M, Young JC, Townsend RN et al (1994) Delayed rupture of the spleen–myths, facts, and their importance: case reports and literature review. J Trauma 36(4):568–571

Liu PP, Liu HT, Hsieh TM, Huang CY, Ko SF (2012) Nonsurgical managment of delayed splenic rupture after blunt trauma. J Trauma 72:1019–1023

Peitzman AB, Richardson JD (2010) Surgical treatment of injuries to the solid abdominal organs: a 50-year perspective from the Journal of Trauma. J Trauma 69:1011–1021

Sizer JS, Wayne ER, Frederick PL (1966) Delayed rupture of the spleen: review of the literature and report of six cases. Arch Surg 92:362–366

Weinberg JA, Magnotti LJ, Croce MA, Edwards NM, Fabian TC (2007) The utility of serial computed tomography imaging of blunt splenic injury: still worth a second look? J Trauma 62(5):1143–1147; discussion 1147–1148

Delayed Stress Disorder

▶ Post Traumatic Stress Disorder

Delayed Stress Syndrome

▶ Post Traumatic Stress Disorder

Delayed Wound Closure

Mahmoud A. Amr
Division of Trauma, Critical Care, and General
Surgery, Mayo Clinic, Rochester, MN, USA

Synonyms

Delayed primary closure; Healing by secondary
and tertiary intention; Negative pressure dressing

Definition

A wound is defined as a disruption of the integrity
of normal anatomic structure with the subsequent
effect on its function (Lazarus et al. 1994).
Healing is a dynamic and interactive process
which aims to restore the anatomic structure and
function. This process is divided into three
phases: inflammatory, proliferative, and tissue
remodeling.

The decision on how to close the wound
depends on the type of wound, mechanism of
injury, and time elapsed from the injury.

In clean surgical wounds, closure is accomplished by primary intention which is performed
by re-approximation of the two edges of the
wound using sutures, staples, or adhesive tapes.

In case of major trauma wherein significant
tissue loss has occurred, primary closure is
contraindicated, and the wound is left open to
be closed by secondary intention, which involves
the formation of granulation tissue and contraction. Healing takes place from the base upward
and from the edges inward (Armitage and
Lockwood 2011). The underlying mechanism of
this process is the interaction between specialized
fibroblasts referred to as myofibroblasts and the
matrix components (Tomasek et al. 2002).

When wounds are presented late, more than 6 h,
or contaminated but are not involved with significant tissue loss, then closure needs to be delayed
for 3–7 days, depending on the severity of injury
and the contamination extent. Prior to closure,
these wounds require frequent debridement and
irrigation to restore as much healthy tissue as
needed to make the closure possible. The extent
of debridement can be determined by the presence
of bleeding which indicates having viable tissue
imminent to be closed safely by primary closure or
secondary intention, depending on the size of the
wound. The reason behind this procedure is to
prevent wound infections and the subsequent complications of abnormal wound healing, especially
wound ulcers.

Delayed wound closure is also applicable in
abdominal wounds after damage control laparotomies, in which primary closure is challenging, with
possible tissue necrosis, fascial dehiscence, and
wound infection. Moreover, primary closure may
cause increased intra-abdominal pressure which
may lead to abdominal compartment syndrome
with the subsequent complications (Howdieshell
et al. 1995). During this period, temporary closure
can be achieved by several methods, such as vacuum packing, silastic sheeting and abdominal fascial prostheses like the Wittmann Patch.

Another application of delayed wound closure
would be in war high-energy injuries. This can be
attained by the utilization of negative pressure
dressing (vacuum-assisted closure) which
facilitates the wound closure while decreasing
the hospital stay, frequency of dressing, and
infection rate. The physiologic benefits of such
a dressing include clearance of wound exudate,
enhanced granulation from local vasodilation,
and mechanical wound contraction because of
pressure differential (Leininger et al. 2006).

Cross-References

▶ ABThera Wound Dressing
▶ Amputation
▶ Debridement
▶ Negative Pressure Dressing

References

Armitage J, Lockwood S (2011) Skin incisions and wound closure. Surgery (Oxford) 29(10):496–501

Howdieshell TR, Yeh KA et al (1995) Temporary abdominal wall closure in trauma patients: indications, technique, and results. World J Surg 19(1):154–158; discussion 158

Lazarus GS, Cooper DM et al (1994) Definitions and guidelines for assessment of wounds and evaluation of healing. Wound Repair Regen 2(3):165–170

Leininger BE, Rasmussen TE et al (2006) Experience with wound VAC and delayed primary closure of contaminated soft tissue injuries in Iraq. J Trauma 61(5):1207–1211

Tomasek JJ, Gabbiani G et al (2002) Myofibroblasts and mechano-regulation of connective tissue remodelling. Nat Rev Mol Cell Biol 3(5):349–363

Delbet Classification

▶ Pediatric Fractures About the Hip

Delegated Choice

▶ Surrogate, Role in Decision-Making

Delirium as a Complication of ICU Care

Lisa D. Burry[1] and Louise Rose[2]
[1]Department of Pharmacy, Mount Sinai Hospital, Toronto, ON, Canada
[2]Lawrence S. Bloomberg Faculty of Nursing, University of Toronto, Toronto, ON, Canada

Synonyms

Acute brain dysfunction; Acute confusion; Agitation; ICU psychosis

Definition

The *Diagnostic and Statistical Manual of Mental Disorders* (DSM-IV) defines delirium as (1) a disturbance of consciousness with inattention, accompanied by (2) acute change in cognition not accounted for by preexisting, established, or evolving dementia; (3) development over a short period of time (hours to days) with fluctuation over time; and (4) evidence that the disturbance is caused by the direct physiological consequences of a general medical condition.

Delirium can be characterized as either *hyperactive* with increased psychomotor activity and agitation; *hypoactive* with somnolence, lethargy, and decreased psychomotor behavior; or *mixed*. The majority of cases present with hypoactive or mixed delirium; purely hyperactive delirium is rare (<2 %) (Girard et al. 2008). Some patients develop subsyndromal delirium, or one or more of the features of delirium, but never meet full diagnostic criteria.

In general, the symptoms of delirium overlap with other psychiatric disorders, making recognition a challenge. Differential diagnoses include delirium tremens, dementia, acute psychiatric syndromes, and severe depression.

Preexisting Condition

Pathophysiology

Despite increasing number of publications describing incidence, prevalence, and etiology of delirium in the ICU in the last decade, the pathophysiology is still poorly understood. Most studies supporting the current theories of etiology have been conducted in noncritically ill patients. Current theories in the critically ill include (Girard et al. 2008):

- Neurotransmitter imbalance – imbalance of synthesis, release, and inactivation of neurotransmitters is thought to result in neuronal instability and unpredictable neurotransmission. In particular, excessive dopamine and depletion of acetylcholine is thought to occur.
- Inflammation – inflammatory mediators produced during critical illness are thought to cross the blood-brain barrier and alter cerebral blood flow and alter neurotransmitter synthesis and transmission.

- Impaired oxidative metabolism – a global reduction of cerebral oxidative metabolism is thought to result in an imbalance of neurotransmission.
- Availability of large neutral amino acids – neurotransmitter levels and function are thought to be affected by altered concentrations of amino acids. For example, large neutral amino acids such as tyrosine and phenylalanine compete with the precursor for serotonin, tryptophan, for transport across the blood-brain barrier. Large uptake of tryptophan and phenylalanine may lead to elevated levels of dopamine and norepinephrine.

Prevalence

Prevalence of delirium in the critically ill ranges from 20 % to 80 %, depending on detection methods and the population evaluated (Girard et al. 2008). Prevalence was 67 % in a cohort of 54 trauma ICU patients and 73 % in 46 surgical ICU patients (Pandharipande et al. 2008), slightly less than the 82 % detected in a study of 224 medical-coronary ICU patients (Ely et al. 2004).

Prognostic Significance

The presence of delirium is consistently associated with multiple complications and adverse outcomes. Delirious patients are at greater risk of self-extubation, accidental removal of other medical devices, and are more likely to be physically restrained. After adjusting for comorbidities and severity of illness, delirium has been associated with increased durations of mechanical ventilation, ICU, and hospital stay, less likely to be discharged home, higher ICU, and hospital costs, and increased 6-month mortality (Ely et al. 2001, 2004). Subsyndromal delirium also has been linked to worse outcomes, including increased mortality compared to patients who do not develop delirium (Ouimet et al. 2007).

Application

Risk Factors

The list of potential risk factors for delirium is long (Table 1). Non-modifiable risk factors

Delirium as a Complication of ICU Care, Table 1 Risk factors for delirium

Non-modifiable	Modifiable
Age	Physical restraints
Gender	Invasive lines and catheters
History of ethanol	Pain
History of smoking	Sleep and sensory deprivation (e.g., nonavailability of hearing devices)
Hypertension	Loss of day-night cycle
Cognitive impairment (e.g., dementia)	Medications (benzodiazepines)
Severity of illness	Infection and sepsis
Depression	Hypoxemia
APO-E4 polymorphism	Dehydration
Vision and hearing impairment	Electrolyte disturbances (hyponatremia, hypocalcemia)
	Azotemia
	Hyperbilirubinemia
	Acidosis
	Anemia
	Urinary retention or constipation

include age, prior nervous system diseases, dementia, smoking or ethanol abuse, and comorbidities such as hypertension. A recent retrospective cohort study of 504,839 trauma patients established the following as independent risk factors for delirium: age >55 years, male gender, intoxication on admission, chronic ethanol use, history of cardiovascular disease, and ICU admission (Branco et al. 2011).

Modifiable risk factors include sleep deprivation, infection, physical restraint use, indwelling catheters, vision impairment, and polypharmacy. Medications with high anticholinergic properties (e.g., antinauseants), sedatives, and opioids may increase the risk of developing delirium (Clegg and Young 2010). Centrally acting anticholinergic medications can cross the blood-brain barrier and block muscarinic receptors resulting in dramatic delirium (e.g., "mad as a hatter"). Medications may be the sole precipitant for 12–39 % of delirium (Clegg and Young 2010). Given the evidence linking delirium to adverse patient outcomes, delirium prevention interventions and risk factor modification are important clinical priorities.

Sedatives and opioids are thought to play a key role in the development of delirium. Interestingly, not only exposure to sedation but also type of sedation may influence development of delirium. In a recent cohort study of trauma ICU patients, the strongest independent risk factor for delirium was midazolam exposure (odds ratio: 2.75) (Pandharipande et al. 2008). Similarly a number of studies involving mixed patient ICU populations identified lorazepam as a weak to moderate risk factor for delirium (Clegg and Young 2010). Furthermore, there may be a dose response, particularly when lorazepam is used to induce coma (Ouimet et al. 2007). Trials with dexmedetomidine, a new α_2-agonist sedative with some analgesic properties, showed more days alive without delirium or coma compared to lorazepam in mixed ICU populations (Pandharipande et al. 2007). Despite this advantage this sedative is not routinely used in clinical practice due to adverse effects such as bradycardia and high acquisition costs.

The link between opiate exposure and delirium has not been consistently demonstrated. For example, Pandharipande and colleagues showed fentanyl to be associated with increased delirium in surgical ICU patients but not trauma ICU patients, while morphine was associated with a lower risk of delirium in both surgical and trauma ICU patients (Pandharipande et al. 2008). Ouimet and colleagues (2007) identified higher mean daily doses of morphine among non-delirious ICU patients. In situations where severe, acute pain is common, lower doses of opioids may be associated with higher risk of delirium inferring that untreated pain contributes to delirium development (Ouimet et al. 2007). In contrast, Dubois and colleagues found morphine to be the strongest predictor of delirium using a multivariable model in mixed ICU population (Dubois et al. 2001).

Recognition of Delirium

Use of a daily screening tool to identify delirium is necessary to prompt investigation and treatment of this condition that may otherwise be missed, particularly for patients with hypoactive delirium. Although this practice is endorsed by various practice guidelines endorsed by professional societies, survey data indicate routine screening has yet to be adopted into clinical practice.

The gold standard to diagnose delirium is a psychiatrist assessment using the Diagnostic and Statistical Manual of Mental Disorders (DSM-IV) criteria, taking approximately 30 min. Multiple screening tools are now available; the two most common are the Confusion Assessment Method for the ICU (CAM-ICU) and Intensive Care Delirium Screening Checklist (ICDSC) (Ely et al. 2001; Bergeron et al. 2001). These screening tools rapidly (<5 min) identify delirium by nonpsychiatrists in ventilated and non-ventilated ICU patients. The CAM-ICU initially evaluates level of consciousness or arousal with the Richmond Agitation-Sedation Scale (RASS), a 10-point scale ranging from −5 (no response to voice or physical stimulation) to +4 (overtly combative or violent) (Ely et al. 2001). Patients with a RASS score > −3 are then assessed for delirium by testing for the four features of delirium ((1) acute change or fluctuation in mental status, (2) inattention, and either (3) disorganized thinking or (4) altered level of consciousness).

Both tools are validated against the gold standard, psychiatrist interview. The CAM-ICU has demonstrated very high sensitivity (93–100 %), specificity (89–100 %), and interrater reliability (k 0.96) in multiple ICU patient populations. The ICDSC also requires assessment of level of consciousness before applying the tool (Bergeron et al. 2001). For non-comatose or stuporous patients, the eight-item checklist is applied. A score of ≥4 (range 0–8) has demonstrated excellent sensitivity (99 %) and good specificity (64 %) in a mixed ICU population. The ICDSC can also identify subsyndromal delirium (score of 1–3).

Prevention

Multicomponent interventions that target modifiable risk factors demonstrate reductions in

Delirium as a Complication of ICU Care, Table 2 Controlled trials evaluating treatment of delirium in the ICU

Author (year)	Study design	Population N	Diagnosis of delirium	Interventions	Significant findings
Girard et al. (2010)	Placebo controlled, double-blind RCT	N = 101 MSICU patients	CAM-ICU	Ziprasidone (oral/IM) versus haloperidol (oral/IM) versus placebo up to 14 days	Primary endpoint:
		Delirium @ study entry: 49 %		Dose of study drug titrated	Days alive without coma or delirium – median: haloperidol (14.0 days, IQR 6.0–18.0) versus ziprasidone (15.0, IQR 9.1–18.0) versus placebo (12.5 days, IQR 1.2–17.2); $p = 0.66$
		Coma @ study entry: 36 %		Method of concomitant sedation: per ICU team, weaned off sedation when patient over-sedated	Average dose of study drug per day, in haloperidol equivalents: ziprasidone 3.8 mg, haloperidol 15 mg
		Mechanical ventilation: 100 %			No difference in serious adverse events
		APACHE II (mean): 26			
Devlin et al. (2010)	Placebo controlled, double-blind RCT	N = 36 MSICU patients	ICDSC	Quetiapine oral versus placebo	Primary endpoint:
		Delirium @ study entry: 100 %	Score ≥ 4	Dose of study drug titrated	Time to first resolution of delirium (ICDSC ≤ 3) – median: quetiapine 1.0 days, IQR 0.5–3 versus placebo 4.5 days, IQR 2.0–7.0; $p = 0.001$
		Coma @ study entry: 0 %		Method of concomitant sedation: per ICU team, weaned off sedation when patient over-sedated	No difference in mortality (quetiapine 11 % vs. placebo 17 %) or ICU median length of stay (quetiapine 16 days vs. placebo 16 days)
		Mechanical ventilation: 81 %			Average dose of study drug per day, in haloperidol equivalents: quetiapine 2.9 mg
		Age (mean): 62 years			No difference in the episodes of QTc prolongation or extrapyramidal effects
		APACHE II (mean): 20			
Strobik et al. (2004)	RCT, no placebo	N = 73 MSICU patients	ICDSC	Olanzapine oral versus haloperidol oral for 5 days	Primary endpoint:
		Delirium @ study entry: 100 %		Dose of study drug not titrated	Delirium severity: In the 5 days after randomization, both the magnitude of delirium severity (ICDSC score) and the proportion of patients administered ≥ 1 dose of a benzodiazepine agent were similar in the two groups

(continued)

Delirium as a Complication of ICU Care, Table 2 (continued)

Author (year)	Study design	Population		Diagnosis of delirium	Interventions	Significant findings
		N				
		Coma @ study entry: 0 %			Method of concomitant sedation: as per ICU team, titrated to desired Ramsey goal	Average dose of study drug per day in haloperidol equivalents: olanzapine 4.5 mg, haloperidol 6.5 mg
		Mechanical ventilation: 78 %				
		Age (mean): 65 years				
		APACHE II (mean): 13				No adverse effects were attributed to olanzapine; 6 patients receiving haloperidol had low Simpson-Angus Scale scores when tests for presence of extrapyramidal symptoms

APACHE II Acute Physiologic and Chronic Health Evaluation, *CAM-ICU* Confusion Assessment Method for the ICU, *ICDSC* Intensive Care Delirium Screening Checklist, *MSICU* medical-surgical ICU, *N/A* not available, *IQR* interquartile range

incidence and delirium duration and improved clinical outcomes, including mortality, in hospitalized geriatric and surgical patients (Lundstrom et al. 2005). Interventions include medication review, sedation minimization, sleep promotion, and restoration of the sleep-wake cycle; frequent reorientation to person-place-time; removal of unnecessary catheters; reintroduction of eye glasses and hearing aids; adequate hydration; correction of electrolytes; and early mobilization. Although the ability of these strategies to modify delirium risk in ICU populations has yet to be confirmed in rigorous trials, strategies should be implemented into clinical practice as they address known risk factors.

Treatment

To date, little evidence is available for treatment of ICU delirium, and there are no trials evaluating pharmacologic treatment in surgical patients (Table 2). The antipsychotic agent haloperidol is endorsed as first-line therapy by professional society practice guidelines; however, evidence for this recommendation arises primarily from non-ICU studies. Girard and colleagues showed similar median duration of days alive without delirium and coma for patients treated with haloperidol, ziprasidone, or placebo and no difference in adverse drug events (Girard et al. 2010). In a pilot study, quetiapine was compared to placebo in 36 patients diagnosed with delirium based on ICDSC screening (Devlin et al. 2010). Quetiapine resulted in faster first resolution of delirium (3.5 days), reduced duration of delirium, and fewer hours of agitation, defined as Sedation-Agitation Scale score ≥ 5.

National and international practice surveys demonstrate increasing use of antipsychotics in the ICU, even in the absence of routine delirium screening, and lack of strong evidence indicating that antipsychotic treatment reduces the duration of delirium or improves outcomes. When delirium occurs, the use of drug interventions only should be considered after a thorough evaluation for predisposing and precipitating risk factors. Clinicians must also consider adverse effects associated with antipsychotics such as extrapyramidal and anticholinergic effects, neuroleptic malignant syndrome, QT prolongation, and increased mortality in elderly patients.

Cross-References

▶ Sedation, Analgesia, Neuromuscular Blockade in the ICU

References

Bergeron N, Dubois MJ, Dumont M et al (2001) Intensive Care Delirium Screening Checklist: evaluation of a new screening tool. Intensive Care Med 27:859–864

Branco BC, Inava K, Bukur M et al (2011) Risk factors for delirium in trauma patients: the impact of ethanol use and lack of insurance. Am Surg 77(5):621–626

Clegg A, Young JB (2010) Systematic review: which medications to avoid in people at risk of delirium. Age Ageing 0:1–7

Devlin J, Roberts RJ, Fong J et al (2010) Efficacy and safety of quetiapine in critically ill patients with delirium: a prospective, multicenter, randomized, double-blind, placebo-controlled pilot study. Crit Care Med 38(2):419–427

Dubois MJ, Bergeron N, Dumont M et al (2001) Delirium in an intensive care unit: a study of risk factors. Intensive Care Med 27:1297–1304

Ely EW, Gautam S, Margolin R et al (2001a) The impact of delirium in the intensive care unit on hospital length of stay. Intensive Care Med 27:1892–1900

Ely EW, Margolin R, Francis J et al (2001b) Evaluation of delirium in critically ill patients: validation of the Confusion Assessment Method for the Intensive Care Unit (CAM-ICU). Crit Care Med 29:1370–1379

Ely EW, Shintani A, Truman B et al (2004) Delirium as a predictor of mortality in mechanically ventilated patients in the intensive care unit. JAMA 14:1753–1762

Girard TD, Pandharipande PP, Ely EW (2008) Delirium in the intensive care unit. Crit Care 12(Suppl 3):S3

Girard T, Pandharipande P, Carson SS et al (2010) Feasibility, efficacy, and safety of antipsychotics for intensive care unit delirium: the MIND randomized, placebo-controlled trial. Crit Care Med 38:428–437

Lundstrom M, Edlund A, Karlsson S et al (2005) A multifactorial intervention program reduces the duration of delirium, length of hospitalization, and mortality in delirious patients. J Am Geriatr Soc 53:622–628

Ouimet S, Kavanagh BP, Gottfried SB, Skrobik Y (2007a) Incidence, risk factors and consequences of ICU delirium. Intensive Care Med 33:66–73

Ouimet S, Riker R, Bergeron N et al (2007b) Subsyndromal delirium in the ICU: evidence for a disease spectrum. Intensive Care Med 33(6):1007–1013

Pandharipande P, Pun B, Herr D et al (2007) Effect of sedation with dexmedetomidine vs. lorazepam on acute brain dysfunction in mechanically ventilated patients. The MENDS randomized controlled trial. JAMA 298(22):2644–2653

Pandharipande P, Cotton B, Shintani A et al (2008) Prevalence and risk factors for development of delirium in surgical and trauma intensive care unit patients. J Trauma 65:34–41

Recommended Reading

Gill SS, Bronskill S, Normand S et al (2007) Antipsychotic drug use and mortality in older adults with dementia. Ann Intern Med 146:775–786

Jackson JC, Gordon SM, Hart RP et al (2004) The association between delirium and cognitive decline: a review of the empirical literature. Neuropsychol Rev 14(2):87–98

Metha S, McCullagh I, Burry L (2009) Current sedation practices: lessons learned from international surveys. Critical Care Clin 25(3):471–488

Peterson JF, Pun B, Dittus RS, Thomason JW et al (2006) Delirium and its motoric subtypes: a study of 614 critically ill patients. J Am Geriatr Soc 54:479–484

Delirium Tremens

▶ Alcohol (ETOH) Withdrawal and Management
▶ Alcohol Withdrawal

Dens Fracture

▶ Fracture, Odontoid

Department of Defense Trauma Registry (DoDTR)

▶ Joint Trauma Registry
▶ Joint Trauma System (JTS)

Department of Defense Trauma System (DoDTS)

▶ Joint Trauma System (JTS)

Depressed Reflexes in Spinal Cord Injury

▶ Spinal Shock

1-Desamino-8-d-Arginine Vasopressin

▶ DDAVP

Desanguination Transfusion

▶ Massive Transfusion and Complications

Desmopressin

▶ DDAVP

Detonation

▶ Explosion

Dexamethasone

▶ Steroids, Use of in Acute Spinal cord Injury

Diabetes Insipidus

Jason Moore
Department of Surgery, Lawnwood Regional
Medical Center, Fort Pierce, FL, USA

Definition

Injuries that affect the brain can interrupt the hypothalamus or pituitary production of hormones. Head injury, brain surgery, mass lesions, infiltrative diseases, vascular or hypoxic injuries, and cerebral infections are all causes of failure of the releasing of pituitary hormones which may result in one or more abnormalities (Falvo and Horst 2008). Diabetes insipidus (DI) is a disorder characterized by excretion of large quantities of dilute urine due to an absolute or relative deficiency of antidiuretic hormone (ADH), referred to as central DI, or renal resistance to the effects of ADH, known as nephrogenic DI. Primary central DI is caused by inherited or idiopathic disorders that reduce the number of hypothalamic nuclei. Secondary central DI is more common and is caused by a variety of pathologic lesion of the neurohypophysis including those mentioned above. The renal resistance to ADH that causes nephrogenic DI may be due to an inherited or acquired disorder, such as drugs, renal damage, hypercalcemia, or hypokalemia. DI may be temporary or permanent depending on the etiology (Veloski and Brennan 2010).

Arginine vasopressin aka ADH is produced in the supraoptic and paraventricular nuclei of the hypothalamus, circulates down the pituitary stalk, and is stored in the posterior lobe of the pituitary gland. ADH works to increase water reabsorption at the level of the renal collecting ducts (Veloski and Brennan 2010). Complications arise when cerebral edema or increased intracranial pressures restrict the blood flow, disrupting the hypothalamic-pituitary axis, and these problems manifest as abnormalities of sodium and water balance (Falvo and Horst 2008).

These imbalances can lead to patients presenting with polyuria (urine output exceeding 3 L/day) secondary to the inability to reabsorb water and concentrate urine. Therefore, these patients are thirsty and dehydrated and may also be hypernatremic (Veloski and Brennan 2010). The diagnosis is made with a urine osmolality of <300 mOsm/kg H_2O and urine specific gravity of <1.005. Urine osmolality of >800 mOsm/kg H_2O excludes DI (Falvo and Horst 2008). A serum osmolarity >295 mOsm/kg H_2O, or serum sodium ≥ 145 mEq/L with continued diuresis of dilute urine in the absence of hyperglycemia or significant renal insufficiency, is highly suggestive of DI. However, when the patient has access to water, the serum osmolality and serum sodium are usually normal or only very slightly elevated (Veloski and Brennan 2010).

The water deprivation test is the principal test to establish the diagnosis and underlying cause of DI, where water intake is withheld and urine output, urine osmolality, and weight are

D

measured hourly and serum sodium and osmolality every 2 h. Water deprivation is continued until one of the following conditions are met: (1) the serum osmolality exceeds 295 mOsm/kg H_2O, (2) urine osmolality reaches 600 mOsm/kg H_2O (normal concentrating function), (3) the urine osmolality does not change over 3 h (impaired concentrating function), or (4) the patient develops hypotension, tachycardia, or body weight decreases by 3 %. At the end of the dehydration period, the serum ADH level is drawn while the serum osmolality is elevated. The diagnosis of DI is confirmed if the urine remains dilute (<200 mOsm/kg H_2O) despite serum hyperosmolality (Veloski and Brennan 2010).

To distinguish between central and nephrogenic DI, 10 mcg of desmopressin (DDAVP) by nasal insufflation or 4 mcg of (DDAVP) subcutaneously is given. Urine osmolality and volume are measured for 2 h. An increase in urine osmolality of >50 % after DDAVP is given indicates central DI, whereas no increase or an increase of urine osmolality of <10 % strongly suggests nephrogenic DI or primary polydipsia. If equivocal, or increase of 10–50 %, the plasma ADH drawn at the end of the dehydration period may help identify the underlying cause of DI (Veloski and Brennan 2010).

Treatment for these patients includes ICU monitoring where careful and frequent measurement of urine output and specific gravity and serial serum sodium and osmolality can be recorded in order to avoid severe hypernatremia and obtundation (Veloski and Brennan 2010). The main element is rehydration by calculating and slowly replacing the free water deficit by giving hypotonic IV fluids or free water enterally (Falvo and Horst 2008; Veloski and Brennan 2010).

Treatment of central DI focuses on treating the cause, if reversible, and supplementing DDAVP 2–4 mcg/day subcutaneously or 10–60 mcg/day intranasally until DI resolves. Frequent electrolytes still need to be drawn since it can cause water retention and hyponatremia (Falvo and Horst 2008; Veloski and Brennan 2010). Patients with nephrogenic DI can be treated with thiazide diuretics and by limiting salt intake. Thiazide diuretics paradoxically reduce urine output by decreasing extracellular volume while increasing proximal tubule water reabsorption, with urine volumes falling 25–50 %. Limiting salt intake reduces solute load and urine output. Indomethacin or other prostaglandin inhibitors may also be effective in reducing urine output by decreasing renal blood flow and glomerular filtration rate (Veloski and Brennan 2010).

Cross-References

▶ DDAVP
▶ Electrolyte and Acid-Base Abnormalities
▶ Head Injury
▶ Intracranial Hemorrhage

References

Falvo AJ, Horst M (2008) Management of endocrine disorders in the surgical intensive care unit. In: Asensio JA, Trunkey DD (eds) Current therapy of trauma and surgical critical care, 1st edn. Mosby/Elsevier, Philadelphia, pp 641–648

Veloski C, Brennan KJ (2010) Critical care endocrinology. In: Criner GJ, Barnette RE, D'Alonzo GE (eds) Critical care study guide text and review, 2nd edn. Springer, New York, pp 638–661

Dialysis

Ashita J. Tolwani[1] and Paul M. Palevsky[2,3]
[1]Division of Nephrology, University of Alabama at Birmingham, Birmingham, AL, USA
[2]Renal Section, VA Pittsburgh Healthcare System, Pittsburgh, PA, USA
[3]Renal–Electrolyte Division, University of Pittsburgh School of Medicine, Pittsburgh, PA, USA

Synonyms

Hemodiafiltration; Hemodialysis; Hemofiltration; Renal replacement therapy; Ultrafiltration

Definition

Dialysis is a generic term for all forms of renal replacement therapy (RRT) that remove solutes (uremic toxins) and excess water from the blood. Solute removal during dialysis occurs by diffusion or convection, whereas fluid removal occurs by ultrafiltration. In diffusion, solutes move across a semipermeable membrane from an area of higher concentration to an area of lower concentration. Diffusive transport of a solute depends on the concentration gradient for the solute between the two compartments, permeability of the membrane to the solute, surface area of the membrane, and molecular weight of the solute. In convection, water is driven across the semipermeable membrane by either a hydrostatic or osmotic gradient, passively entraining solutes as it moves. This process of water flow through the membrane in response to a hydrostatic or osmotic pressure difference is known as ultrafiltration; the fluid removed (ultrafiltrate) has the solute composition similar to plasma water as the result of "solvent drag." Convective movement of a solute depends on the ultrafiltrate rate, membrane permeability, and concentration of the solute in plasma water. While diffusion is most effective at removing mostly small molecular weight solutes, such as urea and creatinine, convection provides effective removal of both small and middle molecular weight solutes.

Dialysis Modalities

The available dialysis modalities are peritoneal dialysis (PD), intermittent hemodialysis (IHD), continuous renal replacement therapy (CRRT), or hybrid therapies such as sustained low-efficiency dialysis (SLED) and extended duration dialysis (EDD), now referred to as prolonged intermittent renal replacement therapy (PIRRT). Selection depends on therapy availability, patient hemodynamic status, patient's comorbid conditions, and the physician's preference. PD requires the placement of an intra-abdominal catheter for dialysis. IHD, CRRT, and PIRRT require placement of a dual-lumen venous catheter in the femoral, jugular, or subclavian vein for access to the circulation.

Peritoneal Dialysis

In peritoneal dialysis (PD), a sterile crystalloid solution, known as dialysate, is infused through a catheter placed into the abdominal cavity. The patient's peritoneum functions as a natural semipermeable membrane for diffusive removal of solutes and uremic toxins. After dwelling in the peritoneum for 1–6 h, the dialysate becomes saturated and is discarded. Fresh dialysate is then reintroduced. Multiple such "exchanges" are performed throughout the day. Fluid removal is achieved by using a high solute concentration in the dialysate (most commonly using high concentrations of dextrose), enabling water to flow from the patient's blood into the peritoneal compartment down an osmotic gradient. The main advantages of PD are that it is readily available, easy to perform without requiring complex technology, does not require anticoagulation, and may be better tolerated hemodynamically than hemodialysis. Its major disadvantages are potentially insufficient solute clearance in hypercatabolic patients, unpredictable ultrafiltration, risk of peritonitis, albumin loss across the peritoneal membrane, and potential respiratory compromise from the increased abdominal pressure during dwelling of the dialysate (Tolwani 2012). Acute PD also requires the insertion of a peritoneal dialysis catheter, which can be complicated by catheter leakage and malfunction and is contraindicated in patients with recent abdominal surgery.

Intermittent Hemodialysis

Intermittent hemodialysis (IHD) removes solutes and water by circulating blood through an extracorporeal system that incorporates a filter, called a hemodialyzer, with a semipermeable membrane. In the hemodialyzer, blood flows in one direction and the dialysate flows in the opposite. Solutes move across the membrane by diffusion and fluid is removed by ultrafiltration driven by a hydrostatic pressure gradient. The counter-current flow of the blood and dialysate maximizes the concentration gradient for solutes between the blood and dialysate along the length of the membrane. In AKI, IHD is typically prescribed for 3–5 h per treatment for 3 or more days per week, with blood flow rates of 300–500 ml/min and dialysate flow rates of 500–800 ml/min. IHD offers the advantage of providing for rapid correction of electrolyte and acid–base disturbances. A major disadvantage is the risk of hypotension due to rapid volume removal and changes in plasma osmolality, which complicates 20–30 % of treatments (Palevsky 2013). Hemodynamically unstable patients may not tolerate the higher ultrafiltration rates and solute fluxes needed to achieve adequate clearance and volume removal in the limited duration of the treatment.

Continuous Renal Replacement Therapy

Continuous Renal Replacement (CRRT) Therapy comprises a variety of renal replacement therapies that provide slower solute clearance and volume removal per unit time as compared to IHD but are applied on a continuous (24 h per day) schedule. Solute removal with CRRT is achieved either by convection (continuous venovenous hemofiltration, CVVH), diffusion (continuous venovenous hemodialysis, CVVHD), or by a combination of both mechanisms (continuous venovenous hemodiafiltration, CVVHDF). In the convective modalities (CVVH and CVVHDF), electrolytes and water that are lost from the blood with high rates of ultrafiltration must be returned back to the patient in the form of "replacement" fluids to "correct" electrolyte depletion, metabolic acidosis, and hypovolemia. Middle molecular weight solutes, such as cytokines, are more efficiently removed using convective as compared to diffusive therapies. At the present time, no study has demonstrated a survival benefit of cytokine or middle molecular weight solute removal (Tolwani and Wille 2012). Therefore, the choice of CRRT modality is based on clinician preference and expertise.

Potential advantages of CRRT over IHD include better hemodynamic tolerability, more efficient solute clearance, better control of volume status, and potentially better clearance of middle molecular weight solutes. Disadvantages include patient immobility, increased nursing support, greater need for anticoagulation as compared to intermittent therapies, and increased cost.

Hybrid Therapies

Hybrid therapies are also known as prolonged intermittent renal replacement therapy (PIRRT) and include sustained low-efficiency dialysis (SLED), and extended daily dialysis (EDD). These therapies use standard hemodialysis machines but provide a slower solute and fluid removal per unit time. The duration of dialysis is extended to 8–16 h with a lower blood flow. Hybrid therapies have been shown to be safe and effective alternatives to treating AKI in critically ill patients and cause less hemodynamic instability than IHD while maintaining excellent solute control (Palevsky 2013). Advantages over CRRT include decreased cost, increased patient immobility, and decreased need for anticoagulation.

Preexisting Condition

Acute kidney injury (AKI) in the intensive care unit (ICU) is often multifactorial, commonly developing in the setting of hypovolemia, sepsis, hemodynamic alterations, and/or nephrotoxic medication use. Additional causes of AKI specific to trauma patients include hemorrhagic shock, abdominal compartment syndrome, and rhabdomyolysis. Specific pharmacologic therapies of AKI are not available, and management is primarily supportive. Dialysis is utilized to control the complications of severe AKI such as fluid overload, acid–base and electrolyte abnormalities, and uremia.

Application

Indications for Initiation of Dialysis

Widely accepted indications for dialysis are based on conditions such as hyperkalemia, metabolic acidosis, and pulmonary edema that are refractory to medical therapy. Beyond these life-threatening indications and dialyzable intoxications, the optimal timing of initiation of RRT for AKI is unknown and dependent on subjective clinical judgment. Observational studies using various cutoff values of serum urea or creatinine as criteria for initiation of dialysis have suggested that earlier initiation based on a lower urea or creatinine level may be associated with better survival (Karvellas et al. 2011). However, virtually all of these studies are retrospective and subject to bias since they focus only on patients who receive dialysis and not those with AKI who die or recover without RRT. In the absence of large randomized controlled trials comparing early to late initiation of RRT, the decision of initiating RRT must take into account the clinical situation of the individual patient. In the trauma patient with AKI, considerations for initiating dialysis earlier than conventional indications should take into account patient fluid balance status, catabolic state, other organ function, and conditions, such as rhabdomyolysis, in which the kidneys do not have the functional capacity to meet the metabolic and fluid demands placed on them.

Selection of Modality

Current studies do not support the use of one dialysis modality of renal replacement therapy over another in patients with AKI. Although CRRT is thought to be superior to IHD in hemodynamically unstable patients, prospective randomized clinical trials have not shown a benefit with regard to survival or recovery of kidney function for CRRT as compared to IHD (Bagshaw et al. 2008). Hybrid therapies have been shown to provide comparable hemodynamic stability and solute control as CRRT. Data comparing survival using hybrid therapies as compared to either IHD or CRRT are limited, but suggest similar outcomes (Palevsky 2013). Modern comparisons of PD to the extracorporeal therapies are also limited, but suggest that similar outcomes can be achieved with PD (Palevsky 2013). However, in trauma patients, PD may not be a viable option in patients with intra-abdominal organ injury or penetrating wounds of the abdomen. In addition, solute clearance with PD may not be sufficient in severely hypercatabolic patients.

Selection of modality should be based on the needs of the patient at the time of initiation. Most clinicians choose IHD for hemodynamically stable patients and CRRT or hybrid therapies for those with hemodynamic compromise, multiorgan failure, or high catabolic states. In a trauma patient with cerebral edema, slower modalities of therapy such as CRRT are preferred (KDIGO 2012). Unlike CRRT, IHD can increase cerebral edema and intracranial pressure from rapid intracellular fluid and solute shifts.

Practical Considerations

Practical considerations for delivering adequate dialysis include anticoagulation and dialysis dose.

Anticoagulation

Anticoagulation is frequently required to prevent clotting in the extracorporeal circuit. Clotting of the filter decreases solute and fluid removal and contributes to blood loss in the dialyzer. Unfractionated heparin is the most common anticoagulant used worldwide. However, heparin is contraindicated in trauma patients who are at high risk of bleeding and in patients with heparin-induced thrombocytopenia. Although IHD can be generally be performed without anticoagulation given the shorter duration of treatment and high blood flow rates used, CRRT often requires anticoagulation. Given the challenges with heparin, use of regional citrate anticoagulation (RCA) for CRRT has increased (KDIGO 2012). Citrate is delivered into the blood at the beginning of the CRRT extracorporeal circuit where it chelates free calcium and inhibits the coagulation cascade. An ionized calcium level less than 0.35 mmol/l in the extracorporeal circuit has been shown to adequately inhibit anticoagulation. As some of the calcium-citrate complex is lost across the filter, a systemic calcium replacement is necessary. The remainder of the calcium-citrate complex enters the systemic circulation, where it is metabolized by the liver to bicarbonate, releasing ionized calcium back into the circulation. By maintaining normal levels of ionized calcium in the systemic circulation, anticoagulation is limited to the extracorporeal circuit.

Complications of RCA may include metabolic alkalosis, hypernatremia when hypertonic citrate solutions are used, and hypocalcemia

(Tolwani and Wille 2012). Thus, frequent monitoring of acid–base status, electrolytes, and ionized calcium in the systemic circulation is necessary. Citrate accumulation may occur in patients who cannot metabolize citrate, such as those with liver failure or severe lactic acidosis, leading to severe hypocalcemia and metabolic disorders. The use of citrate as an anticoagulant in these patients may be contraindicated. Randomized controlled trials comparing low molecular weight heparin or unfractionated heparin to citrate during CRRT have found increased circuit life and fewer bleeding events with citrate, with no increase in metabolic complications (Wu et al. 2012).

Dose of RRT

There are no well-established standard methods for measuring the efficacy of RRT in AKI. The "dose" of treatment in AKI has been assessed by urea clearance in PD, IHD, and SLED, and by effluent volume (a surrogate of urea clearance) in CRRT. Urea clearance in IHD is most commonly quantified as the urea reduction ratio (URR) or fractional urea clearance per treatment, expressed as Kt/Vurea. Solute clearance in CRRT is quantified as the sum of the convective and diffusive clearances, which is defined as the effluent (ultrafiltrate plus dialysate).

The Veteran Affairs/National Institute of Health Acute Renal Failure Trial Network (ATN) study (Palevsky et al. 2008) and the Randomized Evaluation of Normal Versus Augmented Level Renal Replacement Therapy (RENAL) (Bellomo et al. 2009) were large, multicenter, randomized controlled trials that investigated the effect of RRT dose on patient outcomes. The ATN study utilized both intermittent and continuous modalities while the RENAL study only utilized CVVHDF in critically ill patients with AKI. In the ATN study, both treatment strategies used conventional IHD in patients who were hemodynamically stable and either SLED or CRRT in patients who were hemodynamically unstable. IHD and SLED were provided three times per week and CRRT was dosed to provide an effluent rate of 20 ml/kg/h in the less intensive arm and six times per week or 35 ml/kg/h, respectively, in the more intensive arm. The study

demonstrated no difference in the primary outcome, death from any cause. In the RENAL study, patients were randomized to CVVHDF at an effluent rate of either 25 ml/kg/h (lower intensity) or 40 mL/kg/h (higher intensity). The RENAL study failed to detect any survival benefit from more intensive CRRT. Both trials also showed that the prescribed CRRT dose is 10–15 % less than the delivered dose due to treatment downtime. Based on these studies, there is no benefit in providing IHD more frequently than three times per week so long as the delivered dose per treatment is at least a Kt/V of 1.2 (approximately corresponding to a URR of at least 0.70). More frequent treatments may be required in hypercatabolic patients and in patients with high obligate fluid loads who require more aggressive ultrafiltration. In AKI patients treated with CRRT, a minimal effluent flow rate of 20–25 ml/kg/h should be provided, with careful attention to ensure that the target dose of therapy is actually delivered (Vijayan and Palevsky 2012).

Cross-References

▶ Acute Kidney Injury

References

Bagshaw SM, Berthiaume LR, Delaney A, Bellomo R (2008) Continuous versus intermittent renal replacement therapy for critically ill patients with acute kidney injury: a meta-analysis. Crit Care Med 36:610–617

Bellomo R, Cass A, Cole L, Finfer S, Gallagher M, Lo S, McArthur C, McGuinness S, Myburgh J, Norton R, Scheinkestel C, Su S (2009) Intensity of continuous renal-replacement therapy in critically ill patients. N Engl J Med 361:1627–1638

Karvellas CJ, Farhat MR, Sajjad I, Mogensen SS, Leung AA, Wald R, Bagshaw SM (2011) A comparison of early versus late initiation of renal replacement therapy in critically ill patients with acute kidney injury: a systematic review and meta-analysis. Crit Care 15:R72

Kidney Disease: Improving Global Outcomes (KDIGO) Acute Kidney Injury Work Group (2012) KDIGO Clinical Practice Guideline for Acute Kidney Injury. Kidney Int Suppl 2:1–138. http://kdigo.org/home/guidelines/acute-kidney-injury/

Palevsky PM (2013) Renal replacement therapy in acute kidney injury. Adv Chronic Kidney Dis 20:76–84

Palevsky PM, Zhang JH, O'Connor TZ, Chertow GM, Crowley ST, Choudhury D, Finkel K, Kellum JA, Paganini E, Schein RM, Smith MW, Swanson KM, Thompson BT, Vijayan A, Watnick S, Star RA, Peduzzi P (2008) Intensity of renal support in critically ill patients with acute kidney injury. N Engl J Med 359:7–20

Tolwani A (2012) Continuous renal-replacement therapy for acute kidney injury. N Engl J Med 367:2505–2514

Tolwani A, Wille KM (2012) Advances in continuous renal replacement therapy: citrate anticoagulation update. Blood Purif 34:88–93

Vijayan A, Palevsky PM (2012) Dosing of renal replacement therapy in acute kidney injury. Am J Kidney Dis 59:569–576

Wu MY, Hsu YH, Bai CH, Lin YF, Wu CH, Tam KW (2012) Regional citrate versus heparin anticoagulation for continuous renal replacement therapy: a meta-analysis of randomized controlled trials. Am J Kidney Dis 59:810–818

Diaphragm Injuries

Beth Hochman
Division of Traumatology, Surgical Critical Care, and Emergency Surgery, Hospital of the University of Pennsylvania, Philadelphia, PA, USA

Synonyms

Diaphragm rupture; Diaphragm trauma; Diaphragmatic hernia; Thoracoabdominal injury

Definition

The diaphragm is a muscular dome extending anteriorly from the sternum and running along the 6th–12th ribs to the 1st–3rd lumbar vertebral bodies posteriorly. It rises to the level of the nipples (4th intercostal spaces) and scapular tips and descends two rib spaces below the costal margin. The phrenic nerves and vessels, which originate anteromedially, provide its main neurovascular supply (Schuster and Davis 2013).

Traumatic diaphragm injury (incidence 0.8–8 %) occurs most often on the left (60–90 %) and is primarily due to penetrating trauma (61–73 %) (Zarour 2013). Penetrating injuries tend to be smaller (1–4 cm) than blunt injuries (10–15 cm), which usually involve high-energy mechanisms (Bocchini 2012). Among those patients sustaining left thoracoabdominal penetrating injury, the incidence of diaphragm injury is high as 42 % (Murray 1997). Overall mortality ranges from 7 % to 21 % but is primarily due to associated injuries (Liao 2013).

Acute diaphragmatic injury is often asymptomatic or obscured by symptoms reflecting concomitant injuries. Clinical and radiographic evidence is most notable when abdominal contents herniate through the injury, but this may be precluded by injury size or positive-pressure ventilation. Since diaphragm injuries do not spontaneously heal and can expand over time, a missed injury – in particular, of the left diaphragm – risks future herniation and strangulation of abdominal viscera, potentially leading to acute sepsis or cardiovascular collapse up to decades after the initial injury (Friese 2005; Zarour 2013; Bocchini 2012). The natural history of right diaphragm injuries is more benign because of the presence of the liver.

Chest X-ray findings include hollow viscus or nasogastric tube above the diaphragm with 27–68 % sensitivity. In addition to visceral herniation, CT may reveal a diaphragm defect or thickening with 77–100 % sensitivity and 75–100 % specificity. CT sensitivity improves with thin-slice CT and multiplanar reformatting. MRI and ultrasound are of uncertain value in acute trauma settings (Bocchini 2012; Stein 2007; Dreizin 2013). Thoracoscopy or laparoscopy can also be used to identify injury. Diagnostic laparoscopy (87.5 % sensitive, 100 % specific) is strongly recommended in hemodynamically stable patients sustaining left-sided penetrating thoracoabdominal wounds given the 31 % incidence of radiographically missed injury in this population. Isolated injuries can be repaired laparoscopically (Friese 2005; Como 2010).

Primary principles of diaphragm repair include reduction of hernia contents and watertight closure with nonabsorbable sutures (Zarour 2013). Large defects may require synthetic or biologic mesh or autologous tissue flaps. Diaphragm avulsion can be repaired using circumferential stitches around anchoring ribs. Post-op complications include failure of repair, respiratory insufficiency or diaphragm paralysis due to phrenic nerve injury, empyema, and subphrenic abscess (Schuster and Davis 2013).

Cross-References

- ► ABCDE of Trauma Care
- ► Chest Wall Injury
- ► Damage Control Surgery
- ► Delayed Diagnosis/Missed Injury
- ► Diaphragmatic Injuries
- ► Empyema
- ► Fibrothorax
- ► Firearm-Related Injuries
- ► Hepatic and Biliary Injuries
- ► Imaging of Aortic and Thoracic Injuries
- ► Lung Injury
- ► Pneumothorax
- ► Splenic Bed Abscess
- ► Splenic Injury
- ► Thoracic Vascular Injuries
- ► Trauma Laparotomy

References

Bocchini G (2012) Diaphragmatic injuries after blunt trauma: are they still a challenge? Reviewing CT findings and integrated imaging. Emerg Radiol 19(3):225–235

Como JJ (2010) Practice management guidelines for selective nonoperative management of penetrating abdominal trauma. J Trauma 68(3):721–733

Dreizin D (2013) Penetrating diaphragmatic injury: accuracy of 64-section multidetector CT with trajectography. Radiology 268(3):729–737

Friese RS (2005) Laparoscopy is sufficient to exclude occult diaphragm injury after penetrating abdominal trauma. J Trauma 58(4):789–792

Liao CH (2013) Factors affecting outcomes in penetrating diaphragmatic trauma. Int J Surg 11(6):492–495

Murray JA (1997) Penetrating left thoracoabdominal trauma: the incidence and clinical presentation of diaphragm injuries. J Trauma 43(4):624–626

Schuster KM, Davis KA (2013) Diaphragm. In: Mattox LK, Moore EE, Feliciano DV (eds) Trauma, 7th edn. McGraw-Hill, NY, Chap 28

Stein DM (2007) Accuracy of computed tomography (CT) scan in the detection of penetrating diaphragm injury. J Trauma 63(3):538–543

Zarour AM (2013) Presentations and outcomes in patients with traumatic diaphragmatic injury: a 15-year experience. J Trauma 74(6):1392–1398

Diaphragm Rupture

► Diaphragm Injuries

Diaphragm Trauma

► Diaphragm Injuries

Diaphragmatic Hernia

► Diaphragm Injuries

Diaphragmatic Injuries

Stephen D. Gowing[1], Waël C. Hanna[2] and Lorenzo E. Ferri[1]
[1]Department of Thoracic Surgery, McGill University Health Centre, The Montreal General Hospital – Room L9-112, Montreal, QC, Canada
[2]Division of Thoracic Surgery, McMaster University - St. Joseph's Healthcare – Room T2105, Hamilton, ON, Canada

Synonyms

Traumatic diaphragmatic hernia (TDH); Traumatic diaphragmatic injury (TDI); Traumatic diaphragmatic rupture (TDR)

Definition

A tear in the diaphragm secondary to blunt or penetrating thoracoabdominal trauma.

Preexisting Condition

None.

Introduction

Traumatic diaphragmatic injury (TDI) is an uncommon complication of trauma occurring overall in approximately 1 % of traumatic injuries (Hanna et al. 2008; Lewis et al. 2009). TDIs have been reported to occur in approximately 1–7 % of serious blunt and 10–15 % of penetrating traumas requiring hospitalization (Meyers and McCabe 1993; Rosati 1998; Scharff and Naunheim 2007), but these rates likely underrepresent the true value, as up to 8 % of patients undergoing thoracotomy or laparotomy for trauma will have an incidental finding of TDI (Shah et al. 1995). TDI is associated with substantial morbidity and an average mortality of approximately 17–22 % resulting primarily from associated injuries secondary to their trauma (Shah et al. 1995; Hanna et al. 2008; Lewis et al. 2009). The Injury Severity Score, transfusion requirements, need for urgent thoracotomy, and traumatic brain injury are predictors of mortality in TDI patients (Williams et al. 2004; Hanna et al. 2008; Lewis et al. 2009).

TDI can be further classified according to its mechanism of injury as either blunt TDI or penetrating TDI. Recent database reviews in North American Level 1 trauma centers have demonstrated that approximately 60 % of TDIs are penetrating and the remaining 40 % are blunt in origin (Hanna et al. 2008; Lewis et al. 2009). Patients with TDI are predisposed to developing traumatic diaphragmatic hernia (TDH) as a result the physiologic pressure difference between the negative pressure thoracic and positive pressure abdominal cavities. Due to the nature of the mechanism, the overall incidence of TDH is higher in blunt TDI (62 %) versus penetrating TDI (33 %) (Hanna et al. 2008). TDHs secondary to blunt trauma are associated with larger defects than their penetrating TDH counterparts with mean sizes of approximately 10 cm versus 3 cm, respectively (Meyers and McCabe 1993; Hanna et al. 2008). The incidence of left-sided TDI has traditionally been reported in a 3:1 ratio relative to right-sided TDI (Demetriades et al. 1988; Meyers and McCabe 1993; Hanna et al. 2008; Lewis et al. 2009). This has been postulated to be due to the protective effects of the liver on the right hemi-diaphragm and to an area of congenital weakness in the posterolateral left hemi-diaphragm (Andrus and Morton 1970; Boulanger et al. 1993). However some recently published studies indicate a more even distribution between left- and right-sided penetrating TDI (Rosati 1998; Lewis et al. 2009). Herniating organs found in left-sided TDH include the stomach, spleen, liver, small and large bowel, and omentum, while in right-sided TDH the liver is overwhelmingly the most common herniated organ (Hanna et al. 2008; Scharff and Naunheim 2007).

A retrospective review of the literature revealed on average a delayed diagnosis of TDI of 15 %, with 44 % of TDI diagnosed preoperatively and an additional 41 % of injuries diagnosis in the operating room or during postmortem autopsy (Shah et al. 1995). A significant portion of patients presenting with chronic diaphragmatic hernias have a history of blunt or penetrating thoracoabdominal trauma, and it is likely the diagnosis of TDI was missed following their initial injury. Therefore, a high index of suspicion is necessary as a delayed diagnosis of TDI can lead to herniation and strangulation of abdominal organs resulting in increased morbidity and mortality (Feliciano et al. 1988).

Mechanism and Associated Injuries

Patients with traumatic diaphragmatic injury frequently present with multiple concurrent injuries due to both the high-energy trauma of blunt TDI and the anatomic location of the diaphragm in both blunt and penetrating TDIs. Associated organ injuries are present in 55–100 % of patients with TDI (Ward et al. 1981; Payne and Yellin 1982; Meyers and McCabe 1993; Hanna et al. 2008; Lewis et al. 2009). Blunt TDI often is associated with traumatic diaphragmatic hernia and results from high-energy impact trauma. Motor vehicle collisions are typically responsible for 70–90 % of blunt TDI, while fall and crush injuries comprise the remainder (Boulanger et al. 1993; Hanna et al. 2008; Lewis et al. 2009). The currently proposed mechanism for blunt TDI involves a rapid increase in intra-abdominal pressure that overwhelms the compliance of the diaphragm leading to rupture. Negative intrathoracic pressures result in the herniation of intra-abdominal organs into the chest. The liver is thought to mitigate some of this force leading to a decreased incidence of right blunt TDR compared to the left (Reiff et al. 2002). One series of patients who experienced blunt thoracoabdominal trauma following motor vehicle collision highlights the prominent rate of associated injuries in cases of blunt diaphragmatic rupture including: pulmonary contusion (45 %), rib fractures (64 %), thoracic aorta (15 %), spleen (53 %), liver (36 %), and pelvic fracture (42 %) (Reiff et al. 2002). Other studies confirm this and reveal a high incidence of extremity fractures (45 %) (Boulanger et al. 1993), traumatic brain injury (Hanna et al. 2008), and cardiac contusions (Meyers and McCabe 1993). Blunt TDI patients will often require prolonged mechanical ventilation in the intensive care unit and in one clinical series had an incidence of tracheostomy of 25 % (Boulanger et al. 1993). This is not surprising given that loss of function of one hemi-diaphragm results in a 25–50 % decrease in respiratory function (Sabanathan et al. 1990).

The diaphragm rises as high as T4 with full inspiration and descends as low at T8 with full expiration with its lowest lateral attachments to the ribs at T12. Therefore any penetrating injury traversing the thoracoabdominal region within this area can potentially injure the diaphragm. Consequently a stab or gunshot wound below the nipples and above the umbilicus is a risk factor for TDI (Scharff and Naunheim 2007). The associated injuries of penetrating TDI are chiefly related to the anatomic location of the diaphragm at the junction of the thoracic and abdominal cavities. Any impalement or missile traversing this region has a high probability of causing injury to the various organs in the vicinity. Associated injuries in penetrating TDI most commonly include liver (44 %), spleen (30 %), gastrointestinal (30 %), renal (9 %), and major vascular (17 %) injuries (Meyers and McCabe 1993). In a more recent case series, penetrating TDI-associated injuries were classified as thoracic (30 %), heart/aorta (9 %), solid organ – abdomen (56 %), and hollow viscus – abdomen (39 %) (Hanna et al. 2008).

Application

Signs and Symptoms

Patients with traumatic diaphragmatic injury can present with a number of symptoms; however, symptoms are rarely in isolation, and findings are primarily due to associated injuries. Physical exam on auscultation may reveal decreased air entry at the lung bases due to lung compression by diaphragmatic hernia or the presence of audible bowel sounds in the chest. Abdominal tenderness may be appreciated on exam in addition to a scaphoid abdomen if a significant amount of viscera have herniated into the chest (Shah et al. 1995; Nursal et al. 2001). On occasion herniated abdominal viscera may be identified by palpation during chest tube placement (Hanna and Ferri 2009) or even clearly evident on inspection alone (Fig. 1). It is important to keep a high clinical suspicion for TDI based on the mechanism of injury as these patients often have severe concomitant injuries that can obscure the diagnosis (Boulanger et al. 1993).

Imaging

Chest radiographs are the most common initial imaging to screen for thoracic injury in trauma, and careful scrutiny of these initial radiographs is critical. Signs of diaphragmatic injury and/or hernia include atelectasis of the lung bases, pulmonary contusion, obscured view of the diaphragm, irregular contour of the diaphragm,

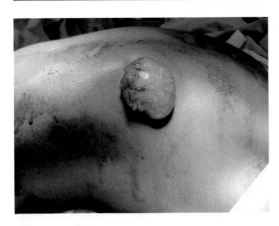

Diaphragmatic Injuries, Fig. 1 Herniated stomach protruding through diaphragmatic defect and chest wall following stab wound to the left chest

diaphragmatic elevation, pleural effusion or hemothorax, rib fractures, air containing viscera in the thorax, and mediastinal shift (Gelman et al. 1991) – (Fig. 2). The presence of a nasogastric tube coiled in the left chest or an intrathoracic air-fluid level is a strong sign of diaphragmatic hernia (Shah et al. 1995; Hanna and Ferri 2009). More elusive right TDIs may only be evident by an obscured or irregular diaphragm contour or elevation of the right hemi-diaphragm (Gelman et al. 1991). Chest radiographs are initially diagnostic of diaphragmatic injury in approximately 23–35 % of patients as they are often initially interpreted by surgical residents and emergency room staff (Nursal et al. 2001; Hanna et al. 2008). However following review by a staff radiologist, this number increases to 44–46 % (Gelman et al. 1991; Hanna et al. 2008). The use of oral contrast can improve the sensitivity of chest radiographs for TDI with an associated hernia (Fig. 3) in patients with chronic TDH; however, the utility in the acute setting is very limited (Payne and Yellin 1982; Rosati 1998).

When chest radiograph is non-diagnostic in hemodynamically stable trauma patients, CT scan has become the imaging modality of choice for evaluating traumatic diaphragmatic rupture in the acute setting. While in the past traditional non-helical CT scanners were poor at detecting traumatic diaphragmatic rupture (sensitivity

0–66 %, specificity 76–99 %), with the advent of newer helical CT and multi-detector CT scanners employing thinner axial cuts and multi-planar image reformatting, their diagnostic accuracy has increased (sensitivity 56–87 %, specificity 75–100 % and sensitivity 71–90 % and specificity 98–100 %, respectively) (Desir and Ghaye 2012). However, in the case of isolated diaphragmatic injury without diaphragmatic hernia, the diagnostic ability of CT scan to detect such injury is greatly diminished (Chen and Wilson 1991).

MRI is a time-consuming and limited access resource for detecting TDI and therefore is often not practical for the acutely injured trauma patient. However some authors have reported the utility of MRI in a small subset of hemodynamically stable patients whom CT scan is non-diagnostic and a high clinical suspicion for TDI remains. Respiratory and cardiac gating in T1-weighted coronal and sagittal images are primarily used (Mirvis and Shanmuganagthan 2007). Importantly visualization of the diaphragm is superior to CT scanning and it is often possible to visualized diaphragmatic defects in the absence of herniation (Boulanger et al. 1992).

Exploratory Laparoscopy/Thoracoscopy

Occasionally imaging studies are negative in hemodynamically stable patients; however, the suspicion for diaphragmatic injury remains high based on the mechanism of injury, particularly in patients with penetrating thoracoabdominal trauma. In this situation exploratory laparoscopy or exploratory thoracoscopy is being increasingly advocated to rule out TDI (Ochsner et al. 1993; Murray et al. 1997; Friese et al. 2005). In a subset of 107 patients with penetrating left thoracoabdominal trauma not requiring trauma laparotomy, exploratory laparoscopy detected an incidence of 42 % of TDI. Among these patients 31 % had no abdominal tenderness and 40 % had normal chest radiography (Murray et al. 1997). Exploratory laparoscopy has a sensitivity of 87.5 %, a specificity of 100 %, and a negative predictive value of 96.8 % for TDI in patients with penetrating thoracoabdominal

Diaphragmatic Injuries,
Fig. 2 Chest radiograph
depicting typical finding of
acute traumatic
diaphragmatic injury with
herniation of stomach into
the left chest following
a motor vehicle crash

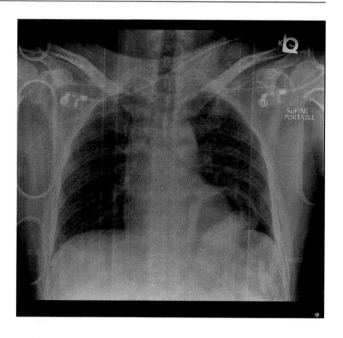

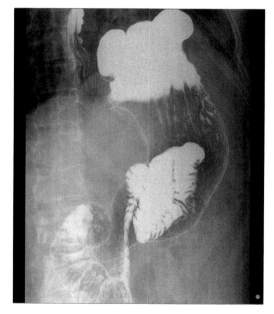

Diaphragmatic Injuries, Fig. 3 Barium contrast upper
GI series demonstrating herniated stomach adjacent, not
through, the esophageal hiatus indicating chronic traumatic diaphragmatic hernia in a patient with a remote
history of a motor vehicle crash

trauma (Friese et al. 2005). Video-assisted
thoracoscopic surgery (VATS) has the advantage
of being able to wash out any retained
hemothorax. Disadvantages include the frequent
need for double lumen endotracheal tube intubation, postoperative tube thoracostomy, and the
inability to adequately visualize the abdominal
cavity for injury (Ochsner et al. 1993; Shaw
et al. 2003). Both VATS and laparoscopy have
been successfully used to repair TDIs in selected
cases (Shaw et al. 2003; Matthews et al. 2003;
Hanna and Ferri 2009). We prefer to perform
laparoscopic examination in patients with
thoracoabdominal penetrating injuries, as it
allows for the inspection of the intra-abdominal
contents, and we find repair of the diaphragm to
be rather facile through this approach.

Treatment

Surgical repair of TDI is mandated due to the risk
of herniation and strangulation of abdominal viscera as well as delayed bowel obstruction (Meyers
and McCabe 1993; Scharff and Naunheim 2007).
The principles of repair include reduction of the
herniated organs if present, a watertight closure to
prevent hernia recurrence, and care to avoid injury
to the phrenic nerves (Scharff and Naunheim
2007). Due to the high incidence of concurrent
intra-abdominal injury, in many series
approaching 100 %, TDI repair is often
approached via a midline laparotomy (Payne and
Yellin 1982; Meyers and McCabe 1993;

Hanna et al. 2008; Lewis et al. 2009). Ultimately the presence and location of associated life-threatening injuries in these patients will dictate the surgical approach used. Many pulmonary injuries due to penetrating trauma can be safely treated with chest tube insertion; however, in the case of massive intrathoracic bleeding or life-threatening thoracic injury, the diaphragmatic repair can be performed via a transthoracic approach (Hanna and Ferri 2009). For patients with significant intrathoracic and intra-abdominal injury, surgical approaches include laparotomy plus thoracotomy, thoraco-abdominal incision, or laparotomy plus median sternotomy (Scharff and Naunheim 2007; Hanna and Ferri 2009). Repair of large right-sided TDHs may be difficult from an intra-abdominal approach alone due to the bulk of the liver and injury to the diaphragmatic attachments to the chest wall. Consequently an approach via thoracotomy, thoracoabdominal incision, or combined laparotomy plus thoracotomy may be required depending on the coexisting traumatic injuries of the patient (Shah et al. 1995; Hanna and Ferri 2009). In the repair of delayed or chronic TDH, a transthoracic approach is usually advisable due to the adhesion of abdominal viscera to intrathoracic contents (Payne and Yellin 1982; Shah et al. 1995).

Permanent suture sizes 0 or 1 are the sutures of choice for repair of diaphragmatic injury due to the constant strain of the repair site with respiration and reduced rates of hernia recurrence compared to repairs with resorbable sutures (Hanna et al. 2008). Although a variety of sutures (monofilament vs. braided) and suturing techniques (continuous vs. simple: single layer vs. double) have been employed, we prefer a single layer of nonabsorbable interrupted braided sutures for all diaphragmatic repairs due to the ease of knot tying, security of repair, and relative absence of tension. In patients with enteric contents within the chest, copious irrigation of the chest cavity is recommended as hollow viscus injury is associated with increased incidence of empyema (Eren et al. 2008; Hanna et al. 2008). Small TDIs may be repaired with simple interrupted sutures. In the case of diaphragmatic avulsion from the chest wall, the repair may be completed using full-thickness horizontal mattress sutures that encircle around the ribs in the submuscular space (Scharff and Naunheim 2007). When it is necessary to incorporate a flail segment of rib into the repair, open reduction and internal fixation of the fracture rib with metal plates and screws is required (Hanna and Ferri 2009) (Fig. 4). For diaphragm repairs under tension in the acute setting, it is advisable to reattach the diaphragm one or two

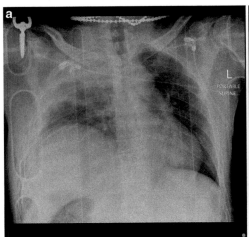
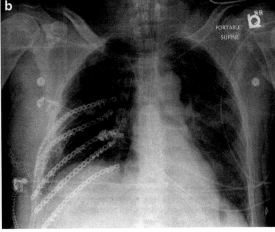

Diaphragmatic Injuries, Fig. 4 Chest radiographs demonstrating an elevated right hemi-diaphragm and rib fractures following a massive crush injury (**a**) indicating a herniated liver and large flail chest. This patient required internal fixation of the chest wall immediately prior to repairing the diaphragm with peri-costal sutures (**b**)

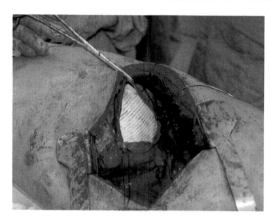

Diaphragmatic Injuries, Fig. 5 Intra-operative image of repair of left chronic traumatic diaphragmatic hernia with the use of prosthetic mesh

rib levels higher rather than using a mesh due to increased rates of foreign body sepsis, especially in the presence of concurrent hollow viscus injury. In general, we avoid the use of prosthetic mesh in the acute setting; however, we find that mesh is frequently required in chronic TDH due to the retraction of the diaphragm (Scharff and Naunheim 2007). In such situations the TDH is frequently approached through a thoracotomy and a nonabsorbable placed (Fig. 5); however, we do employ laparoscopy in selected cases.

References

Andrus CH, Morton JH (1970) Rupture of the diaphragm after blunt trauma. Am J Surg 119:686

Boulanger BR, Mirvis SE, Rodriguez A (1992) Magnetic resonance imaging in traumatic diaphragmatic rupture: case reports. J Trauma 32(1):89–93

Boulanger BR, Milzman DP, Rosati C, Rodriguez A (1993) A comparison of right and left blunt traumatic diaphragmatic rupture. J Trauma 35(2):255–260

Chen JC, Wilson SE (1991) Diaphragmatic injuries: recognition and management in sixty-two patients. Am Surg 57(12):810–815

Demetriades D, Kakoyiannis S, Parekh D, Hatzitheofilou C (1988) Penetrating injuries of the diaphragm. Br J Surg 75(8):824–826

Desir A, Ghaye B (2012) CT of blunt diaphragmatic rupture. Radiographics 32(2):477–498

Eren S, Esme H, Sehitogullari A, Durkan A (2008) The risk factors and management of post-traumatic empyema in trauma patients. Injury 39(1):44–49, Epub 2007 Sep 19

Feliciano DV, Cruse PA, Mattox KL, Bitondo CG, Burch JM, Noon GP, Beall AC Jr (1988) Delayed diagnosis of injuries to the diaphragm after penetrating wounds. J Trauma 28(8):1135–1144

Friese RS, Coln CE, Gentilello LM (2005) Laparoscopy is sufficient to exclude occult diaphragm injury after penetrating abdominal trauma. J Trauma 58(4):789–792

Gelman R, Mirvis SE, Gens D (1991) Diaphragmatic rupture due to blunt trauma: sensitivity of plain chest radiographs. AJR Am J Roentgenol 156(1):51–57

Hanna WC, Ferri LE (2009) Acute traumatic diaphragmatic injury. Thorac Surg Clin 19(4):485–489

Hanna WC, Ferri LE, Fata P, Razek T, Mulder DS (2008) The current status of traumatic diaphragmatic injury: lessons learned from 105 patients over 13 years. Ann Thorac Surg 85:1044–1048

Lewis JD, Starnes SL, Pandalai PK, Huffman LC, Bulcao CF, Pritts TA, Reed MF (2009) Traumatic diaphragmatic injury: experience from a level I trauma center. Surgery 146(4):578–583; discussion 583–584

Matthews BD, Bui H, Harold KL et al (2003) Laparoscopic repair of traumatic diaphragmatic injuries. Surg Endosc 17:254–258

Meyers BF, McCabe CJ (1993) Traumatic diaphragmatic hernia. Occult marker of serious injury. Ann Surg 218(6):783–790

Mirvis SE, Shanmuganagthan K (2007) Imaging hemidiaphragmatic injury. Eur Radiol 17(6): 1411–1421, Epub 2007 Feb 17

Murray JA, Demetriades D, Cornwell EE 3rd, Asensio JA, Velmahos G, Belzberg H, Berne TV (1997) Penetrating left thoracoabdominal trauma: the incidence and clinical presentation of diaphragm injuries. J Trauma 43(4):624–626

Nursal TZ, Ugurlu M, Kologlu M, Hamaloglu E (2001) Traumatic diaphragmatic hernias: a report of 26 cases. Hernia 5(1):25–29

Ochsner MG, Rozycki GS, Lucente F, Wherry DC, Champion HR (1993) Prospective evaluation of thoracoscopy for diagnosing diaphragmatic injury in thoracoabdominal trauma: a preliminary report. J Trauma 34(5):704–709; discussion 709–710

Payne JH Jr, Yellin AE (1982) Traumatic diaphragmatic hernia. Arch Surg 117(1):18–24

Reiff DA, McGwin G Jr, Metzger J, Windham ST, Doss M, Rue LW 3rd (2002) Identifying injuries and motor vehicle collision characteristics that together are suggestive of diaphragmatic rupture. J Trauma 53(6):1139–1145

Rosati C (1998) Acute traumatic injury of the diaphragm. Chest Surg Clin N Am 8(2):371–379

Sabanathan S, Eng J, Mearns AJ (1990) Alterations in respiratory mechanics following thoracotomy. J R Coll Surg Edinb 35(3):144–150

Scharff JR, Naunheim KS (2007) Traumatic diaphragmatic injuries. Thorac Surg Clin 17(1):81–85

Shah R, Sabanathan S, Mearns AJ, Choudhury AK (1995) Traumatic rupture of diaphragm. Ann Thorac Surg 60(5):1444–1449

Shaw JM, Navsaria PH, Nicol AJ (2003) Laparoscopy assisted repair of diaphragm injuries. World J Surg 27:671–674

Ward RE, Flynn TC, Clark WP (1981) Diaphragmatic disruption secondary to blunt abdominal trauma. J Trauma 21(1):35–38

Williams M, Carlin AM, Tyburski JG, Blocksom JM, Harvey EH, Steffes CP, Wilson RF (2004) Predictors of mortality in patients with traumatic diaphragmatic rupture and associated thoracic and/or abdominal injuries. Am Surg 70(2):157–162; discussion 162–163

Diaphyseal Femur Fractures

▶ Femoral Shaft Fractures

DIC

▶ Disseminated Intravascular Coagulation

Died of Wounds

▶ Case Fatality Rate (CFR)

Diffuse Alveolar Damage

▶ Acute Respiratory Distress Syndrome (ARDS), General

Diffuse Alveolar Injury

▶ Acute Respiratory Distress Syndrome (ARDS), General

Diffuse Axonal Injury

▶ Traumatic Brain Injury, Intensive Care Unit Management

Dilutional Coagulopathy

▶ Coagulopathy in Trauma: Underlying Mechanisms

Disaster Management

James D. Kindscher
Department of Anesthesiology, University of Kansas Medical Center, Kansas City, KS, USA

Synonyms

Crisis standards of care; Emergency preparedness; Incident command system; Multiple casualty events; Surge capacity

Definition

Disaster management is the approach by all key stakeholders in responding to catastrophic events that stress the current system of patient management. Disaster management begins in the field at the site of the event, continues during triage and transport, then involves the acute of the victims and ends with secondary management and chronic care of the patients. The disaster, by its very nature, is unpredictable, and the devastation will overwhelm the normal resources used to care for smaller numbers of injured patients. Some key definitions for disaster management, taken from the American College of Surgeons, *Advanced Trauma Life Support Student Course Manual*, 9th ed. (ACS ATLS 2012), are as follows:

> *Area of Operations (Warm Zone)* The geographic subdivision established around a disaster site into which only qualified personnel are permitted.
> *Casualty Collection Point* A sector within the external perimeter of the Warm Zone where casualties who exit the Search & Rescue area (Hot Zone) via a decontamination chute are gathered prior to transport off site.
> *Decontamination Chute* A fixed or deployable facility where hazardous materials are removed

from a patient, and through which the patient must pass before transport, either out of the Search and Rescue area or into a hospital.

Emergency Operations Center The headquarters of Unified Incident Command for a region or system, established in a safe location outside the areas of operation.

External Perimeter The outer boundary of an Area of Operations that is established around a disaster site to separate geographical subdivisions that are safe for the general public from those that are safe only for qualified personnel.

Hospital Incident Command System An organizational structure used chiefly in the Americas to help coordinate an in-hospital disaster response.

Incident Command The final authority and overall coordinator for the management of any disaster response.

Internal Perimeter The outer boundary of a Search & Rescue area that isolates this area from the surrounding Area of Operations.

Minimum Acceptable Care The lowest appropriate level of medical and surgical treatment required to sustain life and limb until additional assets can be mobilized.

Search & Rescue Area (Hot Zone) A sector within the internal perimeter of an area of operations for a disaster in which humans are directly affected by the hazard.

Surge Capacity The extra assets that can actually be deployed in a disaster.

Preexisting Condition

Normally, healthcare delivery focuses on individualized treatments to improve outcome. Elective planning and application of abundant resources allows the care to be maximized for each patient under these circumstances. However in disaster management, major changes in our approach must occur to effectively respond to the overwhelming demand by mass casualties. Resources are likely to be limited, forcing the system to change how it delivers care to patients. The focus changes from individualized care to how best to care for the "community." Constrained resources and limited capacity lead to adopting crisis standards of care and triaging of limited resources (Hanfling et al. 2012b). There are usually four phases of disaster management described by public health authorities (ACS 2012): preparation, mitigation, response, and recovery. Preparation refers to disaster planning

at the national, state, community, hospital, and departmental levels. Mitigation addresses the need to reduce the impact of a disaster on the response and resources required to meet the needs of mass casualties. The response to a disaster begins at the site of harm and includes prehospital, triage, transport, decontamination, and hospital resources. Recovery refers to the phase where the system attempts to return to normal operations, often by transferring patients to other facilities.

Application

Recent disasters, such as the 2001 World Trade Center destruction, US Gulf Coast and upper East Coast hurricanes, the Haitian earthquake, and the Fukushima tsunami/nuclear disaster, demonstrated how mass casualties can quickly overwhelm a system. Even more limited events, such as the Fort Hood, Texas, and Aurora, Colorado, shootings, exposed flaws in our disaster management plans. Disasters often present unique circumstances that must be addressed. The 2001 World Trade Center disaster resulted in large volumes of casualties, many of which were first responders to the disaster, further weakening the response. The Fukushima nuclear disaster added decontamination challenges with radiation exposure. Hurricane Katrina overwhelmed the transportation systems and made evacuation of casualties difficult. The Joplin, Missouri, tornado scored a direct hit on one of the two hospitals in the city, reducing surge capacity and resources.

The initial response to a disaster must be met by the local resources. State and federal agencies will not be available for the first 24–72 h, leaving the brunt of the response to the disaster to be managed by the community. For this reason, it is imperative that hospital, community, and state disaster plans are formulated and disaster drills are conducted.

Planning for disaster management is complex and demanding for a community (Perry and Lindell 2006; Murray 2006). Guidelines have been developed to assist in the preparedness for disasters by the Joint Commission, Institute of Medicine, and Federal Emergency Management Agency (FEMA) (Hanfling et al. 2012a, www. fema.gov/nims). The National Incident Management System is the "…emergency management doctrine used across the United States to coordinate emergency preparedness and incident management response among the public and private sectors" (FEMA 2012). This includes

1. A standardized approach to incident management that is scalable and flexible
2. Enhanced cooperation and interoperability among responders
3. Comprehensive all-hazards preparedness
4. Efficient resource coordination among jurisdictions and organizations
5. Integration of best practices and lessons learned for continuous improvement

Three key elements for disaster management are preparation, command and control, and training.

Preparation for disaster management requires the integration of the local resources to function as a unit. Law enforcement, ambulance services, fire departments, hospitals, public health departments, and county coroners will need to work together in developing the disaster management plan. Members from each of these groups as well as media and public representatives must organize as a committee to oversee the development of the disaster management plan. Protocols, procedures, and plans must be developed that allow application of available resources. It is important to recognize the need to protect the healthcare workers in planning; the Sarin gas attack in Tokyo and SARS outbreak in Asia and Canada resulted in many healthcare workers becoming secondary victims of the disaster.

With the many different agencies responding to the disaster, it is essential that a command and control structure be developed to integrate and coordinate the delivery of care. Communication failures are one of the most important weaknesses identified in analyzing disaster response. The disaster often results in destruction of normal communication infrastructure. Cell phone towers may be destroyed, landlines disrupted, and paging systems rendered inoperable. Redundant communication systems with two-way radios are essential to insure coordinated responses. Communication at the site of the disaster to downstream providers allows for more efficient response and care. Triage must occur at all stages of the response: at the hot zone, during decontamination, in the receiving area of the hospital, and in the presurgical suite. The National Incident Management System describes how to organize this structure (FEMA).

With the limited resources available to care for many injured patients, crisis standards of care must be adopted (Hanfling et al. 2012b). Determining how to apply limited resources to achieve the maximal good requires skilled triage and clear lines of command. This may raise ethical questions and community concerns. Therefore, it is essential to address these issues in the planning stages and involve community leaders and the media, so they can assist in communications.

With the complexity of disaster management and infrequent application of the plan, training and drills are essential in assuring the system will respond appropriately when the actual disaster strikes. These drills should also serve as a mechanism to adapt and revise the plan to meet changing circumstances in the community. Disaster management plans will change as resources and best practices evolve. Therefore, frequent training is needed to insure an up-to-date response to disasters is utilized. The disaster response plan should undergo review and modification on a regular basis.

Cross-References

▶ Emergency Medical Services (EMS)
▶ Disaster Preparedness
▶ Life Support Training
▶ Mass Casualty
▶ Prehospital Emergency Preparedness
▶ Trauma Centers
▶ Triage

References

American College of Surgeons (2012) Advanced Trauma life support student course manual (ACS ATLS), 9th edn. Chicago

FEMA (2012) www.fema.gov/nims. Accessed 26 Nov 2012

Hanfling D, Altevogy BM, Gostin LO (2012a) A framework for catastrophic disaster response. JAMA 308:675–676

Hanfling D, Altevogth BM, Viswanathan K, Gostin LO (2012b) Crisis standards of care: a systems framework for catastrophic disaster response. The National Academies Press, Washington, DC

Murray MJ (2006) Disaster preparedness and weapons of mass destruction. In: Barash P, Cullen B, Stoelting R (eds) Clinical anesthesia, 5th edn. Lippincott Williams & Wilkins, Philadelphia

Perry RW, Lindell MK (2006) Hospital planning for weapons of mass destruction incidents. J Postgrad Med 52:116–120

Disaster Preparedness

George T. Loo[1] and Charles J. DiMaggio[2]
[1]Department of Epidemiology and Biostatistics, School of Public Health, University at Albany, Rensselaer, NY, USA
[2]Department of Anesthesiology and Epidemiology, Mailman School of Public Health, Columbia University, New York, NY, USA

Synonyms

Disaster Management; Emergency Management; Emergency Preparedness; Public Health Preparedness

Definition

While primary prevention is the goal of much of public health, this is often not feasible in the setting of disasters, so a public health approach for disaster preparedness is to minimize consequences by managing risk (Tekeli-Yeşil 2006). Risk can be measured as a factor of the combined input of hazard and vulnerability, where a hazard is the identified occurrence with potential risk and vulnerability is the susceptibility of the infrastructure or inhabitants to sustain consequences of exposure to the hazard. For example, some coastal areas are at *risk* for tropical cyclones and their associated phenomena (storm surge, tornado/high winds). Homes and persons living in the coastal areas would be *vulnerable* to varying degrees if a tropical cyclone were to make landfall. "Disaster preparedness" with an all-hazards approach can help reduce this risk.

Preexisting Condition

The World Health Organization (WHO) collaborating Center for Research on the Epidemiology of Disasters (CRED) defines disasters as "a situation or event which overwhelms local capacity, necessitating a request to a national or international level for external assistance; an unforeseen and often sudden event that causes great damage, destruction and human suffering" (Guha-Sapir et al. 2012). Within this context, disasters can be defined as natural or man-made, intentional or unintentional occurrences resulting in significant damage or destruction to infrastructure, morbidity and mortality to human/animal life, and/or alteration to the environment. Consequences of disasters include damage to established economic, social, and cultural facets of society (Tekeli-Yeşil 2006). According to a CRED report, in 2011 natural disasters resulted in the deaths of 30,773 persons and affected 244.7 million others. Monetary economic losses from natural disasters were calculated to approximate 366.1 billion US dollars (Guha-Sapir et al. 2012). In this brief overview, we discuss the role of hospitals and trauma care systems in disaster preparedness and present some current thinking on approaches to trauma care at the local, state, and national levels.

Application

The concept of resilience generally defined as "the ability to prepare and plan for, absorb, recover from and more successfully adapt to adverse events" (Committee on Increasing National Resilience to Hazards and Disasters et al. 2012) has witnessed a renewed emphasis since being first identified in the handbook Medical Surge Capacity and Capability: A Management System for Integrating Medical and Health Resources During Large-Scale Emergencies (Barbera and Macintyre 2007) as a critical component to guarantee medical surge requirements. Awareness, control, and attenuation of disaster risk strengthen resiliency to disaster consequences. The enhancement of resiliency may be accomplished by practicing basic emergency management principles. A comprehensive emergency management model was first established in the United States as early as the 1970s focusing on four concepts: mitigation, preparedness, response, and recovery. Mitigation is defined as the expectancy and attenuation of the disaster impact. Preparedness is a more complex interaction between advanced planning and management to secure swift and efficient response and recovery efforts. Response comprises direct actions taken to counter a disaster situation. Recovery encompasses measures to resume regular daily operations.

The Role of Hospitals

Hospitals are the backbone of the health-care response to common medical disasters (i.e., mass casualty events that occur with relative frequency, overwhelm a single hospital, and require a community-wide health response) and, in particular, to catastrophic emergencies, such as an influenza pandemic or large-scale aerosolized anthrax attack. The need for hospitals to be prepared to respond to disasters has increasingly become a priority for hospital leaders. They have been influenced by events such as the 2001 terrorist attacks and Hurricane Katrina and the increased emphasis placed by accreditation organizations and regulatory agencies on the importance of such disasters. Trauma care systems need to take an all-hazards approach that addresses all potential hazards and vulnerabilities and is more preferred over planning efforts that focus on single types of incidents or events.

The critical importance of preparedness planning is reinforced by the Joint Commission on the Accreditation of Healthcare Organizations (JACHO) requiring compliance with defined goals and objectives that can be found in a distinct section of their documents.

The US Department of Health and Human Services (HHS) in 2002 established the Hospital Preparedness Program (HPP), originally known as the National Bioterrorism Hospital Preparedness Program (NBHPP), to increase the capability of hospitals and health-care systems to prepare and respond to public health emergencies, such as bioterrorism, pandemic influenza, and natural disasters. The initial mission of the NBHPP was to enhance the capability levels of hospitals and other stakeholders to respond to bioterrorism. As an added benefit, such preparedness activity would enable hospitals and stakeholders to respond to other unintentional disease epidemics. HPP was initially administered by the Health Resources and Services Administration (HRSA). However, the 2006 Pandemic and All-Hazards Preparedness Act (PAHPA) initiated several changes. Major changes were the creation of the Office of the Assistant Secretary for Preparedness and Response (ASPR) within HHS and transferring of the HPP cooperative agreement program administration from HRSA to ASPR. The mission of the NBHPP in conjunction with the DHS National Preparedness Goal was expanded to include all-hazards preparedness. In addition, PAHPA legislation in order to improve surge capacity and strengthen community and hospital preparedness authorized the HHS Secretary to grant competitive funding awards to eligible health-care partnerships by altering a section of the Public Health Service Act, while continuing the original funding formula for HPP cooperative awards to states, territories, and the nation's three largest municipalities.

Funding for the NBHPP was initialized in FY2002 with an influx of approximately $135 million; $125 million was appropriated to hospitals through cooperative agreements with awardees, which included state, municipal, and territorial health departments. Funding award levels for each fiscal year is calculated based on the sum of a fixed amount plus a variable amount that is proportional to each awardee's population. Cooperative agreement awardees determine which hospitals to fund, how many to fund, and the amount of funding for each hospital. From FY2002 to FY2012, the HPP program total yearly funding ranged from $135 million to $515 million with decreases in total yearly funding starting from 2007. HPP cooperative awards are awarded to 62 entities that include the 50 states, the District of Columbia, the nation's three largest municipalities (Chicago, Los Angeles, and New York City), the Commonwealths of Puerto Rico and the Northern Mariana Islands, three territories (American Samoa, Guam, and the US Virgin Islands), Micronesia, the Marshall Islands, and Palau.

This program sought to enhance the ability of health-care facilities and systems by strengthening interoperable communication systems, bed tracking, personnel management, fatality management planning, hospital evacuation planning, bed and personnel surge capacity, decontamination capabilities, isolation capacity, pharmaceutical supplies, training, education, drills, and exercises. In 2012, the US DHHS created a single application process for cooperative agreements under the Hospital Preparedness Program and the Public Health Emergency Preparedness Program. The alignment of cooperative agreements retains separate capabilities that address the specific requirements of each cooperative agreement's mission but now realizes certain shared mission assignments through joint capabilities. HPP capabilities moving forward for the next 5 years 2012–2017 include many of the mentioned activities and have been captured within the eight defined capabilities (Office of the Assistant Secretary for Preparedness and Response 2012).

The Role of Trauma Systems

Beyond the role of US hospitals, a critically important resource for state, regional, and local response to disasters is the US trauma system and its trauma centers. Trauma systems need to be proactively engaged in health-care and public health preparedness planning to ensure that trauma systems themselves are incorporated into the state, regional, and local disaster preparedness and response comprehensive emergency management plans. The trauma center will often be at the forefront of response to a disaster. The challenge exists when the need for assets and resources from the disaster overwhelms the existing capabilities of the trauma care facility, escalating into the activation of a series of actions that cascade the response of additional resources, including resources from the regional and state inventory; very often, these steps are codified in a comprehensive emergency management plan (CEMP).

Although trauma systems are frequently thought of as caring for the individual victim of an injury, their development must incorporate the possibility of a mass casualty disaster. Recent national events have further reinforced the need for disaster preparedness activities to include the involvement of trauma systems and emergency medicine. Trauma system preparedness must include capabilities for victims of weapons of mass destruction including but not limited to nuclear, chemical, and biological weapons. Federal agencies (e.g., USDHS, USDOD, USHHS, USDOT) have interests and authority in this arena, and their input into trauma system development and maintenance is essential. Emergency medicine has contributed by participating with these organizations in disaster preparedness.

A National Highway Traffic Safety Administration (NHTSA) report (US Department of Transportation, National Highway Traffic Safety Administration 2004) highlighted several critical concepts that are paramount for trauma systems to observe for disaster preparedness. They advocated that trauma systems need to be well incorporated into regional and state disaster plans with coordinated incident command efforts that include robust public health infrastructure, emergency medical services, and law enforcement. Education efforts focused on the identification and response to weapons of mass destruction coupled with decontamination efforts in the hospital and prehospital setting. Robust surveillance systems integrating hospital, community, and EMS networks which provide rapid identification of all these threats are needed. Redundant interoperable communication systems that connect across all levels of the response chain and hospital command centers which integrate into the disaster incident command system are crucial communication networks.

Ensuring proper integration of the trauma center and trauma care system into comprehensive emergency plans necessitates the administration of resource assessments of surge capacity. Surge capacity is the ability of a health-care system to meet a sudden increase in demand due to a disaster. This assessment in order to be comprehensive should be based on and tied to a hazard vulnerability analysis and/or gap analysis. To further evaluate the trauma center and the trauma care system's capability to respond to a disaster requires facilitated tabletop or functional exercises. These exercises should then result in Homeland Security Exercise and Evaluation Program (HSEEP) compliant After Action Reports/Improvement Plan (AAR/IPs) with delineated timetables for improvement action execution.

Comprehensive planning and incorporation of the trauma center and trauma care system with related stakeholders/partners (public health, EMS, medical examiner, health-care facilities, OEM) are critically important in the ability of the trauma care system/trauma center to deliver adequate medical care during a disaster crisis. Disasters are by definition chaotic in nature and extensively tax established protocols and resource allocation. Established networks and joint exercise practice with stakeholder/partners ensure urgent and responsive deployment of these assets and support services when a major event/incident does happen (American College of Surgeons Committee on Trauma 2008).

Funding of preparedness activities can be a major commitment, and health-care facilities may be hesitant to commit funding resources to emergency preparedness activities that may or may not be utilized. To respond to these concerns, in the United States, the US Department of Health and Human Services–Assistant Secretary for Preparedness and Response–Hospital Preparedness Program (USDHHS-ASPR-HPP) cooperative agreement provides some resources toward hospital emergency preparedness.

The universal approach to strengthen disaster preparedness capabilities in trauma care systems is to apply a systematically consistent model. One such model is to implement the HPP capabilities as defined in the USHHS Healthcare Preparedness Capabilities Guidance Jan 2012 (Office of the Assistant Secretary for Preparedness and Response 2012). These capabilities cover a wide spectrum of preparedness activities. The issue is whether health-care facilities will be willing to make the necessary expenditures to address gaps covered and/or identified by analysis to approach these capabilities. Trauma care system delivery places an emphasis on satisfying the medical needs of the individual seeking emergency trauma care; this approach differs from the emergency preparedness approach which focuses on satisfying the needs of the greatest number of persons with the available resources, resources which often are finite. This population-based needs approach is not a foreign concept; public health preparedness follows a similar population-based approach. The synthesis of medical and public health emergency preparedness is an ideal model to drive this effort.

Given the hesitation for expenditures in assets and resources that may never be used, innovative concepts in creating the necessary capacities are being fielded. One idea being proposed is Immediate Bed Availability; this concept is most closely aligned with Capability 10 Medical Surge in the Healthcare Preparedness Capabilities Guidance (Office of the Assistant Secretary for Preparedness and Response 2012). The HHS ASPR Immediate Bed Availability concept proposes that a facility make available 20 % of staffed hospital beds to more acute care patients within 4 h of a disaster by classifying and seeking alternate appropriate care for patients with lower acuity; the construct is similar to reverse triage (Kelen et al. 2006, 2009). This is in contrast to alternate models which propose that facilities create an additional 20 % bed capacity by exceeding the daily bed census. The IBA model creates a 20 % surge capacity by decompression of lower acuity patients to alternate appropriate care modalities such as long-term care facilities or other non-acute facilities. This patient transfer can be more readily accomplished by applying another concept, the health-care coalition which is a prescribed function found under Capability 1: Healthcare System Preparedness of the Healthcare Preparedness Capability Guidance (Office of the Assistant Secretary for Preparedness and Response 2012). The concept of health-care coalitions is not new. This concept was described in the handbooks Medical Surge Capacity and Capability: A Management System for Integrating Medical and Health Resources During Large-Scale Emergencies (Barbera and Macintyre 2007) and Medical Surge Capacity and Capability: The Healthcare Coalition in Emergency Response and Recovery (Barbera and Macintyre 2009). An outcome of the health-care coalition is to form a network of health-care systems that share informational situational awareness and can coordinate management of health-care assets. The health-care coalition also prescribes integrated coordination of these efforts within the local incident command system structure. Assets may include long-term care, alternative treatment facilities, dialysis and other outpatient treatment centers, nursing homes and nursing facilities, private physician offices, clinics, and community health centers. Thus, the integrated availability of these assets could facilitate the mission of bed surge by patient decompression and acceptance from one facility to another.

Preparedness has had a long historical presence, and preparedness begins at the individual level by taking efforts to ready one's self. In a disaster or complex crisis, planning at the regional and national level that addresses the population is as crucial as individualized medical/trauma care. Health-care practitioners can contribute to the process by actively engaging in institutional efforts, by adopting common vocabulary and protocols, by providing timely information to help guide interventions, and by familiarizing themselves with local and regional plans.

Cross-References

▶ Disaster Management
▶ Joint Trauma System (JTS)
▶ Mass Casualty
▶ Prehospital Emergency Preparedness
▶ Trauma Centers

References

American College of Surgeons Committee on Trauma (2008) Regional trauma systems: optimal elements, integration and assessments, American College of Surgeons Committee on Trauma: systems consultation guide. A. B. Nathens. American College of Surgeons, Chicago

Barbera JA, Macintyre AG (2007) Medical surge capacity and capability: a management system for integrating medical and health resources during large-scale emergencies. U. S. D. o. H. a. H. Services. The CNA Corporation Institute for Public Research, Washington, DC

Barbera JA, Macintyre AG (2009) Medical surge capacity and capability: the healthcare coalition in emergency response and recovery. U. S. D. o. H. a. H. Services. CNA, Institute for Public Research, Washington, DC

Committee on Increasing National Resilience to Hazards and Disasters et al (2012) Disaster resilience: a national imperative. The National Academies Press, Washington, DC

Guha-Sapir D, Vos F et al (2012) Annual disaster statistical review 2011: the numbers and trends. C. f. R. o. t. E. o. D.-. CRED. Universite Catholique de Louvain, Brussels

Kelen GD, Kraus CK et al (2006) Inpatient disposition classification for the creation of hospital surge capacity: a multiphase study. Lancet 368(9551):1984–1990

Kelen GD, McCarthy ML et al (2009) Creation of surge capacity by early discharge of hospitalized patients at low risk for untoward events. Disaster Med Public Health Prep 3(2 Suppl):S10–S16

Office of the Assistant Secretary for Preparedness and Response (2012) Healthcare preparedness capabilities national guidance for healthcare system preparedness. U. S. D. o. H. a. H. Services, Washington, DC

Tekeli-Yeşil S (2006) Public health and natural disasters: disaster preparedness and response in health systems. J Public Health 14:317–324

US Department of Transportation, National Highway Traffic Safety Administration (2004) Trauma system agenda for the future. A. T. Society, Washington, DC

Discharge Planner

▶ Social Worker

Discharge Planning

John Graffeo
York College Physician Assistant Program, City
University of New York, Jamaica, NY, USA

Synonyms

Aftercare; Post acute phases; Post hospital;
Transfers

Definition

Discharge planning identifies needs and services
to assist patients from one level of care to
another. This can occur in the post-acute phases
with transfer from in-hospital settings to short-
term and long-term facilities (Langstaff and
Christie 2000).

Pre-existing Condition

When a patient is involved in a traumatic accident
usually the last thing on the mind of the first
responders and subsequently the trauma team is
the patient's discharge. The idea of the patient's
discharge from the hospital needs to be placed in
the psyche of the team upon admission. This
could ensure the smooth transition to subsequent
care facilities as well as to home. Ideally the
discharge planner could be a part of the initial
trauma team.

To plan for any patient's discharge from the
hospital setting many factors are taken into consideration. In an attempt to circumvent any delay
the patient and family members need to be
involved in planning. The type of care the
patient will require is always the first consideration and the availability of a receiving facility
in a convenient location for further discharge
planning should be considered. Cost measures
may come into play during the discharge
process.

Application

The most common reasons for admission to
a trauma center are falls, gunshot wounds
(GSW) or motor vehicle accidents (MVA).
These types of injuries may require specific
needs upon discharge (Belcher et al. 2005; Sen
et al. 2009).

Many will need physical therapy, occupational therapy or speech therapy. There may
also be a need for home health assistance with
Activities of Daily Living (ADL) with personal
functions including ambulation, hygiene, feeding, wound care and stoma care.

Two significant issues that need to be considered include patient insurance coverage and
societal assimilation. The initial trauma phase
cost is usually not the issue, but subsequent
care may be delayed until coverage is in
place. Insurance directives may delay the
onset of placement to an alternative facility.
For example, in the United States, a Medicare
patient with a complex plan of care must be
an in-patient for three nights before they can
be discharged to a SNF (Medicare Benefit
Policy Manual 2012). Coordination of care
will decrease length of stay; improve upon
resource utilization and unforeseen discharge
delays.

Societal issues may be more philosophical.
Many injuries occur at inner city or rural locations. Many times discharge and aftercare planning fail to address community violence and
other community problems (Belcher et al.
2005). For instance, a patient with a history
of alcohol abuse (ETOH) and motor vehicle
accidents; an inner city patient with gang
involvement that presents with a gun shot
wound and returns to the same environment. Prior to discharge it is important that
close emphasis on needs requirements are made.
Frequently, readmissions occur because all of
the patient needs were not in place upon discharge. Options that are close to home are best
so that family members can visit and participate
in the patient's physical and psychological
rehabilitation.

Cross-References

▶ Activity Restrictions
▶ Adaptive Equipment
▶ Physical Therapist
▶ Social Worker

References

Belcher J, DeForge BR, Jani JJ (2005) Inner-city victims of violence and trauma care: the importance of trauma-center discharge and aftercare planning and violence prevention programs. J Health Soc Policy 21(2):17–34
Langstaff D, Christie J (2000) Trauma care: a team approach. Elsevier Health Sciences
Sen A, Xia Y, Hu P, Dutton R, Haan J, O'Connor J, Pollak A, Scalea T (2009) Daily multidisciplinary discharge rounds in a trauma center: a little time, well spent. J Trauma 66

Recommended Reading

Medicare Benefit Policy Manual (2012) Coverage of Extended Care (SNF) Services Under Hospital Insurance

---

Discomfort

▶ Pain

Discontinuation of Mechanical Ventilation

▶ Mechanical Ventilation, Weaning

Dislocation, Atlas or Axis

Mari L. Groves and Daniel M. Sciubba
Department of Neurosurgery, The Johns Hopkins University School of Medicine, Baltimore, MD, USA

Synonyms

Atlanto-axial dislocation; Internal decapitation; Occipitoatlantal dislocation

Definition

Atlanto-occipital dislocations (AOD) are unstable injuries that may occur simultaneously with odontoid fractures, likely secondary to disruption of craniocervical ligaments. The basion-dental interval (BDI) and basion-posterior axial line interval (BAI) are the most reproducible and reliable measurements of the upper cervical spine, although other measurements, such as Power's ratio, Lee's lines, McCrae's line, and the Chamberlain line, are well described in the literature (Bono et al. 2007). The BAI measures the horizontal distance between a tangent line to the posterior aspect of axis and the basion and should measure no greater than 12 mm (Fig. 1). The BDI measures the distance between the basion and the tip of the dens and should not exceed 12 mm. (Fig. 1) When either of these measurements exceeds 12 mm, an atlanto-occipital dislocation should be suspected. (Bono et al. 2007).

AOD can present with either minimal neurological deficit or significant bulbar-cervical dissociation that can even result in death due to anoxia and respiratory arrest. AOD should be considered an unstable injury and requires stabilization via an external Halo orthosis or with sandbags. Cervical traction is contraindicated because of the risk of neurologic deterioration. Surgical stabilization via a posterior occipito-cervical fusion is typically indicated when patients have a clear abnormality on MRI that shows disruption of the atlanto-occipital joints, tectorial membrane, or alar or cruciate ligaments as well as any significant findings on CT (Kenter et al. 2001; Labbe et al. 2001; Dickman et al. 1993). In atlanto-occipital dislocation should be immediately immobilized with halo orthosis or with sandbags in patients who are unable to undergo halo stabilization. These dislocations are considered highly unstable and will typically require surgical stabilization or prolonged immobilization. If there is no abnormal CT findings with minimal MRI signal change to indicate less ligamentous injury, the patient may first undergo stabilization through a halo

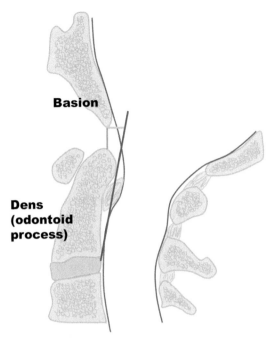

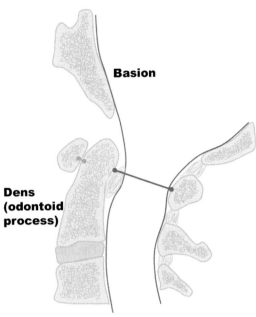

D

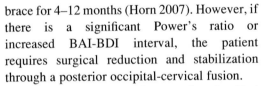

Dislocation, Atlas or Axis, Fig. 1 Illustration of BDI and BAI at the craniocervical junction. The posterior axial line, shown in *red*. The basion-dental interval (BDI) is shown in *blue*. The basion-posterior axial line (BAI) is shown in *green*

Dislocation, Atlas or Axis, Fig. 2 Illustration of ADI and PADI at the craniocervical junction. The atlanto-dental interval (ADI) is shown in *blue*. The posterior atlanto-dental interval is shown in *red*

brace for 4–12 months (Horn 2007). However, if there is a significant Power's ratio or increased BAI-BDI interval, the patient requires surgical reduction and stabilization through a posterior occipital-cervical fusion.

Atlanto-axial subluxation can be classified based on mechanism of injury and include rotatory, anterior, and posterior. Atlanto-axial dissociation involves subluxation, dislocation, and rotary fixation of C1/C2. Measurement of the basion-dens interval (BDI) can identify if there is abnormal displacement between these two vertebrae. BDI > 12 mm is abnormal (Bono et al. 2007) (Fig. 1). The atlanto-dental interval (ADI) and posterior atlanto-dental interval (PADI) have been validated in patients with non-traumatic pathologies in measuring atlanto-axial dislocations. In flexion, the ADI should not exceed 3 mm and the PADI should be no less than 14 mm, as a decrease in the PADI correlates with less space for the spinal cord

(Bono et al. 2007) (Fig. 2). In addition, the Rule of Spence may be applied via an open-mouth odontoid x-ray to assess competency of the cruciate ligaments. If the total overhang of both C1 lateral masses on C2 is greater than 7 mm, the ligament should be considered incompetent. Atlanto-axial dislocation is a highly unstable injury and should be treated with either immediate halo immobilization or posterior fusion.

Cross-References

▶ Fracture, Odontoid
▶ Imaging of CNS Injuries

References

Bono CM, Vaccaro AR, Fehlings M, Fisher C, Dvorak M, Ludwig S, Harrop J, Spine Trauma Study Group (2007) Measurement techniques for upper cervical spine injuries: consensus statement of the Spine Trauma Study Group. Spine (Phila Pa1976) 32(5):593–600

Dickman CA, Papadopoulos SM, Sonntag VK, Spetzler RF, Rekate HL, Drabier J (1993) Traumatic occipitoatlantal dislocations. J Spinal Disord 6(4):300–313

Kenter K, Worley G, Griffin T, Fitch RD (2001) Pediatric traumatic atlanto-occipital dislocation: five cases and a review. J Pediatr Orthop 21(5):585–589

Labbe JL, Leclair O, Duparc B (2001) Traumatic atlanto-occipital dislocation with survival in children. J Pediatr Orthop B 10(4):319–327

Dislocation, Facets

Patricia L. Zadnik and Daniel M. Sciubba
Department of Neurosurgery, The Johns
Hopkins University School of Medicine,
Baltimore, MD, USA

Synonyms

Jumped facets; Locked facets; Perched facets

Definition

Locked facets typically result from severe flexion injuries that reverse the normal "shingled" relationship between the facets and can result from disruption of the facet capsule. This is considered to be an unstable injury, as it includes severe disruption of the posterior ligaments and distraction of the posterior column. Bilateral facet dislocation is caused by hyperflexion and subluxation of adjacent vertebral bodies. Due to the disruption of normal joint integrity, facets may "jump" and become locked or "perched"; the phrase "jumped locked facets" may be used to describe a bilateral facet dislocation (Wheeless III 2013) (Fig. 1). Bilateral facet dislocation often results in neurologic compromise, which may be worsened by disk herniation or an epidural hematoma. CT scans may show a "naked facet sign" when the articular surface of the facet will be seen without the appropriate articulating surface of the facet. MRI should also be performed to rule out traumatic disk herniation, which can be seen in up to 80 % of bilateral locked facets (Rizzolo et al. 1991). Reduction of facet dislocation associated with disk herniation may worsen spinal cord injury (Doran et al. 1993). Closed or open reduction can be applied to reduce subluxation and can be followed by anterior or posterior arthrodesis with fixation (Wheeless III 2013).

Unilateral facet dislocation can result from flexion injuries with a rotational component. These fractures may occur with fracture of either facet or the lateral mass and partial tearing of the posterior longitudinal ligament. Disk herniation may also be seen. These patients may be neurologically intact (19 %), nerve root deficit (22 %), incomplete cord injuries (26 %), or complete quadriplegics (13 %) (Hadley et al. 1992).

Dislocation, Facets, Fig. 1 Axial (**a**) and sagittal (**b**) CT scans demonstrating left sided perched facet (*white arrow*). The contralateral facet is dislocated without superior displacement

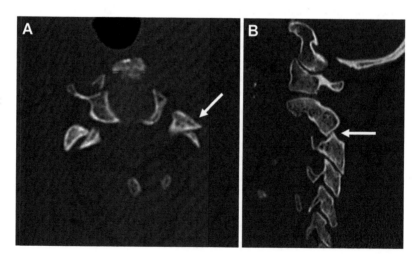

Cross-References

► Fracture, Flexion Injury
► Fractures

References

Doran SE, Papadopoulos SM, Ducker TB, Lillehei KO (1993) Magnetic resonance imaging documentation of coexistent traumatic locked facets of the cervical spine and disc herniation. J Neurosurg 79(3):341–345
Hadley MN, Fitzpatrick BC, Sonntag VK, Browner CM (1992) Facet fracture-dislocation injuries of the cervical spine. Neurosurgery 30(5):661–666
Rizzolo SJ, Piazza MR, Cotler JM, Balderston RA, Schaefer D, Flanders A (1991) Intervertebral disc injury complicating cervical spine trauma. Spine (Phila Pa1976) 16(Suppl 6):S187–S189
Wheeless III CR (2013) "Wheeless Textbook of Orthopedics." Wheeless' textbook of orthopaedics. Duke University Medical Center. http://www. wheelessonline.com/. Accessed 8 Feb 2013

Dismember

► Amputation

Disseminated Intravascular Coagulation

Bryan A. Cotton[1] and Laura A. McElroy[2]
[1]Department of Surgery, Division of Acute Care Surgery, Trauma and Critical Care, University of Texas Health Science Center at Houston, The University of Texas Medical School at Houston, Houston, TX, USA
[2]Department of Anesthesiology, Critical Care Medicine, University of Rochester Medical Center, Rochester, NY, USA

Synonyms

DIC

Definition

Disseminated intravascular coagulation (DIC) is a clinicopathological syndrome characterized by massive systemic activation of the coagulation cascade by a wide range of etiologies, leading to both extensive microvascular thrombi and impaired fibrinolysis with diffuse bleeding from many sites (Ho et al. 2005). DIC, once initiated, requires prompt diagnosis and aggressive resuscitative efforts in order to reverse its rapid progression to death. Recently, two main patterns of activation have been identified: one a systemic inflammatory response leading to cytokine production and coagulation seen most frequently in sepsis and trauma and the other a massive release of prothrombotic material into the circulation (Hess et al. 2008). The second type occurs in obstetrics with amniotic fluid embolism and tumor lysis syndromes with certain types of cancer (Kawano et al. 2013).

Trauma, or more specifically the extensive tissue damage subsequent to traumatic injury, has been recognized as a potential activator of DIC. Endothelial damage, release of phospholipids and fats into the blood stream, and cytokine release are all implicated in activating DIC (Levi and Meijers 2011). Recent investigations have delineated DIC into two distinct phases that follow after a tissue factor (TF)-dependent initiation: an early fibrinolytic subtype manifested clinically as massive bleeding and a later antifibrinolytic subtype that can lead to disseminated thrombus formation and ultimately multiorgan dysfunction syndrome (MODS) (Gando et al. 2013a).

Whether DIC is responsible for the early coagulopathy seen in severely injured patients or represents a point on the spectrum of coagulopathic disorders seen in trauma is unknown and debated at present. Early acute coagulopathy of trauma (ACOT) has received much interest lately, and there is some debate currently whether this is a new clinical entity resulting from global and systemic hypoperfusion and resultant shock or this represents a fibrinolytic phenotype of DIC (Gando et al. 2013b).

Cross-References

► Acute Coagulopathy of Trauma
► Coagulopathy
► Coagulopathy in Trauma: Underlying Mechanisms

References

Gando S, Wada H, Thachil J (2013a) Differentiating disseminated intravascular coagulation (DIC) with the fibrinolytic phenotype from coagulopathy of trauma and acute coagulopathy of trauma-shock (COT/ACOTS). J Thromb Haemost 11(5):826–835. doi:10.1111/jth.12190

Gando S, Saitoh D, Ogura H (2013b) A multicenter, prospective validation study of the Japanese Association for acute medicine disseminated intravascular coagulation scoring system in patients with severe sepsis. Crit Care 20(3):R111(epub ahead of print)

Hess JR, Brohl K, Dutton RP et al (2008) The coagulopathy of trauma: a review of mechanisms. J Trauma 65(4):748–754. doi:10.1097/TA.0b013e3181877a9c

Ho LWW, Kam PCA, Thong CL (2005) Disseminated intravascular coagulation. Curr Anesth Crit Care 16(3):151–161

Kawano N, Kuriyama T, Yoshida S (2013) Clinical features and treatment outcomes of six patients with disseminated intravascular coagulation resulting from acute promyelocytic leukemia and treated with recombinant human soluble thrombomodulin at a single institution. Intern Med 52(1):55–62

Levi M, Meijers JC (2011) DIC: which laboratory tests are most useful. Blood Rev 25(1):33–37. doi:10.1016/j.blre.2010.09.002

Distal Femoral Physeal Fractures

▶ Pediatric Femur Fractures

Distal Femur Fractures

Arun Aneja[1] and Matt L. Graves[2]
[1]Department of Orthopaedic Surgery and Rehabilitation Medicine, University of Chicago Medicine & Biological Sciences, Chicago, IL, USA
[2]Department of Orthopaedic Surgery, Division of Trauma, University of Mississippi Medical Center, Jackson, MS, USA

Synonyms

OTA 33 A-C fracture; Supracondylar femur fractures; Supracondylar-intercondylar femur fracture

Definition

Distal femur fractures involve the distal one third of the femur, consisting of the region between the diaphyseal-metaphyseal junction and the articular surface of the femoral condyles. This is considered to be the terminal 10–15 cm of the distal femur. These injuries make up about 3–7 % of all femur fractures (Court-Brown and Caesar 2006). They occur with a bimodal age distribution. Younger patients typically have higher-energy mechanisms such as motor vehicle collisions, motorcycle crashes, and falls from a considerable height. These mechanisms are characterized by significant fracture displacement, comminution, and occasionally associated vascular injuries and soft tissue compromise (Albert 1997; Schmidt and Teague 2010; Kenneth et al. 2010; Wiss et al. 1996). Elderly patients typically have a lower-energy mechanism such as a fall from standing height. These lower-energy mechanisms create fractures in the elderly secondary to osteopenic or osteoporotic bone quality. The prevalence of distal femur fractures in the elderly patient population is increasing as the number of knee replacement procedures increase, occurring in 0.5–2.5 % of patients with total knee arthroplasty (TKA). The femoral component of the knee prosthesis creates a mismatch between the stiff implant and osteopenic bone creating a stress riser that increases the risk of fracture at the proximal extent of the implant. Risk factors for periprosthetic distal femur fractures include osteopenia, inflammatory arthritis, prolonged corticosteroid use, anterior notching of the femoral cortex, and revision arthroplasty (Chen et al. 1994; DiGioia and Rubash 1991). Regardless of the energy associated with the injury, the mechanism for nearly all distal third femur fractures is an axial load with an angular component (varus/valgus) or an axial rotational component (internal rotation/external rotation).

Anatomy

In order to appropriately manage and treat such injuries, one must truly understand the three-dimensional anatomy of the distal femur which includes both the supracondylar and condylar regions (Fig. 1). The femoral shaft is cylindrically

Distal Femur Fractures, Fig. 1 Anatomy of the distal femur. (**a**) Anterior view. (**b**) Lateral view. The shaft of the femur is aligned with the anterior half of the lateral condyle. (**c**) Axial view. The distal femur is trapezoidal. The anterior surface slopes downward from lateral to medial, the lateral wall inclines 10°, and the medial wall inclines 25° (Adapted from Wiss et al. 1996)

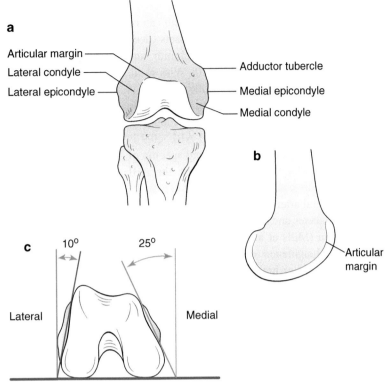

shaped and broadens into two curved condyles distally, separated by an intercondylar groove which articulates with the patella and an intercondylar notch that has the origin of the cruciate ligaments. The medial condyle is more convex, extending more distally than the lateral femoral condyle, creating the apparent anatomic valgus of the knee that measures approximately 8° (variation range from 5 to 12°). The lateral condyle is broader and does not extend as far distally. On lateral views, the anterior half of the condyles is aligned with the femoral shaft while the posterior half protrudes posterior to the posterior cortex of the shaft. When viewing the distal femur end on (i.e., guns' eye view), the condyles form a trapezoid that is wider posteriorly than anteriorly, with an angle of inclination of the medial surface of approximately 25° and an angle of inclination of 10° on the lateral surface. On average, a line bisecting the epicondyles (epicondylar axis) is in 3° of external rotation compared to a line bisecting the posterior axis of the condyles (posterior condylar axis).

The knee joint should be parallel to the ground during ambulation. Radiographs of the contralateral limb are often the best way to define the limb axis of each person and are particularly useful for preoperative planning. The deforming forces acting on a distal third femur fracture include the gastrocnemius which produces an apex posterior deformity at the fracture site in the sagittal plane, while the quadriceps and hamstring insertion cause shortening of the lower extremity in the axial plane (Albert 1997; Schmidt and Teague 2010; Kenneth et al. 2010; Wiss et al. 1996; Court-Brown and Caesar 2006).

Evaluation

Patients presenting with such injuries have pain, swelling, and deformity of the lower thigh and knee with the inability to ambulate. Additional injuries in the same extremity and/or other body parts must be sought after particularly for high-energy mechanism injuries. Distal pulses must be evaluated given the proximity of the popliteal vasculature to the fracture site. Tense swelling, pallor, and inability to palpate distal pulses in the injured versus the non-injured distal limb can be indicative of rupture of the major vessels (deep femoral/popliteal) (Albert 1997; Schmidt and Teague 2010; Kenneth et al. 2010; Wiss et al. 1996; Court-Brown and Caesar 2006). If there is any concern for vascular injury, ankle-ankle (AAI) or ankle-brachial indices (ABI) should be measured. In a healthy patient, an ABI <0.9 is considered to be 100 % sensitive and specific of a significant arterial injury. However, the ABI may be inaccurate and falsely elevated in patients with peripheral arterial disease such as hypertension and diabetes and elderly patients with vessel calcification (Mills et al. 2004). Nonetheless, if there is a heightened concern for a vascular injury, the next step in the algorithm is to proceed with a computed tomography angiogram (CTA) or formal angiogram and enlistment of a vascular surgery consult. The incidence of vascular disruption with isolated supracondylar fractures is between 2 % and 3 %. Open fractures occur in 5–25 % of all distal femur fractures with the traumatic wound usually located anteriorly with partial disruption of the extensor mechanism (Albert 1997; Schmidt and Teague 2010; Kenneth et al. 2010; Wiss et al. 1996). As with all open fractures, early debridement and irrigation along with IV antibiotic administration is critical to avoid infection. In cases of laceration or puncture wounds involving the distal femur, the knee joint may be challenged with 120 cc of saline injected from a remote location to determine continuity of the open wound to the knee joint. This would be witnessed by extravasation of the fluid through the open wound after being injected into the knee joint. CT scanning and radiographs may also show free air in the knee joint prior to saline injection suggesting communication between the open wound and the knee joint. Appropriate anteroposterior (AP) and lateral radiographs of the knee should be obtained in addition to biplanar radiographs of the entire femur. Traction views can help better define the fracture fragments in the case of comminuted distal femur fractures or fractures associated with significant shortening and deformity. Two-dimensional CT scans with coronal and sagittal

reformats are a prerequisite if there is concern for intraarticular involvement (Schmidt and Teague 2010; Kenneth et al. 2010). CT scans delineate fracture fragments and can identify occult fracture fragments such as the coronal plane Hoffa fracture line that can often be missed in plain radiographs (Baker et al. 2002). MRI may be useful when there is concern for associated ligamentous or meniscal injury.

Classification

As with all osseous injuries, the first step in classification is determination of whether the fracture is open versus closed. The level and location of the fracture lines must also be noted to determine whether the fracture is extra-articular (supracondylar), partial articular (lateral or medial femoral condylar), or complete articular (supracondylar intercondylar). This classification scheme can help with treatment planning as articular involvement dictates anatomic reconstruction. The pattern of the fracture can be indicative of the mechanism with an axial load combined with angulation producing an oblique fracture line, torsion resulting in a spiral fracture line, and three-point bending producing a transverse fracture on the tension side and an oblique fracture with or without a wedge on the compression side of the bone (Alms 1961). Factors crucial for treatment planning include articular involvement and the degree and direction of displacement. The Orthopaedic Trauma Association (OTA) classification system distinguishes between extra-articular (Type A), partial articular (Type B), and complete intraarticular (Type C) distal femur fractures (Marsh 2009). There can be a vast array of fracture patterns, and each and every case must be evaluated individually with treatment based on the individual "personality" of the fracture and the patient.

Nonoperative Treatment

The treatment goal is to obtain an anatomic reduction of the articular surface and restore limb length, alignment, and rotation in order to permit early mobilization and fracture union so that the patient can return to normal function (Schatzker and Tile 1991). This makes conservative treatment challenging, as close control of displacement is compromised. Nonoperative treatment is sought for nondisplaced fractures, impacted stable fractures, incomplete fractures, and in patients with advanced underlying medical conditions that preclude them from surgical treatment because of the potential life-threatening anesthetic and operative risks. The involved extremity is placed in a cast brace or long-leg cast with early mobilization and protected ambulation with non-weight-bearing status. If the fracture is significantly displaced, the involved extremity can undergo a closed manipulative reduction and be placed in a cast for 6–12 weeks, with serial cast changes every few weeks. Other nonoperative treatment options for displaced distal femur fractures include skeletal traction that may be combined with a Thomas splint and Pearson attachment. This requires a traction pin placed through the proximal tibia that is maintained for 6–8 weeks until the fracture becomes "sticky" while the patient is bedridden (Albert 1997). Mobilization is begun once pain and swelling subside in order to prevent intraarticular adhesion and fibrosis. Mobilization is facilitated via a cast brace with a molded thigh component contoured around the condyles and extending well above the fracture site connected with hinges to another full contact cast brace section applied to the leg and foot. This cast brace is worn for an additional 6–8 weeks and removed once the patient is able to tolerate full weight bearing. Drawbacks of nonoperative treatment include knee stiffness with prolonged immobilization, residual fracture displacement and angulation, and the need for prolonged hospitalization and bed rest (Mooney et al. 1970).

Operative Treatment

Most displaced distal femur fractures are managed with operative treatment. Indications include open fractures, fractures with vascular injury, ipsilateral lower extremity fracture, polytrauma patients, pathologic fractures, and cases where prolonged immobilization is contraindicated (Johnson and Hickens 1987).

Closed distal third femur fractures can be temporarily immobilized in a bulky cotton dressing and a knee immobilizer or long-leg splint. A tibial traction pin can be placed for significantly shortened fractures to maintain limb length, especially if surgery has to be delayed beyond 72 h. Open fractures require urgent debridement and irrigation along with immediate intravenous antibiotic administration. Temporary stabilization with a knee-spanning external fixator may be used in polytrauma patients or patients that require staged debridements Haidukewych (2002). The external fixator allows for stabilization of the fracture with restoration of alignment and length, limiting secondary soft tissue damage and assisting with pain relief, patient mobilization, and wound care. The external fixator is converted to definitive fixation once the patient is stable, and the soft tissue bed is clean and amenable for definitive fixation. The external fixator is applied with two pins in the proximal femur and two pins in the tibia after undergoing closed reduction with axial traction (Schmidt and Teague 2010).

Due to the vast array of distal femur injuries, there is no single implant that is ideal for all fractures; rather, the "personality" of the fracture and the patient dictates the implant of choice. Certain variables that need to be considered when choosing an implant include (1) the degree of comminution, (2) the involvement of the articular surface, (3) whether the fracture is open, (4) whether the fracture is isolated or one of multiple injuries, (5) the bone quality of the patient, (6) the functional level of the patient including ambulatory status, and (7) the condition of the soft tissue. Key principles to follow during surgical treatment include meticulous soft tissue dissection, maintenance of the blood supply to fragments, and the creation of a logical mechanical construct.

Implant options include isolated screws, a myriad of plates (non-contoured vs. periarticular contoured, conventional vs. locking), intramedullary rods (IMN), definitive external fixation (rare), and total knee arthroplasty (extremely rare) (Fig. 2) (Albert 1997; Schmidt and Teague 2010; Kenneth et al. 2010).

Distal Femur Fractures,
Fig. 2 AP radiographs of
distal femur fractures
treated via various
modalities: (**a**) locked
plating, (**b**) intramedullary
rodding, (**c**) temporizing
external fixation, and (**d**)
megaprosthesis

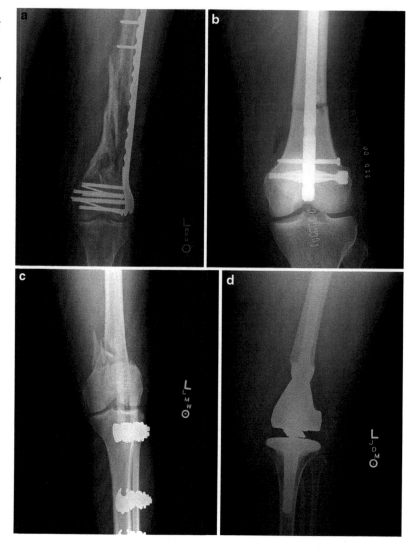

Isolated screws are used only for simple partial articular (lateral or medial femoral condyle) fractures. Even with these simple, partial articular fracture patterns, the surgeon often decides to supplement the lag screws with the addition of a buttress plate to improve the fixation strength. For extra-articular and complete articular fractures, plating and rodding are the mainstay of treatment. Plating is the most generalizable of all techniques. It can be used for the majority of fracture patterns and can be placed through extensile or minimally invasive limited approaches. It can be used to achieve compression across fracture fragments or bridging across

zones of comminution. One advantage of an intramedullary rod is that it can be used for segmental fractures or fractures with diaphyseal extension with minimal soft tissue violation. A prerequisite for all intramedullary rodding procedures is the presence of a distal segment large enough to be captured and stabilized by the relationship between the rod and the distal locking screws. Retrograde starting points are most common when stabilizing distal femur fractures with rodding. Whether the fracture is fixed with an intramedullary rod or plate, the addition of anterior to posterior countersunk lag screws is necessary if coronal plane ("Hoffa") fragments are noted.

Distal femoral replacement with a "megaprosthesis" is an option in elderly patients with preexisting knee arthritis. This form of treatment provides the most rapid return to function, but at a significant cost of bone removal and complication risk. Loosening of the prosthesis in this scenario is hard to overcome functionally.

Treatment of supracondylar fractures after total knee replacement (periprosthetic fracture) is individualized based on the status of the arthroplasty components. The two primary surgical options include revision long-stem arthroplasty for aseptically loose implants and fixation around the components when the components are stable. Plate fixation is used when there is no direct access to the intramedullary canal via the femoral component. Retrograde rodding can be used for open-box femoral component designs. Irrespective of the treatment choice, all distal femur fractures require restoration of angular, translational, and rotational anatomy (Albert 1997; Schmidt and Teague 2010; Kenneth et al. 2010; Wiss et al. 1996; Chen et al. 1994; DiGioia and Rubash 1991; Baker et al. 2002).

Postoperative Management

Postoperative management consists of immediate knee motion with active range of motion exercises to prevent knee contractures. A continuous passive motion machine may be useful in the unconscious patients with prolonged intubation or intensive care unit stay. Weight-bearing status is dependent on the personality of the fracture and the type of implant used to treat the fracture. Non-weight bearing to toe-touch weight bearing with crutches is recommended for fractures treated with ORIF, Ex-fix, or IMN that are axially unstable. Immediate weight bearing is begun for fractures that are axially stable after IMN and TKA. In general, most intraarticular fractures require prolonged non-weight bearing, approximately 3 months, to allow the articular fracture to heal. Weight bearing for these injuries is begun once there is radiographic evidence of healing with most patients bearing substantial weight in the affected extremity by 3 months (Schmidt and Teague 2010; Kenneth et al. 2010; Wiss et al. 1996).

Complications

Potential complications of distal third femur fractures include wound healing problems, infection, thromboembolic disease, malunion, nonunion, nerve or vessel injury, knee stiffness, and posttraumatic arthritis. Malunions can occur from inadequate initial reduction or postoperative loss of reduction associated with hardware failure or implant/bone interface failure. Nonunions are associated with poor patient biology, aggressive surgical dissection, an underlying infection, or early implant failure. Knee stiffness occurs with immobilization and can lead to limitations in extension, flexion, or both. Posttraumatic arthritis is associated with the original chondral injury, incongruent joint surface reductions, and/or malalignment of the mechanical axis (Albert 1997; Schmidt and Teague 2010; Kenneth et al. 2010; Wiss et al. 1996).

Cross-References

▶ External Fixation
▶ Falls from Height
▶ Femoral Shaft Fractures
▶ Knee Dislocations
▶ Open Fractures

References

Albert MJ (1997) Supracondylar fractures of the femur. JAAOS 5(3):163–171

Alms M (1961) Fracture mechanics. J Bone Joint Surg Br 43-B:162–166

Baker BJ, Escobedo EM, Nork SE, Henley MB (2002) Hoffa fracture: a common association with high energy supra-condylar fractures of the distal femur. Am J Roentgenol 178(4):994

Chen F, Mont MA, Bachner RS (1994) Management of ipsilateral supracondylar femur fractures following total knee arthroplasty. J Arthroplasty 9(5):521–526

Court-Brown CM, Caesar B (2006) Epidemiology of adult fracture: a review. Injury 37(8):691–697

DiGioia AM, Rubash HE (1991) Periprosthetic fractures of the femur after total knee arthroplasty: a literature review and treatment algorithm. Clin Orthop 271:135–142

Haidukewych GJ (2002) Temporary external fixation for the management of complex intra and periarticular fracture of the lower extremity. J Orthop Trauma 16(9):678–685

Johnson KD, Hickens G (1987) Distal femur fractures. Orthop Clin North Am 18:115–132

Kenneth E, Kenneth K, Zuckerman J (2010) Handbook of fractures, 4th edn. Lippincott Williams and Wilkins, Philadelphia, pp 420–428

Marsh JL (2009) OTA fracture classification. J Orthop Trauma 23(8):551

Mills WJ, Barei DP, McNair P (2004) The value of the ankle-brachial index for diagnosing arterial injury after knee dislocation: a prospective study. J Trauma 56(6):1261–1265

Mooney V, Nickel VL, Harvey JP, Snelson R (1970) Cast-brace treatment for fractures of the distal part of the femur: a prospective controlled study of one hundred and fifty patients. J Bone Joint Surg Am 52:1563–1578

Schatzker J, Tile M (1991) The rationale of operative fracture care. Springer, New York

Schmidt AH, Teague DC (2010) Orthopaedic knowledge update trauma. American Academy of Orthopaedic Surgeons, Rosemont, pp 445–459

Wiss D, Watson JT, Johnson EE (1996) Fractures of the knee. In: Rockwood CA, Green DP, Bucholz RW (eds) Rockwood and Green's fractures in adults, 4th edn. Lippincott Williams and Wilkins, Pennsylvania, pp 1919–2000

Distal Humerus Fracture

▶ Distal Humerus Fractures

Distal Humerus Fractures

Eric C. Fu and David Ring
Department of Orthopaedic Surgery,
Massachusetts General Hospital, Harvard
Medical School, Boston, MA, USA

Synonyms

Bicolumn humerus fracture; Coronal shear humerus fracture; Distal humerus fracture; Single column humerus fracture; Supracondylar humerus fracture

Definition

Distal humerus fractures are injuries to the elbow which can be extra- or intra-articular.

These injuries require a thorough understanding of the neurovascular status of the extremity, the fracture pattern, and the patient's medical comorbidities before determining treatment. Options for treatment can range from nonoperative to open reduction internal fixation to elbow arthroplasty.

Background

Epidemiology

Fractures of the distal humerus are relatively uncommon, comprising an estimated 2 % of all fractures (Jupiter and Morrey 1993). The age distribution of this injury is bimodal. In a study of patients 12 years and older, Robinson et al. found that distal humerus fractures were most common in young, active patients ages 12–19 years as a result of a high-energy injury (i.e., motor vehicle accident, sporting activity, and fall from height) (Robinson et al. 2003). In the adult, these are most common among osteopenic women after low-energy injury such as a fall from standing.

Anatomy

The elbow is an inherently stable and complex joint composed of three bones (the humerus, ulna, and radius), three articulations (ulnohumeral, radiocapitellar, and proximal radioulnar), as well as capsuloligamentous and musculotendinous attachments.

The ulnohumeral articulation is a simple hinged joint. It is comprised of the trochlear notch of the ulna, which forms a 180° arc around trochlear spool and allows for 140° of flexion and extension at the elbow. The end of the humerus is best conceptualized as a triangle whereby the trochlea is supported by medial and lateral bony columns (Fig. 1; Bucholz and Heckman 2005). Failure to restore one of the limbs of the triangle can lead to mechanical instability and failure of fixation.

The radiocapitellar articulation is formed by the capitellum of the humerus (the rounded, cartilaginous end of the lateral column of the humerus) and the radial head and allows for

Distal Humerus Fractures, Fig. 1 The architecture of the distal humerus is formed by triangle medial and lateral columns which support the trochlear spool (Credit: Rockwood & Green's Fractures in Adults 6th edition (Bucholz and Heckman 2005)

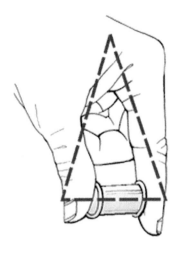 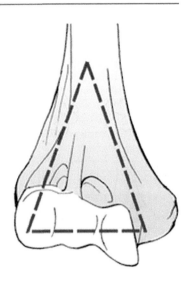

D

rotation of the radius around the ulna. The proximal radioulnar joint consists of the lesser sigmoid notch of the proximal ulna, which accommodates the radial head during rotation.

The radiocapitellar articulation and the articulation between the anteromedial facet of the coronoid and the medial trochlea are the most important bony stabilizers of the elbow. Secondary stabilizers of the elbow include capsuloligamentous structures – the medial collateral ligament (MCL) and the lateral collateral ligament (LCL). The MCL resists valgus stress. The LCL primarily resists varus and posterolateral rotatory stresses.

Fracture Classification

Fractures of the distal humerus are notoriously complex to describe and treat. Traditionally, classification schemes have described these fractures anatomically (i.e., supracondylar, transcondylar, etc.). However, more recent classification systems have adopted column-based descriptions. The AO/OTA Foundation classification divides the fractures into three types: extra-articular (A type), intra-articular with involvement of a single column (B type), and intra-articular involving both columns (C type) (AO Foundation: https://www.aofoundation.org/Documents/mueller_ao_class.pdf). Each type is further subdivided by the location of fracture and degree of metaphyseal and articular comminution. While comprehensive, the AO

classification reliability decreases with the subtype classification of fractures and the subtype nomenclature can be cumbersome for clinician communication.

Davies and Stanley designed a classification system for clinical usage which describes fractures by the location of the major fracture line (Fig. 2; Ruan et al. 2009). Type 1 injuries are extra-articular fractures, type 2 are intra-articular single or two-column fractures, and type 3 are articular surface fractures which do not extend proximally past the olecranon fossa. Although there are numerous classification schemes, the Davies and Stanley classification scheme has demonstrated better inter- and intra-observer reliability compared to other classification systems and has an associated treatment algorithm that derives directly from the classification system (Fig. 2).

Physical Exam

Many patients with a distal humerus fracture will have other injuries; therefore, initial assessment should consist of a thorough trauma evaluation starting with primary survey of the patient's airway, breathing, and circulation. The clinician should avoid being distracted by bony injuries during primary evaluation which may lead to missed vital injuries. After the ABCs of the trauma evaluation have been completed, the clinician can begin their secondary survey of the extremities.

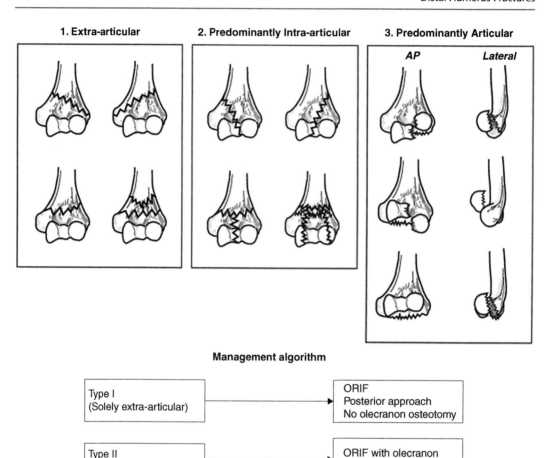

1. Extra-articular   **2. Predominantly Intra-articular**   **3. Predominantly Articular**

Management algorithm

Distal Humerus Fractures, Fig. 2 Classification of distal humerus fractures by Davies. Fractures are described by major fracture lines and proposed treatment algorithm (Credit: Davies and Stanley 2006)

A thorough upper extremity evaluation should consist of assessing the patient's entire shoulder girdle down to the fingertips to rule out an ipsilateral injury. With a distal humerus fracture, the elbow is typically edematous, shortened, and grossly deformed. Careful inspection of the skin, especially posteriorly, is necessary so as not to miss an occult open fracture, which is present in up to one-third of patients. Neurovascular exam including careful evaluation of the radial, ulnar, median, anterior, and posterior interosseous nerves is essential. One study identified ulnar nerve symptoms in 25 % of patients with complete articular fractures, although ulnar neuropathy is generally more of an issue after surgery (Ruan et al. 2009).

Finally, the patient should be questioned about their previous elbow function as well as the extent of their current activities.

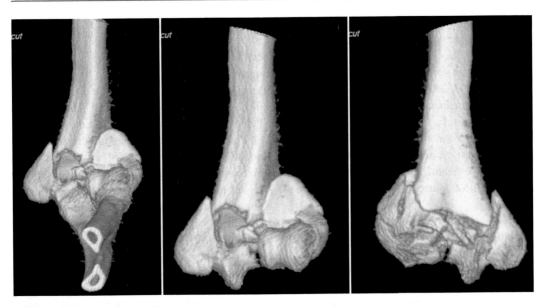

Distal Humerus Fractures, Fig. 3 3D CT reconstruction of distal humerus fracture with and without ulnar subtraction. Ulnar subtraction improves visualization of articular surface

Imaging Evaluation

Initial imaging should consist of dedicated anteroposterior, oblique, and lateral X-rays of the distal humerus as well as full-length humeral and forearm films. With nondisplaced fractures, the fracture line can be difficult to detect on plain radiographs. The clinician should look for evidence of a "fat pad sign" on the lateral radiograph, which is indicative of a hemarthrosis secondary to fracture hematoma and an occult fracture. Intercondylar split fractures are the most common in adults; therefore, the AP and oblique views should also be examined closely for evidence of a vertical split.

In the setting of comminution and displacement, radiographs obtained with axial traction applied to partially reduce the fracture via ligamentotaxis can improve the treating clinician's understanding of the fracture pattern on a radiograph. In practice, traction radiographs are difficult to do without anesthesia and usually obtained in the operating room. CT scans can also help in clarifying the injury pattern especially in the setting of articular comminution. Two-dimensional cross sections of a CT scan can be out of plane and difficult to interpret; therefore, we recommend three-dimensional reconstructions.

These reconstructions have been shown to improve the reliability of fracture classification and subsequent treatment decisions (Doornberg et al. 2006). In particular, they help with difficult fracture patterns such as coronal plane fractures of the trochlea or capitellum. Work with your radiologists to remove the radius and ulna from the image to get an isolated view of the articular surface of the humerus (or you can do it yourself with a software) (Fig. 3).

Treatment

Nonoperative Treatment

Nonoperative treatment can lead to surprisingly good results. Brown and Morgan reported on 11 patients treated with brief immobilization followed by early range of motion who achieved an average of 100° of flexion-extension, a range of motion that is sufficient for most activities of daily living. Mudgal has reported on 5 patients treated with the same method who obtained an average of 113° of flexion-extension and excellent functional outcomes as measured by the Mayo Score and DASH at an average of 3 years after injury (Mudgal, "personal communication"). On the other hand, Robinson et al. compared 273 surgically treated patients and 47 nonoperatively treated patients and found nonoperative treatment was associated with six times greater risk of nonunion (Robinson et al. 2003). We use nonoperative treatment for infirm, inactive patients. For instance, it is difficult to justify the risks of fixation or total elbow replacement in a patient who is so demented that she must be fed. Likewise, the results of nonoperative treatment are good enough that we feel that most infirm patients should not have surgery.

Bicolumnar Fractures: Open Reduction and Internal Fixation

The goal of open reduction internal fixation is to restore native anatomy with a construct stable enough to accommodate active elbow motion. Patients who undergo operative treatment are typically placed in a well-padded posterior elbow splint while awaiting surgery. The skin and neurovascular status should be reexamined prior to anesthesia or peripheral nerve blocks. In the operating room the patient is placed in the lateral decubitus position with the arm supported by a rolled pillow or other padded support.

Approach

A midline posterior incision with medial and lateral full-thickness fasciocutaneous flaps is used most frequently.

There are several options for addressing the ulnar nerve. Once in a while the fracture will result in articular fragments that are large enough that the medial plate does not need to enter the cubital tunnel and the nerve can be left in place. In this uncommon circumstance, we recommend at least an in situ release of the nerve to see and protect it but also because scarring can narrow the tunnel leading to ulnar neuropathy over the years after injury.

Most ulnar nerves will be moved out of the way to realign and repair the fracture. This can be done in one of two ways: either by a standard transposition freeing the nerve and moving it anteriorly or by taking the periosteum of the olecranon, the capsule of the ulnohumeral joint, and the periosteum of the distal humerus with the nerve as

a sleeve. If this latter "subperiosteal" mobilization is performed, the nerve will be returned to the cubital tunnel at the end of the surgery. If the nerve is mobilized on its own, one can either keep it anterior in the subcutaneous tissues or place it back in the cubital tunnel. There is insufficient data to recommend one tactic over another.

Postoperative ulnar neuropathy has been documented in 15–20 % of all patients with bicolumnar fractures, and it would likely be higher if we looked more carefully, for instance, with Semmes-Weinstein monofilament sensibility testing. Techniques to limit stretching and pressure on the ulnar nerve include using a vessel loop rather than a Penrose drain for retraction (less force), avoiding any instruments on the loop, considering temporarily sewing the nerve into a subcutaneous pocket while working, and using oscillating drills to avoid wrapping the nerve up in the drill.

The most common exposures of the fracture are the paratricipital (Alonso-Llames), triceps-splitting (Campbell), and olecranon osteotomy approaches (Fig. 4; Nauth et al. 2011).

The paratricipital approach is best reserved for simple, extra-articular fractures and fractures for which total elbow arthroplasty might be a better option based on age, activity level, articular fracture complexity, and bone quality – the latter two are sometimes uncertain until after exposure. The major benefit of this approach is avoiding disruption of the extensor mechanism. King has described a paratricipital technique where the medial joint is exposed through an interval between brachialis and the medial head of the triceps. The triceps muscle is elevated off the posterior aspect of the humerus and the tendinous insertion into the olecranon is preserved. The lateral window is made through a split at the interval between the ulna and anconeus and extended proximally in the same line leaving a lateral tendinous cuff for repair. Limitations of this approach are inadequate visualization of the distal humeral articular surface; however, it can be easily converted to an olecranon osteotomy.

The triceps-splitting approach is performed through a midline incision in the triceps fascia, which is carried distally onto the ulnar crest of the

D

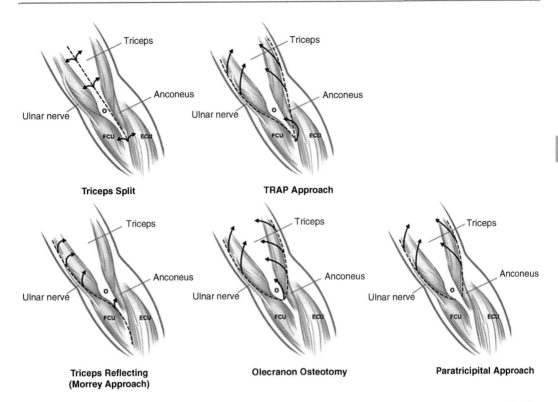

Distal Humerus Fractures, Fig. 4 Schematic representing the different operative approaches to the distal humerus. *O* olecranon, *FCU* flexor carpi ulnaris, *ECU* extensor carpi ulnaris, *TRAP* triceps-reflecting anconeus pedicle (Credit: Nauth et al. 2011)

olecranon (lifting the flexor carpi ulnaris from the ulna). The further distally this dissection is carried, the more the split tendons will sublux anteriorly and improve visualization. The triceps insertion, the periosteum, and the extensor and flexor muscle masses are elevated off of the ulna, leaving the triceps tendon in continuity with the extensor and flexor fascia. The theoretical downside of this approach is the potential for weakening of the extensor mechanism and even triceps rupture, but a study of patients with open fractures showed no differences in triceps strength between patients that had an olecranon osteotomy compared to a triceps split (McKee et al. 2000).

The olecranon osteotomy is the workhorse approach for most intra-articular distal humerus fractures. Wilkinson et al. demonstrated in cadavers that an olecranon osteotomy offers the best exposure of the articular surface (Wilkinson and Stanley 2001). Many surgeons favor a chevron-shaped, apex-distal osteotomy at the center and bare spot of the trochlear groove. There are several options for repair of the osteotomy (screw, intramedullary device, plate), but we still favor a tension band wire technique. Drawbacks to an olecranon osteotomy are the creation of another site of bony healing, potential damage to the articular cartilage during osteotomy, and possible symptomatic prominent hardware.

Fixation

The traditional recommendation is to fix the articular fragments to one another and then secure the distal part to the shaft. Alternatively, one can piece the fracture back together directly on to the shaft, typically placing the least comminuted most stable fractures first. Reduction is held provisionally with smooth Kirschner wires and then exchanged for plates and screws.

Anatomic plates are now widely available and should be placed along the medial and lateral columns in either an orthogonal ("90–90," usually direct medial and posterolateral) or parallel (direct medial and direct lateral) fashion. While the orthogonal orientation is mechanically beneficial, the parallel plating allows for much longer screws, making it superior in some biomechanical studies although both can be considered good options and the treatment can be individualized (Stoffel et al. 2008).

O'Driscoll laid out fundamental rules for fixation of the distal humerus fractures (O'Driscoll et al. 2002):

- Every screw should pass through a plate.
- Every screw in the distal fragment should end in a fragment on opposing side.
- As many screws as possible should be placed in the distal humerus and should interdigitate in the distal segment.
- Screws should be as long as possible.
- The articular segment should be fixed to the metaphysis and diaphysis with compression plating.
- Plates should be strong enough to resist breaking (3.5 mm plates at least; one-third tubular plates are insufficient).

Capitellum and Trochlea Fractures: Open Reduction and Internal Fixation

Apparent capitellum fractures usually involve part of the lateral trochlea and often involve fracture of the lateral epicondyle, impaction of the lateral column, and even fracture of the posterior trochlea. They can also be part of an elbow fracture dislocation with associated avulsion of the MCL from the medial epicondyle.

Dubberley and colleagues classified capitellum and trochlea fractures as follows: (Fig. 5; Dubberley et al. 2006) type I primarily involves the capitellum with or without the lateral aspect of the trochlea; type II involves the capitellum and the trochlea as one fragment; and type III involves both the capitellum and trochlea as separate pieces.

Radiographic evaluation begins with standard AP and lateral radiographs of the elbow. The lateral view is most likely to demonstrate the capitellum fragment. Involvement of the trochlea

is recognized by a "double-arc" sign that represents the displaced fracture fragment composed of the capitellum and lateral ridge of the trochlea (Fig. 6; McKee et al. 1996). CT scans of the elbow can be useful for understanding the fracture characteristics and have been shown to improve intra- and interobserver reliability of fracture classification (Doornberg et al. 2006).

Treatment of these fractures is typically operative. Guitton et al. demonstrated excellent long-term functional outcomes after surgical fixation of these fractures with a median arc of elbow flexion and extension of 119° at a 17-year follow-up (Guitton et al. 2009). In our experience, a lateral skin incision with exposure through an extended lateral Kocher approach is sufficient in most cases. However, if there is a fracture of the posterior trochlea, our preference proceeds with an olecranon osteotomy to expose the articular surface.

Provisional fixation can be obtained with Kirschner wires. Countersunk headless screws (3.5 or 2.7 mm) are placed from anterior to posterior. In cases with metaphyseal comminution, a lateral plate, and even structural corticocancellous bone graft in some cases, is recommended to support the lateral column. For very small fragments, threaded Kirschner wires can be used as small fine screws, but they will migrate if the fracture does not heal.

Operative Treatment: Elbow Arthroplasty

The subset of capitellum and trochlea fractures that are complex and difficult to repair, with intact columns and no more than lateral or medial epicondyle fractures, can be addressed with hemiarthroplasty (replacement of the distal humerus articular surface). There is a prosthesis available for this in other parts of the world but not currently in the United States.

Patients with limited demands and a 10–20 year maximum life expectancy can benefit from total elbow arthroplasty (TEA). TEA is typically reserved for older, infirm, low-demand patients with comminuted osteoporotic articular fractures. Total elbow arthroplasty allows for immediate, independent motion of the elbow. In a randomized trial, McKee et al. demonstrated

Distal Humerus Fractures,
Fig. 5 Dubberley's classification of capitellar and trochlear fractures (Credit: Dubberley et al. 2006)

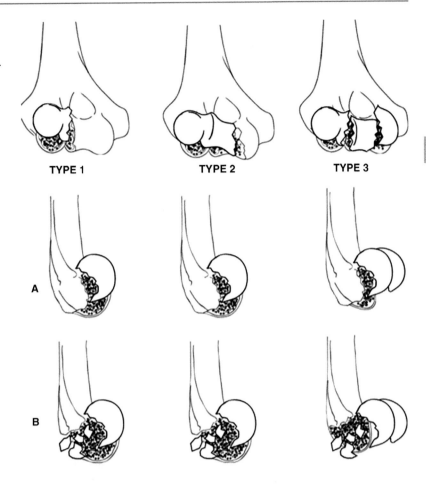

Distal Humerus Fractures, Fig. 6 Clinical radiograph showing the double arc of coronal shear fracture (Credit: McKee et al. 1996)

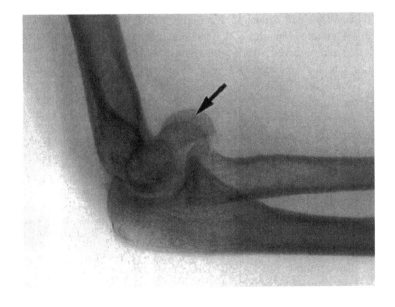

better short-term functional outcomes in elderly patients with displaced, comminuted, intra-articular distal humerus fractures treated with total elbow arthroplasty compared to open reduction and internal fixation (McKee et al. 2000). Drawbacks to total elbow arthroplasty are a lifting limit of five to ten pounds lifting in the operative extremity and higher infection rates than for hip, knee, and shoulder arthroplasty. In addition, complications such as wound problems, infection, and early loosening can be difficult to salvage.

Outcomes

Fracture of the distal humerus is an elbow-changing event. Good or excellent outcomes have been reported in 84–100 % of patients, with most patients regaining 100° arc of flexion-extension (Sanchez-Sotelo et al. 2007; Huang et al. 2005). Strength testing has shown that most patients will regain 75 % of their flexion-extension strength relative to their uninjured side (McKee et al. 2000).

Complications

Postoperative ulnar nerve neuropathy associated with distal humerus fracture has been reported between 0 % and 33 %. The literature on whether or not to transpose the ulnar nerve remains insufficient to recommend one approach over the other. Vazquez et al. reviewed 69 patients who underwent open reduction internal fixation of distal humerus fractures with or without transposition and observed a 16 % ulnar nerve dysfunction rate at a minimum of 1-year follow-up with no protective benefit of transposition of the ulnar nerve (Vazquez et al. 2010).

Heterotopic ossification hinders motion in about 10 % of patients that have operative fixation of distal humerus fractures (Nauth et al. 2011). The role of prophylaxis is debated, and a recent randomized trial of radiation therapy was halted due to increased nonunions in the radiated patients. We tend to emphasize fracture healing and do not use prophylaxis against heterotopic bone.

The nonunion rates with open reduction and internal fixation using modern plating techniques are about 5–10 % (Theivendran et al. 2010). The diagnosis is based largely on loosening or breakage of implants with a persistent fracture line and fracture instability. As long as the implants are not loose and the arm is stable, radiographic and CT appearance probably should not lead to additional surgery, but we need more data on this. Treatment of nonunion is fairly reliable with revision open reduction internal fixation with compression plating and bone grafting with iliac crest autograft.

Cross-References

▶ ABCDE of Trauma Care
▶ Damage Control Orthopedics
▶ Open Fractures
▶ Pediatric Fractures About the Elbow

References

AO Foundation: https://www.aofoundation.org/Documents/mueller_ao_class.pdf

Bucholz R, Heckman JD (2005) Rockwood and green's fractures in adults, 6th edn. Lippincott, Williams & Wilkins, Philadelphia

Davies MB, Stanley D (2006) A clinically applicable fracture classification for distal humeral fractures. J Shoulder Elbow Surg 15:602–608

Doornberg J, Lindenhovius A, Kloen P, van Dijk CN, Zurakowski D, Ring D (2006) Two and three-dimensional computed tomography for the classification and management of distal humeral fractures. Evaluation of reliability and diagnostic accuracy. J Bone Joint Surg Am 88:1795–1801

Dubberley JH, Faber KJ, MacDermid JC, Patterson SD, King GJW (2006) Outcome after open reduction and internal fixation of capitellar and trochlear fractures. J Bone Joint Surg Am 88:46–54

Guitton TG, Doornberg JN, Raaymakers EL, Ring D, Kloen P (2009) Fractures of the capitellum and trochlea. J Bone Joint Surg Am 91:390–397

Huang TL, Chiu FY, Chuang TY, Chen TH (2005) The results of open reduction and internal fixation in elderly patients with severe fractures of the distal humerus: a critical analysis of the results. J Trauma 58:62–69

Jupiter JB, Morrey BF (1993) Fractures of the distal humerus in the adult. The elbow and its disorders, 2nd edn. W.B. Saunders, Philadelphia, pp 328–366

McKee MD, Jupiter JB, Bamberger HB (1996) Coronal shear fractures of the distal end of the humerus. J Bone Joint Surg Am 78-A:49–54

McKee MD, Wilson TJ, Winston L, Schemitsch EH, Richards RR (2000) Functional outcomes following surgical treatment of intra-articular distal humeral fractures through a posterior approach. J Bone Joint Surg Am 82:1701

Nauth A, McKee MD, Ristevski B, Hall J, Schemitsch EH (2011) Distal humeral fractures in adults. J Bone Joint Surg Am 93:686–700

O'Driscoll WH, Sanchez-Sotelo J, Torchia ME (2002) Management of the smashed distal humerus. Orthop Clin North Am 33:19–33

Robinson CM, Hill RM, Jacobs N, Dall G, Court-Brown CM (2003) Adult distal humeral metaphyseal fractures: epidemiology and results of treatment. J Orthop Trauma 17:38–47

Ruan HJ, Liu JJ, Fan CY, Jiang J, Zeng BF (2009) Incidence, management, and prognosis of early ulnar nerve dysfunction in type C fractures of distal humerus. J Trauma 67:1397–1401

Sanchez-Sotelo J, Torchia ME, O'Driscoll SW (2007) Complex distal humeral fractures: internal fixation with a principle-based parallel-plate technique. J Bone Joint Surg Am 89:961–969

Stoffel K, Cunneen S, Morgan R, Nicholls R, Stachowiak G (2008) Comparative stability of perpendicular versus parallel double-locking plating systems in osteoporotic comminuted distal humerus fractures. J Orthop Res 26:778–784

Theivendran K, Duggan PJ, Deshmukh SC (2010) Surgical treatment of complex distal humeral fractures: functional outcome after internal fixation using precontoured anatomic plates. J Shoulder Elbow Surg 19:524–532

Vazquez O, Rutgers M, Ring DC, Walsh M, Egol KA (2010) Fate of the ulnar nerve after operative fixation of distal humerus fractures. J Orthop Trauma 24(7):395–399

Wilkinson JM, Stanley D (2001) Posterior surgical approaches to the elbow: a comparative anatomic study. J Shoulder Elbow Surg 10:380–382

Recommended Reading

Arnander MW, Reeves A, MacLeod IA, Pinto TM, Khaleel A (2008) A biomechanical comparison of plate configuration in distal humerus fractures. J Orthop Trauma 22:332–336, 48

Chen RC, Harris DJ, Leduc S, Borrelli JJ Jr, Tornetta P 3rd, Ricci WM (2010) Is ulnar nerve transposition beneficial during open reduction internal fixation of distal humerus fractures? J Orthop Trauma 24:391–394

Doornberg JN, van Duijn PJ, Linzel D, Ring DC, Zurakowski D, Marti RK, Kloen P (2007) Surgical treatment of intra-articular fractures of the distal part of the humerus. Functional outcome after twelve to thirty years. J Bone Joint Surg Am 89:1524–1532

Schemitsch EH, Tencer AF, Henley MB (1994) Biomechanical evaluation of methods of internal fixation of the distal humerus. J Orthop Trauma 8:468–475

Distal Radius Fractures

John Elfar and W. Lee Richardson
Department of Orthopaedics, University of Rochester, Rochester, NY, USA

Synonyms

Barton fracture; Colles' fracture; Radius fracture; Smith fracture; Wrist fracture

Definition

Distal radius fractures are common injuries seen in the emergency department (Chung and Spilson 2001). Patients typically present in a bimodal distribution as young high-energy injuries or elderly low-energy falls from standing height. It is important to inspect radiographs for intra-articular extension of fracture lines as well as initial displacement of fracture fragments as these will help dictate treatment.

Preexisting Condition

Closed reduction and casting of distal radius fractures remains a treatment mainstay for stable injuries. However, there has been a recent trend towards more aggressive operative fixation of these fractures based on data focusing on cost of treatment (Kakarlapudi et al. 2000; Shauver et al. 2011). Normal distal radius anatomy reveals a volar or palmar tilt of the articular surface of the distal radius in the sagittal plane (Fig. 1).

Fractures of the distal radius may involve the articular surface, or they may fracture only in the metaphyseal bone, sparing the joint. Such joint-sparing fractures are termed extra-articular and have characteristic patterns of displacement. Typically, fractures of the distal radius cause the bone of the articular surface to displace dorsally towards a position first described by Colles (1970) (Fig. 2). If the fracture heals in a dorsally displaced position, the functional range of

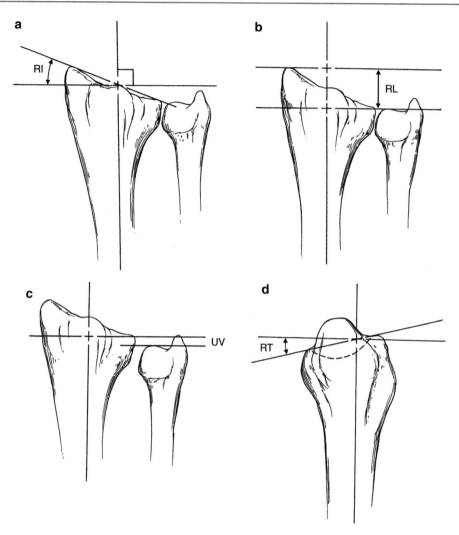

Distal Radius Fractures, Fig. 1 Normal distal radius anatomy. (**a**) Radial inclination (*RI*; normal, 22°). (**b**) Radial length (*RL*; normal, 12 mm). (**c**) Ulnar variance (*UV*; normal, −2 to +2 mm). (**d**) Radial tilt (*RT*; normal, 11° volar) (Graham 1997)

motion of the wrist will change towards extension and there is often malalignment of the distal radioulnar joint which interferes with pronation and supination. The opposite type of fracture, first described by Smith (1847) (Fig. 2), occurs less commonly and results in volar displacement of the articular portion. The goal of treatment in distal radius fractures is to reestablish normal anatomy. However, the amount of malalignment that can be tolerated is currently not known and is likely related to the functional needs of the patient. Normal distal radius anatomy has an average radial height of 11–12 mm, radial inclination of 22–23°, and average volar tilt of 11–12° (see Fig. 1).

Intra-articular fractures may involve both the radiocarpal and distal radioulnar joints. The exact amount of articular displacement which will allow acceptable clinical outcomes remains unclear; however, limiting articular step-off (Fig. 3a) or diastasis (Fig. 3b) is desired. Many radiographic parameters have been used to indicate fracture instability that would benefit from reduction and stabilization. These parameters

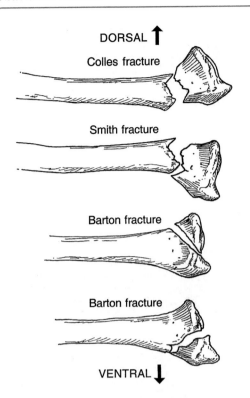

DORSAL ↑

Colles fracture

Smith fracture

Barton fracture

Barton fracture

VENTRAL ↓

Distal Radius Fractures, Fig. 2 Eponyms for typical distal radius fracture patterns (Source: www.studyortho. com/?page_id=108)

include initial dorsal angulation greater than 20°, dorsal comminution of greater than half the anteroposterior diameter of the radial metaphysis, and large intra-articular step-off among others. There is no consensus as to which value is most important, but there is a trend towards surgical stabilization of these fractures (Chung and Murray 2012). To this end operative fixation with volar wrist plate, external fixation with supplemental wire fixation, dorsal bridge plating, and fracture-specific plating are all very common treatment modalities (Fig. 4).

Application

It is important to complete a thorough neurovascular examination focusing special attention on impending traumatic carpal tunnel symptoms (numbness in the thumb, index, and middle digits. At the initial patient encounter,

closed reduction of displaced fracture fragments helps reduce tension on neurovascular structures such as the median nerve). If the patient complains of worsening neurologic symptoms despite reduction of the fracture, then urgent carpal tunnel release may be indicated. Examination of the elbow is also important to exclude injuries which transmit energy from the hand into the upper extremity. Any skin breakage denoting open fracture should be noted and appropriate emergent treatment initiated to minimize the risk of infection.

Initial reduction of the fracture normally takes place in an emergency department or urgent care setting, although reduction can be undertaken in the office as well. Techniques for analgesia and relaxation include hematoma block, conscious sedation, and regional anesthetics such as the bier block. Hematoma block is usually administered as 10–15 mL of 1 % lidocaine injected directly into the fracture site. The practitioner may aspirate hematoma and mix the local anesthetic in and out of the fracture site until it is adequately infiltrated to ensure correct placement. Anesthetic agents such as lidocaine typically require over 8 min to achieve maximal effect, so reduction should be delayed to allow optimal anesthetic action. Conscious sedation in the form of propofol or ketamine administration can be provided in an emergency department setting by practitioners who are comfortable with airway management. Regional anesthetics are also administered by specialized practitioners.

Actual reduction is normally achieved by first recreating and exaggerating the deformity of the fracture and then reducing the fracture to an anatomical alignment. Portable fluoroscopy can be very helpful to confirm adequate reduction before splinting. Fractures that have a great deal of soft tissue swelling or muscle spasm may benefit from traction before reduction to allow the tissues to stretch along with muscle fatigue before the reduction maneuver. This can be achieved by placing the index and middle digits in finger-traps after hematoma block and hanging 5–10 pounds of weight from the arm near the elbow for 15–20 min (Fig. 5). If the first reduction is not adequate, repeated attempts at reduction are often

D

Distal Radius Fractures, Fig. 3 Computed tomography showed (**a**) a 3-mm step-off of the articular surface of the distal radius and (**b**) distal and ulnar migration of the volar fragment (Source: Journal of Hand Surgery 2008; 33:835–840)

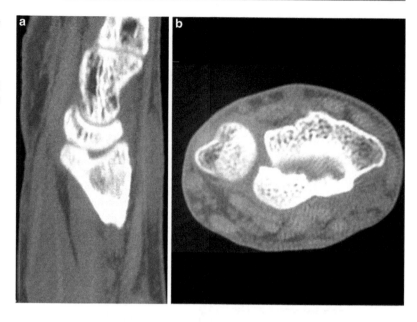

Distal Radius Fractures, Fig. 4 Examples of volar plate fixation, fragment-specific fixation, external fixation with supplemental K-wires, and dorsal spanning plate fixation, respectively (Sources: (**a**) http://www. newyorkinjurycasesblog. com/2013/03/articles/ wrist-injuries/appellate-court-upholds-1250000-pain-and-suffering-verdict-in-wrist-injury-case/ (**b**) www.ortho.hku.hk/ trauma.html (**c**) www. wheelessonline.com (**d**) www.eatonhand.com)

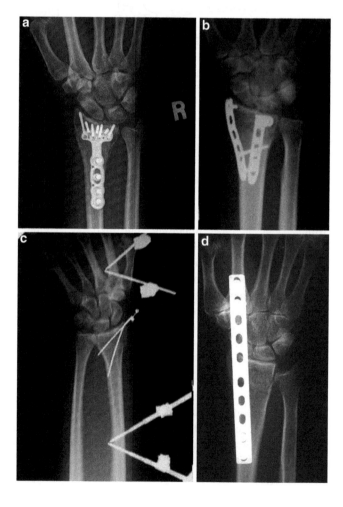

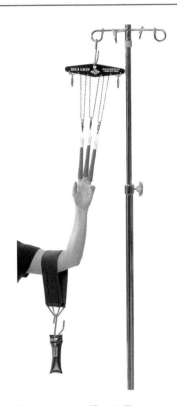

Distal Radius Fractures, Fig. 5 Finger trap traction for distal radius fracture reduction (Source: http://www. isisurgery.com/products/upper-extremity-traction/digigrip/digigrip-system/digigrip-system)

treated conservatively and up to 89 % in patients who are at least 65 years old (Gartland and Werley 1951; Makhni et al. 2008). This and other factors have contributed to a trend towards surgical fixation which is usually accomplished with volar locked plating. The modified Henry surgical approach between the flexor carpi radialis and radial artery allows excellent exposure for volar locked plating of most distal radius fractures. Operative fluoroscopy confirms that the fracture reduction is adequate and that the screws do not penetrate into the radiocarpal joint. Dorsal spanning bridge plate fixation and external fixation act by reducing and stabilizing osseous structures adjacent to the fracture. They can be coupled with supplemental wire fixation and allow for acceptable healing and function.

Complications

Stiffness and loss of range of motion are the most common findings after distal radius fracture; however, most patients tend to do well functionally if the overall alignment of the distal radius and radiocarpal joint is maintained (Aktekin et al. 2010; Azzopardi et al. 2005; Egol et al. 2010; Jupiter et al. 2002). Traumatic carpal tunnel syndrome should be assessed with a careful vigilant eye towards avoiding catastrophic complications. Although the incidence of complex regional pain syndrome associated with distal radius fracture is low, recent literature indicates that it can be decreased further with the use of vitamin C 500 mg per day for 6 weeks (AAOS 2009).

contraindicated by all but the most experienced practitioners because of the potential for complications. This is also true in children with distal radius fractures which involve the physis because permanent physeal injury can lead to growth arrest. If adequate reduction in the emergency department cannot be attained, operative management with either closed or open reduction and fixation may be indicated.

The type of splint used to immobilize the reduced fracture is variable and depends on practitioner preference. Most practitioners immobilize the elbow and wrist during initial treatment after reduction. Vigilant care is taken to ensure that swelling is not confined to a tight cast or splint to avoid catastrophic resultant compartment syndrome.

Virtually all distal radius fractures will heal; however, up to 60 % can lose reduction when

Cross-References

▶ Compartment Syndrome of the Forearm
▶ Complex Regional Pain Syndrome and Trauma
▶ Distal Humerus Fractures
▶ External Fixation
▶ Falls
▶ Principles of Internal Fixation of Fractures
▶ Principles of Nonoperative Treatment of Diaphyseal Fractures

References

AAOS (2009) American Academy of Orthopaedic Surgeons: Clinical Practice Guidelines. Guideline on treatment of distal radius fractures. www.aaos.org/Research/guidelines/DRFguideline.asp. Accessed 10 Aug 2014

Aktekin CN, Altay M, Gursoy Z, Aktekin LA, Ozturk AM, Tabak AY (2010) Comparison between external fixation and cast treatment in the management of distal radius fractures in patients aged 65 years and older. J Hand Surg 35(5):736–742

Azzopardi T, Ehrendorfer S, Coulton T, Abela M (2005) Unstable extra-articular fractures of the distal radius a prospective, randomised study of immobilisation in a cast versus supplementary percutaneous pinning. J Bone Joint Surg Br 87(6):837–840

Chung KC, Murray PM (2012) Hand surgery update, 5th edn. ASSH, Chicago, p. 162. Ebook

Chung KC, Spilson SV (2001) The frequency and epidemiology of hand and forearm fractures in the United States. J Hand Surg 26:908–915

Colles A (1970) On the fracture of the carpal extremity of the radius 1814. Injury 2(1):48–50

Egol KA, Walsh M, Romo-Cardoso S, Dorsky S, Paksima N (2010) Distal radial fractures in the elderly: operative compared with nonoperative treatment. J Bone Joint Surg 92(9):1851–1857

Gartland JJ, Werley CW (1951) Evaluation of healed colles' fractures. J Bone Joint Surg Am 33:895–907

Graham TJ (1997) Surgical correction of malunited fractures of the distal radius. J Am Acad Orthop Surg 5:270–281

Jupiter JB, Ring D, Weitzel PP (2002) Surgical treatment of redisplaced fractures of the distal radius in patients older than 60 years. J Hand Surg 27(4):714–723

Kakarlapudi TK, Santini A, Shahane SA, Douglas D (2000) The cost of treatment of distal radial fractures. Injury 31(4):229–232

Makhni EC, Ewald TJ, Kelly S, Day CS (2008) Effect of patient age on the radiographic outcomes of distal radius fractures subject to nonoperative treatment. J Hand Surg 33A:1304–1308

Shauver MJ, Clapham PJ, Chung KC (2011) An economic analysis of outcomes and complications of treating distal radius fractures in the elderly. J Hand Surg 36(12):1912–1918

Smith RW (1847) A treatise on fractures in the vicinity of the joints, and on certain forms of accidental and congenital dislocations. Dublin J Med Science 3:485–500

Distracted Doctoring

▶ Technology Interfacing, Etiquette, and Electronic Safety

Distribution

▶ Pharmacokinetic and Pharmacodynamic Alterations in Critical Illness

Diuretic

▶ Neurotrauma Management, Osmotherapy

Dizziness

▶ Traumatic Brain Injury, Neurological/Psychiatric Issues

Doctor's Assistant (Dr. Hudson, 1961)

▶ Physician Assistant

Donation After Cardiac Death

▶ Organ Donor Management

Donor Management

▶ Organ Donor Management

Dosing Strategies

▶ Pharmacologic Strategies in Adult Trauma Anesthesia

Drowning

Kathleen Webster
Department of Pediatric Critical Care, Loyola
University Medical Center, Maywood, IL, USA

Synonyms

Fatal drowning; Immersion injury; Nonfatal drowning; Submersion injury

Definition

A uniform definition of drowning was created by a world consensus conference held in 2002. Drowning is defined as "the process of experiencing respiratory impairment from submersion/immersion in liquid" (Branche 2006). This definition has been adopted by the World Health Organization and further classifies drowning as fatal or nonfatal but discourages use of the terms "near drowning," "wet drowning," "dry drowning," or "secondary drowning." A submersion event in which no respiratory embarrassment occurs is termed a "water rescue" (Spilzman et al. 2012).

Preexisting Condition

Epidemiology

Drowning, whether intentional, inflicted, or accidental, is a worldwide problem and has been estimated to be the second leading cause of death worldwide. Statistics by country vary slightly; however drowning remains a leading cause of both morbidity and mortality, with children under 14 years being most greatly affected (Branche 2006). Drowning may occur in natural bodies of water such as lakes, rivers, and oceans, or in free-standing bodies of water such as swimming pools, hot tubs, wells, bathtubs, and even large buckets. In the United States, half of all fatal drowning occur in natural bodies of water and primarily affect older children and adults, whereas the very young are more likely to drown close to home (CDC 2012).

Risk Factors

The biggest risk factor for drowning is age, with the highest rates for drowning events overall occurring in the 5–14-year-old group. Males have a 4–5 times greater risk than females. Lower socioeconomic status, lack of supervision, and high-risk behavior also play a role. Alcohol use, either by the victim or the caregiver, increases the risk of injury, as does a lack of preventive measures such as life guards, flotation devices, and water safety knowledge (Branche and vanBeek 2006; Spilzman et al. 2012). Other predisposing factors may include medical conditions such as epilepsy, cardiomyopathy, and cardiac arrhythmias.

Application

Pathophysiology of Drowning

The drowning victim will resist inflow of fluid into the airways initially by swallowing or spitting, then by holding their breath. When this is no longer possible, a breath is taken and water flows in to the airways. This may trigger a coughing reflex and/or laryngospasm (Spilzman et al. 2012). If water enters the lungs, there can be washout of surfactant either by direct effect of the water or by pulmonary edema fluid caused by disruption of the alveolar capillary membrane. Despite these potential effects, aspiration of water into the lungs requires active inhalation and exhalation. Apnea is the result of severe hypoxemia and a loss of the diving reflex, which can be engaged in sudden immersion in cold water. For these reasons, the volumes of water aspirated are usually low in drowning. The majority of subsequent injury is then caused by the effects of hypoxia (Orlowski et al. 1989; Gelissen et al. 2006).

Fluid and Electrolyte Disturbances

Metabolic acidosis occurs in the majority of patients and is due to lactic acidosis subsequent to hypoxemia (Spilzman et al. 2012). As the volumes of aspirated water are low, there is little impact on fluid and cardiovascular status directly attributable to the aspirated fluid. This has been corroborated in studies showing no differences in fluid and electrolyte status with salt water versus fresh water drowning. The degree of injury is more likely due to renal dysfunction and inflammatory response and indeed has been shown to be equivalent to that seen in anoxic injury alone (Orlowski et al. 1989; Gelissen et al. 2006).

Organ Dysfunction

Pulmonary dysfunction may be associated with surfactant washout, injury to the alveolar capillary membrane, or development of ARDS. Development of massive pulmonary edema may be seen in significant drowning events. Systemic inflammatory response, cardiac dysfunction, renal failure, and neurologic dysfunction may all ensue as a result of the severe hypoxic injury (Spilzman et al. 2012).

Associated Injuries

The incidence of cervical spine injury in most drowning events is low, and only of concern in a high-impact or diving injury (Pepe and Bierens 2006; Spilzman et al. 2012). Associated traumatic injuries should be suspected in cases of car submersions, jumping from a height, or intentional drowning events. In addition, toxicologic ingestion should be considered and evaluated on presentation, particularly in the persistently unresponsive patient (Gelissen et al. 2006; Spilzman et al. 2012).

Pre-Hospital Management

The main sequelae of drowning are related to hypoxia; therefore, early establishment of airway and ventilation is key (Pepe and Bierens 2006; Spilzman et al. 2012). Although resuscitation for adults by bystanders now advocates a "hands-only" approach with early defibrillation and chest compressions, the resuscitation of the asphyxiated victim or any child should still have an early focus on rescue breathing and early

attention to airway and ventilation (Soar et al. 2010). Several studies highlight the importance of bystander resuscitation, with much higher survival rates reported versus those with a delay until emergency personnel arrive (Pepe and Bierens 2006). Although shockable cardiac rhythms are rare in drowning events, automated external defibrillators can be lifesaving, particularly if arrhythmia was the cause of the event.

Hospital Management

Despite the high number of deaths and severe injury from drowning, it is estimated that 4–5 patients are seen in the emergency department for every one death. The majority of patients will present with few or no symptoms. If any cough, hypoxemia or rales are heard on auscultation, the patient should be placed on oxygen and observed for further progression of symptoms. In most cases, the clinical state will normalize in 6–8 h and the patient may be discharged (Spilzman et al. 2012). Obviously any patient with severe hypoxemia or cardiovascular compromise will require intubation and mechanical ventilation with care in an intensive care unit setting. Respiratory support provided to drowning patients has included such therapies as protective ventilation strategies, surfactant administration, and use of inhaled nitric oxide therapy; however there is no clear evidence to promote any consensus recommendations on these therapies (Spilzman et al. 2012). Therapy for both cardiovascular and respiratory systems is generally supportive, in accordance with guidelines for acute hypoxic respiratory failure.

Pneumonia occurs in <12 % of drowning victims and use of prophylactic antibiotics is not routinely recommended (Spilzman et al. 2012). The exception to this would be submersion in dirty water such as sewage plants or swamp water (Pepe and Bierens 2006).

Although most patients with an event severe enough to warrant hospital admission are acidotic, routine use of sodium bicarbonate is not recommended, as the acidosis will generally spontaneously resolve with restoration of systemic perfusion and oxygenation (Spilzman et al. 2012).

Hypothermia

Most drowning victims with severe injury will be hypothermic at presentation. This may be due to the cooling effects of water or due to a prolonged hypoperfusion state. Although generally hypothermia is generally felt to be a poor prognostic sign, there have been case reports of dramatic recovery in patients who have drowned in water less than 21 °C even with prolonged submersion time (Gelissen et al. 2006). The current resuscitation literature challenges the benefit of aggressively warming the post-arrest patient, unless hemodynamic instability exists (Ralston et al. 2006). Hypothermia may be neuroprotective by decreasing the cerebral metabolic demand (Spilzman et al. 2012), and there is a growing body of evidence to support use of hypothermia in certain patient populations (Kochanek 2009). Despite this, severe hypothermia may cause metabolic and cardiovascular compromise, refractory to resuscitation efforts. In these cases, aggressive rewarming can be lifesaving (Coskun et al. 2010). In addition, pediatric drowning victims are the most likely to be hypothermic on presentation, due to their high surface area to body mass ratio. This same characteristic however, makes them most amenable to rapid rewarming by passive means as well (Gelissen et al. 2006). The question remains then as to when to rewarm and if so, how aggressively. Although further studies are to delineate the benefits of hypothermia and the goal temperature to be achieved, some guidelines can be proposed: (1) normothermia should be achieved before terminating resuscitative efforts (Pepe and Bierens 2006, Spilzman et al. 2012) and (2) aggressive rewarming by cardiopulmonary bypass should be reserved for extreme hypothermia only and should be limited to a goal temperature of 32–34 °C (Gelissen et al. 2006; Kochanek et al. 2009).

Prediction of Outcome

Prediction of outcome is difficult, due to the variety of factors which can lead to the final common pathway of drowning. The strongest predictor of outcome is provision of bystander resuscitation (Pepe and Bierens 2006) and mental status of the victim at the scene and in the emergency department (Quan 2006). Submersion time is inversely correlated with likelihood of good outcome. Some studies suggest that a time less than 5 min is most commonly associated with good outcome and submersion time of greater than 10 min has a very low likelihood of intact survival (Spilzman et al. 2012). Hypothermia may be protective in cold-water drowning or a poor prognostic sign after a prolonged arrest state. Reports of dramatic survival, even in patients with poor prognostic factors, make the decision to terminate resuscitative efforts difficult. In general, resuscitative efforts of greater than 25 min in a normothermic adult, or longer than 1 hour in a hypothermic patient are not associated with neurologically intact survival (Pepe and Bierens 2006).

Prevention

The best treatment to reduce the morbidity and mortality of drowning is prevention. Risk of events occurring can be reduced by isolation fencing around swimming pools, separating the pool from the house, use of life jackets and flotation devices, water safety training, and limitation of access to and advertising of alcohol at water-related events. In addition, early rescue can be facilitated by vigilant supervision, lifeguards and training in cardiopulmonary resuscitation for pool owners, and those responsible for supervising swimmers (Branche and vanBeek 2006; CDC 2012; Spilzman et al. 2012).

Cross-References

▶ ARDS, Complication of Trauma
▶ Electrolyte and Acid-Base Abnormalities
▶ Extracorporeal Membrane Oxygenation
▶ Fluid, Electrolytes, and Nutrition in Trauma Patients

► Hypothermia
► Life Support, Withholding and Withdrawal of
► Lung Injury
► Outcomes

References

Branche C, vanBeek E (2006) The epidemiology of drowning. In: Bierens JJLM (ed) Handbook of drowning. Springer Verlag, Berlin, pp 39–76

CDC (2012) Drowning-United States 2005–2009. MMWR 61(19):344–347

Coskun KO, Popov AF, Schmitto JD, Hinz J, Kriebel T, Schoendube FA, Ruchewski W, Tirilomis T (2010) Extracorporeal circulation for rewarming in drowning and near-drowning pediatric patients. Atrif Organs 34(11):1026–1031

Gelissen H, Vincent JL, Thijs L (2006) Hospital treatment. In: Bierens JJLM (ed) Handbook of drowning. Springer Verlag, Berlin, pp 389–432

Kochanek P, Fink EL, Bell MJ, Bayir H, Clark RSB (2009) Therapeutic hypothermia:applications in pediatric cardiac arrest. J Neurotrauma 26:421–427

Orlowski JP, Abulleil MM, Phillips JM (1989) The hemodynamic and cardiovascular effects of near-drowning in hypotonic, isotonic or hypertonic solutions. Ann Emerg Med 18(10):1044–1049

Pepe P, Bierens J (2006) Resuscitation in Handbook of drowning: epidemiology of drowning. Bierens JJLM (ed) Springer Verlag, Berlin, pp 312–385

Quan L (2006) Methods for estimating the burden of drowning, in Handbook of drowning. Section 2 The Epidemiology of drowning. Bierens JJLM ed. Springer Verlag, Berlin, pp 49–53

Ralston M, Hazinski MF, Zaritsky AL, Schexnayder SM (eds) (2006) Pediatric advanced life support provider manual. American Heart Association, Dallas

Soar J, Perkins GD, Abbas G, Alfonzo A, Barelli A, Bierens JJ, Brugger H, Deakin CD, Dunning J, Georgiou M, Handley AJ, Lockey DJ, Paal P, Sandroni C, Thies KC, Zideman DA, Nolan JP (2010) European resuscitation council guidelines for resuscitation 2010 section 8. Cardiac arrest in special circumstances: electrolyte abnormalities, poisoning, drowning, accidental hypothermia, hyperthermia, asthma, anaphylaxis, cardiac surgery, trauma, pregnancy, electrocution. Resuscitation 81(10):1400–1433

Spilzman D, Bierens JJLM, Handley AJ, Orlowski JP (2012) Drowning. N Engl J Med 366:2102–2110

Drug Abuse

► Toxicology

Drug Abuse and Trauma Anesthesia

Michael L. McCartney
Department of Anesthesiology, University of Missouri-Kansas City, Kansas City, MO, USA

Synonyms

Drug addiction; Drug misuse; Illicit drug use; Polysubstance abuse; Prescription drug abuse; Substance abuse

Definition

Drug abuse is the use of a psychoactive substance in a manner that is potentially harmful to the user and may lead to dependence or addiction. It includes the use of drugs that are illegal and the use of legally available drugs in excessive amounts or in ways that are not sanctioned or prescribed by a physician or healthcare provider.

Preexisting Condition

Patients presenting to the hospital as a result of trauma are frequently under the influence of abused substances. Two studies at a major trauma center showed that testing of blood and urine of trauma patients was positive for alcohol or other drugs (not including marijuana) at least 65 % of the time (Bailey 1990). The initial evaluation of all trauma patients must include thorough questioning about substance use, even though patients may not be honest or forthcoming with their answers. Physicians must look carefully for the physical signs and symptoms of chronic substance abuse and acute intoxication. Consideration should also be given to testing of blood and/or urine for the presence of alcohol, drugs, and their metabolites, especially in cases when the patient is unable or unwilling to provide a complete social history. Rapid screening tests can accurately detect the presence of commonly abused substances and help guide the management of the intoxicated trauma patient.

The acute and chronic abuse of drugs and alcohol can have severe deleterious effects on the underlying health of the trauma patient and may leave them vulnerable to dangerous drug-drug interactions with medications administered as part of their anesthesia care. Knowledge of the substances used by the patient may enable the anesthesiologist to counteract some of the harmful side effects and avoid worsening their condition. Additionally, victims of trauma may have further derangement of their physiology as a result of their injuries, e.g., hemorrhage, pneumothorax, and cerebral injury that can make them more susceptible to the dangerous side effects of drugs of abuse.

Application

The management of drug abusing trauma patients is highly variable and depends on which substance or substances are being abused. This portion of the essay will address some of the more commonly abused drugs, aid in recognizing the signs of abuse, point out potential interactions with anesthetic drugs, and offer therapies to prevent or treat the complications due to abused substances.

Alcohol

Alcohol is the most frequently encountered substance of abuse among patients admitted to trauma centers and emergency departments (Bailey 1990; Substance Abuse and Mental Health Services Administration (SAMHSA) and Center for Behavioral Health Statistics and Quality 2012). It is commonly abused in combination with other drugs, often leading to additive or synergistic effects. Chronic heavy alcohol use can lead to gastrointestinal complications including pancreatitis, gastritis, and hepatic dysfunction. The central nervous system (CNS) can be affected by sleep disorders, mood disorders, cerebral atrophy, and seizure disorder.

Patients acutely intoxicated with alcohol are a common sight in trauma centers. They exhibit a range of behaviors dependent, in part, on the level of intoxication. At lower alcohol levels, patients may be pleasant, giddy, and slightly disinhibited. Progression to higher alcohol concentrations may lead to impaired speech and motor control. Still, higher concentrations result in nausea, vomiting, uncooperative or combative behavior, and stupor or even complete loss of consciousness. Alcohol is detected on routine toxicology screening and is easily identified by its characteristic odor on the patient's breath.

Anesthetic management of patients acutely intoxicated from alcohol needs to take into consideration the CNS depressant effects of alcohol. Premedication with an anxiolytic is rarely required and may be dangerous. Patients are usually treated as having a full stomach even if they have recently vomited, and full aspiration precautions are taken. Maintenance of anesthesia will usually require lower concentrations of typical anesthetic drugs, and emergence may be prolonged. Postoperative management may include the treatment of nausea and vomiting and a heightened awareness of the signs of withdrawal, including tachycardia, anxiety, tachypnea, elevated temperature, and even seizures. Early recognition of withdrawal symptoms allows for prompt treatment with small doses of benzodiazepines such as lorazepam and prevention of more severe withdrawal. Chronic alcohol abuse may result in some cross-tolerance to opioids, and patients may require higher than expected doses to achieve satisfactory analgesia.

Marijuana

Among the illegal substances, marijuana is the most commonly used drug and is second only to cocaine in its involvement in drug-related emergency department visits (Substance Abuse and Mental Health Services Administration (SAMHSA) and Center for Behavioral Health Statistics and Quality 2012). Typical usage by smoking results in a quick euphoria and mild sedation along with some mild hallucinogenic effects with a duration of approximately 2–3 h. Users may exhibit conjunctival injection, mildly depressed level of consciousness, tachycardia, and increased cardiac output. At higher levels of intoxication, bradycardia and hypotension are occasionally seen (Hernandez et al. 2005). Chronic use of marijuana by smoking can result in pulmonary changes similar to cigarette smoking such as increased airway reactivity, increased secretions, and even an increased risk of lung cancer. Recent marijuana usage may cause an increased tendency toward laryngospasm and bronchospasm. The mild sedation provided by marijuana may obviate the need for anesthetic premedication with a benzodiazepine, and it can decrease anesthetic requirements and lead to prolonged emergence in procedures of shorter duration. Marijuana also possesses antiemetic properties.

Cocaine

Cocaine is the most frequent cause of death due to drug use, due to its multitude of dangerous cardiovascular and pulmonary effects. The commercially available hydrochloride salt of cocaine can be nasally insufflated ("snorted"), ingested orally, or injected intravenously. The combination of sodium bicarbonate or other basic compound, water and heat, is used to convert cocaine hydrochloride back to its "free base" form also known as "crack" which can be smoked for a much faster and more intense high. Regardless of route of ingestion, cocaine acts to inhibit the presynaptic reuptake of norepinephrine, dopamine, and serotonin which results in a higher free concentration of these neurotransmitters. The endogenous opiate system is also stimulated. Users experience euphoria, excitement, decreased need for sleep, and decreased appetite (Steadman and Birnbach 2003).

Along with these pleasurable CNS effects, cocaine causes a combination of cardiovascular effects that can be fatal. Elevated catecholamines produce tachycardia, a tendency toward tachyarrhythmias, and a marked increase in cardiac output, blood pressure, systemic vascular resistance, and myocardial oxygen demand. Combined with a reduction in myocardial oxygen supply due to intense coronary arterial vasoconstriction, myocardial ischemia is the inevitable result. Cocaine also has an activating effect on the platelets,

which can lead to thrombosis and infarction. In addition to coronary vasoconstriction, cerebral vasoconstriction is common and may result in seizures, stroke, and brain damage. Chronic cocaine users should be considered at high risk for cardiovascular complications. Furthermore, it has been suggested that elective surgery should be postponed until the user has abstained from cocaine for at least 1 week. Effects of cocaine on the pulmonary system may include increased airway reactivity, acute bronchospasm, or hemorrhage (Hernandez et al. 2005; Vroegop et al. 2009).

Management of the acutely intoxicated cocaine user requires decreasing the heart rate and blood pressure and reversing coronary and cerebral vasoconstriction. Benzodiazepines can help decrease agitation, which is often present. These goals must be achieved prior to induction of anesthesia if circumstances permit. Nitroglycerin, sodium nitroprusside, phentolamine, and verapamil are considered drugs of choice to treat tachycardia and provide coronary vasodilation. The traditional recommendation is to avoid isolated beta-blockade due to the resultant unopposed alpha-adrenergic vasoconstriction, but in clinical practice, the use of beta-blockers has been helpful. Induction of anesthesia can be achieved with propofol or thiopental, but ketamine should be avoided due to its additive stimulating effect on the CNS and cardiovascular system. Intraoperative hypotension may be resistant to treatment with ephedrine (likely due to depleted stores of catecholamines), but phenylephrine has been shown to be effective. Cocaine-induced seizures are thought to be dopamine mediated and are therefore typically resistant to GABAergic drugs like benzodiazepines, phenytoin, inhalational anesthetics, and the barbiturates (Steadman and Birnbach 2003). Dexmedetomidine has been shown experimentally to raise the seizure threshold in rats exposed to cocaine and may be beneficial in the treatment of cocaine-induced seizures when given in typical doses used for sedation.

Although polysubstance abuse is always a possibility, physicians should be especially vigilant for the presence of multiple drugs in the setting of cocaine intoxication. The combination of cocaine and alcohol produces an active metabolite called cocaethylene, which intensifies the cardiovascular effects of cocaine, increases the duration of action, and greatly increases the risk of death from a cardiac event (Vroegop et al. 2009). Cocaine is also frequently combined with heroin or benzodiazepines, so reversal agents like naloxone or flumazenil should only be given if the perceived benefit outweighs the risk of side effects such as seizures and arrhythmias which can be dangerous and difficult to treat in the setting of cocaine abuse.

Amphetamines

The prevalence of amphetamine abuse in the United States appears to be increasing through multiple pathways. Methamphetamine ("crystal meth," "crank," and "ice") is easily synthesized from over-the-counter cold remedies containing pseudoephedrine, and its use is rampant in the middle and western USA The popularity of 3,4-methylenedioxymethamphetamine (MDMA, "Ecstasy") as a club drug has led to a 114 % increase in the number of MDMA-related emergency department visits between 2004 and 2010 (Substance Abuse and Mental Health Services Administration (SAMHSA) and Center for Behavioral Health Statistics and Quality 2012). Finally, the proliferation of drugs used to treat attention deficit/hyperactivity disorder such as dextroamphetamine, methylphenidate, and related compounds has allowed their increased diversion for illicit use.

Amphetamines act as CNS stimulants through effects on the neurotransmitters dopamine, serotonin, and norepinephrine and also appear to inhibit monoamine oxidase. Users initially experience increased alertness, euphoria, insomnia, and decreased appetite which may progress to agitation, paranoia, delirium, and violence. Cardiovascular side effects are similar to cocaine, including tachycardia, hypertension, increased cardiac output, and a tendency toward increased risk of tachyarrhythmias, cardiovascular events, seizures, and stroke (Mokhlesi et al. 2004).

Chronic abusers of methamphetamine stereotypically exhibit poor grooming, skin lesions from "picking" and "meth mouth," extensive dental decay often attributed to xerostomia, bruxism, poor dental hygiene, or the caustic effect of the drug itself. Long-term use of amphetamines can also cause nonischemic dilated cardiomyopathy through an as yet unknown mechanism. Refractory or unexplained hypotension may require echocardiographic examination or placement of a pulmonary artery catheter.

Frequently seen in club or party users of MDMA, amphetamines may cause hyponatremia due to diaphoresis, thirst, and excessive freewater intake. The hyponatremia can become severe enough to cause seizures. Hyperthermia caused by the combination of peripheral vasoconstriction and physical exertion (such as dancing for hours) can be life threatening and may even mimic the presentation of malignant hyperthermia. Rhabdomyolysis, metabolic acidosis, renal failure, coagulopathy, and elevated temperature must be treated with aggressive cooling measures, hydration, ventilation, and administration of 100 % oxygen. In the absence of actual malignant hyperthermia, administration of nondepolarizing neuromuscular blocking agents should result in complete muscle relaxation (Steadman and Birnbach 2003; Mokhlesi et al. 2004).

Anesthetic management of the acutely intoxicated amphetamine user may require sedation with benzodiazepines or antipsychotics. A blood chemistry profile can detect electrolyte disturbance and renal function. Hypertension and tachycardia can be treated with adrenergic antagonists, although the same theoretical concern exists with amphetamines regarding unopposed alpha-mediated vasoconstriction. Core temperature monitoring is required to detect hyperthermia and guide its treatment.

Hallucinogens

The hallucinogenic drug phencyclidine (PCP, "angel dust," and "wet") is less frequently detected in trauma patients than cocaine and amphetamines but is still responsible for roughly

5 % of all drug-related emergency department visits (Substance Abuse and Mental Health Services Administration (SAMHSA) and Center for Behavioral Health Statistics and Quality 2012). Most patients under the influence of PCP will exhibit vertical nystagmus, pinpoint pupils, and hypertension (Mokhlesi et al. 2004). Some users of PCP may present with psychosis, violent behavior, decreased pain perception, and an apparent increase in muscular strength, making them difficult to manage if combative. Rapid sedation by intramuscular route is usually necessary to protect the patient and caregivers. Other less common signs exhibited by patients on PCP include dystonia, excessive salivation, seizures, muscle rigidity, even apnea, and cardiac arrest. Ketamine, the familiar anesthetic drug originally derived from phencyclidine, has a very similar presentation (nystagmus and psychotic behavior, hypertension) but tends to cause less sympathetic stimulation than PCP and has a shorter duration of action. Haloperidol has been shown to be an effective sedative in acutely intoxicated users of PCP, and the addition of a benzodiazepine may help expedite the effect. If hypertension and tachycardia persist after agitation is resolved, they can be managed in a similar fashion to the other sympathomimetic drugs of abuse, keeping in mind the potential for unopposed vasoconstriction when beta-blockers are given (Mokhlesi et al. 2004).

Lysergic acid diethylamide (LSD), mescaline, and psilocybin are also potent hallucinogens which may occasionally be encountered but tend to have much less sympathetic stimulation than PCP and ketamine. Antimuscarinic effects of tachycardia, dry mouth and elevated temperature, are usually not severe. Patients experiencing severe dysphoric reactions – "bad trip" – may benefit from low doses of benzodiazepines such as lorazepam.

Prescription Drugs

The abuse of prescription drugs such as benzodiazepines, opioids, and stimulants appears to be on the rise, now accounting for more emergency department visits than illicit drugs of abuse (Substance Abuse and Mental Health Services Administration (SAMHSA) and Center for Behavioral Health Statistics and Quality 2012). Anesthesiologists should already be familiar with the management of patients on opioid and benzodiazepine medications but must also take into account the fact that patients often abuse multiple substances at the same time, and administration of reversal drugs may carry additional risk.

Drug abuse is very common among trauma patients and can present many challenges to the anesthesiologist taking care of them. Correct identification of the presence of abused substances and an understanding of the physiologic effects of those substances are important if one is to prevent some of the complications that could otherwise result when caring for these patients.

Cross-References

▶ Alcohol Withdrawal
▶ Benzodiazepines

References

Bailey DN (1990) Drug use in patients admitted to a university trauma center: results of limited (rather than comprehensive) toxicology screening. J Anal Toxicol 43:22–24

Hernandez M, Birnbach DJ, Van Zundert AAJ (2005) Anesthetic management of the illicit-substance using patient. Curr Opin Anaesthesiol 18:315–324

Mokhlesi B, Garimella PS, Joffe A, Velho V (2004) Street drug abuse leading to critical illness. Intensive Care Med 30:1526–1536

Steadman JL, Birnbach DJ (2003) Patients on party drugs undergoing anesthesia. Curr Opin Anaesthesiol 16:147–153

Substance Abuse and Mental Health Services Administration (SAMHSA), Center for Behavioral Health Statistics and Quality (2012) The DAWN report: highlights of the 2010 drug abuse warning network (DAWN) findings on drug-related emergency department visits. Rockville, 2 July 2012

Vroegop MP, Franssen EJ, van der Voort PHJ, van den Berg TNA, Langeweg RJ, Kramers C (2009) The emergency care of cocaine intoxications. Neth J Med 67(4):122–126

Drug Addiction

▶ Drug Abuse and Trauma Anesthesia

Drug Misuse

▶ Drug Abuse and Trauma Anesthesia

Drug Use

▶ Toxicology

DTs

▶ Alcohol Withdrawal

Duodenal Hematoma

▶ Duodenal Trauma

Duodenal Injury

▶ Duodenal Trauma
▶ Gastrointestinal Injury, Anesthesia for

Duodenal Perforation

▶ Duodenal Trauma

Duodenal Trauma

Zoë Maher[1] and Patrick K. Kim[2]
[1]The Trauma Center at Penn, University of
Pennsylvania, Philadelphia, PA, USA
[2]Division of Traumatology, Surgical Critical
Care and Emergency Surgery, Department of
Surgery, Perelman School of Medicine at the
University of Pennsylvania, Philadelphia,
PA, USA

Synonyms

Duodenal hematoma; Duodenal injury; Duodenal perforation; Pancreaticoduodenectomy; Pyloric exclusion; Small bowel injury; Whipple procedure

Definition

Pancreatic trauma and duodenal trauma are considered together because of the close anatomic relationship, shared blood supply, and frequency of combined injuries. Pancreatico-duodenal injuries carry a high morbidity and mortality owing in part to proximity to major vascular structures, the challenges of both diagnosis and management, and associated injuries. Early identification and treatment of this injury complex reduces associated morbidity and mortality.

Preexisting Condition

The duodenum is a primarily retroperitoneal organ divided into four parts: superior (D1), descending (D2), horizontal (D3), and ascending (D4). The ampulla of Vater is located in D2, and its identification is critical in management decisions for duodenal trauma.

Application

Mechanism

Blunt duodenal trauma is the leading cause of duodenal injury in many regions of the world and presents as duodenal hematoma or perforation following a compression injury to the epigastrium.

The majority of duodenal injuries in the United States are seen in the setting of penetrating trauma and often present concurrently with pancreatic injury.

Diagnosis

Diagnosis of penetrating duodenal injury is nearly uniformly made at laparotomy. Blunt duodenal injury can present a diagnostic challenge due to nonspecific physical exam and laboratory findings.

Computed tomography (CT) is the most widely applied adjunct used in the diagnosis of blunt duodenal injury. Except in the setting of duodenal rupture, which presents as extraluminal air or contrast on imaging, CT findings can be nonspecific for duodenal injury and include periduodenal hematoma and thickening.

Upper gastrointestinal series (UGI) should be performed if CT fails to demonstrate contrast extravasation in patients suspected of blunt duodenal injury. Sensitivity of the test is improved if gastrograffin is followed by barium contrast (Degiannis and Boffard 2000). UGI can demonstrate the "coiled spring" appearance of duodenal obstruction secondary to hematoma or contrast extravasation in the case of duodenal perforation.

There are no specific or sensitive laboratory findings for duodenal injury. Elevation of serum amylase on serial exam can indicate an injury, but normal pancreatic enzyme levels do not rule out duodenal injury (Degiannis and Boffard 2000).

AAST Grade
See Table 1.

Management

Blunt duodenal injury manifest as isolated duodenal hematoma is very uncommon in adults and only slightly more common in children. These

Duodenal Trauma, Table 1 AAST duodenum organ injury scale

Grade[a]	Type of injury	Description of injury	AIS-90
I	Hematoma	Involving single portion of the duodenum	2
I	Laceration	Partial thickness, no perforation	3
II	Hematoma	Involving more than one portion	2
II	Laceration	Disruption of <50 % circumference	4
III	Laceration	Disruption of 50–75 % of circumference of D2	4
III		Disruption of 50–100 % of circumference D1, D3, D4	4
IV	Laceration	Disruption of >75 % of circumference of D2	5
IV		Involving ampulla or distal common bile duct	5
V	Laceration	Massive disruption of duodenopancreatic complex	5
V	Vascular	Devascularization of duodenum	5

Adapted from Moore et al. (1990) with permission
[a]Add one grade for multiple injuries up to grade III

injuries can be managed nonoperatively with nasogastric decompression, bowel rest, and serial examination. Decrease in nasogastric output will indicate resolution of the hematoma. Hematomas found incidentally at laparotomy and those not resolving after a period of 2–3 weeks should be surgically decompressed.

Indications for operative intervention for duodenal injury are peritonitis, hemodynamic instability, penetrating mechanism, and concern for duodenal perforation.

A combination of the Kocher and Cattell-Braasch maneuvers allows for exposure of the duodenum. Lateral duodenal and right colonic peritoneal attachments are released to complete a right medial visceral rotation and to visualize the entirety of D1, D2, and D3 and a portion of D4. Transection of the ligament of Treitz will permit complete exposure of D4.

Operative management is guided by the anatomic location of injury and extent of destruction. There are three basic approaches to surgical management of duodenal injury: primary repair with drainage, primary repair with decompression or diversion, and duodenal reconstruction. Closed suction drains should be placed with any of the approaches.

Debridement of devitalized tissue followed by non-narrowing transverse primary closure in one or two layers is appropriate for the majority of duodenal injuries. If primary closure would narrow the duodenal lumen, consideration should be given to placement of a jejunal serosal patch overlying the injury (Neal et al. 2013).

Primary repair followed by decompression or diversion should be considered for more complex or tenuous repairs. Decompression can be accomplished by two methods: nasogastric and nasoenteric tube placement proximal and distal to the repair or the "triple tube" method. The "triple tube" method involves placement of a gastrostomy tube, a retrograde decompressive jejunostomy tube, and an antegrade feeding jejunostomy tube.

Diversion can be accomplished by two methods: pyloric exclusion or "duodenal diverticularization." Pyloric exclusion can be done via anterior gastrotomy with suture closure of the pyloric outlet or with a noncutting stapler fired immediately distal to the pylorus. Gastrojejunostomy should then be constructed. "Duodenal diverticularization" includes duodenal repair, antrectomy with vagotomy, gastrojejunostomy, tube duodenostomy, and T-tube biliary drain. Both the "triple tube" and "duodenal diverticularization" methods have been largely replaced by their simpler counterparts.

Duodenal reconstruction is reserved for injuries not amenable to primary repair and includes duodenoduodenostomy, duodenojejunostomy, Roux-en-Y reconstruction, and pancreaticoduodenectomy.

Controversy in Management

Primary repair with drainage of duodenal injury versus more traditional and complex repair is still controversial. Advocates of the "less is more" approach cite evidence that major complication rates are equivalent between simple duodenal primary repair with drainage and the more complex traditional approaches, including pyloric exclusion. Data indicate that primary repair with drainage is at least equivalent to primary repair with pyloric exclusion (Seamon et al. 2007). Opposition to this approach cites a lack of high-level data supporting this claim (Talving et al. 2006).

Complications

The major complications of duodenal injury are fistula, duodenal dehiscence, and sepsis. Significant increase in complication rates (up to 64 %) and mortality (up to 40 %) occurs if diagnosis is delayed (Neal et al. 2013).

Cross-References

▶ Damage Control Surgery
▶ Delayed Diagnosis/Missed Injury
▶ Gastrointestinal Injury, Anesthesia For
▶ Imaging of Abdominal and Pelvic Injuries
▶ Pancreatic Trauma
▶ Seatbelt Injuries
▶ Trauma Laparotomy

References

Degiannis E, Boffard K (2000) Duodenal injuries. Br J Surg 87(11):1473–1479, Review

Moore E, Cogbill T, Malangoni M et al (1990) Organ injury scaling, 11: pancreas, duodenum, small bowel, colon, and rectum. J Trauma Acute Care Surg 30(11):1427–1429

Neal MD, Britt LD, Watson G, Murdock A, Peitzman AB (2013) Abdominal Trauma. In: Peitzman AB, Rhodes M, Schwab CW, Yealy DM, Fabian TC (eds) The trauma manual: trauma and acute care surgery, 4th ed. Lippincott Williams & Wilkins, Philadelphia

Seamon MJ, Pieri PG, Fisher CA, Gaughan J, Santora TA, Pathak AS, Bradley KM, Goldberg AJ (2007) A ten-year retrospective review: does pyloric exclusion improve clinical outcome after penetrating duodenal and combined pancreaticoduodenal injuries? J Trauma 62(4):829–833

Talving P, Nicol AJ, Navsaria PH (2006) Civilian duodenal gunshot wounds: surgical management made simpler. World J Surg 30(4):488–494

DVT

▶ Thromboembolic Disease

DVT, as a Complication

Adriana Laser[1] and Khanjan H. Nagarsheth[2]
[1]Department of General Surgery, University of
Maryland Medical Center, Baltimore, MD, USA
[2]R Adams Cowley Shock Trauma Center,
University of Maryland School of Medicine,
Baltimore, MD, USA

Synonyms

Deep vein thrombosis; Deep venous thrombosis;
Economy class syndrome

Definition

Deep-vein thrombosis (DVT) of a vein can be
occlusive or not and occurs within the deep-
venous system. The incidence of DVT in the
surgical population varies by type of patient and
surgical procedure, contributing a significant but
unknown percentile of the overall estimated
250,000 DVTs annually. In a recent meta-analysis, high-risk general surgery patients were found
to have a 20 % risk of having a proximal DVT
(Geerts et al. 2001).

Most DVTs are proximal and are found above
the knee in the iliac, femoral, or popliteal veins.
DVTs below the knee, in any of the three groups
of paired deep calf veins, are of little clinical
significance. Upper extremity DVTs, in the axillary and subclavian veins, account for 5 % of
DVTs and are seen most often in the surgical
patient associated with indwelling catheters or
in patients with malignancy. 30 % of upper
extremity DVTs are estimated to lead to pulmonary embolism (PE).

On the extreme end of DVT consequences,
there are two descriptions to consider.
Phlegmasia alba dolens is a massively swollen
leg with pitting edema, pain, and blanching,
resulting from major venous thrombosis of the
iliofemoral venous system. If this progresses to
compromise arterial inflow, phlegmasia cerulea
dolens, a painful blue leg, can develop.

Preexisting Condition

Risk Factors

Virchow's triad was first described over a century
and a half ago and is still relevant in discussing
the etiology of DVTs in trauma patients. The first
element of the triad is venous stasis which likely
increases the time that activated platelets and
procoagulant factors are in contact with the
endothelial cellular layer. There is also a loss of
the calf-muscle pump, which we see in the
immobilized critically ill patient. The calf
normally fills with blood (100–150 ml) and the
muscle contracts, resulting in feeding perforator
vein valves being thrust closed and then blood is
forced proximally through outflow valves
upward against gravity.

The second part is endothelial injury. Many
studies have shown that injury to veins, such as
microtears within valve cusps, occurs during surgery at distant sites to the operation. Lastly, there
is a known hypercoagulable state that occurs postoperatively. Injured cells release a procoagulant
called tissue factor. Physiologic stress (surgery,
trauma) also has been associated with increases
in platelet count, adhesiveness, changes in the
coagulation cascade, and endogenous fibrinolytic
activity. All three of these factors are actually
present in many victims of trauma.

Other risk factors for DVT include acquired
ones: advanced age, malignancy, immobilization, surgery, trauma, oral contraceptives, hormone replacement, pregnancy, obesity,
neurologic or cardiac disease, prolonged travel,
and inflammatory states. There are also a myriad
of genetic hypercoagulable conditions that may
be simultaneously present in the critically ill
trauma patient: antithrombin deficiency, protein
C and S deficiency, factor V Leiden, prothrombin
20210A, blood group non-O, dysfibrinogenemia,

dysplasminogenemia, hyperhomocysteinemia, reduced heparin cofactor II activity, elevated levels of clotting factors (XI, IX, VII, VIII, X, II), and elevated plasminogen activator inhibitor (PAI-1) (Goldhaber and Bounameaux 2012).

Application

Diagnosis

Routine physical exam often triggers an investigation for DVT. A high index of suspicion is crucial for timely diagnosis of this condition. Signs and symptoms include pain, edema usually of the calf or ankle, and warmth or erythema of the skin over the thrombosis. However, more than 50 % of DVTs are asymptomatic and found solely on imaging.

Duplex ultrasound imaging is highly sensitive has, greater than 95 % specificity, and is reproducible (Douglas and Sumner 1996). It also has the advantages of not needing intravenous contrast, being relatively painless, and being safe pregnant patients. Duplex ultrasonography assesses for thrombus presence, venous dilation, and venous segment incompressibility. Acute versus chronic thrombus is suggested by the absence of spontaneous flow, loss flow variation with respiration, failure to increase flow with distal augmentation, and characterization of the thrombus as having increased echogenicity and heterogeneity. When assessing for pelvic vein and inferior vena cava thrombus, magnetic resonance venography or CT venogram may assist in diagnosis.

Routine surveillance duplex ultrasonography has been used in many trauma centers to assess for DVTs in trauma patients. A recent large retrospective review evaluated the value of routine surveillance ultrasound in the detection of DVTs and found that it is warranted in the highest risk patients. In moderate risk patients, this routine exam does not prove helpful in identifying DVT over obtaining an ultrasound based on clinical suspicion (Bandle et al. 2013).

Laboratory tests such as D-dimer can be useful adjuncts in making the diagnosis of DVT, although this is not as sensitive or specific for the disease as duplex ultrasonography. D-dimer assay test measures cross-linked degradation products. This is used as a surrogate of plasmin's activity on fibrin. As D-dimer is often elevated simply due to trauma or surgery, only a negative result has any clinical relevance in the evaluation of DVT in a surgical patient.

Prophylaxis

Prophylaxis in the perioperative patient has been shown to be significantly effective in reducing the rates of DVTs and PEs. Prophylaxis falls under two categories: pharmacologic and mechanical. Traditionally accepted pharmacologic options include low subcutaneous molecular weight heparin (LMWH; 40 mg daily) which inhibits factor Xa and IIA, and low dose unfractionated heparin (LDUH; 5,000 units three times daily). Adherence to one of these regimens can reduce postoperative DVTs by 68 % from 25 % to 8 % (Geerts et al. 2001).

Mechanical prophylaxis includes primarily intermittent pneumatic compression or sequential compression devices which decreases venous stasis and may increase fibrinolysis. Contraindications to mechanical prophylaxis are few and include active DVT in affected extremity and open wounds. In these cases, compression device may be applied to alternate extremity even an upper limb. Early ambulation can also help in DVT prevention. Indications for prophylaxis include patients who are undergoing major abdominal or orthopedic surgery, have sustained major trauma, or will be immobile for more than 3 days.

Treatment

Treatment for DVT involves mainstay medical therapy with mechanical support. Various less commonly used options are also discussed below. The goal of DVT treatment is to reduce the risk of PE, decrease extension of DVT, and prevent the almost 30 % recurrence rate of an untreated DVT.

Systemic anticoagulation is the mainstay of treatment in patients diagnosed with DVT and PE who do not have a contraindication. The most common choice is unfractionated heparin (UFH) intravenous infusion with warfarin started thereafter. Warfarin must be started only after heparin initiation to reduce the risk of warfarin-induced skin necrosis and the transient hypercoagulable state which is induced by protein C and S levels falling before other vitamin K–dependent factors. Monitoring is required when utilizing this method. Serial lab draws looking at partial thromboplastin time (PTT) is important for patients receiving an intravenous infusion of heparin.

Another common option is low molecular weight heparin (LMWH). Studies have shown there to be a lower bleeding risk than UFH, equal or superior effectiveness in preventing recurrence, decreased mortality, diminished antiplatelet effect, reduced incidence of heparin-induced thrombocytopenia and thrombosis (HITT), less interference with protein C, more predictable bioavailability, lower complement activation, lower risk of osteoporosis, and more predictable dose-response. The mechanism of action includes greater anti-factor Xa and less direct antithrombin inhibition. Traditionally, monitoring was not done; however, some situations are now calling for intermittent measurement of anti-factor Xa levels. These include pediatric patients, pregnant patients, obese patients, and patients with renal insufficiency.

More recently, direct factor Xa inhibitors have come on the market including: rivaroxaban (EINSTEIN Investigators et al. 2010), fondaparinux, and dabigatran. Differentiated from heparin, these agents do not use antithrombin as a mediator. The duration of systemic anticoagulation is typically 3 months for an initial proximal DVT. However, lifelong therapy is recommended after a second VTE or those associated with non-temporary hypercoagulable states such as malignancy or certain genetic diagnoses. Treatment for more distal DVTs in calf veins should also be for 3 months (Hirsch et al. 2008).

Catheter-directed pharmacologic thrombolysis is uncommonly used but when initiated early, within 1 week, it is thought to preserve valve function. This is performed generally with recombinant tPA. Indications include massive iliofemoral DVT, phlegmasia, and thrombosis with ischemia or vascular compromise.

Axillary or subclavian DVTs in young patients with effort thrombosis may increase venous patency and decrease post-thrombotic syndrome. Endovascular and surgical methods are also used infrequently but can include thrombectomy, angioplasty, and stenting.

Patients with DVTs should also be encouraged to wear compression stockings, elevate the extremity at rest, and ambulate frequently. Some patients may require physical therapy if the edema inhibits function and activities of daily living.

Inferior vena cava (IVC) filter placement is another aspect of DVT treatment. They can be placed before a DVT is diagnosed, or after, to prevent PE. The indications for IVC filter placement are recurrent venous thromboembolism while on appropriate and adequate anticoagulation, a new DVT with a contraindication to anticoagulation, complications of anticoagulation treatment, or propagating iliofemoral DVT during anticoagulation. There is an approximate 4 % recurrence rate, and a 95 % patency rate. Retrievable IVC filters can be utilized in multiple trauma victims and in high-risk surgical patients.

Complications of DVT

The natural history of DVTs can take one of several routes. First, they can lead to thromboembolization, a PE, which of course is highly morbid and potentially lethal. Secondly, DVTs can result in luminal recanalization. DVTs can alternatively lead to chronic occlusion with scarring. Partial lumen patency can be restored but intraluminal scarring entraps valves. Valve incompetence and vein wall fibrosis follows with early clinical symptoms of edema, pain, and immobility. Eventually chronic venous insufficiency with valvular dysfunction develops, defined as post-thrombotic syndrome. Other sequelae can be recurrent DVTs or paradoxical emboli (embolus to brain through a patent foramen ovale). There is an overall estimated 9 % case fatality rate after first time DVT (Geerts et al. 2001).

Complications of Treatment

Treatment of DVT is not without complications. There is a reported 10 % risk of bleeding in the first 5 days of UFH administration to therapeutic PTT levels. Heparin-induced [thrombotic] thrombocytopenia occurs 0.6–30 % per year and is caused by heparin-dependent antibody IgG which binds to platelets, causing aggregation. Signs and symptoms typically start 3–14 days after starting heparin and include: >50 % drop in platelets, a drop <100,000, or evidence of new thrombosis while on heparin therapy. Diagnosis is by ELISA for antiheparin antibody. Treatment is to stop heparin, and start a direct thrombin inhibitor like lepirudin or argatroban or a factor Xa inhibitor such as fondaparinux or rivaroxaban for anticoagulation.

Cross-References

▶ Venous Thromboembolism Prophylaxis and Treatment Following Trauma
▶ Venous Thromboembolism Prophylaxis in the Intensive Care Unit

References

Bandle J, Shackford SR, Kahl JE, Sise CB, Calvo RY, Shackford MC, Sise MJ (2013) The value of lower-extremity duplex surveillance to detect deep vein thrombosis in trauma patients. J Trauma Acute Care Surg 74(2):575–580
Douglas MG, Sumner DS (1996) Duplex scanning for deep vein thrombosis: has it replaced both phlebography and noninvasive testing? Semin Vasc Surg 9:3
EINSTEIN Investigators, Bauersachs R, Berkowitz SD, Brenner B, Buller HR et al (2010) Oral rivaroxaban for symptomatic venous thromboembolism. N Engl J Med 363:2499–2510
Geerts WH, Heit JA, Clagett GP et al (2001) Prevention of venous thromboembolism. Chest 119:132S
Goldhaber SZ, Bounameaux H (2012) Pulmonary embolism and deep vein thrombosis. Lancet 12(9828):1835–1846
Hirsch J, Guyatt G, Albers GW, Harrington R, Schunemann HJ (2008) Antithrombotic and thrombolytic therapy American College of Chest Physicians evidence based clinical practice guidelines (8th edition). Chest 133:110S–112S

D

Dynamic Hyperinflation

▶ Auto-PEEP

Dysrhythmia

▶ Supraventricular Arrhythmia Management

E

EACA

▶ Aminocaproic Acid

EAF

▶ Entero-Atmospheric Fistula

e-Aminocaproic Acid

▶ Aminocaproic Acid

Early Coagulopathy of Trauma

▶ Coagulopathy in Trauma: Underlying Mechanisms

Early Intervention

▶ Spinal Cord Injury, Early Management

Early Trauma-Associated Coagulopathy

▶ Acute Coagulopathy of Trauma

Earthquake

▶ Crush Syndrome

Echocardiography in the Trauma Setting

Christopher E. Beck
Department of Anesthesiology, University of Kansas, Kansas City, KS, USA

Synonyms

Focused cardiac ultrasound (FOCUS); Lung ultrasound; Transesophageal echocardiography (TEE); Transthoracic echocardiography (TTE); Ultrasonography

Definition

Medical ultrasonography is a diagnostic tool utilizing reflected sound-waves to visualize

© Springer-Verlag Berlin Heidelberg 2015
P.J. Papadakos, M.L. Gestring (eds.), *Encyclopedia of Trauma Care*,
DOI 10.1007/978-3-642-29613-0

underlying anatomical structures. Transthoracic and transesophageal echocardiography are two types of ultrasound technology used to assess cardiac, pulmonary, and aortic structures. The primary difference is that the probe is placed on the outer thoracic wall for transthoracic echocardiography, whereas the probe is inserted in the esophagus for transesophageal echocardiography.

Preexisting Condition

Recently, the American Society of Echocardiography (ASE) and the American College of Emergency Physicians (ACEP) reaffirmed the importance of the focused cardiac ultrasound (FOCUS) within the emergency/trauma setting (American Society of Echocardiography Consensus Statement 2010). The FOCUS exam assesses cardiac size and overall function, pericardial effusions, intravascular volume, and aids with thoracic/cardiac interventions (Table 1). In addition, the FOCUS exam assists in the diagnosis and treatment of various emergency clinical scenarios such as cardiac trauma, cardiac arrest, hypotension, dyspnea, and chest pain. More complex cardiac injuries or aortic injuries that include various valvular injuries, coronary injuries, or aortic dissection are described in the entry "▶ Cardiac and Aortic Trauma, Anesthesia for." These injuries may be beyond the

scope of transthoracic echocardiogram and may require use of the transesophageal echocardiography (TEE) for adequate assessment.

Application

Pericardial Effusion

The FOCUS exam provides the ability to readily identify pericardial effusions with a very high-level of confidence. In the suspected diagnosis of pericardial effusion, it is important to combine the findings of the FOCUS exam (pericardial fluid, blood, or thrombus) with clinical signs demonstrating hypotension, tachycardia, pulsus paradoxus, and distended neck veins.

Furthermore, the clinical impact of a pericardial effusion must be delineated based on its onset and severity. For example, a large, chronic pericardial effusion may have minimal impact on a patient's hemodynamic status because of gradual compensation, whereas a small, acute pericardial effusion could severely impact a patient's hemodynamic status, leading to catastrophic consequences, even death.

In the case of a hemodynamically significant pericardial effusion, the FOCUS exam has the advantage of being immediately available and assisting with the treatment. The ultrasound probe can be used to assess the size, location, and impact of the pericardial effusion, and guide the pericardiocentesis with fewer complications and greater success.

Echocardiography in the Trauma Setting, Table 1 This is an overview of the goals of the FOCUS examination for a symptomatic emergency department patient (American Society of Echocardiography Consensus Statement 2010)

Goals of the focused cardiac ultrasound in the symptomatic emergency department patient
Assessment for the presence of pericardial effusion and pleural effusion
Assessment of global cardiac systolic functions
Identification of marked right ventricular and left ventricular enlargement
Intravascular volume assessment
Guidance of pericardiocentesis
Confirmation of transvenous pacing wire placement

Global Cardiac Systolic Dysfunction

Although the FOCUS exam has limited utility in examining specific regional wall-motion abnormalities, there is excellent correlation between the ability to identify normal overall cardiac function versus impaired cardiac function with the FOCUS exam. It is easy to recognize myocardial thickening and systolic wall-motion with multiple FOCUS imaging windows and determine the overall cardiac function. Assessment of the global cardiac systolic function is important, because it guides the treatment plan, including further diagnostic testing, necessary pharmacologic treatment, or cardiac-invasive interventions.

Right Ventricular Enlargement

Pulmonary embolism results in a dilated right ventricle with depressed function and a hyperdynamic, underfilled left ventricle. The FOCUS exam's main priority in compromised patients with suspected pulmonary embolism is to determine further diagnostic testing, consider alternative diagnoses, and develop a treatment plan. The FOCUS exam confirms right ventricular dilation, decreased functionality, and the visualization of thrombi; however, other diagnostic studies are usually necessary to confirm the diagnosis. In addition, right ventricular dilatation may be indicative of other pathologic processes, such as chronic pulmonary obstructive disease, obstructive sleep apnea, pulmonary hypertension, right-sided ventricular infarction, and obesity rather than pulmonary embolism.

Volume Assessment

The FOCUS exam measures the inferior vena cava and compares the size and the percentage of collapse during the respiratory cycle to determine volume status and estimate central venous pressure. If there is a greater change in the ratio of the size of the extrathoracic inferior vena cava during inspiration compared to expiration, then the intravascular volume status and central venous pressure can be determined (Table 2). This information is valuable in evaluating a patient's intravascular volume status and determining the treatment plan.

Echocardiography in the Trauma Setting, Table 2 Transesophageal echocardiography can be used to measure the size of the inferior vena cava and its change in size with respirations. These measurements correlate with the central venous pressure (Kircher and Schiller 1990)

IVC measured	Percent collapse (IVC) during inspiration	CVP (mmHg)
<1.5 cm	>50 %	0–5
1.5-2.5 cm	>50 %	5–10
1.5-2.5 cm	<50 %	10–15
>2.5 cm	Little phasicity	15–20

Clinical Applications

The FOCUS exam demonstrates many benefits and impacts the clinical decision-making process in several clinical applications. First, cardiac trauma can be readily assessed with the FOCUS exam. It is possible to diagnose pericardial effusions, evaluate penetrating cardiac and/or thoracic injuries, and determine the necessary medical or surgical management. Since FOCUS evaluates the global cardiac function, the blunt cardiac trauma and cardiac contusions may be diagnosed by decreased wall-motion and contractility.

During cardiac arrests, the FOCUS exam helps determine potential cardiac causes and assist with pharmacologic and surgical interventions. Furthermore, the FOCUS exam evaluates overall cardiac contractility and directs cardiopulmonary resuscitation during pulseless electrical activity or pseudo-pulseless electrical activity. In addition, cardiogenic shock can easily be diagnosed with the FOCUS exam and lead to the use of further pharmacologic support or mechanical assist devices.

Dyspnea can be caused by a pericardial effusion, depressed cardiac function/heart failure, and pulmonary embolism. As previously described, the FOCUS exam evaluates each of these potential diagnoses and helps determine the treatment plan and further diagnostic testing. Recently, there have been further advances in thoracic ultrasound and implementation of the Bedside Lung Ultrasound in Emergency (BLUE) protocol to diagnose pneumothorax, pleural effusion, and alveolar interstitial syndromes (Turner and Dankoff 2012).

Finally, chest pain may be secondary to myocardial ischemia/infarction or aortic dissection. The FOCUS exam is valuable in these circumstances, because it evaluates overall heart function, measures the aorta to determine if there is exaggerated widening of the aortic root/ascending aorta, and diagnoses pericardial or pleural effusions.

Despite the advancement of ultrasonography coupled with the improvement of transthoracic echocardiography, critical information for improving and assisting in patient care may be

E

insufficient with these modalities. Therefore, it may be necessary to diagnose and formulate treatment plans with a more guided tool such as transesophageal echocardiography (TEE). Transesophageal echocardiography is a diagnostic tool that has mainly been implemented in cardiology and surgery specialties. Fortunately, the usefulness of transesophageal echocardiography is recognized and is becoming a resource to treat and diagnose in various settings, especially trauma/emergency situations.

Although there is some limited data available examining the potential uses of transesophageal echocardiography in the trauma/emergency setting, there are practice guidelines for perioperative transesophageal echocardiography that are applicable (American College of Emergency Physicians 2006). The practice guidelines presented by the American Society of Anesthesiologists and the Society of Cardiovascular Anesthesiologists Task Force discuss three distinct areas: Cardiac and Thoracic Aortic Procedures, Noncardiac Surgery, and Critical Care. By examining the recommendations for these three subspecialty areas, a general overview and basis for potential situations to use transesophageal echocardiography in the trauma/emergency setting can be determined (Table 3). Although the expertise necessary to obtain and interpret the transesophageal images is beyond the scope of this entry, the 20 transesophageal echocardiography images have been provided as a reference (Table 4).

Prior to the use of transesophageal echocardiography, some circumstances are considered potential contraindications and limit, or even prevent the ability to safely perform transesophageal echocardiography. Planning is an important consideration for safe performance of a transesophageal echocardiography exam. First, the patient must be assessed to determine the appropriateness for the transesophageal procedure, especially in a trauma/emergency setting because of the potential injuries (i.e., esophageal) that may be undiagnosed. As with any procedure, transesophageal echocardiography has potential risks and those risks must be thoroughly reviewed to ensure that patient safety is uncompromised.

Echocardiography in the Trauma Setting, Table 3 There are several areas that transesophageal echocardiography is a valuable tool and can assist in monitoring and diagnosing multiple medical conditions and potential treatments (American Society of Anesthesiologists 2010)

Potential use of transesophageal echocardiography in trauma/emergency setting	
Cardiac and thoracic	Detect new and unsuspected cardiac, pulmonary, and thoracic pathology (valvular disease, aortic dissection, cardiac/pleural effusion, etc.)
	Transcatheter cardiac and pulmonary procedures (pacemaker)
Noncardiac procedures	Cardiovascular pathology might result in severe hemodynamic, pulmonary, or neurologic compromise
Critical care	Diagnostic information is expected to alter management (ACLS, volume management, etc.)

The contraindications to transesophageal echocardiography are listed in Table 5. Sites of potential injury from the transesophageal probe include oropharyngeal, esophageal, and gastric areas. In addition, cardiovascular and respiratory complications, thermal injury, infectious risks, and chemical complications are other potential risks involved with transesophageal echocardiography. Usually, all of the aforementioned risks are caused by or related to probe placement, probe manipulation, or pressure injury.

There are other significant limitations to the performance of transesophageal echocardiography including both personnel and equipment. All personnel must meet certain requirements and maintain certifications to be licensed to perform transesophageal echocardiograms. Thus, credentialing is a potential limiting factor, because only a certain number of providers might have met the required standards for performing and interpreting transesophageal echocardiography. Plus, each institution may not have personnel readily available. All of these requirements include additional costs, training, and time. Furthermore, the equipment necessary to perform transesophageal echocardiography is always evolving and improving, and each institution

Echocardiography in the Trauma Setting, Table 4 The recommended 20 cross-sectional views of the heart and great vessels with transesophageal echocardiography (Shanewise et al. 1999)

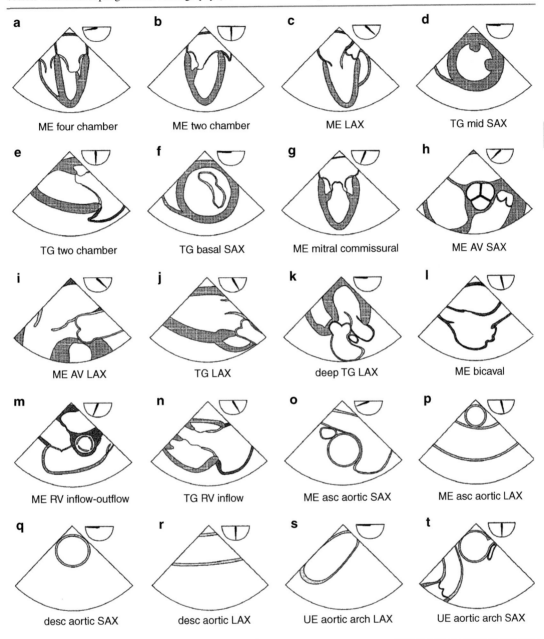

a ME four chamber	**b** ME two chamber	**c** ME LAX	**d** TG mid SAX
e TG two chamber	**f** TG basal SAX	**g** ME mitral commissural	**h** ME AV SAX
i ME AV LAX	**j** TG LAX	**k** deep TG LAX	**l** ME bicaval
m ME RV inflow-outflow	**n** TG RV inflow	**o** ME asc aortic SAX	**p** ME asc aortic LAX
q desc aortic SAX	**r** desc aortic LAX	**s** UE aortic arch LAX	**t** UE aortic arch SAX

Twenty cross-sectional views composing the recommended comprehensive TEE examination. Approximate multiplane angle indicated by the icon adjacent to each view. *ME* mid esophageal, *LAX* long axis, *TG* transgastric, *SAX* short axis, *AV* aortic valve, *RV* right ventricle, *asc* ascending, *desc* descending, *UE* upper esophageal

may have limited resources to maintain current equipment and update the software. Most recently, two-dimensional (2-D) echocardiography equipment is now being replaced by three-dimensional (3-D) echocardiography equipment which will require a far greater financial and personnel commitment to provide optimal patient care.

Echocardiography in the Trauma Setting, Table 5 The absolute and relative contraindications of transesophageal echocardiography (Hilberath et al. 2010)

Contraindications to TEE	
Absolute contraindications	Relative contraindications
Perforated viscous	Atlantoaxial joint disease
Esophageal pathology (stricture, trauma, tumor, scleroderma, Mallory-Weiss tear, diverticulum)	Severe cervical arthritis
Active upper GI bleeding	Prior radiation to chest
Recent upper GI surgery	Symptomatic hiatal hernia
Esophagectomy, esophagogastrectomy	History of GI surgery
	Recent upper GI bleed
	Esophagitis, peptic ulcer disease
	Thoracoabdominal aneurysm
	Barrett's esophagus
	History of dysphagia
	Coagulopathy, thrombocytopenia

Finally, another alternative to transesophageal echocardiography is the use of transthoracic echocardiography. There are similar limitations with transthoracic echocardiography such as availability, certifications, personnel, and equipment. The biggest advantage/disadvantage of transthoracic echocardiography is the ability to perform the exam in the least invasive manner. The advantage is avoiding the potential complications of inserting an echocardiography probe and causing further injury, plus an additional ability to acquire cardiac images from an external source. On the other hand, the external probe may limit the number of views and structures visualized, threaten the sonographer's ability to complete a full exam, and obtain the information necessary to provide appropriate treatment.

Cross-References

▶ Barotrauma
▶ Cardiac and Aortic Trauma, Anesthesia for
▶ Cardiac Injuries
▶ Cardiopulmonary Resuscitation in Adult Trauma
▶ Cardiopulmonary Resuscitation in Pediatric Trauma
▶ Chest Wall Injury
▶ Fat Embolism Syndrome
▶ Fluid, Electrolytes, and Nutrition in Trauma Patients
▶ General Anesthesia for Major Trauma
▶ Heart-Lung Interactions
▶ Hemodynamic Management in Trauma Anesthesia
▶ Hemodynamic Monitoring
▶ Hemorrhagic Shock
▶ Imaging of Aortic and Thoracic Injuries
▶ Lung Injury
▶ Monitoring of Trauma Patients During Anesthesia
▶ Pediatric Trauma, Assessment, and Anesthetic Management
▶ Pneumothorax, Tension
▶ Pulmonary Embolus
▶ Pulmonary Hypertension
▶ Pulmonary Trauma, Anesthetic Management for
▶ Resuscitation Goals in Trauma Patients
▶ Retained Hemothorax
▶ Shock Management in Trauma
▶ Thoracic Vascular Injuries
▶ Ultrasound in the Trauma and ICU Setting
▶ Venous Thromboembolism (VTE)
▶ Venous Thromboembolism Prophylaxis and Treatment Following Trauma
▶ Venous Thromboembolism Prophylaxis in the Intensive Care Unit

References

American College of Emergency Physicians (2006) Emergency ultrasound imaging criteria compendium. Dallas. http://www.acep.org. Accessed 15 Sept 2012

American College of Emergency Physicians (2008) Emergency ultrasound Guidilines. Dallas. http://www.acep.org. Accessed 15 Sept 2012

American Society of Anesthesiologists (2010) Practice guidelines for perioperative transesophageal echocardiography. Anesthesiology 112:1084–1096

American Society of Echocardiography Consensus Statement (2010) Focused cardiac ultrasound in the emergent setting: a consensus statement of the American Society of Echocardiography and American College of Emergency Physicians. Morrisville. Elsevier. J Am Soc Echocardiography 23 (12):1225–1130.

Hilberath J et al (2010) Safety of transesophageal echocardiography. J Am Soc Echocardiogr 23(11):1115–1127

Kircher BJ, Schiller NB (1990) Noninvasive estimation of right atrial pressures from the inspiratory collapse of the inferior vena cava. Am J Cardiol 66:493–496

Shanewise JS et al (1999) ASE/SCA guidelines for performing a comprehensive intraoperative multiplane transesophageal echocardiography examination: recommendations of the American society of echocardiography council for intraoperative echocardiography and the society of cardiovascular anesthesiologists task force for certification in perioperative transesophageal echocardiography. Anesth Analg 89(4):870–884. Print

Turner JP, Dankoff J (2012) Thoracic ultrasound. Emerg Med Clin North Am 30(2):451–473, ix

Recommended Reading

American College of Emergency Physicians (2008) Emergency ultrasound guidelines. Dallas. http://www.acep.org. Accessed 16 Sept 2012

American College of Emergency Physicians. Use of ultrasound imaging by emergency physicians. http://www.acep.org. Accessed 15 Sept 2012

ECLS

▶ Extracorporeal Membrane Oxygenation

ECMO

▶ Extracorporeal Membrane Oxygenation

Economy Class Syndrome

▶ DVT, as a Complication

Elderly Trauma, Anesthetic Considerations for

Venesa Ingold and Mirsad Dupanovic
Department of Anesthesiology, Kansas University Medical Center, The University of Kansas Hospital, Kansas City, KS, USA

Synonyms

Aged person trauma; Centenarian trauma; Geriatric trauma; Nonagenarian trauma; Octogenarian trauma; Older person trauma; Septuagenarian trauma; Sexagenarian trauma; Supercentenarian trauma

Definition

Aging represents a process of progressive decrease in functional capacity of organ systems. Additionally, an organ system may be affected by a pathologic process that will further diminish the end-organ reserve. The onset of aging may vary, but most researchers consider individuals 65 years or greater as elderly. Because of a steady increase in the size of geriatric population, elderly trauma is increasing in volume, complexity of diagnosis, and treatment requirements. Octogenarian trauma is specifically increasing and fares much poorer than the younger aged. Compounding effects of physiologic changes of aging, chronic pathologic changes, and acute trauma often require treatment of elderly trauma patients in the intensive care unit.

Preexisting Condition

The world population is still growing, and the fraction of elderly is continuously increasing. There was a 20-year increase in the average life span during the second half of the twentieth century. Additionally, it is expected that the average life span will be extended another 10 years by 2050 (CDC 2003a). Longer life expectancy is the result of declines in infant/childhood mortality, improvements in adult health care, and better success in treatment of chronic diseases. The average life expectancy in developed countries ranges now from 76 to 80 years (CDC 2003a). Thus, the octogenarian group (persons 80–89 years old) is the fastest-growing segment of the elderly population. The 2010 census showed that age 65 or older accounts for 13 % of the US population. This is projected to almost double by 2030. Despite regional differences in population structure, there is a global trend of progressive aging of the world population.

The physiologic changes associated with aging may increase the susceptibility of elderly to become injured and will often produce an altered response to derangements caused by injury. The elderly have more active lifestyles nowadays. They frequently exercise and/or drive cars. Regular aerobic exercises may help diminish decline of functional capacity caused by the aging process, decrease morbidity, and consequently increase the longevity. However, since elderly may have impaired hearing, vision, and/or coordination, an active lifestyle may place them at risk for falls and car accidents resulting in fractures and/or blunt force trauma. On the other hand, elderly with muscle atrophy, weakness, and osteoporotic changes may suffer fractures caused by a lesser traumatic force. Additionally, the possibility of elder abuse should always be considered when evaluating an injured elderly patient.

The anatomic and physiologic changes associated with aging are presented in relation to trauma and trauma anesthesia-associated risks (Table 1).

The autonomic nervous system and cardiovascular system changes associated with aging result in decreased ability of the sympathetic nervous system to maintain cardiovascular homeostasis despite increased sympathetic tone. The main features are increased norepinephrine levels, the reduction of β- and α_2-receptor-mediated responses, reduction of vagal function, and diminished baroreceptor responsiveness (Miller 2010). There is increased afterload, elevated mean blood pressure, increased pulse pressure, frequently exaggerated changes in blood pressure, and orthostatic hypotension. All these changes result in lower heart rate at baseline, increased left ventricular thickness, decreased diastolic ventricular filling, diastolic dysfunction, decreased cardiac contractile responses, prolonged myocardial contraction, and impaired potential to increase cardiac output. The cardiac index falls off linearly with aging. Thus, atrial contraction becomes increasingly important, and any rhythm other than sinus is poorly tolerated (Miller 2010). A 4-year review of the Washington State trauma registry found in the 13,820 elderly trauma patients that standard physiologic variables like heart rate and blood pressure were poor predictors of injury severity resulting in undertriaging the elderly (Lehmann et al. 2009).

The pulmonary system of the elderly is also changed. Decreased elasticity of the lung leads to progressively increased closing capacity, increased dead space, and decreased alveolar surface area. The functional results are intrapulmonary shunting, decreased diffusion capacity, impaired gas exchange, and decreased arterial oxygen tension. Additionally, decreased airway reflexes may make elderly susceptible to pulmonary aspiration and additional hypoxia.

The aging process affects kidneys resulting in decreased number of nephrons, decreased renal blood flow, and diminished glomerular filtration rate. Fluid and electrolytes are altered. Sodium reabsorption, excretion of potassium, and excretion of hydrogen are decreased. Additionally, renal concentration ability is diminished. Liver volume and hepatic blood flow are decreased. Albumin level is lower than in younger patients. Additionally, total body water is decreased, while fat stores are increased.

Trauma is the seventh leading cause of death in elderly; falls, motor vehicle crashes, and burns are the leading causes of fatalities induced by geriatric trauma (ATLS 2008). Falls are the most common cause of accidental injury in elderly with consequential soft tissue trauma and bone fractures (ATLS 2008). Rib fractures and head injuries may be a consequence of falls as well. Associated brain and/or lung injuries may result in additional complications and

Elderly Trauma, Anesthetic Considerations for, Table 1 Anatomic and physiologic changes associated with aging

Organ system	Aging changes	Trauma-associated risk(s)
Central nervous system	Brain atrophy, lesser coordination, unsteady gait, increased reaction time, memory problems, decreased pain perception	Stretched bridging veins are prone to rupture and bleeding; fall risk, risk of postoperative delirium and cognitive dysfunction, lower analgesic doses
Autonomic nervous system	Increased sympathetic nervous system activity and decreased vagal tone	Hemodynamic instability and inability to meet increased metabolic demands imposed by an acute trauma
Eye	Decreased depth of perception, discrimination of colors, and pupillary response	Fall risk, accidents, risk of perioperative delirium
Auditory system	Diminished hearing	Accidents, risk of perioperative delirium
Airway	Decreased airway reflexes	Pulmonary aspiration, hypoxia
Respiratory system	Impaired gas exchange and decreased arterial oxygen tension	Hypoxia, need for aggressive respiratory support and frequent tracheal intubation
Cardiovascular system	Slowed conduction, diminished heart rate, high afterload state, increased myocardial stiffness, diastolic dysfunction, and diminished cardiac index	Lack of ability to adequately increase cardiac output, susceptibility of injury as a result of hypovolemia and labile blood pressure, sensitivity to volume overload
Hematologic	Decreased total blood volume	Severe hypotension on induction, labile blood pressure during maintenance of anesthesia
Hepatobiliary system	Decreased liver volume, decreased hepatic blood flow	Diminished rate of drug metabolism, slower wake-up
Urinary system	Decreased renal volume and renal blood flow, diminished glomerular filtration rate	Decreased excretion of drugs, susceptibility of kidney injury during stages of hypovolemia
Musculoskeletal system	Degeneration of the joints, stiffness, muscle atrophy, bone demineralization	Fall risk, risk of bone fractures including frequent hip fractures, cervical spine fracture, and injury to spinal cord
Skin	Thinning of the dermis and the epidermis, decreased vascularity and elasticity	Hypothermia due to decreased thermoregulatory ability, risk of skin injuries, impaired wound healing
Body composition	Decreased total body water, decreased circulating albumin level, increased body fat reserves	Smaller central compartment, increased sensitivity to administration of IV drugs, greater volume of distribution, and longer duration of action of fat soluble drugs
Immune system	Decreased immune system competence	Decreased tolerance to infections, risk of failure of multiple organs

disability or death. Elderly undergo more craniotomy and orthopedic procedures than the younger trauma patients (Lehmann et al. 2009). The researchers at Lancaster General Hospital with 2,000 per year trauma volume described the elderly was 36 % of their trauma admissions, many with high-risk indicators (Bradburn et al. 2012). Although elderly have lower incidence of injuries than younger individuals, many studies have showed the elderly to be at increased risk of death from trauma at all levels of Injury Severity Score (ISS). It has been demonstrated that ISS is the best predictor of blunt trauma mortality in the elderly (Knudson et al. 1994). A 2-year review of Pennsylvania trauma registry of 26,300 patients revealed that elderly who receive an ISS >30 use ICU services less due to increased mortality (Taylor et al. 2002). The authors concluded that "age is an independent predictor of outcome in trauma." Octogenarians and older age groups have a high mortality at all injury severity levels. It is very likely that a progressive decrease of end-organ reserve associated with aging, presence of chronic coexisting diseases, and concomitant intake of usually multiple medications can adversely affect trauma outcome. An average elderly patient takes eight different medications daily (Miller 2010). Use of multiple medications may lead to drug interactions. Additionally, narrow therapeutic range in elderly may lead to more frequent side effects. Beta-blocking agents, frequently used in the elderly, limit chronotropic cardiac activity and may mask the symptoms of shock (Neiden et al. 2008). Calcium-channel blockers and ACE inhibitors may prevent peripheral vasoconstriction and contribute to hypotension. Anticoagulant use in the elderly is associated with increased risk of intracranial hemorrhage and traumatic brain injury (Pieracci et al. 2007). Additionally, antiplatelet and anticoagulant agent use may lead to increased blood loss associated with fractures and/or surgery. Therefore, acute traumatic insult that occurs in the setting of altered compensatory response associated with decreased physiologic reserve, chronic disease changes, and frequent polypharmacy may result in atypical clinical presentations, delayed diagnosis, increased risk of complications, and increased morbidity and mortality of elderly patients.

Application

There has been more understanding of particular needs of elderly and progress in their trauma care. Revised in 2006, the American College of Surgeons Committee on Trauma "Guidelines for field triage of injured patients" included age ≥ 55 as a risk factor in the field triage decision scheme. The goal of this new inclusion is to help decrease missed injuries in the elderly by contacting medical control or by transporting these patients to trauma centers (CDC 2003b). It appears that trauma evaluation of elderly should follow a different protocol from that for younger patients. Bradburn et al. applied a high-risk geriatric protocol to help identify high-risk geriatric trauma patients and improve their outcomes. The protocol included geriatric consultation, serial blood gases, lactate levels, and echocardiogram with the aim to diagnose occult shock and increase the sensitivity of diagnosing life-threatening injuries in the elderly. The study showed significantly reduced mortality when this protocol was applied. Therefore, increased vigilance and aggressive triage are needed during the care for elderly trauma patients.

Preoperative Assessment

Trauma management decisions are guided by the history, results of the primary and secondary survey, and the results of initial battery of laboratory, sonographic, and/or radiographic studies. However, since age ≥ 75 significantly increases mortality from injury, a high index of suspicion for injuries common for the specific age group and more aggressive care of elderly trauma patients is necessary to improve survival. Severity of injury, comorbid diseases, and the ASA physical status are the most important determinants of trauma outcome. Additionally, the type of surgery will affect the postoperative outcome. There may be various degrees of surgical urgency that will determine the extent of preoperative assessment and trauma management decisions.

Elderly trauma patients often require aggressive respiratory resuscitation. Tracheal intubation should be considered early in an injured elderly patient presenting with altered level of consciousness, chest wall injury, or in shock. Chest injuries are poorly tolerated by elderly because of frequent respiratory complications such as atelectasis, pneumonia, and pulmonary edema (ATLS 2008). Hemorrhage and aggressive fluid resuscitation are also poorly tolerated not just because of diminished pulmonary reserve but also because of frequently compromised cardiac reserve. Thus, rapid assessment, quick diagnosis, and prompt surgical hemostasis are of great importance. In addition to cardiac and pulmonary conditions, many other common diseases encountered in geriatric population may present trauma risk and may have a significant impact on perioperative management and outcome (Table 2).

Anesthetic Management

Aging is associated with important changes in the pharmacokinetics and pharmacodynamics of

Elderly Trauma, Anesthetic Considerations for, Table 2 Preexisting disease and elderly trauma

Organ system	Preexisting diseases, drugs	Trauma-associated risk(s)
Central nervous system	Stroke, dizziness, vertigo, Parkinson's disease, Alzheimer's disease, depression	Muscle atrophy, use of succinylcholine and hyperkalemia, falls, accidents, decreased ability to make independent decisions, risk of perioperative delirium, higher surgical mortality
Autonomic nervous system	Neuropathy, Parkinson's disease	Accidents, autonomic instability
Eye	Cataract, presbyopia	Falls, car accidents, burns, risk of perioperative delirium
Hearing	Sensorineural hearing loss	Accidents, decreased ability to communicate and make decisions, risk of perioperative delirium
Airway	Poor dentition or lack of teeth, nasopharyngeal fragility, Parkinson's disease	Poor mask fit, difficulty with mask ventilation, nasopharyngeal bleeding, risk of pulmonary aspiration
Respiratory system	COPD	Caution with oxygen administration, increased risk of a respiratory failure, and need for tracheal intubation
Cardiovascular system	Hypertension, coronary artery disease, valvular heart diseases, arrhythmias	Contracted vascular volume, labile blood pressure, myocardial ischemia, diastolic heart failure
Hematologic	Antiplatelet agents, anticoagulants	Intracranial bleeding, increased surgical blood loss
Endocrine system	Diabetes mellitus	Impaired wound healing
Drug abuse	Alcoholism	Falls and accidents
Urinary system	Kidney disease	Fluid overload, decreased drug excretion, electrolyte disturbances
Musculoskeletal system	Arthritis of the spine, larynx, and TMJ; spinal stenosis	Increased risk of spinal cord injury, laryngeal injuries, and difficulty with tracheal intubation

most anesthetic drugs. There is increased brain sensitivity to inhaled anesthetics, midazolam, propofol, and all opiates. The size of the central compartment is decreased. The circulating level of albumin is decreased as well. The initial volume of distribution of thiopental and etomidate is also decreased. These changes result in decreased intravenous drug requirements on anesthetic induction in the range from 30 % to 75 % and decreased inhaled anesthetic requirement during maintenance of anesthesia (MAC decreases approximately 6 % per decade). Additionally, decreases in liver and kidney blood flow result in decreased metabolism, decreased elimination, prolonged duration of action of most intravenous drugs, and slow anesthetic emergence. Coexisting diseases reduce drug requirements even more. Decreases of cardiac output result in slower induction of intravenous anesthesia in the elderly. Thus, anesthetizing elderly patients requires understanding

of these changes, patience, and heightened vigilance.

Anesthetic care should be tailored to the extent of surgery and concurrent comorbid diseases. This includes anesthetic drugs and types of monitors used. It is difficult to exactly determine what constitutes the most optimal physiologic management during anesthetic care of elderly trauma patients. Additionally, the extent of invasive monitoring, the most advantageous mean blood pressure, and the most optimal hemoglobin level are some other controversial issues. The physiologic management should be tailored to the specific patient and the trauma situation. Geriatric trauma patients present in shock more often than the younger trauma patients. "Normal" blood pressure and heart rate may not indicate euvolemia, and limited cardiac output may lead to insufficient cerebral, coronary, or renal perfusion. These early states of hypoperfusion may lead to "inexplicable" sequential organ failure and death in approximately 33 % of elderly patients (ATLS 2008). On the other hand, controlled hypotensive anesthesia may be in order to prevent a large blood loss during critical periods of surgical hemostasis. Thus, in addition to an adequate intravenous access, early placement of an intra-arterial catheter is essential to monitor changes of patient's blood pressure and heart rate as a response to anesthetic drugs and surgery as well as to guide initial fluid resuscitation and potential use of vasoactive drugs. The assessment of pulse pressure variation from arterial pressure wave form will be immediately available. Ability to obtain arterial blood samples in order to monitor and correct acid base and electrolyte abnormalities is additional benefit of an early intra-arterial catheter placement.

Decreased organ perfusion often has a great impact on the postoperative outcome of the elderly patient. Due to the previously described physiologic changes, hypovolemia is more difficult to recognize in the elderly. These patients are sensitive to fluid overload as well. Thus, monitoring the central venous pressure can assist in the care of these fragile patients. Colloid versus crystalloid data is equivocal. Initial hypotension from hypovolemia may result in myocardial ischemia and impaired cardiac performance. Hypovolemic and cardiogenic shock may coexist (ATLS 2008). Such perilous circumstances will dictate not only obtainment of central venous access but also use of additional monitors that can provide more information about the cardiac performance such as pulmonary artery catheter and transesophageal echocardiography. However, pulmonary arterial catheters have not been found to improve the perioperative care of elderly with trauma. Even though the optimal hemoglobin concentration in resuscitation of elderly trauma patients is controversial, hemoglobin should be maintained in the range of 7–10 g/dL to help optimize tissue oxygen delivery in these fragile patients. The current trend toward early replacement of coagulation factors and platelets is most likely highly applicable to elderly trauma patients as well. Anticoagulation and/or antiplatelet agent-induced coagulation deficits should be recognized and corrected early if possible.

Regional anesthesia versus general anesthesia for hip fracture operation in the elderly is equally supported in the literature. Routine thromboembolism prevention and appropriate beta-blockade have reduced risks to the elderly in the perioperative time period. Use of regional anesthesia may reduce surgical blood loss, may decrease risk of postoperative vein thrombosis, and can reduce intravenous opiate use for postoperative pain control. There is no difference in the incidence of postoperative cognitive dysfunction when using regional or general anesthesia in elderly (Miller 2010). When treating acute postoperative pain, priority should be given to multimodal analgesia. When using opiate-based pain management choices, careful approach should be used because of necessary age-related dose adjustments.

Postoperatively, the aged are at increased risk of complications, which are mainly related to respiratory, cardiac, and neurologic systems. The decrease in airway reflexes increases the risk of aspiration in the elderly. Hypoxia is increased in the aged. Atelectasis occurs more often predisposing them to pneumonia during their hospitalization. Postoperative delirium and cognitive dysfunction occurs more frequently in the elderly. Thus, decisions about the length of postoperative intubation, mechanical ventilation, and intravenous sedation are complex.

Awareness of the physiologic changes of aging, impact of chronic diseases, medications, and increased fragility of elderly patients is essential for better outcomes in elderly trauma and should be considered by all care givers. Age-adjusted protocols, a high index of suspicion, close monitoring, and vigilance are particularly important for improved outcomes in geriatric trauma.

Cross-References

▶ ABCDE of Trauma Care
▶ Advance Directive
▶ Burn Anesthesia

► Chest Wall Injury
► Delirium as a Complication of ICU Care
► Falls
► Geriatric Trauma
► Motor Vehicle Crash Injury

References

Advanced Trauma Life Support® for Doctors (ATLS®) (2008). American College of Surgeons Committee on Trauma, Chicago

Bradburn E, Rogers FB, Krasne M, Rogers A, Horst MA, Belan MJ, Miller JA (2012) High-risk geriatric protocol: improving mortality in the elderly. J Trauma Acute Care Surg 73:435–440

Center for Disease Control and Prevention (CDC) (2003a) Public health and aging: trends in aging – United States and worldwide, Feb 14, 2003/52(06):101–106. http://www.cdc.gov/mmwr/preview/mmwrhtml/mm5206a2.htm. Last accessed 18 Dec 2012

Center for Disease Control and Prevention (CDC) (2003b) Guidelines for field triage of injured patients: recommendations of the national expert panel on field triage 2011: Jan 13, 2012. http://www.cdc.gov/mmwr/pdf/rr/rr6101.pdf. Last accessed 18 Dec 2012

Knudson MM, Liebermann J, Morris JA Jr et al (1994) Mortality factors in geriatric blunt trauma patients. Arch Surg 129:448–453

Lehmann R, Beekley A, Casey L, Salun A, Martin M (2009) The impact of advanced age on trauma triage decisions and outcomes: a state wide analysis. Am J Surg 197:571–575

Miller RD (ed) (2010) Miller's anesthesia. Churchill Livingstone, Philadelphia

Neiden T, Lam M, Brasel KJ (2008) Preinjury beta blockers are associated with increased mortality in geriatric trauma patients. J Trauma 65:1016–1020

Pieracci FM, Eachempati SR, Shou J, Hydo LJ, Barle PS (2007) Degree of anticoagulation, but not warfarin use itself predicts adverse outcome after traumatic brain injury in elderly trauma patients. J Trauma 63:525–530

Silverstein JH (2008) Trauma in elderly. In: Smith CE (ed) Trauma anesthesia. Cambridge University Press, New York, pp 391–401

Taylor MD, Tracy JK, Meyer W, Pasquale M, Napolitano CM (2002) Trauma in the elderly: intensive care unit resource use and outcome. J Trauma 53:407–414

Electric Shock

► Electrical Burns

Electrical Burns

Brett Hartman
Department of Surgery, Division of Plastic and Reconstructive Surgery, Indiana University, Indianapolis, IN, USA

Synonyms

Electric shock; Electrical current burns; Voltage burn

Definition

Electrical burns are caused by direct or indirect contact with a certain electrical current. They have the potential to be the most devastating and destructing of all thermal injuries, involving not only the skin but the underlying soft tissues as well. The severity of each electrical burn injury is dependent on a number of factors, including the voltage, type of current, time of contact, and resistance at the point of contact.

Pathophysiology

Electrical burns cause approximately 1,000 deaths per year in the United States. There are two types of circuits over which electrical current can flow: direct current (DC) or alternating current (AC). Over 85 % of electrical burns are caused by commercial alternating current, which is the most common type of electricity in homes and offices producing 60 cycles/second (Hz). This type of current is known to cause muscle contractions secondary to the cyclic flow, which pull the victim toward the source causing prolonged contact and a more severe injury. DC current, on the other hand, tends to catapult or throw the victim away from the source (Herndon 2007).

The terms entrance and exit point are no longer used to describe electrical burn injuries and have been replaced by the term "contact points." The patients may have zero contact points noticed on physical exam or may have many.

Electrical burns have the ability to produce a variety of differing injuries. The most obvious is a true electrical injury caused by current flow. The second is an arc injury triggered as the current passes from the electrical source to an object. The third type is the flash burn in which the current does not enter the body but results in a flash burn typically producing superficial partial-thickness burns. The electrical current also has the possibility of igniting a victims clothing causing a severe flame injury.

The electrical current generates an intense amount of heat causing coagulation necrosis of the tissues. Heat, or power, is defined by Joule's law:

$$\text{Power (Joule)} = \text{Current } (I^2) \times \text{Resistance (R)}$$

There are varying amounts of resistance to electrical current through human tissues. Skin and bone offer the most resistance, whereas nerves and blood vessels offer the least resistance. Therefore, the most severe injuries usually occur in the peri-osseous tissue, specifically between two bones. These peri-osseous injuries are often seen at the wrist and the ankles because the severity of injury is inversely proportional to the cross-sectional area of the tissue carrying the current (Asensio and Trunkey 2008).

Prior to arrival to the hospital, electrical burn victims can pose a significant risk to the rescuer, making it much different than other types of trauma. The patient can become a conductor of electricity if he or she is still in contact with the source, and therefore great care must be taken during the extrication.

Physical Exam

Electrical burn victims must be evaluated according to the Advanced Burn Life Support (ABLS) criteria. Close to 15 % of the victims of electrical burns sustain other traumatic injuries, and it is therefore critical to obtain a full trauma evaluation upon initial presentation. Along with a thorough trauma work-up, serial evaluation of liver, pancreatic, and renal function with appropriate imaging studies as needed is a must in the work-up of an electrical burn.

Cardiovascular System

The most common cause of death at the scene of an electrical injury is cardiac in nature, specifically ventricular fibrillation; however, electrical currents can cause a multitude of arrhythmias, including, but not limited to, atrial fibrillation, sinus tachycardia, and premature ventricular contractions. Indications for cardiac monitoring during hospitalization include a documented cardiac arrhythmia in the emergency department, an abnormal EKG in the ER, a total burn surface area (TBSA) greater than 20 %, or extremes of age. Creatinine kinase enzyme levels including MB fraction have not been found to be reliable indicators of cardiac injury after electrical burns and are therefore not recommended for decision making regarding patient disposition.

Respiratory System

One of the common causes of death in electrical burn injury is respiratory arrest. This is usually not caused by a direct injury to the lungs or the airways but more likely as a result of direct injury to the respiratory control center causing cessation of respiration. A secondary cause could be attributed to tetanic contractions of the respiratory muscles causing suffocation. Pulmonary contusions may also occur secondary to blunt injury to the chest, and as mentioned previously, the mechanism of injury must be determined, and the patient must undergo full trauma evaluation.

Genitourinary System

The kidneys have the potential to incur major damage, not by direct contact but rather through anoxic injury or tubular damage secondary to release of myoglobin and creatinine phosphokinase from muscle necrosis. The presence of pigmented urine indicates significant muscle damage, and these pigments must be cleared rapidly in order to prevent severe damage leading to renal failure. The treatment of pigmented urine is 25 g of IV mannitol, 2 ampules of sodium bicarbonate to alkalinize the urine and minimize pigment precipitation, and Ringer's lactate run at a rate sufficient to produce approximately 1 ml/kg/h of urine output to flush out the pigments (Jeschke and Herndon 2012).

Integumentary System

Cutaneous injuries can range from local erythema to full-thickness burns depending on the intensity of the current, duration of contact, and surface area. To sustain a first-degree burn, the duration of exposure must be at least 20 s to a current of over 20 mA/mm^2. To sustain a second- or third-degree burn, it requires at least 75 mA/mm^2, which is well within range of causing ventricular fibrillation. The skin can almost be completely spared secondary to the resistance of the bony structures, which has the potential to cause surrounding muscular necrosis. High current combined with high temperature has the potential to cause flame burns secondary to the ignition of clothing. Cutaneous burns due to lightening are called Lichtenburg figures (feathering burns) and are considered pathognomonic for lightening-induced injury (Koumbourlis 2002).

Electrical burns in children are most commonly associated with biting of an electrical cord. This burn can cause full-thickness injury to the oral commissure resulting in significant deformity, contracture, and possible microstomia. The labial artery may also be injured causing considerable bleeding. However, this bleed typically does not occur until approximately 2–3 weeks after the injury when the eschar falls off. Suture ligation is often used to control bleeds of this nature, and secondary reconstruction at a later date may be necessary.

Musculoskeletal System

Patients who sustain a high-voltage electrical injury are at great risk for the development of compartment syndrome of the extremities. Compartment syndrome by definition occurs when the pressure within a muscle compartment exceeds the perfusion pressure. Early diagnosis and treatment is paramount to prevent ischemic necrosis of the entire compartment eventually leading to Volkmann contracture. The patients will present with pain out of proportion to the injury with a firm, tense limb. The traditional 5 Ps of acute limb ischemia are fairly unreliable but should be recognized when seen: pain, paresthesia, pallor, poikilothermia, and pulselessness. The earliest sign is pain upon passive extension of the hands or feet. Peripheral pulses as well as capillary refill usually remain normal in the majority of cases of upper extremity compartment syndrome. Compartment syndrome is a clinical diagnosis but obtaining compartment pressure can be used as an adjunct to the physical exam. Compartment pressures of 30 mmHg or above are consistent with acute compartment syndrome. Once a diagnosis is obtained, treatment is aimed at releasing all of the involved compartments. This is accomplished in the operating room by performing four compartment fasciotomies of the lower leg and anterior/posterior fasciotomies of the upper extremities. Wound closure may be obtained primarily with closure of skin only or with split-thickness skin grafting as soon as possible or once the viability of the muscle is no longer compromised.

Fluid Management

Electrical burns are unlike cutaneous burns in that the usual thermal burn resuscitation formulas based on TBSA are inaccurate. The only similarity of the two resuscitations is to establish a minimum amount of volume in order to produce adequate end organ perfusion. The goal of resuscitation is to maintain normal vital signs as well as a urine output of approximately 0.5 ml/kg/h with Ringer's lactate in the absence of myoglobinuria. This fluid rate is then adjusted to meet the aforementioned criteria. Just as in thermal burn resuscitation, it is important to not over- or under-resuscitate the patient because each can cause their own set of complications.

Complications

Electrical injuries have a wide range of complications depending on the severity of the initial injury. The early complications include issues previously mentioned such as renal, cardiac, and neurologic manifestations.

The electrical injury can also cause ocular manifestations in approximately 1–8 % of patients, which present most frequently as cataract formation anywhere from 3 weeks from injury to years afterward.

Tympanic membrane rupture as well as sensorineural hearing loss can occur in up to 50 % of patients.

Neurologic complications following electrical injury are extremely diverse in their presentation and range from simple loss of consciousness to peripheral neuropathies to paralysis. Weakness is the most common clinical finding in a peripheral defect, whereas the primary autonomic manifestation is sympathetic overactivity leading to changes in bowel habits as well as changes in urinary and sexual function.

A common late complication of the skeletal system is heterotopic ossification. Heterotopic bone formation can occur in large joints such as the elbow or the amputation stumps of long bones. This can become painful causing tissue breakdown and the need for eventual stump revision.

Due to the wide array of possible neurologic complications, it is paramount to perform and document a full neurological examination.

Reconstruction

Severe electrical burns can sometimes present a challenge to the plastic reconstructive surgeon. The goal of burn reconstruction is protection, restoration, and maintenance of function. Appearance also plays a role in allowing the patient to return to and become a functional part of society. Depending on the nature and severity of the electrical injury, the patient may require extensive reconstructive surgery of the scalp, face, chest, abdomen, and extremities. This reconstruction includes skin grafting, tissue expansion, adjacent tissue rearrangement, perforator flaps, muscle flaps, musculocutaneous flaps, free flaps, and possible implants and bony rearrangements. The details of the reconstructive aspect are beyond the scope of this entry; however, it is of paramount importance to all burn care providers to recognize early the potential problems encountered in an electrical injury, which will hopefully provide a better quality of life to the burn survivor (Sood and Archauer 2006).

Summary

Electrical burns can cause devastating injuries secondary to the deceptive tissue loss that may go unrecognized if the treating physician is not aware of the pathophysiology. The long-term prognosis depends upon the severity of the initial injury. As previously mentioned, the goals when treating an electrical injury are resuscitation, early debridement, neurovascular decompression if needed, and early wound closure, which may involve free tissue transfer. A large part of treating an electrical burn is the rehabilitation process, which may take months depending on the initial injury. Most electrical injuries are preventable, and the best means to avoid a devastating injury should be done through public education on electrical safety.

Cross-References

▶ Burn Anesthesia
▶ Chemical Burns
▶ Compartment Syndrome of the Forearm
▶ Compartment Syndrome of the Leg
▶ Fasciotomy
▶ Firework Injuries
▶ Flame Burns
▶ Scald Burns

References

Asensio J, Trunkey D (2008) Current therapy of trauma and critical care. Mosby/Elsevier, Philadelphia, p 576
Herndon DN (2007) Total burn care, 3rd edn. Saunders/Elsevier, Philadelphia
Jeschke M, Herndon DN (2012) Chapter 21: Sabiston: textbook of surgery. In: Burns, 19th edn. Saunders/Elsevier, Philadelphia, pp 542–543
Koumbourlis A (2002) Electrical injuries. Crit Care Med 30(Suppl):S424–S430
Sood RJ, Archauer BM (2006) Burn surgery reconstruction and rehabilitation. Saunders/Elsevier, Philadelphia

Electrical Current Burns

▶ Electrical Burns

Electrolyte and Acid-Base Abnormalities

Robert M. A. Richardson
Division of Nephrology, University of Toronto,
University Health Network, Toronto, ON,
Canada

Synonyms

Acute kidney injury; Hyperkalemia; Metabolic acidosis

Definition

This entry reviews hyperkalemia and metabolic acidosis as the important electrolyte and acid-base abnormalities occurring in the trauma patient.

Preexisting Condition

Hyperkalemia

Hyperkalemia is the commonest electrolyte problem encountered in patients with trauma; in one study of 131 patients who were admitted to an intensive care unit with non-crush trauma suffered in military combat, 29 % developed hyperkalemia in the first 12 h (Perkins et al. 2007). Hyperkalemia in trauma patients arises from the convergence of two separate processes: a rapid influx of potassium into the extracellular space and impaired kidney function, limiting potassium excretion.

Normal human kidneys have a large capacity to excrete potassium, exceeding typical daily potassium intake and excretion by a factor of 5 or more; therefore, although in theory, dangerously high serum potassium could come about solely as a result of increased potassium content, it is highly unusual to see severe hyperkalemia in the absence of impaired kidney function.

Metabolic Acidosis

The major focus of studies on acid-base derangements in trauma patients has been metabolic acidosis. Although traditional clinical measures of circulatory function in severely injured patients are important (blood pressure, cardiac output, oxygenation, urine output, etc.), it is recognized that these may be near normal, yet underlying tissue hypoperfusion exists which can lead to irreversible organ failure and death. Tissues receiving inadequate delivery of oxygen and other substrates for normal metabolic activity release a variety of organic acids of which the best known and most easily measured is lactic acid. It has been known for decades that elevated blood lactate predicts poor outcome in patients admitted with critical illness, but more recent studies have shown that lactate does not discriminate well between survivors and non-survivors.

Application

Hyperkalemia

Causes of Impaired Kidney Excretion of Potassium in Trauma

The main requirements for excretion of large amounts of potassium in the urine are aldosterone and urine flow; of the two, adequate urine flow is by far the most critical. Even in patients with deficient aldosterone, or aldosterone blockade by commonly used drugs such as spironolactone, adequate flow of fluid through the collecting ducts of the kidney typically allows sufficient potassium secretion to prevent severe hyperkalemia. In trauma patients, the major factor limiting excretion of potassium is acute kidney injury (acute renal failure) associated with oliguria secondary to hypotension and/or hypovolemia.

The most obvious cause of hypotension/hypovolemia in trauma is blood loss. Another mechanism for hypotension/hypovolemia in trauma patients is redistribution of plasma water into the interstitial compartment. The most common cause of this problem is rhabdomyolysis: muscle damage due to ischemia or crush injury induces muscle edema, which can result in compartment syndrome. The transfer of salt and water from the intravascular to the interstitial compartment of muscle can cause severe blood volume depletion.

While the kidney can manage to maintain glomerular filtration rate over a wide range of mean arterial pressures, as arterial pressure approaches the lower limit of the autoregulatory range, urine volumes begin to decrease because of increased reabsorption of salt and water by the kidney tubules; the decrease in urine flow will impair potassium excretion. When mean arterial pressure falls below the autoregulatory range (mean arterial pressure <70 mmHg in young adults), then GFR falls sharply, and urine flow may fall to <10 ml/h or even cease.

If the acute kidney injury secondary to hypotension/hypovolemia is temporary and mild, it is generally reversible with resuscitation (prerenal acute kidney injury); glomerular filtration rate and urine flow may increase within minutes to hours of restoration of adequate blood pressure/blood volume. However, if hypotension/hypovolemia is more severe, or more prolonged, or associated with nephrotoxins such as myoglobin from muscle injury, or hemoglobin from intravascular hemolysis, then kidney recovery may be delayed for days or weeks (ischemic acute tubular necrosis).

Why Does Serum Potassium Increase?

There are two common mechanisms for potassium addition to the extracellular fluid in trauma patients: tissue damage and blood transfusion.

Potassium in humans exists mainly in the intracellular compartment (98 %). Ischemia or necrosis of cells with loss of function of sodium-potassium-ATPase can result in massive translocation of potassium from the inured tissue into the extracellular space. To a limited extent, the additional potassium may be buffered in healthy tissue, but when these limits are exceeded, and when the ability of the kidney to excrete potassium is reduced, severe acute hyperkalemia may result.

The major store of potassium in the body is skeletal muscle. Widespread skeletal muscle necrosis is called rhabdomyolysis. There are many causes of rhabdomyolysis including exercise in hot humid conditions, drugs, viral infections, hereditary enzyme deficiencies, and of course trauma. Major muscle groups may be injured either by vascular injury, depriving the muscle of adequate blood flow, or by crush injury. The most well-known and classic cause of traumatic rhabdomyolysis is earthquakes: a very significant cause of death in victims trapped under the rubble of collapsed buildings is hyperkalemia due to rhabdomyolysis and associated oliguric acute kidney injury. For example, in the Marmara, Turkey, earthquake of 1999, there were about 17,000 immediate deaths and 24,000 hospital admissions (Erek et al. 2002). Of these, 639 were referred with acute kidney injury, and of this cohort, 42 % had hyperkalemia and 53 % were oliguric. The mean CK in this group of patients was about 23,000 IU/L.

A second, well-documented cause of potassium addition to the extracellular fluid is massive transfusion of stored packed red blood cells (massive meaning more than 10 units within 24 h) (Vraets et al. 2011). The concentration of potassium within red blood cells is approximately 140 mmol/L compared to a plasma level of 4 mmol/L. When red cells are stored, there is a leak of potassium out of cells which is time-dependent; the longer red cells are stored, the higher the extracellular potassium. As a result, when large numbers of red cells are transfused, there is an addition of potassium to plasma which can raise plasma potassium concentration. With time, the stored, transfused red cells can take up potassium again as their metabolic function improves, typically hyperkalemia is mild and reversible. In the study noted above, where 29 % of trauma subjects developed hyperkalemia, administration of blood products was associated with a relative risk of hyperkalemia of 10; the mean number of units of red blood cells in the hyperkalemic group was 15.9.

Diagnosis and Management of Hyperkalemia in Trauma

The most important point about diagnosis is frequent sampling of blood for electrolytes, including potassium, in patients with trauma who have experienced any of the following: oliguria, prolonged hypotension, muscle injury, or transfusion of blood products. Other laboratory tests that will be helpful include a CK (which is normal in the absence of skeletal muscle injury and massively elevated to values 10,000 in rhabdomyolysis). Intermediate values of 1,000–10,000 are rarely associated with important electrolyte or kidney manifestations.

Hyperkalemia over 7.0 mmol/L is a medical emergency as it can cause serious cardiac arrhythmias including heart block, bradycardia, asystole, and death and must be treated within minutes. The treatment of serum potassium values >7.0 mmol/l demands a two-tiered approach. Initial treatment includes the administration of calcium to stabilize the cardiac conducting system and the administration of agents to shift potassium into cells; the second part is removal of potassium from the body to prevent recurrence of hyperkalemia, as shifting potassium into cells is not a permanent solution. Initial emergency management consists of the following:

- 10 ml of 10 % calcium gluconate intravenously
- 20 units regular insulin bolus intravenously
- 25–50 ml 50 % glucose intravenously (unless the patient is hyperglycemic)
- Inhaled β2-agonist such as salbutamol either by metered dose inhaler or nebulizer, for example, 600–800 ug by metered inhaler or 20 mg by nebulizer

Once the above management has been given (and in patients with serum potassium levels of 5.5–7.0 mmol/L who do not require the above urgent management), efforts to prevent further episodes of life-threatening hyperkalemia need to be instituted including:

- Frequent monitoring of serum potassium (every 4–6 h)
- Efforts to increase urine potassium excretion (blood pressure or blood volume support, intravenous furosemide)
- Limitation of red blood cell transfusion rate (if appropriate)
- Attention to the possibility of rhabdomyolysis and its treatment
- Consideration of hemodialysis if more conservative measures fail or are likely to fail

When hyperkalemia occurs in the presence of oliguric acute kidney injury, hemodialysis may be necessary. Conventional hemodialysis is the most efficient means of removing potassium from the body because of very high blood potassium clearance. Continuous renal replacement therapy (CRRT) is much less efficient. Potassium clearance is low in CRRT (50 ml/min with a dialysate/replacement rate of 3.0 L/h) compared to conventional hemodialysis (250 ml/min). Once serum potassium is normalized, CRRT may be sufficient to control hyperkalemia in most cases; simply increasing the dialysate or replacement fluid rate would increase potassium removal proportionately as potassium achieves equilibrium with dialysate. In oliguric patients with severe rhabdomyolysis, conventional hemodialysis may have to be performed repeatedly over 24 h to prevent recurrent episodes of severe hyperkalemia.

Acid-Base Disorders in Trauma

As described above, in addition to the measurement of serum lactate, other measures may be used to evaluate acid-base status. The most obvious and perhaps easiest to obtain, because it can be derived both from arterial or venous blood gas and venous electrolytes, is serum bicarbonate (FitzSullivan et al. 2005). In metabolic acidosis, hydrogen ions produced by ischemic tissue are buffered mainly by bicarbonate in the extracellular fluid and converted to carbon dioxide, thus lowering serum bicarbonate concentration in blood.

E

Closely linked to the serum bicarbonate is the simple estimate of the anion gap, typically calculated as the difference between the major serum cation, sodium, and the two most prevalent anions, chloride and bicarbonate (some include potassium in the calculation). With organic acidosis, the serum bicarbonate falls due to buffering of the hydrogen ion produced with the organic acid, and the anion gap increases. In theory, the anion gap should be somewhat more sensitive to the generation of unmeasured organic acid anions than the bicarbonate alone, because it will not be affected by changes that may occur to the serum bicarbonate concentration that are not due to the production of organic acids (such as bicarbonate administration, bicarbonate loss or gain from body fluids with sodium, or by dilution with bicarbonate-free solutions such as isotonic saline).

Another approach is the use of base excess which is a calculation made by the laboratory on values derived from an arterial blood gas which essentially states how much base must be added to a liter of blood to bring the pH to 7.40 under standard conditions; it correlates strongly with serum bicarbonate.

More recently, there has been interest in even more complex calculations requiring the measurement of not only electrolytes and arterial blood gas but also the cations calcium and magnesium and the anions albumin, phosphate, and lactate. Correcting the anion gap for the anionic charges on albumin and phosphate (which are partly pH-dependent) and including calcium and magnesium yields an entity called the strong ion gap (SIG).

How do these determinations compare? In one excellent study, the area under the receiver operating curve comparing values to mortality gave the following: for pH 0.497, lactate 0.601, base excess 0.626, anion gap 0.818, corrected anion gap (for albumin and phosphate) 0.862, and for SIG 0.959 (Kaplan and Kellum 2008). Clearly, the more sophisticated the estimation of unmeasured anions, the greater the sensitivity and specificity to tissue injury and prognosis.

The anion gap would appear to be the parameter that is simple to determine and relatively accurate in predicting outcome; the SIG is highly predictive of outcome but requires more laboratory testing and a computer algorithm to calculate.

What is not known with any certainty is whether specifically directing therapy at restoring bicarbonate or pH to normal as opposed to restoring circulation and tissue perfusion has additional benefits. Thus, the value of alkali administration in the form of intravenous sodium bicarbonate is controversial.

Cross-References

▶ Acute Kidney Injury
▶ Compartment Syndrome, Acute
▶ Crush Injuries
▶ Dialysis
▶ Fluid, Electrolytes, and Nutrition in Trauma Patients
▶ Massive Transfusion

References

Erek E, Sever MS, Serdengecti K, Vanholder R, Akoglu E, Yavuz M, Ergin H, Tekce M, Duman N, Lameire N (2002) An overview of morbidity and mortality in patients with acute renal failure due to crush syndrome: the Marmara earthquake experience. Nephrol Dial Transplant 17:33–40

FitzSullivan E, Salim A, Demetriades D, Asensio J, Martin MJ (2005) Serum bicarbonate may replace the arterial base deficit in the trauma intensive care unit. Am J Surg 190:941–946

Kaplan LJ, Kellum JA (2008) Comparison of acid-base models for prediction of hospital mortality after trauma. Shock 29:662–666

Perkins RM, Aboudara MC, Abbott KC, Holcomb JB (2007) Resuscitative hyperkalemia in noncrush trauma: a prospective, observational study. Clin J Am Soc Nephrol 2:313–319

Vraets A, Lin Y, Callum JL (2011) Transfusion-associated hyperkalemia. Transfus Med Rev 25:184–196

Electrolyte Disorders

▶ Fluid, Electrolytes, and Nutrition in Trauma Patients

Electronic Safety

▶ Technology Interfacing, Etiquette, and Electronic Safety

Elevated Intra-abdominal Pressure

▶ Abdominal Compartment Syndrome

Elimination

▶ Pharmacokinetic and Pharmacodynamic Alterations in Critical Illness

Embolization

▶ Adjuncts to Damage Control Laparotomy: Endovascular Therapies

Emergency and Trauma Care Education Programs

▶ Academic Programs in Trauma Care

Emergency Care Management

▶ Trauma Emergency Department Management

Emergency Issue Blood

▶ Red Blood Cell Transfusion in Trauma ICU

Emergency Management

▶ Disaster Preparedness

Emergency Medical Services (EMS)

Dennis Allin
Department of Emergency Medicine, University of Kansas School of Medicine, Kansas City, KS, USA

Synonyms

Out of hospital medical care; Prehospital medical care

Definitions

The Emergency Medical Services Systems (EMSS) Act of 1973 defined an EMS as "a system, which provides for the arrangement of personnel, facilities, and equipment for the effective and coordinated delivery in an appropriate geographical area of health care services under emergency conditions (occurring either as the result of the patient's condition or of a natural disaster or similar situations) and which is administered by a public or nonprofit private entity which has the authority and the resources to provide effective administration of the system."

Walz (2002) summarized the components of an EMS system required by the EMSS Act of 1973:

1. Communications
2. Manpower
3. Training of personnel
4. Use of Public Safety Agencies
5. Transportation
6. Mutual Aid Agreements
7. Facilities
8. Accessibility of Care
9. Critical Care Units

10. Transfer of Patients
11. Standard Medical Record Keeping
12. Independent Review and Evaluation
13. Consumer Information and Education
14. Consumer Participation
15. Disaster Linkage

The EMS *Agenda for the Future* (National Highway Traffic Safety Administration 1996) outlined the attributes that would enhance the effectiveness of EMS:

1. Integration of Health Services
2. EMS Research
3. Legislation and Regulation
4. System Finance
5. Human Resources
6. Medical Direction
7. Education Systems
8. Public Education
9. Prevention
10. Public Access
11. Communication Systems
12. Clinical Care
13. Information Systems
14. Evaluation

Preexisting Conditions

In 1966, the National Academy of Sciences, now the NIH, published the now famous "white paper" in response to the lack of coordinated trauma management and the fact that trauma was the leading cause of death in the first half of life (NAS 1966). This report called for a conference on Emergency Services, a national trauma association, community EMS councils, and a national institute of trauma, with the goal of a coordinated United States system of trauma care. The result was the Highway Safety Act that provided federal funding for the development of EMS systems, followed by the 1973 EMS Systems Act which more specifically identified the components of an EMS system as well as mandating each state to develop a lead EMS agency, but left the structure of such an agency up to the states. At the present time, states exert various levels of oversight of EMS operations with most licensing or certifying EMS providers through state-mandated testing as well as licensing ground units and services through inspection processes.

There are over 16,000 ground based EMS providers in the United States [www.the-aaa.org] constituting a mix of paid and volunteer personnel working in systems that range from county owned, hospital owned, private company, and fire based, and encompassing a range from small rural systems to large, complex urban operations. Due to variations in volume and resources, the agencies for which these providers work will staff their vehicles with mixtures ranging from no advance providers to all advanced providers. Most of these providers have trained relative to national standards at one of the following levels:

1. First responder (EMR in newest revision of national scope of practice)
2. EMT-Basic – generally delivers basic life support (BLS) functions
3. EMT-I (AEMT in newest revision) – generally delivers BLS in addition to some advanced procedures such as IV, some medications, and advanced airway procedures
4. EMT-Paramedic – delivers advanced life support procedures

The national standards represent floors of the providers practice, and state-to-state variability exists in the allowed scope of practice especially at the EMT-I, AEMT levels. In most states, providers are certified or licensed through a national, standardized test administered by the National Registry of Emergency Medical Technicians (NREMT).

In addition to ground EMS units, there were over 800 helicopter services functioning as of 2008 [www.aams.org]. These services are generally private, for profit companies that are relatively poorly integrated into the EMS system and are less subject to regulation by the state lead agency. Despite this, the air medical services provide an important service to the EMS system through not only rapid transport of seriously ill and injured patients, but also through the provision of critical care by staff that may include RNs, respiratory therapists, or EMT-Ps who have obtained additional critical care training.

Applications

EMS systems throughout the United States will respond to trauma with a variety of configurations, levels of providers, and capabilities, most working within local, state, or regional trauma systems, with over 40 states currently sponsoring such systems [http://www.aaos.org]. These systems will generally verify, certify, or designate trauma centers as Level 1 (highest capability), through Level 4 utilizing the American College of Surgeons criteria [http://www.facs.org]. In the management of trauma, these EMS providers will focus their evaluations on the primary survey, assessing the patency of the airway, breathing, and circulation along with spinal immobilization and rapid transport to the most appropriate trauma center within the system, utilizing the *Guidelines for Field Triage of Injured Patients* published by the Centers for Disease Control (Sasser et al. 2012) (Fig. 1). Seriously injured patients have been shown to have a 25 % lower mortality when transported to a Level 1 trauma center as compared to non-trauma centers (MacKenzie et al. 2006). Many EMS systems are designed to transport patients meeting step 1 or step 2 criteria to the highest level of trauma center available in the system while transporting the comparatively less injured to the closest trauma center.

The use of air medical transport to a trauma center, particularly rotor-wing, for rapid transport of patients is a subject of debate in the United States but evidence exists for the use of air medical transport in patients meeting step 1 or step 2 criteria of the CDC triage guidelines (Fig. 1), especially those with ground transports of >30 min to a trauma center or those requiring critical care during transport that may not be available through ground transport. Important in the decision to utilize air medical transport is the determination that the critically injured patient will arrive at appropriate definitive care more rapidly than if transported by ground (Thomson and Thomas 2003), which will include factors such as extrication, weather, flight time to the scene, and time required for air medical personnel to evaluate and package the patient.

The management of the trauma airway can range from endotracheal intubation with drug facilitated intubation (DFI), to the use of supraglottic airways such as the King laryngeal tube airway (King LT; King Systems Corp, Noblesville, IN, USA) or the Laryngeal Mask Airway (LMA; LMA North America, San Diego, CA, USA), to the use of the bag-valve-mask (BVM), depending on the level of the responding providers and the medical protocols under which they function. The indications for field invasive airway management include apnea, airway obstruction, hypoventilation, and Glasgow Coma Scale <8, but many ground-based EMS systems will utilize BVM airway management, if the patient can be successfully ventilated and the transport time is not extremely prolonged, due to literature that suggests that field intubation increases both scene time and complications (Hussmann et al. 2011). In patients who are endotracheally intubated, tube placement will be assured by ETCO2 monitoring by colorimetric device or capnography.

In cases of acute breathing compromise, EMS can intervene in a number of ways depending on the level of provider, including early endotracheal intubation in cases of flail chest, but the more common interventions include needle thoracostomy for tension pneumothorax at the midclavicular line of the second intercostal space, and dressing of large sucking chest wounds with dressings designed to allow enough air to escape as to avoid the complication of a tension pneumothorax.

EMS will focus on hemostatic control of external bleeding, usually with the use of compression bandaging but there has been increasing interest in and use of hemostatic dressings (Granville-Chapman et al. 2011) and tourniquets (Doyle and Taillac 2008) by EMS as both have shown efficacy in hemostatic control in the transition from military to civilian practice. Many times, however, the bleeding will be from a more covert source such as intra-abdominal injury, pelvic fracture, and lone bone fracture; therefore, EMS will monitor the patient for blood loss through measurement of pulse rate as well as peripheral circulation, blood pressure, and mental status. If within their scope of practice and allowed by protocol, providers will place peripheral IVs, or alternatively, interosseous

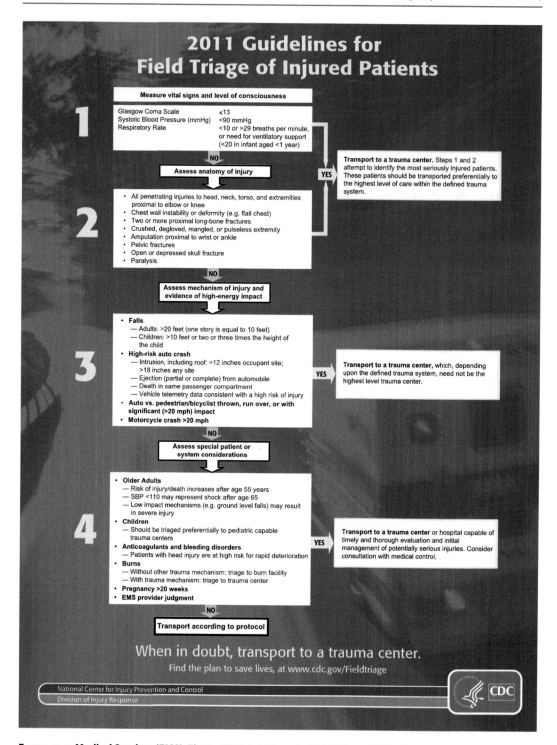

Emergency Medical Services (EMS), Fig. 1 CDC Guidelines for Field Triage of Injured Patients (Source: Sasser et al. 2012)

(IO) access, in patients displaying signs of volume depletion and generally will administer 1–2 L of normal saline (NS) or lactated ringers (LR). The desired result of fluid resuscitation is a matter of debate with Bickell et al. (1994) showing a worse outcome in patients with intra-abdominal bleeding who were resuscitated to normal blood pressure prior to operative control. Questions have arisen as to whether this study population is representative of patients with longer transport times and longer times from injury to the OR, thus most systems will resuscitate shock aggressively but will allow a permissive hypotension as opposed to attempting to achieve normal hemodynamics. Although hypertonic saline (HS) and hypertonic saline with dextran (HSD) have been studied as alternatives to NS or LR as resuscitation fluids, there is currently no convincing evidence of improved outcome with HS or HSD (Holcroft 2011).

Cross-References

▶ Airway Assessment
▶ Airway Equipment
▶ Blood Volume
▶ Hemorrhagic Shock
▶ Motor Vehicle Crash Injury
▶ Prehospital Emergency Preparedness
▶ Trauma Centers

References

Bickell W, Wall M, Pepe P et al (1994) Immediate versus delayed fluid resuscitation for hypotensive patients with penetrating torso injuries. N Engl J Med 331:1105–1109

Doyle GS, Taillac PP (2008) Tourniquets: a review of current use with proposals for expanded prehospital use. Prehosp Emerg Care 12(2):241–256

Granville-Chapman J, Jacobs N, Midwinter MJ (2011) Pre-hospital haemostatic dressings: a systematic review. Injury 42(5):447–459

Holcroft JW (2011) The hypertonic saline trial: a possible downside to the gold standard of double blinding. Ann Surg 253(3):442–443

Hussmann B, Lefering R, Waydhas C, Ruchholtz S, Wafaisade A, Kauther MD, Lendemans S (2011) Prehospital Intubation of the moderately injured patient: a cause of morbidity? A matched-pairs analysis of 1,200 patients from the DGU Trauma Registry. Crit Care 15(5):R207

MacKenzie EJ, Rivara FP, Jurkovich GJ et al (2006) A national evaluation of the effect of trauma center care on mortality. N Engl J Med 354:366–378

National Academy of Sciences (1966) Accidental death and disability: the neglected disease of modern society. Printing and Publishing Office, Washington, DC

National Highway Traffic Safety Administration (1996) Emergency medical services agenda for the future. US Government Printing Office, Washington, DC

Sasser S, Hunt R, Faul M et al (2012) Guidelines for field triage of injured patients. MMWR 61:1–20

Thomson DP, Thomas SH (2003) 2002–2003 air medical services committee of the National Association of EMS physicians. Guidelines for air medical dispatch. Prehosp Emerg Care 7(2):265–271

Walz B (2002) Introduction to EMS systems. Delmar, Albany

E

Emergency Medical Technician (EMT)

▶ Prehospital Emergency Preparedness

Emergency Preparedness

▶ Disaster Management
▶ Disaster Preparedness
▶ Mass Casualty

Emergency Response

▶ Spinal Cord Injury, Early Management

Emergency Surgery

▶ Operating Room Setup for Trauma Anesthesia

Emergent Care of TBI

▶ Traumatic Brain Injury, Emergency Department Care

Empyema

Daniel C. Medina[1], Khanjan H. Nagarsheth[2],
Mayur Narayan[2] and James V. O'Connor[3]
[1]Department of General Surgery, University of
Maryland Medical Center, Baltimore, MD, USA
[2]R Adams Cowley Shock Trauma Center,
University of Maryland School of Medicine,
Baltimore, MD, USA
[3]Shock Trauma Center, University of Maryland
Medical Center, Baltimore, MD, USA

Synonyms

Bacterial pneumonia; Empyema thoracis; Lung
abscess; Parapneumonic effusion; Pleural empyema; Purulent pleuritis; Pyothorax

Definition

Empyema most often refers to a purulent collection
in the space between the lung and the inner surface
of the chest wall. Empyema typically evolves
through exudative, fibrinopurulent, and organizing
phases. This is a life-threatening condition that
may present in the posttrauma setting as a result
of, e.g., pneumonia, iatrogenic contamination from
non-sterile chest tube placement, penetrating
injuries, and post-thoracotomy complications
(O'Connor et al. 2013). *Staphylococcus aureus* is
the most common causative organism identified
from most series, but polymicrobial empyemas
are also seen.

Preexisting Condition

Three to four percent of trauma patients may
develop empyema. In patients requiring tube
thoracostomy after injury, several factors may
be independent predictors for the subsequent
development of empyema. These include pleural
effusion, pulmonary contusion, and the presence
of multiple chest tubes (Eren et al. 2008). Other
factors implicated include chest tube duration,
pulmonary contusion, intensive care length of
stay, retained hemothorax, and exploratory
laparotomy. A recent study revealed that nearly
all patients had sustained thoracic trauma and
95 % had chest tubes prior to the diagnosis of
empyema (O'Connor et al. 2013).

It has been suggested that the bacteriology of
posttraumatic empyema differs from post-
infectious etiologies, with *Streptococcus
pneumoniae* and *Staphylococci* predominating in
the latter (Alfageme et al. 1993). The preponderance of *Staphylococci* and Gram-positive rods
may be explained by the presence and duration
of chest tubes prior to the diagnosis of empyema
(Eren et al. 2008). These conditions allow
the skin flora to access the pleural space and
could account for increased infection rates with
Staphylococcus aureus, coagulase-negative
staphylococci, and gram-positive rods. Although
monomicrobial infections are the offending agents
in some cases, polymicrobial infections are more
likely.

Application

Presentation

The most common causes of empyema for
a trauma victim are: (1) iatrogenic inoculation
of the pleural space through unsterile chest tube
placement, (2) contamination from penetrating
injuries, (3) trans-diaphragmatic colonization
from abdominal and diaphragmatic injury into
the pleural cavity, (4) hematogenous or lym-
phatic dissemination, (5) clot infection, (6) pulmonary contusion, (7) acute respiratory distress
syndrome (ARDS), and (8) trauma-induced
pneumonia (Artom et al. 1977). Empyema will
commonly present with cough, fever, chest pain,
sweating, chills, shortness of breath, and dyspnea. In chronic cases, clubbing may be present
due to the long-standing hypoxia from entrapped
lung lobes. In severe acute cases, patients may
become overtly septic.

Diagnostics

History and physical exam, with attention paid to injury patterns and thoracic procedures, along with clinical suspicion, are important for prompt diagnosis and treatment of empyema. Approximately 2 % of Trauma Critical Care patients necessitating a chest tube eventually develop an empyema – this percentage increases considerably if the patient later undergoes a thoracotomy (Caplan et al. 1984). On physical exam, dullness to percussion with reduced air movement is typical for clinically significant empyema.

In addition to the patient's clinical picture, the diagnosis of posttraumatic empyema relies on advanced imaging and pleural culture. Computed tomography (CT) has emerged as the diagnostic imaging of choice for empyema. Pleural enhancement and air within a pleural collection are suggestive of the diagnosis (Kearney et al. 2000).

Laboratory findings include white blood cell count, C-reactive protein, and erythrocyte sedimentation rate elevation. Thoracocentesis may be performed; purulence usually displays a pH < 7.2, glucose concentrations <60 mg/dL, elevated lactate dehydrogenase and proteins. Bacteria and neutrophils are often present on Gram stains. Gram-positive coccal infections predominate – *S. aureus* is the most common etiology. If Gram-negative cultures grow from an empyema of a posttraumatic patient, then consideration should be given to a *trans*-diaphragmatic process. Microbiological knowledge from cultures and their susceptibility profile should tailor antimicrobial therapy.

Treatment

Historically, the initial therapy for empyema has consisted of pleural drainage and antibiotic therapy, with operative intervention indicated for treatment failure. More recent reports, however, have suggested VATS or thoracotomy should be considered for initial treatment. In a series of 104 patients, Wozniak and colleagues demonstrated the failure of the first intervention was an independent predictor of mortality and proposed early operative management. Additionally, as retained

hemothorax may contribute to the development of empyema, it has been suggested that early VATS (by day five) should be considered (Wozniak et al. 2009).

It has previously been suggested that, while empyema generally evolves slowly, infectious complications can develop in as little as 4 days after trauma, requiring tube thoracostomy (Hoover et al. 1988). The delay created by treatment with thoracostomy tube and antibiotics may contribute to the challenging nature of operations for empyema, as the longer the infectious process continues, the more advanced is the stage and the more dense is the inflammatory response locally.

Once diagnosed, the optimal treatment for empyema involves a combination of surgical source control and antibiotics. Intra-pleural fibrinolytic therapy has been described with varying success. Surgical management options include either traditional open thoracotomy or video-assisted thoracoscopic surgery (VATS). VATS has been used successfully for definitive treatment of empyema (Chan et al. 2007). The use of VATS does, however, have some important potential limitations. Necessary expertise and instruments for adequate decortication must be available. Visibility in the setting of advanced disease may also affect the safety with which an adequate surgical clearance of infection can be conducted. Single lung ventilation can improve visibility and accessibility to the lung surface for decortication during VATS. Video-assisted thoracoscopic surgery is most effective in early stage infections, while thoracotomy is commonly required for adequate clearance of disease in advanced stages.

While optimal management includes adequate resuscitation prior to surgical intervention, stabilization in the face of a significant pleural space infection may not always be possible unless source control is achieved. In this subset of critically ill patients, emergent operation may be necessary if drainage and antibiotics cannot temporarily control pleural sepsis.

Routine postoperative management includes chest tube management, pain control with early mobilization, and directed antimicrobial therapy.

Pain control with either patient controlled analgesia or epidural catheter is recommended and can help facilitate early mobilization and chest physiotherapy. Potential postoperative complications include wound infection, postoperative bleeding, air leaks, bronchopleural fistula, and recurrent empyema. Air leaks, although common, generally resolve by the second postoperative day. Recurrent empyema can be successfully managed by open thoracotomy with or without pleurodesis or image-guided catheter drainage.

Summary

Posttraumatic empyema remains a serious complication of injury, associated with prolonged ICU and hospital lengths of stay and appreciable mortality. Delays in diagnosis may contribute to adverse outcomes. A significant portion of critically ill patients manifesting the sequelae of this infectious process are likely to require surgical intervention, including pleurectomy and pulmonary resection, for clearance of advanced disease. A high index of suspicion, early diagnosis, and an appropriately aggressive management can result in adequate clearance of disease with excellent results.

Cross-References

▶ Retained Hemothorax
▶ Ventilator-Associated Pneumonia

References

Alfageme I, Munoz F, Pena N, Umbria S (1993) Empyema of the thorax in adults. Etiology, microbiologic findings, and management. Chest 103(3):839–843
Artom KV, Grover FL, Richardson JD et al (1977) Post-traumatic empyema. Ann Thorac Surg 23:254
Caplan ES, Hoyt NJ, Rodriguez A, Cowley RA (1984) Empyema occurring in the multiply traumatized patient. J Trauma 24:785
Chan DT, Sihoe AD, Chan S, Tsang DS, Fang B, Lee TW et al (2007) Surgical treatment for empyema thoracis: is video-assisted thoracic surgery "better" than thoracotomy? Ann Thorac Surg 84(1):225–231
Eren S, Esme H, Sehitogullari A, Durkan A (2008) The risk factors and management of posttraumatic empyema in trauma patients. Injury 39(1):44–49
Hoover EL, Hsu HK, Webb H, Toporoff B, Minnard E, Cunningham JN (1988) The surgical management of empyema thoracis in substance abuse patients: a 5-year experience. Ann Thorac Surg 46(5):563–566
Kearney SE, Davies CW, Davies RJ, Gleeson FV (2000) Computed tomography and ultrasound in parapneumonic effusions and empyema. Clin Radiol 55(7):542–547
O'Connor JV, Chi A, Joshi M, Dubose J, Scalea TM (2013) Post-traumatic empyema: aetiology, surgery and outcome in 125 consecutive patients. Injury 44(9):1153–1158
Wozniak CJ, Paull DE, Moezzi JE, Scott RP, Anstadt MP, York W et al (2009) Choice of first intervention is related to outcomes in the management of empyema. Ann Thorac Surg 87(5):1525–1530; discussion 1530–1531

Empyema Thoracis

▶ Empyema

End of Life Care – Terminal Care, End of the Line, Pre-death, Final Hours

▶ End-of-Life Care Communication in Trauma Patients

End-of-Life Care

Younsuck Koh
Department of Pulmonary and Critical Care Medicine, Asan Medical Center, University of Ulsan College of Medicine, Seoul, South Korea

Synonyms

Terminal care; Withholding and withdrawal of life-sustaining therapy

Definition

End-of-life (EOL) care involves a shifting of critical care goals from cure to comfort and begins when death is imminent. Such care reduces unnecessary suffering of both patients and families, as death approaches. EOL care in the intensive care unit (ICU) is receiving a great deal of attention in efforts to improve the overall quality of ICU care.

Background

Dying usually takes some time. Technological advances in life-sustaining measures now allow terminally ill patients to survive longer in hospital, then was previously the case. No one wants to die suffering. Caregivers must optimize the care given to dying patients and their families. Respect for the notion that a patient should be allowed to make personal medical decisions has grown over recent decades. Conflict between caregivers and family members over the level and nature of EOL care is often apparent. The essential features of any debate among caregivers, terminally ill patients, and/or the families of such families remain ill-defined. The clinical benefits of previous or prospective management must be clearly explained by attending physicians.

Ethical Principles of EOL Care

Four ethical principles relevant to EOL care are:

1. The principle of autonomy
2. The principle of beneficence
3. The principle of nonmaleficence ("Do not harm")
4. The principle of distributive justice

Autonomy is the right to make choices about one's life. It can be fully exercised only in the absence of controlling interference by others and by those with intellectual capacity (see "▶ Autonomy"). In clinical situations, the four ethical principles sometimes clash; it may be best to continually redefine the probable best interests of patient as time passes. The doctrine of the "double effect" affords an ethical rationale for relief of pain and other symptoms using sedatives even when this may have the foreseeable (but not intended) consequence of hastening death. The intention of EOL care is to relieve patient suffering and to maintain dignity, and not to facilitate the desire of a patient to die. Thus, neither physician-assisted suicide nor active euthanasia is in play.

Application

Clinical Settings

EOL care is usually considered in clinical practice when the death of a patient appears inevitable. A discussion on the nature and extent of such care should be initiated when application of reasonable available treatment options will almost certainly not afford a patient the option of a meaningful life.

Performance of EOL Care

In EOL care, the goal of treatment shifts from cure to comfort with maintenance of patient dignity (see "▶ Hospice"). The sharing of advance care planning between caregivers and family members (or the patient) minimizes conflicts that may arise when appropriate EOL care is discussed (see "▶ Life Support, Withholding and Withdrawal of"). Advance care planning is a method whereby the autonomy of a patient can be respected when the patient lacks the capacity to make decisions (Colvin et al. 1993). During the giving of EOL care, respect for patient autonomy often requires that a physician elicits patient values and goals relevant to health care (Billings and Krakauer 2011). Physician-given advice is optimal when clinical expertise and compassion are combined with an understanding of the wished of caregivers, the patient, and/or family members. Such advice encourages patients or family members to review EOL care options. The clinical care team should carefully define the health benefits of any life support that is in place or that is a future option. The planned care should address the physical, social, and spiritual needs of the patient. All ICU therapies should be critically evaluated to ensure that patient comfort is maximized. The caregiver team must facilitate pain-free death.

Hospital Ethics Committee (HEC)

If a conflict in terms of EOL care arises between the caregiver teams and patient family members and if further efforts at communication fail to resolve the problem, consultation with ethicists may be helpful. If an HEC supports the caregiver assessment of appropriate EOL care, the HEC may request that clinicians pursue their attempts to reach consensus with the patient or his/her surrogate (Burns and Truog 2007). If the parties are irreconcilable, physicians and the host hospital may seek to transfer the patient to another facility or to request judicial resolution of the dispute. If none of these approaches is successful, and the therapeutic measures demanded by a patient or his/her family seem strongly inappropriate from a medical viewpoint, the HEC could approve the unilateral decline by the hospital to provide the treatment sought. However, this should occur only after the patient and/or family members are informed of the decision and only after sufficient opportunity has been given for legal advice to be taken and (possibly) for a legal challenge, if desired, to be mounted (Burns and Truog 2007).

Outcome

Conflicts between family members and medical staff are not infrequent, when decisions on EOL care are to be done. Patients and families are frequently dissatisfied with the level of EOL care afforded by hospitals. Proactive consultation with ethicists, advance care planning, discussion on possible patient transfer to a hospice, and regular well-planned family conferences all contribute to a sense of family satisfaction. Formal caregiver training in EOL care skills is rare and such care is not standardized in most hospitals. Compassionate EOL care facilitates

the development, within a patient, of a personal relationship with death. Communication skills are paramount: these are used to facilitate EOL decisions (Levy 2001). The use of imprecise or insensitive terminology during family discussions, and poor understanding of family wishes, frequently causes family dissatisfaction. EOL decisions are greatly facilitated if the caregiver is allowed (by the family) to assume the status of a family member. EOL care can best be evaluated by measuring the level of satisfaction experienced by both families and caregiver teams. Encouraging caregivers to view acquisition of EOL skills as a lifelong educational process seems essential to improve the quality of such care. The application of excellent EOL care should lead to a sense of harmony, and not of guilt, distrust, conflict, or fear. The goal of EOL care is to facilitate the successful resolution, by both patients and their families, of the tremendously powerful emotional stresses experienced during dying.

Cross-References

▶ Advance Directive
▶ Autonomy
▶ End-of-Life Care Communication in Trauma Patients
▶ Hospice
▶ Life Support, Withholding and Withdrawal of
▶ Surrogate, Role in Decision-Making

References

Billings JA, Krakauer EL (2011) On patient autonomy and physician responsibility in end-of-life care. Arch Intern Med 171(9):849–853

Burns JP, Truog RD (2007) Futility: a concept in evolution. Chest 132(6):1987–1993

Colvin ER, Myhre MJ, Welch J, Hammes BJ (1993) Moving beyond the Patient Self-Determination Act: educating patients to be autonomous. ANNA J 20(5):564–568

Levy MM (2001) End-of-life care in the intensive care unit: can we do better? Crit Care Med 29(2 Suppl): N56–N61

End-of-Life Care Communication in Trauma Patients

Timothy Rainer[1] and Gavin M. Joynt[2]
[1]Accident and Emergency Department, Prince of Wales Hospital, The Chinese University of Hong Kong, Shatin, Hong Kong, China
[2]Department of Anaesthesia and Intensive Care, The Chinese University of Hong Kong, Hong Kong, China

Synonyms

Communication – interaction, discussion, information transfer, comforting; End of life care – Terminal care, end of the line, pre-death, final hours; Trauma – Wounds and injuries, physical injury

Definition

Trauma: Any injury or damage, whether physically or emotionally inflicted.

End-of-life (EOL) care: In medicine, end-of-life care refers to all medical care and the support of those approaching the end of their lives. This may include a terminal illness or condition that has become advanced, progressive, and incurable.

Communication: Communication is the imparting or exchanging of information by speaking, writing, or using some other medium.

Background

How people die will remain in the lasting memory of relatives and health and social care staff (Michon et al. 2003). It is therefore important that staff recognize their responsibility to provide the best possible care at the end of life. Until recently, life support technology was the limiting factor in the process of healing. Advances are now such that it may be a factor preventing the normal process of death in circumstances where there is little meaningful chance of returning health. Such technology can also unnecessarily prolong suffering for patients, relatives, and staff.

End-of-life care in trauma patients in the Accident and Emergency Department (AED) frequently differs from what is traditionally understood as "EOL care" (Department of Health 2008). Most published EOL knowledge, protocols, and guidance have emerged from the experience gained by those caring for patients suffering with progressive illness such as cancer, where both the patient and the family often have substantial time after diagnosis to digest relevant information and prepare for death. The event leading to death after trauma is usually sudden and totally unexpected and has been described as "unique" (Chan 2004). Clinicians rarely have the advantage of knowing the victims, and are unfamiliar with patients' wishes and values. There is often no time for preparation or adjustment, and the patient is generally in no condition to provide input to the process or decision-making. Therefore, the standard principles supporting the practice of EOL care must be modified accordingly (Mosenthal et al. 2008; Jacobs et al. 2005).

It is therefore helpful to briefly define the different scenarios in which post-trauma end-of-life care may be necessary, to identify key components of EOL care in the trauma setting, and to identify key techniques that may help caregivers effectively manage communication at the end of life.

Literature Search

Entry of the general term "End of life trauma care" into the US National of Medicine National Institutes of Health library which was broken to End[All Fields] AND ("life"[MeSH Terms] OR "life"[All Fields]) AND ("injuries"[Subheading] OR "injuries"[All Fields] OR "trauma"[All Fields] OR "wounds and injuries"[MeSH Terms] OR ("wounds"[All Fields] AND "injuries"[All Fields]) OR "wounds and injuries"[All Fields]) AND care[All Fields] yielded 287 articles for the period between 1975 and 2011, of which 16 were relevant to the subject matter reviewed in this entry. These references will not all be reviewed here in detail, but a selection are included in the references and reading materials as resource for the interested reader.

Application

Identifying Patients Who Require EOL Care

In the early 1980s, Trunkey clearly defined three peaks of death after trauma – immediate deaths that occur within minutes of injury, early deaths which occur within hours of injury (these patients are likely to die in the emergency department), and late or delayed deaths that occur days to weeks or even months after injury (patients likely to die on the ward or in ICU) (Trunkey 1983). End-of-life communication will present different challenges in each context.

A broad range of terminal events may arise after trauma, which include the following:

- Patients with massive blunt trauma, for example, after a motor vehicle crash or a fall from a great height frequently results in death that is sudden and unexpected

There are few EOL decisions to be made, and communication focuses on transferring the information that death has occurred or is imminent, the reason for death, and introduction of strategies to help the relatives to face and respond to this reality.

- Patients whose death is not immediate, but is predicted to occur within the first few hours, or if there is ventilatory support, days after injury

This category includes patients with an abbreviated injury score of 6 (Association for the Advancement of Automative Medicine 1990), which by definition are considered non-survivable. Examples include patients with massive destruction of the skull, brain, and intracranial contents; bilateral destruction of skeletal, vascular, organ, and tissue systems; and torso transection. Under such circumstances, EOL decisions such as limiting life support may be made. Communication focuses on the fact that death is inevitable, on giving the reasons for this inevitability, and on strategies to help the relatives face and respond to this reality.

- Patients with a moderate rather than high likelihood of mortality from the traumatic event, but who have severe preexisting underlying disease such as advanced carcinoma, end-stage organ failure, or severe cognitive dysfunction

In these cases, anticipated survival and quality-of-life outcomes may justify limiting resuscitative measures and subsequent life support. The focus changes from sustaining life to comfort and pain control care. Under these circumstances, the focus is on communicating information that death or a poor quality of life is the likely outcome. Reasons should be given for this conclusion, and then the new goal of care is introduced. The conversation aims to help the relatives to assist in the making of management decisions.

- Patients with parasuicide or attempted suicide, that is, those patients who planned death from the traumatic event

These patients are generally considered not to be in a fit state of mind to decide whether life should be sustained or not. Where the likelihood of a good survival is high, then every attempt should be made to sustain life and to manage the psychological issues later. However, where the likelihood of quality of physical life is extremely poor, then a similar approach to the above should be made. Under these circumstances, the focus is on communicating information that death or a poor quality of life is the likely outcome. Reasons should be given for this conclusion, and then the new goal of care is introduced. The conversation aims to help the relatives to assist in the making of management decisions. The fact that suicide was involved should not play a primary role in the final decision.

Key Components of the End-of-Life Care Process

Prior to the initiation of communication with relatives, and when possible the patient, it is prudent for the management team to have reached a carefully considered consensus regarding the proposed management options for the patient (Bradley and Brasel 2009; Mosenthal et al. 2008).

- Assessment of the patient's clinical condition and a determination that the condition is terminal.
- Determination that life support therapy will be unlikely to provide a net health benefit to the patient.
- Consensus with all relevant management team members that an instituting an EOL pathway is appropriate.
- Achievement of consensus with the patient and/or appropriate surrogate decision makers.
- All medical decisions, the achievement of consensus among team members, the conversation with the family, and their replies and preferences as patient surrogates must to be documented.
- Detailed guidelines have been drawn up for EOL in terminally ill patients in general settings (Department of Health 2008). These may provide guidance for trauma patients; however, there are no internationally recognized EOL care pathways for trauma care.
- The Liverpool care pathway was developed between the Royal Liverpool hospital and the city's Marie Curie hospice in the late 1990s, to transfer practice in the dying phase from hospice to hospital. The Pathway, although developed for cancer patients, has been successfully applied to burns patients whose outlook has been deemed futile (Hemington-Gorse et al. 2011).

End-of-Life Communication

Learning good technique is likely to improve communication success so education is important (Levin et al. 2010). Appropriate training and progressive supervised practice in simulated and clinical settings can enhance communication skills. Relatives face several challenges in the emergency room setting. Apart from the shock of the sudden, catastrophic injury to a loved one, the surroundings are unfamiliar. There is much noise and activity, unfamiliar and frightening procedures such as intubation and resuscitation, and usually restricted access to the loved one, or clear information regarding the minute-by-minute

condition. This creates fear and helplessness, a sense of insignificance, anger, and subsequent depression and stress (Vincent 1997). Better communication is likely to relieve stress, comfort and reassure, and thereby promote trust and decrease subsequent anger and depression.

Communication, just as in every other care process, proceeds much more effectively if there is planning and preparation prior to the communication interface.

Key Issues That Must Be Considered

Planning
- Prepare properly for the interview. The designated communicator should know the patients name, have access to all relevant clinical information, the latest patient status, and management plans.
- Consider making appointments if time allows.
- Identify legal surrogates to be present at interviews, or nominate "senior" representatives of large family groups.
- Be aware of the special requirements that may accompany patients and families from cultures different to those of caregivers (Ball et al. 2010).

Environment
- Inviting relatives to join ward rounds has the advantage of openness and the provision of detailed information, but there are disadvantages. Care must be taken over what is said as you are in the full hearing of patient, and there is a danger of criticism and anxiety-inducing statements.
- Interview rooms should be quiet, comfortable, of *adequate size*, private, with a hand basin, advice and information leaflets, calming pictures, and pleasant aroma.

Staff Demeanor
- Staff should dress appropriately and professionally, and should not display gaiety or superficiality.
- Avoid designating junior, unskilled staff to communicate during EOL or goal of care interviews.

E

- Communicating staff should always identify themselves, and their position of responsibility in relation to the patient's care.

Information Provision

- Communication involves two fundamental areas of information. Giving verbal information on the condition of the patient – the diagnosis, treatment options, and prognosis, and giving and receiving nonverbal communication. The recognition of nonverbal clues to a relative or patient's state, such as facial expression, fidgeting, or tremor may indicate fear or agitation. Similarly, the communicating clinician should utilize facial expression and body language to demonstrate calm and empathy.
- There is some controversy as to how much information should be revealed, and at what time.
  - Patients/relatives should be told everything about their situation, and immediately.
  - Patients/relatives should be told everything about their situation but in stages, depending on their perceived ability to cope with the information.
  - Patients/relatives should be told what they are able to receive and cope with, and this will depend directly upon what questions they ask.
  - Information should be provided with compassion; however, patients are entitled to full disclosure and no attempt should be made to mislead the people concerned or to withhold information that is sought.

Delivering Information

- It is useful to prepare the relative/patient for the delivery of bad news with statements such as "I should inform you that this is going to be a difficult conversation for you because... ." It may be useful to find out what patient already knows. If possible and if appropriate, convey some measure of hope, even if it is to reassure the relative that their loved one's suffering and pain will be controlled. Remember that you are there as a provider of care.

- The language should be simple and direct. Avoid technical diagnostic terminology or medical jargon.
- Information should be given at a pace that can be understood, and often requires repeating.
- Special care should be taken if translation is required. It is important to "check back" to ensure that the patient or relatives have properly understood what has been said.
- Consider the need to provide information in a manner that is sensitive to differences in the recipients' socioeconomic, cultural, and educational condition.
- Use educational tools if appropriate and available (e.g., pamphlets and videos).
- Be prepared to admit uncertainty. For example, it is particularly difficult to provide prognoses with the precision that patients often expect.

Interpersonal Skills

Either verbal or nonverbal information is transmitted and interpreted by involved parties. Techniques that instill confidence in the information provider include the following:

- Maintaining good eye contact.
- Appropriately respond to those receiving the information. Watching the patient or relatives while information is delivered provides an insight into their awareness and emotional state. Listen carefully to what they have to say. Show a courteous demeanor and never appear disinterested or mechanical.
- It is generally better to avoid large physical barriers between the participants in the conversation, and depending on cultural circumstances, it may be useful to sit close to the relative.
- In the appropriate cultural setting, physical contact such as holding a hand, or putting a hand on a forearm, can communicate care and empathy. Empathy is the capacity to recognize, and to some extent to share feelings such as sadness or happiness that are being experienced by another person.
- Demonstrate honesty, and behave with fairness, truthfulness, sincerity, frankness, and freedom from deceit or fraud.

- Communicating staff members should never appear rushed or flustered or in a hurry "to get the interview over with."

Concluding an Interview

- Summarize the discussion both verbally, and when possible, in written form. Occasionally it may be helpful to tape the conversation.
- Allow sufficient time for questions, be open and encourage discussion.
- Patient/relatives should be offered the opportunity to discuss personal needs and preferences with professionals.

Documentation

- All stages of the process should be documented in writing (Thomasson et al. 2011). Additional information may be retained in the form of audio or video recordings.

No training will cover all circumstances. When in doubt, and facing unexpected circumstances for which you are unprepared, a good rule of thumb is to do unto others as you would like them to do to you, if you were in a similar situation.

Special Circumstances in Trauma

There are special and difficult circumstances when unusual or exceptional communication may be considered. For example, in the case of relatives who refuse to accept the futility of continued treatment and the inevitability of death, where threats of litigation are made, and staff face such conflict, it is important to include the most experienced of staff in the discussion, to give as much time as reasonably possible, to document well, and to work with consensus wherever possible.

Another difficult and exceptional circumstance is during major incidents when there may be many critically ill casualties and deaths. Time that normally would be given to communicate with the relatives may be shortened due to the need to treat others with a greater chance of survival. Although communication may be brief, it is important to maintain the attitudes mentioned above wherever possible, to apologize to the relatives because of the brevity of the interview and to reassure them of a fuller discussion as soon as reasonably possible.

Problem Areas

Medical staff in trauma units may be busy, stressed, and sometimes unskilled in communication. Consequently, they may fear blame and an inability to cope. Formal training in communication skills and an understanding of EOL procedures and protocols may serve to alleviate these anxieties and improve performance.

The Kubler-Ross model applies primarily to those with chronic terminal illness. However, the principles involved may apply to any catastrophic life event. Five distinct stages that may occur independently of sequentially are recognized. Denial, anger, bargaining, depression, and acceptance are frequently encountered in patients/relatives at the EOL (Kübler-Ross 1969). The management team members need to understand the different ways in which a relative or patient may respond and allow, to some extent, for inappropriate reactions and there may be some allowance for overreaction and reactionary anger.

End-of-life trauma care is even "more challenging in the acute care setting" where staff are generally focused on saving life, and circumstances where EOL communication is required are relatively infrequent. The availability of intensive care and organ support may make it harder to recognize that the person is dying. Difficult decisions are best made by consensus.

Particular difficulty may be encountered because of the following circumstances:

- The variable time frame within which acute traumatic injuries progress to result in a condition that cannot be reasonably salvaged by medical therapy may lead to a higher incidence of uncertainty regarding non-beneficial therapies.
- Trauma management teams are usually multidisciplinary and all individuals in the management team may not agree on whether continued therapy is likely to result in a net health benefit to the patient.

- In view of the acute and sudden nature of the event, patient's surrogates may more frequently request continued non-beneficial therapy.

These issues may be resolved by repeatedly explaining the rationale, offering a second opinion within or outside the immediate management team or hospital, seeking resolution through a hospital/institutional ethics committee, and as a last resort, seeking resolution through the courts.

Patient's surrogates may rarely request inappropriate discontinuation of therapy. This conflict should be viewed by the treating team in the context that the first duty of care is to the patient. The above pathway of conflict resolution can be followed if necessary.

Conclusions

One of the aims of trauma care is to provide optimal treatment that is in the patient's best interest. This may require the institution of EOL care. Severe traumatic injury is usually sudden and unexpected. Excellent communication skills are required to facilitate the EOL process and deal with potential conflict. Techniques to facilitate communication skills can be learned and should be a part of trauma training programs.

Cross-References

▶ Advance Directive
▶ Autonomy
▶ Brain Death, Ethical Concerns
▶ Futile Care
▶ Life Support, Withholding and Withdrawal of
▶ Surrogate, Role in Decision-Making
▶ Terminal Care

References

Association for the Advancement of Automative Medicine (1990) The abbreviated injury scale, 1990 revision. Association for the Advancement of Automative Medicine, Des Plaines

Ball CG, Navsaria P, Kirkpatrick AW, Vercler C, Dixon E, Zink J, Laupland KB, Lowe M, Salomone JP, Dente CJ, Wyrzykowski AD, Hameed SM, Widder S, Inaba K, Ball JE, Rozycki GS, Montgomery SP, Hayward T, Feliciano DV (2010) The impact of country and culture on end-of-life care for injured patients: results from an international survey. J Trauma 69(6):1323–1333; discussion 1333–4

Bradley CT, Brasel KJ (2009) Developing guidelines that identify patients who would benefit from palliative care services in the surgical intensive care unit. Crit Care Med 37(3):946–950

Chan GK (2004) End-of-life models and emergency department care. Acad Emerg Med 11(1):79–86

Department of Health. End of life care strategy – promoting high quality care for all adults at the end of life. http://www.endoflifecareforadults.nhs.uk/assets/downloads/pubs_EoLC_Strategy_1.pdf. Accessed 2 May 2013

Hemington-Gorse SJ, Clover AJ, Macdonald C, Harriott J, Richardson P, Philp B, Shelley O, Dziewulski P (2011) Comfort care in burns: the burn modified Liverpool care pathway (BM-LCP). Burns 37(6):981–985

Jacobs LM, Jacobs BB, Burns KJ (2005) A plan to improve end-of-life care for trauma victims and their families. J Trauma Nurs 12(3):73–76

Kübler-Ross E (1969) On death and dying. Macmillan, New York

Levin TT, Moreno B, Silvester W, Kissane DW (2010) End-of-life communication in the intensive care unit. Gen Hosp Psychiatry 32(4):433–442

Michon B, Balkou S, Hivon R, Cyr C (2003) Death of a child: parental perception of grief intensity – end-of-life and bereavement care. Paediatr Child Health 8(6):363–366

Mosenthal AC, Murphy PA, Barker LK, Lavery R, Retano A, Livingston DH (2008) Changing the culture around end-of-life care in the trauma intensive care unit. J Trauma 64(6):1587–1593

Thomasson J, Petros T, Lorenzo-Rivero S, Moore RA, Stanley JD (2011) Quality of documented consent for the de-escalation of care on a general and trauma surgery service. Am Surg 77(7):883–887

Trunkey DD (1983) Trauma. Sci Am 249:28–35

Vincent J-L (1997) Communication in the ICU. Intensive Care Med 23:1093–1098

Recommended Reading

Jacobs LM, Burns KJ, Jacobs BB (2010) Nurse and physician preferences for end-of-life care for trauma patients. J Trauma 69(6):1567–1573

Johnson D et al (1998) Measuring the ability to meet family needs in an intensive care unit. Crit Care Med 26:266–271

Ptacek JT, Eberhardt TL (1996) Breaking bad news: a review of the literature. JAMA 276:496–502

Stewart MA (1995) Effective physician-patient communication and health outcomes: a review. Can Med Assoc J 152:1423–1433

End-of-Life Care Decision

▶ Life Support, Withholding and Withdrawal of

End-of-Life Issues

▶ Brain Death, Ethical Concerns

Endotoxemia

▶ Sepsis, Treatment of

Endotracheal Intubation

▶ Airway Management in Trauma, Nonsurgical

End-Tidal CO$_2$

▶ Monitoring of Trauma Patients During Anesthesia

Enhanced Blast Weapon

▶ Explosion

Enteral Nutrition (EN)

▶ Nutritional Deficiency/Starvation
▶ Nutritional Support

Entero-Atmospheric Fistula

Mansoor Khan
Consultant Esophagogastric and Acute Care
Surgeon, Doncaster Royal Infirmary, Doncaster,
South Yorkshire, UK

E

Synonyms

EAF; Entero-cutaneous fistula

Definition

An abnormal epithelialized connection between the gastrointestinal tract, specifically the small bowel and atmosphere.

They are a devastating complication and usually occur in the setting of damage control surgery and have a higher incidence in patients who have an open abdomen; specifically, the longer the abdomen remains open and the more manipulation the small bowel undergoes (Table 1).

There are a spectrum of factors that affect the healing of the fistula: high output (greater than 500 ml/day (Tong et al. 2012)), location in the GI tract (proximal fistulas have a higher morbidity/mortality), presence of an open abdomen, presence of a foreign body (i.e., mesh), or ongoing systemic illness (sepsis/malignancy).

Entero-Atmospheric Fistula, Table 1 Etiology of Entero-atmospheric fistula

Iatrogenic	Operation
	Percutaneous intervention
Trauma	Open abdomen
	Repeated small bowel manipulation
Foreign body	
Inflammatory bowel disease	
Infectious disease	Tuberculosis
	Actinomycosis
Malignancy	

Entero-Atmospheric Fistula, Table 2 Factors affecting fistula healing

Local	Systemic
High output fistula	Malnourished
Foreign body	Sepsis
Proximal location	Malignancy
Local infection	
Distal obstruction	

The mainstay in management of the fistula is to correct local and systemic factors (Table 2).

Treatment depends on a number of factors, and can be divided initially into medical and surgical. Once an EAF occurs, immediate management consists of treatment of sepsis if present; nutrition, fluid, and electrolyte support in the form of parenteral nutrition (PN); and wound/effluent control and protection of surrounding tissues and exposed bowel (Majercik et al. 2012). Medical treatment, which relies on strict absence of oral nutrition, and the initiation of total parenteral initiation; adjuncts to this may be proton pump inhibitors and octreotide. Surgical treatment should be reserved for use after sufficient time has passed from the previous laparotomy to allow lysis of the fibrous adhesion using full nutritional and medical treatment and until a complete understanding of the anatomy of the fistula has been achieved (Lee 2012). It should be noted that Entero-atmospheric fistulas almost never close spontaneously, and definitive repair usually requires major surgical intervention and abdominal wall reconstruction 6–12 months after the original insult (Wright and Wright 2011; Di Saverio et al. 2011).

Cross-References

▶ Prolonged Open Abdomen

References

Di Saverio S, Villani S, Biscardi A, Giorgini E, Tugnoli G (2011) Open abdomen with concomitant enteroatmospheric fistula: validation, refinements, and adjuncts to a novel approach. J Trauma 71:760–762

Lee SH (2012) Surgical management of enterocutaneous fistula. Korean J Radiol Off J Korean Radiol Soc 13(Suppl 1):S17–S20

Majercik S, Kinikini M, White T (2012) Enteroatmospheric fistula: from soup to nuts. Nutr Clin Pract Off Publ Am Soc Parenter Enter Nutr 27(4):507–512

Tong CY, Lim LL, Brody RA (2012) High output enterocutaneous fistula: a literature review and a case study. Asia Pac J Clin Nutr 21:464–469

Wright A, Wright M (2011) Bedside management of an abdominal wound containing an enteroatmospheric fistula: a case report. Ostomy Wound Manage 57:28–32

Entero-Cutaneous Fistula

▶ Entero-Atmospheric Fistula

Epidural Hematoma

▶ Traumatic Brain Injury, Intensive Care Unit Management

Epidural Hemorrhage

▶ Traumatic Brain Injury, Anesthesia for

Eptacog Alfa (Activated)

▶ Adjuncts to Transfusion: Recombinant Factor VIIa, Factor XIII, and Calcium

Escharectomy

▶ Escharotomy

Escharotomy

Mahmoud A. Amr
Division of Trauma, Critical Care, and General
Surgery, Mayo Clinic, Rochester, MN, USA

Synonyms

Escharectomy; Incisional decompression

Definition

Escharotomy is a surgical procedure that is considered as an early management for full-thickness (third-degree) circumferential burns. This procedure concentrates in releasing the inelastic, unviable, and leathery part of the burned skin which is called the eschar that is painless and black, white, or cherry red.

Pre-existing Condition

The effect of circumferential full-thickness burns is dramatic if not managed early. The combination of edema from fluid resuscitation and transcapillary extravasation from the thermal injury will increase the pressure underneath the eschar which becomes restrictive and hence the formation of compartment syndrome. This can be anticipated by several means, the most applicable are the Doppler ultrasound which evaluates the vascular patency and the pulse oximeter which indicates having tissues ischemia when $SO_2 < 95\%$ (Bardakjian et al. 1988).

In addition to the compartment syndrome in the limbs, eschars, when present in the chest, may jeopardize the ventilation by restricting the chest wall movement which may lead to atelectasis and subsequent pneumonia, and when present in the neck, it may cause tracheal obstruction. So in these circumstances escharotomy becomes an emergency procedure.

Application

The need for escharotomy in full-thickness burn patients depends on the site of the burn, the extent of damage, and the type of the burn.

As noted earlier full-thickness burn on the chest and the neck should be managed early to overcome the fatal sequences, without the need to know the exact extent of damage, as the purpose of management here is to maintain the ventilation and to prevent the tracheal obstruction.

As for the limbs, assessment of the extent of damage is rapidly performed to detect the presence of compartment syndrome, first by doing physical examination, looking for the 5 Ps of ischemia: pain, pallor, paresthesia, paralysis, and pulselessness. The next step would be using noninvasive measurements such as Doppler ultrasound and pulse oximetry. The Doppler ultrasound could be misleading as it may show a blood flow in the limb although the blood circulation is not sufficient for the viability of the limb. If still in doubt, and especially in case of electrical injuries, then the utilization of intracompartmental pressure measurements such as manometer would be useful. The values of the manometer are in mmHg; the threshold in which a surgical intervention must be done is 30 mmHg according to Hargens et al. (1979) and 45 mmHg according to Matsen et al. (1980). So, it is necessary to perform escharotomy in the very first hours in order to restore normal blood flow and preventing devitalization of the limbs (Mann et al. 1996).

Technique

The general concept of escharotomy is to do two incisions on both sides of the limb using either a scalpel or electrocautery involving the whole length of the burn, which should be under aseptic technique with the use of anesthesia in case of circumferential deep partial thickness (second-degree) burns; full-thickness burns are insensate and can be managed without anesthesia. The incision should be done until reaching the subcutaneous fat only, so the blood loss would be minimal, and the incidence of infections declines, in comparison to fasciotomy which is deeper and yields higher blood loss and a high incidence of infections.

Limbs: When performing escharotomy, special precautions must be taken when dealing with the upper limbs; the incision should be made medially and laterally with caution not to dissect the ulnar nerve at the elbow or the radial nerve at the wrist. As for the lower limbs, the caution should be for the superficial peroneal nerve near the fibular head, the posterior tibial artery at the ankle, and the lateral popliteal nerve below the knee.

Chest: Escharotomy of the chest is performed to overcome the ventilation interference by the tight eschar. The technique involves bilateral longitudinal incisions in the chest with incisions transversely at the lower and upper parts of the chest, without the need to do the same on the back as the chest expansion mostly occurs anteriorly (Pegg 1992). The caution here is to avoid the breast tissues in females if possible.

Neck: Full-thickness burns in the neck may cause compression of vital parts of the neck especially the carotids, which interfere with the brain oxygenation, in addition to the possibility of tracheal obstruction if the pressure is severe. So emergent escharotomy must be performed in this case, and the incisions must be done laterally and posteriorly to avoid the carotid and jugular vessels (Hedges 2013).

Care of Escharotomy

After releasing the intracompartmental pressure by escharotomy, the incision that was created is considered a wound and has to be managed accordingly to prevent any complication. The first complication to be encountered during escharotomies is bleeding, which can be managed by simple cauterization or compression if not profuse.

Further care of the escharotomy wound is basically the same as dealing with the burn tissue itself. So this requires daily dressing and if extensive then it may require dressing twice daily. The usage of topical antimicrobial agents has been shown to decrease the rate of infections in burns (D'Avignon et al. 2008), so they should be applied to the escharotomy wound as well.

Fasciotomy with Escharotomy

In most of the thermal injuries escharotomy suffices alone, but if the thermal injury is very deep that it involves the muscles as well, or in the case of electrical injury which will affect the muscular tissue, then it is advised and encouraged to do fasciotomy as well to release the muscles and keep them viable by preventing the compartment syndrome. But we should keep in mind all the complications of fasciotomy including bleeding and infections and treat them accordingly.

Summary

Escharotomy is a simple surgical procedure that is used in case of circumferential full-thickness burns, yet the outcomes of utilizing it are remarkable by salvaging the limbs, and in case of chest burns, escharotomy is considered to be lifesaving. Nevertheless, the care of escharotomy must be kept in mind as well by dressing and topical antimicrobial agents.

Cross-References

▶ Burn
▶ Compartment Syndrome
▶ Fasciotomy

References

Bardakjian VB, Kenney JG et al (1988) Pulse oximetry for vascular monitoring in burned upper extremities. J Burn Care Rehabil 9(1):63–65

D'Avignon LC, Saffle JR et al (2008) Prevention and management of infections associated with burns in the combat casualty. J Trauma 64(3 Suppl): S277–S286

Hargens AR, Romine JS et al (1979) Peripheral nerve-conduction block by high muscle-compartment pressure. J Bone Joint Surg Am 61(2):192–200

Hedges R (2013) Roberts and Hedges' clinical procedures in emergency medicine. Saunders/An Imprint of Elsevier, Philadelphia

Mann R, Gibran N et al (1996) Is immediate decompression of high voltage electrical injuries to the upper extremity always necessary? J Trauma 40(4):584–587; discussion 587–589

Matsen FA, Winquist RA et al (1980) Diagnosis and management of compartmental syndromes. J Bone Joint Surg Am 62(2):286–291

Pegg SP (1992) Escharotomy in burns. Ann Acad Med Singapore 21(5):682–684

Esophageal Perforation

▶ Tracheal and Esophageal Injury

Estimated Outcome

▶ Neurotrauma, Prognosis and Outcome Predictions

Estimated Prognosis

▶ Neurotrauma, Prognosis and Outcome Predictions

Ethical Considerations Related to Consent

▶ Refusal of Treatment by Critical Patients

Ethical Issue in Rehabilitation in Trauma Patients

Kyoung Hyo Choi[1] and Ju Seok Ryu[2]
[1]Department of Rehabilitation Medicine, Asan Medical Center, University of Ulsan College of Medicine, Seoul, South Korea
[2]Department of Rehabilitation Medicine, Seoul National University Bundang Hospital, Seoul National University College of Medicine, Seongnam, South Korea

Synonyms

Head trauma rehabilitation; Traumatic brain injury; Traumatic spinal cord injury

Definition

Rehabilitation: To restore to useful life, as through therapy and education or, to restore to good condition, operation, or capacity.

Rehabilitation of people with disabilities is a process aimed at enabling them to reach and maintain their optimal physical, sensory, intellectual, psychological, and social functional levels. Rehabilitation provides disabled people with the tools they need to attain independence and self-determination (WHO).

Background

Prediction of the Prognosis of Rehabilitation in Trauma Patients

There are outcome measures for some issues, but not all of them are identified in qualitative research on surviving trauma patients. In particular, new outcome measures may be required to evaluate experience with the loss of personal identity, satisfaction with the reconstructed identity, and sense of connection with one's body and one's life following traumatic injury (Levack et al. 2010).

Long-term outcomes of trauma patients are important issues. In a study for children 1–2 years after sustained injury, the Child Health Questionnaire can be used to provide information regarding a child's health-related quality of life following injury. On the majority of subscales of the Child Health Questionnaire, study participants recorded scores that were statistically significantly below those of the normal controls. Therefore, injured children are worse off than their counterparts in terms of health-related quality for as long as 2 years following an injury (Davey et al. 2005).

Termination of Treatment

There have been several studies regarding the termination of treatment after traumatic brain injury. Management of patients in irreversible apathy syndrome has been the subject of sustained scientific and moral-legal debate over the last decade. The overall incidence of new apathy syndrome, full-stage cases of all etiology, is 0.5–2/100,000 population per year. Approximately one-third of these injuries are traumatic and two-thirds are non-traumatic cases. The main conceptual criticism is based on the assessment and diagnosis of all of the different apathy syndrome stages based solely on the behavioral findings without knowing the exact or uniform pathogenesis or neuropathologic findings. No special diagnostics and no specific medical management can be recommended for specific classes of apathy syndrome treatment and rehabilitation. As long as there is no single apathy syndrome-specific diagnostic tool and no specific laboratory investigation regimen to be recommended, neuroethical principles demand by all means a humanistic (ethical) activating care even in irreversible, full-stage apathy syndrome cases. Fully acceptable is the only palliative pain therapy with renunciation of maximal therapy (von Wild 2008).

In the last two decades, the minimally conscious state has been distinguished conceptually from the vegetative state, and operational criteria for these diagnoses have been published. Standardized and individualized assessment tools have been developed to assist the diagnosis of severe disorders of consciousness and the measurement of clinical improvement. The natural course of recovery and the importance of key prognostic predictors have been elucidated. Important advances have also been made in defining the similarities and differences in the pathophysiology of these two states, and functional imaging modalities have begun to explain the neural substrate underlying the behavioral features of these disorders. Research on the efficacy of various treatments for severe disorders of consciousness lags behind due to the practical and ethical difficulties in executing large, rigorously controlled clinical trials. The past and future scientific developments in this area provide an important background for continuing discussions of the ethical controversies surrounding end-of-life decision-making and resource allocation (Giacino and Whyte 2005).

Patients' rights regarding cardiopulmonary resuscitation (CPR) are derived from judicially elucidated principles of self-determination, privacy, and liberty interest and are based on the assumption that "every human of adult years and sound mind has a right to determine what shall be done with his/her own body (Caplan et al. 1987). In the head trauma rehabilitation literature, the ethics of CPR and institutional practices regarding resuscitation do not appear to hold the same degree of concern, both medically and from the perspective of medical ethics, as they do outside the field. Nonetheless, TBI facilities and general rehabilitation units can do more to support patients' autonomy by addressing preferences for the future care of the patients who are capable of making decisions and of the surrogates – those who speak for those lacking decision-making capability (Phipps 1998).

TBI rehabilitation and general rehabilitation facilities, like other healthcare institutions, are required by the Patient Self-Determination Act to inquire regarding the presence of advance directives or living wills upon admission. Talking with patients and their families about CPR is complex and brings up many fears. As many patients who experience a severe TBI are at least temporarily unable to participate in decision-making, others might be able to participate, although this would require an assessment of their decision-making capacity. Obviously, assessing a patient's decision-making capacity and preferences for or against resuscitation in many cases of brain injury can be extremely difficult and may not necessarily yield consistent, reliable information; however, this may not be the case with less severe injuries (Phipps 1998).

For the most part, discussion regarding CPR and DNR orders in patients with severe brain injury will take place with family members. Because families view rehabilitation, at least initially, with hopefulness regarding a patient's full recovery, initiating discussion of this topic too early in the rehabilitation process may be considered as too emotionally burdensome to yield an informed decision and may be viewed as counterproductive to establishing trust and rapport.

When the family members are relied on as decision makers, an important controversy concerns the basis for their decisions regarding the patient's treatment. Family members might not know the patient's specific wishes regarding resuscitation. Short of that, medical recommendations regarding the likely outcomes and the benefits and burdens to the patient are key elements in a surrogate's decision regarding CPR. Despite ongoing efforts to educate staff, patients, and their surrogates, DNR status continues to be associated with a dying patient, which in part accounts for its relative absence in the rehabilitation setting where death is not an expected outcome. It is always important to clarify that DNR does not mean Do Not Treat and that other treatments are not automatically affected (Phipps 1998).

Social Integration

Traumatic Brain Injury (TBI)

In recent years there has been a growing trend toward community-based, post-acute rehabilitation for individuals with TBI as opposed to the traditional, medical-center-based model, based on the premise that these individuals will learn more effectively in settings where they usually perform. In a study regarding adult TBI patients, outcomes at 2 years post-injury in 77 individuals with TBI, treated within the community, were compared regarding measures of their activities of daily living (ADL), vocational status, and emotional adjustment with those of 77 TBI patients individually matched for gender, age, education, occupation, post-traumatic amnesia (PTA) duration, Glasgow Coma Scale (GCS) score, and time in inpatient rehabilitation and who had been seen at the hospital for outpatient therapy. There were no significant differences between these groups in terms of employment outcomes or independence in personal or domestic ADL. However, those treated in the community were less likely to be independent when shopping and for their financial management and reported more changes in communication and social behavior. Due to the constraints of time and resources, these patients

had received fewer one-on-one therapy sessions, and therefore, their treatment costs were somewhat lower. Attendant care costs were also lower in the community treatment group (Ponsford et al. 2006).

Spinal Cord Injury (SCI)

Different strategies are necessary for different dimensions of autonomy. Strategies for independence included making independent function for the personal challenge and learning from others with SCI. Strategies for self-determination included keeping oneself informed, setting personal goals, and being assertive. Strategies for participation included making challenges out of barriers, planning and organizing, asking and accepting help, and dealing with reactions from others. Strategies for identification involved taking life as it comes and focusing on the positive aspects of life. Patients can be made aware of strategies for autonomy during the rehabilitation phase.

The relationships between perceived participation and problems in participation and life satisfaction in people with SCI are important issues. In a study using 157 SCI patients, the patients' perceived participation in the five domains of the Impact on Participation and Autonomy Questionnaire (IPA) was significantly correlated with their satisfaction with life as a whole and in most of the eight other domains of life satisfaction in the Life Satisfaction Questionnaire (LiSat-9) IPA. The patients' life satisfaction decreased gradually with the increasing frequency of severe problems in participation, and significant differences were found within patient groups with increasingly severe problems. The level of life satisfaction in respondents who perceived no severe problems with participation was similar to those of a normal population. Therefore, perceived participation and problems in participation are determinants of life satisfaction in people with SCI. The results emphasize the importance of focusing on severe problems with participation in order to optimize life satisfaction during rehabilitation after SCI. Perceived participation and problems in participation are determinants of life satisfaction in people with spinal cord injury (Lund et al. 2007).

E

Application

Ethical Issues in Practice

Neurorehabilitation clinicians are frequently asked to make clinical predictions regarding risk and harm persons with brain injury who are believed to be unable or in whom it is unsafe to conduct normal activities of daily living. Because predictions of risk and harm may ultimately limit a brain-injured person's autonomy, clinicians should be aware of the ethical and empirical issues involved in such determinations. Constraining autonomy can be an ethical problem even when clinicians are actually acting in patients' best interests. Clinicians must consider their ability to make exact risk and harm predictions based on clinical evidence. Clinicians who are aware of contemporary ethical principles will be most prepared to integrate ethical and empirical considerations when determining risk and harm (Macciocchi and Stringer 2001).

A set of ethics regarding relationships for brain injury rehabilitation is described based on three principles: (1) human relationships are important; (2) human relationships are as important as individual survival; and (3) human relationships are important enough to extend throughout the family of humankind. Within the context of these ethics, ethics of relationships, ethical conflict resolution is offered as a process to address disagreements among those involved in brain injury rehabilitation. Ethical conflict resolution provides means to arrive at moral decisions in situations in which people disagree regarding the appropriate course of action because of different values. Ethical conflict resolution recognizes that, although disagreements in brain injury rehabilitation settings can be associated with numerous other factors including disturbed self-awareness, emotions, communication, and interpersonal dynamics, such disagreements may also be value-based either in whole or in part. Ethical conflict resolution invites the professional team to identify the value-based component of these disagreements and provides a rational and supportive process to address disagreements (Malec 1996).

Cross-References

▶ Advance Directive
▶ Autonomy
▶ Withdrawal of Life-Support

References

Caplan AL, Callahan D, Haas J (1987) Ethical and policy issues in rehabilitation medicine. Hastings Cent Rep 17(4):S1–S19
Davey TM, Aitken LM, Kassulke D, Bellamy N, Ambrose J, Gee T et al (2005) Long-term outcomes of seriously injured children: a study using the child health questionnaire. J Paediatr Child Health 41(5–6):278–283
Giacino J, Whyte J (2005) The vegetative and minimally conscious states: current knowledge and remaining questions. J Head Trauma Rehabil 20(1):30–50
Levack WM, Kayes NM, Fadyl JK (2010) Experience of recovery and outcome following traumatic brain injury: a metasynthesis of qualitative research. Disabil Rehabil 32(12):986–999
Lund ML, Nordlund A, Bernspang B, Lexell J (2007) Perceived participation and problems in participation are determinants of life satisfaction in people with spinal cord injury. Disabil Rehabil 29(18):1417–1422
Macciocchi SN, Stringer AY (2001) Assessing risk and harm: the convergence of ethical and empirical considerations. Arch Phys Med Rehabil 82(12 Suppl 2): S15–S19
Malec JF (1996) Ethical conflict resolution based on an ethics of relationships for brain injury rehabilitation. Brain Inj 10(11):781–795
Phipps EJ (1998) Communication and ethics: cardiopulmonary resuscitation in head trauma rehabilitation. J Head Trauma Rehabil 13(5):95–98
Ponsford J, Harrington H, Olver J, Roper M (2006) Evaluation of a community-based model of rehabilitation following traumatic brain injury. Neuropsychol Rehabil 16(3):315–328
von Wild K (2008) Neuroethics with regard to treatment limiting and withdrawal of nutrition and hydration in long lasting irreversible full state apallic syndrome and minimal conscious state. J Med Life 1(4):443–453

Recommended Reading

Bernat JL (2009) Ethical issues in the treatment of severe brain injury: the impact of new technologies. Ann N Y Acad Sci 1157:117–130
Gagnon I, Swaine B, Champagne F, Lefebvre H (2008) Perspectives of adolescents and their parents regarding service needs following a mild traumatic brain injury. Brain Inj 22(2):161–173

Rundquist JM (2002) The right to die–ethical dilemmas in persons with spinal cord injury. SCI Nurs 19(1):7–10

Singh R, Dhankar SS, Rohilla R (2008) Quality of life of people with spinal cord injury in northern India. Int J Rehabil Res 31(3):247–251

Ethical Issues in the Conduct of Clinical Trials in Trauma Patients

Gavin M. Joynt[1] and Timothy Rainer[2]
[1]Department of Anaesthesia and Intensive Care, The Chinese University of Hong Kong, Hong Kong, China
[2]Accident and Emergency Department, Prince of Wales Hospital, The Chinese University of Hong Kong, Shatin, Hong Kong, China

Synonyms

Morality in clinical research; Research integrity

Definition

Ethics: Medical ethics describes a system of moral principles that applies values and judgments to the practice of medicine.

Medical research: Medical research is a systematic investigation designed to contribute to or extend generalizable human medical knowledge.

Clinical trial: Clinical trials involve human subjects and are designed to extend our knowledge of the physical, biological, or social responses of humans to biomedical or behavioral interventions. Typical interventions include investigating the effects of new tests, vaccines, drugs and devices, or new methods of delivery of known interventions on human subjects. Clinical trials should determine whether these biomedical or behavioral interventions are effective and safe.

Background

The ongoing conduct of research and specifically clinical trials relies on the agreement of a conceptual "moral contract" between investigators and society. Both accept that clinical trials are necessary for the advancement of medical knowledge that will benefit individuals in society. Society therefore accepts that some risk to individuals exposed to research can be justified in order to promote a common good. However, this risk should generally be small in magnitude, minimized as much as possible by trial design, and clearly justified by the likely beneficial outcomes, gain in knowledge, expected to be produced by the trial.

Current Western medical bioethics commonly utilizes the moral principles of autonomy, beneficence, non-maleficence, and justice to guide a moral framework within which medicine can be best practiced (Beauchamp and Childress 2001). In brief, *beneficence* recommends that health-care providers should work for the patient's good, *non-maleficence* that health-care providers should do the patient no harm, *autonomy* that health-care providers should respect a patient's right to self-rule, and *justice* that health-care providers should ensure fair allocation of available medical resources. While the strict practical application of these principles often proves difficult (and sometimes impossible), they have been interpreted and specified within the context of clinical research to provide a framework from which currently accepted norms of clinical research can be examined.

Ethical Principles in Clinical Research

The main moral principles that inform us about the ethical conduct of clinical research can be briefly summarized as follows:

1. Every individual participant's *autonomy* should be respected through his or her right of "voluntary informed consent." Persons with diminished autonomy are entitled to special protection, as there is a risk of exploitation of such vulnerable persons in the pursuit of scientific information. Such persons include children, those with diminished mental capacity, and prisoners. Voluntary informed consent has four main components: the participant must have the mental capacity to make the

decision, must receive sufficient information on the proposed experimental intervention in question (including the probability of expected benefits and risks), must be capable of comprehending the information, and must be able to provide his or her consent free of duress or coercion.

2. The principles of *non-maleficence and beneficence* dictate that the clinical trial should do no direct harm to the participant. Thus, clinical trials should be designed such that they maximize possible benefits and minimize risks. While the need to satisfy the principles of non-maleficence and beneficence primarily applies to the exposure risk and the possible benefit to the individual research participant, a limited risk for participants may be reasonably balanced against the gain for society on the basis of the beneficial effect of the knowledge gained from the research. Considering individual risk, in all clinical trials the investigational intervention should always be considered to be at least a par with conventional interventions, so-called clinical equipoise. Regarding societal gain, the principle of beneficence supports research that "makes it possible to avoid the harm that may result from the application of previously accepted routine practices that on closer investigation turn out to be dangerous"(Belmont Report 1979).

3. The principle of *justice*, when applied to the setting of clinical trials dictates that the benefit and burden of research be fairly distributed. In general, research participants should be recruited from those groups who will benefit from research, not convenience populations, especially those that are disadvantaged by local social, demographic, or financial circumstances.

Unfortunately, clinical trial investigators have not always adhered to such apparently sound principles when conducting research. The abuses investigated at the Nuremberg Doctor's trial, the conduct of the Tuskegee trial, the cases brought to light by Beecher in the 1960s, and many others have led to the requirement for greater governance in research (Horner and Minifie 2011). As a result, all clinical trials should be scrutinized

and approved by appropriately instituted Ethical Research Committees prior to commencement. Many jurisdictions have developed clearly documented requirements governing the ethical conduct of clinical trials. Examples include the international ethical guidelines for biomedical research involving human subjects (International Ethical Guidelines for Biomedical Research Involving Human Subjects 2002), the requirements for responsible conduct in research (RCR) in the USA (Basic HHS Policy for Protection of Human Research Subjects. US Department of health and human services 2009), the implementation of good clinical practice in the conduct of clinical trials in Europe (Directive on the Approximation of the Laws 2001), and many others.

Misconduct

It is worth remembering that while professional bodies and IRBs may provide guidance and general ethical oversight to investigators, ultimately it is the investigator that must bear the responsibility for the ethical conduct and reporting of clinical trials. Research misconduct in any form is devastating to society and the scientific and medical community. Research misconduct may be the result of failure to meet the standards referred to above, or breaches of scientific integrity such as the alteration or falsification of original data, plagiarism, unjustified multiple publication, publication suppression, or ghost writing. While the discovery of misconduct may result in the loss of a researcher's reputation, the right to future funding, or even their job, research misconduct continues to occur (Shafer 2010). In addition to personal sanction, there are the potentially harmful consequences of incorrect scientific data being introduced to the scientific community that needs to be considered. Lastly, the loss of the essential trust between scientists and society potentially jeopardizes future research.

Application

The nature of trauma patients sometimes renders the application of all of the above principles to trauma research difficult, or sometimes even impossible, and ethically acceptable methods of resolving the dilemmas must be explored.

Voluntary Informed Consent

The ability of investigators to complete a valid process of voluntary informed consent in the acute trauma setting is often difficult or not feasible. This is because treatment is often by necessity emergent, and time for proper discussion of risks and benefits is lacking. In addition, patients may be distracted by pain, or in a condition of reduced mental capacity as a result of brain injury, the use of recreational drugs, or the presence therapeutic analgesic/sedative drugs. Finally, the desire of the patient for immediate treatment in the trauma setting may unduly influence decision-making regarding consent. Any of these factors may prevent the ability of investigators to obtain valid voluntary informed consent. In addition, these factors also place these patients in a "vulnerable group" category and deserving of special protection in the setting of exposure to possible clinical trials.

Recognizing that individuals in society desire high-quality medical treatments, and that these are in large part developed through knowledge gained through clinical trials, methods to allow the conduct of clinical trials without prior consent in this setting have been explored. There have been several proposed solutions to this dilemma. Securing consent from close relatives or patient advocates is one way of safeguarding some form of autonomy in incapacitated patients; however, timely contact in the emergency trauma setting is seldom realistically achieved, especially given the usual need for rapid therapeutic/investigative intervention. More recently, patients have been entered into clinical trials without consent, but with strict participant safeguards. The specific safeguards implemented in this setting vary from region to region, but are broadly similar. In general to qualify for an exception from obtaining informed consent, clinical trials should meet several strict requirements. The following list summarizes the most commonly cited requirements for exception (International Ethical Guidelines for Biomedical Research Involving

Human Subjects 2002; US Food and Drug Administration 1996; Tri-Council Policy Statement 2010; Thompson 2003):

- The nature of the clinical trial is such that "voluntary informed consent" from the patient or a surrogate decision maker cannot be achieved. This generally means emergency, life-threatening situations in which the patient lacks sufficient capacity to give informed consent, and surrogates cannot be reached within in the time frame that the intervention must be applied.
- The clinical trial must be scientifically sound, and the intervention sufficiently established for justification of trials in critically ill humans.
- The risk to patients from the investigational treatment must be sufficiently small, given the clinical circumstances and standard clinical interventions.
- There should be potential benefit to be gained from the trial by the patient, and the potential knowledge gained for society must be meaningful.
- The trial should be approved by the relevant Clinical Ethics Committee/s and relevant regional authorities.
- Patients or their representatives should always have the opportunity to complete the "voluntary informed consent" process at the earliest opportunity and withdraw from the study if desired.
- An independent Trial/Data Monitoring Board should monitor the progress of the trial.
- Some, but not all, jurisdictions require that the community be informed and consulted about the clinical trial and consent conditions prior to commencement, and formally informed of the results of the trial.

While these conditions seem reasonable, significant problems with practical implementation of these safeguards have been experienced, and considerable time and careful exercise of good judgment is required by investigators, IRBs, and regulatory bodies when exception from informed consent is necessary (McClure et al. 2007).

What is the standard for sufficiently small risk and how is the degree of risk offset against amount of potential benefit? Is it sensible for researchers apply a "reasonable person" standard in deciding which risks potential subjects would agree to? These are difficult questions to answer. It would seem that at a minimum clinical equipoise is necessary if consent is to be waived. Conceptually, clinical equipoise may be accepted as existing "whenever at least a reasonable number of medical professionals believe the experimental treatment would be as good as, or better than the standard treatment, taking risks and benefits into account." In reality, establishing that equipoise exists between standard treatment and an experimental treatment can be a difficult exercise, as existing scientific data can be sparse or a challenge to interpret. As a minimum, it would seem necessary to establish a clearly documented, transparent process for the justification of equipoise, based on a consensus of independent experts, prior to proceeding with the development of clinical trial protocols and seeking of IRB or other regulatory approval (Largent et al. 2010).

Appropriate methods for consulting the community have not yet been developed, and attempts at implementation have resulted in the publication of several reports of the difficulties involved in adequately achieving this goal (Ernst and Fish 2005; Baren and Biros 2007). Nevertheless, it remains a requirement in some regions and it has been suggested that consultation might include meetings with local public officials and community groups, in addition to contacting members of any identifiable populations most likely to be eligible for the research. Use of the media to inform communities has also been suggested, although the success rate of reaching those who will ultimately participate in the research appears poor (McClure et al. 2003).

Justice

Rates of trauma are sometimes higher in countries or regions that are developing but remain historically disadvantaged. The testing of interventions by clinical trials in these populations is potentially problematic. This is especially true if the intervention being tested is likely to be expensive and therefore, if proved to be effective, unlikely to be utilized in the population in which the clinical testing was performed. In emergency trauma research, where exception from informed consent is also required, extra caution would seem prudent to avoid exploitation or the perception of exploitation of vulnerable groups.

Conclusion

Conducting clinical trials in trauma patients presents special challenges, particularly with regard to the conduct of interventional studies in emergency situations. In the absence of the practical ability to get consent prior to entry into the study, the use of additional safeguards to ensure sufficient patient protection is currently considered an acceptable approach to allow emergency research to proceed. Formalized processes incorporating these safeguards have been proposed and successfully used in various regions around the world. Despite this, the detailed requirements of individual bodies vary, sometimes in important dimensions, and in addition, implementation of all safeguards is not always achieved. There does, however, appear to be an increasing consensus that following a detailed system of safeguards devised by reputable professional organizations and supervised by an IRB is sufficient to protect human subjects in this setting.

Cross-References

▶ Autonomy
▶ Evaluating a Patient's Decision-Making Capacity
▶ Surrogate, Role in Decision-Making

References

Baren JM, Biros MH (2007) The research on community consultation: an annotated bibliography. Acad Emerg Med 14:346–352

Beauchamp TL, Childress JF (2001) Principles of biomedical ethics, 5th edn. Oxford University Press, Oxford

Directive on the Approximation of the Laws (2001) Regulations and administrative provisions of the member states relating to the implementation of good clinical practice in the conduct of clinical trials on medicinal products for human use. Directive 2001/20/EC. Offic J Eur Commun :0034–0044

Ernst AA, Fish S (2005) Exception from informed consent: viewpoint of institutional review boards–balancing risks to subjects, community consultation, and future directions. Acad Emerg Med 12:1050–1055

Horner J, Minifie FD (2011) Research ethics I: responsible conduct of research (RCR) – historical and contemporary issues pertaining to human and animal experimentation. J Speech Lang Hear Res 54:S303–S329

International Ethical Guidelines for Biomedical Research Involving Human Subjects. Revised Draft 2002. www.cioms.ch/publications/layout_guide2002.pdf. Accessed 2 May 2013

Largent EA, Wendler D, Emanuel E, Miller FG (2010) Is emergency research without initial consent justified?: the consent substitute model. Arch Intern Med 170:668–674

McClure KB, DeIorio NM, Gunnels MD, Ochsner MJ, Biros MH, Schmidt TA (2003) Attitudes of emergency department patients and visitors regarding emergency exception from informed consent in resuscitation research, community consultation, and public notification. Acad Emerg Med 10:352–359

McClure KB, DeIorio NM, Schmidt TA, Chiodo G, Gorman P (2007) A qualitative study of institutional review board members' experience reviewing research proposals using emergency exception from informed consent. J Med Ethics 33:289–293

Shafer SL (2010) Notice of retraction. Anesth Analg 111(6):1567

The Belmont Report (1979) Ethical principles and guidelines for the protection of human subjects of research. The National Commission for the Protection of Human Subjects of Biomedical and Behavioral Research. http://www.hhs.gov/ohrp/humansubjects/guidance/belmont.html. Accessed 2 May 2013

Thompson J (2003) Ethical challenges of informed consent in prehospital research. Can J Emerg Res 5:108–114

Tri-Council Policy Statement (2010) Ethical conduct for research involving humans (TCPS 2), 2nd edn. Government of Canada, Panel on research ethics. http://www.pre.ethics.gc.ca/eng/policy-politique/initiatives/tcps2-eptc2/Default/. Accessed 2 May 2013

US Department of Health and Human Services (2009) Basic HHS policy for protection of human research subjects. 45 CFR 46. http://www.hhs.gov/ohrp/humansubjects/guidance/45cfr46.html. Accessed 2 May 2013

US Food and Drug Administration (1996) Protection of human subjects; informed consent and waiver of informed consent requirements in certain emergency research. Federal Register 61(192). http://www.fda.gov/ScienceResearch/SpecialTopics/RunningClinicalTrials/ucm118995.htm. Accessed 2 May 2013

Ethical Issues in Trauma Anesthesia

Marko Jukić[1], Iris Dupanović[2] and Mirsad Dupanovic[3]
[1]Department of Anesthesiology, University of Split, Split, Dalmatia, Croatia
[2]University of Missouri, Kansas City, MO, USA
[3]Department of Anesthesiology, Kansas University Medical Center, The University of Kansas Hospital, Kansas City, KS, USA

Synonyms

Bioethics; Biomedical ethics; Clinical ethics; Medical ethics

Definition

Medical ethics represent the application of general moral principles in medicine. These principles should provide a practicing physician with reasonable guidelines for interacting with patients. Bioethical principles are usually incorporated in guidelines issued by national health care authorities around the world. Additionally, ethical codes of professional medical societies provide members with recommendations about generally accepted ethical principles and their duty while caring for patients. The American Society of Anesthesiologists' (ASA) standards of conduct recommend working professionally with all members of the medical team, providing the highest standard of care, and protecting the interests of patients as well as the interests of the broader social community (Guidelines 2012).

Preexisting Condition

Scientists, theoreticians, and philosophers/ethicists have developed basic ethical premises;

they have worked out ethical theories and their application. Their theoretical premises are the result of personal worldviews, religious beliefs, cultural heritage (tradition), political views, and social trends. Pluralistic societies, diversity of cultures, and beliefs might affect moral attitudes, so that something that was moral at one particular time and place can be seen as being immoral at another time and place (Pence 2004; Pellegrino 1993; Jonsen 1992).

In everyday practice, physicians may encounter ethical dilemmas, some of which may be easily resolved, while others require far more consideration and sometimes assistance. A set of six fundamental ethical principles (autonomy, beneficence, non-maleficence, fidelity, justice, utility) should ideally be a moral guide to practicing physicians. Respect for the autonomous decisions of a competent patient about his/her medical care is the cornerstone of contemporary bioethics. Additionally, providing for the patient's benefit, providing truthful communications, preventing harm, respecting the patient's privacy, and protecting personal medical data are other moral responsibilities of physicians. Physicians also have ethical obligations toward society. They should provide the same level of care to all patients, regardless of their social status or immediate availability of resources to pay for the treatment. Physicians should also care for the greater societal good by not wasting available medical resources. In elective situations physicians should have sufficient time to explain and discuss pertinent issues of medical care with patients, their families, colleagues, and even hospital administrators. However, a comprehensive consideration of ethical principles in acute trauma is challenging because of the emergent nature of the disease, the potential presence of life-threatening injuries, the need for immediate invasive interventions, the frequent unconsciousness due to acute intoxication or traumatic brain injury, and the consequent lack of decision-making capacity. Insufficient patient information, absence of family members, limitation of available resources, duty to provide care for others, and possible end-of-life decisions may be additional factors that make quick and sound ethical reasoning in acute trauma not easy and potentially controversial.

Application

Pragmatic Issues in Acute Trauma

An immediate consequence of acute trauma may be mental incapacity and an inability to make autonomous decisions. It would be ideal, from an ethical standpoint, if physicians could wait for the patient to regain his/her decision-making capacity, discuss pertinent medical issues, and then obtain the patient's consent for the necessary medical treatment. However, such an approach is not always feasible from a practical standpoint. Significant deterioration of a patient's condition may occur within minutes, and major harm or death may be the result of reluctance to intervene immediately. This conviction of impending serious harm and certainty that the harm may be reduced by an immediate action, with time as the essential factor for successful resuscitation, dictates the instantaneous actions of the trauma team. Treatment of primary injuries, prevention of secondary injuries, and meaningful survival are the goals of resuscitation. However, since the autonomy of a competent patient is the leading ethical principle, concerns and controversies about the morality of treating trauma patients with invasive procedures but without the patient's informed consent may arise. Emergency medicine physicians, surgeons, and anesthesiologist must be competent and they must work together in a coordinated effort to provide the best possible care. The existence of "the golden hour of trauma care" points toward time as the most important finite resource that needs to be allocated effectively; its poor allocation may have practical and ethical implications. Oftentimes when accidents occur, there may be several people who are injured, or in the case of a mass casualty incident, there may be a great number of people who are injured. In all these situations, treating patients effectively requires an efficient use of time. In such cases, patients may be triaged or categorized based on how urgently they need medical attention and/or on the probability of survival, considering the availability of existing medical resources. The approach to these ethical dilemmas may differ based on the regulations that are in place in different countries.

As already mentioned, resuscitation and treatment of acutely traumatized patients requires a pragmatic approach, making blunt decisions, and teamwork. Physicians should not only posses the knowledge of basic and clinical medical sciences but also be competent in performing life-saving procedures. For anesthesiologists, the approved practice privileges may differ depending on the type and the length of training, as well as the country and the type of legal environment of the medical practice. In general, the professional duties of the anesthesiologist in trauma include, but are not limited to, assistance in initial assessment and resuscitation of a trauma victim, ensuring the optimal functions of the vital organ systems, prevention and/or treatment of traumatic hemorrhagic shock, administration of blood products, delivering appropriate anesthesia and sedation, prevention of secondary injury, and involvement in postoperative care (Merchant et al. 2012).

Application of Ethical Principles in Acute Trauma

Autonomy, Beneficence, Non-maleficence, and Fidelity

Under elective circumstances, the four basic bioethical principles of autonomy, beneficence, non-maleficence, and fidelity are in balance. However, in order to be pragmatic in emergent clinical situations, priority may have to be given to some principles over others. Beneficence and non-maleficence frequently prevail over autonomy and fidelity in major trauma, while utility supersedes social justice in disaster situations.

Patient autonomy represents the culmination of a patient's self-determination and is a dominant ethical principle in Western societies. Autonomy represents the right of a competent patient to make voluntary choices about his/her medical care. It is exemplified in the process of obtainment of informed consent, which represents the authorization of an invasive medical intervention or participation in research. Obtainment of informed consent is an autonomous, open, and voluntary process. It occurs after the explanation of risks and benefits of the procedure. However, the patient's competence to comprehend important issues is a mandatory element for the process to be valid.

Beneficence and non-maleficence are two other fundamental bioethical principles that apply to all doctor-patient encounters (Table 1). In trauma situations, this means that health care providers maintain the highest standards of practice by saving lives, saving vital organs, preventing disability, and alleviating pain. This is based on a principle-based ethical view: Every patient must get the best treatment for him/her at any given time (Gail 2011).

The right of a competent patient to self-determination by making informed and autonomous decisions, based on the truth, about issues pertaining to his/her own health and life may sometimes prevail over beneficence and non-maleficence. However, situations of acute trauma present some of the greatest threats to life and require the highest level of decision-making capacity at a time when patients often become incompetent. Even if conscious, patients may still be mentally shocked after an assault or an accident, may have comprehension difficulties, and temporarily may not be able to make informed and autonomous decisions. Since deterioration of the patient's medical condition in major trauma can occur within minutes, pragmatic choices need to be made by the medical team in order to prevent additional harm. Head injury may result in coma. Severe airway and chest trauma or carbon monoxide intoxication may result in hypoxia and agitation, requiring immediate sedation and tracheal intubation. Additionally, acutely traumatized patients may have severe injuries to the abdomen, pelvis, limbs, or all three. Life-threatening hemorrhages will require immediate use of anesthetic drugs that render the patient unconscious and unaware of life-saving surgical procedures. Since surrogate decision making is not always possible in acute trauma, a patient's autonomy becomes nonexistent. Thus, beneficence and non-maleficence become the dominant

E

Ethical Issues in Trauma Anesthesia, Table 1 Six basic bioethical principles are exemplified in an elective doctor-patient relationship[a] and presented along with challenges of an acute trauma situation[b]

Bioethical principle	Elective doctor-patient relationship[a]	Considerations in acute trauma[b]
Autonomy	Self-determination = the patient knows what is the best for him/her	The patient's decision-making capacity may be diminished or absent; no advance directive or legal surrogate; ultimately paternalistic approach applies (doctors know what is the best for the patient)
Beneficence	Represent the patient's best interest and do only good to patients	Additionally, make resolute decisions, perform quick actions, and utilize multidisciplinary approach in resuscitation and treating primary injuries
Non-maleficence	Do not harm patients	Additionally, prevent secondary injury to the patient and prevent accidental injuries to medical personnel
Fidelity	Patients deserve to know the truth at all times	The patient may have sustained traumatic brain injury, be unresponsive, or be sedated
Justice	All patients deserve the same level of medical care	Utilitarian principle is used in disasters: provide the most good to most patients
Utility	Do not waste available medical resources	Make the most out of available medical resources

decision-making principles and supersede autonomy and fidelity. Ultimately, a paternalistic ethical approach prevails and the consent is implied. It is presumed that if conscious, every patient would agree with a physician's decision for the best medical treatment. However, it is important that under such circumstances physicians adhere not only to the highest standards of medical care but that they also follow the highest standards of ethical care. Basically, the same set of moral rules apply in an elective and an emergency situation, even though the actions may be different (Gert 2005).

Justice and Utility

Generally, justice and utility may be complementary ethical principles; however, in some situations one principle may supersede the other. Faithfulness to a physician's duty and treating all patients fairly according to their medical needs are part of the Hippocratic oath and should always be upheld. Physicians may encounter patients whose political, religious, or moral beliefs radically differ from theirs. However, the same treatment should be provided to all patients. An example of justice represents treating war prisoners.

Utility refers to the practical ethical principle, one that regards the goal of ethical actions as doing what is best for the greater good or what will benefit the largest number of people. Utility is most often used when there are limiting factors involved, such as a limited number of resources. An example of a conflict of resource availability may be a situation in which a patient with an aortic injury undergoing an emergency surgery requires 100 or more units of blood for resuscitation. In this case, the odds of the patient's survival may be very low, and there may be a threat that the resources of the blood bank will be exhausted, endangering the ability to provide care for other patients. Futile treatment is not the purpose of medicine. Strict rationing of hospital resources is a principle utilized during resource-limited disaster situations. However, the same standard may not apply during times of plenty, and mismanagement may lead to significant reduction or total depletion of the vital resources of a hospital or an entire region. The manner in which to approach this ethical dilemma in a practical manner may vary depending on the legal, social, and cultural environment of the physician's practice.

Group Considerations

Care of children may frequently involve ethical controversies related to issues surrounding patient autonomy, beneficence, non-maleficence, and justice (Baines 2008). These issues may be controversial, even in elective situations (e.g., blood transfusion in a Jehovah's Witnesses patient, refusal of chemotherapy because of religious beliefs), and may require legal actions in order to act in the child's best interest. Similar controversies may appear during provision of care to an acutely injured child. Additional ethical conflict will appear if injuries to the child were inflicted by parents or legal caregivers. In most of these situations, physicians will regard the beneficence and non-maleficence of a patient as the highest priorities. However, this may not be the rule in various cultural and legal environments across the globe.

Adolescents are frequent injury victims, especially in traffic accidents. Traumatic brain injury may be a consequence, and it may leave the patient incapacitated for a long time, even for life. Since these injuries typically occur unexpectedly, there has usually not been legal preparation for circumstances of diminished decision-making capacity. These patients will most likely not have an advance health care directive like a living will or durable power of attorney. For that reason, decisions will often have to be made by undesignated surrogates, and the patient's autonomy will be practically nonexistent. There is also ethical controversy about whether the entirety of the circumstances surrounding the trauma should be disclosed to a victim's surrogates. Following a successful recovery, the trauma victim may hold someone liable for disclosing trauma circumstances to surrogates. Additionally, ethical controversy surrounds the determination of an age at which adolescents should be entitled to make their own decisions about their medical care. Should this occur at the same age for all children? (Baines 2008).

Elderly patients may more commonly have a living will, durable power of attorney, or a "do not resuscitate" legal order. However, in an acute trauma situation resuscitation, medical personnel may not have knowledge of any directive and may provide medical care that is in accordance with the current standards of practice, but not in accordance with patient's orders. In this situation, the principles of beneficence and non-maleficence prevail over autonomy and fidelity. Dementia may be another significant factor affecting the autonomy of elderly patients.

Psychiatric conditions and language barriers are additional factors preventing flawless communication of the patient's wishes. In multicultural societies, specific cultural values of patients belonging to a minority culture may be deeply ingrained but may be not in line with the values of the predominant culture in the society. The standard procedures, like full body exposure, performed during the initial trauma assessment, may breach specific cultural and ethical values of certain patients. There may also be a possible conflict between the anesthesiologist's and the patient's cultural values. This may make the above list of ethical controversies in trauma even more complicated.

Jehovah's Witnesses reject receiving blood and blood derivatives on religious grounds. The National Health Service in Great Britain has issued Guidelines on Clinical Management of Jehovah's Witnesses (Guidelines 2005). The American Society of Anesthesiologists has also given recommendations for cases in which the patient does not want to be resuscitated or rejects some therapeutic procedures. In the United States and Western Europe, respecting the patient's autonomy represents the most significant ethical principle. Physicians are obliged to explain the potential medical consequences of refusal of treatment, but the self-determination of a competent patient must be respected. Patients usually provide a special statement confirming their choice. Some other countries may have the same principle-based view but may allow or require the physician to act contrary to the patient's wishes in some situations, such as emergency situations during a life-saving procedure. Hospitals will usually have policies about these issues that should be in accordance with national guidelines. The physician must be well informed about the legal regulations of the country in which he/she works, familiarize himself/herself with the recommendations of professional associations, and know the current policies in his/her work environment (Gail 2011).

Do-Not-Resuscitate (DNR) Orders

A competent patient may produce a legal statement declaring how he/she desires to be treated in case of a life-threatening event that may require resuscitation and use of life-sustaining devices (cardiopulmonary resuscitation, electrical shocks, artificial ventilation, artificial nutrition, blood transfusion, hemodialysis, etc.). The patient may refuse to accept some or all of these or other similar procedures and treatments. It is the patient's basic right to have these decisions respected, not to have his/her agony prolonged, and to be allowed to die with dignity. The surgeon, anesthesiologists, and other team members must be familiar with the directives of the particular DNR order (Gail 2011; Pellegrino 2000). The legal document (a statement with patient's signature and co-signatures of witnesses) is legally binding. In some countries, patients may even wear a DNR bracelet. If such a patient is coming for an elective surgery, the anesthesiologist can usually provide guidance to the patient about the controversial issues of his/her DNR order while under general anesthesia. Those orders are usually created by patients with the intent to prevent prolonged treatment in the intensive care unit in case of a critical illness. Even if identified, a DNR order in case of an acute trauma may be controversial. The anesthesiologist must carefully discuss the pertinent issues with the competent patient or with a legal surrogate, in case of the patient's incompetence. The anesthesiologist must explain the situation, clarify his/her position, and inform the patient or the surrogate about the consequences of refusal of treatment. The anesthesiologist may obtain informed consent from the competent patient or his/her legal surrogate about which procedures to undertake and which to forgo. If the wishes of the patient or the surrogate contradict generally accepted principles or are contrary to the anesthesiologist's worldview, then the anesthesiologist may consider refusing to participate in treatment and may attempt to find a substitute. However, because of practical staffing issues, this is usually not a feasible option in urgent or emergent situations frequently encountered in acute trauma.

Testing Patients for Alcohol, Drugs, Diseases, and Pregnancy

Physicians are morally and legally obligated to observe confidentiality or to uphold the trust and privacy of the patient-physician relationship. Certain ethical conflicts may occur if a patient is unable to give consent and the information gathered is kept strictly confidential. Testing a trauma patient immediately upon arrival to the emergency room for blood level of alcohol, opiates, benzodiazepines, cocaine, and other recreational drugs may be part of the standard battery of tests at many hospitals. In addition, performing a pregnancy test may also be a routine procedure. In some cases of acute trauma, these tests are performed without patient consent and may be seen as a breach of privacy. Whether testing can be done without patient consent depends on the laws of the area. In some areas, even if a patient's capacity is impaired, their consent may be required for testing of these conditions, no matter how urgently these tests need to be conducted. In other areas, patients may be able to be tested without explicit consent if consent is unable to be obtained; however, testing may not be the correct solution in every situation. In this case, a physician must be able to evaluate whether patient care necessitates testing.

There are clear benefits to testing patients, such as the ability to change the course of treatment or to provide counseling and educational resources. However, positive test results for drugs and diseases may have significant implications for the patient, depending on the individual situation, such as loss of a job or their medical care not being covered by insurance.

Summary

The anesthesiologist must be familiar with the principles of medical ethics, his/her legal environment, the recommendations of professional societies, and pragmatic solutions to bioethical dilemmas. A comprehensive application of generally accepted ethical principles may be challenging and/or counterproductive in situations of acute trauma where resolute decisions and quick actions are required. This is even more complicated in disaster situations involving treatment of multiply traumatized patients with various emergent medical needs. A pragmatic approach where beneficence and non-maleficence prevail over autonomy and fidelity should be acceptable in most situations of an incapacitated, acutely traumatized patient. However, the anesthesiologist must remain ethically sensitive and professionally competent when making these important decisions and must adhere to the highest ethical standards of his/her profession.

Cross-References

► Advance Directive
► Autonomy
► Evaluating a Patient's Decision-Making Capacity
► Futile Care
► Informed Consent in Trauma
► Life Support, Withholding and Withdrawal of
► Patient Confidentiality
► Rationing Hospital Resources During Mass Casualty Disasters
► Refusal of Treatment by Critical Patients
► Surrogate, Role in Decision-Making
► Terminal Care
► Triage
► Withdrawal of Life-Support

References

Baines P (2008) Medical ethics for children: applying the four principles of paediatrics. J Med Ethics 34:141–145
Gail AVN (2011) Clinical ethics in anesthesiology (a case-based textbook). Cambridge University Press, New York
Gert JH (2005) How are emergencies different from other medical situations? Mt Sinai J Med 72:216–221
Guidelines for the ethical practice of anesthesiology. Approved by the ASA House of Delegates on October 15, 2003, and last amended on October 22, 2008) http://www.asahq.org/publicationsAndServices/sgstoc.htm. Accessed 1 Nov 2012
Guidelines on Clinical Management of Jehovah's Witnesses. Maidstone and Tunbridge Wells NHS Trust, London, 2005
Jonsen AR (1992) Clinical ethics: a practical approach to ethical decisions in clinical medicine. Macmillan, New York
Merchant R, Chartrand D, Dain S et al (2012) Guidelines to the practice of anesthesia – revised edition. Can J Anesth 59:63–102
Pellegrino ED (1993) The metamorphosis of medical ethics. A 30-year retrospective. JAMA 269(9):1158–1162
Pellegrino ED (2000) Decisions to withdraw life-sustaining treatment: a moral algorithm. JAMA 283(8):1065–1067
Pence GE (2004) Classic cases in medical ethics: accounts of cases that have shaped medical ethics, with philosophical, legal, and historical backgrounds. McGraw-Hill, New York

Ethical Issues Surrounding the Use of New Technology in Trauma Care

Cook-John Lee
Trauma Service, Department of Surgery, Ajou Trauma Center, School of Medicine, Ajou University, Suwon, South Korea

Synonyms

Evolving surgery; New technology; Work ethic

Definition

Ethics are guidelines to influence humans in a manner intended to protect and fulfill the rights of individuals in a society.

Just as a core definition of "ethics of new technology on trauma" is needed, a core definition of "new technology" is needed as well. New technology consists of both a method of treatment and new instruments. Any consistent application of a surgeon's beliefs on the new technology that is supposed to be employed to achieve a purpose should be used for saving trauma victims. New technology is not the goal itself; it is nothing but a tool which is applied to achieve a goal.

Background

Surgeons are often consulted to take care of massively injured patients because they play a pivotal role in managing such victims using emergency procedures or operative techniques. They attempt to arrive at the best solution. In other words, surgeons have a great tendency to discover alternative ways for better treatment; there might be many ways by which the patient arrives at a complete recovery. Surgeons are able to learn new technology from postgraduate surgical residents or fellowship interns by repeating the patient care procedures so that they may confirm their certitude that the procedure is invariable. However, surgeons might be influenced by presentations or theories which have not been confirmed yet. Many new surgical devices, without sufficient evidence of effectiveness and safety, are being marketed. The ethical issues faced by surgeons have never been more challenging than they are today.

Many recent editorials have discussed the dangers of early adoption of new surgical products and methods. Although a manufacturer is supposed to meet all the requirements of a government licensing authority before marketing this product, trauma surgeons should be very careful when employing new techniques. Clearly, there is no second chance on trauma victims!

Introduction

Since human beings first appeared on the planet, trauma issues must have been closely connected to our daily life. Although it is difficult to imagine the struggle of early humans for survival in chronic medical diseases, it is quite clear to see ancient surgeons initially treated injuries by empirical surgical techniques. Meanwhile, surgical procedures have developed. Since then, surgeons are often those who introduce new technologies. Any patient who has been injured is supposed to promptly be transferred to the trauma center where surgeons could evaluate his/her injuries and administer appropriate treatment.

Due to concerns over the new technology in the field of trauma, technological advances have stirred medical controversy. Reflecting on the technological shifts of the past two decades, it is appropriate to address whether new technologies introduce new ethical problems.

There are aspects of applying new technology that have implications in the "ethical" use of technology. New technology is not only expensive but may have unexpected side effects. On the other hand, new technologies might promise the possibility of great economic returns and make surgeons proud.

In contrast to the medical development process, the development of ethical systems to govern new surgical applications is slower for several reasons. The development of ethical guidelines does not take place in a controlled environment, and there is not a real competitive structure in treating patients. The growth of ethical controversies surrounding the new surgical technology illustrates these conditions and ethical guidelines.

These new surgical technologies may offer today's greatest challenges to the trauma surgeons for several reasons. Many of these are closely involved in saving and protecting patients. Controversies over these new surgical technologies are not new, but little progress has been made to prepare us for today's medical capabilities. In addition, the potential for improving outcomes through medical treatment begs the questions of fairness in access and applicability.

Clinical Fields

Every single surgeon should be responsible for establishing his own standards when introducing new technologies. More importantly, the practical implications of these "new technologies" often lead to horrible results as exemplified by current debates over minimal invasive surgery or robotic surgery. There is such false belief that the new must be better. The surgeon should assess the evidence of effectiveness as well as safety of the treatment and as well his own competence in its use. If the surgeon has doubts about either aspect, he should not use the new treatment (Iserson and Chiasson 2002).

Surgeons would like to apply new technologies for many reasons. It is of the utmost importance for surgeons to think of the benefit for patients who receive new technologies as part of surgical procedures. Surgeons tend to think that new procedures would be more effective and safer than conventional methods (Gates 1997; Norton 2006). Surgeons may desire to learn new techniques so that they can be leaders in their field as well (Gates 1997). Lots of new procedures requiring medical devices are getting interest because they tend to be less invasive and seem to have shorter admission days. In addition, the obvious ease of use may lead to adoption by less skilled young surgeons.

The trauma surgeon should stay on the best level of knowledge to make clinical choices rather than adopt new technology so easily. Delay in adoption of new ways of treatment might make a surgeon feel left behind. Frankly speaking, this could be quite a terrible fear for some surgeons. However, patients are the weakest point in the introduction of new medical technology; it is they who will be damaged as the consequences of a new device used inappropriately. Quite different from our common senses, newer technology could not promise absolute improvements over conventional procedures (American College of Obstetricians and Gynecologists Committee on Ethics 2006), and hasty application of new technology might affect objective result of device's effectiveness and safety (Bekelman et al. 2003). Unfortunately, there is no second chance for a trauma victim. Too early adoption into clinical practice of new technology with only limited evidence of effectiveness may lead one to believe that patients do not get a standard of care (Nandi 2000). It could produce terrible results in a trauma setting. As final decision makers of the trauma victims, trauma surgeons maintain the greatest moral and ethical responsibility. The surgeon should bear in mind that, in a trauma setting, trauma patients are mostly unable to choose, or discuss with surgeons, the procedures. The trauma victims cannot truly give informed consent.

Manufacturers

Manufacturers allow themselves to be persuaded by the intensive promotion of new products. One area where the ethical field of new surgical technology has remained backwards is in the industrial aspect. Advances in this field are quickly coming to challenge our application of new surgical products.

With new technologies developing so quickly today, there is the risk of monopolistic giants approaching whose aim is to develop and invent new surgical devices and procedures without proper control over key technologies. Along with the surgeons who are always seeking new technologies, lots of medical device manufacturers are delivering enormous amounts of new medical products.

Consider the rapid spread of the new medical devices industry. Consider the frequency with which robotic surgical instrument has appeared throughout our operating theatres as well. As these new surgical technologies build and are spreading out, they create advantages for patients and companies with special technologies useful to surgeons.

Although the data is provided by manufacturers, still some companies are quite reluctant to carry out expensive multicenter and large-scale clinical trials, which might delay the release and increase the cost of new products. Honestly, carrying out such rigorous randomized trials is definitely complex and costly (Bernstein and Bampoe 2004). There is firm evidence that manufacturers might influence the research findings and how they are published (Winter 2000). Without guidelines on new surgical devices, on which perceptions of trust and justice should be based, manufacturers could not carry on.

The vital aim of companies is to satisfy shareholders with financial success. Finally, there is a pressing need for attention to ethical issues concerning the new device's effectiveness and safety. Even though no company will truly ignore patient safety and satisfaction, most try to build sufficient safeguards into the regulations. In order to meet the ethical obligations of beneficence and non-maleficence, manufacturers should be prepared to cooperate with physicians in the appropriate study of their products before releasing them and showing the objective evidence (Gates 1997). This is a difficult challenge. However difficult, the challenge must be overcome, since it is core in issues of new surgical progress, and once a consensus is built on a reasonable idea basis, it will be easier to find a vehicle for the next consensus. Even from a business development perspective, any complication or side effect of new procedures would add financial uncertainty to the investment required for development and market diffusion.

Application

As new ways of treatment and devices develop, how will they be controlled? Do we have any proper surveillance system?

Government, rather than manufacturers, may be the more powerful and better choice of institution to look toward for guidelines. While debates and efforts regarding governance of new surgical technologies have been active for many decades, much of the debate in the past was based in speculation. Most civilized countries' governments are advising that surgeons are not allowed to adopt new technology until evidence is definitely seen from rigorous randomized clinical trials. There are pressing needs for guidelines in order to avoid malpractice involving new surgical technologies. "Guidelines" do not simply mean laws for specific products. Guidelines also include basic principles of analysis, beliefs, and assumptions about the introduction of new surgical technologies. Significant new technologies often generate a period of initial excitement and euphoria. Even so, at a basic level, there should be a government's exploration of the ethical implications of new surgical technologies.

There are clear ethical roles for hospitals in the introduction of new technologies on elective patients (Iserson and Chiasson 2002). However, as stated earlier, it is impossible to give an appropriate explanation to major trauma victims in most cases. The responsibility of hospitals is to make sure that trauma patients are treated with confident procedures and the review process be followed in every single complicated case (Bernstein and Bampoe 2004). If institutions rely on individual surgeon's opinions rather than careful evaluation of procedures, such institutions will be criticized for failing to fulfill their responsibilities (Iserson and Chiasson 2002; Bernstein and Bampoe 2004). Looking back on history, lots of trials conducted after favorable initial reports sometimes show less benefit than initially predicted or even show harm (Gates 1997) in later trials (Eaton and Kennedy 2007).

As a practical matter, ethical guidelines for new surgical technology must be accepted by surgeons, patients, and manufacturers in order to be effective. Such acceptance requires the development of consensus rooted in the patient's safety and effectiveness in treatment compared to conventional treatments.

Professional societies such as surgical societies should take responsibility in providing guidance, as well. Every single senior member in a surgical society should be careful to not allow themselves to be affected by anything outside of patient's safety issues. Among the concerns of surgical societies, the ethical introduction of new medical treatments and surgical devices must be based on objective reports and very conservative. It is important to keep in mind that managing major trauma patients is quite different than treating elective-based disease patients.

Conclusions

New technologies change our way of treatment, recovery time, and treatment outcome. Today's accelerating pace of technological change exacerbates an ever-widening gap between new technologies and accepted ethical guidelines for their use. The issue we face today is how to improve the process to make it more effective in saving trauma victims. The consensus regarding technological improvements should be created without the influence of manufacturers or the opinions of young surgeons who want to be the first to apply something new. Surgeons, governments, and academic societies should demand properly designed prospective studies from industry to support their decision making. They should also resist the adoption of new devices until appropriate evidence is available (Terry 2007).

Government and academic societies must determine now whether and which new technologies would be allowed, and if the preliminary studies are successful, how we will ethically apply the results to the clinical field. Ultimately, it is the surgeon's job to make the decision to adopt such a new technology by using the available information, the experience of his colleges, and the teaching programs of academic societies.

Proven safety and effectiveness is a key concern in adopting a new technology in trauma surgery, but it should be also a concern for many fields. On average, it will take a new technology at least a couple of years to become accepted as a safe procedure. It is quite clear that the standard of evidence required for new surgical technology is similar to that required for new pharmaceutical products. Furthermore, the standards of evidence required for licensing surgical devices should be as rigorous as those required for licensing medicines. As things currently stand, the early marketing and adoption of surgical devices leads to potential hazards for both patients and surgeons (Norton 2006).

The culture and the prestige of trauma surgery, associated with the treatment of patients, exerts enormous pressures against mistakes which lead to deaths. Trauma surgeons should choose the safest method of treatment until the desired new technology is proven absolutely safe. The field of trauma surgery will remain one of the most conservative areas in all areas of medicine, both ethically and clinically.

Cross-References

▶ Ethical Issues in the Conduct of Clinical Trials in Trauma Patients
▶ Surrogate, Role in Decision-Making
▶ Traumatology

References

American College of Obstetricians and Gynecologists Committee on Ethics (2006) ACOG Committee Opinion No. 352: innovative practice: ethical guidelines. Obstet Gynecol 108(6):1589–1595
Bekelman JE, Li Y, Gross CP (2003) Scope and impact of financial conflicts of interest in biomedical research: a systematic review. JAMA 289(4):454–465
Bernstein M, Bampoe J (2004) Surgical innovation or surgical evolution: an ethical and practical guide to handling novel neurosurgical procedures. J Neurosurg 100(1):2–7
Eaton ML, Kennedy D (2007) The need to ask questions about innovation. In: Eaton ML, Kennedy D (eds) Innovation in medical technology – ethical issues and challenges. John Hopkins University Press, Baltimore, pp 1–22
Gates EA (1997) New surgical procedures: can our patients benefit while we learn? Am J Obstet Gynecol 176:1293–1298
Iserson KV, Chiasson PM (2002) The ethics of applying new medical technologies. Semin Laparosc Surg 9(4):222–229
Norton P (2006) New technology in gynaecologic surgery: is new necessarily better? Am J Obstet Gynecol 108:707–708
Nandi PL (2000) Ethical aspects of clinical practice. Arch Surg 135:22–25
Terry S, Kaplan LJ (2007) Ethical imperatives in staffing and managing a trauma intensive care unit. Crit Care Med 35(2):24–28
Winter RB (2000) Innovation in surgical technique. The story of spine surgery. Clin Orthop Relat Res 378(9):9–14

E

Ethics

▶ Brain Death, Ethical Concerns

Etiquette

▶ Technology Interfacing, Etiquette, and Electronic Safety

ETOH Withdrawal

▶ Alcohol (ETOH) Withdrawal and Management

Evacuants

▶ Bowel Active Agents in the ICU

Evaluating a Patient's Decision-Making Capacity

Jin Pyo Hong[1] and Subin Park[2]
[1]Department of Psychiatry, University of Ulsan College of Medicine, Seoul, Republic of Korea
[2]Department of Psychiatry, Seoul National Hospital, Seoul, Republic of Korea

Synonyms

Competence to consent to treatment; Reasoning in consent capacity

Definition

Decision-making capacity is a medical term that affirms a patient's ability to make informed decisions about his or her health care at a particular point in time (American College of Physicians 2005).

The physician is responsible for explaining the proposed intervention and the reasons for making the recommendation as well as disclosing the risks, benefits, and alternatives. The patient is expected to understand, weigh the options with respect to his or her own values and goals, and express a preference to the physician (Chow et al. 2010).

Background

Any diagnosis or treatment that compromises mental function may be associated with incompetence. Patients with impaired competence are commonly found in medical and surgical inpatient units and most commonly among infectious and neurological patients (Appelbaum 2007). Patients with dementias, stroke, schizophrenia, and bipolar disorder may have high levels of impairment in decision making. In the absence of accompanying cognitive impairment, common medical conditions, such as diabetes mellitus, coronary artery disease, and viral infection, have not been found to be associated with incapacity in decision making.

Patients with neuropsychiatric syndrome due to head trauma have high rates of incompetence. Every patient with head trauma should be evaluated about decision-making capacity.

Common Indications

Assessing a patient's medical decision-making capacity is part of every medical encounter. Without it, there can be no informed consent. Decision-making capacity is always considered to be specific to the certain decision in question (Grisso and Appelbaum 1998). Certain patients may be able to decide some aspects of their care but not others. Furthermore, the level of evidence required to confirm decision-making capacity varies on a continuum with the benefits and risks associated with the clinical circumstances. With respect to the situation in which a patient is refusing the recommended care, circumstances involving lower risk in which the recommended care is of marginal benefit require a lower threshold of decision-making capacity (e.g., drawing serial hematocrits to monitor mild to moderate anemia in the setting of a gastrointestinal bleed). However, circumstances involving high risk (e.g., cardiac catheterization and angioplasty for coronary artery disease) or low or unclear benefit (e.g., the use of an unproven or experimental chemotherapy agent) require the greatest evidence of decision-making capacity (Tunzi 2001; Chow et al. 2010).

Four clinical scenarios are described that should particularly alert physicians to assess a patient's decision-making capacity (Grisso and Appelbaum 1998):

1. When patients have an abrupt change in mental status – This change may be caused by several medical conditions, including an acute neurologic or psychiatric process, hypoxia, infection, and metabolic disturbances or medication.

2. When patients refuse the recommended treatment – Assessing capacity is particularly needed when a patient is not willing to discuss the refusal or when the reasons for the refusal are unclear or irrational.
3. When patients consent to risky or invasive treatment too hastily – Some patients lack the capacity consent to treatment without careful consideration of the risks and benefits.
4. When patients have a known risk factor for impaired decision making – The known risk factors are as follows: a chronic neurologic or psychiatric condition, a significant cultural or language barrier, a low education level, an acknowledged fear of or discomfort with institutional health-care settings, and an age at either end of the adult spectrum (adolescents younger than 18 years or adults older than 85 years).

Application

Physicians may use a directed clinical interview and/or formal tools to assess decision-making capacity. Ancillary tests may be required, depending on the individual circumstances, including a history from therapists or other caregivers, physical assessment, laboratory evaluation, and neuroimaging studies (Tunzi 2001). A cognitive assessment, such as the Mini-Mental Status Examination (MMSE), can be performed to determine whether cognitive impairment may be influencing a patient's thinking and judgment.

Directed Clinical Interview
A directed clinical interview by a well-trained physician may be sufficient to evaluate a patient's decision-making capacity. The patient's abilities that should be assessed are described (Tunzi 2001) based on a literature review (Grisso and Appelbaum 1998; Etchells et al. 1999) as follows:

1. Questions to determine the ability of the patient to understand his/her medical condition and options for care

2. Questions to determine the ability of the patient to appreciate how that information applies to their own situation
3. Questions to determine the ability of the patient to reason with that information in a manner that is supported by the facts and the patient's own values
4. Questions to determine the ability of the patient to communicate and express a choice clearly

Formal Assessment Tools
In addition to or instead of a directed clinical interview, a formal assessment tool can be used to assess capacity. Several assessment tools exist, including the MacArthur Competence Assessment Tool for Treatment (MacCAT-T) (Grisso et al. 1997), the Hopkins Competency Assessment Test (HCAT) (Janofsky et al. 1992), Understanding Treatment Disclosure (UTD) (Pruchno et al. 1995), and the Aid to Capacity Evaluation (ACE) (Etchells et al. 1999). The abilities assessed in these tools are the same as those assessed in a clinical interview.

Among these tools, the ACE is a short and more clinically oriented tool that can be administered and scored in 5–10 min. The ACE can also be found on the website of the University of Toronto Joint Centre for Bioethics: http://www.jointcentreforbioethics.ca/tools/ace.shtml. The instrument consists of eight questions that assess the understanding of the problem, the treatment proposed, treatment alternatives, the option to refuse treatment, possible consequences of the decision, and the effect of an underlying mental disorder on the decision. The instrument includes a scoring manual that provides objective criteria for scoring responses. The sample questions are as follows:

Sample Questions

1. Medical condition:
   • What problem are you having right now?
   • What problem is bothering you most?
   • Why are you in the hospital?
   • Do you have [name problem here]?
2. Proposed treatment:
   • What is the treatment for [your problem]?

- What else can we do to help you?
- Can you have [proposed treatment]?

3. Alternatives:
   - Are there any other [treatments]?
   - What other options do you have?
   - Can you have [alternative treatment]?

4. Option of refusing the proposed treatment (including withholding or withdrawing the proposed treatment):
   - Can you refuse [proposed treatment]?
   - Can we stop [proposed treatment]?

5. Consequences of accepting the proposed treatment:
   - What could happen to you if you have [proposed treatment]?
   - Can [proposed treatment] cause problems/ side effects?
   - Can [proposed treatment] help you live longer?

6. Consequences of refusing the proposed treatment:
   - What could happen if you do not have [proposed treatment]?
   - Could you get sicker/die if you do not have [proposed treatment]?
   - What could happen if you have [alternative treatment]? (If alternatives are available)

7a. The person's decision is affected by depression:
   - Can you help me understand why you've decided to accept/refuse treatment?
   - Do you feel that you are being punished?
   - Do you think you are a bad person?
   - Do you have any hope for the future?
   - Do you deserve to be treated?

7b. The person's decision is affected by psychosis:
   - Can you help me understand why you have decided to accept/refuse treatment?
   - Do you think anyone is trying to hurt/harm you?
   - Do you trust your doctor/nurse?

Final Assessment and Documentation

The clinician's final assessment of whether a patient has medical decision-making capacity depends on whether the clinician believes that the patient is free of significant impaired thinking and possesses a sufficient capacity to make the specific decision in question. Regardless of whether the physician uses a directed clinical interview or a formal assessment tool, he/she must clearly document the assessment process, the final judgment about the capacity of the patient in the specific task requiring a decision, and the reasoning used to reach the final judgment in the medical record.

Cross-References

▶ Cognitive Impairment
▶ Competency
▶ Ethical Issues in the Conduct of Clinical Trials in Trauma Patients
▶ Ethical Issues Surrounding the Use of New Technology in Trauma Care
▶ Glasgow Coma Scale
▶ Informed Consent in Trauma
▶ Trauma Patient Evaluation
▶ Withdrawal of Life-Support

References

American College of Physicians (2005) Ethics manual, 5th edn. ACP Press, Philadelphia, pp 10–12

Appelbaum PS (2007) Assessment of patients' competence to consent to treatment. N Engl J Med 357:1834–1840

Chow GV, Czarny MJ, Hughes MT, Carreses JA (2010) CURVES: a mnemonic for determining medical decision-making capacity and providing emergency treatment in the acute setting. Chest 137(2):421–427

Etchells EP, Darzins P, Silberfeld M, Singer PA, McKenny J, Naglie G, Katz M, Guyatt GH, Molloy DW, Strang D (1999) Assessment of patient capacity to consent to treatment. J Gen Intern Med 14(1):27–34

Grisso T, Appelbaum PS (eds) (1998) Asessing competence to conset to treatment: a guide for physicians and other health professionals. Oxford University Press, New York

Grisso T, Appelbaum PS, Hill-Fotouhi C (1997) The MacCAT-T: a clinical tool to assess patients' capacities to make treatment decisions. Psychiatr Serv 48(11):1415–1419

Janofsky JS, McCarthy RJ, Folstein MF (1992) The hopkins competency assessment test: a brief method for evaluating patients' capacity to give informed consent. Hosp Community Psychiatry 43(2):132–136

Pruchno RA, Smyer MA, Rose MS, Hartman-Stein PE, Henderson-Laribee DL (1995) Competence of long-term care residents to participate in decisions about their medical care: a brief, objective assessment. Gerontologist 35(5):622–629

Tunzi M (2001) Can the patient decide? Evaluating patient capacity in practice. Am Fam Physician 64(2):299–306

Evaluation of Hemodynamics

▶ Hemodynamic Monitoring

Evolving Surgery

▶ Ethical Issues Surrounding the Use of New Technology in Trauma Care

Examination, Neurological

Patricia L. Zadnik and Daniel M. Sciubba
Department of Neurosurgery, The Johns Hopkins University School of Medicine, Baltimore, MD, USA

Synonyms

ASIA score; Frankel neurological performance scale

Definition

The patient's neurological status and evaluation of other distracting injuries should be performed upon arrival as part of the primary and secondary survey. Several grading scores exist for the evaluation of a patient's neurological exam. The American Spinal Injury Association (ASIA) may be used to rapidly assess 10 key motor segments using a scale of 0–5 on the left and the right for a total score of 100 possible points. The ASIA impairment scale is also widely used to assess completeness of spinal cord injury and is separate from the ASIA motor scale. This scale is based on a modified Frankel Neurological Performance scale and grades patients from A, with a complete injury with no preserved motor or sensory function, to E, normal motor and sensory function. In addition to a complete motor and sensory workup, a baseline neurological assessment should be performed to assess for a concomitant brain injury. Rectal tone should also be examined to determine if there is any sensory or tonal loss. Patients who have sustained significant trauma should be followed with close serial exams to monitor for any changes or decline in neurological function for at least 24 h following the incident.

Externally, the examiner should look for signs of trauma to the neck, chest, back, face, and head to assess for spinal cord injury. If the patient is responsive, the examiner should inquire about focal or diffuse pain. Bruising on the forehead is consistent with hyperextension and hyperflexion injury to the spine and strongly suggests a dangerous mechanism of injury. Palpable tenderness or bruising along the posterior aspect of the spine, or a step-off between the spinous processes, is concerning for cervical spine fracture. Penetrating injuries to the neck should be carefully evaluated with adjunct imaging to determine the degree of neural and vascular compromise. If metal fragments are present and MRI is contraindicated, CT myelogram can be performed to assess compromise of the spinal canal or neural foramen. Scarring on the anterior or posterior neck consistent with a previous surgical procedure should also be noted. Vertebral artery injury occurs in 17 % of cervical spine factures, and blunt cervical spine trauma can lead to dissection or vessel rupture, and subsequent cerebral ischemia and stroke (Taneichi et al. 2005). Signs of vertebral artery injury include vertigo, unilateral facial paresthesias, cerebellar signs (coordination deficits), lateral medullary signs (contralateral loss of pain and temperature sensation in the body and ipsilateral loss of sensation in the face), and visual field deficits. Any patient with concern for fracture through the transverse foramina, significant dislocation, or symptoms of cerebral ischemia or stroke should undergo CTA or MRA for evaluation of arterial injury (Daffner and Hackney 2007).

Cross-References

▶ Trauma Patient Evaluation

References

Daffner RH, Hackney DB (2007) ACR appropriateness criteria on suspected spine trauma. J Am Coll Radiol 4(11):762–775

Taneichi H, Suda K, Kajino T, Kaneda K (2005) Traumatically induced vertebral artery occlusion associated with cervical spine injuries: prospective study using magnetic resonance angiography. Spine (Phila Pa1976) 30(17):1955–1962

Exchange of a Supraglottic Airway (or Malfunctioning Endotracheal Tube) for an Endotracheal Tube

▶ Airway Exchange in Trauma Patients

Excision of Devitalized Tissue

▶ Debridement

Expectant Trauma Patient

▶ Pregnant Trauma Patient, Anesthetic Considerations for the

Expected Outcome

▶ Neurotrauma, Prognosis and Outcome Predictions

Expected Result

▶ Neurotrauma, Prognosis and Outcome Predictions

Expertise

▶ Competency

Exploratory Laparotomy

▶ Trauma Laparotomy

Explosion

Craig D. Silverton[1] and Paul Dougherty[2]
[1]Department of Orthopedic Surgery, Henry Ford Hospital, Detroit, MI, USA
[2]Department of Orthopedic Surgery, University of Michigan, Ann Arbor, MI, USA

Synonyms

Blast; Bomb; Detonation; Enhanced blast weapon

Definition

Explosion is caused by the rapid energy release from the chemical conversion of a solid or liquid explosive material into a gas. Explosions can be classified as low intensity or high intensity based on the time it takes to release this energy or blast wave (Wightman and Gladish 2001). Gun powder, pipe bombs, and Molotov cocktails are examples of a low-intensity explosion compared to TNT (2,4,6-trinitrotoluene), C-4, or ammonium nitrate fuel oil which is a high-intensity explosion. The blast wave associated with a low-intensity explosion measures less than 2,000 m/s compared with the high-intensity explosion that has a blast wave of up to 9,000 m/s. This blast wave moves in all directions exerting pressures of up to 700 t. In addition, the incendiary thermal effects of a high-intensity explosion create a "fireball" and intense heat for shorter periods of time compared to the longer-duration lower-intensity heat created by a low-intensity explosion.

The severity of the blast injury is based on three components:

1. The larger the size of the initial charge is associated with a greater peak overpressure (blast wave) and longer duration.
2. The distance from the blast.
3. The surrounding medium. Blast waves propagate further underwater and last longer as compared to air. In addition, closed structures (i.e., buildings) amplify the blast wave as it ricochets off the solid walls.
4. Injury caused by blast overpressure is a pressure versus duration phenomena. The longer the duration of blast wave the amount of injury is increased. Therefore, a threshold for injury is lowered the longer the duration of a pressure wave.

Injuries

Primary blast injuries are a form of barotrauma, unique to explosions. The most susceptible organs are the ears, lungs, and GI tract as they are filled with air. Patients may present with ruptured tympanic membranes, blast lung, abdominal perforation, and most recently TBI (traumatic brain injury) depending on how close they were to the epicenter of the blast. A form of spalling occurs when the shock wave travels through two dissimilar mediums (fluid to air) similar to water thrown into the air during an underwater explosion. This creates microscopic tears at this interface of the lung or bowel causing bleeding and disruption of tissues (Kluger 2003). Many casualties present without external signs of injury; thus the true incidence of primary blast injury is unknown, but should be suspected on any patient with a history of exposure to a significant explosion.

Secondary blast injuries refer to the shrapnel, fragmentation, and perforating trauma caused from the primary explosion. The shrapnel may be as small as 2 mm to large pieces of metal that cause traumatic amputations, perforations, and lethal injuries. This is the leading cause of casualties following an explosion since these fragments can travel great distances from the epicenter of the blast.

Tertiary blast injuries occur when the victim is hurled through the air with a force of 15 g's into a solid structure. Instantaneous death may occur from impalement. Multiple skull and skeletal fractures may be present along with the blunt trauma. Should a building collapse from the explosion, the crushing from falling debris is a part of the tertiary blast effect.

Quaternary blast injuries include flash burns associated with the explosion, inhalation injury as well as breathing problems associated with the toxic fumes. Crush injuries (compartment syndrome and crush syndrome) are included in this category as well as explosion-related injury or illness not directly attributed to the primary explosion effects.

Treatment

Most of the casualties from an explosion present with multiple trauma, including thoracic, and abdominal and head injuries. This accounts for approximately 40 % of the admissions (Kluger 2003). All management follows the latest Advanced Trauma Life Support Guidelines and begins with the ABC's of care. The uniqueness of caring for the victim of an explosion centers on the significant blast exposure. Primary blast lung has the highest morbidity and mortality of any blast injury (Pizov et al. 1999). This may present as a simple tension pneumothorax that initially appears benign. The spalling effect may cause alveolar hemorrhages, peribronchial disruptions, and pneumomediastinum leading to a systemic air embolism. Failure to recognize the significance of this injury leads to a high mortality rate. Pressures of 50–100 psi are associated with pulmonary damage in 50 % of patients (Stein and Hirshberg 1999). Many patients present with minimal symptoms of blast lung

E

and progress to a life-threatening condition within 24–48 h. Supportive treatment is the only therapy for this devastating condition. The modern use of body armor has saved many lives from the fragmentation injuries commonly seen that were lethal in the past; however, it does not change the mortality and morbidity of primary blast injuries. In fact, the use of body armor may exacerbate the blast effect as it appears to act like a wall around the chest cavity (Phillips et al. 1988).

Gastrointestinal, auditory, and neurological injuries unique to an explosion all present a difficult challenge to the treating facility and physicians. Most patients have ruptured tympanic membranes (overpressure of 5 psi) since this organ is the most sensitive to any blast injury. Hearing loss may be permanent in up to 50 % of cases if ossicular injury occurs along with tympanic membrane rupture.

The treatment of secondary blast injuries centers around the ballistic nature of the explosion. Fragmentation injuries can be overwhelming as many are minute in size yet can travel at velocities of up to 3,000 fps. These small fragments easily perforate the abdominal, thoracic, or skull cavities, many having a nearly imperceptible entrance wound. Surgical intervention is key to survival in identifying those life-threatening penetrating fragments. Ballistic injury is the most common form of blast injury seen, because ballistic effects take place farther away from the explosion than burn or overpressure. In confined spaces, such as armored vehicles, thermal and overpressure effects are seen more frequently.

Thermal burns in addition to the above noted injuries significantly increase the mortality rate in explosive-related trauma. Compared to civilian-related burns, the level of temperature far exceeds what is normally seen with the flash burns. The blast heat may exceed 3,000 °C. Standard burn protocols are recommended for treatment.

In summary, injuries caused from an explosion are mostly related to fragmentation injuries (secondary blast injury) and primary blast lung (primary blast injury). These injuries require a detailed physical examination with advanced imaging to determine the extent of damage. The treatment of these injuries caused by explosions is complex based on the multiorgan damage that may be present. Proper diagnosis and supportive care remains the mainstay of treatment.

Cross-References

- ▸ Ballistics
- ▸ Blast
- ▸ Blast Lung Injury
- ▸ Compartment Syndrome
- ▸ Crush Syndrome
- ▸ Damage Control Resuscitation, Military Trauma
- ▸ External Fixation
- ▸ Fragment Injury
- ▸ High-Velocity
- ▸ IED (Improvised Explosive Device)
- ▸ Mass Casualty
- ▸ Tourniquet
- ▸ Triage
- ▸ Spalling

References

Kluger Y (2003) Bomb explosions in acts of terrorism-detonation, wound ballistics, triage and medical concerns. Isr Med Assoc J 5:235–240

Phillips YY et al (1988) Cloth ballistic vest alters response to blast. J Trauma 28:S149

Pizov R, Oppenheim-Eden A, Matot I (1999) Blast lung injury from an explosion on a civilian bus. Chest 115:165–172

Stein M, Hirshberg A (1999) Medical consequences of terrorism. The conventional threat. Surg Clin North A 79:1537–1552

Wightman J, Gladish S (2001) Explosions and blast injuries. Ann Emerg Med 37:664–678

Explosive Formed Projectile (EFP) Devices

- ▸ IED (Improvised Explosive Device)

Exposed Break

▶ Open Fractures

Exsanguination Transfusion

▶ Massive Transfusion and Complications

Extension Avulsion Fracture

▶ Fracture, Extension Injury

Extension Compression Injury

▶ Fracture, Extension Injury

External Chest Compressions

▶ Cardiopulmonary Resuscitation in Pediatric Trauma

External Fixation

Craig D. Silverton[1] and Paul Dougherty[2]
[1]Department of Orthopedic Surgery, Henry Ford Hospital, Detroit, MI, USA
[2]Department of Orthopedic Surgery, University of Michigan, Ann Arbor, MI, USA

Synonyms

Fix ex; Fixateur externe; Hoffman device; Temporary fixation

Definition

Use of external fixation is not new. A practical system of external fixation was developed by the Swiss surgeon Hoffmann in the mid-twentieth century. He also developed a practical fixateur that allowed for the reduction of the fracture site after the application of the external fixateur.

External fixation allows for stabilization of a bone with a minimal physiological impact on the patient, as well as minimal invasiveness of the soft tissues surrounding the bone (Schwechter and Swan 2007).

Temporary external fixation is used to care for patients with severe limb trauma in war and peace (Fig. 1). The current US Military external fixation system today still bears Hoffman's name. The principle and theory have remained essentially the same although the offerings of multiple variations of this device have increased (Behrens 1989). There is no clear external fixateur device that has shown substantially better outcomes as compared to another. Most evaluations of external fixateurs are based on axial, bending, and torsional strengths.

For temporary stabilization of long-bone fractures, there has been no treatment method to date that does not have some degree of limitation. In the field, splinting either with traction or without has been of limited. The evacuation of casualties with any type of traction splinting is difficult at best. Static splinting with various materials has similar problems (Grubor et al. 2011). Plaster casting provides a better method of fracture stabilization; however, this cannot be done in the field and is even slower to apply than traditional temporary splinting. In addition, should the fracture be associated with open wounds, dressing changes become difficult and within a short period of time, the casting material becomes a culture medium for the continuous serious drainage. Splinting generally requires the immobilization of the joint above and below the fracture. External fixation has the advantage of only immobilizing the fractured bone, thus allowing motion of adjacent joints.

E

External Fixation,
Fig. 1 The use of an
external fixator allows easy
access for the treatment of
soft tissue wounds

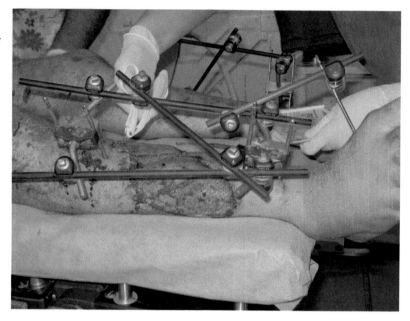

The external fixation device currently is the best method for temporary stabilization of fractures. It is relatively easy to apply, has minimal complications, and provides excellent stability to fractures. It can be used on almost all extremity fractures as well as pelvic fractures. The learning curve to apply this apparatus is short; however, the application of an external fixateur generally requires a trip to the operative suite. The use of an image intensifier is not required; however, it can assist in the ideal placement of pins. In field conditions, local anesthesia and IV sedation have been done with success in applying external fixation devices.

Application

Pins are placed above and below the fracture site. The pins should be as far from the zone of injury as possible but close enough to provide some degree of stability. Generally, a minimum of two pins are placed proximal and two pins distal to the fracture site. They are connected to a long bar and held in place with clamps. There are multiple different external fixateur devices on the market and all function in a similar manner. The use of multiple connectors and bars allow the surgeon the ability to adjust the external fixateur aligning the fracture as best possible with or without image intensification. The principles of all the various external fixateur available remain the same. Additional pins and bars in various planes provide additional stability if needed; however, this increases the time to application and usually is not required for most fracture temporary stabilization. Currently, two bars are recommended for most fractures to provide adequate stability.

Short-term complications of the external fixateur relate mostly to the pin placement. The pins can be inserted with a hand drill or power drill. The pins are usually self-drilling and self-tapping. The concept is to obtain two cortices of the bone for maximum stability. Only obtaining one cortex allows the pin to toggle and offers limited stability. Obtaining fixation in the second cortex requires the operator to limit the amount of pin protrusion since the neurovascular buddle is at risk if the pin protrudes a significant distance. Knowing the "safe zones" for pin placement is critical prior to inserting any external fixation pins. We try and limit this protrusion to less than 5 mm maximum in most extremity fractures. For the occasional surgeon, the power drill may be too aggressive, and although quicker, the chance of having the pin compromise significant structures is higher. The hand drill combined with image intensification may be a safer route.

Longer-term complications center around pin tract infections. Despite best efforts at relieving the pin tract insertion sites and judicious use of pin tract care, this remains a significant problem (Pathak and Atkinson 2001).

Silver nitrate-coated pins and atraumatic insertion techniques including limiting the number of pin sites may help in decreasing infections. Ultimately, many of the pin sites will need to be changed if definitive care is determined to be the use of an external fixation device.

Unstable open-book type pelvic fractures are a life-threatening injury. Temporary stabilization involves the use of circumferential sheets, pelvic clamps, or previously antishock trousers. External fixation provides an alternative to stabilizing the anterior pelvis with two pins into each iliac crest. Connected with two bars, this is an excellent adjunct for temporary stabilization limiting the continual volumetric increase of the pelvic inlet seen with this injury.

For damage control orthopedics in the trauma setting, the application of an external fixateur remains an important tool in the surgeon's armamentarium. It is relatively quick to apply, provides reasonable stability, and allows the patient free access to other diagnostic modalities such as CT or MRI without the cumbersome traction devices previously used.

Cross-References

▶ Compartment Syndrome, Acute
▶ Compartment Syndrome: Complication of Care in ICU
▶ Damage Control Resuscitation
▶ Damage Control Resuscitation, Military Trauma
▶ Damage Control Surgery
▶ Debridement
▶ Explosion

▶ Fasciotomy
▶ Negative Pressure Dressing
▶ Principles of External Fixation

References

Behrens F (1989) General theory and principles of external fixation clinic. Orthop Relat Res 241:15–23

Grubor P, Grubor M, Golubovic I, Stojiljkovic P, Golubovic Z (2011) Importance of external fixation in primary treatment of war wounds of the extremities. Sci J Faculty Med Nis 28(4):225–233

Pathak G, Atkinson RN (2001) Military external fixation of fractures. Aust Def Forces Health 2:24–28

Schwechter EM, Swan KG (2007) Raoul Hoffmann and his external fixateur. J Bone Joint Surg 89-A(3): 672–678

E

External Hemorrhage

▶ Compressible Hemorrhage

External Osteosynthesis

▶ Principles of External Fixation

Extra-articular Tibial Fracture

▶ Tibial Fractures

Extracorporeal Life Support

▶ Extracorporeal Membrane Oxygenation

Extracorporeal Lung Support

▶ Extracorporeal Membrane Oxygenation

Extracorporeal Membrane Oxygenation

Marcelo Cypel
Surgical Director ECLS Program at UHN,
Canada Research Chair in Lung Transplantation,
Assistant Professor of Surgery, Division of
Thoracic Surgery, University of Toronto,
Toronto, ON, Canada

Synonyms

ECLS; ECMO; Extracorporeal life support;
Extracorporeal lung support

Definition

Extracorporeal membrane oxygenators (ECMO)
are membranes made of synthetic material that
are connected to blood vessels through tubes and
cannulas of plastic or silicone materials. The
blood passing through the device is oxygenated
and cleared of carbon dioxide. Because this technology can be applied to patients who do not have
oxygenation problems such as patients with
hypercapnic respiratory failure, or to patients
with severe pulmonary hypertension and right
ventricular failure, the most current term is extracorporeal lung support or ECLS.

Preexisting Condition

In the 1930s the concept of artificial organ support started with the work of Carrel and Lindbergh (Carrel and Lindbergh 1935). However, the
first successful clinical use in humans was
described by Hill et al. using a heart–lung
machine in 1972 on a young man with
posttraumatic respiratory failure (Hill et al.
1972). The patients stayed 75 h on support and
eventually recovered.

Since then, ECLS has been widely used in the
neonate and pediatric population where survival
rates approached 50–60 %. In contrast, clinical

trials in adults demonstrated dismal results
(<20 % survival) (Zapol et al. 1979). However,
in the last decade, improvements in patient selection, a better understanding of ventilator-
associated lung injury, and improvements in
device technologies have made it possible to successfully bridge patients to recovery or to lung
transplantation (LTx) (Lang et al. 2012). Recent
studies have shown more promising results using
ECLS for adults with acute respiratory distress
syndrome (ARDS) with survival rates ranging
from 50 % to 80 %. This includes the experience
from Michigan in 100 patients (Kolla et al. 1997),
the UK CESAR trial (Peek et al. 2009), and
H1N1/ARDS reports (Freed et al. 2010; Davies
et al. 2009).

Indications and Contraindications for ECLS

The main indications for ECLS are:

1. Bridge to recovery in patients with severe
   acute lung injury – ARDS.
2. Bridge to recovery in patients with severe
   primary graft dysfunction after lung
   transplantation.
3. Bridge to lung transplantation in patients with
   end-stage lung diseases (as an extension of life
   until a suitable organ becomes available).
   Patients with end-stage lung disease who are
   not eligible for lung transplantation are generally not candidates for ECLS, although some
   patients may benefit from extracorporeal CO_2
   removal as a weaning strategy.

The three main physiological indications for
the use of ECLS are:

1. Refractory hypoxemia – usually $PaO_2/FiO_2 <$
   80 mmHg despite maximal conventional
   respiratory support
2. Hypercapnia and respiratory acidosis –
   inability to maintain safe levels of pH despite
   high ventilatory plateau pressures
3. Pulmonary hypertension and right ventricular
   dysfunction

Absolute contraindications for the use of
ECLS are currently not clear as with advancements in technology; indications have expanded
over the past few years. However, unfavorable

Extracorporeal Membrane Oxygenation, Fig. 1 The main components of the ECLS system include a membrane oxygenator, a pump, cannulas, and tubing circuits

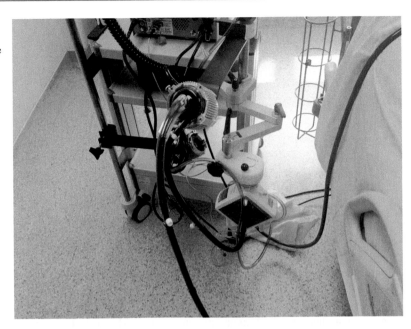

prognostic factors include sepsis, multi-organ dysfunction, acute renal failure, high vasopressor requirements, a long preceding duration of mechanical ventilation (>7 days), advanced age, and obesity.

Application

The main components of the ECLS system include a membrane oxygenator, a pump, and tubing circuits (Fig. 1). In the last decade, several important advancements in technology have contributed to improve management and overall outcomes of these patients, as detailed below.

Development of Polymethylpentene Membranes

In the past, most adult ECLS circuits used silicone membrane oxygenators, and the remainder used polypropylene microporous oxygenators. Both these oxygenators had drawbacks. The introduction of polymethylpentene (PMP) membranes provided several technical advantages. The PMP oxygenator has reduced red blood cell and platelet transfusion requirements, significantly less plasma leakage, better gas exchange, lower resistance, and lower priming volume.

Compared to polypropylene microporous oxygenators, the PMP oxygenator has a reduced rate of oxygenator failure and can be functional for several weeks. The PMP fibers are woven into a complex configuration of hollow fibers through which the oxygenated gas passes. The hollow fibers themselves are then arranged into mats and stacked into a configuration that allows blood to pass between the fibers with low resistance. This provides maximum blood/gas mixing, and gas transfer can take place without direct contact with blood. The low resistance also allows the use of these membranes without the need of an external pump in some cases (pumpless). Examples of new-generation PMP membranes include the Quadrox D (Maquet) and iLA (Novalung).

Introduction of Heparin-Coated Circuits

Heparin-coated circuits led to reduced rates of platelet, complement, and granulocyte activation and also significantly reduced heparin requirements. Importantly, PMP oxygenators can also be readily heparin coated, whereas the silicone membrane oxygenators cannot. Thus, the modern ECLS circuit can be entirely heparin coated and requires less systemic heparinization or no heparin for a few days if patients are bleeding

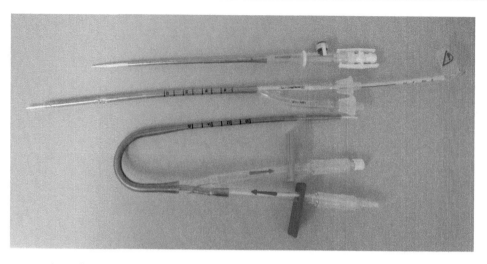

Extracorporeal Membrane Oxygenation, Fig. 2   Dual-lumen cannulas for venous–venous ECLS

(e.g., recent history of trauma or surgery). In contrast, early ECLS circuits required full heparinization, and consequently bleeding complications and daily blood product requirement were high.

Development of a New Generation of Centrifugal Pumps

Compared with traditional roller pumps, the centrifugal pumps have an improved performance and safety profile. They have virtually no risk of tubing rupture, require a smaller priming volume, do not require the use of a reservoir, and in general have a decreased incidence of hemolysis. One of the most used pumps is the new-generation Centrimag (Thoratec). This pump has no bearings but instead uses magnetic levitation. This approach diminishes both hemolysis and the likelihood of mechanical pump failure.

Development of New Cannulas

A major advance in recent years has been the development of new cannulas that can be easily inserted using percutaneous Seldinger techniques. Moreover, dual-lumen cannulas for venous–venous ECLS have been developed and allow ECLS to be run through a single neck port, decreasing risk of infection and allowing patient mobilization as the groin is kept free. The most common cannula used to date is the Avalon Elite

(Maquet). The Novaport Twin (Novalung) and the Hemolung catheter (Alung) are other dual-lumen cannulas currently available (Fig. 2).

Modes of ECLS: Configuration of Device

In addition to the technical advances, device configuration can be individualized and tailored for specific patient ventilatory and hemodynamic requirements. The configuration and mode of ECLS will depend on the specific clinical scenario.

Hypercapnic Respiratory Failure

Refractory hypercapnic respiratory failure and acidosis is a common scenario in patients with cystic fibrosis (CF) waiting for lung transplantation, for example, or patients with COPD. Noninvasive ventilation (NIV) has become an important option as a treatment modality in ARF in CF, avoiding endotracheal intubation with its attendant complications. If a suitable organ does not become available in time, respiratory failure progresses and mechanical ventilation becomes necessary. At that stage, management becomes increasingly difficult as high-pressure ventilation is required and alveolar hypoventilation and hypercapnia often persist despite it. The large amounts of bronchopulmonary secretions in these patients make ventilation even more difficult. Traditionally, patients with hypercapnia and respiratory acidosis required ECLS with the use of a pump. However, the advent of an interventional lung assist device (iLA, Novalung®, Germany) allowed patients to use the iLA in a *pumpless* arteriovenous (A-V) mode (Fischer et al. 2006). This low-resistance (11 mmHg) hollow-fiber polymethylpentene membrane is attached to the systemic circulation (usually femoral artery) and receives only part of the cardiac output (CO) (15–20 %) for extracorporeal gas exchange. This allows prompt and effective CO_2 removal and correction of respiratory acidosis. CO_2 removal rates can be controlled by varying the sweep of gas flow up to 15 L/min. The usual recommended rate of CO_2 clearance is 20 mmHg/hour. In order to use the pumpless device, the patient must have an adequate mean arterial blood pressure to be able to sustain good flows through the device (mean arterial pressure >80 mmHg). Since only a portion of the CO, in the range of one fifth of total, is oxygenated in the membrane, the PaO_2 is only augmented minimally with this mode of ECLS (Fischer et al. 2006); therefore, A-V iLA is not recommended in patients with severe hypoxemia. Cannulation is usually achieved percutaneously using a Seldinger technique (or an open modified Seldinger technique) in the femoral artery (13–15Fr) and femoral vein (17 Fr). Since a centrifugal pump is not required, and the circuit is fully heparin coated, anticoagulation times (ACT) are generally run in the range of 160–200 s, but if there is a concern about bleeding, an ACT of 150–180 s is acceptable.

In the initial publication from Fischer et al., 12 patients were bridged to transplantation using the iLA. The mean duration of iLA support in the 12 patients was 15 ± 8 days (4–32days). Efficient CO_2 removal was rapidly achieved in all patients. Four patients died of multi-organ failure, 2 before LTx and 2 on days 16 and 30 after LTx. Thus, 10 of the 12 patients were successfully bridged to LTx, and 8 of the 10 were alive 1 year posttransplantation (Fischer et al. 2006).

One of the disadvantages of the pumpless iLA is the need for groin arterial cannulation which can lead to vascular complications and also immobilize the patient. As patient mobilization and rehabilitation seem to be an important component of the overall success of artificial lung devices in recent years, many investigators are now using low-flow venous–venous ECLS using a single dual-lumen cannula. The advantage here is the simplicity of insertion and avoidance of groin and arterial cannulation. Most of the time, 1.5 L of VV flows are sufficient to control CO2 and maintain patients without mechanical ventilation. A concept of "respiratory dialysis" has also been proposed with even lower blood flows and smaller catheters using highly efficient membranes. The Hemolung (Alung) and Novalung Petit (Novalung) are examples of such technology.

Hypoxemic Respiratory Failure

Some patients will progress to hypoxemic respiratory failure and a different level of support is required. Whereas CO_2 removal can be achieved with low membrane flows (0.5–1 l/min) (Zwischenberger et al. 2006), substantial oxygenation requires more physiologic flows over the membrane (3–6 l/min). In order to achieve this, venous–venous (V-V) or venoarterial pump-driven ECLS support is required. V-V mode is the preferred choice if the patient is hypoxemic but hemodynamically stable. The advantages of the V-V mode in comparison to V-A mode are the decreased rate of complications such as bleeding, arterial thrombosis, or neurologic complications. Generally, a 22–25Fr cannula is inserted into a femoral vein for drainage and a 17–20 F single-stage cannula inserted into an internal jugular vein percutaneously for patient inflow. More recently, a dual-lumen single-cannula system has been developed for V-V ECLS that has the advantage of simplicity and, importantly, allows for patient mobilization (Garcia et al. 2010). A 27Fr or 31Fr Avalon cannula can be inserted percutaneously. We usually use fluoroscopy as a guide for cannula insertion and positioning. Usual ACTs should range from 160 to 200 s.

Hypoxemic Respiratory Failure and Hemodynamic Compromise

For patients with respiratory failure and significant hemodynamic compromise, V-A ECLS is

E

the recommended option since it provides both cardiac and pulmonary support. In fact, the initial experience with ECLS in LTx was using this mode (The Toronto Lung Transplant group 1985). Usually a femoral vein is cannulated for drainage and a femoral artery cannulated for blood return. Some authors also propose the use of the axillary artery with an interposition graft. Although vascular access is a bit more difficult, the advantages of the axillary artery in this setting are the possibility of better patient mobilization and the low incidence of atherosclerosis in this vessel. Improved upper-body oxygenated perfusion is also an important advantage. Another option to improve central oxygenation is to insert another cannula into the internal jugular vein and convert the circuit to a hybrid V-VA (V, femoral vein – VA, jugular vein and femoral artery) ECLS. This configuration of V-VA ECMO can also be used to provide partial cardiac support when cardiac function is depressed and does not improve with improved oxygenation on V-V support alone. It is important to note that if the primary cause of hemodynamic shock is severe hypoxemia and respiratory acidosis, most of the time it can be readily reversed with V-V support alone.

The use of the traditional femoral venoarterial (V-A) support often fails to correct hypoxemia in patients with somewhat preserved cardiac output. Thus, this mode should be reserved for patients with primary hemodynamic failure such as cardiomyopathy or severe RV dysfunction due to pulmonary hypertension.

Pulmonary Hypertension and Right Ventricular Failure

A novel mode of ECLS that we recently described is pulmonary artery to left atrium (PA to LA) ECLS configuration (Strueber et al. 2009). Although progress has been made for isolated lung failure, no truly effective solution existed for patients with primary pulmonary hypertension (PAH). Compared to patients with lung failure due to isolated lung parenchymal disorders, patients with end-stage PAH develop severe right heart failure. V-A or V-V ECLS does not effectively unload the RV. An atrial septostomy is

sometimes performed as a last-ditch effort; however, this leads to desaturated blood being systemically ejected as a result of the iatrogenic right to left shunt. In this scenario, the connection of a low-resistance gas-exchange device (Novalung[R]) between the main trunk of the pulmonary artery and the left atrium (PA-LA) in a pumpless mode effectively creates an *oxygenating* shunt that pressure unloads the right ventricle much like an atrial septostomy. However, the important advantage in this case is that the membrane oxygenates the blood, and thus the central hypoxia seen with a simple septostomy is avoided. In our experience, patients improve dramatically as soon as flow across the Novalung[R] is instituted (Strueber et al. 2009).

Another innovative ECLS approach to bridge patients with severe PAH to lung transplantation is V-V ECLS with added atrial septostomy. In two studies using adult sheep, right to left atrial shunting of oxygenated blood with VV-ECMO was capable of maintaining normal systemic hemodynamics and normal arterial blood gases during high right ventricular afterload dysfunction (Camboni et al. 2011). The theoretical advantage in comparison to PA-LA mode is the avoidance of sternotomy and central cannulation; however, the use of a pump is required.

Clinical Management

Patients receiving ECLS as a bridge to LTx require clinical management comparable to patients with ARDS. Once ECLS is initiated, the ventilator should ideally be adjusted to "resting" lung settings. The ECLS flow should be maintained to sustain a venous blood saturation of 80–85 % and an arterial saturation of 80–95 %. Diuretics are given if required to maintain adequate urine output and remove excess fluid. If negative fluid balance cannot be achieved with diuretics, hemofiltration should be initiated early. Neurologic status is frequently checked and any deterioration should prompt further investigations. Cannulation sites and limb perfusion status are also frequently checked for bleeding and distal perfusion, respectively. Prophylactic antibiotics are given prior to insertion of cannulas.

Clinical Trials

The only randomized clinical trial in the modern era is the UK CESAR trial. This study randomized 180 patients with severe ARDS to transfer to a specialized center for consideration of ECMO versus usual care. Despite only 75 % of patients (68 of 90) randomized to the intervention group actually receiving ECMO, this group had significantly higher survival as compared to the control group (63 % vs. 47 %, $p = 0.03$). Although the study may not be conclusive on the clinical efficacy of ECMO as compared to conventional mechanical ventilation, it strongly suggests that the referral of patients with severe ARDS to regionalized centers with proven ECLS expertise may be an important consideration in these patients.

Conclusions and Future of ECLS

Despite significant advances and much improved outcomes with the use of ECLS, there are still significant challenges especially for the development of a long-term wearable artificial lung device. There has been ongoing research toward the development of a miniaturized, cell-coated artificial lung for long-term use.

Cross-References

▶ Acute Respiratory Distress Syndrome (ARDS), General
▶ Mechanical Ventilation, Conventional
▶ Mechanical Ventilation, High-Frequency Oscillation

References

Camboni D, Akay B, Pohlmann JR, Koch KL, Haft JW, Bartlett RH (2011) Veno-venous extracorporeal membrane oxygenation with interatrial shunting: a novel approach to lung transplantation for patients in right ventricular failure. J Thorac Cardiovasc Surg 141(2):537–542, 42 e1

Carrel A, Lindbergh CA (1935) The culture of whole organs. Science 81(2112):621–623

Davies A, Jones D, Bailey M, Beca J, Bellomo R, Blackwell N et al (2009) Extracorporeal membrane oxygenation for 2009 influenza A(H1N1) acute respiratory distress syndrome. JAMA 302(17):1888–1895

Fischer S, Simon AR, Welte T, Hoeper MM, Meyer A, Tessmann R et al (2006) Bridge to lung transplantation with the novel pumpless interventional lung assist device NovaLung. J Thorac Cardiovasc Surg 131(3):719–723

Freed DH, Henzler D, White CW, Fowler R, Zarychanski R, Hutchison J et al (2010) Extracorporeal lung support for patients who had severe respiratory failure secondary to influenza A (H1N1) 2009 infection in Canada. Can J Anaesth 57(3):240–247

Garcia JP, Iacono A, Kon ZN, Griffith BP (2010) Ambulatory extracorporeal membrane oxygenation: a new approach for bridge-to-lung transplantation. J Thorac Cardiovasc Surg 139(6):e137–e139

Hill JD, O'Brien TG, Murray JJ, Dontigny L, Bramson ML, Osborn JJ et al (1972) Prolonged extracorporeal oxygenation for acute post-traumatic respiratory failure (shock-lung syndrome). Use of the Bramson membrane lung. N Engl J Med 286(12):629–634

Kolla S, Awad SS, Rich PB, Schreiner RJ, Hirschl RB, Bartlett RH (1997) Extracorporeal life support for 100 adult patients with severe respiratory failure. Ann Surg 226(4):544–564; discussion 65–66

Lang G, Taghavi S, Aigner C, Renyi-Vamos F, Jaksch P, Augustin V et al (2012) Primary lung transplantation after bridge with extracorporeal membrane oxygenation: a plea for a shift in our paradigms for indications. Transplantation 93(7):729–736

Peek GJ, Mugford M, Tiruvoipati R, Wilson A, Allen E, Thalanany MM et al (2009) Efficacy and economic assessment of conventional ventilatory support versus extracorporeal membrane oxygenation for severe adult respiratory failure (CESAR): a multicentre randomised controlled trial. Lancet 374(9698):1351–1363

Strueber M, Hoeper MM, Fischer S, Cypel M, Warnecke G, Gottlieb J et al (2009) Bridge to thoracic organ transplantation in patients with pulmonary arterial hypertension using a pumpless lung assist device. Am J Transplant 9(4):853–857

The Toronto Lung Transplant Group (1985) Sequential bilateral lung transplantation for paraquat poisoning. A case report. J Thorac Cardiovasc Surg 89(5):734–42

Zapol WM, Snider MT, Hill JD, Fallat RJ, Bartlett RH, Edmunds LH et al (1979) Extracorporeal membrane oxygenation in severe acute respiratory failure. A randomized prospective study. JAMA 242(20):2193–2196

Zwischenberger BA, Clemson LA, Zwischenberger JB (2006) Artificial lung: progress and prototypes. Expert Rev Med Devices 3(4):485–497

Recommended Reading

Brodie D, Bacchetta M (2011) Extracorporeal membrane oxygenation for ARDS in adults. N Engl J Med 365(20):1905–1914

Del Sorbo L, Cypel M, Fan E (2014) Extracorporeal life support for adults with severe acute respiratory failure. Lancet Respir Med 2(2):154–164

E

Extremity Compartment Syndrome

▶ Compartment Syndrome: Complication of Care in ICU

Extremity Fractures

▶ Falls

Extremity Hemorrhage

▶ Compressible Hemorrhage

Extremity Injury

▶ Crush Injuries

Eye Injury

▶ Eye Trauma, Anesthesia for

Eye Trauma, Anesthesia for

Amy M. Pichoff
Department of Anesthesiology, University of Kansas Hospital, Kansas City, KS, USA

Synonyms

Blunt ocular injury; Eye injury; Ocular contusion; Ocular injury; Ocular trauma; Open globe; Penetrating ocular injury; Perforating ocular injury; Ruptured globe

Definition

Eye trauma may present as mechanical or burn injury to the cornea and/or the sclera and may include retention of an ocular foreign body. The ophthalmic literature is not consistent in the nomenclature of these injuries. Some terminology seeks to describe the type of injury (blunt vs. penetrating) while others may refer to the object with which injury occurs (blunt vs. sharp object) leading to what may be ambiguous descriptions. The most important clinical distinction is between an "open-globe" injury and a "closed-globe" injury. Penetrating mechanical force results an "open-globe" injury, while blunt mechanical force may result either in a "closed-globe" or an "open-globe" injury.

Preexisting Condition

There are approximately 2 million eye injuries in the United States annually; the economic impact is 1–3 billion dollars per year (Kohli et al. 2007). Patients who sustain traumatic eye injuries are at high risk for pulmonary aspiration, have an increased incidence of acute intoxication, and may have accompanying facial fractures, cervical spine fractures, and closed head injury.

Anatomy and Physiology of the Eye
The eye is an extension of the central nervous system and is comprised of the sclera, uveal tract, and retina. The sclera is a fibrous structure that gives shape to the eye. The uveal tract is made of the iris (divides eye into anterior and posterior chambers), ciliary body (site of aqueous humor production and accommodation of the lens), and the choroid plexus (arterial network). Finally, the retina is responsible for receiving light and converting it to neural impulses. Vascular supply to the eye is derived from branches of the carotid artery and venous drainage is via the cavernous sinus (Fig. 1) (Kohli et al. 2007).

Intraocular pressure (IOP) is impacted by physiologic and pharmacologic alterations; it can be thought of quite similarly to intracranial pressure. The eye's choroidal plexus undergoes

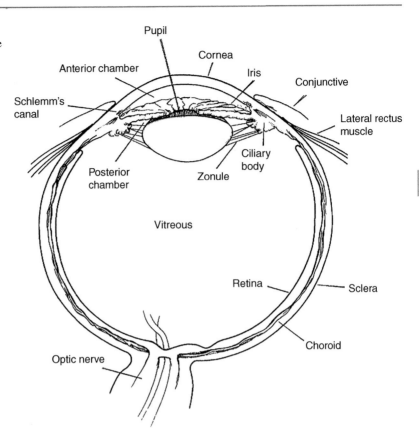

autoregulation to maintain near-constant pressures over a range of arterial blood pressures. Normal IOP ranges from 10 to 22 mmHg with normal variations occurring throughout the day. Activities such as supine positioning, blinking, eye rubbing, and Valsalva maneuvers (coughing, bucking, and vomiting) can increase IOP as much as 40 mmHg (Jaffe et al. 2004). The major determinant of intraocular pressure is the production and elimination of aqueous humor within the eye. In addition, choroidal blood volume (which increases with hypercarbia and hypoxia), central venous pressure (which increases with Valsalva), and extraocular tone also impact IOP (Chidiac et al. 2006; Miller et al. 2005; Kohli et al. 2007).

Classification

Subsequent to initial evaluation and stabilization, an eye examination should be performed by an ophthalmologist. Several ocular injury classification systems have been described. Mechanism of injury, anatomic structures involved, presence of pupillary defect (a measure of retinal and optic nerve function), and grade of injury (measure of visual acuity) are among the most common features assessed (Pieramici et al. 2003). An important consideration is the possibility of vision salvage or certainty of full visual loss.

Application

Operative Procedure

Goals of surgery include replacement of extruded intraocular contents, removal of any existing foreign bodies, and repair of defects (Jaffe et al. 2004). If visual salvage is possible, management of IOP becomes critical.

Anesthetic Implications

Adequate depth of anesthesia is the most important factor in minimizing anesthesia-related ocular complications. An analysis of the ASA Closed Claims Database revealed that most claims derived from ophthalmic procedures were due to inadequate anesthesia or patient movement (Bhananker et al. 2006). Minimizing the risk of vitreous expulsion is vital and can best be achieved by cautious application of the face mask during preoxygenation (to minimize external pressure on the globe), avoiding Valsalva maneuvers, and optimizing hemodynamics as well as arterial oxygen and carbon dioxide partial pressures (Kohli et al. 2007).

Topical Anesthesia

Topical anesthesia is rarely a viable option for patients with open-globe injuries. The risks associated with topical anesthesia are minimal but its use is limited by lack of eye akinesis, the limited anatomic coverage, and the need for patient cooperation. On the other hand, topical and local anesthesia may be viable options for repair of isolated lacerations of the eyelid, conjunctiva, and the cornea.

Regional Anesthesia

There are injuries amenable to regional anesthesia (i.e., retrobulbar block) in the setting of appropriate patient selection (Kohli et al. 2007). Patients with smaller, more anterior defects and favorable presenting visual acuity are more likely to undergo regional anesthesia than their counterparts with larger, posterior defects or those presenting with a greater visual loss (Chidiac et al. 2006). Patients with significant comorbid medical and/or traumatic conditions may be at higher risk for undergoing general anesthesia.

A significant disadvantage of retrobulbar block is it may increase the risk of extrusion of globe contents as local anesthetics in significant volumes exert external pressure on the eye. Thus, regional ophthalmic blocks should only be performed by skilled providers with adequate training. There is a link between provider inexperience and complication rates associated with regional anesthesia.

General Anesthesia

Premedication

Benzodiazepines and narcotics have been demonstrated to reduce IOP. There is some concern about the use of narcotics due to the side effects of nausea and vomiting that may occur. Antisialagogues (atropine, glycopyrrolate) given intravenously have little to no effect on IOP and can be used as necessary. However, when given topically these drugs will increase IOP due to mydriasis (Kohli et al. 2007).

Induction Agents

Most intravenous induction agents provide acceptable conditions in the setting of an open globe. However, there is some controversy surrounding the use of ketamine and etomidate. Ketamine can increase IOP, which may be blunted when benzodiazepine premedication is given (Kohli et al. 2007). It is the least favorable agent in the setting of eye trauma. Etomidate has been used successfully and lowers IOP (Kohli et al. 2007); however, a case report of etomidate-induced myoclonus linked to expulsion of vitreous material has been published (Berry et al. 1989). Propofol has been shown to reduce IOP by relaxation of extraocular muscles and reduction of aqueous humor production (Kohli et al. 2007) and is favored over the use of ketamine, and possibly etomidate, for patients with open-globe injuries. Ensuring adequate anesthesia prior to airway instrumentation to prevent coughing or bucking is of utmost importance regardless of the anesthetic agent chosen. Patient comorbid medical conditions, additional areas of injury, and salvageability of the eye warrant consideration in devising an optimal plan for airway management.

Muscle Relaxation

Succinylcholine has received much scrutiny in the setting of open-globe injuries. The controversy surrounding its use dates back to the 1950s when two studies on intraocular physiology concluded that succinylcholine increased IOP.

These were accompanied by anecdotes of vitreous extrusion when succinylcholine was used. With time the prevailing sentiment within anesthesia literature, until as recently as the late 1990s, was to avoid succinylcholine in open-globe injuries (Vachon et al. 2003).

More recent literature advocates for cautious use of succinylcholine in appropriate settings (pulmonary aspiration risk, anticipated difficult intubation). The rationale for this shift in practice is multifactorial. First, most studies looking at increased IOP associated with succinylcholine are in patients with an intact globe and no ocular disease. Once the globe is compromised ("open globe"), ocular contents are at atmospheric pressure and modalities typically associated with increases in IOP have a less significant impact (Kohli et al. 2007; Brinkley et al. 2004). Second, the morbidity and mortality associated with pulmonary aspiration is significant and must be adequately addressed and managed. Succinylcholine remains the gold standard for rapid sequence induction as other currently available neuromuscular blockers do not have the speed of onset nor short duration afforded by succinylcholine. Third, there are still no published studies linking loss of vitreous contents to use of succinylcholine (Kohli et al. 2007). In fact, commentary has been published from several high-volume eye trauma centers citing good outcomes (no vitreous expulsion) with succinylcholine (Libonati et al. 1985; Chidiac et al. 2006).

Of note, while increasing IOP may be less concerning with "open-globe" injuries (due to atmospheric intraocular pressure), the muscular fasciculations that occur with succinylcholine will cause simultaneous contraction of extraocular muscles which increase external pressure exerted on the open globe. This could, in theory, lead to extrusion of ocular contents; however, this has never been documented clinically (Brinkley et al. 2004).

Attenuation of Succinylcholine Response

With the historical controversy that surrounds use of succinylcholine, multiple studies have been published attempting to elucidate the mechanism of IOP increase and evaluate various methods of attenuating this response. One study of patients undergoing enucleation evaluated IOP after extraocular muscles to the operative eye were severed and succinylcholine had been administered. IOP increase was the same in the eye undergoing enucleation as the non-diseased eye suggesting perhaps a vascularly mediated mechanism (Chidiac et al. 2006). Medications studied to minimize IOP increases related to succinylcholine include benzodiazepines, narcotics, alpha-2 agonists, and the use of "de-fasciculating" doses of non-depolarizing muscle relaxants and "priming" doses of succinylcholine. The results have been inconsistent. It is important to reemphasize that succinylcholine-induced vitreous expulsion has not been reported in the literature (Kohli et al. 2007).

Emergence

Use of anticholinesterase medications along with their anticholinergic adjuncts for reversal of neuromuscular blockade has been used with no adverse effect on IOP (Kohli et al. 2007). The goal is a smooth emergence to minimize coughing, bucking, retching, or vomiting.

Cross-References

▶ ABCDE of Trauma Care
▶ Airway Trauma, Management of
▶ Burn Anesthesia
▶ Multi-trauma, Anesthesia for
▶ Spinal Cord Injury, Anesthetic Management for
▶ Traumatic Brain Injury

References

Berry J et al (1989) Etomidate myoclonus and the open globe. Anesth Analg 69:256–259
Bhananker S et al (2006) Injury and liability associated with monitored anesthesia care- a closed claims analysis. Anesthesiology 104:228–234

Brinkley J et al (2004) Role of extraocular pressure in open globe injury. Anesthesiology 100:1036

Chidiac E et al (2006) Succinylcholine and the open eye. Ophthalmol Clin N Am 19:279–285

Jaffe R et al (2004) Surgical procedures, 3rd edn. Chapter 2

Kohli R et al (2007) The anesthetic management of ocular trauma. Int Anesth Clin 45(3):83–98

Libonati M et al (1985) The use of succinylcholine in open eye surgery. Anesthesiology 62:637–640

Miller R et al (2005) Miller's anesthesia, 6th edn. Chapter 65

Pieramici D et al (2003) The prognostic significance of a system for classifying mechanical injuries of the eye (globe) in open-globe injuries. J Trauma 54(4):750–754

Vachon C et al (2003) Succinylcholine and the open globe. Anesthesiology 99:220–223

F

Facial Burn

▶ Airbag Injuries

Factor I Concentrate

▶ Adjuncts to Transfusion: Fibrinogen Concentrate

Factor IX Complex Concentrate

▶ Adjuncts to Transfusion: Prothrombin Complex Concentrate

Factor VIIa

Harvey G. Hawes[1], Bryan A. Cotton[1] and Laura A. McElroy[2]
[1]Department of Surgery, Division of Acute Care Surgery, Trauma and Critical Care, University of Texas Health Science Center at Houston, The University of Texas Medical School at Houston, Houston, TX, USA
[2]Department of Anesthesiology, Critical Care Medicine, University of Rochester Medical Center, Rochester, NY, USA

Synonyms

NiaStase; Novoseven; Recombinant factor VIIa; rFVIIa

© Springer-Verlag Berlin Heidelberg 2015
P.J. Papadakos, M.L. Gestring (eds.), *Encyclopedia of Trauma Care*,
DOI 10.1007/978-3-642-29613-0

Definition

Factor VII is a vitamin K-dependent enzyme of the serine protease class that acts as the initiating factor in the extrinsic arm of the human coagulation cascade (Broze and Majerus 1980). Following blood vessel damage, FVII leaves the circulation and comes into contact with tissue factor (TF) expressed on tissue-factor-bearing subendothelial cells including stromal cells and leukocytes in response to cellular injury. The binding of TF and FVII forms an activated complex (TF-FVIIa) that begins the amplification of the coagulation cascade (Pallister and Watson 2010). Recombinant factor VIIa, expressed in baby hamster kidney cells, was initially developed for use in individuals with hemophilia A who developed antibodies to factor VIII (Parameswaran et al. 2005).

The success of factor VIIa in stemming hemophiliac bleeding has led to the exploration of its potential efficacy in life-threatening hemorrhage from trauma, cardiac surgery, liver failure, and intracranial hemorrhage secondary to anticoagulants. Two early randomized controlled trials in patients with severe blunt trauma showed a significant reduction of the number of units of RBCs needed in the factor VIIa arm (Boffard et al. 2005), but they showed no difference in mortality between the two groups. Subsequent studies in non-hemophiliac populations have shown limited, if any, benefit of factor VIIa and have raised questions about the possibility of harm.

An analysis of 35 randomized controlled trials where factor VIIa was used in an off-labeled fashion showed a significant increase in arterial thromboembolic events (Levi et al. 2010), and a retrospective study of almost 1,500 ICU patients who were administered factor VIIa was found to have more than 2-fold increase in mortality vs. matched controls who did not receive factor VIIa (Brophy et al. 2013). The efficacy of rFVIIa is known to decrease up to 90 % when pH drops from 7.4 to 7.0, and in data from 10 years collected in New Zealand and Australia with >2,000 trauma patients, the single biggest predictor of factor VIIa effect on mortality was pH (James and John 2010). This pH-dependent effectiveness, combined with its increasing risk profile, extreme expense (up to $75,000 per patient), and no well-established dosing schedule, have led the World Trauma Congress and other societies to move away from advocating its use even as a last resort in trauma (Mamtani et al. 2012).

Cross-References

▶ Factor I Concentrate

References

Boffard KD, Riou B, Warren B et al (2005) Recombinant factor VIIa as adjunctive therapy for bleeding control in severely injured trauma patients: two parallel randomized, placebo-controlled, double-blind clinical trials. J Trauma Inj Infect Crit Care 59:8–18

Brophy GM, Candeloro CL, Robles JR et al (2013) Recombinant activated factor VII use in critically ill patients: clinical outcomes and thromboembolic events. Ann Pharmacother 47:447–454

Broze GJ, Majerus PW (1980) Purification and properties of human coagulation factor VII. J Biol Chem 255(4):1242–1247

James I, John M (2010) Australia and New Zealand haemostasis registry. Monsah University, Melbourne

Levi M, Levy JH, Andersen HF et al (2010) Safety of recombinant activated factor VII in randomized clinical trials. N Engl J Med 363(19):1791–1800

Mamtani R, Nascimento B, Rizoli S et al (2012) The utility of recombinant factor VIIa as a last resort in trauma. World J Emerg Surg 22(7 Suppl 1):S7. doi:10.1186/1749-7922-7-S1-S7

Pallister CJ, Watson MS (2010) Haematology. Scion Publishing, London, pp 336–347. ISBN 1-904842-39-9

Parameswaran R, Shapiro AD, Gill JC et al (2005) Dose effect and efficacy of rFVIIa in the treatment of haemophilia patients with inhibitors: analysis from the Hemophilia and Thrombosis Research Society Registry. Haemophilia 11(2):100–106

Factor XIII

▶ Adjuncts to Transfusion: Recombinant Factor VIIa, Factor XIII, and Calcium

Falls

Jan Gillespie
Trauma Program Manager, Loyola University Medical Center, Maywood, IL, USA

Synonyms

Extremity fractures; Falls from heights; Falls from standing; Hip fractures; TBI (traumatic brain injury); Vertebral column injuries

Definition

The definition for "falls" varies throughout the literature. For this chapter, the definition utilized is found in http//:dictionary.reference.com/browse/falls 2014. As stated, two characterizations for "falls" are pertinent to the chapter: (1) to drop or descend under the force of gravity, as to a lower place through loss or lack of support, and (2) to come or drop down suddenly to a lower position, especially to leave a standing or erect position suddenly, whether voluntarily or not. Simply put, a fall is categorized as descending, unintentionally or intentionally, under the force of gravity, to a lower place.

Introduction

Falls are a conundrum for trauma, as each fall will yield different results for different patients. In 2010, falls accounted for 424,000 deaths worldwide (WHO 2012). Since only trauma centers report data, the true number of falls and types of those falls remains approximate. One of the biggest concerns is the aging population and their propensity for falls, some seemingly insignificant.

For the sake of continuity, this chapter will be divided into three sections: pediatrics aged 1–14 (SafeKIDS 2004), adults 16–59, and the elderly ≥60 years of age (WHO 2012). Each section will discuss falls with specific mechanisms. Common signs and symptoms with appropriate treatment will be explored. All types of falls are predicated on the use of the primary and secondary surveys, as discussed in ATLS, Advanced Trauma Life Support (ACS-COT 2012); TNCC-P, Trauma Nursing Core Course (Gurney and Westergard 2014); and ATCN, Advanced Trauma Care for Nurses (ACS-COT 2012).

Primary: Looking for Life Threats
- Airway: Is the airway obstructed? Immobilize the C-Spine if appropriate; alertness can also be observed at this time.
- Breathing: What type of breathing are they exhibiting? Administer oxygen.
- Circulation: Stop external hemorrhage; start IV access.
- Disability: Neurological check; use the Glasgow Coma Scale (GCS).
- Environment: Strip/flip/keep warm; look for visible injuries and check the back.

Secondary: Looking for All Injuries
- Full set of vitals/adjuncts: Cardiac monitor, SpO$_2$ monitor, naso- or orogastric tube if not contraindicated, Foley catheter if not contraindicated, labs, and family presence.
- Give comfort measures: Non-pharmacological and pharmacological.
- History: Event and patient.
- Head to toe: Look, listen, and feel – start with the head and move downward.

- Diagnostics and labs if not done with full set of vitals.
- Admission/transfer.

Pediatrics

Etiology
More than 2.3 million children ages 14 and under are treated annually at hospital emergency rooms (Safe KIDS 2004). Falls injure more children 14 and under than any other unintentional injury.

The causes of pediatric falls are varied and many. In the younger child, supervision is the main reason children fall. Falls also occur as part of "growing up" where a child may be encouraged to try risky behaviors, i.e., riding a bike, climbing a tree, or jumping off of elevated playground equipment. In the older child, who is seeking independence, poor choices are the reasons for their falls. Infants are more likely to fall from furniture, baby walkers, and downstairs. Toddlers tend to fall from windows. Other children fall more often from playground equipment (Safe KIDS 2004). Prevention is the key to decreasing any of these types of falls.

Kinematics
Historically, pediatric falls from elevations 2–3 times the height of the child, or falls greater than 15 ft (Murray et al. 2000), have been used as criteria for transport to trauma centers. These falls would include, but not be limited to, falls from second-story windows, falls from balconies, and falls down a flight of stairs. However, falls from less than 15 ft have been found to also have significant injuries (Murray et al. 2000). These falls would include, but not be limited to, falls from baby walkers and playground equipment (CDC 2012). A high index of suspicion is required in injuries associated with falls, as more than one system may have been damaged. A small external injury could have life-threatening internal impairment.

Anatomy and Physiology Considerations
Remember, children are not small adults. They have anatomical and physiological differences. The head is larger in proportion to body size

and as such will lead the way during falls. Significant brain injuries have been reported. The airway is smaller, the trachea is more anterior, the tongue is large, and the uvula is "floppy," so airway considerations are important. When in a supine position, a child's large head will flex the airway forward, causing an airway obstruction. The cricoid rings are not well formed. A surgical cricothyrotomy should not be the first choice for young children who have difficult airway access. The neck muscles do not provide much support in the young child and a SCIWORA (spinal cord injury without radiologic abnormality) must always be considered (Gurney and Westergard 2014). The ribs are soft and pliable, so rib fractures in children are significant. Children have poor pulmonary reserve. Their intercostal muscles are weak and they are unable to increase their tidal volume, so you will see an increased respiratory rate in a stressed child (Tuggle and Kreykes 2013). The cardiac system is immature and they rely on heart rate to maintain cardiac output. The abdominal muscles are not well formed, and the abdomen itself is protuberant, thus not protected by the ribs. The bones are pliable. Internal organs are not fully mature and injury can again be substantial.

Falls That Will Be Covered

- Falls from heights varying in degrees of elevation – balconies, windows, trees, stairs, baby walkers, and playground equipment.
- Falls from bicycles, scooters, and skateboards will **not** be included in this chapter.

Falls from Heights

Falls from heights, varying in degrees of elevation, should always have a high index of suspicion for injury. In several studies, falls from heights varying in degrees of elevation had some of the same injuries and also different injuries. The falls from heights 2–3 times the height of the child may produce traumatic brain injury and extremity injuries (CDC 2012). The brain injuries also include skull fractures. Internal organ injury must be suspected. The lower-level falls will result in more significant brain injuries and fewer extremity injuries (Murray et al. 2000).

All falls need to be prospectively evaluated to ensure that critically injured children are triaged to the appropriate trauma center.

Signs and Symptoms

Look at the mechanism of injury. How are did the child fall? What kind of surface did the child land on? What part of the child's body landed first? Knowing this information will give you an idea of what to expect during assessment.

Complete your primary and secondary surveys (ACS-COT 2012). Listed below is an example of a primary and secondary assessment tool you may want to use:

- **Airway:** Is it clear? Immobilize C-spine if appropriate. An obstructed airway is a life threat – be sure the patient is in a sniffing position and their head is not flexed forward; alertness should also be noted at this time.
- **Breathing**: Look, listen, and feel; bilateral breath sounds indicate good ventilation and oxygenation – life threats would include a tension pneumothorax, open pneumothorax, flail chest, or massive hemothorax. A flail chest is rare in a pediatric patient.
- **Circulation:** Stop the bleeding – check pulses; bradycardia is an ominous sign in pediatric patients. Establish IV access and give appropriate fluid – remember a child's liver hasn't fully matured and you need to add glucose to maintenance fluid.
- **Disability:** Neurological exam; based on the pediatric Glasgow Coma Scale, the earliest sign of a head injury in a pediatric patient is the patient's inability to recognize their primary caregivers.
- **Environment:** Take off their clothes, check for external injuries, look at their back, and keep them warm.
- **Full set of vitals:** Remember blood pressure is one of the most unreliable signs of homeostasis in the pediatric patient.
- **Adjuncts:** Put the patient on the cardiac monitor, use the SpO_2 monitor, place a naso-/orogastric tube unless contraindicated, insert a Foley catheter unless contraindicated, and draw labs.

- **Give comfort measures:** Pain management – both non-pharmacological and pharmacological.
- **History:** Make sure you know if there are any disabilities or comorbid factors.
- **Head to toe survey:** Look for additional injuries – if the patient is in need of an operation, the secondary survey may not be finished.
- **Inspect the back**, if it is not already completed.
- **Diagnostics:** Tests you will need – at what point will plain films be used or CT scans appreciated?

Appropriate Care

During the primary and secondary surveys, you will find life threats, which are treated immediately, and other injuries which may be treated later. Appropriate care is based on patient diagnosis, which should rely on kinematics and clinical assessment. For example, if there is an airway issue, immediately you would use an airway adjunct such as a nasal airway for the conscious patient or an oral airway for the unconscious patient. Pediatric patients must have appropriately sized airway adjuncts. Definitive care would include intubation. When other life threats are discovered, they must be taken care of immediately. Covering an open pneumothorax with a three-sided occlusive dressing and then placing a chest tube is lifesaving. A tension pneumothorax is definitively taken care of with a chest tube and should be determined clinically before any films are taken. The massive hemothorax needs a chest tube and possibly a thoracotomy, if the origin of the bleeding needs to be determined. A flail chest is extremely painful, and if the patient is unable to take deep breaths, intubation with positive pressure ventilation should be considered. A flail chest is very rare in the pediatric population. External hemorrhage must be controlled and IV access attained. Once the patient is stabilized, the secondary survey can be completed. Pediatric patients are resilient, but depending on age and maturity, all systems must be considered when assessing falls. The most important challenge you have is

making sure you identify "what will kill your patient right now."

Tips

- If you are having difficulty hearing breath sounds on the anterior chest, listen at the midaxillary area. By doing this, you will not hear "gurgling" stomach sounds.
- Keep the head/neck/chest in line (sniffing position) by placing a folded blanket/towel under the patient's shoulders.
- A tension pneumothorax needs an immediate chest tube.
- Maintain a logical manner of assessment.
- Never discount the possibility of a spinal cord injury.
- Remember the anatomical and physiological parameters for children of all ages, as this age group goes from 1 to 15.

Prevention is paramount to avoiding these injuries. Prevention can include but not be limited to safety fairs for children, teen hot lines, and parenting classes.

Adult

Etiology

The study of falls in adults between 15 and 60 has been remote (Friedland et al. 2013). Falls from heights have been studied more than falls from standing. The other caveat is to be able to look at the percentage of people with an elevated alcohol level and discern whether alcohol had an impact on the injury itself and subsequently the recovery (Friedland et al. 2013).

Kinematics

The adult patient, from 16 to 44 years of age, is the most prone to deadly trauma (CDC 2012). Car crashes lead this group as the number one reason for fatalities. Falls from different elevations are also a risk for this age group, and traumatic brain injuries (TBI) are of most concern. Spinal cord injuries will also occur in this age group (Como et al. 2009). Remember, when looking at kinematics, how far did the patient fall, on what kind of surface did they land, and what body part hit the surface first? As an example, a fall from a third-story window may be a head first, feet first, buttocks first, or side first, all of which may provide an axial load injury.

Anatomy and Physiology Considerations

The adult will have reached maturity and will maintain a physiological reserve. Care needs to be taken with comorbidities and disabilities. This group is heading for the elder population.

Falls That Will Be Covered

- Falls from heights: Porches, stairs, roofs, trees, and cherry pickers
- Falls from standing

Signs and Symptoms

Assess the patient using the primary and secondary surveys (ACS-COT 2012). Once you establish a logical assessment practice, determining life threats will become more routine. The primary and secondary survey tool is listed below as a refresher:

- **Airway:** Is it clear? Immobilize C-spine if appropriate; an obstructed airway is a life threat – alertness should also be noted at this time (alert, verbal, painful stimuli, unresponsive – AVPU) (Gurney and Westergard 2014); consider the need for an airway adjunct and/or intubation.
- **Breathing:** Look, listen, and feel; bilateral breath sounds indicate good ventilation and oxygenation – life threats would include a tension pneumothorax, open pneumothorax, flail chest, or massive hemothorax; each one needs to be taken care of before moving on.
- **Circulation:** Stop the bleeding – check pulses; bradycardia is an ominous sign. Establish IV access – give appropriate fluid.
- **Disability:** Neurological exam; based on the Glasgow Coma Scale, the earliest sign of a head injury is the patient's inability to recognize their significant others – although a space-occupying lesion may need evacuation, each patient will be individually evaluated for immediacy.

- **Environment:** Take off their clothes, check for external injuries, take them off of the backboard, and keep them warm.
- **Full set of vitals:** Remember blood pressure is one of the most unreliable signs of homeostasis.
- **Adjuncts:** Put the patient on the cardiac monitor, use the SpO_2 monitor, place a naso-/orogastric tube unless contraindicated, insert a Foley catheter unless contraindicated, and draw labs.
- **Give comfort measures:** Pain management – both non-pharmacological and pharmacological.
- **History:** Make sure you know if there are any disabilities or comorbid factors. Confirm the kinematics of the fall – distance, landing, and body.
- **Head to toe survey:** Look for additional injuries, and start at the head and work down – look, listen, and feel; if the patient is in need of an operation, the secondary survey may not be finished.
- **Inspect the back**, if it is not already completed.
- **Diagnostics**: Tests you will need – at what point will plain films be used or CT scans appreciated?

Appropriate Care

The mechanism of injury is paramount. How far did the patient fall and on what kind of surface did they land? Did they hit any objects during the fall? Did they lose consciousness? If the fall was from standing, knowing the reason is important – did they lose their balance, did they have a syncopal episode, and did they trip? Those will help determine the injuries. Remember falls from standing can produce a severe traumatic brain injury (TBI) and extremity injuries will be less. Falls from heights can produce a TBI, spinal cord injury, torso injuries, and extremity injury.

Life threats must be identified and resolved immediately. Listed below are the life threats:

1. Airway: Open and intubate. Use a surgical airway, if needed.
2. Tension pneumothorax: Chest tube.

3. Massive hemothorax: Chest tube – possible thoracotomy.
4. Open pneumothorax: 3-sided occlusive dressing followed by a chest tube.
5. Flail chest: May require intubation and positive pressure ventilation.
6. Uncontrolled hemorrhage: Stop the bleeding – may need immediate OR – crystalloids/blood.
7. TBI: Is there uncontrolled bleeding? Does the patient need to go immediately to the OR, for such focal injuries as an epidural and/or a subdural hematoma?

Consults should be called as soon as a diagnosis reveals immediate need.

Tips

- Reassessment is the key to a successful resuscitation.
- Vitals need to be trended to be meaningful – obtaining a blood pressure is important, and a narrowing pulse pressure may indicate continued bleeding versus a widening pulse pressure which may indicate a brain injury. Keep track of pulses, as sustained tachycardia could indicate the need for more intense resuscitation. Respirations will reveal good ventilation/oxygenation and may indicate the need for intubation.
- Transfers should be accomplished as soon as the need has been identified. Obtaining more diagnostics could delay transfer and put the patient at risk for secondary injury.

Again, prevention is the key to decreasing fall injuries.

Elderly

Etiology

The major causes for fall-related hospital admissions are hip fractures, traumatic brain injuries, and upper limb injuries (WHO 2007). In addition, 20 % of those patients with hip fractures die within a year of the incident (WHO 2007). Falls account for 36.8 per 100,000 population in the United States (CDC 2012). Fall fatalities for both men and women increase exponentially with age. More women sustain hip fractures, but mortality with a hip fracture is greater in men (CDC 2012).

By 2050 more people worldwide will be over 60 than children under the age of 14 (WHO 2007). This will be a historical event. There are four major risk factors for the elderly to consider – biological, behavioral, environmental, and socioeconomic (WHO 2007). Biological risks consist of age, gender, and race which are not able to be modified. Behavioral risks are those things over which we have control, such as medications, alcohol use, and a lifestyle that doesn't contain much movement (WHO 2007). Environmental risks consist of hazardous elements of a personal environment, such as narrow steps, loose carpeting, and poor lighting (WHO 2007). The public environmental challenges could include slippery floors, uneven walking surfaces, and poor building design (WHO 2007). Behavioral and environmental risks can be reduced. Socioeconomic issues are challenges for the person and community which may consist of low-income areas, a population with low education, and housing that is not adequate.

Kinematics

Elderly falls can be an enigma, as each patient will be unique. People do not age in the same fashion and the aging population in the United States is growing. Falls from standing are truly a puzzle and can make diagnosis and treatment a challenge. The simple hip fracture may also include a traumatic brain injury, such as a subdural hemorrhage or epidural hemorrhage and/or a spinal cord/vertebral column injury. The decision to operate or transfer the patient should be made quickly during the primary survey (ACS-COT 2012).

Anatomy and Physiology Considerations

The aging population will have anatomical and physiological changes which directly affect trauma outcomes of falls. The hallmark of aging is the lack of reserve NOT confusion. In other words, the elder trauma patient will not rebound like a pediatric or adult patient. Their length of stay in the hospital will be longer, they have the potential for an elevated number of morbidities, and comorbid factors will play a role in healing.

The cardiovascular system is slowing, with the SA node not conducting as it normally should. Atrial fibrillation and AV heart blocks are not uncommon. The vessels are stiffening and the elderly are less responsive to catecholamines. The work of breathing increases, especially if the patient has respiratory comorbidities such as COPD or emphysema. The brain begins to atrophy, with the bridging veins being stretched. The stretched bridging veins are labile and easily torn resulting in chronic and acute subdural hematoma formation. Cognition is diminished, autoregulation is impaired, and motor changes may be seen. The renal system diminishes in size, and the kidneys begin to lose function. The musculoskeletal system is affected with decreased lean muscle. Bone mass decreases, leading to osteoporosis. The immune system slows down and the elderly are at more risk for infection and sepsis.

Falls That Will Be Covered
- Falls from standing/sitting
- Falls from heights – porches, ladders, stairs, and roofs

Common Symptoms
Understanding the kinematics of the incident is paramount in making the correct diagnosis. How far did the patient fall? What kind of surface did they land on? What body part hit the surface first? Assess the patient using the primary and secondary surveys (ACS-COT 2012). Once you establish a logical assessment practice, determining life threats will become more routine. The primary and secondary survey tool is listed below as a refresher:

- **Airway:** Is it clear? Immobilize C-spine if appropriate – an obstructed airway is a life threat. Dentures might be the reason for the obstruction – remove them – alertness should also be noted at this time (AVPU).

- **Breathing:** Look, listen, and feel; bilateral breath sounds indicate good ventilation and oxygenation – life threats would include a tension pneumothorax, open pneumothorax, flail chest, or massive hemothorax. These need to be taken care of immediately.

- **Circulation:** Stop the bleeding, and check pulses; bradycardia is an ominous sign. Establish IV access, give appropriate fluid, and avoid overhydration and attempt euvolemia.

- **Disability:** Neurological exam: based on the Glasgow Coma Scale, the earliest sign of a head injury is the patient's inability to recognize their significant others or family members – although a space-occupying lesion may need evacuation, each patient will be individually evaluated; the elder patient may not be a candidate for surgical intervention due to increased risk of surgery and the type or volume of bleeding. Anticoagulation medications and their reversibility will play a role in determining surgical intervention.

- **Environment:** Take off their clothes and check for external injuries. Take them off the backboard and inspect their back; keep them warm. Skin breakdown can occur within 15 minutes of patients being placed on the backboard.

- **Full set of vitals:** Remember blood pressure is one of the most unreliable signs of homeostasis.

- **Adjuncts:** Put the patient on the cardiac monitor, use the SpO_2 monitor, place a naso-/orogastric tube unless contraindicated, insert a Foley catheter unless contraindicated, draw labs, and have family presence.

- **Give comfort measures:** Pain management – both non-pharmacological and pharmacological. Just repositioning a patient may give them great relief. Remember the elder patient may have a different response to pain medication due to many factors, including loss of lean muscle.

- **History:** Make sure you know if there are any disabilities, comorbid factors, and medications they are taking – include over-the-counter medications. Again it is important to determine if they are taking anticoagulant medication.

- **Head to toe survey:** Look for additional injuries – if the patient is in need of an operation, the secondary survey may not be finished. Start at the head and proceed downward, using the look, listen, and feel method. One of the most common vertebral column injuries is a fracture of the odontoid process at cervical vertebrae 2.
- **Inspect the back**, if it is not already completed.
- **Diagnostics:** Tests you will need – at what point will plain films be used or CT scans appreciated? Remember the literature suggests that the only plain film to be taken should be a chest x-ray (Como et al. 2009).

Appropriate Care

Mechanism of injury is extremely important. Was their fall from a height or from standing? On what type of surface did they land? Remember a simple hip fracture can also be combined with a TBI, spinal cord/vertebral injury, or extremity trauma. Torso trauma should also be explored.

Again, rely on the primary survey for life threats and the secondary survey to define all other injuries. Consider the anatomical and physiological changes which occur with aging.

Life threats must be identified and resolved immediately. Listed below are the life threats:

1. Airway: Open and intubate. Use a surgical airway, if needed.
2. Tension pneumothorax: Chest tube.
3. Massive hemothorax: Chest tube – possible thoracotomy.
4. Open pneumothorax: 3-sided occlusive dressing followed by a chest tube.
5. Flail chest: May require intubation and positive pressure ventilation.
6. Uncontrolled hemorrhage: Stop the bleeding – may need immediate OR – crystalloids/blood.
7. TBI: Is there uncontrolled bleeding? Does the patient need to go immediately to the OR for such focal injuries as an epidural and/or subdural hematoma?

Consults should be called as soon as a diagnosis reveals immediate need. It is important to note that the elder population needs the resources of trauma centers when the injury has more than one system involved. Example: An elder patient with a simple hip fracture turns out to also have a TBI and a vertebral column challenge. This patient needs a trauma center with adequate resources to care for the elder trauma patient.

Tips

- Determine the patient's normal mental and physical status: Did it change after the traumatic incident? Confusion is not normal.
- Loss of reserve function is the hallmark of aging. They won't rebound as quickly.
- Speak slowly and clearly, wait for several seconds for an answer, and don't rush the patient.
- There are no "simple" falls with the elder trauma patient; always have an index of suspicion for injury other than the obvious one.
- All systems are aging; never rely on the "normals" for the aging patient – a normal blood pressure in an elder patient may indicate shock rather than normalcy.
- The vertebral column is always at risk with a fall. The odontoid fracture commonly occurs in the elder patient. The mnemonic "A brain injury is a neck injury until proven otherwise and a neck injury is a brain injury until proven otherwise" will prove helpful during assessment.
- Transfers should be decided on as soon as a diagnosis is made that would require a transfer.

Prevention will reduce the number of elder falls. The prevention may include, but not be limited to, wellness checks; having the homes checked for possible hazards such as loose rugs, uneven steps, or floors; and accepting resources to maintain living in the home versus going to a nursing home.

Summary

Falls continue to occur for many different reasons and from many different heights. The three questions that need to be asked for all falls are as follows: (1) From what height did they fall? (2) On what type of surface did they fall? (3) What part of the body hit the surface first? It is imperative to look at the age and condition of your patients. Using the primary and secondary tools for assessment will make diagnoses, admission, and transfer, if indicated, a more logical, reasonable, and successful mechanism for patients who have fallen, no matter how young or old they are. Prevention is the key to avoiding these potentially life-threatening injuries.

Cross-References

▶ Airway Management in Trauma, Nonsurgical
▶ Alcohol (ETOH) Withdrawal and Management
▶ Bicycle-Related Injuries
▶ Clearance, Cervical Spine
▶ Distal Femur Fractures
▶ Distal Humerus Fractures
▶ Distal Radius Fractures
▶ Examination, Neurological
▶ Falls from Height
▶ Femoral Shaft Fractures
▶ Fluid, Electrolytes, and Nutrition in Trauma Patients
▶ Fracture, Odontoid
▶ Fracture, Axis (C2)
▶ Geriatric Trauma
▶ Hip Dislocations and Fracture-Dislocations
▶ Imaging of Spine and Bony Pelvis Injuries
▶ Interpersonal Violence
▶ Mechanical Ventilation, Conventional
▶ Neurotrauma, Introduction
▶ Neurotrauma, Pediatric Considerations
▶ Neurotrauma, Prognosis and Outcome Predictions
▶ Open Fractures
▶ Pedestrian Injuries
▶ Pediatric Fractures About the Hip
▶ Pelvis Fractures
▶ Principles of Internal Fixation of Fractures
▶ Principles of Nonoperative Treatment of Diaphyseal Fractures
▶ Proximal Femoral Fractures
▶ Shock
▶ Shock Management in Trauma
▶ Spinal Shock
▶ Tibial Fractures

References

American College of Surgeons Committee on Trauma (2012) Initial assessment and management. In: Advanced trauma life support, 9th edn. American College of Surgeons Committee, Chicago, pp 2–22

Centers for Disease control and Prevention (2012) Falls among older adults: an overview. Atlanta. Retrieved from www.cdc.gov/Falls/adultfalls.html

Centers for Disease Control and Prevention, National Center for Injury Prevention and Control (2012) Playground injuries: fact sheet. (Updated, March). Centers for Disease Control and Prevention, National Injury Prevention and Control printing office, Atlanta. Retrieved from www.cdc.gov/homeandrecreationalsafety/Play-ground-injuries/playgroundinjuries-factsheet.htm

Como J, Diaz J, Dunham M, Chiu W, Duane T, Capella J, Holevar M, Winston E et al (2009) Cervical spine injuries following trauma. J Trauma 67(3):651–659

Dictionary.com (2014) Definition of FALL. Retrieved from http//:dictionary.reference.com/browse/falls. 26 May 2014

Friedland D, Brunton I, Potts J (2013) Falls and traumatic brain injury in adults under the age of sixty. Springer, New York

Gurney D, Westergard A (2014) Initial assessment. In: Gurnee D (ed) Trauma nursing core course, 7th edn. Emergency Nurses Association, Des Plaines, pp 39–54

Murray JA, Chen D, Velmahos GC, Alo K, Belzberg H, Demetriades D, Berne V (2000) Pediatric falls: is height a predictor or injury and outcome? Am Surg 66(9):863–865

National SAFE KIDS Campaign (NSKC) (2004) Falls fact sheet. NSKC, Washington, DC

Tuggle D, Kreykes N (2013) Chapter 43. The pediatric patient. In: Mattox K, Moore E, Feliciano D (eds) Trauma, 7th edn. McGraw Hill, New York, pp 859–873

World Health Organization (2007) WHO global report on falls prevention in older age. WHO Press, Geneva, pp 1–47. Printed in France

Recommended Reading

Allerman D (2007) Considerations in pediatric trauma. Retrieved from www.emedicine.medscape.com/article455031. 26 May 2014

American College of Surgeons (2012) [ST-65] Statement on concussion and brain injury. Bull Am Coll Surg 97(12)

Children's Hospital of Pittsburg of UPMC (2012) Fall-injury statistics and incidence rates. Children's Health A-Z, Pittsburg. Retrieved from www.chp.edu/CHP/PO2974. 7 May 2014

Claridge J, Banerjee A (2014) Immunoligic. In: Yelon J, Luchette F (eds) Geriatric and critical care. Springer, New York, pp 45–54

Currie L (2011) Chapter 10. Fall and injury prevention. In: Patient safety and quality: an evidence-based handbook for nurses. Columbia University School of Nursing, New York, pp 1–24

Esposito T, Brasel K (2013) Chapter 2 Epidemiology. In: Mattox K, Moore E, Feliciano D (eds) Trauma, 7th edn. McGraw Hill, New York, pp 18–35

Farrah J, Martin S, Chang M (2014) Cardiovascular physiology. In: Yelon J, Luchette F (eds) Geriatric and critical care. Springer, New York, pp 11–20

Hunt J, Marr A, Stuke L (2013) Chapter 1, Kinematics. In: Mattox K, Moore E, Feliciano D (eds) Trauma, 7th edn. McGraw Hill, New York, pp 8–15

MedlinePlus (2013) Falls. Retrieved from www.nim.nih.gov/medlineplus/falls.html. 27 May 2014

NIH Senior Health (2013) About falls. Retrieved from www.nihseniorhealth.gov/falls/aboutfalls/01.html. 16 May 2014

Staudenmayer K (2013) Seniors with serious injuries often don't receive specialized care. American College of Surgeons, news release, Chicago. Accessed 1 May 2014

World Health Organization Media Centre (2012) Falls, Fact sheet N°344. Retrieved from mediainquiries@who.int. 1 May 2014

World Health Organization (2012) Violence and injury prevention, falls. Retrieved from www.who.int/violence_injury_prevention/other_injury/falls/en/index.html. 1 May 2014

Yelon J (2013) Chapter 44, the geriatric patient. In: Mattox K, Moore E, Feliciano D (eds) Trauma, 7th edn. McGraw Hill, New York, pp 874–895

Falls from Elevation

▶ Falls from Height

Falls from Height

Elizabeth K. Powell
Department of Emergency Medicine,
Hospital of the University of Pennsylvania,
Philadelphia, PA, USA

Synonyms

Falls from elevation; Jumper injuries; Vertical deceleration injuries

Epidemiology

Falls from height effect a wide demographic and can occur in many different settings. Falls can be due to either unintentional circumstances or suicide attempts and can also be associated with drugs, alcohol, and psychiatric illness. In the occupational setting, falls from height are the most common cause of accidents (Jeong 1998). Out -of-hospital mortality from falls comprises 70 % of all fall mortality (Lapostolle et al. 2005).

Both pediatric and elderly patients are at particular risk for falls. Pediatric falls are a frequent source of emergency department visits and hospitalizations. Falls among children and adolescents account for more than three million emergency department visits each year, and more than 40 % occur among infants, toddlers, and preschoolers (Schermer 2002).

Falls from height account for 29 % of injury-related deaths among adults aged 65 and older (CDC 2002). Older patients are also more likely to die from falls (Lapostolle et al. 2005) and are also five times more likely to be hospitalized after a fall then younger patients (Alexander et al. 1992). Elderly patients tend to have poorer muscle tone, vision problems, and medication use that make them more prone to falls (CDC 2002). Falls in the home from standing can also be due to lack of handrails and poor lighting conditions as well as rugs. Elderly patients are also more likely to be on anticoagulation medications which predispose to greater injury from less height.

Anatomy of Injury

Similar to motor vehicle crashes, falls from height cause injury through an abrupt deceleration injury. However, unlike motor vehicle crashes which cause injury from horizontal deceleration, falls cause injury from vertical deceleration (Buckman and Buckman 1991). Several factors can affect injuries after a fall. When considering potential injury from a fall, the patient's age, height of fall, what the patient struck when falling, and what body part first struck the ground are all predictors of prognostic factors in a patient with a fall from height. Distance fallen can predict serious injury after a fall. Impact (v) is related to height fallen (h) and acceleration due to gravity (g) (Goodacre et al. 1999):

$$v = \sqrt{2gh}$$

The median height of falls in patients who died was 15 m which corresponded to five floors (Lapostolle et al. 2005). Though patients who fall from greater heights are at greater risk for serious injury, falls from shorter heights can also lead to serious injury depending on additional factors such as the use of blood thinners or preexisting medical conditions.

The location on the body that strikes the ground first is another predictor of serious injury. Individuals who strike their feet first on any presenting surface are at less risk for major injury then those who strike head first. Also, those who land on their heads had a greater risk of injury (Lapostolle et al. 2005). Children are particularly at risk for striking head first as their head weight is a greater proportion of their body than in adults. Due to the relatively greater weight of the child's head, they are more likely to have cranial trauma from falls resulting in increased mortality (Lapostolle et al. 2005). Death due to falls is generally from a head injury (Hall et al. 1989). The majority of falls occurs in the home from windows or balconies (Lallier et al. 1999). In children under age 5, falls of less than 2 m rarely result in death, and severe injuries reported from these heights should be further investigated (Reiber 1993).

Landing head first is life-threatening while landing feet first has the potential for lower extremity injuries which are not typically life-threatening though transmitted energy can travel up the spine, leading to fractures. In ventral impacts, there is a 57 % mortality compared to 23 % mortality in dorsal impacts (Lapostolle et al. 2005). In vertical deceleration injuries, fractures and extremity injuries are seen more commonly than in horizontal deceleration injuries where intra-abdominal injuries are more common. However, aortic lacerations do also occur in vertical deceleration injuries. In patients with

a fracture in the foot, two thirds also had a lumbar spinal fracture (Scalea et al. 1986). Patients with feet-first falls can also have head, neck, and pelvis injuries from throw-back injuries. Pelvic fractures are most commonly seen in buttock and feet-first falls. Pelvic fractures occur 20–30 % of the time with falls from height and have an increasing prevalence with increasing height of fall (Scalea et al. 1986). Cervical spine fractures are rarely seen in falls but can be observed with feet-first falls with flexion of the neck.

The impact surface also plays a role in traumatic injuries. Soft impact surfaces such as snow with maximum deformity can be life-saving unlike concrete where deceleration forces are more severe and ground deformity is much less (Lapostolle et al. 2005). Water also offers greater deformability and increased deceleration times, lessening injury. Feet-first impact into water also allows decreased deceleration forces when compared to lateral impacts.

Clinical Impact

Trauma Triage Significance
When triaging and considering possible injuries from falls from height, it is important to consider the age of the patient, the height of the fall, structures stuck during the fall, and the surface that the patient lands on in addition to the part of the body that first strikes the ground. Patients with falls are also at risk for spinal injuries, so full immobilization should be performed. Considering these factors will lead to appropriate triage, stabilization, and treatment of these patients.

Clinical Evaluation/Care Caveats
Initial clinical evaluation should first involve a primary assessment and determination of adequacy of airway, breathing, and circulation. An initial GCS should also be determined and the patient should be fully exposed to assessment for any hidden injuries. All patients should be fully immobilized for transport as neurologic injuries should always be assumed until the patient can be fully assessed. Patients that are intoxicated,

unconscious, or who have any distracting injuries should receive head and c-spine imaging in addition to further patient specific imaging as these patients can have multiple injuries.

Cross-References

▶ ABCDE of Trauma Care
▶ Falls
▶ Head Injury
▶ Imaging of Abdominal and Pelvic Injuries
▶ Imaging of Aortic and Thoracic Injuries
▶ Imaging of CNS Injuries
▶ Imaging of Spine and Bony Pelvis Injuries
▶ Trauma Patient Evaluation

References

Alexander BH, Rivara FP, Wolf ME (1992) The cost and frequency of hospitalization for fall-related injuries in older adults. Am J Public Health 82(7):1020–1023

Buckman RF, Buckman PD (1991) Vertical deceleration trauma: principles of management. Surg Clin North Am 71:331–344

CDC (2002) Centers for Disease Control and Prevention, Injury Research Agenda: Preventing Injuries at Home and in the Community. National Center for Injury Prevention and Control

Goodacre S, Than M, Goyder EC, Joseph AP (1999) Can the distance fallen predict serious injury after a fall from a height? J Trauma 46(6):1055–1058

Hall JR, Reyes HM, Horvat M et al (1989) The mortality of childhood falls. J Trauma 29(9):1273–1275

Jeong BY (1998) Occupational deaths and injuries in the construction industry. Appl Ergon 39(5):355–360

Lallier M, Bouchard S, St-Vil D et al (1999) Falls from heights among children: A retrospective review. J Pediatr Surg 34(7):1060–1063

Lapostolle F, Gere C, Borron SW, Pétrovic T, Dallemagne F, Beruben A, Lapandry C, Adnet F (2005) Prognostic factors in victims of falls from height. Crit Care Med 33(6):1239–1242

Reiber GD (1993) Fatal falls in childhood: How far must children fall to sustain fatal head injury? Report of cases and review of the literature. Am J Forensic 14(3):201–207

Scalea T, Goldstein A, Phillips T (1986) An analysis of 161 falls from a height: the jumper syndrome. J Trauma 26:706–711

Schermer C (2002) Falls from heights. Injury Prevention and Control. American College of Surgeons. Online 17 Oct 2002. https://www.facs.org/quality-programs/trauma/ipc/falls

Falls from Heights

▶ Falls

Falls from Standing

▶ Falls

Family Preparation for Organ Donation

Pamela Lipsett and Albert Chi
Department of Surgery, The Johns Hopkins Hospital, Baltimore, MD, USA

Synonyms

Close friend; Guardian; Health-care advocate; Relative; Spouse

Definition

Family refers to any spouse, relative, or close friend who is interested in the health, life, and well-being of an injured or critically ill patient and for whom the "family" may be asked to provide consent for organ donation. Family preparation for organ donation refers to the process of a families' understanding of the injuries, the process of dying and brain death, and the option of organ donation.

Introduction

Perhaps the most difficult task a trauma/critical care practitioner must face is that of end-of-life decision making. Conversations which are related to brain death, withdrawal of support, and organ donation during a time of stress can be overwhelming for family members as well as staff.

In addition, despite all of the training and preparation of critical situations, most physicians are ill prepared to help facilitate the complex intellectual and emotional needs of the family, especially when approaching for organ donation (Williams et al. 2003). Most hospital personnel are also uncomfortable and lack sufficient training necessary in order to present all of the options of organ donation to families. End-of-life decision making for families during a time of complicated grief carries significant consequences long after the death of the loved one. As the decision to donate is limited by time, it is imperative that the discussion between medical staff and family be a decision that is not regretted later while maximizing the donation opportunity.

Background

Organ Donation Shortage

Due to improvements in transplant medicine, survival rates and the quality of life continually improves for patients who have undergone solid organ transplantation. Successful organ transplantation reduces health-care costs and allows transplant recipients to return to the workforce who would otherwise be debilitated. All of these factors have fueled the demand for transplantable organs (Gortmaker et al. 1996). The current demand for solid organs for transplantation far exceeds the number of organs that is available. The need for solid organ transplants is increasing at an annual average rate of 16 %, while the number of actual donors has not changed. Despite efforts to inform the public and professionals about organ donation, and the increased emphasis on documentation for organ donation intention and governmental policies, it has been consistent that more than half of families of potential donors refuse consent.

Application

Elements to Successful Donation

In efforts to increase organ donation, the United States Health Care Financing Administration (HCFA) changed the federal Conditions of Participation (CoP) for organ donation and required hospitals to notify local organ procurement organizations (OPO) for patients in which death is imminent. Families would be approached by trained donation requestors and be presented with the options of organ and tissue donation.

Several key elements have been identified to help in the conversion of potential organ donors to actual organ donors (Williams et al. 2003; Siminoff et al. 2001, 2007). The most successful requests for donation (1) are made in a private setting; (2) allow the family to comprehend death before discussing organ donation, a process known as decoupling; and (3) involve the OPO transplantation coordinator in the consent process.

All three of these factors significantly and independently increase the consent rate from potential organ donors. The consent rate is 2.5 times higher when all three elements are present compared to when none are present (Siminoff et al. 2001, 2007). Despite identifying these key elements to success, still less than 1/3 of all organ donation requests have all three elements present and overall OPO donor efficiency is approximately 35 % within the USA from medically suitable donor candidates. Even with multidisciplinary approaches including involvement of the intensive care unit physicians, OPO staff, pastoral care, and social services, organ procurement rates are staggering in the face of the present overwhelming need (Table 1).

In-House Coordinators

The utilization of in-house coordinators (IHCs), who are often OPO staff but located directly within the donor hospital, has been shown to increase donations (Shafer et al. 2003). The IHCs are employed by the OPO and help to manage all donor cases. IHC duties include coordinating consent, making the donation request, providing assistance and advice regarding donor management, and ensuring best practices are implemented in all cases. The use of IHCs increased donor referral, consent, and conversion rates in all racial and ethnic groups with the largest in minority populations.

Family Preparation for Organ Donation, Table 1
Practice suggestions for discussing organ donation with families

Focus processes of care on supporting families of all potential donors, consistent with end-of-life care principles
Consider having families present during brain death examinations
Decouple discussions of brain death from the organ donation request
Give families time to comprehend brain death before discussing organ donation
Offer the option of organ donation to all families
Make organ donation requests in a private setting
Involve the organ procurement organization transplantation coordinator in the consent process
Coordinate the efforts of the intensive care unit team and organ procurement organization staff
Provide special training to all persons who request organ donation

The IHC model has proven effective in both large level I trauma centers as well as smaller community hospitals.

Much has been written of the "Spanish model" which consists of a decentralized structure of organ procurement in which "transplant coordinators" located within the hospital manage the entire donation process (Martinez et al. 2001). Managing organ donation from within rather than cultivating a referral-response system from an outside organization resulted in an increase of 14.3 donors per million population in 1989 to 33.6 donors per million per population in 1999 in Spain. The reason identified for the success of the Spanish model, lies in the sense of involvement and accountability for performance held by hospital transplant coordinators. It is now widely accepted that the main cause of the dramatic increase of organ donation is due to the position and personal responsibility of the in-house transplant coordinators.

Family Factors Affecting Donation

Families' hospital experiences significantly affect their decisions to donate organs. There are often striking differences between donor and nondonor families (Rodrigue et al. 2006). Nondonor families are often less satisfied with the donation request process. Specifically, nondonor families are less likely to believe sufficient time and privacy were provided to make their decision, the perceptions that the staff making the request was insensitive to the families' needs. Overall, only 66 % of nondonor families expressed satisfaction with their decision regarding organ donation. About of third of the family members of nondonors, when subsequently interviewed, suggested they would not make the same decision again. Donor families however have a much clearer understanding of brain death and were much more satisfied with the process for requesting donation. Overall 94 % of donor families expressed satisfaction with their decision.

Assessing Family Readiness

Several improvements in the approach to organ donation have been noted by clinical experience (Simpkin et al. 2009). An innovative approach using the transtheoretical model (TTM) to assess the family readiness for donation may prove useful to enhance family satisfaction as well as improve consent rates (Robbins et al. 2001). TTM research is based that in order to change behavior, people pass through a series of defined stages of change: precontemplation, contemplation, preparation, action, and maintenance (Table 2). In the precontemplation stage, individuals are not ready to take action. They are aware of an issue, but may be misinformed or hold beliefs against it and consequently underestimate the benefits of taking action and overestimate the cost. In the contemplation stage, individuals are thinking of taking action, but the advantages and disadvantages are balanced. Individuals in the preparation stage have decided to take action and make small steps towards the goal. Individuals in the action stage actively engage in modifying behaviors and acquire new health-promoting behaviors. In the maintenance stage, they strive to maintain the change and prevent relapse. Progress through the stages has been found to be cyclic rather than linear as most people revert to earlier stages of change several times before making a successful behavior change. TTM also defines a set of outcomes or

Family Preparation for Organ Donation, Table 2
Stages of change for organ donation consent

Stage category	Staging item
Precontemplation	I was opposed to organ donation
Precontemplation	I was NOT considering organ donation as an option
Contemplation	I was considering the option of organ donation but was not yet ready to make that decision
Preparation	I was ready to choose the option of organ donation and needed more information on the process to go ahead
Action	I had already decided to donate and only needed to move the donation process along

Family Preparation for Organ Donation, Table 3
Pros and cons

Pros	Organ donation is an important way to help somebody else
	Organ donation allows something positive to come out of my loved one's death
	Organ donation might prevent another family from losing a loved one
	My family approves of organ donation
	Organ donation helps people cope with the loss of a loved one
	Consenting to organ donation helps bring meaning to the death of a loved one
	People who consent to organ donation can feel proud of what they have done
Cons	My loved one has suffered enough already and shouldn't have surgery for organ donation
	Organ donation will cause my family more emotional distress
	If I consent to organ donation, the doctors will not try to save my loved one's life
	The physicians may take my loved one's organs before he/she is really dead
	Consenting to organ donation means you can't have an open casket for your loved one
	Hospitals could bill donor families for the costs of organ donation
	Consenting to organ donation will delay my loved one's burial

immediate variables that includes decisional balance, a subjective weighting of the pros and cons of the behavior change (Table 3).

Both stage of change and the decisional balance inventory were strongly associated with the donation decision. Individuals who consented were significantly more likely to be in the preparations or action stages for consent when first meeting with the donation specialist. Donor family members also rated the pros as much more important compared to nondonor family rating the cons as more important. As complex as the physiological factors plays in any decision-making tools such as the TTM models may aid in appropriateness, the timing of approaching the family, and improving sensitivity perceptions. Successful donation may require several preassessments for readiness as well as following practice guidelines (Table 1).

Conclusions
It is our responsibility to be mindful of the significance of family satisfaction with hospital care and successful donation. There are both intellectual and emotional components which are involved in this endeavor. From the intellectual side, a clear explanation of brain death which is decoupled from the discussion of donation is vital. Staff should provide clear information about their loved ones condition and involve specialized OPOs for the organ donation process.

From an emotional standpoint, we also must be cognizant of the timing of the donation request, allow the family time to bring up concerns with staff, not pressure the family to make a decision, and always show respect and compassion. Realize that acceptance of organ donation may be a dynamic process that may cycle from precontemplation to action. By being aware of the complexity of all of the emotional issues, we improve the family's overall hospital experience and optimize our chance of a successful interaction.

Although the goal of increasing the consent rate and procuring more organs is desirable, the more important goal is the implementation process that focuses on the families of potential donors.

When the focus is on the process and not the outcome, either decision becomes acceptable, simultaneously preserving and promoting the goals of the families and organ donation system.

Cross-References

▶ Surrogate, Role in Decision-Making
▶ Terminal Care
▶ Withdrawal of Life-Support

References

Gortmaker SL et al (1996) Organ potential and performances: size and nature of the organ donor shortfall. Crit Care Med 24(3):432–439

Martinez JM, Lopez JS, Martin A et al (2001) Organ donation and family decision-making within the Spanish donation system. Soc Sci Med 53:405

Robbins ML et al (2001) Assessing family members' motivational readiness and decision making for consenting to cadaveric organ donation. J Health Psy 6(5):523–535

Rodrigue JR, Cornell DL, Howard RJ (2006) Organ donation decision: comparison of donor and nondonor families. Am J Transplant 6:190–198

Shafer TJ et al (2003) Location of in-house organ procurement organization staff in level 1 trauma centers increases conversion of potential donors to actual donors. Transplantation 75(8):1330–1335

Siminoff LA et al (2001) Factors influencing families' consent for donation of solid organs for transplantation. JAMA 286(1):71–76

Siminoff LA, Mercer MB, Graham G et al (2007) The reasons families donate organs for transplantation: implications for policy and practice. J Trauma 62:969

Simpkin AL, Robertson LC, Barber VS, Young JD (2009) Modifiable factors influencing relatives' decision to offer organ donation: systematic review. BMJ 338:b991

Williams MA et al (2003) The physician's role in discussing organ donation with families. Crit Care Med 31(5):1568–1573

Fascial Bridge Closure

▶ Mesh Temporary Closure

Fasciotomy

David S. Morris
Division of Trauma, Critical Care, and General Surgery, Mayo Clinic, Rochester, MN, USA

Synonyms

Compartment release, aponeurotomy

Definition

Fasciotomy refers to a procedure wherein a closed anatomical fascial compartment is surgically opened, typically to relieve increased pressure within the compartment or to prevent the development of, or to treat acute compartment syndrome. This increased pressure most commonly results from injury, but may also be a result of ischemia and reperfusion. Providers should have a high suspicion for acute compartment syndrome, as failure to promptly diagnose and treat may lead to devastating dysfunction, limb loss, or even death. The most frequently performed fasciotomies will be briefly described here along with key anatomic considerations.

Lower Leg

The lower leg is comprised of four fascial compartments: anterior, lateral, deep posterior, and superficial posterior. Fasciotomy can be accomplished by either a double or single incision approach, although the single incision, four-compartment fasciotomy is more technically demanding and is less frequently performed (Azar 2013). The double incision fasciotomy is performed by releasing the anterior and lateral compartments through a lateral incision, and the posterior compartments through a medial incision.

Fasciotomies through minimal skin incisions have been described but should be avoided in trauma patients. The amount of tissue edema may exceed the capacitance afforded by fascial release alone without also opening the overlying skin.

Forearm

Similar to the lower leg, the forearm contains four fascial compartments, the dorsal, the lateral – also known as the "mobile wad" – and the superficial and deep volar. The volar compartments are approached via a curvilinear incision on the forearm which avoids major neurovascular structures. The deep volar compartment fascia can be divided after the superficial muscles are retracted to either side.

Unlike the lower leg, acute compartment syndrome of the forearm is often relieved with release of the volar compartments alone; pressures in the lateral and dorsal compartments can be measured after volar release and if concern for high pressures still exists, dorsal release can be performed through a single linear incision.

Thigh

The thigh contains three compartments: anterior, posterior, and medial. Release of the anterior and posterior compartments can be achieved through a single lateral skin incision. The anterior compartment is released by dividing the fascia lata and the posterior compartment is release by retracting the vastus lateralis medially and identifying the posterior septum. A medial incision can be performed to release the adductor compartment.

Other types of fasciotomies, including those of the hand, foot, buttock, or upper arm, are less frequently required.

Fasciotomy incisions should be left open until the cause of the increased pressure within the compartment is reversed. Negative pressure wound dressings are often employed. When primary closure is not possible, split-thickness skin grafting may be necessary (Watson and Lee 2008).

Cross-References

▶ Compartment Syndrome
▶ Compartment Syndrome of the Forearm
▶ Compartment Syndrome of the Leg

▶ Compartment Syndrome, Acute
▶ Compartment Syndrome: Complication of Care in ICU

References

Azar FM (2013) Chapter 48. Traumatic disorders. In: Canale ST, Beaty JH (eds) Campbell's operative orthopaedics, 12th edn. Mosby, Philadelphia
Watson GA, Lee JC (2008) Chapter 34. Compartment syndrome. In: Peitzman AB, Rhodes M, Schwab CW, Yealy DM, Fabian TC (eds) The trauma manual: trauma and acute care surgery, 3rd edn. Lippincot, Williams & Wilkins, Philadelphia

FAST

▶ Imaging of Aortic and Thoracic Injuries
▶ Ultrasound in the Trauma and ICU Setting

Fat Embolism

▶ Fat Embolism Syndrome

Fat Embolism Syndrome

Khanjan H. Nagarsheth
R Adams Cowley Shock Trauma Center,
University of Maryland School of Medicine,
Baltimore, MD, USA

Synonyms

Fat embolism; Fatty embolism

Definition

Fat embolism (FE) is the presence of fat globules in the peripheral circulation and lung tissue. The vast majority of these cases occur after trauma and specifically boney injuries. Even though FE is a relatively common phenomenon, fat embolism syndrome (FES) is not a common occurrence. Gurd and colleagues noted that the classic presentation of cerebral confusion, respiratory distress and a petechial rash of the skin and mucosa are not always observed (Gurd and Wilson 1974). Gurd went on to say that the pathologic finding of pulmonary fat emboli was of questionable value when the features of FES were not present. FES is most commonly associated with long bone fractures and pelvic fractures and more prevalent in closed fractures as opposed to open. Johnson et al. demonstrated that the likelihood of developing FES increased with the number of fractures present. For example, a single long bone fracture resulted in a 1–3 % risk of developing FES but bilateral closed femur fractures had a risk of almost 33 % for developing FES (Johnson and Lucas 1996). There is a wide range reported in the literature as the exact incidence of FES, ranging from 0.9 % when clinically relevant criteria are used to make the diagnosis to 20 % in postmortem studies (Georgopoulos and Bouros 2003).

Preexisting Condition

Pathophysiology
There are two major theories concerning the pathophysiology of FES. The first was touted by Glossing et al. and has come to be known as the "mechanical" theory of FES (Glossing and Pellegrini 1982). This theory rests on the observation that patients with long bone fractures and marrow disruption have a higher incidence of FES. When a fracture occurs, tears in the venules within the bone marrow occur. These tears are suspended open by their boney attachments, so now the adipose in the bone marrow and the surround fatty tissues have an entry point into the systemic circulation. Once in the pulmonary circulation, some of these droplets become fixed and cause local ischemic reactions and some pass through arteriovenous shunts up to the brain where they become lodged in end-capillaries and cause ischemia.

The second theory is called the biochemical theory. This belief rests on the idea of embolized adipose tissue being degraded into free fatty acids (FFAs). These FFA molecules have been shown to experimentally result in severe Acute Respiratory Distress Syndrome (ARDS) in experimental models. Some feel that FFAs are made by pneumocyte induced hydrolysis of embolized fat molecules when they reach the pulmonary capillary beds. From here, these FFA can travel throughout the circulatory system and cause end-organ dysfunction almost anywhere in the body (Baker et al. 1971).

Application

Diagnostics
The traditional method of diagnosing FES was based on clinical signs and ruling out other possible sources. Gurd et al. created a list of major and minor criteria to rule in FES. The diagnosis was based on the presence of at least one major and four minor criteria. The major criteria on their list were: petechial rash, respiratory insufficiency, and cerebral involvement. The minor criteria as they described them were: tachycardia, fever, retinal changes, jaundice, kidney injury, thrombocytopenia, lipomacroglobulinemia, elevated erythrocyte sedimentation rate (ESR), and anemia (Gurd and Wilson 1974).

Laboratory anomalies have been mentioned and include: elevated ESR, anemia, and thrombocytopenia. Another more specific finding will involve presence of an increased pulmonary shunt on arterial blood gas. This will usually be temporally related by 24–48 h to the preceding trauma. Identifying fat cells on peripheral smear and in urine microscopic analysis may point to the diagnosis of FE but are not sensitive for the diagnosis and their absence does not effectively remove this from the differential diagnosis (Van den Brande et al. 2006).

Both chest X-ray (CXR) and chest computed tomography (CT) scans have been used to identify and follow bilateral pulmonary infiltrates. The appearance can range from fluffy infiltrates, have the appearance of lung contusion, or have the appearance of severe ARDS. CT scan of the brain is useful when neurologic alterations have occurred to rule out a traumatic brain injury with delayed presentation (Van den Brande et al. 2006).

Treatment

Treatment of FES is aimed at supportive care with the aggressive use of mechanical ventilation when necessary in order to ensure adequate tissue oxygenation (Habashi et al. 2006). Treatment of the patient with FES in a critical care unit is necessary as is the maintenance of stable hemodynamics, adequate nutrition, restoring circulating blood volume and prophylaxis against gastrointestinal bleeding and deep venous thrombosis. There is a belief that restoring volume with albumin is beneficial in these patients as the albumin is thought to bind with FFA and may decrease the extent of injury to the rest of the body (Habashi et al. 2006). There is significant work on both sides as to the validity of using corticosteroids and heparin and as such, neither can be fully recommended in treatment of FES.

Early operative fixation of long bone and pelvic fractures is beneficial in patients with multiple injuries as it allows for early mobilization of the patient. There has long been controversy as to the ideal method of fixation of long bone fractures: whether there is less FES associated with plates and screws versus intramedullary nailing. EH Schemitsch et al. looked at the pulmonary effects of plate versus intramedullary nailing of long bone fractures in a canine model. They found there was no significant difference in amount of intravascular fat that remained in the lungs, kidneys, or brain 24 h after pressurizing the intramedullary canal, regardless of fixation technique. They also concluded that fracture fixation had no effect on pulmonary artery pressure and that the development of FES is likely dependant on many other factors, not the method of fixation (Schemitsch et al. 1997).

Summary

FE is the presence of fat globules in the peripheral circulation and lung tissue. Over 95 % of cases of FE are associated with trauma, in particular long bone or pelvic trauma. FES is a constellation of symptoms that is most often diagnosed based on the clinical criteria set forth by Gurd et al. This involves the presence of one or more major signs such as cerebral involvement, petechial rash, and respiratory dysfunction as well as minor criteria such as tachycardia, anemia, and elevated ESR. Several imaging adjuncts like CXR and brain and chest CT scan are helpful in ruling out other causes for the symptoms but cannot by themselves make the diagnosis. Treatment is supportive care with aggressive MV when indicated to maintain adequate tissue oxygenation and restoration of stable hemodynamics.

Cross-References

▶ Acute Respiratory Distress Syndrome (ARDS), General
▶ ARDS, Complication of Trauma

References

Baker PL, Paxel JA, Pettier LF (1971) Free fatty acids, catecholamine and arterial hypoxia in patients with fat embolism. J Trauma 11:1026–1030

Georgopoulos D, Bouros D (2003) Fat embolism syndrome clinical examination is still the preferable diagnostic method. Chest 123:982–983

Glossing HR, Pellegrini VD Jr (1982) Fat embolism syndrome: a review of pathology and physiological basis of treatment. Clin Orthop Relat Res 165:68–82

Gurd AR, Wilson RI (1974) The fat embolism syndrome. J Bone Joint Surg Br 56:408–416

Habashi NM, Andrews PL, Scalea TM (2006) Therapeutic aspects of fat embolism syndrome. Injury 37(suppl 4): S68–S73

Johnson MJ, Lucas GL (1996) Fat embolism syndrome. Orthopedics 19:41

Schemitsch EH, Jain R, Turchin DC et al (1997) Pulmonary effects of fixation of a fracture with a plate compared with intramedullary nailing. A canine model of fat embolism and fracture fixation. J Bone Joint Surg Am 79:984–996

Van den Brande FG, Hellemans S, De Schepper A, De Paep R, Op De Beeck B, De Raeve HR et al (2006) Post-traumatic severe fat embolism syndrome, with uncommon CT findings. Anaesth Intensive Care 34:102–106

Fatal Drowning

▶ Drowning

Fatty Embolism

▶ Fat Embolism Syndrome

FDP

▶ Fibrinogen Split Products (Test)

Federal Emergency Management Agency (FEMA)

▶ Prehospital Emergency Preparedness

Feldsher (Russia)

▶ Physician Assistant

Fellow

▶ Postgraduate Education

Femoral Head Fracture-Dislocation

▶ Hip Dislocations and Fracture-Dislocations

Femoral Shaft Fractures

Ryan P. Ficco and Peter J. Nowotarski
Department of Orthopaedic Surgery, Erlanger
Hospital, University of Tennessee College of
Medicine-Chattanooga, Chattanooga, TN, USA

Synonyms

Diaphyseal femur fractures

Definition

Contemporary management of femoral shaft fractures emphasizes early surgical stabilization and rapid mobilization of the patient. The standard treatment of an isolated femoral shaft fracture is intramedullary nailing performed with minimal soft tissue disruption, allowing for early weight-bearing. Nonoperative treatments including prolonged skeletal traction, splinting, bracing, and spica casting have a limited role in modern definitive treatment of adult femoral shaft fractures. Other than their use in provisional stabilization, these modalities are reserved only for patients medically unfit for surgical treatment. The morbidities of prolonged immobilization including skin breakdown, pneumonia, thromboembolism, joint stiffness, and deconditioning are minimized by early surgery, joint motion, and ambulation.

Preexisting Condition

The majority of femoral shaft fractures occur secondary to high energy mechanisms such as motor vehicle crashes, motorcycle accidents, and falls from heights. As such, many of these patient's require formal trauma evaluation by ATLS protocol to evaluate for non-orthopedic injuries including head trauma, thoracic injury, and visceral injury. A secondary survey of the entire musculoskeletal system should be

F

performed with radiographs taken of any area with deformity, crepitus, swelling, or large abrasions. Femoral shaft fractures typically present with visible deformity and swelling of the thigh. Examination for open wounds is critical as these define open fractures requiring immediate intravenous antibiotic treatment and expedient debridement in the operating room. A great deal of energy is required to cause an open femur fracture and extensive underlying soft tissue injury should be expected. Vigilance must be maintained for compartment syndrome, in which excessive swelling and pressure within the thigh prohibit normal tissue perfusion. If present, urgent compartment releases are indicated. After 6 h, progressive irreversible tissue damage occurs. A neurologic and vascular exam of the affected extremity must also be performed. Any discrepancy in pulses requires further workup to rule out vascular injury.

Application

Radiographic evaluation of femoral shaft fractures must include both anteroposterior (AP) and lateral images of the injured femur. As with all musculoskeletal injuries, the joint above and below should be imaged. An AP pelvis, usually required as part of the routine trauma evaluation, should be scrutinized for injuries to the pelvic ring and acetabulum. Ipsilateral hip dislocations can occur, requiring urgent reduction within 6 h of injury to minimize the risk of permanent disruption to the blood supply of the femoral head. An AP and cross table lateral image of the hip should be assessed for associated femoral neck or proximal femur fractures. A fine cut CT scan of the pelvis with sagittal and coronal reformats should be strongly considered even if radiographs of the hip are normal to ensure that no femoral neck fracture is present (Tornetta et al. 2007). A missed femoral neck fracture can have devastating consequences for the patient and surgeon.

In the field prior to hospital arrival, patients with suspected femoral shaft fractures are often treated with traction bracing using Hare or Sager traction splints. Unless immediate surgical

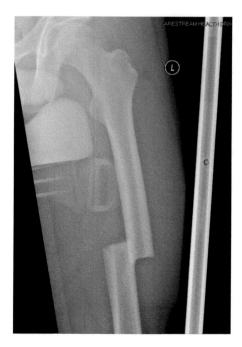

Femoral Shaft Fractures, Fig. 1 An AP image of the proximal two-thirds of the femur demonstrating a transverse non-comminuted midshaft fracture with approximately 2 cm of shortening and 100 % medial translation of the distal fragment. The patient had been placed in Hare traction in the field as evidenced by the radiopaque metallic bar seen laterally

intervention is planned, skeletal traction in the distal femur or proximal tibia should be applied in the trauma bay or emergency room. Up to one sixth of patient body weight can be applied. Skeletal traction improves patient comfort and reduces additional tissue damage by limiting motion at the fracture site. The amount of bleeding that occurs into the thigh, which can be substantial, is limited through a tamponade effect. Subsequent surgical intervention, particularly if delayed several days, is also facilitated as the fracture is maintained at proper length during this time (Fig. 1).

Though not a surgical emergency, expedient fixation of femoral shaft fractures is recommended. Fixation within 24 h is ideal if resources are available and the patient's resuscitation status and medical condition allow in order to facilitate patient mobilization and recovery.

Intramedullary nailing is the treatment of choice for the vast majority femoral shaft fractures.

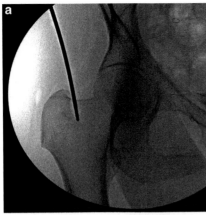 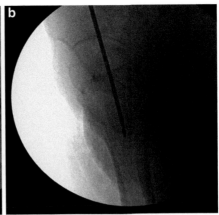

Femoral Shaft Fractures, Fig. 2 Intraoperative AP (**a**) and lateral (**b**) fluoroscopic images of initial guidewire placement into the piriformis fossa for subsequent placement of a piriformis nail. This starting point is directly in line with the canal of the femur

F

Modern nails are constructed with titanium alloy, as this is a durable material that closely mimics the stiffness of bone. A cannulated design allows for insertion over a pre-placed guidewire, which also facilitates reaming. A bow with a 150–300 cm radius of curvature (when viewed from the lateral side) is incorporated in order to correspond to the anterior bow or convexity of the native femur (see Fig. 3c). Nails that do not incorporate this bow have a high risk of perforating the anterior cortex of the distal femur during insertion. There are varying degrees of lateral bend, or valgus, in the proximal nail to correspond with the different entry point utilized. In general, a nail diameter of 10 mm or more is desired to provide adequate canal fill and stability during fracture healing.

Nailing can be performed in an antegrade fashion starting at the level of the hip and directing the implant toward the knee or conversely via a retrograde technique (Ostrum et al. 2000). Surgeon preference and fracture configuration affect specific implant selection, but general principles apply. Antegrade nailing is particularly useful for femoral shaft fractures are more proximal in location or extend into the subtrochanteric region (within 5 cm of the lesser trochanter). Drawbacks of antegrade nailing include the possibility of hip or proximal thigh pain and injury to the hip abductor musculature.

There are multiple entry site options for antegrade nailing with correspondingly designed nails. Patients can be positioned supine on a fracture/traction table with traction applied to the extremity through a boot or a trans-osseous traction pin/wire. Alternatively, a free-legged technique on a radiolucent table in the supine position with a bump under the ipsilateral hip or in the lateral decubitus position can be utilized.

The piriformis entry point is directly in line with the intramedullary canal of the femur and thus a "straight" nail without any valgus bend is used (Figs. 2 and 3). A major advantage of utilizing this entry point is that a correctly inserted nail helps with reduction of the fracture, particularly if it is proximal in location. The piriformis entry site is relatively medial and thus can be difficult to access in muscular or obese patients. This can be mitigated by positioning the patient in a lateral position or placing a large bump under the ipsilateral hip so that the leg can be adducted to improve access. Piriformis entry nails should be avoided in skeletally immature patients as the blood supply to the femoral head is vulnerable with this approach in patients of this age group.

Trochanteric entry nails incorporate a 5–7° valgus bend into the proximal nail to correspond to the path of a nail placed with an entry point through the tip of the greater trochanter, which lies lateral to the piriformis fossa. Though access

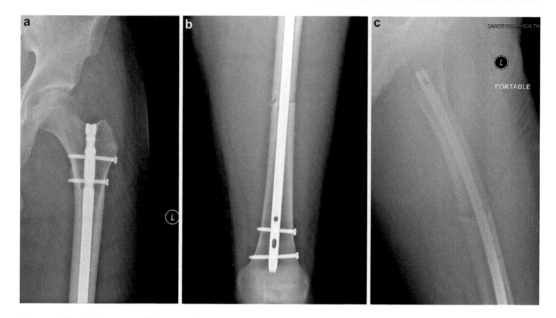

Femoral Shaft Fractures, Fig. 3 (**a**, **b**) show the fracture from Fig. 1 after reamed piriformis entry intramedullary nailing with two proximal and two distal interlocking screws. The postoperative AP hip (**a**) should be inspected closely to ensure that no femoral neck fracture is present. Anatomic reduction has been obtained. Note the anterior bow of the femur and corresponding nail design on the lateral image seen in (**c**) from a similarly treated fracture

is easier, failure to obtain a proper starting point may predispose to fracture malreduction, particularly in proximal fractures. A classic error is making the entry point too lateral or reaming laterally into the greater trochanter resulting in a varus deformity of the fracture after nail insertion. Furthermore, anatomic variation in the location of the tip of the trochanter exists. In some cases, starting several millimeters medial to the tip will better match nail geometry.

"Lateral entry" nails with higher levels of valgus bend and an entry point lateral to the tip of the greater trochanter are available. Advantages are ease of entry point access and avoidance of the hip abductor musculature insertion on the greater trochanter. Vigilance is required to avoid fracture malreduction as when trochanteric entry nails are utilized.

Retrograde nails are inserted with the patient in the supine position with a small bump under the ipsilateral hip. Relative indications for this approach include obesity, polytrauma (easier positioning), and distally located fractures. The entry point is located in the center of the femoral

notch on the AP view and 1–2 mm anterior to Blumensaat's line on the lateral fluoroscopic image (Fig. 4). Concerns include an entry point that violates knee joint cartilage and the potential for lingering knee pain. Retrograde nailing is not suitable for patients with open distal femoral growth plates.

Regardless, of entry point selected, general surgical principles are as follows. After the entry point is established with an awl or guidewire, an entry reamer is used to gain access to the femoral canal. A long ball tipped guidewire is then advanced into the canal and across the fracture. Reduction of the fracture facilitates guidewire passage and must be maintained throughout the reaming process to avoid malalignment once the nail is placed. Correct fracture length, alignment in the AP and lateral projections, and rotation must all be obtained. Traction is a key component of maintaining reduction during surgery.

There has been some controversy regarding unreamed versus reamed nailing. Unreamed nails can be placed more quickly and with less

Femoral Shaft Fractures, Fig. 4 Intraoperative AP (**a**) and lateral (**b**) fluoroscopic images of initial guidewire placement in the center of the femoral notch on the AP and 1–2 mm anterior to Blumensaat's line on the lateral view for subsequent placement of a retrograde femoral nail

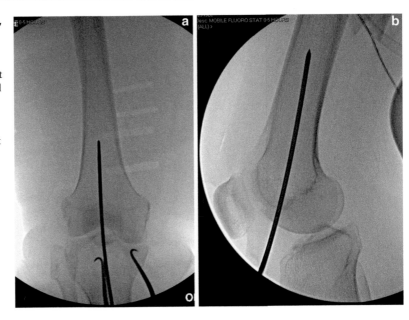

blood loss. However, standard practice is to place a reamed nail as this allows placement of a larger diameter nail and leads to increased healing rates (Tornetta and Tiburzi 2000). Reaming is performed by advancing progressively larger cutting tipped devices through the femoral canal over the guidewire, sequentially removing a small amount of endosteal bone. Reaming is generally performed to 1–2 mm larger than the anticipated nail diameter in order to facilitate nail passage. Reamer flutes should be sharp to avoid thermal necrosis of the bone. Reamers with deep flutes and a narrow shaft diameter are desirable to allow egress of marrow contents and avoid excessive intramedullary pressure during reaming. After the nail is advanced into the canal, one to two interlocking screws are placed through the bone into the proximal and distal aspects of the nail to provide control of length and rotation (Brumback et al. 1988). In all cases, the femoral neck should be evaluated after nail placement on AP and lateral fluoroscopic imaging. Dynamic fluoroscopy should be utilized to ensure that no femoral neck fracture is present. Cannulated screws can be placed around or proximal to the nail if a femoral neck fracture is found (Fig. 5). A ligamentous exam of the knee, clinical assessment of rotation compared to the uninjured side,

and evaluation of distal pulses are also required prior to leaving the operating room.

The Winquist classification stratifies fractures according to the amount of comminution present. A fracture with Winquist one comminution is represented by a single fracture line without comminution; thus, the ends of the bone should be in 100 % contact after fixation (as seen in Figs. 1 and 3). A Winquist four fracture has circumferential cortical comminution, representing a segmental fracture. Consideration may be given to placing two or more interlocking screws in higher Winquist level fractures as well as potentially restricting weight-bearing on the involved extremity during the initial postoperative period (Winquist et al. 1984).

In the setting of polytrauma, head injury, thoracic/pulmonary injury, hemodynamic instability, or bilateral femoral shaft fractures, external fixation should be considered in the acute setting to limit the additional physiologic insult from surgery (Pape et al. 2002). Reaming for nail placement leads to increased blood loss and surgical time. It also forces varying amounts of medullary fat and reaming debris into the patient's circulation. An increased systemic inflammatory response accompanied by diminished pulmonary function can ensue, exemplified

Femoral Shaft Fractures,
Fig. 5 AP (**a**) and lateral
(**b**) images showing two
cannulated screws placed
anterior to a femoral nail
for a femoral neck fracture
identified after nail
insertion

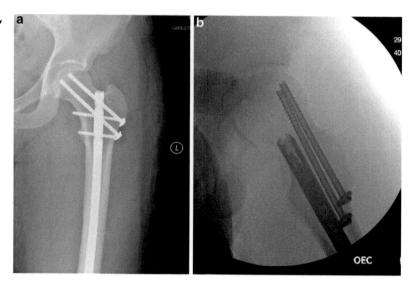

by the fat embolism syndrome. External fixation can be performed quickly and with minimal blood loss to stabilize femur fractures and allow for further resuscitation until definitive fixation is appropriate (Fig. 6). Nailing can safely be performed for up to 2 weeks after an external fixator has been placed on a femur (Nowotarski et al. 2000). Keeping the fracture out to length with the fixator greatly facilitates subsequent nailing. Occasionally, an external fixator may be used for definitive treatment. Close radiographic follow-up is recommended to ensure that satisfactory alignment is maintained.

Plate fixation of femur fractures can be considered if there is preexisting deformity or obliteration of the femoral canal that precludes intramedullary nail placement. Periprosthetic femur fractures around ipsilateral hip and knee arthroplasty components are becoming endemic with our expanding senior population. These fractures most often require plate fixation since the femoral canal is blocked or occupied by the intramedullary implants. Dissection can be minimized with submuscular, minimally invasive techniques (Zlowodski et al. 2007). A long, 4.5 mm plate with four screws on each side of the fracture contributes to optimal construct stability.

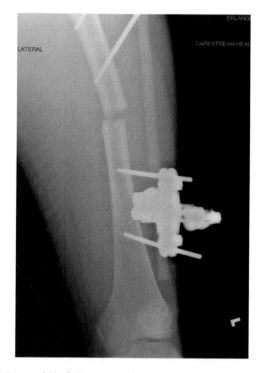

Femoral Shaft Fractures, Fig. 6 A postoperative image after external fixation of a femoral shaft fracture in a polytrauma patient. Two bicortical 5 or 6 mm pins are placed in both the proximal and distal fracture fragments taking care to avoid the zone of injury. Fracture reduction is imperfect, but length has been maintained

Locking screws can be used in the setting of poor bone quality. Protected weight-bearing is required until fracture healing is seen in order to avoid plate failure.

Special Considerations

Concomitant injuries to the extremity can affect treatment decisions for femoral shaft fractures. In the case of ipsilateral femoral neck and shaft fractures, the standard is to first reduce and stabilize the femoral neck. Fixation preference varies: some may choose a screw and side plate implant, some may choose cannulated screws for the neck with either a retrograde nail or a plate for the shaft, while others prefer an antegrade "recon" nail that allows for placement of two screws across the femoral neck through the nail.

Similarly, proximal or distal fractures of the femur may require plate fixation. A concomitant shaft fracture can be treated by utilizing a longer plate across the shaft fracture or by placing a nail for the shaft and overlapping the plate (Fig. 7).

The "floating knee" knee injury occurs with femoral shaft and tibial shaft fractures are present on the same extremity. Stabilization is frequently performed with a retrograde femoral nail and tibial nail inserted through the same incision at the knee.

Pathologic fractures, or fractures through weakened bone, can occur with metastatic or primary bone tumors, metabolic bone disease, severe osteopenia, or prolonged bisphosphonate use. If a pathologic femoral shaft fracture is diagnosed, strong consideration should be given to prophylactic fixation of the femoral neck with an antegrade recon nail with two interlocking screws placed across the femoral neck and into the femoral head.

For patients nearing skeletal maturity but with open physes, lateral entry or trochanteric entry nails are an option to avoid the main proximal and distal femoral growth plates. Piriformis entry nails endanger the femoral head blood supply in this group of patients and retrograde nails cross the distal femoral physis. For slightly younger patients, flexible nailing or plate fixation are treatment options.

Nonunion, or failure of fracture healing, occurs in less than 5 % of femoral shaft fractures treated with modern techniques. These patients may have persistent pain with attempted weight-bearing

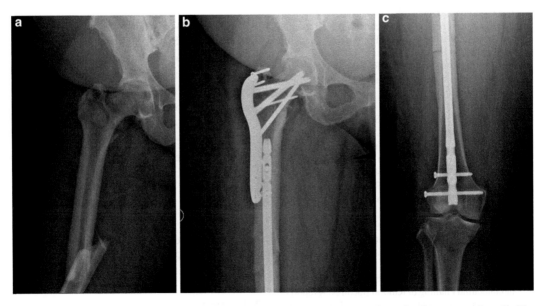

Femoral Shaft Fractures, Fig. 7 Preoperative (**a**) and postoperative (**b**, **c**) images of ipsilateral femoral pertrochanteric and shaft fractures treated with a proximal plate and overlapping retrograde nail. The implants must overlap to minimize the risk of fracture occurring between the implants

beyond 4–6 months. The presence of an infection must be definitively ruled out and a CT scan can assist with diagnosis. Exchange nailing can be performed with nail removal and reaming up by two or more millimeters for placement of a larger sized nail. Plate fixation of femoral nonunions previously treated with IM nailing is an excellent treatment option with high success rates. Bone grafting can be considered, particularly if a bone defect is present.

Cross-References

▶ External Fixation
▶ Pediatric Femur Fractures
▶ Proximal Femoral Fractures

References

Brumback RJ, Uwagie-Ero S, Lakatos RP, Poka A, Bathon GH, Burgess AR (1988) Intramedullary nailing of femoral shaft fractures. Part II: fracture healing with static interlocking fixation. J Bone Joint Surg Am 70(10):1453–1462
Nowotarski PJ, Turen CH, Brumback RJ, Scarboro JM (2000) Conversion of external fixation to intramedullary nailing for fractures of the femur in multiply injured patients. J Bone Joint Surg Am 82(6):781–788
Ostrum RF, Agarwal A, Lakatos R, Poka A (2000) Prospective comparison of retrograde and antegrade femoral intramedullary nailing. J Orthop Trauma 14(7):496–501
Pape HC, Hildebrand F, Pertschy S, Zelle B, Garapati R, Grimme K, Krettek C, Reed RL (2002) Changes in the management of femoral shaft fractures in polytrauma patients: from early total care to damage control orthopedic surgery. J Trauma 53(3):452–461
Tornetta P, Kain MS, Creevy WR (2007) Diagnosis of femoral neck fractures in patients with a femoral shaft fracture. Improvement with a standard protocol. J Bone Joint Surg Am 89(1):39–43
Tornetta P, Tiburzi D (2000) Reamed versus nonreamed anterograde femoral nailing. J Orthop Trauma 14(1):15–19
Winquist RA, Hansen ST Jr, Clawson DK (1984) Closed intramedullary nailing of femoral fractures. A report of five hundred and twenty cases. J Bone Joint Surg Am 66(4):529–539
Zlowodski M, Vogt D, Cole PA, Kregor PJ (2007) Plating of femoral shaft fractures: open reduction and internal fixation versus submuscular fixation. J Trauma 63(5):1061–1065

Recommended Reading

Nork SE (2005) Fractures of the shaft of the femur. In: Rockwood CA, Bucholz CM, Court-Brown CM, Heckman JD, Tornetta P, Rockwood CA, Bucholz CM, Court-Brown CM, Heckman JD, Tornetta P (eds) Rockwood and Green's fractures in adults, 6th edn. Lippincott Williams and Wilkins, Philadelphia, p 1847
Smith RM, Giannoudis PV (2008) Femoral shaft fractures. In: Browner BD, Jupiter JB, Levine AM, Trafton PG, Krettek C (eds) Skeletal trauma, 5th edn. WB Saunders, Philadelphia, p 2035

Fibrin Breakdown Products

▶ Fibrinogen Split Products (Test)

Fibrin Stabilizing Factor

▶ Adjuncts to Transfusion: Recombinant Factor VIIa, Factor XIII, and Calcium

Fibrinogen (Test)

Bryan A. Cotton[1,2] and Laura A. McElroy[2]
[1]Department of Surgery, Division of Acute Care Surgery, Trauma and Critical Care, University of Texas Health Science Center at Houston, The University of Texas Medical School at Houston, Houston, TX, USA
[2]Department of Anesthesiology, Critical Care Medicine, University of Rochester Medical Center, Rochester, NY, USA

Synonyms

Clauss fibrinogen assay; Prothrombin-derived fibrinogen test (PT-fg)

Definition

Fibrinogen level determination provides important information for clinicians regarding acquired and inherited clotting defects, but it represents a challenge for medical laboratories. Many direct and indirect methods of determining fibrinogen levels exists, each with their own advantages and difficulties, but the most common is the modified Clauss fibrinogen assay, followed by the prothrombin-derived fibrinogen test (PT-fg) (Mackie et al. 2003).

The Clauss assay is performed either manually or via automated system with prepared reagents along with prothrombin (PT) and partial thromboplastin time (PTT) assays. A high concentration of thrombin reagent is added to a diluted, spun platelet-poor ($<10 \times 10^9$ platelet count) plasma test sample and incubated at 37 °C with calcium and phospholipids. The time to clot formation is then measured by either electromechanical or photo-optic means. This time is then compared to serial dilutions of reference plasma for which the fibrinogen level is known. The manual Clauss assay requires significant operator skill, and automated systems are now more common.

PT-fg assays are an attractive appearing alternative to the Clauss method because they use the same equipment used to measure PT and aPTT, but they are an indirect test of fibrinogen levels. PT is determined via the photo-optical method and then referenced against serial dilutions of plasma with known fibrinogen levels generating a graph to which the test plasma is compared. This test is dependent on the quality of the reference plasma used for calibration, notably with respect to turbidity. Results from the PT-fg assay are consistently higher than those returned from the Clauss method, making comparisons between laboratories difficult (Jennings et al. 2009). In addition, the PT-fg methods' consistent overestimation leads to missed diagnoses in patients with dysfibrinogenemia, which makes it unsafe to use in those populations (Cunningham et al. 2008).

Cross-References

► Fibrinogen (Test)
► Fibrinogen Split Products (Test)
► Partial Thromboplastin Time
► Prothrombin Time

References

Cunningham MT, Olsen JD, Chandler WL et al (2008) External quality assurance of fibrinogen assays using normal plasma. Arch Pathol Lab Med 136:789–795

Jennings I, Kitchen DP, Woods T et al (2009) Differences between multifibrin U and conventional Clauss fibrinogen assays: data from the UK National External Quality Assessment Scheme surveys. Blood Coagul Fibrinolysis 20(5):388–390. doi:10.1097/MBC.0b013e328329e446

Mackie IJ, Kitchen S, Machin SJ et al (2003) Guidelines on fibrinogen assays. Br J Haematol 121(3):396–404

Fibrinogen Degradation Products

► Fibrinogen Split Products (Test)

Fibrinogen Replacement

► Cryoprecipitate Transfusion in Trauma

Fibrinogen Split Products (Test)

Harvey G. Hawes[1], Bryan A. Cotton[1] and Laura A. McElroy[2]
[1]Department of Surgery, Division of Acute Care Surgery, Trauma and Critical Care, University of Texas Health Science Center at Houston, The University of Texas Medical School at Houston, Houston, TX, USA
[2]Department of Anesthesiology, Critical Care Medicine, University of Rochester Medical Center, Rochester, NY, USA

Synonyms

FDP; Fibrin breakdown products; Fibrinogen degradation products; FSP

Definition

Fibrinogen is a soluble 340 kDa plasma glyco-protein that is synthesized in the liver. By the Clauss method, normal ranges of fibrinogen in plasma range from 200 to 400 mg/dL. In normal secondary hemostasis, fibrinogen is converted to fibrin by the action of thrombin leading to an unstable clot. These fibrin strands are then cross-linked by factor XIII to produce a stable clot. Factor XIIIa then further stabilizes fibrin by helping incorporate alpha-2-antiplasmin and thrombin-activatable fibrinolysis inhibitor (TAFI). Fibrinogen can also bind platelets via their GpIIb/IIIa surface membrane proteins (McKee et al. 1970).

Along with the prothrombotic pathway, there exists a balancing fibrinolytic pathway, where both the precursor fibrinogen and fibrin (cross-linked or not) are broken to their constituent parts by the action of plasmin. This fibrinolysis produces both fibrinogen and fibrin degradation products (FDP) and cross-linked fibrin degradation productions (XDP).

Cross-linked fibrin degradation products can be differentiated from fibrinogen and non-cross-linked fibrin products; however, the latter two cannot. There exist both semiquantitative and quantitative method assays for measuring FDP levels. The quickest and most common test is the semiquantitative latex bead agglutination assay. This test uses a monoclonal antibody, which binds to an epitope exposed on the D fragment left in plasma after fibrinogen is cleaved to fibrin, but not on intact fibrinogen (Mirshahi et al. 1986). This test cannot differentiate between fibrin degradation products cleaved by thrombin or plasmin. More specific and quantitative assays that can determine the difference between split products from the thrombotic or fibrinolytic pathways are available if needed (Connaghan et al. 1985).

Cross-References

▶ Fibrinogen (Test)

References

Connaghan DG, Francis CW, Lane DA et al (1985) Specific identification of fibrin polymers, fibrinogen degradation products, and crosslinked fibrin degradation products in plasma and serum with a new sensitive technique. Blood 65(3):589–597

McKee PA, Mattock P, Hill RL (1970) Subunit structure of human fibrinogen, soluble fibrin, and cross-linked insoluble fibrin. Proc Natl Acad Sci USA 66(3):738–744

Mirshahi M, Soria J, Soria C et al (1986) A latex immunoassay of fibrin/fibrinogen degradation products in plasma using a monoclonal antibody. Thromb Res 44(6):715–728

Fibrinous Pleural Effusion

▶ Fibrothorax

Fibrogammin®-P (Coagulation Factor XIII Made from Pooled Human Plasma)

▶ Adjuncts to Transfusion: Recombinant Factor VIIa, Factor XIII, and Calcium

Fibrothorax

Jason Moore
Department of Surgery, Lawnwood Regional Medical Center, Fort Pierce, FL, USA

Synonyms

Fibrinous pleural effusion

Definition

Fibrothorax is a condition characterized by accumulation of fibrous tissue in the pleural cavity in reaction to undrained pleural fluid, where a thick "peel" can form on either pleural surface, preventing the lung from completely expanding (Birdas and Keenan 2009).

Preexisting Conditions

Some of the more common non-trauma-related causes of fibrothorax include empyema, undrained pleural effusion, recurrent effusions after open-heart surgery, chronic pneumothorax, and tuberculosis (Birdas and Keenan 2009). For the purposes of this publication, the most common trauma-related cause of fibrothorax is hemothorax.

The main insult is the presence of an undrained pleural effusion that may result from any of the above named conditions. This results in an inflammatory response in the pleural space that causes fibrin deposition, followed by infiltration of macrophages and fibroblasts and eventually formation of a collagen-rich "peel" covering both the parietal and visceral pleurae, and the diaphragm, encapsulating the initial fluid collection (Birdas and Keenan 2009). Not only does the undrained pleural effusion already have a space-occupying effect compressing the lung parenchyma, inducing atelectasis, but with continued organization of the fibrotic peel, these atelectatic portions of the lung become trapped (Birdas and Keenan 2009). This process results in the pathophysiologic restrictive pattern of lung disease where hypoxic pulmonary vasoconstriction limits blood flow and results in ventilation/perfusion mismatches. Hypoxia may be absent at rest; however, desaturation can be seen with exercise (Birdas and Keenan 2009).

Patients usually present with a recurrent or persistent pleural effusion that can be easily correlated with a traumatic event and/or injury. Depending on the degree of parenchymal involvement, symptoms may vary. The most common symptom is exertional dyspnea, followed by chest discomfort and nonproductive cough. Clinicians may detect signs such as decreased chest wall movement, decreased breath sounds, and dullness to percussion (Birdas and Keenan 2009).

Application

Upon the suspicion of fibrothorax, imaging is the next step. The standard chest radiograph may demonstrate obliteration of the costophrenic angle and thickened pleural surfaces seen over the diaphragmatic surface and the lateral chest wall. This may progress superiorly and eventually obliterate the pleural space. The intercostal spaces may be narrowed, and the overall size of the hemithorax may be reduced. Pleural calcifications, when present, can help to determine the thickness of the parietal peel (Birdas and Keenan 2009). The superior imaging technique for evaluating fibrothorax is CT scan. The thickness of the peel, the presence of loculations, the status of the underlying lung parenchyma, and potential differentiation from other lung disorders are revealed, such as tuberculous lesions, bronchiectasis, and underlying lung malignancies. Also, a reasonable estimation of the effectiveness of the decortication can be made based on the extent of diseased lung parenchyma, which usually limits the postoperative expansion (Birdas and Keenan 2009).

Managing fibrothorax is not so straightforward. The most effective treatment of fibrothorax is prevention, where early treatment of hemothorax and recurrent pleural effusions may avoid the formation of the thick fibrous peel (Birdas and Keenan 2009). This can be accomplished with chest tube drainage or thoracoscopy within the first few weeks of injury. On the other hand, when these methods fail or the patient presents in a delayed fashion, management strategies become more complicated. Now the surgeon has to decide if a thoracotomy and decortication is warranted and if so, when the ideal time would be to perform the surgery. Before any further thought goes into this process, there are certain diseases and conditions that preclude performing a decortication. They include malignant pleural disease, endobronchial disease preventing lung expansion, extensive ipsilateral parenchymal disease, significant operative risk, chronic debilitation, and fibrothorax with limited subjective or objective impairment (Birdas and Keenan 2009). If the patient has none of the above conditions, the decision to proceed with a decortication depends on several factors. The degree of involvement of the disease has to be such that it causes significant symptomatology and objective physiologic pulmonary impairment. Most patients requiring decortication are those with at least 50 % compression of the lung (especially with apical involvement), those with unsuccessful attempts at evacuation of pleural fluid or blood, and those with lack of improvement after 6 weeks of conservative management (Birdas and Keenan 2009). In the case of hemothorax, control of coagulation disorders must be addressed before extensive surgery. If the initial intervention has been with a chest tube, an early decision, within 1 week, should be made regarding the necessity of more aggressive surgical evacuation (Birdas and Keenan 2009).

The traditional method of decortication is via a posterolateral thoracotomy through the sixth intercostal space, which allows exposure not only to the lung but also the diaphragm. The main goal is to achieve as much re-expansion of the lung as possible by removing the peel off the surfaces of the lung, chest wall, and diaphragm and removing all loculations. In doing so, one can expect a significant amount of bleeding. When removing the visceral peel, inadvertent removal of the visceral pleura may sometimes be unavoidable and can cause small air leaks, but these usually heal on their own. On the other hand, there may be areas where decortication cannot be performed without causing significant parenchymal injury, including formation of a large air leak or a bronchopleural fistula, and thus should be left alone. Upon completion of the procedure, the chest is irrigated thoroughly and hemostasis is achieved. Two to three chest tubes may be placed in multiple positions.

The less traditional approach to decortication is by thoracoscopy, and this may be best performed on patients with thinner peels. Thoracoscopy may allow for better visualization of the lung base and diaphragm, but depending on surgeon technique, this approach may take longer.

Postoperative care is routine management of chest tubes. The main findings that deserve attention are air leaks and chest tube output and resolution of both. If desired, a CT scan may be obtained to look for any undrained collections prior to chest tube removal.

Overall, the operative mortality for decortication is 0–5 %, which is usually predetermined by the patient's preexisting comorbid diseases. The most common complications include intra- and postoperative bleeding, prolonged air leaks, empyema, and wound infection. Inability to achieve a satisfactory outcome is usually due to one of three factors: underlying parenchymal disease, incomplete operation, or development of postoperative complications (Birdas and Keenan 2009).

Cross-References

▶ Delayed Diagnosis/Missed Injury
▶ Empyema
▶ Lung Injury
▶ Retained Hemothorax

References

Birdas TJ, Keenan RJ (2009) Chapter 112, Fibrothorax and decortication. In: Sugarbaker DJ, Bueno R, Krasna MJ, Mentzer SJ, Zellos L (eds) Adult chest surgery. McGraw-Hill, New York. http://www.accesssurgery.com/content.aspx?aID=5297306. Accessed 13 Oct 2012

Firearm Wound

▶ Gunshot Wounds to the Extremity

Firearm-Related Injuries

Ellen C. Omi
Division of Trauma and Critical Care,
Department of Surgery, Advocate Christ Medical Center, Oak Lawn, IL, USA
Division of Critical Care, Department of Surgery, The University of Illinois, Chicago, IL, USA

Synonyms

Bullet wound; Gunshot wound injuries; Handgun injuries; Penetrating injuries; Revolver injuries; Rifle injuries; Shotgun wound injuries

Definition

An injury caused by a firearm. Firearms are weapons capable of firing a missile or other projectile(s) propelled by an explosive force.

Preexisting Condition

There are various types of firearms from pistols and revolvers (collectively known as handguns) to rifles, machine guns, and shotguns. Each is designed for a different purpose and a different type of target at different ranges.

Handguns are typically for combat, civilian or military, but are simple in design and use. Rifles have long barrels cut with a spiral groove to spin the bullet. The spin provides stability and accuracy. The machine gun is an automatic weapon that will keep firing as long as the trigger is held and there is ammunition to fire. Shotguns contain cartridges that have lead pellets that are propelled and spread depending on the bore and the length of the barrel. There are various types of ammunition that are designed for each of the weapons with different ranges and different characteristics in behavior of the missile once a target is hit. For example, full metal jacket ammunition causes a deep penetrating wound. Hollow point bullets allow for expansion of the round upon impact with a larger amount of energy transfer to the tissue. Soft point bullets allow for rapid expansion of the missile at lower velocities and create a wide wound (Brooks et al. 2011).

Firearm-related injury is a result of kinetic energy transfer from the projectile to the human body. The tract of the bullet through the tissues is called the permanent cavity, and the surrounding blast cavity is referred to as the temporary cavity. Figure 1 is adapted from *Emergency War Surgery* (Burris et al. 2004). The figure illustrates the interaction between the projectile and the tissue it enters. With penetration, a temporary and a permanent cavity are created. Also leading the bullet is the sonic shock wave, which can inflict damage to the tissues. The permanent cavity causes damage from direct contact to the missile. The temporary cavity is a transient damage that can become permanent and is a result of the lateral displacement of energy and the rebound from the energy transfer. Different organs react variably to the energy transfer. Solid organs such as the bone, the liver, and the spleen can fracture, and softer organs such as the bowel and lung will tear or leave very little temporary cavity. The kinetic energy transfer from the bullet to the tissues is influenced by the course, diameter, shape, yaw, fragmentation, and velocity of the bullet.

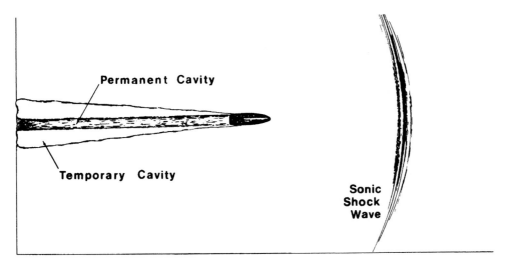

Firearm-Related Injuries, Fig. 1 Projectile-tissue interaction, showing components of tissue injury: permanent cavity, temporary cavity, and sonic shock wave (Source: Burris et al. (2004), Chapter 1, Fig. 1–1, p. 1.2)

All of these characteristics have an effect on the extent of the injury incurred to the patient. International humanitarian law states that all bullets that are used in armed military conflict should remain intact with the intention to wound and not kill. Ammunition which has a full metal jacket is designed to stay intact when it penetrates the human body. Bullets used for hunting are designed to deform and kill quickly as to more "humanely" kill large animals. The bullets used in civilian conflict do not have such restrictions and various bullets are used in domestic conflict (Giannou and Baldan 2009). A full description on the study and details of the behavior of bullets can be found in the ballistics chapter.

Application

Firearm Homicide and Suicide

Across the world, firearms are used in conflict, both civilian and military, recreationally, and for hunting. Privately owned guns globally outnumber passenger vehicles by 29 % and there are enough rounds of ammunition manufactured annually to shoot every person on earth twice (Sydney School of Public Health, University of Sidney 2013). In a special report published in 2010 by The World Health Organization (WHO), *Injuries and Violence: The Facts*, after road traffic collisions, homicide and suicide are the leading causes of death globally from injuries. Eight times more people die of homicide or suicide than war-related deaths per year globally (World Health Organization, Department of Violence and Injury, Prevention and Disability 2010).

In 1996, the World Health Organization declared violence as a major public health issue and published a world report on violence and health in 2002. Worldwide, the availability of data with regard to the incidence of violent deaths is variable, especially in areas where the political and social conflict is the greatest. In some areas of the world, the homicide and suicide rate is high, but due to poverty and other political reasons, the collection and recording of good mortality data is compromised. Poor data with regard to the numbers of suicides and homicides often make it

difficult to tease out the violent deaths that are related to firearms in many countries. Because not all gun violence is fatal, it is even more difficult to estimate how many nonfatal injuries are related to firearms. Of the millions of people that die every year from injuries related to firearms worldwide, the mortality is only a small fraction of those that are injured or suffer morbidity related to firearms. As an estimate, it is thought that about 20–40 people are treated for nonfatal violence for every death. Again, it is difficult to quantify how many of those violent acts involve firearms (Krug et al. 2002).

According the WHO Report on Violence in 2002, between 1985 and 1994 the increase in gun violence attributed to the increase in the youth homicide rate for people aged 10–24 in many parts of the world. Homicide is most prevalent in youth of this age range globally, and, in general, there is a dominance of men over women dying from homicide and suicide. There tend to be close links between committing violent acts and the exposure to violence such as witnessing violence in the home, physical or sexual abuse, and prolonged exposure to armed conflicts. Youths with a history of exposure to violence in turn adopt violence as a means of resolution of conflict. They have been taught no other outlets of managing stress, anxiety, revenge, or anger, and violence becomes a familiar means of dealing with these emotions (Krug et al. 2002).

It is difficult to separate the characteristics of homicide and suicide from any cause and homicide and suicide related to firearms. The demographics behind the violence tend to be the same in that it involves male youths that tend to have poor coping mechanisms from a lack of social, emotional, and educational support. The weapon that is used to commit the violent act, however, can vary between societies. For example, there is very little civilian gun ownership in Russia, but the murder rate was at one point three times the rate of the United States. In the 1970s the murder rate in both the United States and Russia doubled, but Russia did not see the increase in the number of civilians owning guns, while the United States saw a rapid increase in the number of guns owned. Recent data shows that Russia currently has more murders per year than the United States but only about one tenth of the number of guns in possession of its citizens (Sydney School of Public Health, University of Sidney 2013). If guns are not available, it is thought that people will find other means to commit homicide and suicide. It can sometimes be seen that those areas of the world with the highest criminal rates often have the most strict gun laws. This demonstrates the multifactorial effects that social, economic, and cultural factors that contribute to crime rates (Kates and Mauser 2007).

It has not been proven that more gun possession in a given society correlates with more crime, nor that gun control will improve violent crimes. Studies looking at this in many different countries observe various trend, but no consistent trend that allows one to conclude that there is any consistent effect of gun possession in a positive or negative way on the rate of violent crime in a society (Kates and Mauser 2007). Looking at gun possession in the European continent and comparing the rate of gun ownership and the rate of murder demonstrate this lack of correlation. In Fig. 2, there is a comparison of different countries in Europe. It demonstrates the estimated rate of legal and illegal civilian firearm possession per 100 population and the rate of homicide and suicide from any cause compared to homicide and suicide as a result of firearms per 100,000 population. Figures 3 and 4 demonstrate the same data for the Americas and Asia, Pacific, Middle East, and Africa. Countries such as Russia and China are conspicuously omitted from the graphs because of lack of available data to compare. The data is from various years ranging from 2004 to 2011 depending on the most recent availability of homicide, suicide, and gun-related injury numbers for each country (Sydney School of Public Health, University of Sidney 2013). Trinidad and Tobago has a higher rate of homicides by firearm than the total number of homicides because the data was from two different years but is the most recent available data. The rate of civilian gun possession in some countries may be an over- or underestimate and not accurate, depending on the means of each country to

accurately count these numbers. It also does not take into account the number of military-owned guns. In some of the heavily militarized states, the number of military-owned guns may account for high rates of gun homicides despite low numbers of civilian-owned guns. This is demonstrated in countries such as Venezuela, Honduras, El Salvador, and Colombia. It is clearly demonstrated that the number of homicides does not correlate with the number of guns possessed by the citizens of the country. For example, Lithuania has a very low rate of firearm possession but the largest rate of both homicide and suicide compared to other countries in Europe. The United States, which decidedly has the largest amount of gun possession per capita in the world (101.05 firearms per 100 people), has a relatively low murder and homicide rate compared to other countries in North, Central, and South America. Data for Asia, Pacific, the Middle East, and Africa is very limited.

Suicide is a leading violent killer in youth that cannot be overlooked. In some countries, the number of suicides outnumbers the homicides. In 2000, 815,000 people died from suicide globally. Cultural and gender differences exist in the prevalence of firearms as the weapon used for the suicide attempt (Krug et al. 1998). In Fig. 4, most of the Asian countries have a much higher suicide rate than homicide rate but they rarely involve firearms. In a study done on United States service men and women from 1998 to 2011, firearms were the predominant weapons of choice in both genders (Armed Forces Health Surveillance Center 2012). There is a larger proportion of males over females in most cultures that commit suicide. Individuals that are exposed to violence as soldiers or civilians who live in areas of military conflict are particularly susceptible to suicide and often display signs and symptoms. In Israel, soldiers are the only population of citizens with easy access to firearms, and it is the most common suicide instrument. In the general population in Israel, guns are used in suicides 1.6 per 100,000 compared to 25.2 per 100,000 in military suicides. This number decreased with the restriction of gun possession in off-duty soldiers (Rosenbaum 2013).

F

Firearm-Related Injuries, Fig. 2 Europe. Firearm possession, homicide, and suicide. (**a**) Number of firearms per 100 population by country. (**b**) The number of homicide of any cause and number of homicide related to firearms per 100,000 population. (**c**) The number of suicide of any cause and number of suicide related to firearms per 100,000 population (Source: Data from www.gunpolicy.org)

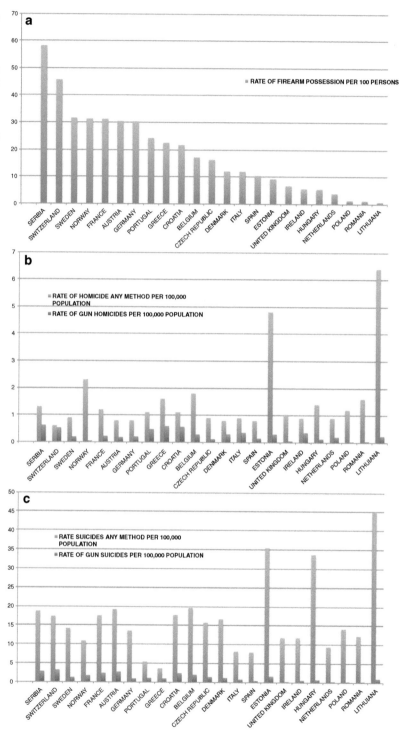

Firearm-Related Injuries, Fig. 3 North, Central, and South America. Firearm possession, homicide, and suicide. (**a**) Number of firearms per 100 population by country. (**b**) The number of homicide of any cause and number of homicide related to firearms per 100,000 population. (**c**) The number of suicide of any cause and number of suicide related to firearms per 100,000 population (Source: Data from www.gunpolicy.org)

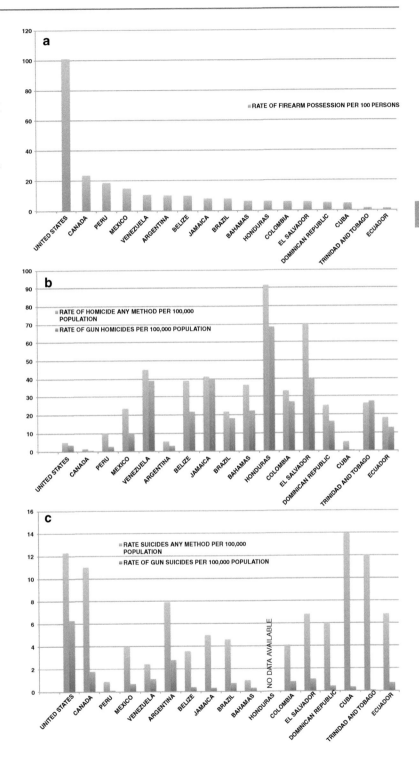

F

Firearm-Related Injuries,
Fig. 4 Asia, Pacific,
Africa, and Middle East.
Firearm possession,
homicide, and suicide. (**a**)
Number of firearms per 100
population by country. (**b**)
The number of homicide of
any cause and number of
homicide related to
firearms per 100,000
population. (**c**) The number
of suicide of any cause and
number of suicide related to
firearms per 100,000
population (Source: Data
from www.gunpolicy.org)

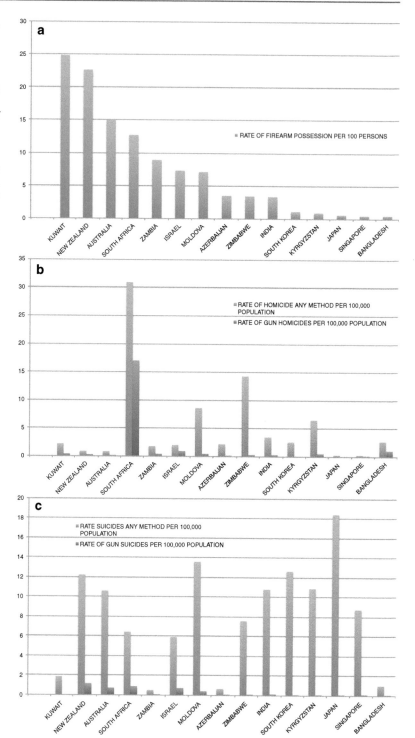

Mental disorders such as depression and anxiety, substance abuse, societal and environmental factor, major life events, and even genetics can predispose one to suicide. As such, it takes a multidisciplinary approach from the community, family, and social structure and educational, religious, and mental health resources to collectively prevent suicide rates (Krug et al. 2002). It appears to be a trend that the proportion of suicides involving firearms is directly related to the availability of the firearms in a given population. Like homicides, the availability of firearms has made their use in suicide more prevalent, but overall number of suicides does not often change.

Prevention

Prevention of gun violence can be approached from three aspects: primary, secondary, and tertiary prevention. Primary prevention aims at preventing firearm-related death and injury before they happen. Secondary prevention aims at the access to care and treatment for firearm-related injuries. Tertiary prevention aims at preventing the long-term physical and psychological effects that can accompany firearm-related injury and death. It extends not only to the individual that was killed or injured but to the family, support structure, and the community in which that person lives.

The aim of primary prevention is to prevent the violent acts from firearms before they happen. Primary prevention tends to be the most challenging. Programs often need to be customized to the societal and cultural and even to the individual family support structure and communities in which those susceptible to violent crime preside. Depending on the culture and the societal situation, anything from gender equality, limitation of firearms, educational improvement, community outreach, and support of family structure can contribute to the primary prevention of firearm-related violence. Important factors with primary prevention in suicide is recognizing the signs and symptoms and seeking treatment. Homicidal signs and symptoms are often more difficult to identify early, but history of violence in the past and social support is one important factor that can contribute among many other cultural and biologic factors.

Gun control is a very controversial and is questionably a means of primary prevention. It is thought by some to be one way to prevent firearm-related injuries and death, but there has been no consistent proof that gun control or the rate of gun ownership in civilians has changed the rate of mortality and morbidity of firearm-related injuries. There has been some isolated success with primary gun control to reduce rates of firearm-related deaths. In 1996, Australia responded to a mass casualty event where 35 people were shot dead and 18 wounded. The government prohibited semi-automatic and pump-action rifles and shotguns and set up a federal government buyback program with the recovery of more than 700,000 guns from civilians. A study done by Chapman et al. in 2006 looked at the reduction in mass shooting incidents in Australia. Prior to 1996, there were 13 mass shootings where 112 people died and 52 were wounded. In the 10.5 years following the gun laws, no mass shootings had occurred. Prior to the introduction of the gun laws, firearm-related deaths were decreasing by about 3 % per year and this doubled to about 6 % per year after the gun laws. Gun-related suicides also decreased at a higher rate after the gun laws. To date, Australia has had one of the world's largest programs for the collection and destruction of firearms (Chapman et al. 2006). It has to be considered that there were many social factors working at this time that are not able to be quantified and may also have contributed to the decrease in firearm-related deaths. Most firearm-restrictive programs do not have the success demonstrated in Australia. In the United States, the Brady Handgun Violence Prevention Act was established to require firearms dealers to observe a waiting period and initiate a background check for handgun sales. In a study published in 2000, the only effect the law had on firearm-related deaths was that suicide rate in people over 55 years of age decreased. However, there were no reductions in homicide rates or overall suicide rates (Ludwig and Cook 2000). The overall suicide and homicide rate stability suggests that the number of guns does not affect the violent crime but perhaps just the means in which it is committed.

F

There are several European countries that have liberal gun possession laws and have consistently had low crime rates. Other countries with very strict gun control laws have very high violent crime rates. There has been no evidence that the isolated application of gun control has shown consistent decreases in the rate of gun-related violent crime. This also speaks to the multifactorial nature of violent crime, especially suicide and homicide. In the United States, a study was done that compared the firearm-related fatalities to the strength of the firearm legislation in each of the states from 2007 to 2010. Those with more laws had lower suicide and homicide rates in comparison to states with fewer laws (Fleegler et al. 2013). It is thought that gun control laws are stricter in these regions because they are a response to an already violent society and not the cause of increased violent crime. It can be argued that there is no correlation of gun ownership to murder. It has not been proven that less gun possession in a given society correlates with more crime nor that gun control will improve violent crimes. Studies looking at this in many different countries observe various trends, but no consistent trend allows one to conclude that there is any reproducible effect of gun possession in a positive or negative way on the rate of violent crime in a society (Kates and Mauser 2007). It is also not necessarily the case that the more guns that are available, the more murders and suicides occur in a given country related to firearms. Some even argue that the more guns that are possessed by civilians, the more crime is reduced. Focusing on the root cause of violence in a society will guide countries and communities to decrease the amount of firearm-related violent crime.

Secondary prevention measures aim to focus on the treatment of those who sustain firearm-related injuries. This includes the prehospital and the in-hospital treatment of patients. In many countries, emergency services are designed to get patients to where they will be appropriately treated, but in many poor and rural countries, the prehospital transport and care is a very large obstacle. In addition, it takes specialized trauma surgeons, emergency room doctors, and multiple physicians and support from various other specialties to care for the patient with firearm-related injuries.

The care of the patient involved in a firearm-related injury tends to be very expensive and requires many resources.

In 1976, an American orthopedic surgeon witnessed his family receive inadequate and disorganized care after a plane crash. It was this experience that caused him to help standardize care of the trauma patient and create Advanced Trauma Life Support. Prehospital Trauma Life Support (PHTLS) and Advanced Trauma Life Support (ATLS) are international courses sponsored by the American College of Surgeons Committee on Trauma. PHTLS aims to train any prehospital care provider with the tools to most effectively assess, treat, and transport patients sustaining traumatic injuries. ATLS aims to teach first-responding physicians proven, systematic and concise treatment methods in the care of the traumatically injured patient. Currently, ATLS and PHTLS are taught worldwide with the aim of improving the care of the civilian traumatically injured patient. The military has perfected the multiple levels of transport of patients from the front line of conflict, to specialized transportation capable of care of the critically injured patient, and finally to post-care rehabilitation (American College of Surgeons 2012).

Tertiary prevention aims at lessening the burden of the long-term effects of firearm-related injury. Depending on the type of injury, people can live full productive lives or be permanently physically and/or mentally disabled as a result of their injuries. Firearm-related injury is a major cause of disability in the youth of the world. Post-traumatic stress disorder (PTSD) can be encountered by both those involved in military conflict and civilians that are exposed to violence. Some groups of injured individuals are more vulnerable than others, and injuries as a result of firearms and violence can lead to depression, anxiety, chronic pain syndromes, and behavioral changes which may lead to risky behavior (e.g., drug use, alcohol abuse, smoking, unsafe sexual practices). Many preventative measures aim in preventing the "cycle of violence" that can occur when youth are victims of violence and thus are taught to use violence as a means of revenge, anger, and conflict resolution. Prevention at this level varies as much as cultures vary worldwide, but most focus on support by families, counselors, and support systems to nurture those affected by firearm-related violence through the psychological and social effects of their exposure and impact of the firearm violence. Firearm injuries also include the scope of the treatment and prevention of suicide, and the details are beyond the scope of this entry. Psychological treatment, early detection, and psychological support are all preventative measures (World Health Organization, Department of Violence and Injury, Prevention and Disability 2010).

In summary, firearm-related injuries are difficult to quantify worldwide but are often related to the number of firearm-related deaths in many countries. Access to guns can increase the rate of suicides and homicides caused by firearms, but often restriction of guns will not change the rate of violent deaths. Multiple factors contribute to the rates of injuries and deaths in different communities and the prevention and treatment needs to be multidisciplinary. Providing quality treatment and support for the individual injured by firearms can prevent fatalities, reduce short- and long-term disabilities, and help those that are affected cope with the impact of the injury and the potential act of violence that often accompanies injuries inflicted by firearms (World Health Organization, Department of Violence and Injury, Prevention and Disability 2010).

Cross-References

▶ Ballistics
▶ Gunshot Wounds to the Extremity
▶ Post Traumatic Stress Disorder

References

American College of Surgeons Committee on Trauma (2012) Advanced trauma life support student course manual, 9th edn. American College of Surgeons, Chicago

Armed Forces Health Surveillance Center (2012) Deaths by suicide while on active duty, active and reserve components US Armed Forces 1998–2011. Med Surveill Mon Rep 19:7–10

Brooks AJ, Clasper J, Midwinter MJ, Hodgetts TJ, Mahoney PF (eds) (2011) Ryan's ballistic trauma, 3rd edn. Springer, London

Burris DG, Dougherty PJ, Elliot DC, FitzHarris JB et al (2004) Emergency war surgery, third United States revision. Borden Institute, Walter Reed Army Medical Center, Washington, DC

Chapman S, Alpers P, Agho K, Jones M (2006) Australia's 1996 gun law reforms: faster falls in firearm deaths, firearm suicides and a decade without mass shootings. Inj Prev 12:365–372

Fleegler EW, Lee LK, Monteaux MC et al (2013) Firearm legislation and firearm-related fatalities in the United States. JAMA 173:732–740

Giannou C, Baldan M (2009) War surgery. International Committee of the Red Cross, Geneva

Kates DB, Mauser G (2007) Would banning firearms reduce murder and suicide? A review of international and some domestic evidence. Harv J Law Public Policy 30:649–694

Krug EG, Powell KE, Dahlberg LL (1998) Firearm-related deaths in the United States and 35 other high- and upper middle-income countries. Int J Epidemiol 27:214–221

Krug EG, Dahlberg LL, Mercy JA, Zwi AB, Lozano R (eds) (2002) World report on violence and health. World Health Organization, Geneva

Ludwig J, Cook PJ (2000) Homicide and suicide rates associated with implementation of the Brady Handgun Violence Prevention Act. JAMA 284:585–591

Rosenbaum J (2013) Gun utopias? Firearm access and ownership in Israel and Switzerland. J Public Health Policy 33:46–58

Sydney School of Public Health, University of Sidney (2013) www.GunPolicy.org. Web 5 Dec 2013

World Health Organization, Department of Violence and Injury, Prevention and Disability (2010) Injuries and violence: the facts. World Health Organization, Geneva

Firearm-Related Injury

▶ Gunshot Wounds to the Extremity

Firearms

▶ Ballistics

Firework Blast Injuries

▶ Firework Injuries

Firework Explosions

▶ Firework Injuries

Firework Injuries

Anthony J. Baldea and Thomas J. Esposito
Loyola University Medical Center, Maywood,
IL, USA

Synonyms

Firework blast injuries; Firework explosions; Firework ocular injuries

Definition

Firework injuries can encompass a wide range of traumatic effects, with clinical sequelae often involving trauma to the skin, soft tissue, and ocular regions. The majority of trauma is secondary to significant thermal and blast injury effects. Significant firework injuries are often noted to occur in proximity to festivals and other celebratory events. Due to public safety concerns about the appropriate use of fireworks and the potential for sustaining serious injuries, a significant amount of legislation from both federal and state jurisdictions has been passed (Hall 2013).

A substantial percentage of injuries sustained by firework injuries involve thermal injuries to the skin and soft tissues. In a large study of firework trauma (Wang et al. 2014), burn injuries were reported in approximately 66 % of patients injured by fireworks, most commonly involving the hands and fingers (32.0 %), head and neck (28.3 %), and trunk (22.4 %). The majority of burn injuries were minor, with 96.4 % of the burn injuries involving 1–10 % of the patient's total body surface area. The majority of patients were also noted to be male (87.9 %).

The initial evaluation of a patient involved in a trauma from a firework explosion should start with the assessment of their airway, since substantial burns to the head and neck region can lead to a significant amount of soft tissue edema, and a resultant possibly compromised airway. For substantial burn injuries, intravenous access should be obtained, and fluid resuscitation should be commenced, preferably using a crystalloid regimen. For burns greater than 20 % total body surface area, many fluid resuscitation formulas have been described to estimate the amount of fluid resuscitation needed; the most commonly utilized is the Parkland formula, which estimates 24-h fluid resuscitation needs with the formula: Fluid administered over 24 h $= 4 \times (\%\text{TBSA}$ burn) $\times$ (weight in kg). It is important to recognize that this represents an estimate of the fluid resuscitation requirements and that actual fluid administered should be tailored based on the patient's urine output. Wound care should involve exposing all involved areas of thermal injury, removing any soiled clothing, and covering the burn wounds to minimize further insensible fluid losses.

The second most common injury from fireworks is lacerations and soft tissue injuries (34.3 %). Lacerations and soft tissue defects should be irrigated and sutured close if the injury has occurred within 6 h. Significant soft tissue defects should be referred to a burn or plastic surgeon for definitive management.

Firework injuries also carry the potential to cause significant ocular injuries. In a large systemic literature review of 7,752 ocular injuries (Wisse et al. 2010), the majority of the trauma was minor, with the incidence rates of corneal abrasions (42.2 %) and globe contusions (25.9 %). Severe ocular trauma was present in approximately 18.2 % of patients, with visual loss in 16.4 % and enucleation in 3.9 % of patients. Countries that had passed restrictive legislation against firework use had an 87 % decrease in ocular injuries. If ocular injury is suspected, the eye should be copiously irrigated with saline, and an ophthalmology consultation should be requested.

Cross-References

References

Hall J (2013) Fireworks. Resource document. National Fire Prevention Association. http://www.nfpa.org/~/media/Files/Research/NFPA%20reports/Major%20Causes/osfireworks.pdf. Accessed 10 Dec 2013

Wang C, Zhao R, Du WL et al (2014) Firework injuries at a major trauma and burn center: a five-year prospective study. Burns 40(2):305–310

Wisse RP, Bijlsma WR, Stilma JS (2010) Ocular firework trauma: a systematic review on incidence, severity, outcome and prevention. Br J Ophthalmol 94(12):1586–1591

Firework Ocular Injuries

First Responder

First-Degree Burn

Fix Ex

Fixateur Externe

Fixation Failure

Flak Jacket, Protective Body Armor

Flame Burns

Jennifer K. Plichta and Michael J. Mosier
Department of Surgery, Loyola University Medical Center, Maywood, IL, USA

Synonyms

Burn; Flame injury; Thermal injury

Definition

A flame burn is incurred when the skin is exposed to and injured by a flame. This contact may be brief or prolonged and result in minor to life-threatening injuries.

Preexisting Condition

In the USA, an estimated 450,000 people receive medical treatment for a burn injury each year, resulting in 45,000 hospitalizations and 3,500 deaths (American Burn Association 2012b). Of these, more than 40 % are specifically caused by a flame and will be the focus of this entry.

Burn injuries are more common among males and frequently occur at home. Flame burns may result from careless smoking, improper use of flammable liquids, automobile collisions, space heaters, gas stoves, or starting charcoal fires with gasoline or kerosene. Following burn injury, it is critical to evaluate the extent of the wounds, determine appropriate wound management, and assess the need for additional clinical intervention. The overall mortality rate for all burn injuries is roughly 3 %, and increases with age, burn size, and the presence of inhalation injury (American Burn Association 2012). These three parameters can further be used to calculate a revised Baux score, which has been shown to be associated with mortality (American Burn Association 2012). The revised Baux score is calculated as follows: Age + % Burn + 17 * (Inhalation Injury, 1 = yes, 0 = no) (Osler 2010).

Pathophysiology

The severity of a thermal injury depends upon the size of the burn, depth of injury, and the area of the body affected. While smaller burns are often limited to a local cutaneous response, larger burns trigger a systemic response. More specifically, burn injuries ≥ 20 % total body surface area (TBSA) result in a significant, generalized capillary leak, leading to a decrease in intravascular volume. The resulting decrease in cardiac output and hypovolemic state, combined with a robust sympathetic response, lead to hypoperfusion of the skin and viscera, further affecting the depth of the burn. Furthermore, depression of the central nervous system (CNS), acute renal failure, and cardiovascular collapse will ultimately ensue if aggressive and adequate fluid resuscitation is not provided.

Initial Clinical Evaluation

The depth of the burn injury depends on the temperature, duration of exposure, and specific characteristics of the affected skin. Although wound depth can be indeterminate initially, monitoring the response to wound care for several days can aid in the determination of a wound's true depth of injury.

Burn wounds are commonly classified as: first degree, superficial partial thickness, deep partial

thickness, and full thickness. Burns limited to the epidermis are considered superficial (i.e., first degree), and most heal within 3–4 days following desquamation and without significant scarring. They do not blister, are often erythematous and painful, and, thus, are treated with soothing lotions that frequently contain aloe vera to optimize epithelialization and provide patient comfort. In contrast, superficial partial thickness burns characteristically involve the upper layers of the dermis, form blisters, and are quite painful. Following blister debridement, the wound typically appears pink and moist, is hypersensitive to touch, demonstrates increased perfusion, and blanches with pressure. Healing requires re-epithelialization from the skin appendages (i.e., hair follicles, sweat glands, and sebaceous glands) and wound perimeter, which usually occurs within 2–3 weeks without functional impairment. Deep partial thickness burns extend into the deeper dermal layers, but also blister. They are a mottled pink to white color, dry, and variably painful. Capillary refill and sensation to light touch are diminished. Without surgical intervention, healing usually occurs within 3–8 weeks and results in severe scarring, contraction, and risk for loss of function. Full-thickness burns extend through the entire dermis, and thus are white (or black), dry, leathery, firm, and insensate to touch. Classically, the dead and denatured dermis remains structurally intact, forming an eschar. Similar to deep partial thickness burns, operative intervention is required to avoid significant wound contracture and delayed healing.

While burn depth plays a crucial role in wound management, the most important feature in predicting mortality is the overall burn size as a percentage of the victim's TBSA (American Burn Association 2012). Most commonly, the "rule of nines" is utilized to provide a preliminary estimate of a burn size. In adults, each upper extremity and the head and neck account for 9 %, while each lower extremity, the anterior torso, and the posterior torso each account for 18 % (Fig. 1). For smaller burns, one can use the palm of the patient's hand to represent 1 % TBSA and calculate the burn size accordingly.

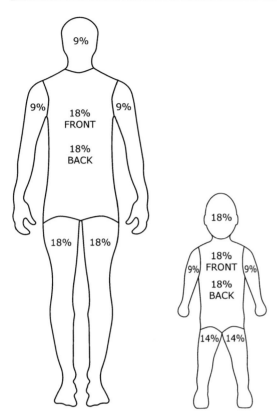

Flame Burns, Fig. 1 The rule of nines. The total body surface area affected by a burn injury can be roughly estimated using the rule of nines, which is based on the Lund-Browder charts. Slight adjustments are made when estimating the burn size in children, as compared to adults

Application

Patient Management

The majority of burn injured patients do not require hospitalization and may be managed as outpatients with local wound care. For more significant injuries, hospital admission or transfer to a burn center should be considered (Table 1) (American Burn Association 2012). Specifically, it is important to assess what level of support is required given the size or depth of injury, patient comorbidities, and the need for monitoring or support of altered physiology.

Airway management – For unconscious patients, basic life support measures and standard ABCs as advocated in ATLS and ABLS are followed, and the airway should be immediately addressed. This may include supplemental

Flame Burns, Table 1 Burn center referral criteria (American Burn Association criteria for referral to a burn center, www.ameriburn.org American Burn Association 2012)

Burn injuries that should be referred to a burn center.	
1.	Partial thickness burns >10 % TBSA.
2.	Full-thickness burns (any size, any age).
3.	Electrical burns, including lightning injury.
4.	Chemical burns.
5.	Inhalation injuries.
6.	Burn injuries involving the face, hands, feet, genitalia, perineum, or major joints.
7.	Burn injured patients with comorbidities that could complicate management, prolong recovery, or affect mortality.
8.	Any patient with burns and trauma (such as fractures) in which the burn injury poses the greatest risk of morbidity or mortality.
9.	Burn injured children in hospitals without the necessary, qualified personnel or equipment.
10.	Burn injured patients who may require specific social, emotional, or rehabilitative intervention.

oxygen via face mask or intubation based upon the extent of injury and mental status. However, minor burn injuries sparing the respiratory tract rarely affect the airway, oxygenation, or ventilation, and supplemental oxygen is likely unnecessary.

Inhalation injury – Inhalation injuries occur in approximately one third of all major burns and significantly increase mortality (American Burn Association 2012). Similar to cutaneous burn injury, inhalation injury is a graded phenomenon and can be separated into three distinct components: carbon monoxide (CO) poisoning, upper airway thermal burns, and inhalation of products of combustion. Diagnosis of inhalation injury relies upon a thorough history and physical exam, and is often suggested by exposure to fire in a closed space, carbonaceous sputum, and an elevated carboxyhemoglobin (COHb). It rarely results from outdoor exposure to fire and smoke. All patients involved in a fire within a closed space should be evaluated for an inhalation injury and administered 100 % supplemental oxygen via a tight-fitting mask or an endotracheal tube, as the oxygen rapidly accelerates the dissociation of CO from hemoglobin. Early clinical signs and symptoms of inhalation injury include copious mucus production, carbonaceous sputum, and hoarseness. The characteristic airway damage results in wheezing, air hunger, atelectasis, and, in severe cases, airway edema and acute respiratory distress syndrome (ARDS). Symptoms may appear immediately or up to 12–48 h following injury, although more severe disease is associated with earlier onset of symptoms. Work-up includes a CXR and arterial blood gas with a COHb level. More severe injury is commonly associated with a decreased partial pressure of oxygen to fractional inspiration of oxygen ratio (PaO_2:FiO_2) and may require mechanical ventilatory support. Elevated COHb levels often cause neurologic symptoms, which sequentially worsen with increasing levels ranging from a simple headache to confusion, lethargy, coma, and eventually death (Mosier and Gibran 2011). Conversely, the absence of neurologic deficits correlates with a good prognosis. Hyperbaric oxygen remains controversial in the treatment of CO poisoning. It may be appropriate in the patient with severe neurologic impairment, as it can more rapidly lower COHb levels. However, the risks of barotrauma, isolation from nursing staff, and the ability to perform critical care may be too significant for a patient with combined burn injury undergoing resuscitation.

We utilize fiber-optic bronchoscopy to verify the diagnosis of inhalation injury and to assess the degree of airway edema, microbial contamination, and mucosal damage, although some argue that it should only be performed when the diagnosis is in question. Regardless, oxygen and supplemental airway and ventilator support is the mainstay of treatment. Mild cases of smoke poisoning can be managed with humidified air, pulmonary toilet, and bronchodilators. More severe cases with significant oropharyngeal edema and face and neck burns require early intubation before it becomes emergent and oral airway access is not obtainable (Fig. 2). Once an endotracheal tube is placed, it should typically remain for 2–5 days, allowing for the edema to subside. The patency of the airway can be verified by testing for a cuff leak around the endotracheal tube when the cuff is deflated. In the absence of

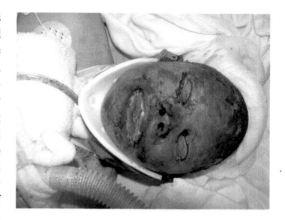

Flame Burns, Fig. 2 Facial burn and edema. Significant facial burns and edema suggest possible concurrent inhalation injury and airway edema, and thus immediate intubation should be undertaken

a cuff leak, significant airway edema may still be present. In isolated inhalation injury or with an associated small burn injury, a short course of corticosteroids may be considered to decrease airway edema and facilitate extubation.

Resuscitation – The massive shifts of fluid and electrolytes from the intravascular to the extravascular space, associated with burns $\geq$ 20 % TBSA, begin immediately following burn injury, while reversal typically initiates on postburn day 3 and may not be completely restored until 7–10 days following injury. Resuscitation can be achieved using a variety of algorithms, which target maintaining normal renal, cardiac, and respiratory functions. The initial resuscitation requirements for patients with $\geq$ 20 % TBSA burns are most commonly calculated using the Baxter (or Parkland) formula. Specifically, the predicted first 24-h fluid requirements are equal to 4 mL/kg body weight/%TBSA burn. Half of the volume is administered over the first 8 h post injury, and the remainder over the next 16 h. The subsequent ongoing resuscitation is then modified according to the patient's clinical status, including blood pressure, heart rate, central venous pressure, and urine output. The urine output, in particular, remains the simplest and most reliable indicator of the resuscitation's adequacy in patients with preserved renal function. We target a urine output of 30–50 mL/h measured by Foley catheter in adult patients and 0.5–1 mL/kg/h for children. For patients with larger burn injuries, colloid solutions should be considered to decrease complications associated with large volume resuscitation. While some institutions utilize high dose vitamin C and FFP, we find 5 % albumin works well in maintaining euvolemia without worsening systemic edema.

Wound Management

As a part of the initial wound assessment, the burn injury should be cleansed thoroughly with soap and water, and then dried with a clean towel. Some wounds can be managed at the bedside, while others may require the use of a shower table to adequately address the initial cleaning. Small blisters can be left intact, while large, flaccid blisters should be debrided. Debridement of dead skin and blisters can be achieved with forceps and scissors.

Escharotomy – During the initial wound evaluation, the burn depth, TBSA involved, and adequacy of perfusion should all be determined. For full-thickness burns involving the circumference of an extremity, the extremity should be elevated to decrease edema, and distal pulses must be routinely and continually monitored. Furthermore, substantial burn injuries to the torso may significantly impair chest wall compliance and effective ventilation. While it appears structurally similar to intact skin, eschar no longer retains the natural elasticity of healthy skin and contributes to an increased pressure. Following burn injury, the accumulation of local edema may eventually exceed capillary and venous pressure and approach arterial pressure, resulting in distal hypoperfusion and ischemia. Compartment syndrome is present in a tense and edematous extremity with pallor, pain, paresthesias, and pulselessness. Pulses may be monitored via palpation, but faint or non-palpable pulses should be more thoroughly evaluated using a Doppler. If clinical suspicion escalates or Doppler signals weaken, escharotomy should be performed. Escharotomy is performed by incising the insensate eschar using either a scalpel or electrocautery. Releasing incisions along the medial and lateral aspects of an extremity should be

performed with attention to the degree of release that is achieved. In extreme cases, fasciotomies may be required as well if compartment pressures are not sufficiently improved following escharotomy. If the burn injury involves the majority of the trunk, a chest wall escharotomy via incisions along the bilateral anterior axillary lines, with subcostal and subclavicular connections, may improve pulmonary function and decrease intra-abdominal pressure (Fig. 3).

Daily burn wound care – Once a wound has undergone its initial cleansing, a topical agent and dry gauze should be placed. The dressing should cover the entire wound, protect the body, keep the wound moist, prevent evaporative heat and water loss, and allow for maximum mobility. Often the initial topical agent of choice, silver sulfadiazine is soothing to the wound, has broad-spectrum antimicrobial activity, does not penetrate eschar, and has minimal systemic absorption. Mafenide acetate is also commonly used, provides reliable Gram-negative coverage, penetrates eschar well, and is our preferred topical agent following excision and grafting. Superficial wounds may be covered with bacitracin, neomycin, or polymyxin B in conjunction with basic ointments or lotions to maintain a moist and optimal environment for re-epithelialization. Methicillin-resistant *Staphylococcus aureus* (MRSA) wound colonization may be treated with mupirocin. Regardless of the topical agent or type of dressing used, wound mobility must be maintained, and involved extremities should be consistently elevated. Wounds with modest drainage should undergo daily dressing changes, while those with significant drainage likely require two changes daily. Routine dressing changes remove debris and promote re-epithelialization with minimal scarring. When the depth of injury is indeterminate, routine dressing changes may continue for several days before the final determination of the need for surgical intervention is made.

Surgical burn wound management – Operative debridement is often necessary for deep partial thickness burns and full-thickness burns. The decision to operate often hinges on the determination of how quickly a wound would heal

Flame Burns, Fig. 3 Burn wound escharotomy. Burn injuries involving a significant area of the torso may require escharotomy in order to improve respiratory function

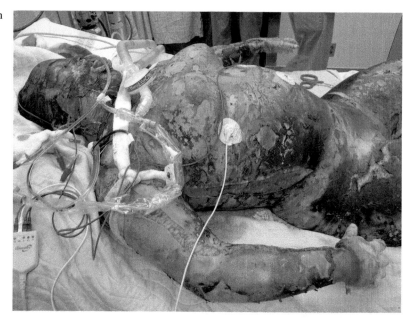

without surgery. The acceptable timeframe is typically estimated at 2–3 weeks, while surgical intervention is preferred in wounds requiring longer. However, early excision of the eschar and skin grafting is often essential for optimal healing by decreasing inflammation and the risk for hypertrophic scarring. Early burn excision and grafting is the single largest advancement in burn care, improving survival, reducing infection rates, and shortening hospital stays (Mosier and Gibran 2009). The standard of care today includes early excision, as early as post-injury day 3, and coverage with autografts (Mosier and Gibran 2009; Kagan et al. 2009; Sterling et al. 2011). The two main surgical approaches to burn wound excision are fascial excision and tangential excision. Fascial excisions yield a well-vascularized wound bed and tend to readily accept grafts, although at a cost of significant cosmetic deformities. Tangential excisions are often more cosmetically appealing, but they can be difficult to assess suitability for graft acceptance. With either approach, hemostasis is crucial and can be achieved using a variety of techniques, including use of tourniquets, clysis with dilute epinephrine solution under the burn wound, and topical measures such as laparotomy pads soaked in thrombin and epinephrine solution, pressure,

and selective use of cauterization. When necessary, temporary coverage with a biologic dressing or cadaveric allograft can be performed until autografting can be achieved.

Once the wound bed has been adequately prepared, skin grafts are the gold standard for definitive wound closure and should yield a > 90 % success rate. Full-thickness skin grafts produce fewer contractions and are typically used to cover small defects on the hand or face. However, they also create a larger donor wound, may lengthen healing time, and increase the risk of hypertrophic scarring. In contrast, split-thickness skin grafts are at a higher risk for contraction (the thinner the graft, the higher the risk), but the resulting donor site wound is less substantial. Depending on the distribution of the burn injury, the anterolateral thigh is often the preferred donor site. Once harvested, skin grafts can be applied as a sheet (or unmeshed) graft, or they can be meshed by varying ratios (1:1 to 4:1). The advantages to meshing include the ability to cover larger areas from a smaller starting donor site and allowance of spontaneous drainage from the wound (decreasing the incidence of seromas and hematomas and consequently improving graft survival). Once the autograft is secured, an overlying dressing should be placed to prevent shearing.

Options include wet dressings, greasy gauze, a non-adherent dressing (i.e., Conformant) with an outer antimicrobial wet dressing, or negative pressure wound therapy. For wounds crossing joints, we utilize splints to improve immobilization of the wound and simultaneous mobilization of the extremity, while awaiting graft adherence. Once graft acceptance has been demonstrated, physical therapy becomes the focus of the recovery process.

Supplemental Considerations

Significant burn injuries create a hypermetabolic state with greater alteration to systemic physiology than any other condition or injury. A multidisciplinary team approach to care utilizing a nutritionist, pharmacist, social worker, and physical and occupational therapy in addition to the intensivist burn surgeon, as is provided in verified burn centers, is uniquely suited to deliver high quality care of the burn injured patient (Mosier and Gibran 2011). Additional concerns beyond the burn wound include nutrition, infection prevention, thermoregulation, and pain management.

Nutrition – Early supplemental nutrition is crucial in order to adequately compensate for the increased metabolic demands of patients with larger burn injuries. Although smaller burns do not require significant changes in a patient's normal intake, patients with moderate (10–29 %TBSA) to large (>30 % TBSA) burns require oral supplements, and temporary feeding tubes should be strongly considered. Nutritional requirements should be assessed within hours of injury and plans initiated shortly thereafter. Oral diets and supplements serve as the primary source of nutrition, as the injury itself rarely results in a contraindication to enteral feeding. The addition of tube feedings, even for short intervals, can easily and quickly improve caloric and protein intake. Furthermore, tube feedings can be cycled at night in order to allow for oral intake during the day. They can also be adjusted to meet the specific metabolic needs of each individual patient. For patients with extended hospital stays, nutritional lab values should be considered to assess the adequacy of the dietary regimen.

Infection – Significant progress has been made toward reducing infection rates in burn patients. In addition to the improved surgical treatment paradigm, the development and understanding of antimicrobials has also expanded. However, the risk of infection remains a constant threat to any burn patient and can affect any number of sites, including the wound, lungs, and urinary tract. Pneumonia, cellulitis, and urinary tract infections were the most prevalent complications in burn centers in 2012 (American Burn Association 2012). While specifically identified infections require appropriate antimicrobial coverage, the routine use of prophylactic systemic antibiotics promotes development of multidrug resistant organisms, has not been shown to reduce infection rates, and is not recommended. Topical antimicrobials, however, deliver high concentrations of antimicrobial agents to the wound surface and, thus, have become the gold standard for treating the wound.

Temperature regulation – Intact skin not only serves as a physical barrier important to prevent water loss and evaporation, but also as a means of thermoregulation. When the barrier is disrupted by a significant burn injury, the body immediately begins to lose substantial amounts of heat and water via evaporation, which normally serves as a means of cooling in non-injured skin. Although heat and water loss cannot be completely prevented, the application of wound dressings, linens, and warming blankets can all serve as adjuncts to help restore and maintain normothermia. In addition, ambient temperatures should be adjusted to a higher baseline, which is especially important during wound care and operative interventions to prevent hypothermia.

Pain management – Pain from large burn injuries can typically be controlled with narcotics. Although minor burns may only require acetaminophen, more significant injuries often necessitate the use of morphine or hydromorphone. Once oral intake has been established, oral pain medications can and should be administered. Pain medications should target background pain, breakthrough pain, and procedural pain. Thus, patients undergoing routine dressing changes should receive supplemental pain medications at that time, and patients with significant background pain benefit from use of long-acting pain medications. It is not uncommon for substantial doses of narcotics and anxiolytics to be required when burn injuries are large or involve sensitive areas of the body.

Cross-References

▶ ABCDE of Trauma Care
▶ Burn Anesthesia
▶ Cardiopulmonary Resuscitation in Adult Trauma
▶ Cardiopulmonary Resuscitation in Pediatric Trauma
▶ Chemical Burns
▶ Debridement
▶ Electrical Burns
▶ Escharotomy
▶ Fasciotomy
▶ Fluid, Electrolytes, and Nutrition in Trauma Patients
▶ ICU Management
▶ Nutritional Support
▶ Resuscitation Goals in Trauma Patients
▶ Scald Burns
▶ Systemic Inflammatory Response Syndrome
▶ Ventilatory Management of Trauma Patients

References

American Burn Association. Advanced burn life support. Burn center referral criteria. http://www.ameriburn.org/BurnCenterReferralCriteria.pdf. Accessed 28 Oct 2012

American Burn Association (2012) National burn repository: report of data from 2002–2011. www.ameriburn.org/2012NBRAnnualReport.pdf. Accessed 28 Oct/2012

Kagan RJ, Peck MD, Ahrenholz DH, Hickerson WL, Holmes JH, Korentager RA, Kraatz JJ, Kotoski GM (2009). American burn association white paper: surgical management of the burn wound and use of skin substitutes. http://www.ameriburn.org/WhitePaperFinal.pdf. Accessed 28 Oct 2012

Mosier MJ, Gibran NS (2009) Surgical excision of the burn wound. Clin Plastic Surg 36(4):617–651

Mosier MJ, Gibran NS (2011) Section 7, chapter 14: Management of the patient with thermal injuries.

In: Souba WW, Fink MP, Jurkovic GJ, Pearce WH, Pemberton JH, Soper NJ (eds) American college of surgeons: principles and practice, 6th edn. BC Decker Incorporated, New York

Osler T, Glance LG, Hosmer DW (2010) Simplified estimates of the probability of death after burn injuries: extending and updating the baux score. J Trauma 68(3):690–697

Sterling JP, Heimbach DM, Gibran NS (2011) Section 7, Chapter 15: Management of the burn wound. In: Souba WW, Fink MP, Jurkovic GJ, Pearce WH, Pemberton JH, Soper NJ (eds) American college of surgeons: principles and practice, 6th edn. BC Decker Incorporated, New York

Recommended Reading

Ahrenholz DH, Cope N, Dimick AR et al (2001) Practice guidelines for burn care. J Burn Care Res 22 (suppl):1S–69S

Granick M, Boykin J, Gamelli R et al (2006) Toward a common language: surgical wound bed preparation and debridement. Wound Rep Reg 14:S1–S10

Klein MB, Hayden D, Elson C et al (2007) The association with fluid administration and outcome following major burn: a multicenter study. Ann Surg 245:622–628

Mosier MJ, Heimbach DM (2012) Part 3, Chapter 13: Emergency care of the burned victim. In: Auerbach PS (ed) Wilderness medicine, 6th edn. Mosby, Philadelphia

Mosier MJ, Pham TN, Klein MB et al (2010) Acute kidney injury predicts progressive renal dysfunction and mortality. J Burn Care Res 31:83–92

Mosier MJ, Pham TN, Park DR et al (2012) Predictive value of bronchoscopy in assessing inhalation injury. J Burn Care Res 33:65–73

Pham TN, Cancio LC, Gibran NS (2008) American burn association practice guidelines burn shock resuscitation. J Burn Care Res 29:257–266

Flame Injury

▶ Flame Burns

Fleet Surgical Teams (FSTs)

▶ Forward Surgical Teams and Echelons of Care

Fleischner Lines

▶ Atelectasis

Flexion Contractures

▶ Contractures

Flight Medic

▶ Critical Care Air Transport Team (CCATT)

Flight Nurse

▶ Critical Care Air Transport Team (CCATT)

Floating Shoulder

▶ Scapula Fractures

Fluid Resuscitation

▶ Fluid, Electrolytes, and Nutrition in Trauma Patients

Fluid, Electrolytes, and Nutrition in Trauma Patients

Imad Btaiche
Department of Pharmacy Practice, School of Pharmacy, Lebanese American University, Byblos, Lebanon

Synonyms

Electrolyte disorders; Fluid resuscitation; Nutrition

Definition

Fluid and electrolyte disturbances are common in traumatic injury patients. These may due to increased or decreased intake, losses, shifts, underlying clinical conditions and disease states, and drug therapy. Trauma patients are also at risk for malnutrition, and therefore, proper nutritional intervention is necessary to promote healing.

Preexisting Condition

Hemorrhage and excessive fluid losses in severe trauma patients may lead to hypovolemic shock, tissue hypoperfusion, and cell death. Fluid resuscitation aims at maintaining tissue perfusion by restoring the intravascular volume and stabilizing circulatory hemodynamics. Fluid management should be individualized and titrated to the patient's clinical condition along with close monitoring of vital signs, urine output, cardiac output, mental status, and oxygen consumption.

Electrolyte abnormalities are common in critically ill trauma patients. The assessment and management of electrolyte disorders should account for serum electrolyte concentrations, electrolyte intake and elimination, renal function, acid–base status, underlying diseases and clinical status, medications, and response to therapy. Regular monitoring of serum electrolyte concentrations is necessary for the timely and appropriate management of electrolyte disorders.

Patients with severe trauma are at risk for malnutrition and delayed recovery unless adequate nutrition is provided. Severe stress or injury such as critical illness, trauma, burns, or sepsis triggers a metabolic response mediated by counterregulatory hormones (e.g., catecholamines, cortisol, glucagon, growth hormone), cytokines (e.g., tumor necrosis factor-α), interleukins (e.g., interleukins 1 and 6), and other immune mediators that cause hypermetabolism and hypercatabolism. Therefore, timely nutrition is necessary to prevent malnutrition, support the immune system, and promote healing. Enteral nutrition is the mainstay of nutrition support in patients with a functional gastrointestinal tract who cannot or should not eat and are who are at risk for malnutrition. Enteral nutrition modulates the metabolic response to stress, increases intestinal blood flow, and maintains gut mucosal integrity and function. Parenteral nutrition is not indicated unless the patient is malnourished and the gastrointestinal tract cannot be used for feeding and when oral or enteral nutrition is not tolerated for more than 7–10 days in well-nourished patients. Although supplemental parenteral nutrition to enteral feeding improves energy delivery, there is no clear indication for its benefits in improving patient outcomes. As compared to enteral nutrition, parenteral nutrition is associated with a higher risk of hyperglycemia and increased infectious complications (McClave et al. 2009; Heyland et al. 2003).

Application

Fluids

Crystalloids (e.g., saline, lactated Ringer's) and colloids (e.g., albumin, hetastarch, dextran) are used in the fluid resuscitation of hemodynamically unstable patients, along with blood products to replace blood loss. However, the timing, volume, and type of fluid used for resuscitation remain debatable. Crystalloids are most commonly used in trauma patients. Typically, the volume of crystalloids infused is three times the volume lost because about one-third of the administered fluid remains in the intravascular space and the remaining two-thirds cross into the tissues. Infusion of large fluid volumes should be avoided as it can be lead to peripheral and pulmonary edema, brain swelling, heart failure, gastrointestinal ischemia, hypothermia, and acid–base and electrolyte disturbances (Perel et al. 2013).

Colloids are larger molecules than crystalloids and are therefore more easily and longer retained in the intravascular space. However, there is concern about the possibility of increased mortality with the use of human albumin as a resuscitation fluid in traumatic brain injury patients. Also, high doses of hetastarch and dextran are associated with increased bleeding risk. Further, colloids are more expensive and there is no evidence that they reduce the risk of mortality in trauma patients as compared to crystalloids (Perel et al. 2013; Reinhart et al. 2012).

Electrolytes

Electrolytes are involved in many enzymatic, biochemical, and hormonal reactions, neurotransmission, muscle contraction, cardiovascular function, bone composition, cell membrane structure and function, and fluid and acid–base regulation. Electrolyte disorders affecting sodium, potassium, magnesium, calcium, phosphorus, and chloride are discussed below.

Sodium

Sodium is the most abundant cation in the body that is mostly found in extracellular fluids. Serum sodium concentration largely determines plasma osmolality, and sodium and water disturbances are closely interrelated. Hyponatremia is the most common sodium and water disorder in critically ill patients. It is mainly due to relative water excess as compared to sodium or excessive sodium loss in the urine or gastrointestinal tract. Hyponatremia is classified as hypotonic (hypovolemic, isovolemic, or hypervolemic), isotonic (pseudohyponatremia), or hypertonic. Hyponatremia in neurotrauma patients is mostly due to cerebral salt wasting syndrome, syndrome of inappropriate antidiuretic hormone (SIADH) secretion, or mannitol therapy that causes hypertonic hyponatremia. The treatment of hyponatremia depends on the diagnosis and symptoms. Isotonic or hypertonic saline may be given along with restriction of hypotonic fluids. Diuresis is used in patients with edema (Kraft et al. 2005).

Hypernatremia is classified as hypovolemic (e.g., diarrhea, burns, lactulose, osmotic diuresis) which is the most common form of hypernatremia, isovolemic (e.g., diabetes insipidus), or hypervolemic. Mannitol therapy in brain trauma patients may cause hypernatremia as a result of volume contraction. The treatment of hypernatremia mainly consists of hypotonic fluids (e.g., hypotonic saline, dextrose solutions). In patients with volume depletion, therapy should aim at first restoring the intravascular volume with proper fluid resuscitation and then at correcting the water deficit (Kraft et al. 2005).

In case of sodium disturbances, serum sodium concentrations should be slowly corrected at a rate not exceeding 1–2 mEq/L/h or 12 mEq/L/24 h in order to avoid potential development of cerebral edema in the case of hypernatremia or central pontine myelinolysis in the case of hyponatremia (Kraft et al. 2005).

Potassium

Potassium is the second most common cation in the body and is mostly located intracellularly. Potassium is primarily excreted via the kidneys with smaller losses that occur via the gastrointestinal tract and sweat. Patients with traumatic brain injury have increased urinary potassium losses. Mannitol therapy further enhances renal potassium elimination. Loop diuretics and aminoglycosides cause urinary potassium loss, and large insulin doses for the management of hyperglycemia in critically ill trauma patients cause intracellular potassium redistribution. Hypokalemia is corrected with the use of oral and/or intravenous potassium chloride. Oral potassium causes gastrointestinal intolerance. Intravenous potassium is typically infused at a rate of 10 mEq/h. Higher infusion rates require the patient to be on a cardiac monitor. Maximum potassium infusion rates should not exceed 40 mEq/h. Intravenous potassium solution concentrations exceeding 10 mEq/100 mL may cause phlebitis when infused via a peripheral vein and therefore should be infused via a central vein. Because hypokalemia and hypomagnesemia may coexist, magnesium deficiency should be corrected in order to correct hypokalemia (Kraft et al. 2005).

Hyperkalemia is mainly caused by decreased renal function. Serum potassium concentrations exceeding 6.5 mEq/L may be associated with severe cardiac abnormalities that are aggravated by concomitant hypocalcemia. Hyperkalemia in trauma patients may result from the release of intracellular potassium following muscle injury, tissue breakdown, hypercatabolism, or impaired renal function. Treatment of hyperkalemic emergencies requires the discontinuation of any potassium sources or potassium-retaining medications, intravenous administration of calcium (calcium gluconate 1–2 g) to symptomatic patients or those with ECG abnormalities, and administration of regular insulin (5–10 units with dextrose) or beta-2 agonists (e.g., albuterol nebulization 10–20 mg) to shift potassium intracellularly. In non-emergent cases, the administration of sodium polystyrene sulfonate resin (15–60 g) orally or rectally increases fecal potassium elimination (removes potassium at 0.5–1 mEq per 1 g of sodium polystyrene sulfonate). The additional use of loop diuretics or dialysis will further remove potassium from the body (Kraft et al. 2005).

Magnesium

Approximately two-thirds of total body magnesium is in the bones, about one-third is intracellular, and only about 2 % is extracellular. Hypomagnesemia is a common complication in trauma patients and an incidence of 43 % reported with blunt trauma (Frankel et al. 1999). Causes of hypomagnesemia may include lower intestinal losses (e.g., diarrhea, fistula), renal losses (e.g., loop and thiazide diuretics, aminoglycosides), sepsis, and insulin therapy. The treatment of hypomagnesemia relies on oral or intravenous magnesium supplements. Because oral magnesium supplementation is limited by diarrhea, intravenous supplementation is the mainstay of magnesium supplementation in hospitalized patients. Magnesium sulfate is the intravenous magnesium salt of choice. Based on the severity of hypomagnesemia and the patient's clinical status and renal function, individual doses of magnesium sulfate 1–4 g (8–32 mEq) are typically infused at a rate of 1 g/h in asymptomatic patients, with a maximum daily dose not exceeding 12 g. In symptomatic patients, magnesium sulfate up to 4 g can be administered over 4–5 min along with close patient monitoring. Magnesium sulfate 1–2 g intravenous push is used in patients with polymorphic ventricular tachycardia including torsades de pointes (Kraft et al. 2005).

Hypermagnesemia is mainly due to decreased renal magnesium elimination such as in renal failure or to excessive magnesium intake (e.g., magnesium-containing antacids or laxatives, intravenous or oral magnesium). Treatment of hypermagnesemia starts with discontinuing magnesium sources and administration of intravenous calcium in symptomatic patients to reverse the cardiovascular and neuromuscular toxicity (Kraft et al. 2005).

Calcium

Most body calcium is in the bones. Calcium plays a role in bone metabolism, blood coagulation, platelet adhesion, neuromuscular activity, endocrine and exocrine secretory functions, and regulation of the electrophysiology of heart and smooth muscles. Hypocalcemia in critically ill patients is mostly due to hypoalbuminemia considering that calcium is 45 % bound to plasma proteins, primarily albumin. Because of poor correlation between active calcium and total calcium concentrations in patients with severe hypoalbuminemia and acid–base imbalances, direct measurement of ionized calcium (unbound calcium is the free biologically active calcium) is recommended. Other causes of hypocalcemia may also include hypoparathyroidism, malabsorption (calcium and vitamin D malabsorption), hyperphosphatemia (reciprocal relationship between calcium and phosphorus), hypomagnesemia, medications (e.g., furosemide), liver and renal disease (decreased vitamin D synthesis), pancreatitis (possible calcium saponification or parathyroid hormone suppression), vitamin D deficiency, or citrated blood transfusions (citrate calcium binding). Oral and intravenous calcium salts can be used to treat hypocalcemia. High doses of oral calcium cause constipation. Intravenous forms of calcium salts include calcium chloride (13.6 mEq elemental calcium/1 g) and calcium gluconate (4.5 mEq elemental calcium/1 g). Calcium chloride should only be infused via a central vein due the risk of severe thrombophlebitis and tissue necrosis. Calcium gluconate can be safely infused via a peripheral vein and is the most commonly used intravenous calcium salt in hospitalized patients. In asymptomatic patients, individual calcium gluconate dose is 1–2 g mixed in 100 mL saline of 5 % dextrose solution and infused over 30–60 min. Calcium infusion rates should not exceed 0.75–3 mEq/min in order to avoid cardiotoxicity (Kraft et al. 2005).

Hypercalcemia in hospitalized patients is mainly caused by malignancy due to bone metastases and humoral factors. Immobilization in bedridden patients is another common cause of hypercalcemia. Symptomatic hypercalcemia is a medical emergency and requires hydration with 0.9 % sodium chloride (rate 200–300 mL/h) along with treatment using a loop diuretic to increase renal calcium elimination and hemodialysis as clinically indicated (Kraft et al. 2005).

Phosphorus

Phosphorus is the major intracellular anion with about 85 % of total body phosphate stores in the skeleton. Hypophosphatemia is a common occurrence in multi-trauma patients likely due to increased urinary phosphorus excretion especially in the immediate posttraumatic period. Other causes of hypophosphatemia may include refeeding syndrome following starvation or severe malnutrition, malabsorption, vitamin D deficiency, or increased excretion (e.g., hyperparathyroidism, hypercalcemia, recovery from severe burns). Severe hypophosphatemia may cause acute respiratory failure, tissue hypoxia, decreased myocardial contractility, paralysis, weakness, paresthesias, neurologic dysfunction, seizures, and death. As phosphorus provides energy-rich bonds as adenosine triphosphate (ATP) that is required in metabolic functions, critically ill patients who may often be hypermetabolic have higher phosphorus requirements. For instance, critically ill patients on ventilator support who have sustained hypophosphatemia have difficulty weaning off the ventilator (Daily et al. 1990). Phosphate dosing should take in consideration the patient's renal function as phosphorus is mainly eliminated by the kidneys. Individual phosphate doses range from 0.25 to 1 mmol/kg repeated every 6–12 h as needed depending on the severity of hypophosphatemia (Brown et al. 2006). Mild to moderate hypophosphatemia can be treated with oral phosphate supplements. However, gastrointestinal intolerance is the main side effect of oral phosphates. Intravenous phosphate supplements include potassium phosphate (1 mmol of potassium phosphate provides 1.47 mEq of elemental potassium) and sodium phosphate (1 mmol sodium phosphate provides 1.33 mEq of elemental sodium). Phosphate infusion rate should not exceed 7 mmol of phosphate/h (Kraft et al. 2005).

Hyperphosphatemia mainly results from decreased renal function, hypoparathyroidism, or cell lysis (e.g., rhabdomyolysis). The use of phosphate binders (e.g., calcium acetate, sevelamer) is the mainstay of treatment of hyperphosphatemia along with dialysis as clinically indicated (Kraft et al. 2005).

Chloride

Chloride is mostly an extracellular anion and its serum concentrations are usually proportionate to sodium. Hypochloremia may be caused by renal (e.g., overdiuresis) or gastrointestinal losses (e.g., vomiting, nasogastric tube drainage). Plasma volume and chloride depletion increase renal sodium and bicarbonate resorption that result in metabolic alkalosis. Saline infusion is used to treat chloride-responsive metabolic alkalosis. Hyperchloremia is typically caused by excessive saline administration or secondary to volume depletion. Serum chloride concentrations exceeding 130 mEq/L may cause hyperchloremic metabolic acidosis.

Nutrition

Energy requirements in critically ill adult patients can be estimated at 25–30 kcal/kg/day or by applying predictive equations for resting energy expenditure. Considering the rapidly changing clinical status, underlying disease states, and drug therapy that affect the metabolic rate of critically ill patients, indirect calorimetry is the gold standard for measuring energy expenditure in intensive care unit patients. In a study of severe head injury with controlled normothermia and sedation, predictive energy expenditure equations overestimated measured energy expenditure by 13 % (Osuka et al. 2012). In mechanically ventilated multi-trauma patients, energy expenditure did not correlate with the severity of injury, and the modified Harris-Benedict predictive equation for trauma patients overestimated total energy expenditure (Brandi et al. 1999). In order to promote tissue healing

and nitrogen retention in trauma patients, protein doses in adults typically range from 1.5 to 2 g/kg/day in the absence of renal or liver disease.

Early enteral nutrition initiation within the first 24–36 h of injury in critically ill patients has been shown to reduce infectious complications. In trauma patients with an open abdomen without bowel injury, enteral nutrition is associated with more rapid fascial closure, decreased abdominal abscess infection, and lower risk for fistula formation. Further, early enteral nutrition in patients with traumatic brain injury has shown beneficial effects on patients' hormonal profile (Burlew et al. 2012). Because traumatic brain injury patients have a high incidence of dysphagia and delayed gastric emptying that precludes adequate oral intake or gastric feeding, small bowel feeding can be successfully initiated at continuous low rates (10–20 ml/h) and slowly advanced to nutritional goal with the occasional use of prokinetic agents (e.g., erythromycin, metoclopramide). In critically ill and severe trauma patients, frequent interruptions of enteral nutrition may occur as a result of high gastric residual volumes, mechanical feeding tube problems, procedures, and vomiting. High gastric residual volumes are of concern because of the associated risk of aspiration pneumonia. The Society of Critical Care Medicine (SCCM) and the American Society for Parenteral and Enteral Nutrition (A.S.P.E.N.) Guidelines for the Provision and Assessment of Nutrition Support Therapy in the Adult Critically Ill Patient recommend not to holding enteral feeding in critically ill adult patients as long as gastric residual volumes are lesser than 500 ml in the absence of other signs of intolerance. Elevating the head of the patient's bed to 30–45 ° angle, using postpyloric continuous feeding, and treating with prokinetics can be implemented with gastric residual volumes of 200–500 ml (McClave et al. 2009).

More data are emerging on the positive role of immune-modulating enteral nutrition on the outcome of critically ill patients. Trauma or surgical injuries and malnutrition are associated with increased expression of T-helper 2 lymphocytes that cause impairment of cell-mediated immunity. Further, decreased lymphocyte function may result from arginine deficiency. Immune-modulating nutrients include L-glutamine, L-arginine, nucleic acids, omega-3 fatty acids, and antioxidants. Under metabolic stress, L-glutamine is a conditionally indispensable amino acid that is also a preferential fuel to enterocytes and immune cells. Similarly, L-arginine is a conditionally indispensable amino acid that may improve immune response and wound healing. Nucleotides are required for many metabolic processes and may also be important to rapidly growing and replicating cells. Omega-3 fatty acids are precursors of the three-series eicosanoids and five-series leukotrienes that decrease inflammation and improve the immune system. Clinical studies have shown benefits of immune-modulating formulas in specific patient populations leading to fewer infections, shorter days on mechanical ventilation, and shorter length of stay in the intensive care unit. Immune-modulating enteral formulas containing arginine and omega-3 fatty acids may reverse many immune-mediated changes and decrease the number of adverse outcomes after major surgery and trauma. Supplementation of enteral glutamine at 0.3–0.5 g/kg/day in 2–3 divided doses may also provide trophic effect on the intestinal mucosa and gut integrity (Marik and Zaloga 2010). The SCCM/A.S.P.E.N. guidelines state that immune-modulating enteral nutrition formulations should be used only for appropriate patients such as those following major elective surgery, trauma, thermal injury, head and neck cancer, and critically ill patients on mechanical ventilation. At least 50–65 % of daily energy requirements should be provided from the immune-modulating formulas in order to achieve therapeutic benefits. The guidelines however caution about the use of immune-modulating formulas in patients with severe sepsis (McClave et al. 2009).

Trace elements are essential for normal metabolism, are normally abundant in the human body, and are physiologically required in relatively small amounts. During stress, tissue trace element redistribution occurs, which may lead to low serum trace element concentrations without necessarily indicating trace element deficiencies. Vitamins are also essential micronutrients for substrate metabolism, body immunity, and tissue repair. Adequate amounts of trace elements and multivitamins should be provided to trauma patients. Higher zinc intake, vitamin C, vitamin A, and other antioxidants may improve wound healing, although their optimal doses to promote wound healing effect remain unknown.

Critically ill and severe trauma patients are at high risk for hyperglycemia as a result of stress-induced gluconeogenesis, glycogenolysis, and insulin resistance mediated by the increased release of counterregulatory hormones and cytokines. Because of the detrimental effects of uncontrolled hyperglycemia on patient outcomes, careful monitoring of serum glucose concentrations and adjustment of carbohydrate intake along with treatment with insulin are necessary measures to maintain serum glucose concentrations between 140 and 180 mg/dl (McMahon et al. 2013).

Conclusion

Fluid and electrolyte abnormalities in trauma patients should be adequately addressed in order to avoid complications. Providing optimal nutrition support to trauma patients promotes healing and improves patient outcomes.

Cross-References

▶ Cerebral Salt Wasting
▶ Electrolyte and Acid-Base Abnormalities
▶ Hemodynamic Monitoring
▶ Intensive Insulin Therapy in Surgery/Trauma
▶ Lean Body Mass Wasting
▶ Nutritional Deficiency/Starvation
▶ Nutritional Support
▶ Shock Management in Trauma

References

Brandi LS, Santini L, Bertolini R, Malacarne P, Casagli S, Baraglia AM (1999) Energy expenditure and severity of injury and illness indices in multiple trauma patients. Crit Care Med 27:2684–2689

Brown KA, Dickerson RN, Morgan LM, Alexander KH, Minard G, Brown RO (2006) A new graduated dosing regimen for phosphorus replacement in patients receiving nutrition support. J Parenter Enteral Nutr 30:209–214

Burlew CC, Moore EE, Cuschieri J, The WTA study group et al (2012) Who should we feed? Western trauma association multi-institutional study of enteral nutrition in the open abdomen after injury. J Trauma Acute Care Surg 73:1380–1387

Daily WH, Tonnesen AS, Allen SJ (1990) Hypophosphatemia: incidence, etiology, and prevention in the trauma patient. Crit Care Med 18:1210–1214

Frankel H, Haskell R, Yong Lee S, Miller D, Rotondo M, Schwab CW (1999) Hypomagnesemia in trauma patients. World J Surg 23:966–969

Heyland DK, Dhaliwal R, Drover JW, Gramlich L, Dodek P, Canadian Critical Care Clinical Practice Guidelines Committee (2003) Canadian clinical practice guidelines for nutrition support in mechanically ventilated, critically ill adult patients. J Parenter Enteral Nutr 27:355–373

Kraft MD, Btaiche IF, Sacks GS, Kudsk KA (2005) Treatment of electrolyte disorders in adult patients in the intensive care unit. Am J Health Syst Pharm 62:1663–1682

Marik PE, Zaloga GP (2010) Immunonutrition in high-risk surgical patients: a systematic review and analysis of the literature. J Parenter Enteral Nutr 34:378–386

McClave SA, Martindale RG, Vanek VW, A.S.P.E.N. Board of Directors, American College of Critical Care Medicine, Society of Critical Care Medicine et al (2009) Guidelines for the provision and assessment of nutrition support therapy in the adult critically Ill patient: Society of Critical Care Medicine (SCCM) and American Society for Parenteral and Enteral Nutrition (A.S.P.E.N.). J Parenter Enteral Nutr 33:277–316

McMahon MM, Nystrom E, Braunschweig C et al (2013) A.S.P.E.N. clinical guidelines: nutrition support of adult patients with hyperglycemia. J Parenter Enteral Nutr 37:23–36

Osuka A, Uno T, Nakanishi J, Hinokiyama H, Takahashi Y, Matsuoka T (2012) Energy expenditure in patients with severe head injury: Controlled normothermia with sedation and neuromuscular blockade. J Crit Care 28:218.e9–218.e13

Perel P, Roberts I, Ker K (2013) Colloids versus crystalloids for fluid resuscitation in critically ill patients. Cochrane Datab Syst Rev (2). Art. No.: CD000567. doi:10.1002/14651858.CD000567. pub6

Reinhart K, Perner A, Sprung CL et al (2012) European society of intensive care medicine consensus statement of the ESICM task force on colloid volume therapy in critically ill patients. Intensive Care Med 38:368–383

Fluoroscopy

▶ Imaging of Aortic and Thoracic Injuries

Focused Cardiac Ultrasound (FOCUS)

▶ Echocardiography in the Trauma Setting

Foot

▶ Compartment Syndrome

Formula-Driven Transfusion

▶ Plasma Transfusion in Trauma

Forward Resuscitative Surgical System (FRSS)

▶ Forward Surgical Teams and Echelons of Care

Forward Surgical Team (FST)

▶ Forward Surgical Teams and Echelons of Care

Forward Surgical Teams and Echelons of Care

Charles A. Frosolone
Medical Department, USS Nimitz CVN-68, Everett, WA, USA

Synonyms

Fleet Surgical Teams (FSTs); Forward Resuscitative Surgical System (FRSS); Forward Surgical

Team (FST); Mobile Field Surgical Team (MFST); Mobile Shipboard Surgical Suite (MSSS); Shipboard Surgical System (SSS)

Definition

Forward Surgical Teams (FST*) are US military surgical assets that are small teams, of slightly varying compositions in each service, which stay close to the battle, and can advance with the ground forces, setting up quickly anywhere to receive casualties needing immediate surgery. Being close to the point of wounding, these teams can save wounded who otherwise would have died or had increased morbidity due to delay if evacuated further back to a larger more capable medical asset.

Preexisting Condition

The concept of forward surgical teams is not new to modern warfare. In WW 1, Depage deployed mobile surgical units termed *postes avances des hospitaux du front* to sites within 3 km of the trenches. These advance hospital posts consisted of several automobiles and a trailer that served as the operating room. The units were designed to treat emergent chest and abdominal injuries, as well as to control massive hemorrhage, in soldiers who would not survive transport to a field hospital. Small surgical teams were utilized in WW 2 in North Africa by the British and later throughout the war by British and American forces to decrease the distance and time from wounding to surgical treatment. Auxiliary surgery groups (ASGs), consisting of small detachments of surgeons, anesthesiologists, surgical nurses, and technicians from larger US Army evacuation hospitals, were created during WW 2 to provide resuscitative surgical support a few miles from the front lines (Schoenfeld 2012). The US Navy outfitted landing ships (LSTs) so that after off-loading, they would stay on the beach and act as forward surgically capable casualty-receiving ships.

During the post-WW 2 "Cold War" until after the Gulf War, American military surgical assets mostly were a part of larger facilities; examples are combat support hospitals CSH (Army) and fleet hospitals (Navy). These hospitals were more capable and large (a Desert Storm-era CSH had 296 beds) (Beekley 2006), and they took considerable transportation assets to move and up to weeks to fully set up. It was felt they were too cumbersome to meet the mobility needs of the modern combat maneuver elements and too heavy to airlift. Frequently they were left in the far rear of the advancing ground forces, lengthening evacuation times and distances to surgical treatment. These hospitals were decommissioned after Desert Storm, and more mobile smaller surgical teams were developed and utilized in the Iraqi and Afghanistan conflicts.

The US Army has FSTs (forward surgical teams), the US Air Force MFSTs (mobile field surgical teams), and the US Navy FRSSs (forward resuscitative surgical systems), FSTs (fleet surgical teams on large (big deck) amphibious warfare ships) for care of US Marine Corps, and SSS (shipboard surgical systems)/MSSS (mobile shipboard surgical suite) deployed forward on smaller naval ships. The compositions of these teams vary, with the Army's FST being the largest and the Navy's SSS the smallest. All teams have at least a general surgeon, anesthetist, operating technician, nurses, and usually an orthopedic surgeon, and this composition can be changed to meet mission requirements (Fig. 1).

Application

Ogilvie said in 1944 ". . . an important aspect of forward surgery, particularly in mobile war, is that without early and expert operation, the majority of patients die. . . .though shock may be temporarily alleviated by transfusion, it cannot be arrested or overcome; resuscitation divorced from surgery is folly" (Ogilvie 1944).

To better appreciate the forward surgical teams' utilization, we should review the levels of care in the theater of military operations. There are five levels of care, once referred to as echelons, but today called "roles" by NATO and

Forward Surgical Teams and Echelons of Care, Fig. 1 USN forward resuscitative surgical system team in Afghanistan. *Back row*: OR techs × 2, critical care RN, general surgeon, orthopedic surgeon, anesthetist; *front row*: medical evacuation RNs × 2

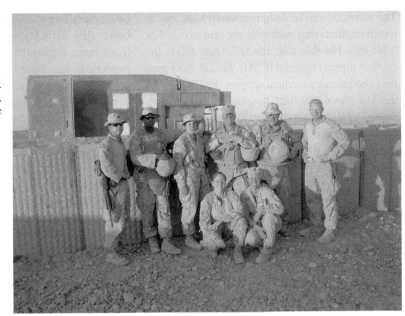

allied countries (Emergency War Surgery 2004). These levels should not be confused with the American College of Surgeon designated levels for trauma centers. The capabilities change with roles, being most basic at role 1 and increasing to role 5. The lower the role number, the closer it is to the front of operations. Minor injuries can be taken care of at roles 1 or 2, but more severely injured need to be evacuated to higher roles. Each level has the capability of the level forward of it and expands on that capability (Beekley 2006).

Role I

Medical care at role 1 is delivered at or very close to the site of wounding by one of three ways: (1) first aid and immediate life-saving measures provided by self-aid, buddy aid from another team/squad member, or a "combat lifesaver" (nonmedical team/squad member trained in enhanced first aid); (2) care by the trauma specialist (combat medic, corpsman) assigned to the team or squad; and (3) role I medical treatment facility (MTF) commonly referred to as the battalion aid station (BAS) or USMC shock trauma platoon (STP), both of which provide triage, treatment, and evacuation. These BAS/STPs have no surgical capability and minimal to no holding capacity and are staffed by physicians, physician assistants, and medics.

Role 2

Role 2 has increased medical capability and limited inpatient bed space. Role 2 can have primary care, mental health, optometry, dental, laboratory, and X-ray and is the lowest level where surgical care may be available. This is the role at which the forward surgical teams are usually utilized. Without surgical capability, they are designated as role 2A, with surgical capability role 2B (or 2+). In the US Navy, casualty-receiving and treatment ships (CRTS), which are the amphibious transport ships carrying USMC forces, act at role 2+ after disembarkation of Marines.

Role 3

Role 3 is the highest level of medical care available within the combat theater, with most inpatient beds located at this level. They have subspecialty care available (neurosurgery, otolaryngology, urology, oral maxillofacial surgery, etc.) and other services such as CT scans, increased blood bank and laboratory capability, and ICU beds, but take a large "footprint."

The wounded can be fully recovered here, but in recent conflicts they generally are sent to role 4 or 5 for this. For this role, the US Army fields the combat support hospital (CSH), the US Air Force the expeditionary medical support (EMEDS), and the US Navy the fleet hospital which is now termed expeditionary medical units (EMU) and the two hospital ships the (TAH)-USNS Mercy and USNS Comfort which function as a 1,000-bed floating hospital.

Role 4

Role 4 is a full-service medical center outside the combat theater and is for patients requiring more intensive treatment, rehabilitation, or special needs. In the recent conflicts for the USA, role 4 has been Landstuhl Army Regional Medical Center in Germany.

Role 5

Role 5 is military or veterans hospitals in the USA that can offer the full spectrum of medical, surgical, rehabilitative, and convalescent care.

The goal of FST*s is to give surgical capability close to the point of wounding. Bellamy's studies of causes of death on the battlefield in Vietnam (Bellamy 1984) showed that most victims who died did in less than 1 h of wounding. Ten percent of victims had surgically correctable torso injuries that could have survived with appropriate early surgery. Another 9 % died from extremity exsanguination, some of which would have required surgical control, noncompressible hemorrhage. Putting the surgical capability truncal closer to the point of wounding can potentially save these lives. Plus there are other benefits of having surgical capability further up front that will be discussed later.

Forward surgical teams (FST*) can act alone, but are usually placed at a role 2 augmenting it to a role 2B/2+ providing surgical treatment to an area of combat operations that is a small "footprint." FST*s can set up and move quickly. By doctrine (policy), FST*s can be set up in climate-controlled tents or other available shelters to start performing operations within 1 h. They can be transported by a number of means (HMMWVs (Humvees) and trailer, trucks,

helicopters, fixed wing, or even on the providers' backs (the MFST)) and also can be airborne (parachute) deployable. They can operate independently, but have limited holding capacity postoperatively, so they are usually collocated with additional medical resources (FST with a medical company, MFST with a small portable expeditionary aeromedical rapid response (SPEARR) team, and FRSS with an STP) (Emerg War Surg 2004) (Figs. 2 and 3).

The mission of the FST*s is twofold: to perform damage control surgery (Gawande 2004) close to the front and to often provide elective and semi-elective surgery (appendectomy, abscess drainage, etc.) without compromising care to the patient, allied military, or local national civilians. However, the FST*'s main mission is damage control surgery to provide noncompressible (truncal) hemorrhage control, control of enteric contamination, and restoration of extremity perfusion (temporary vascular shunting) close to the point of wounding to save the lives of wounded who would not tolerate the delay if they had to be evacuated to a higher role (Rhee et al. 2008).

The mobility of the FST*/role 2B which is an asset also creates deficiencies. There is some lack of sterility in surgery, certain subspecialties, blood banking capabilities, blood components (FFP, cryoprecipitate, and platelets), CT scans, and long-term ICU care. Some deficiencies can be overcome, for example, utilizing a walking blood bank, training general surgeons with nontraditional surgeries (e.g., craniotomies), and utilizing ultrasound for imaging (portable X-ray is often available here). Overall the role 2B care is reserved for damage control or minor outpatient type surgeries. The patients whose injuries fall between these two extremes, if they can tolerate the delay, should best be evacuated to a role 3 facility for more definitive care. Though per study by Eastridge despite the operational and logistic challenges that burden the FST, this level of surgical care confers equivalent battlefield injury outcome results compared with the role 3 CSH (Eastridge et al. 2009).

If the role 3 cannot receive casualties, due to patient load, tactical or weather situations, or non-availability of evacuation assets, the patients

Forward Surgical Teams and Echelons of Care, Fig. 2 USN FRSS in Afghanistan

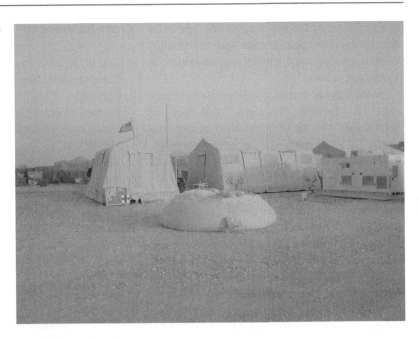

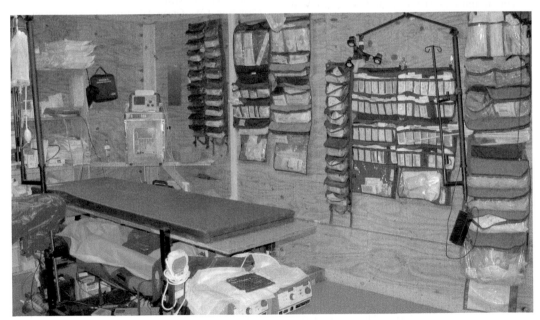

Forward Surgical Teams and Echelons of Care, Fig. 3 FRSS operating theater setup

can receive care at the role 2b to temporize them or downgrade patient status from an urgent transport to a routine. Though not optimal, this usually suffices for patient survival.

The FST*s are best utilized in maneuver warfare, when there is lack of air superiority, or for special contingencies of anticipated casualties. Once the theater has become static (like in the later part of the Iraq and Afghanistan campaigns), when air superiority has been attained, and level III surgical assets are established and are robust, such that most evacuation times are less than 1 h, FST* volume should be looked at closely. Teams that are underutilized should be redeployed or used to augment the role 3 facilities or reserved for contingencies such as planned missions anticipating appropriate casualties or special operations.

These forward teams do not operate free from risk. The forward positioning and lack of hard shelter puts the team members at risk, and deaths of team members, including surgeons, have occurred. So when no longer needed forward and if hard facilities (e.g., already standing local medical facilities) are available, teams are moved to more secure and capable facilities.

Though firepower has increased in these recent campaigns, lethality for allied wounded has decreased. The mortality rates of wounded US troops in Iraq and Afghanistan are the lowest in the history of warfare. Lethality of war wounds in current conflicts is 10 %, compared to 24 % for Vietnam and Desert Storm and 30 % for WW 2 (Gawande 2004). There are a number of factors that are responsible for this: the effectiveness and wearing of body armor, mine protected vehicles, use of effective new design tourniquets in the field, better training of role 1 on up providers, the FST*s, changes in transfusion policy, combat support hospitals, air force critical care transport teams, efficient medevac system, and others. However, there is little doubt that when role 3 care was more than an hour away, FST*s contributed much to this lower mortality rate especially with hemorrhage not able to be controlled in the field.

It is difficult to give a number to the lives that were saved by the utilization of FST*, but data from Chambers et al. on their small forward team experience showed the mortality of victims they treated were comparable to civilian trauma center care (Chambers et al. 2006). They demonstrated that they could deliver capable surgical trauma care even in austere conditions. In this same paper, it was determined that there were no preventable deaths once the wounded reached their FRSS. Referencing Bellamy's data on preventable deaths from truncal hemorrhage, treatment of these wounds in a prompt fashion with FST*s undoubtedly contributed to this change in lethality of war wounds.

Cross-References

- ▶ CASEVAC
- ▶ Compressible Hemorrhage
- ▶ Corpsman
- ▶ Damage Control Surgery
- ▶ Joint Trauma System (JTS)
- ▶ MEDEVAC
- ▶ Noncompressible Hemorrhage
- ▶ Shunt, Vascular

References

Beekley AC (2006) United States military surgical response to modern large-scale conflicts: the ongoing evolution of a trauma system. Surg Clin N Am 86:689–709

Bellamy RF (1984) The causes of death in conventional land warfare: implications for combat casualty care research. Mil Med 149(2):55–62

Chambers LW, Green DJ, Bruce L, Gillingham BL, Sample K, Rhee P, Brown C, Brethauer S, Nelson TJ, Narine N, Baker B, Bohman HR (2006) The experience of the US Marine Corps' surgical shock trauma platoon with 417 operative combat casualties during a 12 month period of operation Iraqi freedom. J Trauma 60:1155–1164

Eastridge BJ, Stansbury LG, Stinger H, Blackbourne L, Holcomb JB (2009) Forward Surgical Teams provide comparable outcomes to combat support hospitals during support and stabilization operations on the battlefield. J Trauma 66(Suppl 4):S48–S50

Emergency War Surgery (2004). Third United States Revision. Chapter 2. Levels of medical care. Borden Institute, Washington, DC

Gawande A (2004) Casualties of War — military care for the wounded from Iraq and Afghanistan. N Engl J Med 351:2471–2475

Ogilvie WH (1944) Abdominal wounds in the Western desert. SG&O, March 1944

Rhee P, Holcomb J, Jenkins D (2008) Modern combat casualty care. In: Moore EE, Feliciano DV, Mattox KL (eds) Trauma, 6th edn. McGraw Hill, New York, Chapter 55

Schoenfeld AJ (2012) The combat experience of military surgical assets in Iraq and Afghanistan: a historical review. Am J Surg 204(3):377–383

Foundations

- ▶ Trauma Associations

Four Wheeler

▶ ATV Injuries

FP24

Bryan A. Cotton[1] and Laura A. McElroy[2]
[1]Department of Surgery, Division of Acute Care Surgery, Trauma and Critical Care, University of Texas Health Science Center at Houston, The University of Texas Medical School at Houston, Houston, TX, USA
[2]Department of Anesthesiology, Critical Care Medicine, University of Rochester Medical Center, Rochester, NY, USA

Synonyms

Frozen plasma; PF-24; Plasma frozen within 24 hours of phlebotomy

Definition

FP24 is a plasma product that is prepared within 24 h from whole blood that has been kept at 4 °C after collection. It is then stored in 200–250 ml aliquots at −18 °C until it is thawed for administration to patients (Eder and Sebok 2007). FP24 was created to cope with increasing plasma demand and the noted incidence of Transfusion Related Lung Injury (TRALI), with its suspected association with plasma from multiparous women having elevated anti-HLA and anti-neutrophil antibodies. As a result, many blood banks now discard the plasma fraction from women during whole blood preparation. FP24 is an attractive alternative as it greatly increases the plasma source from remote donation sites and can include plasma produced during the buffy coat method of platelet concentrates. In 2006 FP24 made up about 15 % of the total amount of plasma transfused in the United States (Yazer 2010).

FP24 is produced by the same methods as FFP and is stored and thawed identically. Studies comparing FP24 to FFP have shown the two products have comparable levels of most clotting factors (Yazer et al. 2010), except FP24 has lower levels of factors VIII and V (Scott et al. 2009). Both FP24 and FFP can therefore be used to combat single or multiple clotting factor deficiencies. Labeling in the United States disallows the use of FP24 specifically for FV or FVIII deficiencies (Benjamin and McLaughlin 2012).

FP24 and FFP are both prepared for use by thawing units from 30 °C to 37 °C. Units not used within the first day are labeled Thawed Plasma (TP). The liquid portion of the thawed units can be stored at 1–6 °C for an additional 4 days with good preservation of most clotting factors except for factor VIII, which quickly degrades (Yazer et al. 2008). Although there are no specific guidelines for this practice with FP24, in practice many blood blanks will label FP24 as TP as well.

Cross-References

▶ Plasma Transfusion in Trauma

References

Benjamin RJ, McLaughlin LS (2012) Plasma components: properties, differences, and uses. Transfusion 52(Suppl 1):9S–19S. doi:10.1111/j.1537-2995.2012.03622.x
Eder AF, Sebok MA (2007) Plasma components: FFP, FP24, and thawed plasma. Immunohematology 23(4):150–157
Scott E, Puca K, Heraly J et al (2009) Evaluation and comparison of coagulation factor activity in fresh-frozen plasma and 24-hour plasma at thaw and after 120 hours of 1 to 6 degree Celsius storage. Transfusion 49(8):1584–91. doi:10.1111/j.1537-2995.2009.02198.x
Triulzi DJ, Kleinman S, Kakaiya RM et al (2009) The effect of previous pregnancy and transfusion on HLA alloimmunization in blood donors: Implications for a transfusion related acute lung injury (TRALI) risk reduction strategy. Transfusion 49(9):1825–1835. doi:10.1111/j.1537-2995.2009.02206.x
Yazer MH (2010) The how's and why's of evidence based plasma therapy. Korean J Hematol 45(3):152–157. doi:10.5045/kjh.2010.45.3.152

F

Yazer MH, Cortese-Hassett A, Triulzi DJ (2008) Coagulation factor levels in plasma frozen within 24 hours of phlebotomy over 5 days of storage at 1 to 6 degrees C. Transfusion 48(12):2525–2530. doi:10.1111/j.1537-2995.2008.01913.x

Yazer MH, Triulzi DJ, Hassett AC et al (2010) Cryoprecipitate prepared from plasma frozen within 24 hours after phlebotomy contains acceptable levels of fibrinogen and VIIIC. Transfusion 50(5):1014–1018.   doi:10.1111/j.1537-2995.2009.02535.x

Fracture Bracing

▶ Principles of Nonoperative Treatment of Diaphyseal Fractures

Fracture Complications

▶ Compartment Syndrome of the Leg

Fracture Fixation

▶ Principles of Internal Fixation of Fractures

Fracture Healing

▶ Principles of Nonoperative Treatment of Diaphyseal Fractures

Fracture of the Os Calcis

▶ Calcaneus Fractures

Fracture Stability

▶ Principles of Nonoperative Treatment of Diaphyseal Fractures

Fracture, Atlas (C1)

Mari L. Groves and Daniel M. Sciubba
Department of Neurosurgery, The Johns Hopkins University School of Medicine, Baltimore, MD, USA

Synonyms

Atlas fracture; C1 fracture

Definition

There are three types of C1 fractures: type I that involves a single arch; type II, a classic Jefferson burst fracture; and type III, lateral mass fractures. Other fracture types include isolated horizontally oriented avulsion fractures, fracture of the transverse process of C1 (excluding the joint), Jefferson fractures of the anterior and posterior arch (Fig. 1) caused by axial loading of the head and subsequent compression and lateral displacement of the C1 lateral masses (Pratt et al. 2008). These fractures typically require external orthosis for stabilization either through a Miami J or SOMI collar. For fractures through both the anterior and posterior rings, halo stabilization may also be considered. Ligamentous injury is best assessed on MRI, but may be suspected if a small fragment of bone appears displaced at the site of ligamentous attachment. Unstable C1 fractures include comminuted lateral mass fractures, and displaced anterior arch fractures with anterior displacement of the dens (Plough fracture). These patients will typically require C1-2 stabilization.

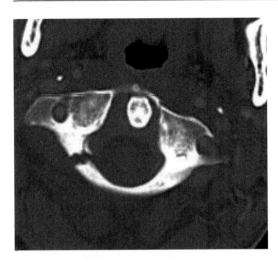

Fracture, Atlas (C1), Fig. 1 Jefferson fracture through the anterior and posterior arch of C1

C1 fractures do not typically cause neurologic deficits as the spinal canal is wide in this region (Pimentel and Diegelmann 2010). Fracture of C1 occurs in 2–13 % of cervical spine injuries (Resnick 1995). Congenital clefts of the C1 arch may appear as non-displaced, corticated midline clefts in the posterior arch (Pratt et al. 2008). These should not be confused with fractures, which are displaced and often occur bilaterally. Axial loading following blunt force to the apex of the head, such as in diving into a shallow pool, or hyperextension injuries can cause compression fractures of C1 (Pratt et al. 2008; Wheeless III 2013). The transverse ligament is the most important determinant of stability, and fractures through bony architecture are typically stable. Treatment for fractures through C1 relies upon the integrity of the transverse atlantal ligament. If the transverse ligament is intact, the fracture can be considered stable and will typically heal on its own with simple external orthosis through a rigid cervical collar. If the transverse ligament is disrupted, the fracture is less likely to heal and these are more typical with Type II fractures that extend through both the anterior and posterior arches. However, these can still be managed through a rigid collar or halo vest stabilization. If the fracture has not healed on follow-up imaging, surgical stabilization is indicated. Conversely, these lesions may be fused through a posterior C1-2 fixation.

Cross-References

▶ Imaging of CNS Injuries
▶ Imaging of Spine and Bony Pelvis Injuries

References

Pimentel L, Diegelmann L (2010) Evaluation and management of acute cervical spine trauma. Emerg Med Clin North Am 28(4):719–738

Pratt H, Davies E, King L (2008) Traumatic injuries of the c1/c2 complex: computed tomographic imaging appearances. Curr Probl Diagn Radiol 37(1):26–38

Resnick D (1995) Diagnosis of bone and joint disorders. W.B. Saunders, Philadelphia

Wheeless III CR (2013) "Wheeless Textbook of Orthopedics." Wheeless' textbook of orthopaedics. Duke University Medical Center. http://www.wheelessonline.com/. Accessed 8 Feb 2013

Fracture, Axis (C2)

Mari L. Groves and Daniel M. Sciubba
Department of Neurosurgery, The Johns Hopkins University School of Medicine, Baltimore, MD, USA

Synonyms

C2 fracture; Hangman's fracture

Definition

Acute fractures through C2 account for roughly 20 % of cervical spine fractures, although the majority of these do not cause neurological injury (Pratt et al. 2008). Fracture of the ring of C2, the laminae, the interior or superior articular facets,

F

the pedicles or pars interarticularis are typically bilateral and are described by the Levine/Effendi classification (Levine and Edwards 1985; Effendi et al. 1981). Odontoid process fractures are discussed in a separate entry in this encyclopedia. Levine and Effendi fractures are Type I non-angulated, non-displaced, or minimally displaced fractures less than 2–3 mm with normal C2/C3 disk and are caused by axial loading and extension (Table 1). These are typically caused by hyperextension and lateral bending and can be associated with spinal canal compromise and paralysis. Type II fractures are anteriorly displaced or angulated fractures of the C2 vertebral body with C2/C3 disruption and fracture of the C2 pedicles from axial loading and extension with rebound flexion. Type IIA fractures are obliquely oriented, either tracking from anterior to inferior or posterior to superior. These lesions are typically caused by flexion distraction and are rare. Traction is contraindicated for type IIA fractures as it can cause increased angulation and widening of disk space. Type III fractures are type II fractures with bilateral C2-3 facet capsule disruption as the posterior arch is free floating and the C2/3 facets may be subluxed or locked (Pratt et al. 2008) (Fig. 1).

The Francis grading system is based on the degree of angulation and displacement (Francis et al. 1981). This system correlates with the Levine/Effendi classification as Francis Grade I lesions are similar to Levine Type I. Further, Francis Grade IV fractures are similar to Levine Type III (Table 1).

3 body width/b < 0.5 Frances Grade I lesions are similar to Levine Type I. Frances Grade IV are similar to Levine Type III. end.

The hangman's fracture refers to bilateral fractures through the pars interarticularis of C2 with subsequent traumatic subluxation due to hyperextension with axial loading. In judicial hangings, forceful hyperextension of the head and neck causes bilateral C2 pedicle fractures, and subsequent distraction of the head causes disruption of the C2-C3 disk and ligaments (Pratt et al. 2008; Wheeless III 2013). In "hangman's" fractures associated with motor vehicle accidents and falls, bilateral pedicle fracture is characteristic; however, the C2/C3 disk and ligaments may not be completely disassociated. These fractures can be stable without neurological deficit. However, if there is disruption of the C2-3 disk, the fracture is considered unstable. Most patients do well with

Fracture, Axis (C2), Table 1 Classification of Levine/Effendi and Francis grading systems

Classification	Angulation	Displacement	Disk involvement	Stability
Levine/Effendi grade				
I	Non-angulated	Minimally displaced <2–3 mm	None	Stable
II	Angulated fracture of C2 pedicles	Anterior displacement	C2/C3 disk disruption	Unstable
IIA	Oblique	Anterior displacement	C2/C3 disk disruption	Unstable
III	Severe angulation	Uni-/bilateral C2-C3 facet capsule disruption	C2/C3 disk disruption	Unstable
Francis grade				
I	<11	D < 3.5 mm	None	Stable
II	>11	D < 3.5 mm	None	Unstable
III	<11	D > 3.5 mm and displacement/C3 body width < 0.5	None	Unstable
IV	>11	D > 3.5 mm and displacement/C3 body width < 0.5	None	Unstable
V	Any	Any	Disk disruption	Unstable

Fracture, Axis (C2), Fig. 1 Illustration showing axis (C2) in sagittal view for demonstration of Levine/Effendi classification of C2 fractures. *Arrows* indicate angulation. *Dashed line* indicates non-displaced fracture

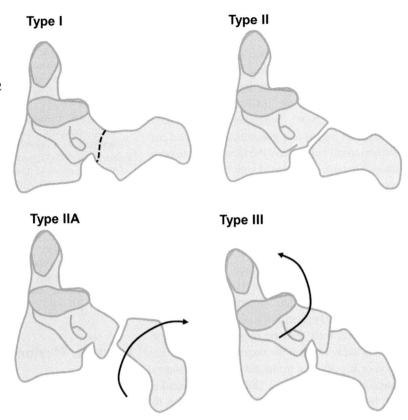

Type I

Type II

Type IIA

Type III

F

halo immobilization for 8–14 weeks unless there is significant mal-alignment or in the case of unstable fractures.

Cross-References

▶ Fracture, Odontoid
▶ Imaging of CNS Injuries
▶ Imaging of Spine and Bony Pelvis Injuries
▶ Strangulation and Hanging

References

Effendi B, Roy D, Cornish B, Dussault RG, Laurin CA (1981) Fractures of the ring of the axis. A classification based on the analysis of 131 cases. J Bone Joint Surg Br 63-B(3):319–327

Francis WR, Fielding JW, Hawkins RJ, Pepin J, Hensinger R (1981) Traumatic spondylolisthesis of the axis. J Bone Joint Surg Br 63-B(3):313–318

Levine AM, Edwards CC (1985) The management of traumatic spondylolisthesis of the axis. J Bone Joint Surg Am 67(2):217–226

Pratt H, Davies E, King L (2008) Traumatic injuries of the c1/c2 complex: computed tomographic imaging appearances. Curr Probl Diagn Radiol 37(1):26–38

Wheeless III CR (2013) "Wheeless Textbook of Orthopedics." Wheeless' textbook of orthopaedics. Duke University Medical Center. http://www.wheelessonline.com/. Accessed 8 Feb 2013

Fracture, Extension Injury

Mari L. Groves and Daniel M. Sciubba
Department of Neurosurgery, The Johns Hopkins University School of Medicine, Baltimore, MD, USA

Synonyms

Extension avulsion fracture; Extension compression injury

Definition

The most common extension compression injury involves lateral mass or facet fractures. There are four types of lateral mass fractures: separation, comminuted, split, or traumatic spondylolysis (Kotani et al. 2005). Separation fractures occur through the lamina and ipsilateral pedicle and permit horizontal migration of the facet. This can occur through extension combined with compression and rotation, and patients will typically present with a neurologic deficit. Comminuted fractures can also be associated with lateral angulation. Split fractures are coronally oriented vertical fractures in one lateral mass, with invagination of the superior articular facet of the level below into the fracture site. Traumatic spondylolysis are bilateral horizontal fractures through the pars interarticularis separating the anterior and posterior spinal elements. In cases of unilateral facet fracture, nonoperative management is likely to fail if the fragment is greater than 1 cm or is >40 % of the height of the contralateral lateral mass (Spector et al. 2006). These fractures can be managed through a posterior approach for fusion as well as possible decompression.

Extension avulsion fractures make up 19 % of C2 injuries by some estimates, but can occur at any level (Resnick 1995). This fracture occurs secondary to a hyperextension injury, and a triangular bone fragment is avulsed anteriorly by the anterior longitudinal ligament. The fragment typically has a vertical height equal to or greater than its transverse dimension (Pratt et al. 2008; Wheeless III 2013). These lesions are not associated with malalignment, fracture, or loss of height of the vertebral bodies. There should also be no prevertebral soft tissue swelling at the level of the fragment or disruption of the posterior elements. These should be distinguished from teardrop fractures. These fractures are typically managed with a rigid cervical collar.

Cross-References

▶ Central Cord Syndrome
▶ Imaging of CNS Injuries
▶ Imaging of Spine and Bony Pelvis Injuries

References

Kotani Y, Abumi K, Ito M, Minami A (2005) Cervical spine injuries associated with lateral mass and facet joint fractures: new classification and surgical treatment with pedicle screw fixation. Eur Spine J 14(1):69–77

Pratt H, Davies E, King L (2008) Traumatic injuries of the c1/c2 complex: computed tomographic imaging appearances. Curr Probl Diagn Radiol 37(1):26–38

Resnick D (1995) Diagnosis of bone and joint disorders. W.B. Saunders, Philadelphia. Print. Null

Spector LR, Kim DH, Affonso J, Albert TJ, Hilibrand AS, Vaccaro AS (2006) Use of computed tomography to predict failure of nonoperative treatment of unilateral facet fractures of the cervical spine. Spine (Phila Pa1976) 31(24):2827–2835

Wheeless III CR (2013) "Wheeless Textbook of Orthopedics." Wheeless' textbook of orthopaedics. Duke University Medical Center. http://www.wheelessonline.com/. Accessed 8 Feb 2013

Fracture, Flexion Injury

Mari L. Groves and Daniel M. Sciubba
Department of Neurosurgery, The Johns Hopkins University School of Medicine, Baltimore, MD, USA

Synonyms

Anterior subluxation; Quadrangular fracture; Teardrop fracture; Wedge fracture

Definition

Teardrop fractures typically result from hyperflexion or axial loading at the vertex of the skull, while the neck is flexed (Pratt et al. 2008; Wheeless III 2013). There are varying degrees of severity with the most severe form affecting all the ligaments, facet joints, and intervertebral disks (Harris et al. 1986). In some large series, these lesions occur in 5 % of patients and presentation may range from neurologically intact to quadraparesis. Anterior cord syndrome may also arise secondary to hyperflexion of the spinal column that creates compression on the

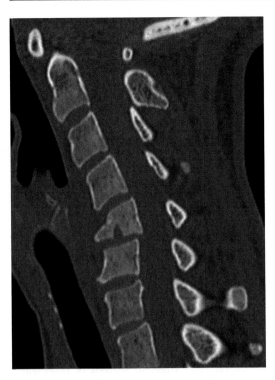

Fracture, Flexion Injury, Fig. 1 Sagittal CT scan demonstrating wedge fracture at C5. A local kyphotic deformity can be seen at C5

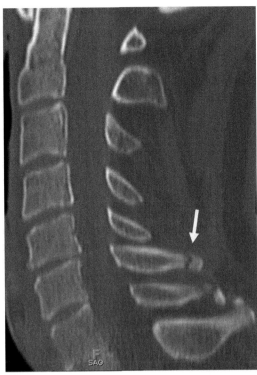

Fracture, Flexion Injury, Fig. 2 Clay shoveler's fracture of the spinous process of C6 (*white arrow*)

anterior spinal artery, resulting in profound ischemia. A teardrop fracture must be differentiated from a simple avulsion fracture and is typically more involved on imaging. These fracture patterns include a fracture through the sagittal plane of the vertebral body, triangular fragment of the anterior inferior vertebral body, a wedge defect, or retrolisthesis of a vertebral body fragment into the spinal canal. There is typically prevertebral soft-tissue swelling, disruption of the adjacent disk space, and disruption of the facet joints or posterior ligaments. The disk space and ligaments should be assessed with MRI and surgical stabilization should be considered if there is disruption. Severe injuries with canal compromise require decompression and stabilization either through an anterior, posterior, or combined approach.

Quadrangular fractures are oblique vertebral body fractures that pass from the anterior-superior cortical margin to the inferior end plate. There is typically angular kyphosis and

posterior subluxation of the superior fragment of vertebral body on the inferior fragment. There is disruption of the disk space, anterior and posterior ligaments that requires fixation through often a combined anterior/posterior approach.

Wedge fractures are caused by forceful hyperflexion or axial loading (Wheeless III 2013) (Fig. 1). Anterior wedge fractures are unstable if there is loss of greater than 50 % of vertebral body height, greater than 20° of angulation at the level of fracture, if there is associated neurologic impairment, if greater than 50 % of the spinal canal is compromised, or if adjacent levels are similarly fractured (Wheeless III 2013).

Burst fracture in the cervical spine is associated with axial loading and a vertical fracture through the vertebral body (Wheeless III 2013). Loss of anterior vertebral body height may be seen with an anterior wedge fracture. On axial and sagittal CT imaging, retropulsed bone fragments will likely be visible. This is an unstable injury and is worsened with axial loading. Clay shoveler's fracture is a stable fracture of the spinous process caused by hyperflexion, most commonly at C6-C7 (Wheeless III 2013) (Fig. 2). Occult fractures may be present, and CT imaging can help to rule out associated facet fractures or locked facets.

Anterior subluxation in the cervical spine is typically associated with hyperflexion injury and may be purely ligamentous. When subluxation is associated with a fracture, or when myelopathy is present, it is an unstable injury (Green et al. 1981). On imaging, localized angulation at the level of injury, anterior translation of a superior, adjacent vertebral body, narrowing of the disk space, and dislocation of the facet joints may be present (Green et al. 1981; Greene et al. 1997) (Fig. 3).

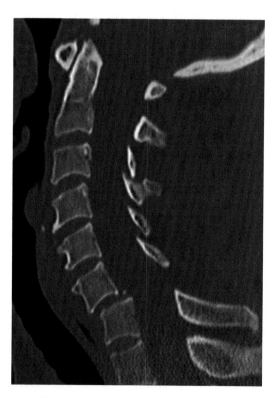

Fracture, Flexion Injury, Fig. 3 Anterior subluxation of C6

Cross-References

▶ Anterior Cord Syndrome
▶ Imaging of CNS Injuries
▶ Imaging of Spine and Bony Pelvis Injuries

References

Green JD, Harle TS, Harris JH (1981) Anterior subluxation of the cervical spine: hyperflexion sprain. AJNR Am J Neuroradiol 2(3):243–250

Greene KA, Dickman CA, Marciano FF, Drabier JB, Hadley MN, Sonntag VN (1997) Acute axis fractures. Analysis of management and outcome in 340 consecutive cases. Spine (Phila Pa1976) 22(16):1843–1852

Harris JH, Edeiken-Monroe B, Kopaniky DR (1986) A practical classification of acute cervical spine injuries. Orthop Clin North Am 17(1):15–30

Pratt H, Davies E, King L (2008) Traumatic injuries of the c1/c2 complex: computed tomographic imaging appearances. Curr Probl Diagn Radiol 37(1):26–38

Wheeless III CR (2013) "Wheeless Textbook of Orthopedics." Wheeless' textbook of orthopaedics. Duke University Medical Center. http://www.wheelessonline.com/. Accessed 8 Feb 2013

Fracture, Odontoid

Patricia L. Zadnik and Daniel M. Sciubba
Department of Neurosurgery, The Johns Hopkins University School of Medicine, Baltimore, MD, USA

Synonyms

Dens fracture; Odontoid process fracture

Definition

Fracture of C2 involves the odontoid process in 55 % of fractures and constitutes 10–15 % of cervical spine fractures (Pimentel and Diegelmann 2010). These fractures typically result from a flexion injury, which can lead to anterior displacement of C1 on C2. In younger

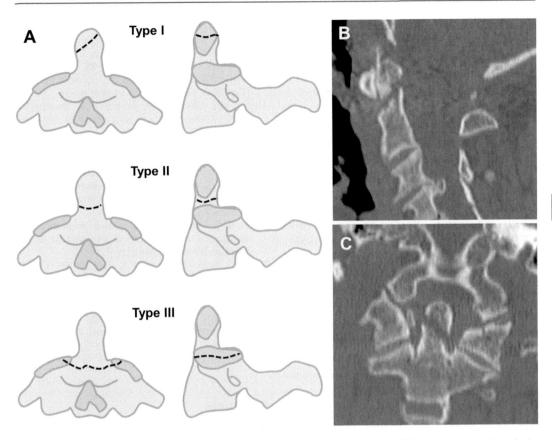

Fracture, Odontoid, Fig. 1 Odontoid fractures. (**a**) Illustration of Anderson classification of odontoid fractures. Type I fractures pass through the tip of the odontoid process. Type II fractures involve the base of the odontoid, while type III fractures pass through the body of C2. (**b**) Sagittal and (**c**) coronal CT scan demonstrating type II fracture through the base of the odontoid process

individuals, they require a great deal of force and as a result can present with significant canal compromise or neurological deficit. In the elderly population, an odontoid fracture may result from relatively minor trauma and can be missed on initial evaluation.

Odontoid fractures have been classified into three types by Anderson and D'Alonzo (Anderson and D'Alonzo 1974): Type I involves the tip of the odontoid and has historically been considered stable. However, Type I fractures could be a marker for atlanto-occipital dislocation or disruption of the transverse ligament, which would then be unstable. Type II fractures run through the base of the odontoid process and are unstable. Type IIA is similar to type II, but has large bone chips at the fracture site (Hadley et al. 1988). Type III fractures pass through the

cancellous bone of the superior body of C2 and are usually stable (Fig. 1). In one series, 70 % of patients with type II fractures were neurologically intact and 18 % presented with significant deficit such as neuroparesis or quadriplegia (Hadley et al. 1985). It has been estimated that 25–40 % of fractures result in fatalities at the time of injury (Crockard et al. 1993).

Type I and III fractures can be managed conservatively with external cervical immobilization through a rigid cervical collar or halo vest (Polin et al. 1996). Isolated type II odontoid fractures in adults greater than 50 years of age should be considered for surgical stabilization and fusion as older individuals have an increased nonunion rate with halo vest immobilization that is 21-fold greater than a younger patient (Lennarson et al. 2000). Surgical fixation should be considered for any fracture with >5 mm of displacement, a comminuted pattern, or an inability to maintain alignment at the fracture site with external fixation.

Surgical options include both an anterior or posterior approach. In patients where the transverse ligament is intact and there is not significant posterior displacement, an anterior odontoid screw can be placed. C1-2 arthrodesis and fusion may also be performed with adequate results. Halo vest immobilization can have a fusion rate as high as 72 % (Hadley et al. 1989) and appears superior to a rigid collar (53 %; (Polin et al. 1996; Hadley et al. 1989)). For type II fractures, up to 90 % will heal with external immobilization through either halo (100 %) or rigid cervical collar (50–70 %) for 8–14 weeks (Hadley et al. 1989; Sonntag and Hadley 1988). If there is movement at the fracture site despite halo vest immobilization, then the patient will require surgical stabilization. In older patients with Type II fractures who are not adequate surgical candidates, arguments have been made for rigid cervical orthosis and calcitonin therapy (Darakchiev et al. 2000). These patients are at risk of nonunion and late myelopathy may develop in as many as 77 % of patients with nonunion (Crockard et al. 1993; Paradis and Janes 1973).

Cross-References

► Fracture, Atlas (C1)
► Fracture, Axis (C2)

References

Anderson LD, D'Alonzo RT (1974) Fractures of the odontoid process of the axis. J Bone Joint Surg Am 56(8):1663–1674
Crockard HA, Heilman AE, Stevens JM (1993) Progressive myelopathy secondary to odontoid fractures: clinical, radiological, and surgical features. J Neurosurg 78(4):579–586
Darakchiev BJ, Bulas RV, Dunsker SB (2000) Use of calcitonin for the treatment of an odontoid fracture. Case report. J Neurosurg 93(1 Suppl):157–160
Hadley MN, Browner CM, Sonntag VK (1985) Axis fractures: a comprehensive review of management and treatment in 107 cases. Neurosurgery 17(2):281–290
Hadley MN, Browner CM, Liu SS, Sonntag VK (1988) New subtype of acute odontoid fractures (Type IIA). Neurosurgery 22(1 Pt 1):67–71
Hadley MN, Dickman CA, Browner CM, Sonntag VK (1989) Acute axis fractures: a review of 229 cases. J Neurosurg 71(5 Pt 1):642–647
Lennarson PJ, Mostafavi H, Traynelis VC, Walters BC (2000) Management of type II dens fractures: a case–control study. Spine (Phila Pa1976) 25(10):1234–1237
Paradis GR, Janes JM (1973) Posttraumatic atlantoaxial instability: the fate of the odontoid process fracture in 46 cases. J Trauma 13(4):359–367
Pimentel L, Diegelmann L (2010) Evaluation and management of acute cervical spine trauma. Emerg Med Clin North Am 28(4):719–738
Polin RS, Szabo T, Bogaev CA, Replogle RE, Jane JA (1996) Nonoperative management of types II and III odontoid fractures: the Philadelphia collar versus the halo vest. Neurosurgery 38(3):450–456 discussion 456–7
Sonntag VK, Hadley MN (1988) Nonoperative management of cervical spine injuries. Clin Neurosurg 34:630–649

Fractures

► Principles of Nonoperative Treatment of Diaphyseal Fractures

Frag or Fragmentation Injury

► Fragment Injury

Fragment Injury

Sara J. Aberle
Department of Emergency Medicine, Mayo School of Graduate Medical Education – Mayo Clinic, Rochester, MN, USA

Synonyms

Frag or fragmentation injury; Penetrating blast injury; Secondary blast injury

Definition

Fragmentation or secondary blast injuries occur as a result of flying fragments of any type, associated with a blast or explosion, which can affect every part of the body. These injuries are the most common cause of death in blasts, (CDC 2006) as well as the most common survivable injuries that require immediate attention. The effects of flying fragments, no matter how small, can be devastating.

The airborne fragments that cause these injuries can be pieces of the actual exploding device, which may be designed with many various types of projectiles (such as nails, nuts, ball bearings, etc.) within the device itself, or may be from nearby debris that is picked up along with the blast. Any hole in a patient from a flying fragment can be linked to major injury. Much research has been gone into these types of injuries, and an underlying theme has been found: When patients are injured by an explosion, the effects of flying fragments are similar to gunshot wounds, (Navarro et al. 2012; Champion et al. 2010; Ramasamy et al. 2008; Peleg et al. 2004; Bala et al. 2008) though some research has shown that gunshot wounds had a higher likelihood of surgical intervention than explosion-related injuries (Navarro et al. 2012). Also similar to gunshot wounds, the mantra "trajectory determination equals injury identification" can also apply in the case of penetrating fragmentation injuries. Establishing the trajectory of fragments, by looking at entry and exit wounds if present, can help identify what tissues may be injured between those two points.

Despite advancements in body armor and ballistics protection, the extremities and junctional regions (such as the neck, axilla, and groin) are still quite vulnerable to this type of injury. Because of this, early hemorrhage control continues to be a mainstay of acute trauma management for blast injuries (Eastridge et al. 2012). Types of hemorrhage control methods that are commonly used in the care of fragmentation injuries include tourniquets, pressure dressings, hemostatic agents (such as gauze that is impregnated with pro-coagulant substances), specialized vascular clamps and related devices, remote damage control resuscitation with early transfusion capabilities, and definitive surgical management (Gerhardt et al. 2010; Morrison et al. 2011).

Cross-References

▶ Adaptive Equipment
▶ Ballistics
▶ Blast
▶ Body Armor
▶ Cardiopulmonary Resuscitation in Adult Trauma
▶ Cardiopulmonary Resuscitation in Pediatric Trauma
▶ Compressible Hemorrhage
▶ Damage Control Resuscitation, Military Trauma
▶ Damage Control Surgery
▶ Explosion
▶ Exsanguination Transfusion
▶ Extremity Injury
▶ Fluid, Electrolytes, and Nutrition in Trauma Patients
▶ IED (Improvised Explosive Device)
▶ Military Trauma, Anesthesia for
▶ Noncompressible Hemorrhage
▶ Orthopedic Trauma, Anesthesia for
▶ Phantom Limb Pain
▶ Shock Management in Trauma
▶ Tactical Combat Casualty Care
▶ Tourniquet

References

Bala M, Rivkind AI, Zamir G, Hadar T, Gertsenshtein I, Mintz Y et al (2008) Abdominal trauma after terrorist bombing attacks exhibits a unique pattern of injury. Ann Surg 248(2):303–309

CDC (2006) Bombings: injury patterns and care. Blast curriculum: one-hour module. http://www.bt.cdc.gov/masscasualties/bombings_injurycare.asp. Accessed 28 July 2013

Champion H, Holcomb JB, Lawnick MM, Kelliher T, Spott MA, Galarneau MR et al (2010) Improved characterization of combat injury. J Trauma 68(5):1139–1150

Eastridge BJ, Mabry RL, Seguin P, Cantrell J, Tops T, Uribe P et al (2012) Death on the battlefield

(2001–2011): implications for the future of combat casualty care. J Trauma Acute Care Surg 73(6): S431–S437

Gerhardt RT, Mabry RL, Delorenzo RA, Butler F (2010) Fundamentals of combat casualty care. Combat casualty care: lessons learned from OEF & OIF. DVD. Pelagique, LLC, Los Angeles

Morrison CA, Carrick MM, Norman MA, Scott BG, Welsh FJ, Tsai P et al (2011) Hypotensive resuscitation strategy reduces transfusion requirements and severe postoperative coagulopathy in trauma patients with hemorrhagic shock: preliminary results of a randomized controlled trial. J Trauma 70:652–663

Navarro SR, Abadía de Barbará AH, Gutierrez OC, Bartolome CE, Lam DM, Gilsanz RF (2012) Gunshot and improvised explosive casualties: a report from the Spanish role 2 medical facility in Herat, Afghanistan. Mil Med 177(3):326–332

Peleg K, Aharonson-Daniel L, Stein M, Michaelson M, Kluger Y, Simon D et al (2004) Gunshot and explosion injuries: characteristics, outcomes, and implications for care of terror-related injuries in Israel. Ann Surg 239(3):311–318

Ramasamy A, Harrisson SE, Clasper JC, Stewart MP (2008) Injuries from roadside improvised explosive devices. J Trauma 65(4):910–914

Fragmentation

▶ Spalling

Frankel Neurological Performance Scale

▶ Examination, Neurological

Fresh Frozen Plasma (FFP) Transfusion

▶ Plasma Transfusion in Trauma

Frozen Plasma

▶ FP24

Frozen Plasma (FP) Transfusion

▶ Plasma Transfusion in Trauma

FSP

▶ Fibrinogen Split Products (Test)

Full-Thickness Burn

▶ Scald Burns

Fulminate Hepatitis

▶ Hepatic Failure

Fungal Infections

Archana Bhaskaran and Shahid Husain
Division of Infectious Diseases and Multi-Organ Transplantation, University Health Network/ University of Toronto, Toronto, ON, Canada

Synonyms

Aspergillus; Candida; Intensive care unit; Mold; Trauma

Definition

Fungi are ubiquitous in the environment. Hence breach in the innate barriers, skin or mucosa, and inoculation of environmental material, fundamental to trauma, are predisposing factors to fungal infections especially in the immune-competent host. The predominating issue with severe injuries are hemodynamic, anatomical, and mechanical, but these patients are susceptible to nosocomial fungal infections due to their intensive care unit stay. We will briefly summarize fungal infections in trauma patients owing to paucity of data and focus on fungal infections in the intensive care unit.

Preexisiting Condition

Fungal Infections in Trauma Patients

Post trauma patients may acquire fungal spores from the environment, secondary to tissue necrosis, and ischemia may develop local fungal disease with any mold. The largest series of invasive mold infections in trauma patients is from US military personnel in Afghanistan (Warkentien et al. 2012). The diagnostic criteria were well defined with 20 proven, 4 probable, and 13 possible invasive mold infections. Between June 2009 and December 2010, the incidence per quarter ranged from 0.5 % to 3.5 %. All injuries were secondary to explosive blasts and involved extremities with 78 % requiring amputation at the time of injury or first surgery. Most patients had hypotension at the time of presentation and developed fever at the time of diagnosis. Over 50 % of the molds were *Aspergillus* or mucormycosis. The median number of surgeries after the first was 11 consisting of debridement and amputation revisions. In the proven and probable categories, median time from injury to diagnosis was 10 days; median duration of antifungal treatment was 34 days, and mortality was 17 %. Findings were similar with traumatic mucormycosis in tornado victims in Joplin, Missouri, in 2011 (Neblett Fanfair et al. 2011).

Non-severe injuries can result in mold infections as well; fungal corneal ulcers are common in agricultural areas; eumycetoma and chromoblastomycosis of extremities occur after inconspicuous injuries predominating again in agrarian areas. *Pseudallescheria boydii* (*Scedosporium apiospermum*) infection in near-drowning incidents has been well described. Patients with burns despite lack of penetrating trauma have lost the most important protecting barrier. *Candida* which is rarely a causative pathogen in other traumatic injuries is very important in this setting. *Aspergillus*, *Fusarium*, and other hyaline and dematiaceous molds and mucormycosis are gaining importance with high mortality rates. Detailed review of these topics is beyond the scope of this article, and suggested readings are provided below.

Fungal Infections in the Intensive Care Unit

Infections are common in the intensive care unit (ICU). Bacterial infections are the norm, but lately fungal infections have also entered the scene. In a point prevalence study involving 1,265 intensive care units from 75 countries in 2007, 51 % of ICU patients were considered infected based on the International Sepsis Forum definition of infections in the ICU (Calandra et al. 2005). Sixteen percent of the infected patients were on an antifungal medication, and 17 % of the positive microbial isolates in infected patients were fungi (Vincent et al. 2009). The commonest invasive fungi were *Candida* and *Aspergillus* at incidence of 19–20 and 2–3 per 10,000 hospital discharges, respectively, between 1996 and 2003 in the United States (Pfaller and Diekema 2007).

Candida

Candida is the fourth most common nosocomial blood stream infection in the United States, and half of all candidemia occur in the ICU. The incidence of candidiasis rose dramatically in the 1980s and 1990s. This was likely due to extensive use of antimicrobials and intravascular devices, increasing population of susceptible individuals due to better medical care, immunosuppression, or transplantation.

Candida is a commensal of the human intestinal tract. Invasive candidiasis (IC) most commonly manifests as candidemia, but it also includes endophthalmitis, endocarditis, meningitis, peritonitis, and hepatosplenic candidiasis. Pulmonary candidiasis is very rare and is noted in the setting of extension of pleural *Candida* infection. Candidemia is usually a result of catheter-related infection although dissemination from endogenous colonizing source is possible. More than 90 % of IC is caused by *Candida albicans*, *C. glabrata*, *C. krusei*, *C. tropicalis*, and *C. parapsilosis*. *Candida albicans* is the most common among them, but its frequency varies geographically.

Clinical presentation of IC is nonspecific. 2–16 % of patients with candidemia have eye involvement. The ophthalmoscopic findings are classical, and an exam is warranted in every patient with candidemia due to sight-threatening consequences and variation in eye penetration of antifungal agents.

Diagnosis is usually delayed until the laboratory identifies the organism as yeast which might take a few days. Blood cultures are crucial for identifying candidemia. In general *Candida* in blood culture is not considered a contaminant. Earlier studies with the older blood culture systems had a low sensitivity of ∼45 % when compared to autopsy findings. The newer blood culture systems with improved techniques should be better but have not been compared with autopsy findings. However when compared with PCR, blood cultures did not detect any of the suspected cases of invasive candidiasis in contrast to 56 % detected by PCR (Ahmad et al. 2002). PCR however is only a research tool and has not made it to the commercial market yet. Contrastingly other methodologies to improve turnaround time for species identification of *Candida* (as antimicrobial susceptibilities differ) have been developed, and the newer ones include probes directly from blood culture bottles. β D-glucan is a commercially available antigen detection test that has a sensitivity of 81 % with a cutoff value of 60 pg/ml. A combination of antigen and antibody detection test for *Candida* is also available in the commercial market. Diagnosis of IC is usually made by blood culture though commercially available serum β D-glucan is increasingly used.

Several risk factors for IC in nonimmunocompromised individuals have been identified. Prior antibiotic use, central venous or urinary catheters, total parenteral nutrition, surgery and fungal colonization are a few. However, many ICU patients have these risk factors, and moreover the clinical presentation of IC is nonspecific. Therefore, to identify patients at risk for IC, a *Candida* score was developed. The categories for the scoring system include severe sepsis, >1 fungal colonizing site, TPN, and surgery. A score of >3 may necessitate empiric anti-candida treatment (Leroy et al. 2011).

Amphotericin B with its limiting renal toxicity was the only anti-candida treatment available earlier. All *Candida* species except rarely occurring *C. lusitaniae* are susceptible to amphotericin. Fluconazole has better tolerability but is not active against all *Candida* species: *C. krusei* is intrinsically fluconazole resistant. Echinocandins as a class (caspofungin, micafungin, and anidulafungin) have activity against all Candida species. In 2002 caspofungin, an echinocandin was shown to be as efficacious as amphotericin for candidemia but with fewer side effects. Subsequently micafungin and anidulafungin too proved to be non-inferior to amphotericin and fluconazole, respectively, for candidemia.

C. glabrata in general has high MICs (minimum inhibitory concentration) to fluconazole; hence, candidemia with *C. glabrata* is traditionally treated with an echinocandin. Caspofungin, micafungin, and anidulafungin are similar except that anidulafungin does not undergo hepatic metabolism and hence presumed to have less drug interactions. Candida chorioretinitis and endophthalmitis are treated with systemic fluconazole, parenteral amphotericin, or intravitreal amphotericin injections as echinocandins do not penetrate the central nervous system well. In an ICU patient suspected of IC, empiric antifungal treatment is recommended (Fig. 1), which should be tapered based on the culture and susceptibility report.

Mortality from candidemia was consistently around 50 % in the 1990s. In this past decade, there has been a trend towards lower but persistently significant mortality of around 30 % despite advancements in antifungal therapy and medical progress.

Table 1 lists the salient features of invasive candidiasis.

Fungal Infections, Fig. 1 Empiric therapy in non-neutropenic ICU patient

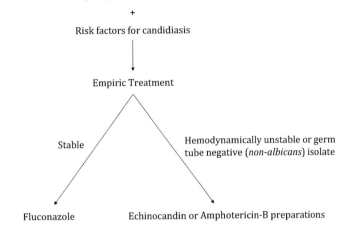

Persistent systemic inflammatory response unresponsive to 4-7 days antibiotic therapy

+

Risk factors for candidiasis

Empiric Treatment

Stable

Hemodynamically unstable or germ tube negative (*non-albicans*) isolate

Fluconazole

Echinocandin or Amphotericin-B preparations

Fungal Infections, Table 1 Summary, invasive candidiasis

Epidemiology	Presentation	Diagnosis	Treatment	Mortality
1. Most common IFI	1. Nonspecific	1. Blood or sterile site cultures	1. Echinocandins, fluconazole, or amphotericin B formulations may be used	~30 % despite advancements in antifungal therapy and medical progress
2. *C. albicans* is the commonest candida	2. If eye is involved – classic retinal changes	2. Blood cultures may miss some candidemia	2. *C. glabrata* has higher MICs to fluconazole than other candidas	
	3. Every patient with candidemia needs a retinal exam	3. Antigen and antibody tests for candida have variable sensitivities and specificities	3. *C. krusei* is resistant to fluconazole	
			4. *C. lusitania* is resistant to amphotericin B	
			5. Consider empiric anti-candida treatment when candida score >3	

IFI invasive fungal infections

Aspergillus

Aspergillus is the second most common invasive fungal infection in hospitalized patients. The incidence of invasive aspergillus infection in the ICU ranges from 0.33 % to 5.7 %. To give further perspective, invasive aspergillosis (IA) is the fourth most common misdiagnosis in the ICU based on several autopsy series. The traditional risk factors for IA include neutropenia, hematopoietic, and solid organ transplantation. However in the ICU, apart from the traditional risk factors, chronic obstructive pulmonary disease (COPD) and receipt of >700 mg of corticosteroids in the previous 3 months are significantly associated

Fungal Infections, Table 2 Summary, invasive aspergillosis in ICU

Epidemiology	Risk factors and presentation	Diagnosis	Treatment	Mortality
1. Second most common IFI	1. COPD with prolonged antibiotic use, >370 mg of accumulated steroid use	1. EORTC/MSG criteria modified by Blot et al. –92 % sensitivity and 61 % specificity	1. First line – Voriconazole	70–80 % likely due to low suspicion and critical illness
2. *A. fumigatus* is the most common species	2. Receipt of >700 mg steroids in the preceding 3 months	2. BAL *Aspergillus* galactomannan sensitivity 88 %	2. Salvage:	
			a. Amphotericin B and its formulations	
			b. Caspofungin or Micafungin	
			c. Itraconazole	
			d. Posaconazole	
	3. Antibiotic-resistant pneumonia		3. *Aspergillus terreus* is resistant to amphotericin	
	4. Tracheobronchitis on bronchoscopy			

IFI invasive fungal infections, *COPD* chronic obstructive pulmonary disease, *EORTC/MSG* European Organization for Research and Treatment of Cancer/Mycoses Study Group (National Institute of Allergy and Infectious Diseases), *BAL* bronchoalveolar lavage

with IA. Invasive aspergillosis has also been described as case reports and series in patients with end-stage renal and hepatic disease. In COPD patients admitted to the ICU, risk factors include prolonged duration of antibiotics and steroids with an accumulated mean steroid dose of 370 mg. Outbreaks of IA can occur in the ICU as elsewhere in the hospital from aerosolization of spores during periods of construction.

A. fumigatus is the most common *Aspergillus* species causing IA followed by *A. flavus, A. niger*, and *A. terreus*. Pulmonary invasive aspergillosis is the commonest manifestation. Signs to raise suspicion for invasive aspergillosis in this patient population are an antibiotic-resistant pneumonia and findings of tracheobronchitis on bronchoscopy.

The diagnosis of IA is difficult in patients without traditional risk factors because of low suspicion and nonspecific findings. The EORTC/MSG criteria are usually used for diagnosis of IA, but it includes only traditional risk factors and classic imaging abnormality (De Pauw et al. 2008). The characteristic halo and air crescent sign is seen only in 5 % of ICU patients with probable and proven IA.

Therefore, the EORTC/MSG criteria were modified to include any kind of imaging abnormality and in the absence of traditional risk factors to satisfy both criteria – bronchoalveolar lavage fluid smear positive for hyphae and aspergillus growth on culture. The modified criteria in a multicenter center study had a sensitivity and specificity of 92 % and 61 %, respectively, with histopathology as gold standard (Blot et al. 2012).

Aspergillus galactomannan has been found to be very useful in the diagnosis of IA in the neutropenic and transplant population. In the study by Meersseman et al. published in 2008, the sensitivity of *Aspergillus* galactomannan in the BAL and serum for proven IA in ICU patients were 88 % and 42 %, respectively. In patients with proven IA, only 58 % had a positive *Aspergillus* culture and/or cytological smear positive for hyphae.

Amphotericin B and its lipid formulations was the drug of choice for IA until voriconazole emerged in 2002. *Aspergillus terreus* is resistant to amphotericin but is isolated uncommonly. In a randomized unblinded controlled trial (Herbrecht et al. 2002), more subjects in the voriconazole arm responded to treatment

(53 vs. 32 %) with fewer deaths (71 vs. 58 %) and side effects compared to amphotericin B deoxycholate. Caspofungin received FDA approval as salvage therapy for patients with invasive aspergillosis who are refractory or intolerant of standard therapy. Due to poor treatment response of IA, combination antifungal treatment is used in clinical practice if monotherapy fails.

The mortality of IA in critically ill patients is 80 % in contrast to 38 % in the transplant and neutropenic population, likely due to lower suspicion and the underlying critical illness. Table 2 summarizes invasive aspergillosis in the ICU.

Application

In conclusion, *Candida* and *Aspergillus* species are the predominant fungal pathogens in the post-injury patient followed by other molds. These infections are associated with a high mortality, and hence a heightened index of suspicion is required to improve outcomes.

Cross-References

▶ Catheter Associated Urinary Tract Infection
▶ Catheter-Related Infections
▶ Infection Control
▶ Surgical Site Infections
▶ Systemic Inflammatory Response Syndrome
▶ Tetanus
▶ Ventilator-Associated Pneumonia

References

Ahmad S, Khan Z, Mustafa AS, Khan ZU (2002) Seminested PCR for diagnosis of candidemia: comparison with culture, antigen detection, and biochemical methods for species identification. J Clin Microbiol 40(7):2483–2489

Blot SI, Taccone FS, Van den Abeele AM, Bulpa P, Meersseman W, Brusselaers N, Dimopoulos G, Paiva JA, Misset B, Rello J, Vandewoude K, Vogelaers D, AspICU Study Investigators (2012) A clinical algorithm to diagnose invasive pulmonary Aspergillosis in critically ill patients. Am J Respir Crit Care Med 186(1):56–64

Calandra T, Cohen J, International Sepsis Forum Definition of Infection in the ICU Consensus Conference (2005) The international sepsis forum consensus conference on definitions of infection in the intensive care unit. Crit Care Med 33(7):1538–1548. Review

De Pauw B, Walsh TJ, Donnelly JP, Stevens DA, Edwards JE, Calandra T, Pappas PG, Maertens J, Lortholary O, Kauffman CA, Denning DW, Patterson TF, Maschmeyer G, Bille J, Dismukes WE, Herbrecht R, Hope WW, Kibbler CC, Kullberg BJ, Marr KA, Muñoz P, Odds FC, Perfect JR, Restrepo A, Ruhnke M, Segal BH, Sobel JD, Sorrell TC, Viscoli C, Wingard JR, Zaoutis T, Bennett JE, European Organization for Research and Treatment of Cancer/Invasive Fungal Infections Cooperative Group; National Institute of Allergy and Infectious Diseases Mycoses Study Group(EORTC/MSG) Consensus Group (2008) Revised definitions of invasive fungal disease from the European organization for research and treatment of cancer/invasive fungal infections cooperative group and the national institute of allergy and infectious diseases mycoses study group (EORTC/MSG) consensus group. Clin Infect Dis 46(12):1813–1821

Herbrecht R, Denning DW, Patterson TF, Bennett JE, Greene RE, Oestmann JW, Kern WV, Marr KA, Ribaud P, Lortholary O, Sylvester R, Rubin RH, Wingard JR, Stark P, Durand C, Caillot D, Thiel E, Chandrasekar PH, Hodges MR, Schlamm HT, Troke PF, de Pauw B (2002) Invasive fungal infections group of the European organisation for research and treatment of cancer and the global Aspergillus study group. Voriconazole versus amphotericin B for primary therapy of invasive Aspergillosis. N Engl J Med 347(6):408–415

Leroy G, Lambiotte F, Thévenin D, Lemaire C, Parmentier E, Devos P, Leroy O (2011) Evaluation of "Candida score" in critically ill patients: a prospective, multicenter, observational, cohort study. Ann Intensive Care 1(1):50

Meersseman W, Lagrou K, Maertens J, Wilmer A, Hermans G, Vanderschueren S, Spriet I, Verbeken E, Van Wijngaerden E (2008) Galactomannan in bronchoalveolar lavage fluid: a tool for diagnosing Aspergillosis in intensive care unit patients. Am J Respir Crit Care Med 177(1):27–34

Neblett Fanfair R, Benedict K, Bos J, Bennett SD, Lo YC, Adebanjo T, Etienne K, Deak E, Derado G, Shieh WJ, Drew C, Zaki S, Sugerman D, Gade L, Thompson EH, Sutton DA, Engelthaler DM, Schupp JM, Brandt ME, Harris JR, Lockhart SR, Turabelidze G, Park BJ (2011) Necrotizing cutaneous mucormycosis after a tornado in Joplin, Missouri, in 2011. N Engl J Med 367(23):2214–2225

Pfaller MA, Diekema DJ (2007) Epidemiology of invasive candidiasis: a persistent public health problem. Clin Microbiol Rev 20(1):133–163. Review

Vincent JL, Rello J, Marshall J, Silva E, Anzueto A, Martin CD, Moreno R, Lipman J, Gomersall C,

Sakr Y, Reinhart K, EPIC II Group of Investigators (2009) International study of the prevalence and outcomes of infection in intensive care units. JAMA 302(21):2323–2329

Warkentien T, Rodriguez C, Lloyd B, Wells J, Weintrob A, Dunne JR, Ganesan A, Li P, Bradley W, Gaskins LJ, Seillier-Moiseiwitsch F, Murray CK, Millar EV, Keenan B, Paolino K, Fleming M, Hospenthal DR, Wortmann GW, Landrum ML, Kortepeter MG, Tribble DR, Infectious Disease Clinical Research Program Trauma Infectious Disease Outcomes Study Group (2012) Invasive mold infections following combat-related injuries. Clin Infect Dis 55(11):1441–1449

Recommended Reading

Branski LK, Al-Mousawi A, Rivero H, Jeschke MG, Sanford AP, Herndon DN (2009) Emerging infections in burns. Surg Infect (Larchmt) 10(5):389–397. doi:10.1089/sur.2009.024. Review

Gopinathan U, Garg P, Fernandes M, Sharma S, Athmanathan S, Rao GN (2002) The epidemiological features and laboratory results of fungal keratitis: a 10-year review at a referral eye care center in south India. Cornea 21(6):555–559. Review

Lichon V, Khachemoune A (2006) Mycetoma: a review. Am J Clin Dermatol 7(5):315–321. Review

Lu S, Lu C, Zhang J, Hu Y, Li X, Xi L (2013) Chromoblastomycosis in mainland China: a systematic review on clinical characteristics. Mycopathologia 175(5–6): 489–495

Futile Care

Hitoshi Arima[1] and Akira Akabayashi[2]
[1]Graduate School of Urban Social and Cultural Studies, Yokohama City University, Yokohama, Japan
[2]Department of Biomedical Ethics, The University of Tokyo Graduate School of Medicine, Tokyo, Japan

Synonyms

Non-beneficial care

Definition

Futile care or treatments are those care or treatments that are believed, usually by physicians, to be of little or no benefit to their patient. Paradigmatic examples include cardiopulmonary resuscitation attempted in an unconscious, aged patient who appears to have little chance of recovery or artificial nutrition and hydration used to sustain the life of a patient in a persistent vegetative state. Ethical problems arise when physicians judge certain care to be futile, while the patient or the patient's family insists that the care be provided nonetheless. How and whether the concept of futile care can reach a clear-cut definition is a matter of controversy, as will be explained below, and it is difficult to demarcate futile and non-futile or meaningful.

Background

Judicial Controversy

Treatments considered futile typically concern terminal care and end-of-life decision making. Previously, legal and ethical debates regarding terminal care were mostly devoted to the issue of a patient's right to death. In the USA, two landmark court cases on this issue occurred between the 1970s and 1980s: the Quinlan case and the Cruzan case. In both cases, a young woman was kept alive in a persistent vegetative state; her family requested that the treatment be terminated, whereas the attending physicians insisted on continuing care. The court eventually ruled in favor of the families, allowing them to make the final decision (Quinlan 1976; Cruzan 1990). After these and several other similar cases, the idea that patients have the right to refuse unwanted medical treatment, even if it would result in death, has gained wide acceptance in both legal and ethical considerations.

The futility debate starkly contrasts with the previous debate on a patient's right to death, in that the role of physicians and that of patients are seemingly reversed. In the futility debate, it is health-care professionals who refuse to provide care that they believe is futile, while patients or their families request continued treatment.

Court opinions on this more recent issue have thus far been divided. The most important legal cases include the Wanglie case and the Baby K case. The former case involves Ms. Wanglie, a well-educated 87-year-old lady who was left in a persistent vegetative state following cardiac arrest. Although the patient did not have a living will, she had occasionally discussed with her family about the meaning of life and the use of life-sustaining treatments while she was still capable. When the attending physician suggested that Ms. Wanglie's ventilator should be turned off on the grounds of futility, the patient's husband opposed, and thus, the case went to the court. In 1991, the Minneapolis District Court ruled by appointing the husband as the patient's guardian on the basis that it would best serve the patient's interest (Wanglie 1991).

The second legal case concerned a baby ("Baby K" as referred to by the court) who was born with anencephaly, leaving her permanently unconscious. Baby K had difficulty breathing and therefore was connected to a ventilator immediately after birth. The hospital staff and its ethics committee recommended that ventilator treatment should be ended for the reason that it is futile. As the baby's mother opposed this recommendation, attending clinicians eventually filed a petition asking for the court's approval to terminate treatment. The request was rejected by a federal district court in Virginia (Baby 1994).

While both cases supported the family's wish to continue treatment that clinicians found futile, a later case reached a different conclusion. In the Gilgunn case, which took place in Massachusetts in 1995, the court found that neither the hospital nor its physicians were negligent for removing mechanical ventilation from a female patient who was unconscious against the wishes of the patient's daughter (Gilgunn 1995). These cases illustrate that there is no clear legal consensus regarding the futility debate to this day.

Application

Ethics of Futile Care

Heated moral debates have revolved around the questions of how the concept of futility should be defined and of whether health-care providers have the ultimate authority to forgo treatments that are considered futile. Often, these questions concern a physician's decision to write a do-not-attempt-resuscitation (DNR or DNAR) order in the patient's chart. When a DNR order is placed, cardiopulmonary resuscitation (CPR) will not be instituted even if the patient suffers a serious arrhythmia or cardiac arrest. Are physicians allowed to make unilateral decisions to withhold resuscitation by writing a DNR order and, if so, under what conditions?

The significance of these questions must be understood in the context of the mainstream thinking in contemporary biomedical ethics, in which the principle of respect for patient autonomy is considered paramount. The worry often voiced is that entitling physicians with such power may spark the resurgence of the old paternalism. Many are also wary of the strong possibility that the power will be abused; it is all too easy to foresee that unless a clear and unambiguous definition is given to the concept of futile care, more treatments may be withheld by physician's discretion than is ever legitimate.

Against these worries, a number of commentators advanced various arguments in defense of the physician's ultimate authority to forgo treatments that are determined futile. Four such arguments are discussed below.

Conceptual Definitions

In the first place, some scholars attempt to erase the worry about abuse by defining the concept of futility in clearer terms. Among different types of definitions proposed to date, three merit a special attention to this effect. First, it is suggested that care should be considered futile if it would not attain the goals of treatment to recover a desired physiological state. A classic example of futile care in terms of this understanding is prescribing an antibiotic to a patient with viral infection. Futility in this sense is normally referred to as physiological futility.

Second, it is claimed that whether care should be deemed futile or not depends upon the likelihood of the care achieving the targeted condition. For example, Lawrence Schneiderman and his colleagues proposed that physicians should regard a treatment as futile if that treatment has never been successful in the last 100 cases (Schneiderman et al. 1990). Futility defined in such terms is called quantitative futility or probability futility. Finally, the third definition implies that care should be considered futile when the condition achieved with the care is of no value or not worth the effort. For example, it may be considered worthless to live a few days longer with constant pain and agony or to live any longer once rendered permanently unconscious. If this was the case, according to the third definition, care is considered futile, as its only aim is to sustain life (Schneiderman et al. 1990). Futility, as thus understood, is commonly referred to as qualitative futility.

All three definitions described above have the advantage of being relatively free of ambiguities; hence, it is argued that physicians can employ these definitions for futility judgment, on the basis of which they can forgo certain care without patient consent.

This type of argument, however, has been severely criticized. For one thing, setting the physiological futility aside, it is inevitable that a given definition of futility care, which demarcates what is futile from meaningful, would still leave the impression that such demarcation seems arbitrary, no matter how that line is drawn. For example, why is care deemed quantitatively futile when it had failed in the last 100 trials instead of 100 and ten trials? A related but more important point is that any judgment to draw a line as such is at least partially a value judgment. It is clear that a judgment on qualitative futility (e.g., "it is worthless to extend one's life with constant pain a few days longer") holds value. Similarly, with regard to quantitative futility, one may judge that a CPR attempt on a patient at hand is futile based on the fact that success rate for patients in similar conditions is lower than x%. This can be rephrased as a palpably value-laden judgment that it is not worth attempting CPR in this case because the success rate in other similar cases is below x%.

To put it succinctly, futility judgments in either of these cases signify the idea that, if a patient has a low chance of survival or a low quality of life after survival, it is not worth providing care. The problem here is that both cases involve a value judgment. Some critics have thus come to claim that any futility judgments other than those pertaining to physiological futility include a value judgment and therefore should not be used as a basis for decisions to withhold treatment without patient consent (Youngner 1998). Furthermore, some claim that the use of the expression "futility" should be abandoned in this context, as the expression insinuates that relevant judgments can be entirely medical by concealing their value-laden nature (Wicclair 2006). These criticisms have led most people to believe that the dispute cannot be settled simply by defining the concept of futility.

Medical Integrity

A second argument that supports the idea that physicians can unilaterally decide when to withhold treatments considered futile appeals to the concept of medical integrity. According to this argument, the value-laden nature of futility judgment does not necessarily bar physicians from using such judgments to justify their unilateral decision to forgo treatment.

The first thing to note here is the fact that there is virtually no treatment choice that is entirely free of value judgment. As Tom Tomlinson and Howard Brody once suggested, even a judgment pertaining to physiological futility, which itself is solely medical in nature, must be combined with some value judgment, if it should generate a treatment choice (Tomlinson and Brody 1990). For example, although antibiotics cannot combat a viral infection – a notion that is not always understood by patients – prescribing antibiotics may nonetheless make patients with viral infections happy. Now, physicians do not normally prescribe antibiotics for this purpose because they believe it is inappropriate to do so; however, this latter belief is clearly a value judgment. What this implies is that if we accept the claim that physicians should never withhold care solely based on the assessment of futility, then apparently unacceptable conclusions will follow: physicians will have no reason to refuse patients who ask for antibiotics for viral infections.

Tomlinson and Brody propose that physicians should be able to refuse to provide such treatment by appealing to the values inherent to medicine as a professional practice. A plausible understanding of medicine as a practice is that it aims to promote a patient's right and health – a goal that sets moral standards for medical practitioners. Thus, medical practitioners are to make judgments as to what is reasonable in their treatment choices in accordance with such standards, as well as to take responsibility for treatment outcome. It is asserted that depriving them of the opportunity to behave as a moral agency will undermine their integrity (Tomlinson and Brody 1990).

One particularly noteworthy point connected to this issue is the distinction between the positive and negative rights of patients and its relation to the principle of autonomy. While the principle of respect for patient autonomy has established nearly an absolute status in contemporary biomedical ethics, the practical implication of this principle is normally understood as patients retaining the negative right to refuse all unwanted treatments (or at best a weak positive right only to choose from treatment options offered by medical providers). The negative right in this sense is distinguishable from the strong positive right to demand any and all treatments they may desire. The latter kind of right will not be logically derivable from the former (Cranford and Gostin 1992).

Many consider that the argument from the point of medical integrity has a certain force to justify physician authority to forgo futile care. However, even this argument is not free of criticism. One important opposing opinion is offered by Robert Veatch and Carol Spicer. Admitting that any treatment choice includes a value judgment and that a patient's positive right to demand every treatment cannot be derived from the principle of patient autonomy, Veatch and Spicer claim that patients retain the right to demand care that physicians consider futile. Their rationale focuses on minority rights in the society. Medical professionals are licensed by the society and thereby granted the power to exercise exclusive control over the use of medical technology. A demerit of granting such power without any preconditions is that minorities in the society might be deprived of the opportunity to have their unique opinions regarding use of technology to be accepted. Given that any individual may someday become a minority in this regard, it is more rational for society to grant the power to medical professionals only on the condition that minority's opinions, whatever they may be, will be heard. With this understanding of the principle of physician's authority, physicians will always have to accede to the minority's opinion on use of technology (Veatch and Spicer 1993).

Process Approach

Another popular approach to this problem, which is essentially compatible with the idea of medical integrity introduced in the previous section, is called process approach. Prominent features of this more recent approach include, firstly, that it is founded on the recognition that since futility judgments are mostly value-laden, no universal consensus can be expected on people's judgments in this regard. Secondly, the approach takes into account the legitimate fear that allowing physicians to make unilateral decisions on what constitutes futile care may invite abuse. Hence, this approach aims to specify a procedure that people can engage to solve moral disputes concerning futility judgments without providing the necessary and sufficient conditions for a care to count as futile (Rowland 2006).

When medical providers and the patient (or the patient's family) disagree over whether a given treatment is futile or should be stopped, the process approach recommends both parties to engage in a conversation. Physicians will be given an opportunity to explain why they believe the treatment at hand would be futile, as well as to understand the reasons for the patient's refusal. The patient or the patient's family is also informed of the right they possess to obtain a second opinion from another physician or to consult the hospital's ethics committee. The point of such conversation is to attempt to negotiate an understanding between both parties through frank discussion. Furthermore, the conversation with physicians will help eliminate patient fears that physicians may exercise their power improperly and withhold care without legitimate reasons (Brody 1997).

The due process approach has also been espoused in various guidelines and legal documents. In 1999, the American Medical Association published an ethical policy entitled "Medical Futility in End-of-Life Care," which recommends a process approach to futility problems (Council on Ethical and Judicial Affairs, American Medical Association 1999). In the same year, the State of Texas passed the Texas Advance Directives Act (TADA), which also incorporates a due process standard for futility dispute resolution. According to TADA, when the family of a terminally ill patient who is currently incapacitated insists on a treatment that the attending physician believes is futile, the physician is allowed to request a formal meeting for dispute resolution. At the meeting, the hospital's ethics committee will hear the opinions of both sides, and if the committee eventually agrees with the physician, the family will be informed accordingly by letter. Most families reportedly change their mind and stop asking for treatment continuation at some point during this process. However, if the family remains unpersuaded, referral to another physician will be carried out, or if transfer to another physician is not possible, the law permits the attending physician to stop treatment (Fine 2009).

A prevailing opinion on this issue today seems that the process approach is both ethically sound and effective in dispute resolution. However, concerns have been raised over this approach as well. A most notable criticism argues that the approach is not as tolerant of the diversity of values as it initially appeared. Commenting on TADA, Robert Troug notes that an ethics committee is normally composed of a variety of clinicians, so when the attending physician's opinion conflicts with that of the family, the committee is most likely to agree with the former over the latter. This suggests that, when the family's request is one that the majority of clinicians find unreasonable, the procedure will only help to impose the majority's value on the family. The minority viewpoint, on the other hand, is systematically overridden (Troug 2007). Troug's criticism echoes the concerns expressed by Veatch and Spicer over the idea that physicians are allowed to make futility judgments in accordance with the values inherent to medicine as a professional practice.

Expenditure of Scarce Resources

The last argument in defense of the physician's power to unilaterally decide to forgo futile treatments pertains to the fair distribution of scarce medical resources. Most treatments addressed in futility debates are very costly. If we stop spending enormous amount of medical resources on patients who have little prospect of recovery, we may also be able to help other needy patients. One may think that such consideration provides sufficient reason to allow (or oblige, perhaps) physicians to withhold care when they think the care is futile.

Most scholars, however, do not accept this argument today. It is certainly true that the question of fair distribution of medical resources (i.e., who should receive care when not all can) is of great importance. At the same time, this is not the type of question that should be answered by individual physicians at the bedside. The question rather belongs to those involved in policy making and should be properly addressed in a wider context which allows for comparisons to be made among patients with various needs and where different prospects of recovery can be made.

Cross-References

▶ Autonomy
▶ Cardiopulmonary Resuscitation in Adult Trauma
▶ Cardiopulmonary Resuscitation in Pediatric Trauma
▶ End-of-Life Care Communication in Trauma Patients
▶ Evaluating a Patient's Decision-Making Capacity

References

Baby K (1994) Matter of, 16 F.3d 590 (4th cir. 1994)

Brody H (1997) Medical futility: a useful concept? In: Zucker M, Zucker H (eds) Medical futility and the evaluation of life-sustaining interventions. Cambridge University Press, Cambridge, UK, pp 1–14

Cranford R, Gostin L (1992) Futility: a concept in search of a definition. Law Med Health Care 20(4):307–309

Cruzan (1990) v. Director, Missouri Dept. of Health, 497 U.S. 261, 110 S.Ct. 2481, 111 L.Ed.2d 224 (1990)

Council on Ethical and Judicial Affairs, American Medical Association Medical (1999) Futility in End-of-Life-Care: Report of the Council on Ethical and Judicial Affairs. JAMA. 281(10): 937–941

Fine R (2009) The Texas advance directives act effectively and ethically resolves disputes about medical futility. Chest 136(4):963–967

Gilgunn (1995) v Massachusetts General Hospital, No 92–4820 (Mass Super Ct Civ Action Suffolk So April 22, 1995).

Quinlan, Matter of, 70 N.J. 10, 355 A.2d 647 (N.J.1976)

Rowland B (2006) Communicating past the conflict: solving the medical futility controversy with process-based approaches. Univ Miami Int Comp Law Rev 14(2):271–310

Schneiderman L, Jecker NS, Jonsen A (1990) Medical futility: its meaning and ethical implications. Ann Intern Med 112(12):949–954

Tomlinson T, Brody H (1990) Futility and the ethics of resuscitation. JAMA 264(10):1276–1280

Troug RD (2007) Tackling medical futility in Texas. N Engl J Med 357(1):1–3

Veatch R, Spicer CM (1993) Futile care: physicians should not be allowed to refuse to treat. Health Prog 74(10):22–27

Wanglie (1991) In re, No. PX-91-283 (Minn. 1991)

Wicclair M (2006) Medical futility: a conceptual and ethical analysis. In: Mappes T, DeGrazia D (eds) Biomedical ethics, 6th edn. McGraw Hill, Boston, pp 345–349

Youngner S (1998) Who defines futility? JAMA 260:2094–2095

F

G

Gastric Injury

▶ Gastrointestinal Injury, Anesthesia for

Gastric Necrosis from Short Gastric Embolization

Mansoor Khan
Consultant Esophagogastric and Acute Care
Surgeon, Doncaster Royal Infirmary, Doncaster,
South Yorkshire, UK

Mansoor Khan
Consultant Esophagogastric and Acute Care
Surgeon, Doncaster Royal Infirmary, Doncaster,
South Yorkshire, UK

Synonyms

Post embolization gastric necrosis

Definition

Gastric necrosis that is a direct result of embolization, and may be contributed by an overall global hypoperfusion of the stomach.

Cases of extensive gastric necrosis after therapeutic transcatheter embolization of the gastric arteries (Bradley and Goldman 1976; Bookstein et al. 1974; Tadavarthy et al. 1974) have been reported with more severe outcomes associated with embolization of the left gastric artery (Brown et al. 1989). However, they are very rare, due to the extensive blood supply of the stomach.

Studies have demonstrated that in order for gastric necrosis to occur, you have to ligate the right and left gastric arteries, as well as the right and left gastroepiploic arteries and 80 % of collaterals. There is a higher chance of necrosis to occur if both arteries and veins are ligated (Somervell 1945; Babkin et al. 1943). However, cases have been reported where high-dose intra-arterial vasopressin has caused necrosis (Alves et al. 1979).

Diagnosis is usually delayed due to the relative rarity of the condition. The patient may have signs of peritonism, increasing nasogastric tube output, shock, and/or worsening acidosis. Imaging modalities, which may prove useful, are an erect chest radiograph or a supine abdominal radiograph, which may demonstrate subphrenic air or air in the stomach wall. This can be confirmed by contrast-enhanced CT which may demonstrate pneumoperitoneum, decreased uptake of contrast in the stomach wall, gastric pneumatosis (Abboud et al. 2006), or intra-biliary air.

If gastric necrosis is suspected, then empiric physiological resuscitation must take place, this includes intravenous fluids and antibiotics, and expeditious transfer to the operating room. Operative interventions can vary from local wedge resections, but invariably require major resection.

© Springer-Verlag Berlin Heidelberg 2015
P.J. Papadakos, M.L. Gestring (eds.), *Encyclopedia of Trauma Care*,
DOI 10.1007/978-3-642-29613-0

References

Abboud B, Mchayleh W, Sleilaty G, Yaghi C (2006) Gastric pneumatosis as a manifestation of ischemic infarction of the stomach. Report of a case and review of the literature. Leban Med J (Le Journal Medical Libanais) 54:217–220

Alves M, Patel V, Douglas E, Deutsch E (1979) Gastric infarction: a complication of selective vasopressin infusion. Dig Dis Sci 24:409–413

Babkin BP, Armour JC, Webster DR (1943) Restoration of the functional capacity of the stomach when deprived of its main arterial blood supply. Can Med Assoc J 48:1–10

Bookstein JJ, Chlosta EM, Foley D, Walter JF (1974) Transcatheter hemostasis of gastrointestinal bleeding using modified autogenous clot. Radiology 113:277–285

Bradley EL 3, Goldman ML (1976) Gastric infarction after therapeutic embolization. Surgery 79:421–424

Brown KT, Friedman WN, Marks RA, Saddekni S (1989) Gastric and hepatic infarction following embolization of the left gastric artery: case report. Radiology 172:731–732

Somervell TH (1945) Physiological gastrectomy. Br J Surg 33:146–152

Tadavarthy SM, Knight L, Ovitt TW, Snyder C, Amplatz K (1974) Therapeutic transcatheter arterial embolization. Radiology 112:13–16

Gastritis

Jason Moore
Department of Surgery, Lawnwood Regional Medical Center, Fort Pierce, FL, USA

Synonyms

Hemorrhagic gastritis; Stress erosive gastritis; Stress gastritis; Stress ulcerations

Definition

Gastritis in the setting of traumatic injury that may or may not require intensive care unit therapy is best described as acute stress gastritis. This disease is characterized as superficial erosions in the stomach and can usually develop within hours or the first 2 days of a major traumatic injury (Newman et al. 2011). They begin in the proximal acid-secreting portion of the stomach and progress distally.

Preexisting Conditions

Some predisposing conditions that can exacerbate stress gastritis include multiple traumatic injuries, hypotension, massive blood transfusion, sepsis, acute respiratory distress syndrome (ARDS), multiple organ failure, burn injuries (aka Curling's ulcer), use of steroids, and central nervous system disease or injury (aka Cushing's ulcer) (Newman et al. 2011; Mercer and Robinson 2008).

Application

The exact pathophysiologic mechanism for stress gastritis is not yet fully understood; however, a multifactorial etiology is suspected. The gastric lesions appear in the presence of acid. Other factors that can weaken the stomach's mucosal defense mechanisms are a reduction in mucous secretion, bicarbonate secretion by mucosal cells, or a decrease in the endogenous prostaglandins (Mercer and Robinson 2008). The element of stress is considered a necessary factor as it is considered present when there is tissue hypoxia, sepsis, or organ failure. When it occurs, tissue ischemia becomes responsible for the breakdown of the normal defense mechanisms mentioned above. Then, luminal acid is able to damage the already compromised mucosal lining (Mercer and Robinson 2008).

The way most patients with stress gastritis present is a painless upper GI bleed that may have a delay in onset. Most patients will experience this within the first 2 days of the traumatic injury. The bleeding is usually slow, intermittent, and may be detected by an unexplained drop in hemoglobin or some small clots of blood after vomiting. If there is a large bleed, then there may be frank hematemesis and hypotension. On the other hand, there may be no overt upper manifestations, but there may be lower signs including guaiac-positive stools or melena (Mercer and Robinson 2008).

When suspicious of gastritis, the initial test should be nasogastric tube lavage and decompression. If there is bleeding, a lavage with 1 l of cold saline may be enough to stop it. This works well for a majority of cases. The best method to truly diagnose stress gastritis or stress ulcers is to perform endoscopy. This will confirm the diagnosis of stress gastritis or other pathologic entities that cause upper GI bleeding (Mercer and Robinson 2008).

Prevention is paramount when discussing stress gastritis. High-risk trauma patients are more likely to progress from a normal state to a massive upper GI bleed. One of the first priorities needs to be correcting any perfusion abnormalities resulting from sepsis, blood loss, or other systemic malfunction. Sepsis, the leading causes of stress gastritis, requires source control and antibiotic therapy. Other conditions that may or may not coexist with sepsis that need correction include systemic acid–base abnormalities and electrolyte imbalances. Of note, providing nutrition, preferably by the enteral route, is associated with fewer infectious complications and stress ulcer bleeding (Mercer and Robinson 2008; Swift et al. 2010).

Sucralfate, histamine-2 (H2) receptor antagonists, and proton pump inhibitors (PPIs) have been shown to be effective for prophylaxis against stress gastritis. Sucralfate and H2 receptor antagonists, specifically, have been shown to have an efficacy rate in the 90–97 % range (Mercer and Robinson 2008). Sucralfate works by forming a protective barrier by binding to exposed epithelial cells and ulcer craters. It is given usually orally or via nasogastric tube at 1 g every 6 h. It is considered safe and inexpensive; however, it can interfere with the absorption of a number of medications including ciprofloxacin, phenytoin, and ketoconazole; thus, they must be given at least 2 h ahead of time. Also, sucralfate requires acid for activation and tissue binding and therefore cannot be given while receiving H2 receptor blockers (Swift et al. 2010).

H2 receptor antagonists are considered the most popular method of providing stress gastritis

prophylaxis. These are designed to inhibit gastric acid production by blocking the histamine receptor for acid production and are equally effective orally or intravenously. There are several H2 receptor blockers available including cimetidine, ranitidine, and famotidine; however, the side effect profiles vary but commonly include thrombocytopenia, delirium, and interference of cytochrome P450 that causes other potential drug interactions. Famotidine appears to have the most favorable side effect profile (Swift et al. 2010).

PPIs, used more for known or documented upper GI bleeding, peptic ulcer disease, GERD, and erosive esophagitis, should theoretically reduce the risk of bleeding from stress gastritis. PPIs are very effective in reducing acid secretion by preventing the release of hydrogen ions in activated parietal cells that are both vagally and histamine-mediated. Even though the final pathway of acid secretion is inhibited, there is currently no data to suggest that PPIs have any additional benefit over H2 receptor antagonists in preventing stress-related mucosal disease (Swift et al. 2010).

Finally, the way stress gastritis is treated depends on the severity of the disease. First and foremost, the patient has to be adequately resuscitated to restore organ perfusion. Large bore intravenous access must be obtained. Crystalloid can be utilized; however, blood products are likely needed if there is evidence of significant acute blood loss anemia. Second, the correction of any coagulopathy is required with the use of fresh frozen plasma and/or factor VII, as well as treating platelet deficiencies with platelet transfusion.

Third, as mentioned before, nasogastric decompression is helpful as it removes noxious substances that may be harmful to the gastric mucosa, and saline lavage can stop bleeding in up to 80 % of cases (Mercer and Robinson 2008).

One of the benefits of endoscopy is that it is both diagnostic and therapeutic. Upon diagnosis of stress gastritis, cautery or injection can be used to stop bleeding. If bleeding persists, the next step would be angiographic embolization of the left gastric artery or infusion of vasopressin. These methods have been proven to decrease blood transfusion requirements, but mortality still persists (Newman et al. 2011).

Surgery is the last resort and should be considered when bleeding recurs after other treatments or it persists and requires six or more units of blood to be transfused. There are a few techniques and their use depends on severity of bleeding. One way is to make an anterior gastrotomy, find the bleeding area, and place a few deep figure-of-eight sutures. Another necessary approach is a partial gastrectomy with vagotomy or, in even more dire cases, a near-total gastrectomy. An alternative approach that does not require any surgical resection is gastric devascularization where all major blood vessels that supply the stomach except for the short gastrics are ligated. This procedure may be ideal in patients who are unstable since it may be performed faster than a near-total gastrectomy (Newman et al. 2011).

In conclusion, stress gastritis is found most commonly in acutely ill, poly-trauma patients who are prone developing systemic conditions such as sepsis. This should alert the physician to counteract the deleterious effects of weakened mucosal defense mechanisms by attempting to keep patients normotensive and start prophylactic therapy with sucralfate, H2 blockers, or PPIs and initiate enteral nutrition as soon as possible. Endoscopy is the best method for accurate diagnosis and treatment; however, if bleeding is refractory, angio-embolization or surgery may be indicated to definitively control ongoing blood loss.

Cross-References

▶ Acute Coagulopathy of Trauma
▶ Acute Respiratory Distress Syndrome (ARDS), General
▶ Curling's Ulcer
▶ Cushing's Ulcer
▶ Flame Burns
▶ Gastrointestinal Bleeding: Indications for Prophylaxis Post-trauma and Treatment
▶ Gastrointestinal Hemorrhage
▶ Hypoxemia, Severe

▶ Infection Control
▶ Multiorgan System Failure (MOF)
▶ Nutritional Support
▶ Sepsis, General Mechanism of
▶ Sepsis, Treatment of
▶ Shock

References

Mercer DW, Robinson EK (2008) Stomach. In: Townsend CM, Beauchamp RD, Evers BM, Mattox KL (eds) Sabiston textbook of surgery, 18th edn. Saunders/Elsevier, Philadelphia, pp 1223–1277

Newman NA, Mufeed SM, Makary MA (2011) The stomach. In: Cameron JL, Cameron AM (eds) Current surgical therapy, 10th edn. Saunders/Elsevier, Philadelphia, pp 63–92

Swift AE, Wynkoop WA, D'Alonzo GE (2010) Prophylactic regimens in the intensive care unit. In: Criner GJ, Barnette RE, D'Alonzo GE (eds) Critical care study guide text and review, 2nd edn. Springer, New York, pp 1173–1192

Gastrocutaneous Fistula

Mansoor Khan
Consultant Esophagogastric and Acute Care Surgeon, Doncaster Royal Infirmary, Doncaster, South Yorkshire, UK

Definition

A gastrocutaneous fistula (GCF) represents a fistula connecting the stomach and the skin. By definition, it consists of an internal orifice (gastric outlet), an external orifice (cutaneous outlet), and a tract (usually covered by epithelium) (Table 1).

In order to manage a GCF, its proper recognition is necessary. Both internal and external orifices should be appropriately identified, as well as the topographic relations and the trajectory of the fistula tractus.

Diagnosis is relatively straightforward, with a plain x-ray after taking oral contrast being more than adequate.

Gastrocutaneous Fistula, Table 1 Etiology of GCF

Iatrogenic	Operative complication
	Drain erosion
	Failure of PEG site to close
Chronic inflammation	
Foreign body	
Carcinoma	
Radiotherapy	

GCFs close spontaneously in only 6 % of cases, and the mortality rate is about 35 % among patients with normal body weight who underwent recent gastric surgery and the mortality rate is higher in patients who have undergone bariatric surgery (Papavramidis et al. 2004).

The optimal approach to the management of gastrocutaneous fistulas remains controversial. Conservative management consists of adequate time (Janik et al. 2004), adequate drainage, control of infection and sepsis, gastric decompression, gastric acid inhibition, bowel rest, and parenteral nutrition is preferred before surgical intervention. Surgery in some cases has resulted in total gastrectomy (Martin-Malagon et al. 2011).

The mainstay of therapy for gastrocutaneous (GC) fistulas has been surgical intervention. However, endoclips (Kothari et al. 2012; Sobrino-Faya et al. 2011) and fibrin sealant have been used for management of perforations and fistulas (Gonzalez-Ojeda et al. 2004; Lorenzo-Rivero et al. 2012; Bratu and Bharmal 2011).

Cross-References

▶ Entero-Atmospheric Fistula
▶ Prolonged Open Abdomen

References

Bratu I, Bharmal A (2011) Incidence and predictors of gastrocutaneous fistula in the pediatric patient. ISRN Gastroenterol 2011:686803

Gonzalez-Ojeda A, Avalos-Gonzalez J, Mucino-Hernandez MI, Lopez-Ortega A, Fuentes-Orozco C, Sanchez-Hochoa M, Anaya-Prado R, Arenas-Marquez H (2004) Fibrin glue as adjuvant treatment for gastrocutaneous fistula after gastrostomy tube removal. Endoscopy 36:337–341

Janik TA, Hendrickson RJ, Janik JS, Landholm AE (2004) Analysis of factors affecting the spontaneous closure of a gastrocutaneous fistula. J Pediatr Surg 39:1197–1199

Kothari TH, Haber G, Sonpal N, Karanth N (2012) The over-the-scope clip system–a novel technique for gastrocutaneous fistula closure: the first North American experience. Can J Gastroenterol (Journal Canadien de Gastroenterologie) 26:193–195

Lorenzo-Rivero S, Rosen PD, Moore RA, Stanley JD (2012) Closure of gastrocutaneous fistula using autologous blood product sealant. Am Surg 78:313–315

Martin-Malagon A, Rodriguez-Ballester L, Arteaga-Gonzalez I (2011) Total gastrectomy for failed treatment with endotherapy of chronic gastrocutaneous fistula after sleeve gastrectomy. Surg Obes Relat Dis Off J Am Soc Bariatr Surg 7:240–242

Papavramidis ST, Eleftheriadis EE, Papavramidis TS, Kotzampassi KE, Gamvros OG (2004) Endoscopic management of gastrocutaneous fistula after bariatric surgery by using a fibrin sealant. Gastrointest Endosc 59:296–300

Sobrino-Faya M, Macias-Garcia F, Souto-Rodriguez R, Lesquereux-Martinez L, Dominguez-Munoz JE (2011) Percutaneous endoscopic suturing is an alternative treatment for persistent gastrocutaneous post-PEG fistula. Revista Espanola de Enfermedades Digestivas: Organo Oficial de la Sociedad Espanola de Patologia Digestiva 103:328–331

Gastrointestinal Bleeding

▶ Gastrointestinal Hemorrhage

Gastrointestinal Bleeding: Indications for Prophylaxis Post-trauma and Treatment

Melissa R. Pleva and James T. Miller
Department of Pharmacy Services, University of Michigan Hospitals and Health Centers and University of Michigan College of Pharmacy, Ann Arbor, MI, USA

Synonyms

Gastrointestinal hemorrhage; Stress gastritis; Stress-related mucosal damage; Stress-related mucosal disease; Stress ulceration; Stress ulcer bleeding; Upper gastrointestinal bleeding

Definition

Upper gastrointestinal (GI) bleeding is defined as any bleeding proximal to the ligament of Treitz. Stress-related mucosal disease (SRMD) is an acute erosive gastritis that is a common complication of critical illness and can lead to upper GI bleeding.

Preexisting Condition

Normal GI Mucosal Lining Function

The gastric mucosa is characterized by its secretion of a variety of functional and protective substances. Parietal cells exchange potassium for hydrogen via the H,K-ATPase, yielding a highly acidic environment in the gastric lumen, which assists in digestion. In order to protect itself from this environment, glands in the stomach secrete alkaline mucus that lines the wall. Additionally, chief cells secrete pepsinogen, the inactive zymogen of pepsin which aids in the breakdown of ingested protein. Histamine (stimulated by gastrin) and somatostatin are also secreted from cells in the gastric mucosa. Pepsin, histamine, and somatostatin maintain homeostasis of the gastric luminal environment. Disruption of these processes by critical illness can lead to mucosal damage.

Mechanisms of Stress-Induced Gastrointestinal Bleeding

Critical illness places the patient at increased risk of stress-related mucosal damage (SRMD) of the upper GI tract. SRMD can occur both in the stomach and the duodenum. Common causes of intensive care unit (ICU) admission such as hypovolemia and hypotension; increased circulating catecholamines and pro-inflammatory cytokines associated with the systemic inflammatory response; and compromised cardiac output lead to splanchnic hypoperfusion as the body shunts blood flow to the vital organs (Stollman and Metz 2005). These factors can be disease related or iatrogenically induced (e.g., medications, positive pressure ventilation). Ischemic conditions prevent the normal protective functions of the cells lining the GI tract. The alkaline mucus produced by these cells is one of the primary barrier functions of the stomach. Bicarbonate secretion from the pancreas is disrupted, leaving the duodenum exposed to high concentrations of gastric acid. Finally, GI motility is impaired. Each of these is a factor contributing to the development of SRMD and ulceration.

Incidence and Consequences of Gastrointestinal Bleeding

SRMD-related overt GI bleeding occurs in approximately 1.5–2.5 % of critically ill patients (Cook et al. 1994). While this incidence is relatively low, overt GI bleeding has a significant impact on patient outcomes. In a large, prospective observational study, clinically important GI bleeding was found to be associated with an increased absolute risk for mortality between 20 % and 30 % (relative risk for mortality of 1–4). These authors also reported an increase in ICU length of stay (LOS) of 4–8 days (Cook et al. 2001). Thus, appropriate prophylaxis is a vital component of supportive care in the ICU for patients at risk.

Application

Prophylaxis

Risk Factors

A landmark multicenter prospective cohort study of 2,252 patients identified mechanical ventilation for greater than 48 h and coagulopathy as the two factors placing patients at the highest risk for SRMD (odds ratios [OR] of 15.6 and 4.3, respectively) (Cook et al. 1994). Additional risk factors identified include hypotension, sepsis, hepatic failure, renal failure, and glucocorticoid administration. However, this landmark trial included only 18 patients with multiple trauma and 28 patients with head injury. Smaller studies have identified recent major surgery, major trauma, head injury, spinal cord injury, and severe thermal injury as other factors that may also increase the risk of SRMD. Studies have shown that risk increases as the number of risk factors present in a single patient increases. Gastric enteral nutrition may contribute to decreasing the risk of SRMD, but this protective effect is not significant enough to constitute adequate prophylaxis for patients with mechanical ventilation or coagulopathy.

Indications for Prophylaxis

Prophylaxis against SRMD is indicated in patients receiving mechanical ventilation or who are coagulopathic. Prophylaxis is likely also indicated in patients with multiple other risk factors. However, no studies have clearly delineated how many risk factors, or particular combinations of risk factors, require prophylaxis. Lack of gastric enteral nutrition in the absence of other risk factors does not necessarily warrant use of prophylactic mediations. A survey evaluating institutional practices related to stress ulcer prophylaxis in trauma patients found that $\geq 85\%$ of institutions surveyed routinely prescribed stress ulcer prophylaxis in patients with head injury, spinal cord injury, or multiple trauma (Barletta et al. 2002).

Pharmacologic Prophylaxis Agents

Pharmacologic agents that have been used for stress ulcer prophylaxis include antacids, sucralfate, histamine-2 receptor antagonists (H2RAs), and proton pump inhibitors (PPIs). Of these, H2RAs have the most supporting evidence and have been the most widely used agents (Barletta et al. 2002; Lin et al. 2010). Intravenous (IV) ranitidine was shown to be superior to sucralfate in preventing upper GI bleeding in 1,200 mechanically ventilated patients (Cook et al. 1998).

Since the introduction of PPIs to the market, their use for stress ulcer prophylaxis has been increasing. Studies using maintenance of gastric pH > 4 as the primary endpoint have demonstrated that PPIs are more effective than H2RAs. However, studies have failed to definitively show that this translates into lower rates of clinically significant bleeding. A meta-analysis of seven trials, including 936 patients, failed to demonstrate a significant difference in rates of stress-related upper GI bleeding between patients receiving PPIs and those receiving H2RAs (Lin et al. 2010). Due to the relatively low incidence of GI bleeding related to SRMD, the sample size required to conduct an adequately powered clinical trial comparing H2RAs and PPIs would be prohibitively large.

Doses of H2RAs used for prophylaxis of SRMD are relatively well established (famotidine 20 mg IV or enterally twice daily, ranitidine 50 mg IV every 8 h or 150 mg enterally every 12 h). Continuous infusion H2RA regimens have also been studied, but have not been shown to be superior to intermittent dosing strategies. Due to the heterogeneity of the few small clinical trials available, dosing regimens for PPIs are more widely varied (ranging from the equivalent of pantoprazole 40 mg once daily to 80 mg twice daily). Subgroup analyses of the recent meta-analysis comparing PPIs and H2RAs did not find any difference in efficacy based on route or dose of PPI used (Lin et al. 2010).

Adverse Effects of Prophylactic Agents

Both H2RAs and PPIs are well tolerated. Increased bacterial growth in the stomach due to reduction of gastric acid has been hypothesized to lead to a higher risk of pneumonia and *Clostridium difficile*-associated diarrhea (CDAD). Some studies have demonstrated higher rates of pneumonia (OR 1.3) and CDAD (OR 2.6) in patients receiving acid suppression, especially PPIs (Herzig et al. 2009; Dial et al. 2004). Other studies have failed to find a difference in incidence of these infectious complications. The Lin meta-analysis did not demonstrate a difference in rates of pneumonia between patients receiving PPIs and H2RAs and did not examine rates of CDAD.

In patients at high risk of SRMD and stress ulcer-associated GI bleeding, the benefit of acid suppression to reduce GI bleeding and the associated morbidity and mortality outweighs the risks. Risks such as pneumonia and CDAD may be minimized by reserving use of stress ulcer prophylaxis for patients with clear, high-risk indications (e.g., mechanical ventilation and coagulopathy), discontinuing prophylaxis as soon as the risk factors are no longer present,

G

and avoiding discharging patients from the ICU and/or hospital on acid suppression without an indication.

Treatment

Pharmacologic Treatment

Evidence-based strategies for the pharmacologic treatment of acute GI bleeding related to SRMD rely primarily on data from patients with bleeding peptic ulcers. Various treatment modalities have been used, including somatostatin and analogues, H2RAs, and PPIs. Somatostatin inhibits gastrin secretion and the formation of gastric acid and has been used as an adjunct therapy in the treatment of bleeding peptic ulcers. However, in a randomized study comparing somatostatin to PPI after endoscopy, somatostatin was found to be inferior (Tsibouris et al. 2007).

H2RAs have been compared to PPI therapy. One trial found H2RA therapy to be no more effective than placebo, but did not utilize endoscopic treatment of the lesion (Walt et al. 1992). Several studies have shown H2RAs to be as effective as PPIs, but large well-designed clinical trials suggest that PPI therapy is superior. A large multicenter randomized controlled trial (n = 1,256) compared high-dose PPI to high-dose H2RA (bolus followed by continuous infusion) after endoscopy. Outcomes were similar, but PPI appeared to be superior to H2RA in the subgroups of patients with gastric ulcers and spurting lesions (van Rensburg et al. 2009).

In a randomized, placebo-controlled trial of 240 patients by Lau et al., a high-dose regimen of IV proton pump inhibitor (omeprazole 80 mg IV bolus followed by infusion of 8 mg/h for 72 h) was superior to placebo at preventing rebleeding episodes after endoscopic hemostasis. The incidence of rebleeding was significantly less in the PPI group at 3, 7, and 30 days after endoscopy. Additionally, patients who received PPI therapy were more likely to have a successful endoscopic retreatment if indicated, had a shorter hospital LOS (unless bleeding developed while an inpatient), and required less blood transfusion after endoscopy. Mortality was not affected (Lau et al. 2000).

Faced with acute GI bleeding, most clinicians use the treatment regimen prescribed by Lau et al. However, there is recent data that suggests that the dose of PPI may not be the factor that determines efficacy. In a randomized study of nearly 500 patients, intensive therapy (80 mg IV bolus, 8 mg/h IV infusion for 72 h) was compared to a standard regimen of 40 mg IV daily. Investigators were allowed to use either omeprazole or pantoprazole. Rates of rebleeding were no different between the intensive group and the standard regimen (11.8 vs. 8.1 %, $p = 0.18$). Another study by Chen et al. found similar results with the same regimen. The dose of PPI was not related to outcome, but end-stage renal disease (ESRD), hematemesis, and chronic obstructive pulmonary disease were independent predictors of rebleeding. Of note, *Helicobacter pylori* infection was protective against rebleeding. Nonetheless, a consensus statement from the International Consensus Upper Gastrointestinal Bleeding Conference Group (Greenspoon et al. 2012) recommends the intensive regimen as studied by Lau et al. (2000).

Procedural Treatment

Although some peptic ulcer bleeds resolve spontaneously, the risk of rebleeding and the adverse outcomes related to it are high. Therefore, endoscopic therapy is indicated in most patients with acute upper GI bleeding. Endoscopic treatment strategies include epinephrine injection, thermal coagulation, and hemoclip application. Injection therapy with epinephrine alone is associated with unacceptable rates of rebleeding, so it is recommended that it be combined with either thermal coagulation or the application of hemoclips. A large meta-analysis concluded that combination therapy including epinephrine or monotherapy with either thermal coagulation or hemoclip application was superior to epinephrine alone (Laine and McQuaid 2009). It should be noted that due to the diffuse nature of the lesion in bleeding related to SRMD, endoscopic therapy may not be effective. Most clinicians utilize the high-dose PPI regimen even if endoscopic therapy is unsuccessful.

Cross-References

▶ Coagulopathy
▶ Gastritis
▶ Gastrointestinal Hemorrhage
▶ Hypocoaguability
▶ Nutritional Support
▶ Ventilatory Management of Trauma Patients

References

Barletta JF, Erstad BL, Fortune JB (2002) Stress ulcer prophylaxis in trauma patients. Crit Care 6:526–530

Cook DJ, Fuller HD, Guyatt GH et al (1994) Risk factors for gastrointestinal bleeding in critically ill patients. N Engl J Med 330:377–381

Cook D, Guyatt G, Marshall J et al (1998) A comparison of sucralfate and ranitidine for the prevention of upper gastrointestinal bleeding in patients requiring mechanical ventilation. N Engl J Med 338:791–797

Cook DJ, Griffith LE, Walter SD et al (2001) The attributable mortality and length of intensive care unit stay of clinically important gastrointestinal bleeding in critically ill patients. Crit Care 5(6):368–375

Dial S, Alrasadi K, Manoukain C, Huang A, Menzies D (2004) Risk of clostridium difficile diarrhea among hospital inpatients prescribed proton pump inhibitors: cohort and case–control studies. Can Med Assoc J 171:33–38

Greenspoon J, Barkun A, Bardou M et al (2012) Management of patients with nonvariceal upper gastrointestinal bleeding. Clin Gastroenterol Hepatol 10(3):234–239

Herzig SJ, Howell MD, Ngo LH et al (2009) Acid-suppressive medication use and the risk for hospital-acquired pneumonia. JAMA 301:2120–2128

Laine L, McQuaid KR (2009) Endoscopic therapy for bleeding ulcers: an evidence-based approach based on meta-analyses of randomized controlled trials. Clin Gastroenterol Hepatol 7(1):33–47

Lau JYW, Sung JJY, Lee KKC et al (2000) Effect of intravenous omeprazole on recurrent bleeding after endoscopic treatment of bleeding peptic ulcers. N Engl J Med 343:310–316

Lin PC, Chang CH, Hsu PI, Tseng PL, Huang YB (2010) The efficacy and safety of proton pump inhibitors vs histamine-2 receptor antagonists for stress ulcer bleeding prophylaxis among critical care patients: a meta-analysis. Crit Care Med 38:1197–1205

Stollman N, Metz DC (2005) Pathophysiology and prophylaxis of stress ulcer in intensive care unit patients. J Crit Care 20:35–45

Tsibouris P, Zintzaras E, Lappas C et al (2007) High-dose pantoprazole continuous infusion is superior to somatostatin after endoscopic hemostasis in patients with peptic ulcer bleeding. Am J Gastroenterol 102(6):1192–1199

van Rensburg C, Barkun AN, Racz I et al (2009) Clinical trial: intravenous pantoprazole vs. ranitidine for the prevention of peptic ulcer rebleeding: a multicentre, multinational, randomized trial. Aliment Pharmacol Ther 29(5):497–507

Walt RP, Cottrell J, Mann SG, Freemantle NP, Langman MJS (1992) Continuous intravenous famotidine for hemorrhage from peptic ulcer. Lancet 340:1058–1062

G

Gastrointestinal Hemorrhage

Andrew S. Brock and Joseph Romagnuolo
Division of Gastroenterology and Hepatology,
Medical University of South Carolina,
Charleston, SC, USA

Synonyms

Gastrointestinal Bleeding; GI Bleeding; GI Hemorrhage

Definition

Gastrointestinal (GI) hemorrhage is defined as bleeding from the GI tract, anywhere from the mouth to the anus. Traditional terminology uses the ligament of Treitz to demarcate upper from lower GI bleeding. The advent of technologies capable of accessing the small intestine, however, has led to the addition of "mid-gut" bleeding, whereby upper, mid-, and lower sources refer to areas accessible to esophagogastroduodenoscopy (EGD), enteroscopy, and colonoscopy, respectively. Thus, upper GI bleeding now refers to lesions proximal to the papilla of Vater, mid-GI bleeding includes lesions distal to the papilla of Vater to the terminal ileum, and lower GI bleeding refers to lesions in the colorectum and anus.

Preexisting Condition

Epidemiology

Gastrointestinal hemorrhage represents a significant health problem worldwide. In 2009, the annual incidence of hospitalizations in the United States for upper and lower GI bleeding was 60.6/100,000 and 35.7/100,000, respectively (Laine et al. 2012). This represents a decline over the past decade, though the reason for this decline is not clear.

Etiology

There are multiple causes of gastrointestinal hemorrhage (Table 1). Peptic ulcer disease is the number one cause of upper GI hemorrhage and diverticular disease the number one lower source. This has remained steady over the last decade.

Presentation

Patients with GI hemorrhage may present in a variety of ways, from fulminant, life-threatening bleeding to slow, occult oozing over many months resulting in unexplained iron deficiency anemia. Vomiting blood is diagnostic of an upper source, while small amounts of bright red blood per rectum in the absence of changes in hemodynamics or hemoglobin represent an anorectal source. Melena typically indicates an upper or mid-gut source, but can also result from a right colon lesion. Lower GI bleeding usually presents with hematochezia, but it also can represent a brisk upper or mid-gut source.

Clues to the source of bleeding may be elicited from the medical history. Patients with cirrhosis or risk factors for liver disease may have a portal hypertensive etiology of hemorrhage, such as varices or gastric antral vascular ectasia (GAVE). Recent nonsteroidal anti-inflammatory drug (NSAID) use predisposes to peptic ulcer disease. Use of anticoagulants, such as warfarin or clopidogrel, should be noted. Patients who have undergone gastrointestinal surgery are at risk for anastomotic hemorrhage. Aortic stenosis and renal failure are risk factors for angioectasia. Malignant GI tumors can hemorrhage. Patients with aortic grafts or aneurysms can develop

Gastrointestinal Hemorrhage, Table 1 Causes of GI hemorrhage by location

Upper	Midgut	Lower
Ulcer	Angioectasia	Diverticulosis
Varices	Erosions	Colitis (ischemia, IBD, radiation)
Gastritis	Tumor	Hemorrhoids
Esophagitis	Polyp	Tumor
Mallory-Weiss tear	Ulcer	Post-polypectomy
Dieulafoy	Dieulafoy	Angioectasia
Angioectasia	Crohn's disease	Polyp
GAVE	Celiac disease	Ulcer
Cameron's erosions	Meckel's diverticulum	Dieulafoy
Tumor	Diverticulosis	
Hemobilia	Aortoenteric fistula	
Hemosuccus pancreaticus		
Polyp		
Portal hypertensive gastropathy		

GAVE gastric antral vascular ectasia, *IBD* inflammatory bowel disease

aortoenteric fistulae. A history of retching might indicate a Mallory-Weiss tear. Recent endoscopic polypectomy or biliary/pancreatic sphincterotomy should raise suspicion for bleeding from those sites.

Five percent of patients will have obscure GI bleeding (OGIB). This is defined as bleeding that is not identified on EGD and colonoscopy. OGIB is subdivided into obscure occult and obscure overt bleeding, with the former referring to bleeding from the GI tract resulting in iron deficiency anemia and the latter as recurrent melena or hematochezia. The majority of patients with OGIB will have small bowel lesions, though approximately 25 % of patients will have lesions within reach of EGD or colonoscopy.

Application

Initial Management

Vital signs must be monitored closely, with consideration for intensive care unit monitoring, especially for patients with active bleeding, hemodynamic compromise, high-risk lesions on endoscopy, suspected varices, advanced age, or major comorbidities. Lab work should include, at minimum, a complete blood count, basic metabolic panel, hepatic panel, and prothrombin time with international ionized ratio (INR). A physical exam should be performed, including a rectal exam to assess stool color. Intravascular volume may be gleaned from the vital signs; resting tachycardia, orthostasis, and hypotension are reflective of depleted stores. Prognostic scales such as the Blatchford (pre-endoscopy) and Rockall (clinical and endoscopic) scores can aid in triaging patients by stratifying them into high- and low-risk categories (Barkun et al. 2010). Placement of a nasogastric tube (NGT) has not been shown to improve outcomes; further, up to 15 % of patients without bloody aspirate will have high-risk lesions. However, NGT can help distinguish upper and lower sources in patients with hematochezia with significant hemoglobin drop and/or mild hypovolemia.

Two large-bore peripheral intravenous (IV) catheters or a single central catheter should be inserted. Patients with signs of intravascular depletion should be resuscitated with crystalloids and blood products as needed. Transfusion should also be given to patients with a hemoglobin less than 7.0 g/dL, though the threshold in patients with underlying coronary artery disease or signs of impaired myocardial perfusion may require hemoglobin levels as high as 10.0 g/dL. Care must be taken to avoid overtransfusion in patients with known or suspected varices, as this can increase portal pressures, thus worsening bleeding; a target hemoglobin of 8.0 g/dL is appropriate in these patients.

Anticoagulants and antiplatelet agents should be held. Coagulopathy should be reversed if safe to do so, aiming for a platelet count of greater than 50 and INR less than 1.5. However, if unsafe, endoscopy can generally be performed in patients with therapeutic coagulopathy. INR in patients with cirrhosis is not predictive of bleeding; thus, attempts at correction may simply lead to excessive volume expansion.

Consideration of platelet transfusion should also be given to patients on antiplatelet agents such as aspirin or clopidogrel who present with life-threatening bleeding. In high-risk situations, such as mechanical valves or newly placed coronary stents, consultation with a cardiologist should be undertaken.

Medical Therapy

The most important life-saving medical treatment for GI hemorrhage is proper resuscitation and maneuvers to protect the airway; this should precede endoscopy and most other therapies. Patients with significant upper GI hemorrhage suspected of having a high-risk lesion on endoscopy should receive high-dose IV proton pump inhibitor (PPI) therapy (Dorward et al. 2006). High-dose therapy includes omeprazole, esomeprazole, or pantoprazole in a bolus dose of 80 mg followed by a continuous infusion dose of 8 mg/h for 72 h. This has been shown to downstage high-risk lesions when given prior to endoscopy and reduce rebleeding, the need for surgery, and mortality after endoscopic therapy of high-risk lesions. This likely has little to no benefit in non-high-risk lesions. H2 receptor blockers have not led to improved outcomes and thus are not indicated for acute upper GI bleeding. Use of a promotility agent such as erythromycin or metoclopramide can reduce the need for repeat endoscopy by clearing the stomach of blood and, thus, should be considered (Gralnek et al. 2008). IV octreotide can be added in selected patients with ongoing bleeding (Imperiale and Birgisson 1997).

Patients suspected of having variceal bleeding should receive IV octreotide with a bolus of 50mcg followed by an infusion at 50mcg/h for 3–5 days (Burroughs 1994). Patients with cirrhosis and GI bleeding should receive IV antibiotics as prophylaxis for spontaneous bacterial peritonitis. Acceptable choices include cephalosporins, such as ceftriaxone, and fluoroquinolones such as ciprofloxacin. These should initially be given IV, but transition can be made to oral administration once the patient is stabilized to complete the recommended 7-day course.

Endoscopic Treatment

Consultation with a gastroenterologist should be made for all significant bleeds. Once the patient has been hemodynamically stabilized, including endotracheal tube placement if necessary, endoscopy can be undertaken. Early endoscopy, defined as within 24 h of presentation, is recommended for patients with acute upper GI bleeding (Barkun et al. 2010). Patients with brisk lower GI bleeding may also warrant inpatient endoscopy, particularly if the bleeding persists. Patients with self-limited hematochezia can undergo outpatient colonoscopy.

The role of endoscopy in patients with GI hemorrhage is to diagnose the source of bleeding, risk stratify the patient, and treat the source lesion if necessary. Lesions at low risk of rebleeding include peptic ulcers with a clean base or flat spot, Mallory-Weiss tear, gastritis, esophagitis, and non-bleeding angioectasia. Healthy patients at low risk of rebleeding can be discharged after endoscopy. Endoscopic hemostasis should be attempted in patients with high-risk lesions, including ulcers with active bleeding or visible vessel, Dieulafoy lesions, bleeding angioectasias, diverticula with bleeding or visible vessel, and varices amenable to endoscopic therapy. All ulcers with clots should be irrigated, but treatment of ulcers with an adherent clot that does not easily wash with gentle irrigation is at the discretion of the endoscopist, where either endoscopic therapy or medical therapy is acceptable. Tumors are at high risk of rebleeding, but are rarely amenable to endoscopic therapy. Other lesions may warrant non-endoscopic therapy; for example, aortoenteric fistulae require surgery, hemosuccus pancreaticus may necessitate angiography, and persistent bleeding from tumors may require angiographic or radiation therapy.

There are various modalities of endoscopic therapy that may be used. Band ligation is the recommended first-line endoscopic therapy for esophageal varices, though sclerosants such as sodium morrhuate may be used when band ligation is not feasible (Garcia-Tsao et al. 2007). Cyanoacrylate glue has recently been introduced for the treatment of bleeding gastric varices, though it is only available at a limited number of United States institutions at this time.

The armamentarium is broader for non-variceal hemorrhage. For peptic ulcers with high-risk stigmata such as active bleeding or non-bleeding visible vessel, there are three basic categories of therapy: injection therapy, thermal, and mechanical. Injection therapy generally consists of normal saline or epinephrine, which works by a tamponade or vasoconstrictive effect, respectively. Injection therapy should not be used alone as rebleeding rates are significantly lower when it is applied concurrently with either thermal or mechanical therapy. Contact thermal techniques include bipolar electrocautery (e.g., Gold probe, Microvasive Boston Scientific, Natick, MA, and BICAP, Circon ACMI, Stamford, CN) and heater probe (Olympus Corp., Lake Success, NY). These methods work by coaptive coagulation, whereby the probe is applied directly to the lesion (coaptation) and an electrical current is applied (coagulation). This compression of the vessel with subsequent cautery enables effective hemostasis. Mechanical hemostasis for ulcers consists of hemostatic clips, which work by grasping the vessel to cut off blood flow. The decision to use thermal therapy versus clipping is based on position of lesion and endoscopist preference, as one has not been shown to be superior to the other. Further, whether one combines injection therapy with either thermal or mechanical therapy or uses the thermal or mechanical technique alone is at the discretion of the endoscopist as there is no evidence these approaches result in different rebleeding rates. A common approach is to use injection therapy first when there is active bleeding (to clear the views) or into an adherent clot before removal (for prophylaxis against bleeding).

The above techniques may also be used for other sources of GI hemorrhage. For example, bleeding diverticula and Dieulafoy lesions may be treated with any of the techniques mentioned for ulcer hemorrhage, or by band ligation. Endoscopic clipping is often effective for

Mallory-Weiss tears. Angioectasia can be treated with thermal techniques, clipping, as well as argon plasma coagulation (APC). APC is a noncontact technique that uses a monopolar current. It is most effective for angioectasia, GAVE, and radiation proctitis. Hemospray (Cook Medical Inc, Winston-Salem, NC) is a promising new technique that has not yet received approval from the Food and Drug Administration. This technique involves directly spraying a nanopowder onto the source of bleeding, with good efficacy in preliminary trials (Sung et al. 2011).

Aspirin therapy should be restarted in less than 5–7 days, as soon as the cardiac risk outweighs rebleeding risk. Helicobacter pylori should be eradicated and NSAIDS avoided in both upper and lower bleeding sources.

Other Therapy

If rebleeding occurs once after successful endoscopic hemostasis, randomized trial data shows repeat endoscopy to be safer than surgery. Second or third rebleeding episodes should have other options considered. If endoscopic therapy fails, or the lesion is not amenable to endoscopic therapy, other modalities may be used. For example, transjugular intrahepatic portosystemic shunting (TIPS) is used in appropriate patients with variceal bleeding, with its most feared adverse event being encephalopathy (30 %). Angiography-guided hemostasis can be performed for hemorrhage from ulcers, Dieulafoy, angioectasia, and diverticula, with contrast-induced nephropathy being the most important adverse event. As noted above, radiation therapy can be used for tumor hemorrhage. Surgery is now considered a last resort for any form of GI bleeding and is rarely needed currently due to improvements in medical and endoscopic therapy. An exception is hemorrhage from a recent anastomosis, which may require surgical revision; also, the air and stress on the anastomosis from endoscopy are generally contraindicated.

Patients with OGIB (negative EGD and colonoscopy) should undergo capsule endoscopy after consideration is given to repeating EGD and/or colonoscopy. Repeat standard endoscopy is particularly useful in cases where views on initial procedures were compromised due to blood, poor prep, or other factors. It remains unclear if non-bleeding diverticula on colonoscopy in a patient with hematochezia defines a "negative" colonoscopy or not, given it is the most common lower source. If a lesion is identified on capsule endoscopy, or the patient continues to bleed from an unknown source, enteroscopy may be undertaken. The form of enteroscopy is driven by lesion location, with the options being push enteroscopy or deep enteroscopy. Deep enteroscopy consists of double-balloon enteroscopy, single-balloon enteroscopy, and spiral enteroscopy and may be approached from an antegrade (per oral) or retrograde (per anus) direction. Hemostatic capabilities mirror those of standard endoscopy discussed above, except banding, which cannot be accommodated by enteroscopes. However, the efficacy of enteroscopic therapy is less clear, and randomized outcome data are lacking. Asian and younger cohorts have a higher incidence of small bowel tumors, which may require surgery after localization.

Hemodynamically unstable patients with OGIB should undergo angiography. Other tests for patients without a bleeding source identified include radionuclide scan, Meckel's scan, computed tomographic (CT) angiography, CT enterography (CTE), and the newer triple-phase CTE. Intraoperative enteroscopy is reserved for patients with life-threatening small bowel hemorrhage that is not responsive to more conservative therapies, as this operation carries significant morbidity and mortality.

Cross-References

▶ Curling's Ulcer
▶ Cushing's Ulcer
▶ Gastritis
▶ Gastrointestinal Bleeding: Indications for Prophylaxis Post-trauma and Treatment

► Hemorrhage
► Hemorrhagic Shock
► Transfusion Thresholds

References

Barkun AN, Bardou M, Kuipers EJ et al (2010) International consensus recommendations on the management of patients with nonvariceal upper gastrointestinal bleeding. Ann Intern Med 152:101–113

Burroughs AK (1994) Octreotide in variceal bleeding. Gut 35:S23–S27

Dorward S, Sreedharan A, Leontiadis GI et al (2006) Proton pump inhibitor treatment initiated prior to endoscopic diagnosis in upper gastrointestinal bleeding. Cochrane Database Syst Rev CD005415(7)

Garcia-Tsao G, Sanyal AJ, Grace ND et al (2007) Prevention and management of gastroesophageal varices and variceal hemorrhage in cirrhosis. Hepatology 46:922–938

Gralnek IM, Barkun AN, Bardou M (2008) Management of acute bleeding from a peptic ulcer. NEJM 359:928–937

Imperiale TF, Birgisson S (1997) Somatostatin or octreotide compared with H2 antagonists and placebo in the management of acute nonvariceal upper gastrointestinal hemorrhage: a meta-analysis. Ann Intern Med 127:1062–1071

Laine L, Yang H, Chang S-C, Datto C (2012) Trends for incidence of hospitalization and death due to GI complications in the United States from 2001 to 2009. Am J Gastroenterol 107:1190–1195

Sung JJ, Luo D, Wu JC et al (2011) Early clinical experience of the safety and effectiveness of Hemospray in achieving hemostasis in patients with acute peptic ulcer bleeding. Endoscopy 43:291–295

Gastrointestinal Injury, Anesthesia for

Kathleen R. Marzluf and Sarah J. Clutter
University of Kansas Medical Center, Kansas City, KS, USA

Synonyms

Colon injury; Duodenal injury; Gastric injury; Intestinal injury; Rectal injury; Small bowel injury; Stomach injury

Definition

The abdomen is anatomically divided into four compartments, each with its respective organs:

1. Thoracoabdominal compartment: stomach, first part of duodenum, transverse colon, diaphragm, liver, spleen
2. Peritoneal cavity: small intestine, parts of ascending and descending colon, sigmoid colon, omentum, gravid uterus, dome of distended bladder
3. Retroperitoneal abdomen: duodenum – second and third parts, parts of ascending and descending colon, pancreas, abdominal aorta, inferior vena cava, kidneys, and ureters
4. Pelvic space: rectum, bladder and urethra, iliac vessels, uterus, and ovaries

The mechanism of abdominal injury can be blunt or penetrating. Knowing the mechanism and location of the injury can help to predict what organs are more likely to be injured.

Blunt Abdominal Trauma

Two types of forces are involved: compression and deceleration. Compression injury is caused by the compression of the abdominal cavity against a fixed object such as a safety belt or steering wheel. Deceleration injuries are those that cause shearing and stretching of those structures located between fixed and mobile objects. The organs most injured during blunt trauma are the spleen and liver. This is due to the fact that these organs are fixed in place whereas the intestines are free to move and are more likely to slide out of the way during the impact in blunt trauma.

Penetrating Abdominal Trauma

The size of the object, the location of the wound, and the force transmitted by the object determine severity and organ injured. The most commonly injured organs during penetrating trauma are the small bowel – due to the large volume it encompasses, followed by the stomach, then colon (Kaslow and Kettler 2012). The focus of this entry will be the gastrointestinal abdominal trauma.

Preexisting Conditions

Gastric, Duodenal, and Small Intestine Injury

Any penetrating injury to the thoracoabdominal compartment or true abdomen can cause damage to the stomach or small intestine, resulting in spillage of the gastric or intestinal contents into the abdominal cavity. Initial physical exam may be relatively nonspecific, i.e., generalized abdominal pain; however, if not treated in a timely manner, the patient can develop peritonitis that can progress to severe sepsis and septic shock. The most common initial findings for gastric injury are blood in the mouth or nasogastric tube. Also, on physical exam, the following abnormalities should raise the suspicion for gastric or small intestinal injury: external signs of injury (seat belt bruising, steering wheel imprint), abdominal distension, or signs of peritonitis (guarding, rebound tenderness). Gastric/intestinal injuries can be seen on CT, if available, which would show the injury, extravasation of oral contrast, and/or free fluid in the abdomen. A chest x-ray may show free air under the diaphragm. If a diagnostic peritoneal lavage is performed, elevated amylase and alkaline phosphatase may be seen (Wilson 2008).

These injuries require emergent exploratory surgery to determine extent of injury, guide repair, and minimize damage incurred to other organs by visceral contents. Indications for exploratory laparotomy are pneumoperitoneum on chest radiograph or signs of peritonitis on physical exam, unexplained hypotension or shock, gunshot wound (GSW) to abdomen, ruptured diaphragm, evisceration of bowel or omentum, or uncontrolled hemorrhage. Anesthetic management will be directed at the extent of injury and the hemodynamic stability of the patient at the time of presentation and surgery.

Injury to the duodenum is fortunately relatively uncommon but presents a special set of complications due to its partially retroperitoneal location (second and third portions) and its proximity to the pancreas. The types of injury most commonly seen are perforations, hemorrhage, and combined pancreaticoduodenal injuries.

Suspected perforations, by clinical deterioration of the patient's condition, or known perforations, determined by retroperitoneal free air or oral contrast extravasation viewed on CT, require exploratory surgery. Again, anesthetic management will be determined by the presenting state of the patient and the extent of the injury. Most duodenal injuries are the result of GSW and can be managed with primary repair. The most commonly injured portion of the duodenum is the second part. The most serious injuries involve disruption of either 50–75 % of the circumference of the second part of the duodenum or 50–100 % of the circumference of the 1st, 3rd, or 4th parts, or are involving some part of the pancreas. These particular injuries can have significant consequences and have a much higher incidence of morbidity and mortality (Bozkurt et al. 2006) – including pancreatic salvage surgery, i.e., pancreaticojejunostomy or pancreaticogastrostomy and possible roux-en-y duodenojejunostomy (duodenum to jejunostomy anastomosis). The need for any of these surgeries places the patient at the risk of prolonged operating room time. Anesthetic management will be based around hemodynamic stability of the patient during the prolonged procedure, including need adequate fluid management, blood transfusion, and potential need for use of vasopressors in the face of septic shock not amenable to fluid resuscitation.

Colon and Rectum Injuries

Gunshot wounds are one of the most common causes of penetrating trauma to the colon. While significant blood loss can be seen in the face of damage to iliac and mesenteric vessels, symptoms are more commonly due to spillage of bowel contents. Peritonitis is more frequent following colorectal injury compared to small bowel injury due to the large bacterial load that can be released. Management of colorectal injury is dependent on location of injury and time-elapse since injury and can be one of the three repairs: primary repair, end-colostomy with mucous fistula/Hartman's pouch, or primary repair with diverting loop ileostomy. According to a 15-year review by Sharpe et al. (2012), larger, more destructive lesions are best treated with resection and diversion whereas smaller, less destructive lesions can be safely treated with resection and primary anastomosis with acceptable levels of morbidity and mortality.

Rectal injuries, though less common, can present a challenge as far as recognition and treatment due to a significant portion being in an extraperitoneal location. Diagnosis of injury can be difficult on physical exam alone and may require proctosigmoidoscopy and/or laparotomy. Repair is also determined by location. The upper two-thirds of the rectum has serosa on the anterior and lateral aspects and is considered intraperitoneal; the lower one-third and the posterior side are lacking serosal covering and are considered to be extraperitoneal. Peritoneal contamination and abscess formation are more likely to be seen in injuries that occur intraperitoneally (McGrath 1998). Options for repair include loop sigmoid colostomy, loop ileostomy, or primary repair. According to a study by Navsaria et al. (2007), extraperitoneal GSWs can safely be repaired by fecal diversion (loop sigmoidcolostomy) without pre-sacral drainage, and most intraperitoneal injuries can be repaired by primary closure with or without fecal diversion.

Applications

Prior to transport to the hospital, the Emergency Medical Service will assess patency of the airway and supply supplemental oxygen as well as make the patient as hemodynamically stable as possible for transport without delaying transport to the hospital. If the patient has any signs of respiratory failure, he or she needs to be intubated prior to transfer to the hospital (Wilson 2008).

Following arrival to the trauma bay, the Advanced Trauma Life-Support primary survey is used to thoroughly assess the patient and address any life-threatening injuries. A history and physical exam from EMS, police, and patient, if conscious, can help to lead the examiners in the detection of any possible injury. During this time, close monitoring of ECG, O_2 saturation, heart rate, and blood pressure should

continue. The hemodynamically stable patient will need an initial set of labs, a type and cross of blood, as well as a blood gas to determine adequacy of ventilation. Once identification of possible abdominal injuries has been made, the stability of the patient determines if the patient can undergo further studies, such as CT scan or ultrasound, versus emergency exploratory laparotomy.

Once the decision for surgery has been made and the patient has been taken to the OR, the non-intubated patient will need to undergo a rapid-sequence intubation with careful choice and titration of an induction agent, attempting to avoid any significant reductions of blood pressure from attenuation of the sympathetic response, followed by a rapid-acting muscle relaxant. Anesthesia can then be maintained with a volatile anesthetic and non-depolarizing muscle relaxants. Nitrous oxide is contraindicated in acute trauma because of the potential to expand air-filled cavities.

The anesthetic goals for abdominal trauma should be to maintain hemodynamic stability, maximize surgical exposure, limit hypothermia, help limit blood loss and coagulopathy, and limit complications to other systems (Wilson 2008). If not already placed, at least two large size peripheral IVs are placed, followed by arterial line placement, which can occur pre- or intraoperatively. A central venous access may be needed if peripheral IV access is inadequate. Prior to surgical incision, blood products need to be made available including packed red blood cells, plasma, and platelets. In case of a massively bleeding patient, massive transfusion protocol needs to be initiated. The patient also needs to be given a broad-spectrum IV antibiotic to cover both gram-positive and gram-negative bacteria as sepsis from peritonitis is of serious concern in this population of trauma patients. The patient may have already received a significant amount of crystalloid and blood products prior to transport to the OR; however, too much IV fluid should be avoided as this can lead to bowel edema. Whether to use warmed blood products versus warm IV fluids will be dictated by laboratory studies such as stat ABG/H&H.

With isolated visceral organ injury, extensive blood loss is less likely when compared to solid organ injury. Ideally, the use of vasopressor agents should only be a temporizing measure until fluid or blood administration by the anesthetic team can stabilize hemodynamic parameters of the patient. When intraoperative central venous pressure monitoring, pulse pressure variation, and clinical signs indicate that the patient is intravascularly repleted but is still unable to maintain hemodynamic stability, inotropic and/or vasopressor agents may be necessary for a short period of time until the patient has gotten past the shock phase.

In addition to monitoring hemodynamic parameters, the anesthesiologist should also be frequently monitoring urine output, core body temperature, peak airway pressures, tidal volumes, peripheral pulses, coagulation studies, ionized calcium, and blood gases, and output from nasogastric tubing. What about monitoring of lactate? Close communication between the anesthesia and the surgical team should be maintained. Spillage of bowel contents into the abdomen can lead to a septic response by the patient, making the maintenance of normal hemodynamic parameters difficult without use of multiple vasoactive agents. Excessive use of vasopressors can have the adverse affect of end-organ damage – most commonly, acute kidney injury. In the event that the anesthesiologist cannot maintain hemodynamic stability – whether due to blood loss or sepsis – packing-off of the abdomen should take place until hemostatic resuscitation occurs or the patient gets through the septic phase. This requires stopping the surgery and implementing "damage control."

Damage control surgery, as described by Hirshberg and Mattox (1995), involves three phases: initial control, stabilization, and delayed reconstruction. Following initial control in the OR, the stabilization phase takes place in the ICU where the patient's hemodynamic status, metabolic derangements, and coagulopathies can be optimized. The patient is then typically taken back to the OR at a later time for completion of intestinal reconstruction and any other repairs that need to be addressed.

Tracheal Extubation

Many factors go into the decision of postoperative extubation. For patients who have suffered from gastrointestinal injury and subsequently needed surgery, we still need to follow the standard criteria for extubation:

– Subjective clinical criteria: follows commands, clear oropharynx, intact gag reflex, sustained head lift for 5 s, minimal end-expiratory concentration of inhaled anesthetics
– Objective criteria: vital capacity ≥ 10 mL/kg; peak voluntary negative inspiratory pressure >20 cm H_2O; Tidal Volume >6 cc/kg; sustained tetanic contractions (5 s); train-of-four ratio >0.7 (Rosenblatt and Sukhupragarn 2009).

We also need to keep in mind that the trauma population has its own set of trauma-related issues associated with extubation that will commonly lead to a prolonged intubation, i.e., TBI, preoperative alcohol intoxication, maxillofacial trauma, pulmonary contusion, pneumothorax, spine fractures, etc. Also, patients who have had exploratory laparotomy will have significant pain issues that can cause hypoxemia and decreased respiratory effort. If the patient has had significant blood loss with subsequent blood transfusion and increased fluid administration, edema of the airway is a real possibility, as well as pulmonary edema. If damage control surgery has been instituted and the patient will be going back for multiple procedures, he or she is usually left intubated to circumvent the complications associated with multiple re-intubations.

Pediatric Considerations

Penetrating and visceral injuries are less common in the pediatric population than solid organ (liver and spleen) injuries. Anatomic considerations must be taken into account when treating this population. Abdominal organs are much larger relative to the space they occupy when compared to the adult, the musculature is not as well developed, and the rib cage is much more flexible. Intestinal injury will need to be addressed immediately with exploratory laparotomy to minimize contamination by bowel contents.

Comparatively, when a pediatric patient has solid organ injuries but is hemodynamically stable, operative intervention may be avoided (Loy 2008).

Cross-References

▶ Abdominal Solid Organ Injury, Anesthesia for
▶ Airway Equipment
▶ Damage Control Resuscitation
▶ Damage Control Surgery
▶ Delayed Wound Closure
▶ Fluid, Electrolytes, and Nutrition in Trauma Patients
▶ Massive Transfusion
▶ Massive Transfusion Protocols in Trauma
▶ Monitoring of Trauma Patients during Anesthesia
▶ Pediatric Trauma, Assessment, and Anesthetic Management
▶ Shock Management in Trauma

References

Bozkurt B, Ozdemir BA, Kocer B, Unal B, Dolapci M, Cergiz O (2006) Operative approach in traumatic injuries of the duodenum. Acta Chir Belg 106:405–408
Hirshberg A, Mattox KI (1995) Planned reoperation for severe trauma. Ann Surg 222(1):3–8
Kaslow O, Kettler R (2012) Anesthetic considerations for abdominal trauma in essentials of trauma anesthesia. Cambridge University Press, Cambridge
Loy J (2008) Pediatric trauma & anesthesia in Trauma Anesthesia. Cambridge University Press, Cambridge
McGrath V, Fabian TC, Croce MA, Minard MD, Pritchard FE (1998) Rectal trauma: management based on anatomic distinctions. Am Surg 64:12
Navsaria PH, Eclu S, Nicol AJ (2007) Civilian extraperitoneal rectal gunshot wounds: surgical management made simpler. World J Surg 31:1345–1351
Rosenblatt WH, Sukhupragarn W (2009) Airway management in clinical anesthesia. Lippincott Williams & Wilkins/Wolters/Kluwer, Philadelphia
Sharpe JP, Magnott LJ, Weinberg JA, Parks N, Maish GO, Bhahan CP, Fabian TC (2012) Adherence to a simplified management algorithm reduces morbidity and mortality after penetrating colon injuries: a 15-year experience. J Am Coll Surg 214(4):591–597
Wilson W (2008) Anesthesia considerations for abdominal in trauma anesthesia. Cambridge University Press, Cambridge

GCS

▶ Neurotrauma, Pre-hospital Evaluation and Care

General Anesthesia for Major Trauma

Patrick Braun
Department of Anesthesiology and Critical Care Medicine, Innsbruck Medical University, Innsbruck, Austria

Synonyms

Airway management; Anesthesia; Anesthesia induction; Anesthetic drugs; Oxygenation; Ventilation

Definition

General anesthesia may be lifesaving in severely traumatized or critically ill patients, but it increases morbidity and mortality, if not performed properly. For instance, a patient with an acute severe respiratory insufficiency, due to trauma, may benefit from emergency anesthesia and ventilatory support. Likewise, a patient with a traumatic brain injury and a GCS < 8 may profit from prehospital emergency anesthesia and intubation. On the other hand outcome is also depending on factors such as transfer time to the next suitable trauma center and anesthesia including airway-management skills of the attending healthcare personnel. Possibly some injured patients with acute respiratory insufficiency benefit even more from pain management and noninvasive ventilatory support with continuous positive airway pressure (CPAP) mask or helmet, instead of insufficient anesthesia attempts. The pros and cons of emergency anesthesia, airway management, fluid, and vasopressor therapy are intensively debated. When should a patient be anesthetized and the airway secured invasively? Which airway is appropriate for the actual clinical situation? Which anesthetic should be administered? Recently, impressive progress has been made in the fields of anesthesia drugs and airway management. The aim of this essay is to offer an overview on general anesthesia in major trauma.

Preexisting Condition

The decision to anesthetize a traumatized patient in the field is based on sound clinical judgement. Severely traumatized patients with apnea or rapidly deteriorating and insufficient, exhausting breathing patterns require a secured airway for oxygenation and ventilation. Additional indications are hypoxemia with oxygen saturation below 90 % despite oxygen insufflation and after exclusion of tension pneumothorax, severe traumatic brain injury with a Glasgow Coma Scale (GCS) <9, trauma-associated hemodynamic instability with a systolic blood pressure <90 mmHg, and severe chest trauma with respiratory insufficiency (Braun et al. 2010). Apart from this, the decision to anesthetize a patient in the prehospital setting or later in the emergency department depends on further deliberations. These include the mechanism of injury, surgical urgency, progression of disease, and long transport time to the trauma center. Indications and prospects of successful prehospital anesthesia should be critically evaluated. Prosperous anesthesia will only be possible with experienced team members and the entire emergency anesthesia equipment including monitoring, drugs, airway-management tools, and ventilation devices. A safe and appropriate environment including terrain, temperature, and light should be ensured, if possible. Also, contraindications and possible outcome deterioration, due to prehospital anesthesia, when compared to anesthesia induction in the emergency department should be kept in mind. For instance, mortality and pneumonia rate may be increased with prehospital anesthesia in comparison to anesthesia performed in the emergency department. Pneumonia as a result of aspiration during anesthesia induction will affect the outcome in multiple trauma. However, many study results are difficult to extrapolate from one emergency medical system to another, because of different structures. For example, in an urban vs. a rural emergency medical system, transfer time is short and anesthesia induction therefore may be delayed until hospital arrival. This may be safer for a patient, because logistics, personnel resources, and equipment in the emergency department are complete.

Differences in Emergency Medical Systems and in Anesthesia Skills

Different structures and anesthesia training levels in several emergency medical systems lead to significant differences in medical outcome. For example, in France, airway-management-experienced emergency physicians reported problems in only 3 % of all analyzed prehospital intubations (Tentillier et al. 2008). In contrast to these data, paramedics from Miami (USA) encountered intubation difficulties in about 30 % of the patients and were not able to intubate 10 % of the cases (Cobas et al. 2009). In a German study on prehospital intubations, which was performed by emergency medical system (EMS) physicians with widely varying airway-management skills, a 15 % rate of esophageally or bronchially positioned tubes was reported. Mortality rate in patients with esophageally misplaced tubes was near 80 % compared to 20 % for the overall study cohort (Timmermann et al. 2007). In 2009 the Association of Anesthetists of Great Britain and Ireland published safety guideline for prehospital anesthesia and recommended prehospital anesthesia only for appropriately trained and competent practitioners. Studies on intubation recommendations have provided conflicting results, mainly attributable to variable study setting parameters such as different patient cohorts (e.g., blunt vs. penetrating trauma), profession groups (e.g., anesthesiologist vs. EMS physician vs. nurse vs. paramedic), skill levels (e.g., anesthesiologist vs. general practitioner), and hospital transfer time. Anesthesia and airway strategies of a rescuer have to be adapted to his or her skill level. For example, a paramedic with regular clinical experience may have a higher skill level than an EMS physician with rare airway-management practice. A highly skilled and trained rescuer could decide freely how to oxygenate, anesthetize, and ventilate a patient. A moderately skilled rescuer with constant training could try endotracheal intubation twice and then switch to an alternative supraglottic airway device or bag-valve-mask ventilation. A less skilled rescuer should completely refrain from anesthesia induction and endotracheal intubation. Focus should be on optimal noninvasive oxygenation, fast hospital transfer, and the use of supraglottic airway devices or bag-valve-mask ventilation only in life-threatened patients, due to respiratory insufficiency.

Application

Before anesthesia induction the patient should be placed in a supine position, with a pad beneath the occiput to align the oral, pharyngeal, and laryngeal axes of the upper airway during laryngoscopy. This sniffing position provides visibility of the laryngeal structures. This may be especially helpful in patients with obesity or a stiff cervical spine. In infants, a support under the chest may counteract the anterior head flexion caused by the large occiput. The patient should be monitored with ECG, blood pressure measurement, and pulse oximetry. At least one reliable intravenous line should be available and well fixed, to avoid extravenous injection and dislocation during anesthesia induction and maintenance. Further peripheral intravenous lines should be contemplated in every severely traumatized patient, if possible. Involved personnel have to be experienced in anesthesia induction and treatment of side effects. All drugs for anesthesia induction, maintenance, treatment of side effects, and advanced life support (ALS) must be prepared. A suction device with a large diameter tube has to be ready. All emergency patients have to be treated like non-fastened, with increased risk of regurgitation, or traumatic bleeding.

General Anesthesia for Major Trauma, Table 1 Devices for oxygenation and preoxygenation. Oxygen flow (L/min) and resulting inspiratory oxygen fraction (FiO_2) are given

Oxygenation device	O_2 flow (L/min)	Maximum inspiratory oxygen fraction (%)
Nasal cannula	1–6	24–44
Face mask	8–10	40–60
Face mask with reservoir	6–10	60–100
Anesthesia bag-valve-mask device	12	50
Anesthesia bag-valve-mask device with reservoir	12	100

An emergency is not a playing ground for testing new drugs or techniques. Patients are too sick to tolerate errors based on inexperienced rescuers. Drugs and techniques should be sufficiently trained in a controlled environment with noncritically ill or injured patients under expert supervision before being used in emergencies.

Anesthesia Induction Starts with Preoxygenation

Body oxygen stores should be filled up with oxygen in spontaneously breathing patients, in order to avoid oxygen desaturation during anesthesia induction. Preoxygenation must be performed before anesthesia induction starts. Several preoxygenation techniques are able to fill up the oxygen stores in the body. Optimally, oxygen should be applied with a tightly fitting face mask with reservoir and high oxygen flow (e.g., 10 L/min, Table 1), approaching an inspiratory oxygen fraction of nearly 100 %. Functional residual capacity can be increased with continuous positive airway pressure (CPAP) up to 10 cm H_2O, by elevating the chest by 25°, or a sitting position, if applicable with the present hemodynamics and trauma patterns such as spine injuries. However, during hemorrhage with unstable circulation, CPAP may destabilize hemodynamics. Also, fear and pain should be treated to decrease excessive oxygen demand (Mort 2005). In case of sufficient spontaneous breathing, 3 min or eight deep breaths of 100 % oxygen denitrogenize the lungs. Efficiency of preoxygenation can be monitored with an end-expiratory oxygen fraction, measured by an anesthetic monitor. End-expiratory oxygen fraction should exceed values of 80 % oxygen. The pulse oximetry target value should be ≥99 %. Many factors can influence the effectiveness of preoxygenation. Oxygen stores may be reduced due to traumatic lung contusion, hemato- and pneumothorax, the combination of both, or even pneumonia. All these disorders lead to decreasing functional residual capacity in critically ill patient and an increasing right-to-left shunt. In trauma patients hemoglobin may be low because of hemorrhage. Therefore, preoxygenation may be less effective in some patients, but it should be employed without exception, because of increased safety margins during airway management and anesthesia induction in general. Nevertheless, a short induction time with provision of a definite airway is a key factor in the prevention of a hypoxemia-related secondary organ injury (Russo et al. 2010).

Drugs in Emergency Anesthesia

All the applied drugs must be highly familiar to the user. Tables 2–6 give an overview of commonly used hypnotics, analgetics, neuromuscular blockers, and antagonists.

Etomidate is a carboxylated imidazole derivative with anesthetic and amnestic properties. It was discovered in 1964 and was introduced as an intravenous agent in 1972 in Europe and in 1983 in the United States. It has a rapid onset of action and a relatively safe cardiovascular risk profile and is therefore known to cause a less significant drop in blood pressure than other induction agents. In recent times, administration of etomidate in critically ill patients has been questioned, because of its inhibitory effect on steroid genesis, even after a single administration (Jabre et al. 2009).

Today, propofol is widely used for induction and maintenance of anesthesia. It has largely replaced other hypnotics like sodium thiopental for these indications. Apart from many advantageous characteristics of propofol, it should be avoided in hemodynamically unstable patients, because of dose-dependent cardiocirculatory depression. In addition to low blood pressure and transient apnea following an induction dose, one of propofol's most frequent side effects is pain during intravenous injection, especially in smaller veins.

General Anesthesia for Major Trauma, Table 2 Generic name, analgesic potency, indications, doses (i.v.), mean duration of action after single dose, and side effects of commonly used opioids

Generic name	Analgesic potency	Indications	Dose (i.v.)	Duration of action	Side effects
Morphine	1	• Analgesia	• 20–100 µg/kg	~3–5 h	• Respiratory depression • Cardiocirculatory depression • Histamine release → asthma bronchiale
Fentanyl	~100	• Anesthesia induction in hemodynamically stable patients • Anesthesia maintenance	• Anesthesia induction: 1–5 (µg/kg) • Maintenance: 1–3 (µg/kg) as repetitive bolus	~20–30 min	• Respiratory depression • Cardiocirculatory depression
Sufentanil	~1,000	• Anesthesia induction in hemodynamically stable patients • Anesthesia maintenance	• Anesthesia induction: 0.3–1.0 (µg/kg) • Maintenance: 0.5–1.5 (µg/kg/h) continuously or 0.15–0.7 (µg/kg) as repetitive bolus	~30 min	• Respiratory depression • Cardiocirculatory depression

G

General Anesthesia for Major Trauma, Table 3 Indications, doses (i.v.), duration of action after single dose, and side effects of ketamine and (S+)-ketamine

Generic name	Indications	Dose (i.v.)	Duration of action (min)	Side effects
Ketamine	• Anesthesia induction in hemodynamically fragile or unstable and asthma bronchiale patients • Anesthesia maintenance	• Analgesia: 0.25–0.5 (mg/kg) • Anesthesia induction: 1–2 (mg/kg), in combination with midazolam • Maintenance: 0.3–1.0 (mg/kg/h) continuously or 0.5–1 (mg/kg) as repetitive bolus, in combination with midazolam	• 5–15	• Dissociative anesthesia • Psychotropic properties • Hypersalivation
(S+)-Ketamine	• Anesthesia induction in hemodynamically fragile or unstable and asthma bronchiale patients • Anesthesia maintenance	• Analgesia: 0.125–0.25 (mg/kg) • Anesthesia induction: 0.25–0.5 (mg/kg), in combination with midazolam • Maintenance: 0.15–0.5 (mg/kg/h) continuously or 0.25–0.5 (mg/kg) as repetitive bolus, in combination with midazolam	• 5–15	• Dissociative anesthesia • Less psychotropic properties • Hypersalivation

General Anesthesia for Major Trauma, Table 4 Indications, doses (i.v.), mean duration of action after single dose, and side effects of commonly used hypnotics

Generic name	Indications	Dose (i.v.)	Duration of action (min)	Side effects
Etomidate	• Anesthesia induction in hemodynamically fragile or unstable patients	• Induction: 0.15–0.3 (mg/kg)	• 3–5	• Superficial anesthesia • Inhibitory effect on steroid genesis
Propofol	• Anesthesia induction in hemodynamically stable patients • Anesthesia maintenance	• Induction: 1.5–2.5 (mg/kg) • Maintenance: 2–6 (mg/kg/h) continuously or 0.5–2 (mg/kg) as repetitive bolus	• 4–6	• Cardiocirculatory depression • Arterial hypotension • Respiratory depression
Thiopental	• Anesthesia induction in hemodynamically stable patients • Status epilepticus	• Induction: 3–7 (mg/kg)	• 5–10	• Histamine release → asthma bronchiale • Tissue necrosis of extravasation
Midazolam	• Anesthesia induction in hemodynamically fragile or unstable patients → Co-induction with ketamine • Anesthesia maintenance	• Induction: 0.1–0.2 (mg/kg) • Maintenance: 0.03–0.1 (mg/kg/h) continuously or 0.03–0.2 (mg/kg) as repetitive bolus	• ~45	• Slow onset • Superficial anesthesia

Ketamine is exceptional with its analgetic and hypnotic properties and does not compromise spontaneous breathing and circulation. It was originally developed in 1965 as a derivative of phencyclidine. It seems to be the beneficial drug for anesthesia induction in hemodynamically unstable patients (Morris et al. 2009). Also, propofol co-induction with 0.1 mg/kg midazolam

General Anesthesia for Major Trauma, Table 5 Indications, doses (i.v.), onset, mean duration of action after single dose, and side effects of neuromuscular blockers used in emergency anesthesia

Generic name	Dose (i.v.)	Onset (s)	Duration of action (min)	Side effects
Suxamethonium	1–1.5 mg/kg	60–90	7–12	• Malignant hyperthermia • Anaphylactic reactions • Intraocular pressure increase • Hyperkalemia
Rocuronium	0.5–1.2 mg/kg	90–180	30–40	• Anaphylactic reactions

General Anesthesia for Major Trauma, Table 6 Indications, doses (i.v.), mean duration of action after single dose, and side effects of commonly used antagonists in adults

Generic name	Indications	Dose (i.v.)	Duration of action	Side effects
Naloxone	• Reversal of opioid effects (e.g., respiratory depression)	1 µg/kg fractional, repetition until required effect	~30–45 min	• Rebound effects (e.g., re-respiratory depression)
Flumazenil	• Reversal of benzodiazepine effects	0.2 mg initial, repetition with 0.1 mg until required effect, maximum 1 mg	~5–15 min	• Rebound effect
Sugammadex	• Reversal of steroidal non-depolarizing muscular relaxants (e.g., rocuronium)	16 mg/kg (emergency dose)	Inactivation of steroidal non-depolarizing muscular relaxants	• None known

or 0.5 mg/kg ketamine compared to propofol alone is resulting in less hemodynamic depression, which may be advantageous in unstable patients, despite slower onset in the propofol-midazolam combination. For analgesia during anesthesia induction, fentanyl or sufentanil in hemodynamically stable and ketamine in hemodynamically unstable patients may be the agents of choice because of fast onset and acceptable analgesic effect and duration.

Adding neuromuscular block to emergency anesthesia induction is hotly debated. Some argue that the presence of a neuromuscular block offers the best possible intubation condition and should always be applied in emergency anesthesia induction. Others point out that with neuromuscular blockade an esophageally placed endotracheal tube inevitably leads to death, as spontaneous breathing is impossible. Therefore, some EMS services do not recommend administration of neuromuscular blockers when performing an emergency anesthesia induction. Suxamethonium (1–1.5 mg/kg) is still the most widely employed neuromuscular block agent and has surely saved a lot of lives. However, some refrain from using this drug because of several, potentially lethal, drawbacks, such as malignant hyperthermia, hyperkalemia, intraocular pressure increase, and muscle pain. Recently, the relatively new noncompetitive rocuronium antagonist sugammadex has been introduced into clinical practice. With an emergency dose of 16 mg/kg of sugammadex, rocuronium-induced neuromuscular block reversal is faster than spontaneous muscular recovery after suxamethonium administration. Accordingly, rocuronium up to 1.2 mg/kg might have the potential to become the first-line neuromuscular blocking agent in emergency anesthesia.

Rapid Sequence Induction, Tracheal Intubation, and Ventilation

Anesthesia induction in emergencies should always be performed as rapid sequence induction (RSI), in order to have definite airway control as fast as possible. After preparation of the patient, the equipment, and preoxygenation, all selected drugs are administered in a fast array. Endotracheal intubation (ETI) is performed immediately after sufficient onset of anesthesia. Endotracheal intubation is known to be the most reliable technique to ventilate a patient and to provide a best possible security to the airway, if performed properly. However, it may be especially challenging in traumatized patients. Trauma or bleeding in the airway, in the craniofacial region, as well as trauma of the cervical spine may lead to aggravated intubation conditions. After initial immobilization of the cervical spine by a cervical collar, temporary removal of a cervical collar may be necessary for ETI. In this case, the cervical spine needs to be immobilized by means of manual in-line stabilization when securing the airway. One new option to make tracheal intubation safer could be a suction laryngoscope, which rendered esophageal intubations less likely when laryngoscopists with less experience were performing airway management in a simulated severe airway bleeding. Flexible bronchoscopy may be an excellent tool to intubate a patient with a known difficult airway. However, it will be hardly accessible in the field and for an efficient use more training is required than with other intubation techniques. Beyond that, the use of optical devices may be restricted, due to blood or secretions in the airway. In case of difficult direct laryngoscopy, a backward-upward-rightward-pressure (BURP) maneuver may improve laryngoscopy and tracheal intubation. Cricoid pressure (Sellick maneuver) has been widely advocated to prevent reflux of gastric content during RSI. Recently, several studies suggested that it does not prevent aspiration. Additionally, bag-valve-mask ventilation, laryngoscopy, and tracheal intubation may be hindered (Steinmann and Priebe 2009). Therefore, the Sellick maneuver cannot be recommended in emergencies anymore. To facilitate intubation, a tracheal tube should always be equipped with a guide wire. In small children, employing a cuffed vs. an uncuffed endotracheal tube may result in fewer tube exchange rates with a comparable frequency of side effects.

Verifying Endotracheal Tube Position

Only two details guarantee a correct endotracheal tube position and should be checked immediately: As far as direct laryngoscopy is possible, the endotracheal tube should be seen passing in between the vocal cords. Furthermore, end-expiratory carbon dioxide should be confirmed with capnography. Capnography is obligatory to confirm correct placement of the endotracheal tube and to monitor ventilation as well as tube dislocations in the prehospital and hospital setting. However, during cardiac arrest, in low-blood-flow states, e.g., hemorrhagic shock, or chest trauma, capnography may be not reliable, respectively false-negative. In these situations chest auscultation, besides visual control, may be the only method to validate correct tracheal tube placement (Takeda et al. 2003). Bronchial intubation should be considered in case of diminished compliance, unilateral ventilation sounds, chest movements, and low oxygen saturation.

How to Proceed After a Failed Intubation Attempt

Sometimes endotracheal intubation within one attempt is not possible. At least after 30 s of intubation attempts, bag-valve-mask ventilation should be resumed and efforts made to improve intubation conditions. An oropharyngeal or nasopharyngeal tube may be employed to improve upper airway patency and therefore bag-valve-mask ventilation. In patients with frontobasal trauma patterns, nasopharyngeal tubes should be avoided. Bag-valve-mask ventilation is sufficient if the chest rises clearly during positive pressure ventilation and recedes during expiration. Additionally, bag-valve-mask ventilation may be monitored with capnography. Bag-valve-mask ventilation should be performed as cautiously as possible to avoid adverse effects of excessive stomach inflation, such as regurgitation and impaired ventilation conditions, due to rising intra-abdominal pressures. In some rare cases an abdominal compartment syndrome can be triggered by excessive stomach inflation. Venous return to the heart may diminish, decreasing cardiac output and contributing to final outcome. Gut ischemia in a patient with excessive stomach inflation has been described. If three intubation attempts have been unsuccessful, even an experienced healthcare provider should refrain from further attempts. Bag-valve-mask ventilation should be resumed, or if not possible ventilation should be achieved with a supraglottic airway device and a senior help should always be called early. Some scientific societies in Europe and North America have developed difficult airway algorithms. Similarly, emergency medical systems (EMS) should develop algorithms for an expected and an unexpected difficult airway, adapted to local conditions

Alternative Airway Devices

Direct laryngoscopy and conventional tracheal intubation may not be possible in some patients, despite optimal performance in all arrays. In this case, an alternative airway device may be the best way to ventilate and eventually to perform endotracheal intubation. Established tools for blind or optical guided tracheal intubation are the laryngeal mask airway (LMA) Fastrach and the LMA CTrach, both devices allow ventilation and further intubation. The Airtraq device seems to be another promising intubation tool. Many supraglottic airway devices allow ventilation without securing the airway comparable to tracheal intubation. Adverse effects of ventilation might resemble those of bag-valve-mask ventilation. Therefore, ventilation has to be performed cautiously. Most of the supraglottic airway experience has been gathered with the LMA Classic and the LMA ProSeal. Literature refers that insertion of the LMA Classic seems to be easier, but the LMA ProSeal offers a higher airway leakage pressure, thus higher ventilation pressures may be provided. Insertion of the LMA ProSeal may be most efficient when performed the with help of a laryngoscope and guided with a gum elastic bougie. Ventilation quality with the laryngeal tube suction (LTS) is overall comparable to the LMA ProSeal; the LTS requires a higher cuff pressure compared to the LMA ProSeal, which may cause pressure sores and macroglossia. The Combitube allows supraglottic or tracheal ventilation, depending on its position after insertion. However, the Combitube may be more traumatic that other devices. Mucosal injuries and even life-threatening esophageal ruptures are reported. Therefore the Combitube is less frequently employed today. All mentioned airway devices may be used for training during routine anesthesia, except for the Combitube.

Anesthesia Maintenance and Monitoring

Once the airway is under control and the patient is being ventilated, anesthesia has to be maintained until definitive treatment. Long-acting anesthetic drugs with almost inert hemodynamic properties are favorable and should be administered as repetitive doses or as continuous infusion (Tables 2–6). During transport, monitoring with ECG, automated blood pressure measurement, pulse oximetry, and capnography should be performed. Capnography has to be employed in every ventilated patient. The goal of ventilation is to achieve normocapnia. However, in a patient with severe chest trauma, arterial partial carbon dioxide pressure is more reliable than capnography, due to an increased alveolo-arterial carbon dioxide pressure gradient. Also, capnography should be interpreted cautiously in a patient with severe traumatic brain injury and ventilation adjusted according to arterial partial carbon dioxide pressure. Extended hemodynamic monitoring can be applied from the moment the patient reaches the emergency department.

Side Effects of Anesthesia

Acute hypoxemia, arterial hypotension, and hypothermia with detrimental effects on outcome are possible side effects of general anesthesia and should be avoided, if possible. For instance, a brain-injured patient may be at risk of hypoxia- and hyperventilation-induced secondary brain injury. Also, in hemodynamically unstable trauma patients, ventilation rate >10/min and positive end-expiratory pressure should be avoided, because mortality may be increased (Herff et al. 2008). In a ventilated patient with a sudden drop of arterial oxygen saturation, **DOPES** should be considered as causes: (tube-) **D**islocation, (tube-) **O**bstruction, (tension-)

Pneumothorax, Equipment failure, and Stomach distension. One should keep in mind that positive pressure ventilation may lead to fast development of a tension pneumothorax, especially in patients with thorax trauma. Opportunities for decompression must be available and effectively controlled by healthcare personnel providing emergency anesthesia.

Clinical Treatment

Clinical treatment of severely traumatized patients is interdisciplinary therapy from the moment the patient reaches the emergency department. Vital functions have to be stabilized before further diagnostic and therapeutic measures can be achieved. Definite treatment of the airway like final positioning of the endotracheal tube, tracheotomy, double-lumen endobronchial intubation, and specific ventilatory support according to the trauma pattern may be necessary. In addition to this, improvement of anesthetic care, such as choice of drugs (Tables 2–6), hemodynamic monitoring, infusion, vasopressor application, transfusion, coagulation therapy, and early antibiotic supply, may have to be implemented. Further diagnostic and therapeutic decisions have to be based on the clinical situation. The anesthetic goal should be to keep the patient in a physiological homeostasis with continuation of diagnostic and therapeutic requirements. This may include surgical and other specialized treatments and intensive care medicine.

Training in Anesthesia

No patient should die or suffer damage because of a healthcare provider's lack of anesthesia and airway-management skills. A healthcare provider has to be familiar with all locally available conditions, such as anesthetics, monitoring, and alternative airway devices. Management of anesthesia and securing the airway depends more on the experience of the rescuer than on a given airway device. Regular training with manikins, simulation courses, and practice in the operating theater are essential.

Recently, the Association of Anesthetists of Great Britain and Ireland stated that a high training level and simple techniques are the key factors to successful anesthesia and airway management. Healthcare personnel providing prehospital anesthesia "should have the same level of training and competence that would enable them to provide unsupervised rapid sequence induction in the emergency department." Unfortunately, this desirable highest training level seems to be unrealistic in many emergency medical systems worldwide.

Summary

General anesthesia can be lifesaving in severely traumatized patients. On the other hand it increases morbidity and mortality, if it is not performed properly. The pros and cons of emergency anesthesia are hotly debated. The decision to anesthetize a traumatized patient in the field is based on sound clinical judgement. Severely traumatized patients with insufficient breathing patterns require a secured airway for oxygenation and ventilation. A highly skilled and trained rescuer can decide freely how to oxygenate, anesthetize, and ventilate a patient. A moderately skilled rescuer with constant training could try endotracheal intubation twice and switch to an alternative supraglottic airway device or bag-valve-mask ventilation, if intubation fails. A less skilled rescuer should completely refrain from anesthesia induction and endotracheal intubation. Focus should be on optimal noninvasive oxygenation, fast hospital transfer, and the use of supraglottic airway devices or bag-valve-mask ventilation only in life-threatened patients, due to respiratory insufficiency. Before any anesthesia induction, the patient should be placed in a supine position, with a pad beneath the occiput. The patient should be monitored with ECG, blood pressure measurement, and pulse oximetry. At least one reliable intravenous line has to be available and well fixed and a suction device with a large diameter tube should be ready. Preoxygenation should be employed without exception, because of increased safety margins during anesthesia induction and airway management in general. It is most effective when performed with high-flow oxygen delivered through a tight-fitting face mask with a reservoir. Ketamine may be the induction agent of choice in patients with unstable circulation. Endotracheal intubation is known to be the most reliable technique to ventilate a patient and to provide a best possible security to the airway. Only two details guarantee a correct endotracheal tube position and should be checked immediately: As far as direct laryngoscopy is possible, the endotracheal tube should be seen passing in between the vocal cords. Furthermore, end-expiratory carbon dioxide should be confirmed with capnography. The goal of ventilation is to achieve normocapnia. When intubation fails three times, ventilation should be performed with an alternative supraglottic airway or a bag-valve-mask device. Senior help should be called early. In a "can-not-ventilate, can-not-intubate" situation, a supraglottic airway should be employed, and if ventilation is still unsuccessful, a surgical airway should be performed. In a ventilated patient with a sudden drop of oxygen saturation, **DOPES** should be considered as causes: (tube-) **D**islocation, (tube-) **O**bstruction, (tension-) **P**neumothorax, **E**quipment failure, and **S**tomach distension. Regular training with manikins, simulation courses, and clinical practice in the operating theater are essential to retain general anesthesia in major trauma patients.

Acknowledgments The author has no conflict of interest to declare. Sincere thanks to Peter Paal, Volker Wenzel, Sebastian G. Russo, and Ulrich Braun.

Cross-References

- ▶ Airway Anatomy
- ▶ Airway Assessment
- ▶ Airway Equipment
- ▶ Airway Exchange in Trauma Patients
- ▶ Airway Management in Trauma, Cricothyrotomy
- ▶ Airway Management in Trauma, Nonsurgical
- ▶ Airway Management in Trauma, Tracheostomy
- ▶ Airway Trauma, Management of
- ▶ Benzodiazepines
- ▶ Burn Anesthesia
- ▶ Emergency Medical Services (EMS)
- ▶ Hemodynamic Management in Trauma Anesthesia
- ▶ Hemodynamic Monitoring
- ▶ Mechanical Ventilation, Conventional
- ▶ Monitoring of Trauma Patients during Anesthesia
- ▶ Pneumothorax, Tension
- ▶ Pulmonary Trauma, Anesthetic Management for
- ▶ Ventilatory Management of Trauma Patients

References

Braun P, Wenzel V, Paal P (2010) Anesthesia in prehospital emergencies and in the emergency department. Curr Opin Anaesthesiol 23(4):500–506. doi:10.1097/ACO.0b013e32833bc135

Cobas MA, De la Pena MA, Manning R, Candiotti K, Varon AJ (2009) Prehospital intubations and mortality: a level 1 trauma center perspective. Anesth Analg 109(2):489–493. doi:109/2/489 [pii] 10.1213/ane.0b013e3181aa3063

Herff H, Paal P, von Goedecke A, Lindner KH, Severing AC, Wenzel V (2008) Influence of ventilation strategies on survival in severe controlled hemorrhagic shock. Crit Care Med 36(9):2613–2620. doi:10.1097/CCM.0b013e31818477f0

Jabre P, Combes X, Lapostolle F, Dhaouadi M, Ricard-Hibon A, Vivien B, Bertrand L, Beltramini A, Gamand P, Albizzati S, Perdrizet D, Lebail G, Chollet-Xemard C, Maxime V, Brun-Buisson C, Lefrant JY, Bollaert PE, Megarbane B, Ricard JD, Anguel N, Vicaut E, Adnet F (2009) Etomidate versus ketamine for rapid sequence intubation in acutely ill patients: a multicentre randomised controlled trial. Lancet 374(9686):293–300. doi:S0140-6736(09)60949-1 [pii] 10.1016/S0140-6736(09)60949-1

Morris C, Perris A, Klein J, Mahoney P (2009) Anaesthesia in haemodynamically compromised emergency patients: does ketamine represent the best choice of induction agent? Anaesthesia 64(5):532–539. doi: ANA5835 [pii] 10.1111/j.1365-2044.2008.05835.x

Mort TC (2005) Preoxygenation in critically ill patients requiring emergency tracheal intubation. Crit Care Med 33(11):2672–2675. doi:00003246-200511000-00033 [pii]

Russo SG, Zink W, Herff H, Wiese CH (2010) Death due to (no) airway. Adverse events by out-of-hospital airway management? Anaesthesist 59(10):929–939. doi:10.1007/s00101-010-1782-y

Steinmann D, Priebe HJ (2009) Cricoid pressure. Anaesthesist 58(7):695–707. doi:10.1007/s00101-009-1548-6

Takeda T, Tanigawa K, Tanaka H, Hayashi Y, Goto E, Tanaka K (2003) The assessment of three methods to verify tracheal tube placement in the emergency setting. Resuscitation 56(2):153–157. doi:S0300957202003453 [pii]

Tentillier E, Heydenreich C, Cros AM, Schmitt V, Dindart JM, Thicoipe M (2008) Use of the intubating laryngeal mask airway in emergency pre-hospital difficult intubation. Resuscitation 77 (1):30–34. doi:S0300-9572(07)00529-1 [pii] 10.1016/j.resuscitation.2007.06.035

Timmermann A, Russo SG, Eich C, Roessler M, Braun U, Rosenblatt WH, Quintel M (2007) The out-of-hospital esophageal and endobronchial intubations performed by emergency physicians. Anesth Analg 104(3):619–623. doi:104/3/619 [pii] 10.1213/01.ane.0000253523.80050.e9

Geriatric Injuries

▶ Geriatric Trauma

Geriatric Trauma

Mark Hawk
Adult-Gerontology Acute Care Nurse Practitioner Speciality (Retired), School of Nursing University of California, San Francisco, CA, USA
Trauma Nurse Practitioner (Retired), San Francisco General Hospital, San Francisco, CA, USA

Synonyms

Geriatric injuries; Gerotrauma; Injuries in older adults; Trauma in older adults

Definition

Geriatric trauma refers to injury to bodily tissue in the older adult population from an external object or force. The most common mechanism is blunt trauma of which 75 % is the result of falls. Motor vehicle crashes (MVC), including pedestrian versus auto crashes (PVA), account for all

but 4 % of the remaining mechanisms (Bonne and Schuerer 2013). There is no standardized age limit in the trauma literature at which a person is defined as being "older." For trauma research purposes, the term "older adult" has been defined as ranging from a lower threshold of 55 years to 70 years of age; however, it is routinely defined as ≥65 years of age in the majority of trauma literature. This is also the definition accepted by the United States (US) Senate Special Committee on Aging, the American Association of Retired Persons, the Federal Council on Aging, and the US Administration on Aging (Hawk et al. 2012).

In the year 2007, 12.6 % of the US population (37.9 million people) was ≥65 years old. By 2030, this number will grow to 72.1 million (19.3 % of US population). Those aged ≥ 85 years are the fastest growing subgroup of older adults, and their number will double from five million in 2005 to nine million in 2030 (Hawk et al. 2012).

Preexisting Condition

Age-associated physiologic changes to the respiratory, cardiovascular, neurological, renal, musculoskeletal, and immune systems predispose older adults to higher morbidity and mortality from injury. Comorbidities are present in 82 % of older adults, with hypertension and heart disease being present in >50 % and >30 %, respectively. Other common comorbidities include history of stroke, COPD, diabetes, osteoporosis, dementia, renal disease, liver disease, and cancers. Mortality is significantly increased in injured, older adults with each comorbid condition present at the time of injury. This has prompted revisions in some prehospital triage criteria to recommend transport of injured, older adults with any comorbidities to a trauma center (Werman et al. 2011).

The use of anticoagulants and β-blockers for treatment of heart failure can increase the risk of death from trauma in this group by five to ten times due to hemorrhage and masking of normal physiologic responses. Medication used to treat other conditions may interfere with examination of the neurologic and musculoskeletal systems, as well as interfere with wound healing (Bonne and Schuerer 2013; Hawk et al. 2012).

Application

Currently, trauma is the fifth leading cause of death in adults ≥65 years of age, and this group accounts for 23 % of hospital admissions related to trauma (Keller et al. 2012). It is projected that by the year 2050, 39 % of all trauma-related hospitalizations will be in those ≥65 years of age (MacKenzie et al. 1990).

Current treatment guidelines for injured adults ≥65 years of age recommend judicious prehospital triage to designated trauma centers, early recognition of comorbidities, identification and reversal of anticoagulation within 2 h of injury, trauma activation and admission to ICU for older adults with GCS <15 or a serum base deficit ≤6 mEq/L, and reassessment of treatment options in the setting of continued GCS of ≤8 after 72 h in the absence of sedation (Calland et al. 2012). Vital sign parameters used in assessing injury severity also require adaptation in the older population. Systolic blood pressures less than 110 mmHg have been shown to be indicative of increased mortality in injured, older adults. Fluid resuscitation should be guided by cardiac index measurements, base deficit trends, and the use of pulmonary artery catheters which may be beneficial in this population (Bonne and Schuerer 2013).

Mortality in older patients with head trauma rises with increasing age. CT scanning should be rapidly initiated as significant intercranial bleeding can occur despite minor injury mechanisms or inconclusive or even non-focal presenting neurological examinations. Cervical spine injuries also occur more frequently in this population compared to younger trauma patients with similar minor mechanisms due to degenerative disease and stenosis. Atypical presentations and lack of neurological symptoms or cervical pain are not uncommon, and a high index of suspicion should be maintained until cervical injury can be entirely ruled out through physical examination via tertiary survey once obvious injuries have been addressed. Thoracic and lumbar spinal injuries should also be carefully ruled out given the changes associated with aging of the skeletal system and atypical physical examination findings.

Blunt chest trauma occurs in 25 % of older adults involved in MVCs with an increase in morbidity and mortality from respiratory complications seen with three or fewer rib fractures. Properly applied lap/shoulder belt restraints can contribute to chest injuries because of the physiologic changes that occur to the thoracic cage of older adults. Hospital admission is strongly encouraged with ≥2 fractured ribs with ICU admission recommended for fracture of >6 ribs (Bonne and Schuerer 2013; Hawk et al. 2012). The presence of flail chest with pulmonary contusions has been shown to double mortality rates (Clark et al. 1988). The use of epidural analgesia or spinal regional blocks is encouraged if not contraindicated.

Pelvic fractures in older adults occur more commonly in lateral compression patterns as compared to younger patients. The use of angiography should be routinely considered as occult bleeding is often not seen on routine radiological studies and often accompanies the presence of long-bone fractures in older trauma patients (Bonne and Schuerer 2013).

Knowledge of the assessment and management of acute pain in older adults is critical in the management of not only thoracic injuries but should be a primary consideration when managing all aspects of injury care in this population. Older adults often have persistent pain prior to their new injury, are reluctant to report pain, use a wide vocabulary to describe the sensation of pain, and may not be comfortable using commonly used pain intensity assessment tools. Healthcare providers lack knowledge and understanding of both acute and persistent pain management in this segment of the population.

Finally, the use of geriatric trauma consult services and the creation of geriatric trauma-specific hospital units have shown decreases in length of hospital and ICU stays; significant decrease in complications such as urinary tract infections, respiratory failure, pneumonia, acute renal failure, and delirium; and decreased admissions to long-term care facilities (Lenartowicz et al. 2012; Mangram et al. 2012).

Cross-References

▶ Acute Pain Management in Trauma
▶ Advance Directive
▶ ARDS, Complication of Trauma
▶ Atelectasis
▶ Chest Wall Injury
▶ Delirium as a Complication of ICU Care
▶ Discharge Planning
▶ Elderly Trauma, Anesthetic Considerations for
▶ End-of-Life Care Communication in Trauma Patients
▶ Ethical Issue in Rehabilitation in Trauma Patients
▶ Evaluating a Patient's Decision-Making Capacity
▶ Falls
▶ Fluid, Electrolytes, and Nutrition in Trauma Patients
▶ Hemodynamic Monitoring
▶ ICU Management
▶ Life Support, Withholding and Withdrawal of
▶ Motor Vehicle Crash Injury
▶ Pain
▶ Pedestrian Struck
▶ Resuscitation Goals in Trauma Patients
▶ Trauma Centers

References

Bonne S, Schuerer DJ (2013) Trauma in the older adult: epidemiology and evolving geriatric trauma principles. Clin Geriatr Med 29(1):137–150
Calland JF, Ingraham AM, Martin N, Marshall GT, Schulman CI, Stapleton T, Barraco RD (2012) Evaluation and management of geriatric trauma: an Eastern Association for the Surgery of trauma practice management guideline. J Trauma Acute Care Surg 73(5 Suppl 4):S345–S350

Clark GC, Schecter WP, Trunkey DD (1988) Variables affecting outcome in blunt chest trauma: flail chest vs. pulmonary contusion. J Trauma 28(3):298–304
Hawk M, Cataldo J, Puntillo K, Miaskowski C (2012) Blunt thoracic injury in older adults: application of Haddon's phase-factor matrix model. J Gerontol Nurs 38(2):14–27
Keller JM, Sciadini MF, Sinclair E, O'Toole RV (2012) Geriatric trauma: demographics, injuries, and mortality. J Orthop Trauma 26(9):e161–e165
Lenartowicz M, Parkovnick M, McFarlan A, Haas B, Straus SE, Nathens AB, Wong CL (2012) An evaluation of a proactive geriatric trauma consultation service. Ann Surg 256(6):1098–1101
MacKenzie EJ, Morris JA, Smith GS, Fahey M (1990) Acute hospital costs of trauma in the United States: implications for regionalized systems of care. J Trauma 30(9):1096–1101
Mangram AJ, Mitchell CD, Shifflette VK, Lorenzo M, Truitt MS, Goel A, Dunn EL (2012) Geriatric trauma service: a one-year experience. J Trauma Acute Care Surg 72(1):119–122
Werman HA, Erskine T, Caterino J, Riebe JF, Valasek T (2011) Development of statewide geriatric patients trauma triage criteria. Prehosp Disaster Med 26(3):170–179

Gerotrauma

▶ Geriatric Trauma

GI Bleeding

▶ Gastrointestinal Hemorrhage

GI Hemorrhage

▶ Gastrointestinal Hemorrhage

Glasgow Coma Scale

▶ Traumatic Brain Injury, Intensive Care Unit Management

Glenoid Fracture

▶ Scapula Fractures

Glucose Control

▶ Intensive Insulin Therapy in Surgery/Trauma

Gluteal

▶ Compartment Syndrome

Glycemic Control

▶ Intensive Insulin Therapy in Surgery/Trauma

Gravid Trauma Patient

▶ Pregnant Trauma Patient, Anesthetic Considerations for the

Grenade

▶ Mortars

Guardian

▶ Family Preparation for Organ Donation

Guidelines

▶ Resuscitation Goals in Trauma Patients

Gunshot Wound Injuries

▶ Firearm-Related Injuries

Gunshot Wounds to the Extremity

Craig Bartlett, Bryan Monier, Michael Wright
and Alex Lesiak
Department of Orthopaedics and Rehabilitation,
University of Vermont/Fletcher Allen
Healthcare, Burlington, VT, USA

Synonyms

Ballistic trauma; Bullet wound; Firearm-related injury; Firearm wound; Penetrating trauma from firearm

Definition

A wound made by the penetration of an extremity (arms or legs) by a bullet or other missile projected by a firearm is commonly marked by a small entrance wound and a larger exit wound. The injury can result in damage to blood vessels, bones, muscle, and other tissues, and there is a risk of infection caused by exposure of the injured tissue to the external environment and debris carried inside the body by the bullet. Additional complications depend on the part of the body wounded. To some degree, gunshot wounds to the extremity are defined by the type of firearm, projectile velocity, and projectile mass. Each of these variables contributes to the kinetic energy delivered by the bullet and to the resultant damage to the musculoskeletal tissue. The projectile mass and its velocity can be used to calculate the amount of kinetic energy that could be delivered by the projectile ($KE = 1/2mv^2$). Typically, bullet wounds are classified as low or high velocity. Low-velocity wounds are considered less severe, are more common in the

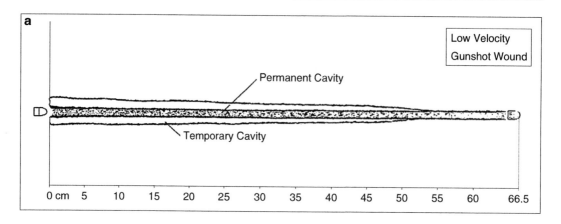

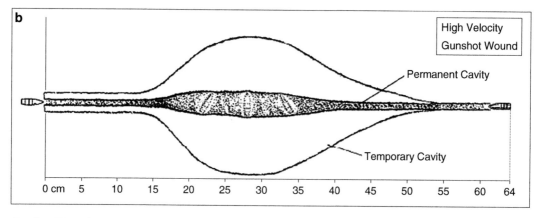

Gunshot Wounds to the Extremity, Fig. 1 (**a**) Low-velocity path of injury. (**b**) High-velocity path of injury (Credit Bowen and Bellamy (1988))

civilian population, and result from projectiles with muzzle velocities less than 2,000 ft per second. Tissue damage usually is more substantial with higher-velocity (>2,000 ft/s) military and hunting weapons. Figures 1a, b demonstrate the temporary cavity created by low- and high-velocity gunshot wounds, respectively.

Preexisting Condition

Extremity gunshot wounds may represent life-threatening injury, especially when associated with vascular injury. While these are sometimes isolated injuries, additional orthopedic injuries and at least one non-orthopedic injury were present in 41 % and 52 % of patients, respectively (Brown et al. 1997).

Application

While the type of weapon plays a role in treatment, it is the amount and type of tissue damage that plays the primary role in dictating the treatment of gunshot wounds. In general, the higher the impact velocity, the greater the size of the entrance wound and the larger the wound channel (Tian-Shun et al. 1988).

General Considerations
An initial trauma evaluation should occur first starting with the ABCs. Gunshot wounds should be evaluated for entrance and exit wounds with concern for injury to surrounding structures. Clothing, wadding and other debris may get transported deep into the wound and can be missed on first glance. Detailed evaluation of the extremities is critical as there are many

traversing neurovascular structures along with the possibility for joint involvement. Some studies have shown an overall 17 % incidence of vascular injury in gunshot wounds of the extremities (Ordog et al. 1994). Physical exam findings such as a pulse deficit, cold, lifeless extremity, cyanosis distal to a wound, a bruit or thrill, pulsatile or uncontrollable bleeding, or expanding hematoma should alert the provider to a vascular injury. Doppler ultrasonography and ABIs (ankle brachial indexes – <1.2 concerning for arterial injury) can be used along with arteriography if a vascular injury is suspected. Clear clinical findings of vascular injury may not need to be confirmed with arteriography and can be treated with operative intervention. Arterial injury should also alert the practitioner to possible nerve injury as well as they often run in conjunction. Nerve injuries should be evaluated and documented but do not generally benefit from early intervention as most are neuropraxic and improve over time. EMGs in the early post injury period cannot distinguish between a neuropraxic lesion and a transection. Imaging should involve radiographs of the injured area along with the joint above and below. Joint involvement should be considered when the wounds are in proximity to a major joint and can often be predicted by the fracture pattern on plain radiographs. Other clues include air in the joint, intra-articular hematoma, and an intra-articular fracture. Aspiration or injection with saline and methylene blue or a CT scan may also aid in the diagnosis. Joint involvement requires surgical exploration as bullets or fragments can cause mechanical trauma leading to arthritis and loss of function as well as lead toxicity due to absorption through the synovium. Most authors recommend routine antibiotic prophylaxis especially in grossly contaminated wounds. Tetanus prophylaxis is required for those who are incompletely immunized or who are uncertain of their immunization history. Table 1 summarizes the recommended Tetanus prophylaxis for gunshot wound patients.

Low-Velocity Gunshot Wound

Low-velocity injuries (<2,000 ft/s) can usually be treated non-operatively with local wound care,

Gunshot Wounds to the Extremity, Table 1 Tetanus prophylaxis recommendations for gunshot wound patients

Number of previous tetanus vaccinations	Give Td	Give TIG
Uncertain or <3	Yes	Yes
3 or more	No	No

Adapted from Recommendations of the Immunization Practices Advisory committee on (ACIP) (2011)
For adults and children 7 years of age or older, Td is preferred to tetanus toxoid alone. For children less than 7 years of age, DTP (DT, if pertussis vaccine is contraindicated) is preferred to tetanus toxoid alone. If only 3 doses of fluid toxoid have been received, a fourth dose of toxoid, preferably an adsorbed toxoid, should be given. A booster should be given if more than 5 years since the last dose
Td adult-type tetanus and diphtheria toxoid, *TIG* tetanus immune globulin

irrigation and debridement and dressing in the emergency department, with or without antibiotics, immobilization of fractures, and outpatient follow-up management (Brettler et al. 1979). Low-energy, uncontaminated wounds of the skin, subcutaneous tissue, and muscle and fractures that can be treated non-operatively fall into this category. Tetanus prophylaxis is required for those who are incompletely immunized or who are uncertain of their immunization history. Fractures may be treated as they normally would in other traumatic settings.

High-Velocity Gunshot Wound

High-velocity injuries and grossly contaminated wounds mandate aggressive irrigation and debridement, including a thorough search for foreign material (Hampton 1961). Open fracture protocols including external fixation or intramedullary nailing and intravenous antibiotics for 48–72 h should be instituted. The surgical treatment of patients with gunshot wounds, significant vascular trauma, and unstable fracture should involve a discussion between the orthopedic and vascular surgeons regarding the optimal timing of procedures for that particular patient. In this setting, vascular exploration and repair are often performed after prompt fracture stabilization (Koval 2009).

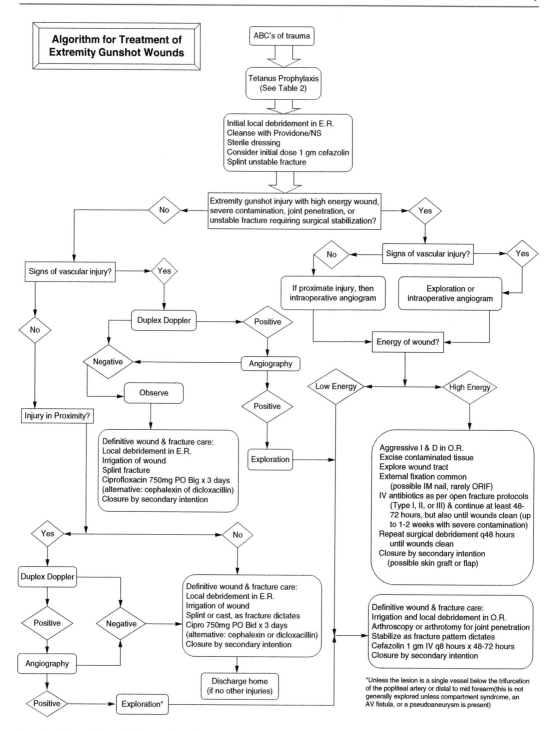

Gunshot Wounds to the Extremity, Fig. 2 Algorithm for treatment of extremity gunshot wounds. *ABC* airway, breathing, circulation, *BID* twice daily, *E.R.* emergency room, *gm* gram, *I&D* irrigation and debridement, *IM* intramedullary, *IV* intravenous, *NS* normal saline, *O.R.* operating room, *ORIF* open reduction and internal fixation, *PO* by mouth, *q48* every 48

Shotgun Wounds

Shotgun injuries are unique in that the wounds and management are often dependent on the range of the weapon and resulting injuries. Damage is based on the range, barrel length (federal law requires a minimum of 18 in.), smoothbore, choke, load, type of ammunition, wadding, and powder charge used. Shot pellets generally separate approximately 1 in. per yard as they travel from 2 to 100 yards. This allows the practitioner to estimate the range of the wound depending on the spread of the shot on the patient. Shotgun wounds are graded from Type 0 to Type III as follows: Type III range <3 yards with extensive soft tissue destruction and bacterial contamination. They are best treated aggressively with irrigation and debridement, antibiotics, and hospitalization. Type II range <3–7 yards and are almost as severe due to the pellets penetration deep to fascia. They also require aggressive treatment as it has been shown that Type II–III wounds are associated with high rates of comminuted fractures (32–48 %), major soft tissue disruption (43–59 %), vascular injury (23–35 %), and peripheral nerve damage (21–58 %) (Bartlett et al. 2000). Type I wounds are from ranges >7 yards and often do not produce major soft tissue disruption due to the scatter of the pellets. Because these pellets only penetrate the subcutaneous tissues and deep fascia, they can be treated as low-velocity wounds with local wound care and outpatient follow-up. Type 0 are >20 yards and cause very minimal damage.

Conclusion

Occasionally a high-velocity injury in flexible tissue results in a through and through injury without much collateral damage, while a low-velocity injury can lead to significant bone and tissue damage depending on the area of involvement and range. While identification of the type of projectile (low or high velocity) is useful, it is important to remember that the clinician should concentrate on treating the wound rather than the weapon (Lindsey 1980).

As the surface wound often represents the "tip of the iceberg," it is essential that the surgeon approaches each injury with the same attention to detail to ensure proper treatment. Figure 2 provides an algorithm that can guide decision-making when a patient with a gunshot wound is encountered.

Cross-References

▶ Ballistics
▶ Blast
▶ Damage Control Orthopedics
▶ Extremity Injury
▶ Open Fractures

References

Bartlett CS, Helfet DL, Hausman MR, Strauss E (2000) Ballistics and gunshot wounds: effects on musculoskeletal tissues. J Am Acad Orthop Surg 8(1):21–36, PubMed PMID: 10666650

Bowen TE, Bellamy RF (1988) Emergency war surgery-NATO handbook, US rev. Government Printing Office, Washington, DC

Brettler D, Sedlin ED, Mendes DG (1979) Conservative treatment of low velocity gunshot wounds. Clin Orthop Relat Res 140:26–31, PubMed PMID: 477080

Brown TD, Michas P, Williams RE, Dawson G, Whitecloud TS, Barrack RL (1997) The impact of gunshot wounds on an orthopaedic surgical service in an urban trauma center. J Orthop Trauma 11(3):149–153, PubMed PMID: 9181495

Hampton OP Jr (1961) The indications for debridement of gun shot (bullet) wounds of the extremities in civilian practice. J Trauma 1:368–372, PubMed PMID: 13711136

Koval KJ (2009) Gunshot wounds and open fractures. AAOS Compr Orthop Rev 1:533–537

Lindsey D (1980) Letter: the idolatry of velocity, or lies, damn lies, and ballistics. J Trauma 20:1068–1069

Ordog GJ et al (1994) Extremity gunshot wounds: part one. Identification and treatment of patients at high risk of vascular injury. J Trauma 36(3):358–368

Recommendations of the Immunization Practices Advisory committee on (ACIP) (1991) Diphtheria, tetanus, and pertussis: recommendations for vaccine use and other preventive measures. MMWR 40(RR-10):1–28

Tian-Shun F, Yuyuan M, Rong-Xiang F, Ming L (1988) The wounding characteristics of spherical steel fragments in live tissues. J Trauma 28(Suppl 1):S37–S40

G

Gut Mucosal Atrophy

Indraneil Mukherjee[1] and
Khanjan H. Nagarsheth[2]
[1]The Southeastern Center for Digestive
Disorders & Pancreatic Cancer, Advanced
Minimally Invasive & Robotic Surgery,
Florida Hospital Tampa, Tampa, FL, USA
[2]R Adams Cowley Shock Trauma Center,
University of Maryland School of Medicine,
Baltimore, MD, USA

Synonyms

Intestinal epithelial apoptosis; Starvation-induced small bowel atrophy

Definition

Mucosal atrophy is defined as anatomical changes in the intestinal mucosa such as reduced number of cells, decreased surface area, and shortened villous height and crypt depth, with subsequent loss of intestinal function.

Preexisting Condition

The gut mucosa starts at the vermilion border at the lip and extends to the dentate line at the anus. The intestinal mucosa, in particular, serves many functions, including digestion and nutrient absorption; it serves as a barrier and has immunological properties as well. It is also adaptable to many situations like starvation, metabolic diseases, and intestinal surgery.These adaptations can be either proliferative or atrophic.

Enterocytes are the dominant cells that form the intestinal brush border. The microvilli at their luminal end are the functional component containing the enzymes and the glycocalyx coat

---

The original version of this entry was revised. An erratum can be found at http://dx.doi.org/10.1007/978-3-642-29613-0_1010

that acts as a physical barrier. The mucosal surface forms villi by extensions of the lamina and then the submucosa folds to form the plicae circulares. This specific anatomical feature increases the surface area. The mucosa is formed by crypt-villus units which include the stem cells, which give rise to the progenitor cells. These progenitor cells further differentiate into absorptive and secretory cells. The stem cells are present throughout life in the crypts; their proliferation is regulated via multiple signals ranging from external diet to hormones and immunity.

In proliferation there is an increase in villus height, crypt depth, and surface area. In the augmentation of intestinal function, there is increased function of not only the epithelial cells but also the deeper cells, such as blood vessels and secretory cells.

Finally, the last kind of adaptation is atrophy. It usually is a result of starvation which reduces enteral nutrition. Supporting the patient with adequate parenteral nutrition has been unsuccessful in preventing atrophy. The atrophic changes result in a failure of the adaptive functions of proliferation, augmentation, and differentiation as well as increased apoptosis.

Multiple animal studies have found that mucosal atrophy is characterized by a decrease in intestinal weight and nitrogen content. The intestine has fewer Peyer's patches and T cells, thereby decreasing the immunological capabilities. The mucosal hypoplasia is mediated by an alteration in the tumor necrosis factor (TNF)-α/EGF signaling pathway. The use of total parenteral nutrition (TPN) may actually cause enterocyte apoptosis and stimulation of ion secretion, via intra-epithelial lymphocyte-derived interferon-gamma, causing a decrease in the barrier function of the mucosa. Direct contact with luminal food and chyme has also been found to be important for mucosal integrity (Shaw 2012).

Mucosal atrophy is a significant problem in the setting of starvation. In the milieu of modern-day healthcare, it is a major problem in the setting of trauma. In these scenarios, gut mucosal atrophy increases sepsis rates dramatically (Kudsk et al. 1992). It is also evident in prolonged starvation for various medical conditions like pancreatitis and short bowel syndrome. Short bowel syndrome is usually secondary to intestinal resections for inflammatory bowel disease, ischemia, and obstruction. In the pediatric age group, it is mostly seen in cases of necrotizing enterocolitis, intestinal malrotations, and atresias. Total parenteral nutrition is used to manage prolonged starvation but may not be beneficial in this regard (Sax 2010). These can be significant enough to cause "intestinal failure" and failure to thrive. It is seen when the absorptive surface is so low that patients have diarrhea, dehydration, malnutrition, and electrolyte disturbance.

Application

Total parenteral nutrition has been the mainstay of management for intestinal failure. This form of nutrition is critical in the short term and in many cases is needed on a chronic basis to maintain homeostasis and electrolyte balance. Total parenteral nutrition should only be used for long-term therapy in extreme cases. There are many known side effects and complications associated with chronic parenteral nutrition use. These complications include catheter malfunctions, infections, and liver failure. In such situation serious consideration should be made about small bowel transplant and management by an multidisciplinary team (Modi et al. 2008).

The therapy in this situation should be geared towards reversing mucosal atrophy and promoting adaptations by proliferation, augmentation, and differentiation.

Even small amounts of enteral nutrition can improve intestinal epithelial growth, motility, and absorption (Perdikis 1997). Lipids in the diet as well as its use in parenteral nutrition add significant benefit. Luminal lipids have been shown to increase adaptation and function of the mucosa. Short-chain fatty acids are shown to reduce mucosal atrophy and promote adaptation. Proteins and amino acids like glutamine improves gut mucosal health by enhancing mucosal function and retards atrophy. Supplements like retinoic acid and ornithine α-ketoglutarate have also shown to improve adaption. Antibiotics may reduce malabsorption and reverse mucosal atrophy by reducing bacterial overgrowth. Epidermal growth factor and glucagon-like peptide-2 have also been used in many controlled settings to improve adaptation. Experimental therapies using leptin, bombesin, and ghrelin may be used in the future for this purpose.

Cross-References

▶ Nutritional Deficiency/Starvation
▶ Nutritional Support

References

Kudsk KA, Croce MA, Fabian TC, Minard G, Tolley EA, Poret HA, Kuhl MR, Brown RO (1992) Enteral versus parenteral feeding. Effects on septic morbidity after blunt and penetrating abdominal trauma. Ann Surg 215:503–511, discussion 511–513

Modi BP, Langer M, Ching YA, Valim C, Waterford SD, Iglesias J, Duro D, Lo C, Jaksic T, Duggan C (2008) Improved survival in a multidisciplinary short bowel syndrome program. J Pediatr Surg 43(1):20–24. doi:10.1016/j.jpedsurg.2007.09.014

Perdikis DA, Basson MD (1997) Basal nutrition promotes human intestinal epithelial (Caco-2) proliferation, brush border enzyme activity, and motility. Crit Care Med 25:159–165

Sax HC (2010) Management of short bowel syndrome. In: Cameron JL, Cameron AM (eds) Current surgical therapy, 10th edn. Elsevier, Philadelphia

Shaw D, Gohil K, Basson MD (2012) Intestinal mucosal atrophy and adaptation. World J Gastroenterol 18(44):6357–6375

H

Haemocomplettan®

▶ Adjuncts to Transfusion: Fibrinogen Concentrate

Handgun Injuries

▶ Firearm-Related Injuries

Hangman's Fracture

▶ Fracture, Axis (C2)

Harm

▶ Interpersonal Violence

Head Injuries

▶ Bicycle-Related Injuries

Head Injury

▶ Neurotrauma, Anesthesia Management
▶ Neurotrauma, Prognosis and Outcome Predictions

▶ Traumatic Brain Injury, Anesthesia for
▶ Traumatic Brain Injury, Emergency Department Care
▶ Traumatic Brain Injury, Mild (mTBI)
▶ Traumatic Brain Injury, Severe: Medical and Surgical Management

Head Trauma

▶ Neurotrauma, Introduction
▶ Traumatic Brain Injury, Mild (mTBI)

Head Trauma Rehabilitation

▶ Ethical Issue in Rehabilitation in Trauma Patients

Head-On Crashes

▶ Motor Vehicle Crashes (MVC), Frontal Impact

"Head-Ons"

▶ Motor Vehicle Crashes (MVC), Frontal Impact

© Springer-Verlag Berlin Heidelberg 2015
P.J. Papadakos, M.L. Gestring (eds.), *Encyclopedia of Trauma Care*,
DOI 10.1007/978-3-642-29613-0

Healing by Secondary and Tertiary Intention

▶ Delayed Wound Closure

Health Associate

▶ Physician Assistant

Health Care Etiquette

▶ Technology Interfacing, Etiquette, and Electronic Safety

Health-Care Advocate

▶ Family Preparation for Organ Donation

Health-Care-Associated Infection

▶ Surgical Site Infections

Heart-Lung Interactions

John Granton
Division of Respirology at University
Health Network, Mount Sinai
Hospital and Women's College Hospital,
Toronto, ON, Canada
Department of Medicine, and Interdepartmental,
Division of Critical Care, Faculty of Medicine,
University of Toronto, Toronto, ON, Canada

Synonyms

Cardiopulmonary interactions

Definition

Heart-lung or cardiopulmonary interactions relate to the effect of lung inflation on cardiac function. In critical care, this usually relates to the effects of positive pressure ventilation. The effect of positive pressure ventilation on cardiac function is mediated through several mechanisms (Table 1). The consequence of these mechanisms depends on the mechanical properties of the lung and thorax as well as the volume status and baseline cardiac function of the patient.

For purposes of this entry, I will focus upon the effects of continuous (non-phasic) pressure applied in the airway either invasively or noninvasively upon cardiac function. The rules:

1. The effects of positive airway pressure on cardiac function depend upon lung, chest wall, and abdominal mechanics.
2. The effects of changes in airway pressure on cardiac function depend upon intravascular and cardiac volume status and intrinsic function of the heart.

Changes in airway pressure affect cardiac function in many ways. However, the most important affect is via changes in intrapleural (Ppl) pressure. It is important to recognize that in order for Ppl to increase with the application of airway pressure (at the mouth or the end of an endotracheal tube), lung inflation must occur against a less compliant thorax (e.g., chest wall, abdomen). As a result, the degree to which a given airway pressure changes Ppl depends upon the compliance of the lung and thorax. Therefore, a patient with a stiff thorax will experience a greater increase in Ppl than a patient with a compliant thorax for a given

Heart-Lung Interactions, Table 1 Factors that mediate the effects of the lung on cardiac function

Changes in alveolar pressure
Changes in pleural/pericardial pressure
Changes in lung inflation
Changes in alveolar oxygen tension
Changes in arterial blood gases
Changes in intra-abdominal pressure

level of airway pressure. Similarly, a patient with reduced lung compliance, an increase in airway pressure will have less influence on Ppl (assuming that the lungs are not already hyperinflated) than a patient with normal chest compliance.

Changes in airway pressure can have a positive or negative effect on oxygen delivery. In patients with hypoxemia, the application of PEEP can lead to an increase in oxygen saturation and arterial oxygen content. However, higher levels of PEEP may be associated with worsening oxygen delivery owing to negative effects on cardiac function. These effects are mediated through changes in heart rate, as well as stroke volume. The changes in stroke volume are primarily mediated through effects on ventricular preload and afterload. For purposes of this entry, I will only focus upon the effects of positive pressure ventilation on loading conditions of the heart. At least in the acute setting, there is unlikely any immediate effect on contractility. In developing the principles of cardiopulmonary interactions, it is useful to consider the effects of positive pressure on the right ventricle (RV) and left ventricle (LV) separately.

Preexisting Condition

Right Ventricular Preload

The most important principle to consider is the effect of positive airway pressure on RV preload. Increases in Ppl mediated by changes in airway pressure and ensuing lung inflation generally leads to a reduction in venous return. This is mediated through an increase in right atrial pressure (essentially reducing compliance of that structure). As flow is dependent upon the pressure gradient between the resting circulatory pressure (venous pressure external to the thorax) and right atrial pressure (RAP), as RAP increases, venous return is reduced (Fig. 1a). This effect on venous return may be overcome by either increasing resting circulatory volume (and pressure) by fluid loading or increasing venous tone. This effect on venous return may also be overcome through an increase in intra-abdominal pressure resulting from descent of the diaphragm. As illustrated by a study in normal patients after cardiac bypass, the increase in intra-abdominal pressure mediated by descent of the diaphragm was capable of negating the effects on Ppl and RAP – an

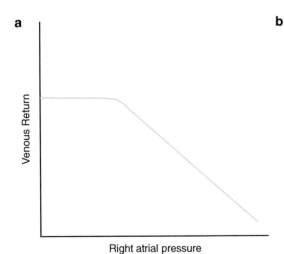

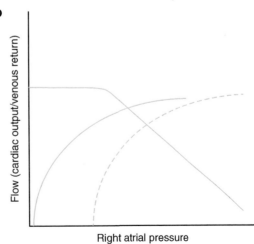

Heart-Lung Interactions, Fig. 1 (**a**) The relationship between right atrial pressure and venous return. As right atrial pressure is increased (as might occur with an increase in intrathoracic pressure), venous return is reduced. (**b**) The influence of venous return on cardiac function depends upon where it intersects the cardiac function curve. Changes in venous return will not have a significant influence along the flat portion of the cardiac function curve (solid line). Conversely, changes in venous return will have a significant influence if it intersects with the steep portion of the curve (dashed line)

effect analogous to the hepato-jugular reflux maneuver (van den Berg et al. 2002). This paper serves to emphasize that the effects of intrapleural pressure on venous return are highly dependent upon the volume status of the patient, resting intra-abdominal compliance, and venous tone. For example, the hypovolemic and septic patient who is placed on positive pressure ventilation may be very susceptible to the ensuing reduction in venous return. Furthermore, they may be incapable of responding through the recruitment of blood volume to their central circulation by changes in venous tone. Diaphragmatic descent may worsen venous return in a patient with intra-abdominal hypertension.

It is important to recognize that changes in venous return on cardiac function are dependent upon the resting loading conditions of the heart. Specifically, it is dependent upon the point at which the venous return curve intersects the cardiac function (Starling) curve. If the venous return curve intersects the steep portion of the cardiac function curve, there will be minimal effect. However, if it intersects the steeper portion of the cardiac function curve, changes in venous return will have an influence on stroke volume (Fig. 1b).

Right Ventricular Afterload

The effects of an increase on right ventricular afterload are complex. In classical physiology teaching, there is a parabolic relationship between lung volume and pulmonary vascular resistance (PVR). As the lung moves toward low lung volumes (residual volume), pulmonary vascular resistance may be increased through loss of patency of extra-alveolar blood vessels. As the lung expands beyond functional resting capacity, PVR increases as the alveolar blood vessels and capillaries are narrowed through stretch or in the case of positive pressure ventilation – direct compression – in effect causing a West Zone I condition where pulmonary blood flow becomes dependent upon alveolar pressure and not the pulmonary arterial to pulmonary venous pressure gradient. For this reason, many feel that the use of positive airway pressure in patients with failing RVs is contraindicated. In reality, this application

of classic physiology to the critical care setting may be an oversimplification. In an elegant series of experiments, Duggan et al. demonstrated that animals with lung injury that developed atelectasis developed severe RV dysfunction – presumably due to an increase in RV afterload caused by hypoxic pulmonary vasoconstriction (Duggan et al. 2003). In animals that underwent lung recruitment, through the application of positive airway pressure, the RV function returned to normal. Consequently, the effects of positive airway pressure on RV afterload depend upon where you start and where you finish. If it leads to alveolar recruitment, there may be a beneficial effect. However, if there is overdistention or if alveolar pressure becomes excessive, RV dilation or dysfunction may develop. The relevance is illustrated in a recent paper that evaluated the effects of high frequency oscillation on RV size (Guervilly et al. 2012). At higher levels of mean airway pressure, the RV became dilated. Although there were no measurements of RV function, higher levels of mean airway pressure were associated with systemic markers of hypoperfusion. Though the clinical relevance of these findings remains to be seen relative to the potential benefits of HFO on ventilator induced lung injury, the paper serves to illustrate the potential adverse effects of high airway pressure on cardiac function.

Left Ventricular Preload

The extent to which the application of positive airway pressure changes RV output will have an effect on LV preload. In essence, the LV gets what the RV delivers. Additionally, an increase in intrathoracic pressure directly decreases left ventricular end-diastolic volume by producing constraint on the left atrium and left ventricle. However, if positive pressure leads to RV dilation, then there may be an additional influence upon LV preload through septal shift. It is well known that RV dilation in the setting of high RV afterload (as seen in patients with pulmonary arterial hypertension) may adversely affect LV preload. In a study by Mitchell et al., the effects of positive airway pressure on venous return and ventricular interaction were evaluated in a closed

Heart-Lung Interactions, Fig. 2 Effects of intrathoracic pressure on left ventricular afterload. The application of positive pressure at the airway will cause an increase in intrapleural pressure. As a result, *transmural pressure* is reduced

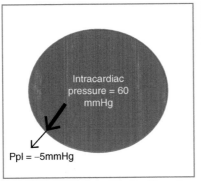

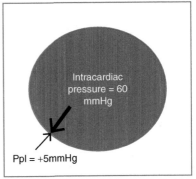

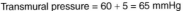

Transmural pressure = 60 + 5 = 65 mmHg   Transmural pressure = 60 − 5 = 55 mmHg

chest dog model (Mitchell et al. 2005a). Here positive pressure ventilation led to RV dilation and decreased left ventricular end-diastolic volume by leftward septal shift.

Left Ventricular Afterload

Increases in intrapleural pressure (more positive) during positive pressure ventilation lead to a reduction in LV afterload. This effect is felt to be mediated by a reduction in transmural myocardial pressure. As seen in Fig. 2, in the resting state, intrapleural pressure is negative. The transmural pressure is therefore the mean LV pressure less Ppl or 65 mmHg. With the application of positive airway pressure, Ppl increases and transmural pressure is reduced: in this example, to 55 mmHg. In a normal ventricle, this degree of reduction in LV afterload will have little effect. However, a failing left ventricle is exquisitely sensitive to changes in afterload. Consequently, even subtle reductions in LV afterload may lead to an improvement in stroke volume.

Application

The potential influence of airway pressure and lung volume on cardiac function is important to consider in a critically ill patient for several reasons. First, a rise in airway pressure may lead to a deleterious effect on stroke volume in a hypovolemic patient. Consequently, efforts to reduce Ppl may lead to an improvement in venous return and stroke volume. An adverse increase in Ppl may be seen in patients with large pleural effusions, ascites, chest wall edema, obesity, scars across the chest wall. Consequently, pleural drainage, patient positioning, and escarotomy may lead to reductions in Ppl and improve venous return. As discussed, increases in alveolar volume and pressure may lead to an adverse increase in RV afterload and impair RV ejection and potentially LV filling via septal influence if the RV dilates. This effect may be observed in patients with high mean airway pressures. In a study by Guervilly et al., higher levels of mean airway pressure during high frequency oscillation led to RV dilation and evidence of systemic hypoperfusion. Recognition of this effect should prompt the clinician to reduce mean airway pressure.

Conversely, increases in airway pressure may be therapeutic. CPAP and PEEP have been shown to lead to an improvement in LV function during acute congestive heart failure (Peter et al. 2006). This beneficial effect may be mediated through a reduction in LV preload (via reduction in venous return – similar to the effect of diuresis) as well as reductions in LV afterload. The application of CPAP may also be beneficial in the postoperative state by reducing atelectasis and both the resultant hypoxemia and adverse influence of atelectasis on RV function. In a recent series of experiments, McCaul et al. presented the potential influence of positive pressure on outcome in an animal model of cardiac arrest (McCaul et al. 2009). The beneficial effect was felt to be secondary to improvements in cardiac function as opposed to oxygenation.

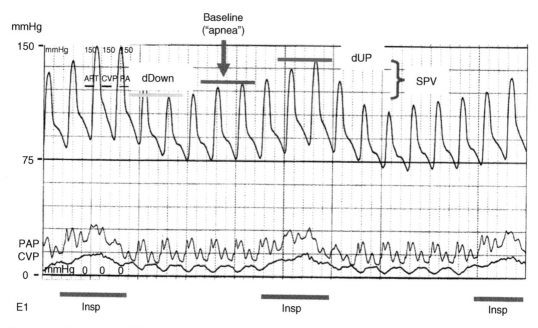

Heart-Lung Interactions, Fig. 3 An example of respiratory variation in arterial pressure. Reprinted with permission of the American Thoracic Society. Copyright © 2013 American Thoracic Society. Magder (2004). During a positive pressure breath, the pulmonary artery pressure (*PAP*) and central venous pressure (*CVP*) increase. The dUp and dDown components of the arterial pressure tracing represent the aggregate influence of the changes in intrapleural and intrathoracic pressure on cardiac function. The *bars* at the bottom indicate inspiration. The *arrow* at the point marked "apnea" represents the end-expiration value for determining dUp and dDown

Finally, variation in positive airway pressure – as occurs during the cycles of mechanical ventilation – may be used to evaluate volume status (Magder 2004). Systemic systolic and pulse pressure variation has been shown to be a useful method to assess volume status and fluid responsiveness. During inspiration (positive pressure), systemic blood pressure initially increases (Fig. 3). This initial increase has been attributed to: (1) movement of blood from the alveolar vessels into the LV, (2) a reduction in LV afterload, and (3) rightward septal shift accommodating LV filling (Mitchell et al. 2005b; Magder 2004). During inflation, however, the effects of a reduction in venous return on LV filling eventually prevail. This reduction in venous return as well as a leftward shift of the intraventricular septum likely leads to the observed reduction in systolic pressure (Mitchell et al. 2005a). The difference in the peak to nadir systolic pressure and pulse pressure has been advocated as a measure of

volume status. Additionally, a reduction in the pulse pressure and systolic pressure variability with fluid bolus has been shown to reflect a volume responsive state. Indeed, these measures appear to be superior to more conventional measurements such as CVP (Marik et al. 2009). However, in addition to volume status of the patient, the effect also depends upon the magnitude of the intrathoracic pressure change. In this regard, a large variation in thoracic pressure (as might be seen with a large pleural effusion) may artificially lead to a "false positive" (Mesquida et al. 2011). Furthermore, a small change in intrathoracic pressure – as might occur with the use of a low tidal volume, lung protective strategy in ARDS may not provide a sufficient change in Ppl – leading to a "false negative" test (Lakhal et al. 2011).

It is worth emphasizing, however, that the presence of pulse pressure variation does not necessarily imply that fluid is required. As emphasized by Magder, it is important to consider the ongoing need for fluid administration as well as the effects of fluid administration on cardiac function and systemic perfusion. Indeed excess fluid administration has been associated with worse outcomes in ARDS and sepsis (National Heart, Lung, and Blood Institute Acute Respiratory Distress Syndrome (ARDS) Clinical Trials Network et al. 2006; Maitland et al. 2011).

Cross-References

▶ Abdominal Compartment Syndrome as a Complication of Care
▶ ARDS, Complication of Trauma
▶ Atelectasis
▶ Fluid, Electrolytes, and Nutrition in Trauma Patients
▶ Pulmonary Embolism
▶ Ventilatory Management of Trauma Patients

References

Duggan M et al (2003) Atelectasis causes vascular leak and lethal right ventricular failure in uninjured rat lungs. Am J Respir Crit Care Med 167(12):1633–1640
Guervilly C et al (2012) Right ventricular function during high-frequency oscillatory ventilation in adults with acute respiratory distress syndrome. Crit Care Med 40(5):1539–1545
Lakhal K et al (2011) Respiratory pulse pressure variation fails to predict fluid responsiveness in acute respiratory distress syndrome. Crit Care 15(2):R85
Magder S (2004) Clinical usefulness of respiratory variations in arterial pressure. Am J Respir Crit Care Med 169(2):151–155
Maitland K et al (2011) Mortality after fluid bolus in African children with severe infection. N Engl J Med 364(26):2483–2495
Marik PE et al (2009) Dynamic changes in arterial waveform derived variables and fluid responsiveness in mechanically ventilated patients: a systematic review of the literature*. Crit Care Med 37(9):2642–2647
McCaul C et al (2009) Positive end-expiratory pressure improves survival in a rodent model of cardiopulmonary resuscitation using high-dose epinephrine. Anesth Analg 109(4):1202–1208
Mesquida J, Kim HK, Pinsky MR (2011) Effect of tidal volume, intrathoracic pressure, and cardiac contractility on variations in pulse pressure, stroke volume, and intrathoracic blood volume. Intensive Care Med 37(10):1672–1679
Mitchell JR, Sas R et al (2005a) Ventricular interaction during mechanical ventilation in closed-chest anesthetized dogs. Can J Cardiol 21(1):73–81
Mitchell JR, Whitelaw WA et al (2005b) RV filling modulates LV function by direct ventricular interaction during mechanical ventilation. Am J Physiol Heart Circ Physiol 289(2):H549–H557
National Heart, Lung, and Blood Institute Acute Respiratory Distress Syndrome (ARDS) Clinical Trials Network et al (2006) Comparison of two fluid-management strategies in acute lung injury. N Engl J Med 354(24):2564–2575
Peter JV et al (2006) Effect of non-invasive positive pressure ventilation (NIPPV) on mortality in patients with acute cardiogenic pulmonary oedema: a meta-analysis. Lancet 367(9517):1155–1163
van den Berg PCM, Jansen JRC, Pinsky MR (2002) Effect of positive pressure on venous return in volume-loaded cardiac surgical patients. J Appl Physiol 92(3):1223–1231

Heat Injury

▶ Burn Anesthesia

Hematobilia

▶ Hemobilia

Hemobilia

Mansoor Khan
Consultant Esophagogastric and Acute Care Surgeon, Doncaster Royal Infirmary, Doncaster, South Yorkshire, UK

Synonyms

Hematobilia; Hemobilia: hematobilia; Hemorrhage in bile

Definition

Hemorrhage into the biliary tree.

Hemobilia, Table 1 Etiology of hemobilia

Hepatobiliary trauma	Penetrating
Iatrogenic	Blunt
	Cholecystectomy
	ERCP
	Biopsies
Inflammatory biliary disease	
Arteriovenous malformations	
Tumor	
Coagulopathy	

Hemobilia is a rare (Kim and Kim 2012) cause of upper gastrointestinal bleeding, but has become widely recognized due to an increased clinical awareness of the disorder and to improvements in diagnostic techniques. Also, the growing use of percutaneous liver puncture for the diagnosis of and therapy for hepatobiliary diseases and the increased incidence of both blunt and penetrating hepatic trauma have contributed to a rising incidence of hemobilia (Merrell and Schneider 1991).

The most common cause (Table 1) is iatrogenic with the commonest non-iatrogenic causes of hemobilia being hepatobiliary malignancies, and the majority of patients presenting with jaundice and abdominal pain (Kim and Kim 2012).

The characteristic presentation, also known as Quincke's triad, consists of upper abdominal pain, upper gastrointestinal hemorrhage, and jaundice. Initial attempts must be made to stabilize and correct the patient's coagulopathy, if present. The majority of cases of bleeding will be self-limiting. Endoscopy has been advocated, especially after sphincterotomies to attempt cautery and hemostasis, and can also be used to place a stent preventing clot obstruction (Kim and Kim 2012; Singh 2007; Schouten van der Velden et al. 2010).

In severe cases, angiographic occlusion is recommended as initial treatment to control hemobilia and to render the patient stable in preparation for elective and definitive surgery. Surgery becomes necessary when nonoperative attempts to stop the bleeding fail and is required for tumors and parasitic disease (Bloechle et al. 1994).

References

Bloechle C, Izbicki JR, Rashed MY, El-Sefi T, Hosch SB, Knoefel WT, Rogiers X, Broelsch CE (1994) Hemobilia: presentation, diagnosis, and management. Am J Gastroenterol 89:1537–1540

Kim KH, Kim TN (2012) Etiology, clinical features, and endoscopic management of hemobilia: a retrospective analysis of 37 cases. Korean J Gastroenterol (Taehan Sohwagi Hakhoe chi) 59:296–302

Merrell SW, Schneider PD (1991) Hemobilia–evolution of current diagnosis and treatment. West J Med 155:621–625

Schouten Van der Velden AP, De Ruijter WM, Janssen CM, Schultze Kool LJ, Tan EC (2010) Hemobilia as a late complication after blunt abdominal trauma: a case report and review of the literature. J Emerg Med 39:592–595

Singh V (2007) Endoscopic management of traumatic hemobilia. J Trauma 62:1045–1047

Hemobilia: Hematobilia

▶ Hemobilia

Hemodiafiltration

▶ Dialysis

Hemodialysis

▶ Dialysis

Hemodynamic Management in Trauma Anesthesia

Joseph Dooley
Department of Anesthesiology, University of Rochester, Rochester, NY, USA

Synonyms

Cardiovascular system management in trauma anesthesia

Definition

The hemodynamic management of patients with trauma undergoing anesthesia is largely like the management of these patients on surgical floors, on step-down units, and on ICUs. Clearly, the management in these areas is determined by the type and severity of the trauma as well as coexisting illnesses. The specifics of hemodynamic management of the various types of trauma are addressed in detail in other entries in this publication. This entry will focus on the hemodynamic management of trauma patients undergoing surgery whose vital functions are compromised by the anesthetic and hypovolemia due to the traumatic event. The effects of anesthesia on the hemodynamic parameters of trauma patients and how this affects the anesthesiologist's choices when administering anesthesia will be explored. Lastly, strategies for the hemodynamic management of patients undergoing general anesthesia will be examined.

Preexisting Condition

Administering anesthesia for patients with acute traumatic injuries with either compromised or potentially compromised vital functions is a common situation for anesthesiologists, especially for those in tertiary care centers and trauma centers. These patients often present with multiple trauma. The most common anesthetic for these patients is general anesthesia. There are multiple reasons for this. Common reasons include but are not limited to the following:

- Multiple injuries not limited to the lower extremities or a single upper extremity precluding a regional technique.
- Patient agitation resulting from intoxication, head injury, or both. In these cases, the patient is unable to cooperate during block placement and/or is unable to stay still during the procedure.
- Pending airway compromise requiring airway control.
- The need for painful, invasive procedures for access and monitoring. Placing large-bore intravenous access for resuscitation or intra-arterial catheters for monitoring for these cases usually needs to be done expeditiously and is often done simultaneously with the surgical procedure.

For these reasons, regional techniques such as neuraxial anesthesia and extremity blocks are much less commonly used than general anesthesia for trauma cases. With the exception of the extremity blocks, all anesthetics can have significant effects on cardiovascular physiology.

Agents used for general anesthesia (induction agents and the volatile agents) depress myocardial contractility and reduce systemic vascular resistance. Induction agents, such as propofol and the barbiturates, are especially prone to cause these effects. Etomidate is considered to be the most hemodynamically stable induction agent. It must be remembered, however, that if the patient's blood pressure is being maintained by endogenous catecholamines produced by the patient's sympathetic response to pain and stress, removing the sympathetic response by rendering the patient unconscious with etomidate can result in profound hypotension. In addition, there is concern that even a single dose of etomidate can cause significant adrenal suppression resulting in hemodynamic compromise throughout the patient's hospital course. Ketamine causes the release of endogenous catecholamines. This masks the cardio-depressant effect of the drug and usually causes increased heart rate and blood pressure when the drug is administered. However, in the setting of extreme stress or prolonged stress, the patient's endogenous catecholamines can be depleted leading to hypotension on induction. This effect can be similar to the effect seen with the barbiturates and with propofol. In addition, ketamine is relatively contraindicated in major trauma with concerns that it can increase ICP in head trauma and can increase bleeding in vascular trauma. For these reasons, etomidate is usually the induction agent of choice for major trauma, but it is not ideal.

The volatile agents (isoflurane, desflurane, sevoflurane, etc.) are inhalation agents used for anesthesia maintenance and can cause varying

H

degrees of myocardial depression and vasodilatation. The degree of myocardial depression is directly related to the inhaled concentration of the drug. Nitrous oxide is an inhaled agent that has fairly minimal direct effects on hemodynamics. However, due to its low solubility, nitrous oxide can rapidly expand in trapped gas spaces in conditions such as pneumothorax or obstructed bowel. Nitrous oxide can exacerbate both. In most traumas, there is at least potential for either or both of these conditions, making nitrous oxide relatively contraindicated.

Other agents used for maintenance of anesthesia can also compromise hemodynamic stability. The narcotic agents cause venodilation (which reduces preload) and also blunt the sympathetic response to pain. Both of these effects can be especially problematic in the setting of hypovolemia. Several common anesthetic agents can cause histamine release. This can lead to hypotension and bronchospasm. These include morphine sulfate (a narcotic) and atracurium (a non-depolarizing neuromuscular blocker). The hypotension can be profound especially in the setting of hypovolemia or when given with other agents associated with hemodynamic depression such as propofol or a barbiturate.

Neuraxial anesthetic techniques can also have significant hemodynamic implications. Depending on the spinal level, these techniques can have significant effects on sympathetic tone. This results in increased venous capacitance (reducing preload) and diminished systemic vascular resistance. If the spinal level reaches T 4 and above, there can be significant effects on myocardial contractility and the ability of heart rate (and cardiac output) to compensate for hypotension.

In summary, the hemodynamic effects of general anesthesia and neuraxial anesthesia can profoundly exacerbate the deleterious effects of hypovolemia, abdominal compartment syndrome, cardiac tamponade, tension pneumothorax, etc. All of these conditions can be seen in varying degrees in trauma cases. Ideally, these conditions would be identified and treatment initiated prior to presenting to the operating room. Sometimes, the clinical situation, such as uncontrolled hemorrhage, precludes correction of these conditions, and the patient is taken directly to the operating room. This forces the anesthesiologist to accept these conditions and manage profound hemodynamic instability while inducing and maintaining anesthesia. Key to successful management of these cases is preparation and having adequate personnel.

Application

Preparation
A "trauma room" should be prepared for each call night. This includes setting up the anesthesia machine with a circuit and airway equipment. Standard anesthetic drugs and resuscitation drugs should be readily available. Equipment and kits for central access and arterial access should be stored in the room. A large-volume blood/fluid warming and administration system (such as the Level I, Smiths Medical) with unopened IV fluids and disposables should be readily available. As soon as possible after a trauma patient arrives in the Emergency Department, one or more members of the anesthesia team should start evaluating the patient and determine potential patient needs. There should be communication with the blood bank especially if a massive transfusion is anticipated or if O negative or type-specific blood is needed. Decisions about the need for calling in additional anesthesia or nursing personnel should be made. Last-minute room preparation such as warming the room, spiking IV bags, and opening disposables for the IV fluid administration system should be done. Ideally, a member of the anesthesiology team should accompany the patient from the Emergency Department to the operating room. This team member may also assist in obtaining IV access and starting resuscitation in the Emergency Department. If time and conditions permit, consideration to placing an arterial line should be made. This would greatly facilitate management during and shortly after induction of anesthesia.

Intraoperative Management
The hemodynamic management of trauma anesthesia is a broad topic. This publication

covers a wide range of trauma conditions which are seen during anesthesia for trauma surgery. The condition may be the one being surgically addressed or may be the coexisting problem. An example would be a multiple trauma patient with a splenic laceration and closed head injury (cerebral contusions) presenting for exploratory laparotomy. This entry examines the anesthetic effects of anesthesia on the generic trauma patient suffering from hypovolemia. Although the cardiovascular effects of these agents are constant over a variety of traumas, the treatment may be different. Such conditions include intracranial hypertension due to head injury, cardiac tamponade, and tension pneumothorax. The cardiovascular effects of the anesthetic agents must be considered and taken into account when managing the patient.

When the patient arrives in the room, care should be taken to minimize the time that the patient is "off monitors." Transfer monitors (ECG, blood pressure, pulse oximetry, etc.) should be removed, and operating room monitors applied in a stepwise fashion. This avoids having the patient being completely off monitors at any given time. If the patient has not been intubated up to this point, preoxygenation with 100 % inspired oxygen in preparation for airway management should be started. When the patient is fully preoxygenated and all monitors are functioning, a determination needs to be made whether or not conditions are optimal to proceed with induction, and if not, whether the surgical procedure can be reasonably delayed in order to improve conditions. A common scenario is hypovolemia due to hemorrhage, and whether or not there is time to correct this.

When it is time to proceed with induction of general anesthesia, several decisions need to be made. One question is whether or not the patient needs a rapid sequence induction. This technique is used when the patient either has a full stomach or is at risk for full stomach. The American Society of Anesthesiologists (ASA) standard is 8 h of fasting. Since the stress of trauma can delay gastric emptying, the duration of fasting ends at the time of trauma. Therefore, if a patient was involved in an MVA at 10 p.m. after eating dinner at 7 p.m., his fasting time is 3 h even if he is presenting to the operating room at 6 a.m. the following day. During a rapid sequence induction, induction agents are given quickly in a sequential fashion while applying pressure to the patient's neck at the level of the cricoid cartilage. During this time, the patient is not ventilated. The intent is to avoid insufflation of gas into the patient's stomach. This along with the application of cricoid pressure is designed to minimize the risk of gastric contents entering the oropharynx and then the lungs, which can cause aspiration pneumonia. If the patient's cervical spine is not cleared, "in-line stabilization" should be applied. Care should be taken to minimize cervical spine motion during intubation. If the cervical spine is known to be unstable, consideration could be given to performing an awake, fiberoptic intubation or alternative airway management technique designed to minimize cervical spine motion. These decisions are largely made based on the patient's ability to cooperate with the technique. In general, at least some degree of hypovolemia is assumed, and induction drugs are chosen and doses titrated to keep the induction period and hemodynamic effects to a minimum. A typical combination of drugs (in order) includes fentanyl, lidocaine, etomidate, and succinylcholine. Fentanyl (2–5 mcg/kg) is a potent, short-acting narcotic agent. It is a potent analgesic which also blunts the sympathetic response and pain response to laryngoscopy, the traumatic injury, and the surgical procedure. It does not cause histamine release and works rapidly. Lidocaine serves two roles. Etomidate can cause significant burning pain during infusion. The local anesthetic effect decreases the pain. Also, at a 0.1 mg/kg dose, lidocaine blunts the sympathetic response to laryngoscopy. Etomidate is probably the most stable induction agent. During rapid sequence induction, the goal is to make the patient unconscious quickly and stay unconscious during laryngoscopy; therefore, an induction dose (0.2–0.3 mg/kg) is used. Equipotent induction doses of either propofol or sodium pentothal can have a much more profound effect on blood pressure. Lastly, succinylcholine, a depolarizing neuromuscular blocking agent, is used to paralyze the patient and to facilitate intubation.

Succinylcholine has no appreciable hemodynamic effects. It has rapid onset (approximately 30 s after a 1.5 mg/kg dose) and rapid offset (spontaneous breathing within approximately 10 min of dosing). This minimizes the period of apnea with a rapid sequence induction and minimizes the time that the patient will be unable to spontaneously breathe. This is especially important if the anesthesiologist is unable to ventilate the following attempted intubation. Succinylcholine is contraindicated if the patient has a burn or significant neurologic injury (CVA, spinal cord injury, large nerve injury) that is greater than 24 h old. This is because a large number of extrajunctional acetylcholine receptors can be formed within 72 h of the neurologic injury or burn injury. This can result in significant and potentially life-threatening hyperkalemia during induction. Succinylcholine is also contraindicated for patients with elevated ICP, open-globe injuries, preexisting hyperkalemia (which occurs in conditions such as renal failure and rhabdomyolysis), and family history (or personal history) of malignant hyperthermia. In this case, a 1.2 mg/kg dose of rocuronium is indicated. At this dose, intubating conditions are achieved in approximately 60 s. However, reversal of neuromuscular blockade may not be possible for approximately 1 h.

Despite these efforts, induction can result in significant and perhaps severe hypotension. In this case, large-volume isotonic fluids should be administered. The patient may require temporary pharmacologic support to achieve an acceptable blood pressure. Choices include ephedrine, which is an indirect alpha- and beta-receptor-stimulating agent. Other options include appropriate dosing of direct alpha- and beta-receptor agonists such as epinephrine, norepinephrine, and dopamine. Many would use phenylephrine, which is a pure alpha-receptor agonist. Phenylephrine will usually improve the patient's blood pressure. However, with few exceptions, phenylephrine has not been shown to improve end-organ perfusion and may result in end-organ ischemia (especially bowel) if the patient is hypovolemic (Thiele et al. 2011b).

After induction of anesthesia and intubation, anesthesia must be maintained. The goal of the anesthesiologist is to keep the patient unconscious and amnestic during the surgical procedure. Other considerations include keeping the patient immobile and providing adequate muscular relaxation. The neuromuscular blocking agents will keep the patient immobile and provide muscular relaxation. They also have little or no effect on heart rate and pulse. Even neuromuscular blocking agents associated with histamine release (such as atracurium) are tolerated well if the patient is on an infusion or receives small bolus doses to maintain adequate paralysis. However, these agents do not have any CNS effects. They do not produce unconsciousness, amnesia, or analgesia. With no other agents, the patient will be aware, unless he or she is severely encephalopathic. The volatile agents are the usual agents used for anesthesia maintenance. However, at concentrations needed to reasonably assure unconsciousness and amnesia, the effects on blood pressure can be significant. This is known as 1 MAC (minimum alveolar concentration) of anesthesia. Isoflurane, desflurane, and sevoflurane all used at an approximately 1 MAC concentration are all reasonable choices. Intravenous agents can also be used but may be problematic. Propofol infusions at anesthetic doses (approximately 100–150 mcg/kg/min) will usually have a greater effect on blood pressure than the volatile agents administered at a 1 MAC concentration. High-dose benzodiazepine agents, such as midazolam, can be used but have relatively long half-lives. This will limit the ability to emerge the patient at the conclusion of the procedure and also limit the ability to obtain meaningful neurologic exams in the immediate postoperative period. Clearly this is not ideal for patients who need to be monitored for significant neurologic injuries.

Often, the anesthesiologist will accept low levels of inhaled and intravenous anesthetic agents in order to preserve hemodynamic stability. This approach increases the risk of the patient having awareness and feeling pain during the procedure. However, it may be the only option to preserve the patient's life while the acute trauma issues are being addressed surgically. During such situations, a monitor to measure level of consciousness, such as the bispectral index (BIS, Aspect Medical Systems) can be used. Nevertheless, it is wise to warn patients and/or their families preoperatively that awareness, although rare, is much more common in trauma cases because of these issues.

The ongoing hemodynamic management of trauma patients is most often the management of hemorrhage or hypovolemia. Determining the patient's volume status is not always straightforward. As noted earlier, the anesthetic can have significant effects on heart rate and blood pressure. Chronic medications such as ACE inhibitors, angiotensin receptor blockers, and beta-blockers can also affect the patient's vital signs. It is important not to weigh any one parameter too heavily. A general approach is to evaluate the heart rate and blood pressure. Are they normal? If not, is there an explanation. Examine the patient as much as possible. Is the patient pale or is the skin mottled? Both suggest shunting of blood away from the skin and muscles as the patient's autonomic nervous system responds in an attempt to preserve central blood volume. Provided the patient has intact renal function and has not received a diuretic, urine output is a reasonable indicator of volume status. However, it is not a very useful indicator when making acute decisions about volume management. Oliguria resulting from hypovolemia or improved urine output from appropriate resuscitation may take a relatively long time to become apparent. Measuring blood loss is also useful as long as there is not unmeasured bleeding such as internal bleeding or blood loss not captured in the suction canister or on sponges. Another strategy is to assess the hemodynamic response to an IV fluid challenge. Specifically, the hemodynamic response to a 10–20 cc/kg IV fluid challenge can give a lot of information about the volume status of the patient.

Other noninvasive methods include the use of an esophageal Doppler and echocardiography. Management with an esophageal Doppler involves an algorithmic approach following corrected flow time (FTc) and the percentage change in stroke volume (SV) (Gan et al. 2002). Transesophageal and transthoracic echocardiography exams can give a rapid, qualitative

assessment of left ventricular filling, left ventricular function, right ventricle volume, right ventricle pressure, and whether or not tamponade physiology exists. This exam can quickly give or confirm the diagnosis for hypotension in the vast majority of cases. Training to achieve this basic level of competency with echocardiography is relatively easy to accomplish and is now being offered by a number of training programs.

There are invasive methods of determining volume status. An arterial line is usually relatively easy to place and can be used to monitor a continuous arterial pressure. The arterial pressure wave form can be analyzed to assess pulse pressure variation. Pulse pressure variation less than 9 % has been demonstrated to indicate a low probability of improved cardiac output to an IV fluid volume challenge (fluid nonresponsiveness), whereas pulse pressure variation greater than 13 % has been associated with improved cardiac output in response to an IV fluid challenge (fluid responsiveness). Fluid management when the pulse pressure variation is between 9 % and 13 % is less clear. In this range, more information should be used when deciding whether or not to administer an IV fluid challenge (Cannesson et al. 2011).

A pulmonary artery catheter can be placed. The pulmonary artery occlusion pressure (wedge pressure) and, to a less extent, the pulmonary diastolic pressure can be used to give information about left ventricular filling pressure. However, caution should be taken when interpreting the data. The assumption is that left ventricular filling pressure correlates with left ventricular volume. This assumes that there is no gradient across the mitral valve at end diastole and that the left ventricle has normal compliance. Noncompliant left ventricles can be seen in the setting of ventricular hypertrophy and ischemic heart disease. Modern pulmonary artery catheters can give continuous cardiac output values and mixed venous oxygen saturation. Both are used to make inferences about cardiac performance and tissue oxygen delivery. The relative difficulty of placing a pulmonary artery catheter, especially for urgent trauma surgery, makes it less valuable than other methods for assessing intravascular volume status. In addition, placement carries risks such as pneumothorax, intraventricular conduction block, and pulmonary artery rupture.

The treatment for hypovolemia is to administer IV fluids (isotonic IV crystalloid solutions or albumin) and blood products. The amount of volume to administer is important. The goal is to reestablish euvolemia. Too little volume leads to under-resuscitation with resultant end-organ hypoperfusion, possible ischemia, and lactic acidosis. Excessive volume leads to volume overload, edema, and possibly respiratory insufficiency. These issues can lead to impaired wound healing, delayed return of gastric motility, and respiratory insufficiency. All can contribute to increased morbidity, increased days on mechanical ventilation, increased ICU days, and increased hospital days. This approach of treating to predetermine goal using methods such as the esophageal Doppler or pulse pressure variation has been described as goal-directed therapy (Bundgaard-Nielsen et al. 2007). The continuous IV fluid rate should be approximately the patient's maintenance rate with boluses (10–20 cc/kg) as needed.

Emergence and the Immediate Postoperative Period

Transitioning the patient from an anesthetic to the ICU or PACU can present a hemodynamic challenge. Significant hemodynamic aberrations can be seen during emergence and in the immediate postoperative period. As the cardiac depressant effects and vasodilatory effects of the maintenance agents (volatile agents or intravenous agents) wear off, significant hypertension and tachycardia can be seen. If the patient requires acetylcholinesterase inhibitors for reversal of neuromuscular blockade, anticholinergics (such as glycopyrrolate and atropine) are used to minimize the cholinergic effects. This can lead to significant tachycardia. Lastly, inadequately controlled pain can cause significant tachycardia and hypertension as the patient emerges from anesthesia. When hypertension and tachycardia are caused by pain, it should be rapidly treated for the reason of compassion. Beyond our goal of reducing pain and suffering, hypertension and

tachycardia can cause significant morbidity including cardiac ischemia, stoke, and bleeding. For these reasons, the etiology for hypertension and tachycardia should be rapidly assessed and aggressively treated.

Cross-References

- ▶ Abdominal Major Vascular Injury, Anesthesia for
- ▶ Abdominal Solid Organ Injury, Anesthesia for
- ▶ Acute Abdominal Compartment Syndrome in Trauma
- ▶ Awareness and Trauma Anesthesia
- ▶ Blood Component Transfusion
- ▶ Blood Volume
- ▶ Damage Control Resuscitation
- ▶ Damage Control Resuscitation, Military Trauma
- ▶ Drug Abuse and Trauma Anesthesia
- ▶ Fluid, Electrolytes, and Nutrition in Trauma Patients
- ▶ General Anesthesia for Major Trauma
- ▶ Hemodynamic Monitoring
- ▶ Hemorrhage
- ▶ Hemorrhagic Shock
- ▶ History of Trauma Anesthesia and Resuscitation
- ▶ Massive Transfusion
- ▶ Military Trauma, Anesthesia for
- ▶ Monitoring of Trauma Patients During Anesthesia
- ▶ Multi-trauma, Anesthesia for
- ▶ Operating Room Setup for Trauma Anesthesia
- ▶ Orthopedic Trauma, Anesthesia for
- ▶ Pediatric Trauma, Assessment, and Anesthetic Management
- ▶ Pharmacologic Strategies in Adult Trauma Anesthesia
- ▶ Pneumothorax
- ▶ Pneumothorax, Tension
- ▶ Pregnant Trauma Patient, Anesthetic Considerations for the
- ▶ Rapid Sequence Intubation
- ▶ Resuscitation Goals in Trauma Patients
- ▶ Shock Management in Trauma
- ▶ Spinal Cord Injury, Anesthetic Management for

References

Bundgaard-Nielsen M, Holte K et al (2007) Monitoring of perioperative fluid administration by individualized goal-directed therapy. Acta Anaesthesiol Scand 51:331–340

Cannesson M, Le March Y et al (2011) Assessing the diagnostic accuracy of pulse pressure variation for the prediction of fluid responsiveness, a "gray zone" approach. Anesthesiology 115:231–241

Gan TJ, Soppitt A et al (2002) Goal-directed intraoperative fluid administration reduces length of stay after major surgery. Anesthesiology 97:820–826

Thiele R, Nemergut E, Lynch C (2011a) The physiologic implications of isolated alpha 2 adrenergic stimulation. Anesth Analg 113:284–296

Thiele R, Nemergut E, Lynch C (2011b) The clinical implications of isolated alpha 2 adrenergic stimulation. Anesth Analg 113:297–304

Hemodynamic Monitoring

Diana Catalina Casas Lopez and Andrew C. Steel
Faculty of Medicine, Department of
Anesthesiology and Interdepartmental, Division
of Critical Care Medicine, Toronto General
Hospital, University of Toronto, Toronto,
ON, Canada

Synonyms

Cardiovascular monitoring; Evaluation of hemodynamics; Hemodynamic parameters

Definition

Monitoring of hemodynamics, which literally means the observation, and recording of "blood power" (Greek etymology) or "blood movement." It is the method by which we obtain qualitative and quantitative data related to the cardiovascular system and therefore the blood flow in the cardiovascular system. Noninvasive or indirect hemodynamic monitoring means that the data are collected by tools that do not physically penetrate the body. Invasive or direct hemodynamic monitoring means that the introduction of a catheter into a vein or artery is needed. Penetration of the body is required and therefore associated with a relative risk to the patient. Minimally invasive denotes that there is a need for a small incision or catheter in a peripheral location and is associated with less morbidity. Regular clinical assessment is an essential part of hemodynamic monitoring. "No monitoring device, no matter how accurate or insightful its data, will improve outcome. Unless it is coupled to a treatment intervention which itself improves outcome" (Michael Pinsky) (Pinsky and Payen 2005).

Preexisting Condition

The cardiovascular system is composed of one main organ, the heart, and two parallel networks of blood vessels. The pulmonary circulation moves deoxygenated blood from the heart to the lungs and returns oxygenated blood back to the heart. The systemic circulation moves oxygenated blood from the heart to all the tissues and returns deoxygenated blood from the body back to the heart.

The major physiological determinants of hemodynamics are the preload, afterload, and contractility of the heart and the vascular resistance or tone of the blood vessels. Ultimately the objective of hemodynamic monitoring is to optimize these physiologic determinants and ensure adequate perfusion, or oxygen delivery, to all tissues to sustain aerobic metabolism.

Critically ill and trauma patients often present with complex hemodynamics secondary to occult (or evident) hypovolemia, myocardial disease, sepsis, or a combination of pathologies. The trauma patient faces a rapid and often vast alteration in physiologic status, resulting in shock. Shock is more than simply hypotension and is defined as a life-threatening, generalized maldistribution of blood flow resulting in failure to deliver and/or utilize adequate amounts of oxygen, leading to tissue dysoxia (Antonelli et al. 2007).

It has been proposed that the multiorgan dysfunction syndrome (MODS) of the critically ill is, in part, a consequence of inadequate oxygen delivery. This is often exacerbated by microcirculatory injury, increased tissue meta-bolic demands (distributive hypoxia), and further compounded by mitochondrial dysfunction (cytopathic hypoxia). With oxygen debt, high concentrations of lactic acid are generated, as it is the final product of the anaerobic cycle for the production of energy. Lactate and base deficit in trauma patients are used to identify shock; the correction of metabolic acidosis is an end point goal of resuscitation (serum lactate < 2 mEq/L). The principle tenet of resuscitation of the trauma patient is to normalize or optimize the fluid status and cardiac output of the patient, thus ensuring optimal oxygen delivery to the tissues.

Many devices have been used for hemody-namic monitoring. All of them assess perfusion in a different way, and the data obtained needs to be interpreted and correlated to the method from which they are derived and the medical history and clinical state of the patient. The goal should be to carry out early and aggressive resuscitation of the patient in order to limit and/or reverse tissue hypoxia and progression to organ failure, thereby improving outcomes (Rivers et al. 2001).

The practice of following tissue dysfunction as a guide to resuscitation requires understanding of the concept of *upstream* and *downstream* indi-cators of organ perfusion (Table 1). The tradi-tional markers of a patient at risk or critically ill include systemic blood pressure, heart rate, cen-tral venous pressure, pulmonary capillary wedge pressure, and cardiac output – the upstream indi-cators. The downstream indicators are those that demonstrate improving tissue perfusion and con-sequently oxygen delivery; these are urine out-put, serum lactate, base deficit, SvO_2, $ScvO_2$, $SvCO_2$, and tissue CO_2 levels.

Application

In every critically ill patient, there are standard hemodynamic indices that should be available at all times, and they include the heart rate (HR) and rhythm, obtained from 5-lead electrocardiogram (ECG), and automated noninvasive blood pres-sure (NIBP) with the calculated mean arterial blood pressure (MAP).

Hemodynamic Monitoring, Table 1 Variables used to assess hemodynamic status

Upstream indicators	Downstream indicators
Assess flow and pressure in the heart and great vessels. They are the traditional variables used to assess the hemodynamic status of the critically ill and at-risk patient	*Account for alterations in the microvasculature when oxygen and metabolic needs vary during the disease course. Such variables estimate adequacy of cardiac output and perfusion pressure*
Systemic blood pressure	Urine output
Heart rate	Serum lactate
CVP	Base deficit
PCWP	SvO_2
Cardiac output	$SvCO_2$
	Tissue CO_2 levels

Systemic blood pressure can be monitored indirectly, or noninvasively, by a sphygmoma-nometer or automated, intermittent oscillometric device. In the ICU, ER, and OR, it is also directly, invasively measured by the insertion of an arte-rial line and transducing the pressure. Invasive monitoring is indicated in patients with all forms of shock and hemodynamic instability, patients with vasoactive medication, and those in which frequent blood tests, especially gas analysis, are required. Therefore, almost all severely injured patients in an ICU will benefit from an arterial line. The arterial waveform varies according to hydrostatic pressure, arterial stiffness, and pressure wave reflection that change according to individual characteristics, disease state, and vasoactive drugs. The most frequently used location for arterial cannulation is the radial artery, followed by the brachial, femoral, dorsalis pedis, and axillary arteries. The pressure waveforms, transmitted by a column of saline, provide the systolic blood pressure (SBP), diastolic blood pressure (DBP), and calculated mean arterial pressure (MAP) [MAP = diastolic pressure + 1/3(systolic pressure − diastolic pressure)]. The MAP is considered the true driving pressure and determinant of the periph-eral tissue blood flow. It is the same throughout the arterial tree and least dependent upon either the site of measurement or technique.

There is not a universal accepted target for MAP, but guidelines for resuscitation in septic shock include a target MAP greater than 65 mmHg (Dellinger et al. 2008; Rivers et al. 2001). It is unclear if this can be extrapolated to include trauma patients, but certainly hypoperfusion and over-resuscitation must both be avoided (Dutton et al. 2002). There are complications associated with line insertion, and these must be balanced with the benefit. The most common complications are infection, hemorrhage, thrombosis and distal ischemia, skin necrosis, embolization, hematoma, and neurologic injury. The femoral is considered a central artery with higher risk of infection due to its proximity to the perineum and higher risk of mechanical complications such as hemorrhage and thromboembolism.

The central venous pressure (CVP) is obtained with a catheter that is introduced through a major vein, usually jugular or subclavian vein with its tip at the atrial-caval junction. It can be simplified that CVP is equivalent to right atrial pressure and is an indicator of the preload of the RV. Central venous lines are primarily placed as secure and reliable routes for administration of drugs, nutrients, and fluids. They are vital for this purpose; however, the hemodynamic data provided should not be undervalued.

The CVP waveform (Fig. 1) is characterized by three inflections (peaks) and two deflections (descents): the *a wave* is the highest peak and results from atrial contraction. The atrial contraction ends with a slight relaxation, the z *point* or plateau, prior to the ventricle contraction. The *a wave* will disappear in the presence of atrial dysrhythmias and will be greatly exaggerated in the presence of tricuspid incompetence or heart block. It coincides with the p wave on the ECG. The *c wave* occurs during ventricular contraction as the tricuspid valve bulges into the atrium and towards the transducer. This correlates with the QRS on the ECG. The *x descent* is a result of the ejection of the RV and is seen before the T wave on the ECG. The *v wave* is the result of atrial filling, and finally the *y descent* is the opening of the tricuspid valve. When diastole is long, the *y descent* is often followed by a small, brief,

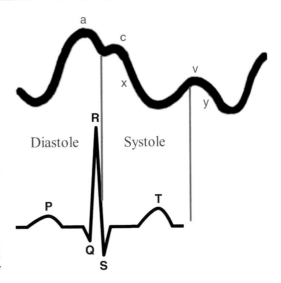

Hemodynamic Monitoring, Fig. 1 Central venous pressure waveform. *a* – RA contraction, *c* – isovolumetric ventricular contraction forces TV into RA, *x* – RAP falls as TV is pulled away from the atrium during RV ejection, *v* – RA filling continuing into late ventricular systole, *y* – TV opens and RA empties into RV during early diastole

positive wave, the *h wave* or *h plateau*, which occurs just prior to the next *a* wave.

For many years the CVP has been regarded as a tool to monitor intravascular volume status, when there is no underlying valvular or pulmonary disease. The trend of this parameter, rather than a single value, is useful in directing treatment. Low systemic BP together with low CVP suggests hypovolemia. The 2006 International Consensus Conference on hemodynamic monitoring in shock proposed that low filling pressures should result in immediate fluid resuscitation and that a fluid challenge should be performed (250 mL over 10 min) to predict fluid responsiveness with the intention of achieving an increase in CVP of greater than 2 mmHg (Antonelli et al. 2007). The pressure at the onset of the *c wave* is the one that best represents the filling pressure of the ventricle. According to Rivers et al. in septic shock the goal should be a CVP between 8 and 12 mmHg for ventilated patients. There are many factors affecting the CVP measure, for example, the rise in intrathoracic pressure, high PEEP, and increased intrapericardial pressure, and the complications of having a central line are thrombosis,

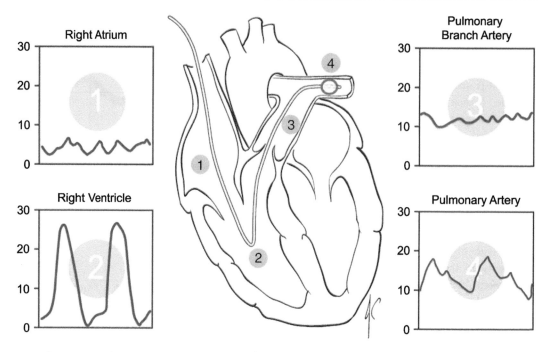

Hemodynamic Monitoring, Fig. 2 Waveforms and measured pressures normally elicited during the passage of the pulmonary artery catheter through the heart and great vessels (With permission of J. Crossingham)

thromboembolism, infection (sepsis or endocarditis), arrhythmias, and hydrothorax.

The gold standard technique to measure cardiac output (CO), against which all new cardiac output measuring devices are compared, is still the pulmonary artery flotation catheter or Swan-Ganz catheter (Vincent 2011). Originally Adolph Fick described the first method of cardiac output estimation in 1870. This method was the reference standard until the introduction of the pulmonary artery catheter (PAC) in the 1970s. The PAC is introduced through 8.5Ch introducer cannula placed in a central vein; it has a small 1.5 ml balloon on the tip, a thermistor near the tip, and two different ports: a distal port placed on the tip and a proximal port 30 cm from the tip. This catheter is introduced through the cannula and advanced until the CVP in the right atrium is acquired. By inflating the aforementioned balloon, the catheter can be flow directed through the tricuspid valve, right ventricle, pulmonic valve, and finally the main pulmonary artery. The catheter can be advanced a few centimeters more to a branch of the pulmonary artery to transduce the pulmonary artery occlusion pressure (PAOP) or pulmonary capillary wedge pressure (PCWP), which approximates to the left atrial pressure and correlates to the filling pressures on the left side of the heart (Fig. 2). The balloon is then deflated and the principal pulmonary artery tracing should then return. In most patients PCWP can be found 50–60 cm from the internal jugular vein insertion point. The PAC is an invasive technique that is associated with significant, inherent risks: acute arrhythmias, air embolism, arterial puncture, bleeding, hemothorax, and pneumothorax. The most serious complication is rupture of the pulmonary artery, which is fatal in up to 70 % of instances and is most frequently caused by PAOP measurement or repositioning. In patients with abnormalities of the tricuspid valve and especially abnormal right ventricle anatomy placement of a PA catheter can be technically challenging or impossible. Unfortunately it is often in the management of these patients where the data from this device will be most useful.

Cardiac output can be calculated using the Stewart-Hamilton principle of intermittent pulmonary thermodilution. An input signal of 10 cm^3 of cold saline is injected through the proximal port of the catheter and is sensed at the distal thermistor. A thermodilution wash-out curve is created from which the intermittent cardiac output values are then calculated. The original design of the catheter has been modified to afford the continuous measurement of CO, as well as mixed venous oxygen saturation (SvO$_2$) with the addition of an oximeter at the tip.

Venous oximetry is a measure of the saturation of hemoglobin from a sample taken from pulmonary artery (SvO$_2$) and the superior vena cava (ScvO$_2$). These two results are similar but not identical, with the ScvO$_2$ measurement lower compared to the SvO$_2$. Reinhart et al. were able to demonstrate that ScvO$_2$ changed in parallel with SvO$_2$ in 90 % of instances. The Fick equation *Cardiac output (CO) = VO$_2$/(CaO$_2$ − CvO$_2$)* holds implicit that if oxygen consumption and oxygen content are constants, then the venous saturation is representative of CO. The value of venous saturation by itself does not indicate the etiology of decreased tissue perfusion, but alerts the clinician to the problem. There are data now in the literature supporting the use of venous oximetry both as a measure of the severity of shock and to guide resuscitation in trauma patients. Using this scientific rationale, a target SvcO$_2$ is greater than 70 %.

Today there is a growing need to have real-time, accurate data, derived from less invasive monitoring, to diagnose and treat patients. Compared with traditional, highly invasive, interrupted bolus thermodilution, the new, minimally and non-invasive, cardiac output monitoring devices use one of four main technologies to determine cardiac output: pulse contour analysis, Doppler ultrasound technology, applied Fick principle, and electrical bioimpedance or bioreactance (Table 2).

Pulse contour analysis systems derive their data from the arterial line waveform. This waveform of pressure versus time is interpreted and mathematically assesses force of ejection from the heart and the impedance, compliance, and resistance of the arterial system (Fig. 3). Such systems depend upon the position, reliability, and accuracy of the arterial line waveform. They are not therefore recommended in patients with dysrhythmias, intra-aortic balloon pumps, and ventricular assist devices. Monitors that use pulse contour analysis can be further classified according to whether they employ a self-calibrating algorithm (e.g., Flotrac™) or require a transpulmonary dilution calibration process for the data. The two available calibrated systems are PiCCO™ (Pulse index Continuous Cardiac Output) and LiDCO™ (Lithium Dilution Cardiac Output). PiCCO™ is calibrated with 15–20 cm^3 of cold normal saline that is injected through a central venous line and needs a thermistor-tipped catheter placed in a large central arterial line (brachial, axillary, or femoral). LiDCO™, as its name suggests, is calibrated with small, subtherapeutic doses of lithium through a central or peripheral vein. A lithium dilution curve is generated by analyzing the entire arterial waveform with an external lithium-sensitive electrode. An advantage of using lithium is that there is no significant loss during lung passage; however, a disadvantage is that lithium is not licensed for this use in all countries. Both systems recommend recalibration every 8–12 h and after major hemodynamic changes. The indices derived from these systems are CO, SV, systemic vascular resistance (SVR), and the indexed values: cardiac index (CI), stroke volume index (SVI), and systemic vascular resistance index (SVRI). PiCCO™, uniquely, calculates two additional parameters: the global end-diastolic volume (GEDV) and extravascular lung water (EVLWI) – a surrogate measure of pulmonary edema.

Increases in pleural pressure associated with intermittent positive-pressure ventilation (IPPV) decrease the venous return to the heart. Reduced RV preload and increased afterload thereby decreases stroke volume. This reduction in RV ejection leads to a decrease in LV filling after a phase lag of two or three heartbeats. Consequently, SV, CO, and SBP all fall during each mechanical breath (Fig. 4). Pulse contour analysis monitors use the magnitude of the respiratory change in left ventricular stroke volume to assess fluid responsiveness. Decreased venous return with positive-pressure ventilation is most marked in hypovolemic patients. Both experimental and

Hemodynamic Monitoring, Table 2 A comparison of the available technologies for assessment of cardiac output

Technology	Advantages	Disadvantages
Pulmonary artery catheter	Familiarity	Pulmonary artery rupture
	Measures right heart and pulmonary artery pressures	Dysrhythmias
	SvO$_2$ assessment	Infection
		Valvular trauma
Transpulmonary thermodilution, e.g., PiCCO	Uses existing CVC	Unclear what to do with additional indices, e.g., post-lung transplant
	Cold thermodilution calibration	
	Additional data points, e.g., extravascular lung water	Requires central arterial line of 14G or 16G, can cause complications (3 %)
	Not influenced by respiratory cycle	
	Suitable in pediatric patient	
Esophageal Doppler	Simple to use	Inter-user variability in critical positioning of probe
	No intravascular component	Increased risk of VAP
	Indices of inotropy and ventricular filling	Risk in liver failure because of incidence of varices
		Discomfort for awake patient
Lithium dilution, e.g., LiDCO	Used with existing standard arterial line and CVC	Lithium use unlicensed in some jurisdictions, e.g., Canada
	Calibrated with lithium or not (LiDCO *rapid*)	Cumbersome calibration process
	Displays stroke volume variation and easy comparison of SVR and CO contribution to BP	Requires recalibration after use of some drugs, e.g., atracurium, change in Hb. or Na, and at least q6hr
Pulse contour analysis, e.g., Flotrac-Vigileo, LiDCO, PiCCO	Used with existing standard arterial line and CVC	SVV most accurate in mechanically ventilated patients
	Stroke volume variation (SVV) used to predict volume status	SVV accurate only in sinus rhythm
	Flotrac "self-calibrates"	Dependent upon quality of arterial waveform
Mixed and central venous oximetry	Can be performed continuously	Very high values difficult to interpret, e.g., cytopathic hypoxia vs. high cardiac output
	CVC oximetric catheter can be combined with PiCCO or Flotrac pulse contour analysis technology	PAC required for SvO$_2$
Bioreactance technology, e.g., NICOM-Cheetah	Completely noninvasive	
	Overcomes limitations of bioimpedance and is more accurate	
	Electrodes not position dependent	
	Comparable sensitivity and specificity to Flotrac and PAC	
Thoracic ultrasound, e.g., USCOM	Determines CO by continuous wave Doppler U/S probe placed on the chest to measure the transaortic or transpulmonary blood flow	Suitability in high and low cardiac output states still requires validation

clinical studies suggest that large variations (>12 %) in systolic, or pulse pressure, are predictive of increasing cardiac output with fluid loading. This dynamic test of "recruitable cardiac output" is highly reproducible and more accurate than traditional hemodynamic indices (Fig. 5) (Michard et al. 2000). However, this analysis has only been validated for controlled tidal

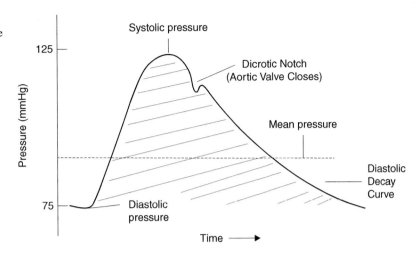

Hemodynamic Monitoring, Fig. 3 Pulse contour analysis

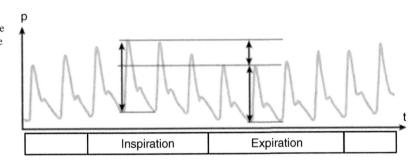

Hemodynamic Monitoring, Fig. 4 Pulse pressure variation with the respiratory cycle during mechanical ventilation

volumes between 8 and 15 ml/kg, not in spontaneous breathing patients, high-frequency oscillation ventilation, or where there is decreased chest compliance, e.g., prone positioning.

Electrical impedance uses stimulation with a constant current that will be impeded through the body proportionally with the volume changes of the cardiac cycle. Electrodes are placed on the thorax or whole body. The disadvantage of this system is that its accuracy deteriorates with fluid shifts, dysrhythmias, and ventilation – all evident in a critical care patient. Bioreactance is a newer application of this technology that has been recently validated for its accuracy in the ICU. When an AC current is applied to the chest, the pulsatile blood flow taking place in the large thoracic arteries causes the amplitude of the applied voltage to change. In addition, it causes a time delay or *phase shift* between the applied current and the measured voltage. Research suggests that these phase shifts are tightly correlated

with stroke volume and that they are less susceptible to interference from fluid shifts, patient movement, or dysrhythmia.

Doppler ultrasound and echocardiography rely upon a fundamental principle that a moving object creates a shift in frequency proportional to the relative velocity between it and the observer. This principle is employed by several cardiac output monitors, e.g., CardioQ™ and Hemosonic™. An ultrasound probe is introduced via the nose or mouth into the mid-esophagus and positioned (blindly) to measure the blood flow velocity in the ascending part of the aorta. Using either the patient demographics or m-mode, respectively, these devices will calculate cardiac output. They have the advantage of being simple to use in an intubated patient with sinus rhythm and have been recommended by the National Institute for Clinical Excellence (NICE) in the UK for postoperative fluid management. However, the esophageal probe is

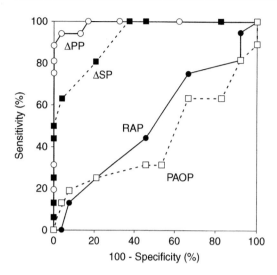

Hemodynamic Monitoring, Fig. 5 Predicting fluid responsiveness. Receiver operating characteristic (*ROC*) curves comparing the ability of *ΔPp* pulse pressure, *ΔPs* systolic pressure, *Pra* right atrial pressure, and *Ppao* pulmonary artery occlusion pressure to discriminate responders (ΔCI > 15 %) and nonresponders to a fluid challenge. The area under the ROC curve for ΔPp was greater than for ΔPs, Para, and Ppao ($p < 0.01$) (From Michard et al. 2000)

Hemodynamic Monitoring, Table 3 Indications for echocardiography in the ICU

Indication	
Hemodynamic instability	Ventricular failure
	Hypovolemia
	Vasodilatation
	Acute valvular dysfunction
	Cardiac tamponade
	Pulmonary embolism
	PA pressure estimation
Aortic dissection	
Infective endocarditis	
Source of systemic embolus	
Unexplained hypoxemia	e.g., intracardiac shunt
Positioning of ECLS cannulae	

uncomfortable for the alert patient, and inter-user variability introduces inaccuracy into the monitoring over time.

Transthoracic echocardiogram (TTE) has become an important tool for hemodynamic monitoring in the intensive care unit. It is a fast and noninvasive means to accurately assess hemodynamic function and circulating volume status (Ferrada et al. 2011). Clinically relevant and management changing views can be gained from more than 90 % of ICU patients with a focused ECHO exam. This differs significantly from a comprehensive echocardiography examination in that the principal aim of the focus approach is rapid, bedside real-time assessment to identify major entities. The objectives are to exclude obvious pathology and assess the wall thickness and size of the chamber (volume) and contractility (Table 3). The acquisition of images of the heart in four scanning positions (subcostal view, apical view, parasternal view, and pleural) is easy to achieve. However, despite the widespread use and popularity of transthoracic

echocardiography in the ICU, there remains a real need for formal training and certification of the intensivist operator.

Cross-References

▶ Cardiopulmonary Resuscitation in Adult Trauma
▶ Central Line Associated Blood Stream Infection
▶ Heart-Lung Interactions
▶ Postoperative Management of Adult Trauma Patient
▶ Sepsis, Treatment of
▶ Shock
▶ Shock Management in Trauma
▶ Trauma Intensive Care Management
▶ Vasoactive Agents in the ICU

References

Antonelli M, Levy M, Andrews PJ et al (2007) Hemodynamic monitoring in shock and implications for management. International consensus conference, Paris, France, 27–28 April 2006. Intensive Care Med 33:575–590
Dellinger RP, Levy MM, Carlet JM et al (2008) Surviving sepsis campaign: international guidelines for

management of severe sepsis and septic shock: 2008. Crit Care Med 36:296–327

Dutton RP, Mackenzie CF, Scalea TM (2002) Hypotensive resuscitation during active hemorrhage: impact on in-hospital mortality. J Trauma 52:1141–1146

Ferrada P, Murthi S, Anand RJ, Bochicchio GV, Scalea T (2011) Transthoracic focused rapid echocardiographic examination: real-time evaluation of fluid status in critically ill trauma patients. J Trauma 70(1):56–62; discussion −4

Michard F, Boussat S, Chemla D et al (2000) Relation between respiratory changes in arterial pulse pressure and fluid responsiveness in septic patients with acute circulatory failure. Am J Respir Crit Care Med 162:134–138

Pinsky MR, Payen D (2005) Functional hemodynamic monitoring. Crit Care 9:566–572

Rivers E, Nguyen B, Havstad S, Ressler J, Muzzin A, Knoblich B, Peterson E, Tomlanovich M (2001) Early goal-directed therapy collaborative group: early goal-directed therapy in the treatment of severe sepsis and septic shock. N Engl J Med 345:1368–1377

Vincent JL (2011) Annual update in intensive care and emergency medicine, vol 1. Springer, Berlin. doi:10.1007/978-3-642-18081-1

Hemodynamic Parameters

▶ Hemodynamic Monitoring

Hemofiltration

▶ Dialysis

Hemorrhage

Caitlin A. Jolda, Khanjan H. Nagarsheth and Mayur Narayan
R Adams Cowley Shock Trauma Center, University of Maryland School of Medicine, Baltimore, MD, USA

Synonyms

Acute blood loss anemia; Blood loss; Hemorrhagic shock; Shock

Definition

Exsanguinating hemorrhage is the most common preventable cause of death after trauma. The acute loss of blood leads to a cascade of severe life-threatening problems including shock, inflammation, and coagulopathy (Kauvar et al. 2006). The American College of Surgeons identifies four categories of acute blood loss based on the percent of blood volume:

Class I: loss of 15 % or less of total blood volume or up to 750 cm^3 EBL. Clinical findings are minimal or absent as the body compensates and maintains blood volume by transcapillary refill.

Class II: loss of 15–30 % of blood volume or 750–1,500 cm^3 EBL. Clinical findings may include tachycardia and decrease in urine output below 30 mL/h. However, blood pressure and perfusion of vital organs may be maintained by sympathetic vasoconstriction.

Class III: loss of 30–40 % of blood volume. At this stage, the vasoconstrictor response to hemorrhage is no longer able to sustain blood pressure and vital organ perfusion, therefore leading to decompensated hypovolemic shock. Clinical signs include hypotension and markedly reduced urine output (<15 mL/h).

Class IV: loss of >40 % of blood volume. When blood loss exceeds 40 % of blood volume, the effects on the body and organ failure may be irreversible. Profound hypotension and oliguria (urine output <5 mL/h) are the most common clinical signs (Marino 2007).

Preexisting Condition

Hemorrhagic Shock

Severe hemorrhage with large decreases in circulating blood volume can result in decreased cardiac output and perfusion pressure. This leads to a state of shock as the delivery of oxygen and nutrients to tissues becomes inadequate to maintain aerobic metabolism (Gutierrez et al. 2004). When the level of oxygen delivery is unable to sustain the level of oxygen uptake by the cells, tissues turn to anaerobic sources of energy. Anaerobic metabolism leads to the

H

buildup of acids and metabolic acidosis. Some tissues such as skeletal and smooth muscles are more resistant to hypoxia and irreversible damage may not occur until after several hours of ischemia, but other tissues such as the brain and intestinal mucosa sustain permanent damage after only a few minutes of hypoxia. Failure to reverse severe hemorrhage will lead to uncompensated shock and subsequent multisystem organ failure and death (Gutierrez et al. 2004).

Recognition of Hemorrhagic Shock

Early diagnosis can lead to early intervention. The importance of the clinical physical exam should be stressed. All trauma patients should be evaluated with the airway (A,) breathing (B), circulation (C), disability (D), and exposure (E) approach prescribed by the Advanced Trauma Life Support course (ATLS). Evaluating a patient's color, temperature, and pulse exam can give quick clues to the presence of hemorrhagic shock. The five major cavities that can hide major blood loss leading to hemorrhagic shock include the chest, abdomen and pelvis, retroperitoneum, long bones, and the street. Each of these should be evaluated by physical exam and a quick adjunctive study such as x-ray or ultrasound. Hypotensive patients with a positive ultrasound exam in the pericardium should proceed to pericardiocentesis, pericardial window, or sternotomy. Hypotensive patients with a positive ultrasound in the abdomen should proceed directly to diagnostic laparotomy. In this scenario, additional diagnostic information with CT scan is not warranted and can lead to delays in management and occasionally death of the patient.

Application

Compensatory Responses in Acute Hemorrhage

Hemorrhage results in a number of compensatory responses by the body to maintain adequate blood volume and tissue perfusion. The initial response is movement of interstitial fluid into the capillaries. Up to 15 % of blood volume can be replenished with transcapillary refill, but it results in an interstitial fluid deficit. Hemorrhage also leads to activation of the renin-angiotensin-aldosterone system. This results in sodium conservation by the kidneys and maintenance of the interstitial fluid deficit. Increased production of red blood cells does not occur until several hours after onset of hemorrhage and the response takes place very slowly, over weeks to months. Therefore, volume replacement is almost always necessary when blood loss exceeds 15 % of blood volume (Marino 2007).

Resuscitation

The main goal of therapy is to rapidly control the source of bleeding and to restore the circulating blood volume. Intravascular fluid must be replaced to prevent impaired tissue oxygenation. Even with low hemoglobin concentrations, as long as circulating volume is maintained, adequate tissue oxygenation may be maintained. Goals of fluid resuscitation should be guided by hemodynamic parameters including blood pressure, heart rate, cardiac output, central venous pressure, pulmonary artery wedge pressure, and mixed venous saturation (Gutierrez et al. 2004). Measures of hemoglobin and hematocrit in a bleeding patient are inappropriate because acute blood loss involves the loss of whole blood, with proportional decreases in the volume, plasma, and erythrocytes. Therefore, in the period of acute blood loss, the hematocrit may not change significantly. Newer resuscitation markers, in addition to traditional lab values and urine output, such as lactate and base deficit, are now routinely obtained to guide resuscitation efforts (Marino 2007).

Resuscitation strategies have evolved over the past 20 years. Normalizing blood pressure is no longer an accepted treatment goal as overaggressive fluid resuscitation may increase the blood flow to injuries and perfusion pressures, increasing the risk of "popping the clot," causing recurrent bleeding, or increasing ongoing blood loss (McSwain and Barbeau 2011). In addition, large volumes of fluid may also result in significant third-spacing, causing complications such as bowel edema and anastomotic leaks, abdominal compartment syndrome, and acute respiratory distress syndrome (Schnuriger et al. 2011).

Permissive hypotension strategies that minimize fluids to preserve cerebral perfusion while maintaining systolic blood pressures above a threshold value of 70–80 mmHg are now aggressively being promoted. Proponents of permissive hypotension suggest that administration of crystalloid may aggravate the inflammatory response, increase blood loss before definitive hemostasis, and increase transfusion requirements, which could further exacerbate early inflammation and late immunosuppression. Rapid surgical correction in the setting of a lower target blood pressure will prevent the large inflammatory response seen with traditional massive resuscitation strategies (Kobayashi et al. 2012).

Coagulopathy

Coagulopathy is one of the many complications of hemorrhage that leads to poor outcomes. Classically, trauma-induced coagulopathy has been explained by a combination of several factors including dilution due to resuscitation fluids, hypothermia, and acidemia-associated dysfunction of or consumption of coagulation proteases. However, more recent evidence suggests that acute coagulopathy is a result activation of anticoagulant and fibrinolytic pathways rather than a dysfunction of the coagulation proteases. Activation of these pathways is initiated by hypoperfusion from acute hemorrhage and results in systemic anticoagulation and hyperfibrinolysis (Gruen et al. 2012).

A precise assessment of acute coagulopathy in the trauma patient is difficult to obtain. The tests most commonly used to assess coagulopathy, prothombin time (PT), and partial thromboplastin time (PTT) can take 20–60 min to process in most trauma centers and their accuracy in trauma patients with massive hemorrhage is unknown (Brohi et al. 2007). More recently, methods such as thromboelastography (TEG) or thromboelastometry (ROTEM) have been found to more accurately guide coagulation management in trauma patients. Thromboelastometry measures the viscoelastic properties of the clot and provides information on speed of coagulation initiation, kinetics of clot growth, and clot strength and breakdown. The full test results of thromboelastometry can also be obtained within 10–20 min, with preliminary test results available within 5 min after starting analysis (Schochl et al. 2010).

In order to prevent or treat the effects of coagulopathy in a patient with hemorrhage, transfusion of products that not only increase fluid and blood volume but also contain clotting factors is required. Massive transfusion protocols now recommend transfusion of red blood cell, fresh frozen plasma, and platelets in a ratio of 1:1:1. The addition of transfusion products such as fibrinogen concentrate, recombinant activated factor VII, and prothrombin complex concentrate guided by assessment of coagulopathy with methods such as thromboelastometry has been shown to improve outcomes (Schochl et al. 2010). Newer agents such as tranexamic acid have also been studied and shown to improve survival by mitigating mild to moderate bleeding.

Summary

Exsanguinating hemorrhage is the most common preventable cause of death after trauma. Worldwide, it is the cause of approximately one third of the almost six million trauma deaths per year. Key strategies involve early diagnosis, balanced resuscitation, and aggressive surgical or percutaneous intervention to stop the bleeding. In addition, newer strategies to address the problem of acute traumatic coagulopathy and drugs such as factor VII, prothrombin complex concentrate, and tranexamic acid have also started to be implemented.

Cross-References

▶ Acute Coagulopathy of Trauma
▶ Hemorrhagic Shock
▶ Shock Management in Trauma
▶ Transfusion Strategy in Trauma: What Is the Evidence?

References

Brohi K, Cohen M, Davenport R (2007) Acute coagulopathy of trauma: mechanism, identification and effect. Curr Opin Crit Care 13:680–685

Gruen RL, Brohi K, Schreiber M, Balogh ZJ, Pitt V, Narayan M, Maier RV (2012) Haemorrhage control in severely injured patients. Lancet 380(9847): 1099–1108

Gutierrez G, Reines H, Wulf-Gutierrez M (2004) Clinical review: hemorrhagic shock. Crit Care 8:373–381

Kauvar DS, Lefering R, Wade CE (2006) Impact of hemorrhage on trauma outcome: an overview of epidemiology, clinical presentations, and therapeutic considerations. J Trauma 60:S3–S11

Kobayashi L, Costantini TW, Coimbra R (2012) Hypovolemic shock resuscitation. Surg Clin North Am 92(6):1403–1423

Marino P (2007) The ICU book, 3rd edn. Lippincott Williams & Wilkins, Philadelphia

McSwain N Jr, Barbeau J (2011) Potential use of prothrombin complex concentrate in trauma resuscitation. J Trauma 70(Suppl 5):S53–S56

Schnuriger B, Inaba K, Wu T et al (2011) Crystalloids after primary colon resection and anastomosis at initial trauma laparotomy: excessive volumes are associated with anastomotic leakage. J Trauma 70(3):603–610

Schochl H, Nienaber U, Hofer G, Voelckel W, Jambor C, Scharbert G, Kozek-Langenecker S, Solomon C (2010) Goal-directed coagulation management of major trauma patients using thromboelastometry (ROTEM)-guided administration of fibrinogen concentrate and prothrombin complex concentrate. Crit Care 14:R55

Recommended Reading

Cotton BA, Guy JS, Morris JA Jr et al (2006) The cellular, metabolic, and systemic consequences of aggressive fluid resuscitation strategies. Shock 26(2):115–121

Cotton BA, Reddy N, Hatch QM, LeFebvre E, Wade CE, Kozar RA, Gill BS, Albarado R, McNutt MK, Holcomb JB (2011) Damage control resuscitation is associated with a reduction in resuscitation volumes and improvement in survival in 390 damage control laparotomy patients. Ann Surg 254(4):598–605

Dutton RP (2012) Resuscitative strategies to maintain homeostasis during damage control surgery. Br J Surg 99(Suppl 1):21–28

Hemorrhage in Bile

▶ Hemobilia

Hemorrhage Resuscitation

▶ Whole Blood

Hemorrhagic Gastritis

▶ Gastritis

Hemorrhagic Shock

▶ Hemorrhage
▶ Shock Management in Trauma

Hemostatic Adjunct

Frank K. Butler
Department of the Army, Committee on Tactical Combat Casualty Care, U.S. Army Institute of Surgical Research, Fort Sam Houston, TX, USA
Department of the Army, Prehospital Trauma Care, Joint Trauma System, U.S. Army Institute of Surgical Research, Fort Sam Houston, TX, USA

Synonyms

Hemostatic agent; Junctional pressure device; Tourniquet; Tranexamic acid

Definition

Hemostatic adjuncts are dressings, medications, or devices that assist the medical provider in gaining control of hemorrhage.

Preexisting Condition

External hemorrhage.

Tourniquets
One of the signature successes in combat casualty care to emerge from the conflicts in Afghanistan

and Iraq has been the widespread use of pre-hospital tourniquet use to manage life-threatening extremity bleeding. The CAT and the SOFT-T are the most frequently used tourniquets at present. Kragh's papers (2008, 2009) on tourniquet use on the battlefield have both documented the success of these devices in saving lives and led to several refinements in battlefield tourniquet use: (1) In the Care Under Fire phase, tourniquets should be placed clearly proximal to the site of hemorrhage, applied over the casualty's uniform, and tightened as necessary to stop the bleeding; (2) in the Tactical Field Care phase, the wound should be re-evaluated, the tourniquet applied directly to the skin 2–3 in. above the bleeding site and tightened sufficiently to stop the distal pulse; (3) tourniquets should be rechecked frequently, especially when the casualty is moved, to ensure that bleeding is still controlled; (4) tourniquets should be left in place without attempts to transition to other methods of hemorrhage control if evacuation is expected to take 2 h or less; (5) tourniquets should be used for all traumatic amputations; (6) tourniquets should be left in place if the casualty is in shock; and (7) tourniquet application time should always be noted on the TCCC casualty card (Butler 2009).

Tourniquet use in the past has been considered a treatment modality of last resort when extremity hemorrhage cannot be controlled by any other means. The concern was that ischemic damage to the extremity caused by the tourniquet would necessitate a subsequent amputation. This misconception has now been definitively refuted (Kragh 2008, 2009). There is an emphasis in TCCC training on using tourniquets only to control extremity bleeding that is life-threatening. Evacuation times in Afghanistan and Iraq have typically been an hour or less in recent years after these theaters had matured. Casualties arrive at Role II or Role III facilities in time for surgeons to obtain definitive control of the injured vessel and then perform temporary shunting or revascularization procedures as needed. The success of tourniquets on the battlefields of Afghanistan and Iraq has led to increasing tourniquet use in the civilian sector in the United States (Butler 2012).

Hemostatic Dressings

There were no hemostatic dressings in widespread use among US forces at the start of the conflicts in Afghanistan and Iraq. The chitosan-based HemCon dressing and the granular zeolite agent QuikClot were fielded early in these conflicts. Improved hemostatic agents were subsequently developed and tested at the US Army Institute of Surgical Research (USAISR), the Naval Medical Research Center (NMRC), and other medical research facilities. These studies found Combat Gauze™ and WoundStat™ to be consistently more effective than HemCon® or QuikClot® (Kheirabadi 2009). As a result, the Committee on TCCC (CoTCCC) voted to recommend Combat Gauze as the first line treatment for life-threatening hemorrhage that is not amenable to tourniquet placement. WoundStat™ was recommended as the backup agent. The primary reason for this order of priority was that combat medical personnel on the CoTCCC expressed a strong preference for a gauze-type hemostatic agent rather than a powder or granule. This preference is based on field experience that powder and granular agents do not work well in wounds in which the bleeding vessel is at the bottom of a narrow wound tract or in windy environments (Butler 2009). WoundStat™ was later removed as a backup agent because of concerns about embolic and thrombotic complications noted in further animal testing (Kheirabadi 2010).

Junctional Pressure Devices

The increasing use of pressure-activated improvised explosive devices (IEDs) by insurgent forces in Afghanistan has produced an injury complex that has been designated dismounted complex blast injury (DCBI). This injury pattern is characterized by severe injuries to one or both lower extremities, often accompanied by upper extremity, urogenital, pelvic, and abdominal trauma. Multiple amputations are common in this injury pattern (Caravalho 2011). Lower-extremity amputations may be quite proximal, soft tissue damage is typically massive, and control of hemorrhage is often difficult to achieve with tourniquets and Combat Gauze.

H

This has led to the development of devices such as the Combat Ready Clamp (CRoC), which is designed to apply sustained pressure to large arteries in the groin. The CROC applies both anterior and posterior pressure to the injured area and has been shown to work in swine and perfused cadaver models (Dubick 2012). If a lower-extremity wound is not amenable to tourniquet application and bleeding is not controlled by hemostatic dressings, the CRoC or other junctional pressure devices may be considered (Dickey and Jenkins 2011a).

Tranexamic Acid (TXA)

Noncompressible hemorrhage remains one of the leading causes of potentially preventable deaths among combat casualties (Kelly 2008). A potential means for reducing the mortality in casualties suffering from noncompressible hemorrhage is found in the CRASH-2 study. The authors reported a reduction in the risk of death due to bleeding. Subgroup analysis suggested that the benefit of TXA was greater in patients treated within 3 h of injury compared to those treated later and in patients with a presenting systolic blood pressure of ≤ 75 mmHg. There was no difference in rate of vascular occlusive events between the two arms of the study. No unexpected adverse events were reported.

Further subgroup analysis of the CRASH-2 data found that the greatest benefit of TXA administration is obtained when patients receive the medication within 1 h of injury. Patients receiving TXA within this 1-h time window had a reduced risk of death from exsanguination compared to controls (5.3 % vs. 7.7 %, $p < 0.0001$). In this analysis, TXA given between 1 and 3 h post-injury also reduced the risk of death due to bleeding (4.8 % vs. 6.1 %). TXA given more than 3 h after injury was observed to increase the risk of death due to bleeding (4.4 % vs. 3.1 %) (CRASH-2 2011).

The findings of the CRASH-2 study were compelling, but the application of this data to combat casualties was uncertain. The different mechanisms of wounding, differences in injury patterns, delays to evacuation, and differences in trauma systems made it less than obvious that

TXA would provide similar benefits to individuals wounded in combat. A registry-based study of combat casualties receiving blood at the Bastion Role 3 facility in Afghanistan during the period January 2009 to December 2010 has confirmed the benefit of TXA in this population. In a review of 896 combat casualties treated at Bastion during the study period, 32.7 % ($N = 293$) received TXA (mean dose: 2.3 g) while 67.2 % ($N = 603$) did not. The TXA group was more severely injured (mean ISS: 25.2 vs. 22.5; $p < 0.001$), required more blood (mean 11.8 vs. 9.8 units of pRBCs; $p < 0.001$), had a lower Glasgow coma score (GCS) (mean 7.3 vs. 10.5; $p < 0.001$) and a lower initial systolic blood pressure (mean 112 vs. 122.5 mmHg). Despite being more severely injured, the TXA group had a lower unadjusted mortality than the no-TXA group (17.4 % vs. 23.9 %; $p = 0.028$). In the massive transfusion cohort ($N = 321$; mean 24-h transfusion: 21.9 $\pm$ 14.7 pRBC; 19.1 $\pm$ 13.3 FFP and 3.5 $\pm$ 3.2 apheresis platelet units), mortality was markedly lower in the TXA group compared to the no-TXA group (14.4 % vs. 28.1 %; $p = 0.004$). In a multivariate regression model, TXA use in the massive transfusion cohort was independently associated with survival (odds ratio: 7.28). For all patients requiring at least one unit of blood after combat injury, patients receiving TXA had higher rates of DVT (2.4 % vs. 0.2 %, $p = 0.001$) and PE (2.7 % vs. 0.3 %, $p = 0.001$), but casualties who received TXA were also more likely to have injury patterns associated with a higher risk of thromboembolic events: higher mean ISS (25 vs. 23, $p < 0.001$) and more severe extremity injuries (Morrison 2011).

The CRASH-2 and MATTERs findings support the use of TXA in combat casualties who are in hemorrhagic shock or at significant risk of hemorrhagic shock (Dickey and Jenkins 2011b).

Preexisting Condition

Hemorrhage is the preexisting condition that necessitates the use of hemostatic adjuncts.

Hemorrhage may be the result of motor vehicle accidents, falls, or criminal violence in the civilian setting. In the military setting, it is typically the result of small-arms fire or explosions secondary to grenades, artillery rounds, or IEDs.

Application

Tourniquets are not the intuitively simple devices that they might seem. Thanks to the work of Kragh and others, TCCC has developed a set of detailed guidelines that describe when to use tourniquets, how to apply them, and when to remove them (Butler 2010a).

Likewise, Combat Gauze must be applied in the recommended manner to be effective. Simply applying the gauze without maintaining pressure is not adequate. After 3 min of direct manual pressure, a pressure dressing may be applied over the wound to cover the wound and the agent, as well as to maintain a degree of pressure (Butler 2010a).

TXA must be given early after injury in order to be effective at reducing mortality (CRASH-2 2011). It is less effective after 1 h and may actually increase mortality if given after 3 h (CRASH-2 2011).

Cross-References

▶ Abdominal Major Vascular Injury, Anesthesia for
▶ Abdominal Solid Organ Injury, Anesthesia for
▶ Acute Coagulopathy of Trauma
▶ Adjuncts to Transfusion: Antifibrinolytics
▶ CASEVAC
▶ Compressible Hemorrhage
▶ Corpsman
▶ Damage Control Resuscitation
▶ Damage Control Resuscitation, Military Trauma
▶ Exsanguination Transfusion
▶ Fluid, Electrolytes, and Nutrition in Trauma Patients
▶ FP24
▶ Hemorrhage

▶ Hypothermia
▶ IED (Improvised Explosive Device)
▶ Monitoring of Trauma Patients During Anesthesia
▶ Noncompressible Hemorrhage
▶ Packed Red Blood Cells
▶ Plasma Transfusion in Trauma
▶ TACEVAC
▶ Tactical Combat Casualty Care
▶ Tourniquet
▶ Tranexamic Acid

References

Butler FK (2010) Tactical combat casualty care: update 2009. J Trauma 69:S10–S13

Butler FK, Giebner SD, McSwain N, Salomone J, Pons P (eds) (2010) Prehospital trauma life support manual, 7th edn – Military Version, Nov 2010

Butler F, Carmona R (2012) Tactical combat casualty care: from the battlefields of Afghanistan to the streets of America. The Tactical Edge

Butler FK Tactical combat casualty care: update 2009; J Trauma. 2010;69:S10–S13

Caravalho J (2011) OTSG dismounted complex blast injury task force; Final report, 18 June 2011, pp 44–47

CRASH-2 Collaborators (2011) The importance of early treatment with tranexamic acid in bleeding trauma patients: an exploratory analysis of the CRASH-2 randomized controlled trial. Lancet 377:1096–1101

Dickey N, Jenkins D (2011) Combat ready clamp. Defense Health Board Memo 23, Sep 2011

Dickey N, Jenkins D (2011) Tranexamic acid. Defense Health Board Memo 23, Sep 2011

Dubick M, Kragh JF (2012) Evaluation of the combat ready clamp to control bleeding in human cadavers, manikins, swine femoral artery hemorrhage model and swine carcasses. U.S. Army Institute of Surgical Research Technical Report, June 2012

Kelly JF, Ritenhour AE, McLaughlin DF et al (2008) Injury severity and causes of death from operation Iraqi freedom and operation enduring freedom: 2003–2004 versus 2006. J Trauma 64:S21–S27

Kheirabadi BS, Edens JW, Terrazas IB et al (2009) Comparison of new hemostatic granules/powders with currently deployed hemostatic products in a lethal model of extremity arterial hemorrhage in swine. J Trauma 66:316–328

Kheirabadi B, Mace J, Terrazas I et al (2010) Safety evaluation of new hemostatic agents, smectite granules, and kaolin-combat gauze in a vascular injury wound model in swine. J Trauma 68(2):269–278

Kragh JF, Walters TJ, Baer DG, Fox CJ, Wade CE, Salinas J, Holcomb JB (2008) Practical use of emergency tourniquets to stop bleeding in major limb trauma. J Trauma 64:S38–S50

Kragh JF Jr, Walters TJ, Baer DG, Fox CJ, Wade CE, Salinas J, Holcomb JB (2009) Survival with emergency tourniquet use to stop bleeding in major limb trauma. Ann Surg 249:1–7

Morrison JJ, Dubose JJ, Rasmussen TE, Midwinter MJ (2011) Military application of tranexamic acid in trauma emergency resuscitation study (MATTERs). Arch Surg published online 17 Oct 2011

Hemostatic Agent

▶ Hemostatic Adjunct

Hemostatic Resuscitation

▶ Blood Therapy in Trauma Anesthesia
▶ Plasma Transfusion in Trauma
▶ Resuscitation Goals in Trauma Patients
▶ Transfusion Strategy in Trauma: What Is the Evidence?

Hemostatic Transfusion Strategy

▶ Cryoprecipitate Transfusion in Trauma

Heparin-Induced Thrombocytopenia

Nadine Shehata
Departments of Medicine and Pathology and Laboratory Medicine, Mount Sinai Hospital, Institute of Health Policy Management and Evaluation, Li Ka Shing Knowledge Institute University of Toronto, Toronto, ON, Canada

Synonyms

Heparin-induced thrombocytopenia (HIT); Heparin-induced thrombocytopenia and thrombosis (HITT)

Definition

Heparin-induced thrombocytopenia is an immune-mediated adverse drug reaction to heparin. Patients develop platelet-activating IgG antibodies against platelet factor 4 (PF4)/heparin complexes, resulting in platelet aggregation and the release of procoagulant platelet-derived microparticles (Linkins et al. 2012). Thrombocytopenia (a platelet count less than 150×10^9/L) is the most common primary indicator of HIT, but bleeding or petechiae rarely occur (Linkins et al. 2012); rather HIT is a prothrombotic syndrome that manifests most commonly as venous or arterial thrombosis. Venous thrombosis is the most common complication occurring in 17–55 % of untreated patients who present with thrombocytopenia (Linkins et al. 2012). Arterial thrombotic events, such as limb artery thrombosis, thrombotic stroke, and myocardial infarction, occur less frequently, 3–10 % (Linkins et al. 2012), the exception being cardiac surgery where the majority of HIT-related thrombotic events are arterial (Linkins et al. 2012). Acute systemic reactions such as erythematous skin lesions at heparin injection sites, anaphylactic reactions, venous limb gangrene, and adrenal hemorrhagic necrosis are also indicative of HIT but occur less commonly. The mortality associated with HIT is high, from 5 % to 10 %, and is usually a result of thrombotic complications (Linkins et al. 2012).

Preexisting Condition

Frequency

Precise estimates of the frequency of HIT are limited by the challenges in disease diagnosis and factors that alter the rates of developing HIT such as the patient population and the heparin product (i.e., unfractionated heparin (UFH) compared to low molecular weight heparin (LMWH)). The risk of HIT is estimated to be highest in patients undergoing cardiac or orthopedic surgery (1–5 %) compared to medical or obstetrical patients (0.1–1 %) (Linkins et al. 2012). Women have twice the risk as men (Linkins et al. 2012; Warkentin 2012).

Heparin-Induced Thrombocytopenia, Table 1 The frequency of heparin-induced thrombocytopenia in relation to the type of prophylactic heparin in the trauma population (Lubenow et al. 2010)

Patient population	Incidence of HIT	Proximal VTE or PE
Major trauma UFH (n = 100)	4 %	8 %
Major trauma LMWH (n = 124)	0.8 %	8.9 %
Minor trauma UFH (n = 189)	0	0.53 %
Minor trauma LMWH (n = 148)	0	0

LMWH low molecular weight heparin, *PE* pulmonary embolism, *UFH* unfractionated heparin, *VTE* venous thromboembolism

Nondrug factors such as the severity of trauma have also been shown to alter the frequency of HIT (Lubenow et al. 2010). Patients undergoing major trauma surgery (defined as fracture of the humerus, hip or pelvis, femur, head of tibia, tibia or knee endoprosthesis) had a higher frequency of HIT compared to patients having minor surgery (defined as surgery involving the lower arm or hand, shoulder, spine, knee, ankle joint, foot, removal of metal, or tendon injury (Table 1)) (Lubenow et al. 2010). Development of HIT also differed in these patients according to the heparin product, higher with UFH compared to LMWH in patients undergoing major trauma, but no difference in patients undergoing surgery for minor trauma (Table 1) (Lubenow et al. 2010). Several other studies describe a higher frequency of HIT with UFH (2.6 %) compared to LMWH (0.2 %), and serologic investigations demonstrate much lower frequencies of anti-PF4/heparin antibody formation with LMWH compared with UFH consistent with an underlying plausible explanation that larger, and presumably more immunogenic, PF4/heparin complexes are formed with UFH than with LMWH (Levine et al. 2006; Martel et al. 2005; Warkentin and Greinacher 2007). This difference in the rates of HIT with the heparin products, however, may be more pronounced in the surgical setting (Warkentin and Greinacher 2007, Morris et al. 2007), as this difference has been predominately described in surgical populations, e.g., orthopedic surgery (Levine et al. 2006), compared to the medical population, and there are some reports that do not describe a difference in the rates of HIT with different heparin products (Warkentin and Greinacher 2007, Morris et al. 2007).

Application

Diagnosis

Prompt recognition of the pattern of thrombocytopenia that heralds HIT is key to the management of patients with HIT. Thrombocytopenia, a platelet count less than 150×10^9/L, is the most common clinical manifestation of HIT and occurs in 85–90 % of patients (Linkins et al. 2012). The platelet count may not need to fall below this number to be classified as HIT, however, as a 50 % or greater drop in platelet count even if the nadir remains more than 150×10^9/L is also suggestive of HIT, particularly in the postoperative patient population (Warkentin et al. 2003).

In the absence of prior exposure to heparin, the characteristic onset of decline in the platelet count is 5–10 days after initiation of heparin (Linkins et al. 2012; Warkentin 2012). An abrupt decline in platelet count that occurs within 24 h is seen in patients who already have circulating HIT antibodies because of recent exposure to heparin (usually within 30 days and occasionally as long as 100 days prior to exposure) (Linkins et al. 2012). Infrequently, thrombocytopenia may occur as long as 3 weeks after cessation of heparin (Linkins et al. 2012). Although the most common presenting characteristic of HIT is thrombocytopenia, in up to 25 % of patients with HIT, thrombosis precedes the development of thrombocytopenia (Linkins et al. 2012).

The diagnosis of HIT relies on (1) clinical probability and (2) laboratory testing (Warkentin 2011). Clinical assessment plays a critical role in the diagnosis of HIT because management decisions must be made immediately (the rate of thrombosis prior to treatment is approximately 5 % per day), and there is commonly a delay before the results of laboratory testing for HIT are available. Scoring tools have been developed

Heparin-Induced Thrombocytopenia, Table 2 The 4T score for heparin-induced thrombocytopenia (Linkins et al. 2012)[a]

4T	Thrombocytopenia	Timing of platelet count fall	Thrombosis or other sequelae	Other causes for thrombocytopenia
2 points	>50 % decline in platelets and platelet nadir ≥20 and no surgery within 3 days prior to the decline	Platelet decline 5–10 days after the start of heparin or platelet decline within 1 day of starting heparin and prior exposure to heparin within 5–30 days	Confirmed new venous or arterial thrombosis or skin necrosis at heparin injection site or anaphylactic reaction to intravenous unfractionated heparin bolus or adrenal hemorrhage	None
1 point	50 % decline in platelets but surgery within prior 3 days or 30–50 % decline or nadir of 10–19 or nadir and decline that does not fit criteria for score 2 or 0	Consistent with a decline days 5–10 but not clear (e.g., missing platelet counts) or platelet decline after day 10 or decline with 1 day of start of heparin and prior exposure to heparin in the past 31–100 days	Progressive or recurrent thrombosis in a therapeutically anticoagulated patient or erythematous skin lesions at heparin injection sites or suspected thrombosis (not proven)	Possible
0 points	Platelet decline <30 % or platelet nadir <10	Platelet decline ≤4 days without exposure to heparin in the past 100 days	Suspected	Probable other cause

[a]Adapted from Linkins LA, Dans AL, Moores LK, Bona R, Davidson BL, Schulman S, Crowther M, American College of Chest Physicians (2012) Treatment and prevention of heparin-induced thrombocytopenia: antithrombotic therapy and prevention of thrombosis, 9th ed: American College of Chest Physicians Evidence-Based Clinical Practice Guidelines. Chest 141(2 Suppl):e495S–e530S with permission

to estimate the pretest probability of HIT as there are many other causes of thrombocytopenia, and HIT is commonly overdiagnosed – only 10 % of patients suspected of having HIT are shown to have this diagnosis (Warkentin 2011). The most common scoring systems are the 4T score based on the mnemonic (Thrombocytopenia, Timing, Thrombosis, lack of oTher Explanations (Table 2)) and the more recent score, the HIT Expert Probability (HEP) score, based on eight features, namely, the magnitude of fall in platelet count, timing of fall in platelet count, nadir platelet count, thrombosis, skin necrosis, acute systemic reaction, bleeding, and other causes of thrombocytopenia (Linkins et al. 2012; Cuker et al. 2010). Patients with a low 4Ts score (≤3) have a very low probability of HIT (0–3 %). Yet, many patients (24–61 %) with a high 4Ts score prove not to have HIT (Linkins et al. 2012). The HEP score has been estimated to have a sensitivity of 100 % and specificity of

60 % for determining the presence of HIT but further validation is warranted to establish its accuracy (Cuker et al. 2010).

Because of the difficulty in clinical diagnosis, laboratory testing plays a vital role in the diagnosis of HIT. The two types of assays that are available are the immunological assays, i.e., enzyme immunoassay (EIA) that detects anti-PF4/heparin antibodies, and functional assays that detect platelet activation (e. g., the ^{14}C-serotonin release assay (SRA) and heparin-induced platelet activation (HIPA) assay) (Linkins et al. 2012). The EIA is the most commonly used assay. Correlation between the strength of the reaction with EIA is measured using optical density (OD) – a higher optical density is a marker of higher antibody levels and corresponds to a greater risk of HIT (Warkentin 2011). An OD level of more than 2.5 units indicates a high probability, more than 90 % of true HIT. For patients with weak

(0.45–0.99) or moderate (1.00–1.99) OD levels, referral of patient serum for a washed platelet activation test, e.g., SRA, should be considered (Warkentin 2011).

EIAs are very sensitive, but as only a minority of anti-PF4/H antibodies are platelet activating, the assay frequently detects irrelevant antibodies and has limited specificity and poor positive predictive value (Linkins et al. 2012; Warkentin 2011). However, EIAs have a high negative predictive value, i.e., negative test essentially rules out HIT (Warkentin 2011). The reference standards are the functional assays, the SRA, and the HIPA as they are sensitive and specific and are useful in the confirmation of HIT (Linkins et al. 2012). These assays are restricted to reference laboratories because of challenging technical requirements so that results are not readily available.

A diagnosis of HIT should only be made if (1) the clinical picture coincides with this diagnosis (i.e., 4 points or more in the 4T scoring system), with the presence of platelet-activating anti-PF4/H antibodies (EIA/SRAs), and (2) there should be no other diagnosis that provides a better explanation for the patient's clinical course. If only an EIA test result is available, a negative test may be interpreted as excluding HIT; and routine repeat testing is not required (Linkins et al. 2012; Warkentin 2011).

Management

The crucial first step in the treatment of HIT is the discontinuation of all forms of heparin and LMWH (including heparin flushes and heparin-coated catheters). Discontinuation without additional anticoagulation with a non-heparin product is inadequate as (1) the risk of thrombosis in patients who are not treated with a non-heparin anticoagulant is in the range of 17–55 %; (2) hypercoagulability is intensified from day 7 to 14, despite stopping heparin (Warkentin 2012); and (3) the risk of thrombosis in patients with isolated HIT who have heparin discontinued or substituted by a vitamin K antagonists (VKA) is approximately five times that of patients with isolated HIT who receive lepirudin or argatroban (Linkins et al. 2012). Standard treatment consists

of parenterally administered direct thrombin inhibitors (DTIs) such as lepirudin or desirudin (recombinant hirudin), argatroban, or bivalirudin, or indirect factor Xa inhibitors, such as danaparoid or fondaparinux (Tables 3 and 4) (Linkins et al. 2012). As there are no high-quality prospective head-to-head trials comparing one agent with another, cost (the cost of argatroban is approximately US$5,000 for a 5-day course), comorbid illnesses (renal or hepatic insufficiency that could affect clearance), bleeding risk (18–16 % with the DTIs), and availability (danaparoid was withdrawn from US market in 2002 by the manufacturer) guide the selection of these agents (Linkins et al. 2012). The new oral thrombin and factor Xa inhibitors (e.g., dabigatran, rivaroxaban) are promising, but their efficacy and safety have not yet been established in the treatment of HIT.

Vitamin K antagonists are initiated once the thrombocytopenia has recovered to 150×10^9/L as there is a potential risk of thrombosis if thrombocytopenia has not resolved (Linkins et al. 2012). VKAs should be started at a low dose, i.e., 5 mg, as rapid initiation of VKA in patients with HIT results in reduction in the natural anticoagulant protein C faster than the reduction in prothrombin levels and may lead to a prothrombotic state such as is manifested with warfarin-induced skin necrosis or venous limb gangrene (Linkins et al. 2012). Non-heparin anticoagulants generally overlap with VKAs for a minimum of 5 days. As the DTI argatroban also increases the INR (Table 3), the therapeutic level at which argatroban should be discontinued is when the INR is more than 4. The minimum duration of treatment of HIT with thrombosis follows recommendations of treatment of provoked VTE, i.e., 3–6 months. For patients with a diagnosis of HIT in the absence of thrombosis, consideration should be given to 4 weeks of anticoagulation as there is a high risk of thrombosis within the 2–4 weeks after treatment is initiated (Linkins et al. 2012).

Spontaneous bleeding is uncommon with HIT; thus, platelet transfusion is not routinely recommended as the safety of platelet transfusion has not been established (Linkins et al. 2012).

Heparin-Induced Thrombocytopenia, Table 3 Characteristics of anticoagulants used to treat HIT (Linkins et al. 2012)[a]

Characteristic	Lepirudin	Argatroban	Danaparoid	Bivalirudin	Fondaparinux
Target	Thrombin	Thrombin	Factor Xa	Thrombin	Factor Xa
Half life	80 min	40–50 min	24 h	25 min	17–20 h
Dosing	Prophylactic and therapeutic regimens	Prophylactic and therapeutic regimens	Prophylactic and therapeutic regimens	Prophylactic and therapeutic regimens	Prophylactic and therapeutic regimens
Elimination	Renal	Hepatobiliary	Renal	Enzymatic (80 %) Renal (20 %)	Renal
Approved for patients with HIT	Treatment	Treatment	Treatment	PCI/cardiac surgery	No
Method of administration	IV, SC	IV	SC	IV	SC
Monitoring	aPTT	aPTT	Anti-Xa	aPTT	Anti-Xa
Effect on INR	Increases INR	Increases INR	No effect	Increases INR	No effect
Antidote available	No	No	No	No	No
Dialyzable	High-flux dialyzers	20 %	Yes	25 %	20 %

aPTT activated partial thromboplastin time, *INR* international normalized ratio, *IV* intravenous, *SC* subcutaneous
[a]Adapted from Linkins LA, Dans AL, Moores LK, Bona R, Davidson BL, Schulman S, Crowther M, American College of Chest Physicians (2012) Treatment and prevention of heparin-induced thrombocytopenia: antithrombotic therapy and prevention of thrombosis, 9th ed: American College of Chest Physicians Evidence-Based Clinical Practice Guidelines. Chest 141(2 Suppl):e495S–e530S with permission

Heparin-Induced Thrombocytopenia, Table 4 Doses of direct and indirect thrombin inhibitors (Linkins et al. 2012)

Anticoagulant	Dosage
Argatroban	Omit the bolus. Infuse at $\leq 2\,\mu$ g/kg/min intravenously. Infuse from 0.5 to 1.2 μ g/kg/min for patients who have heart failure, multiple organ system failure, severe anasarca, or following cardiac surgery
	Target aPTT 1.5–3 times patient's baseline
Danaparoid[a]	Intravenously; bolus (weight, 60 kg: 1,500 units; 60–75 kg: 2,250 units; 75–90 kg: 3,000 units; 90 kg: 3,750 units) followed by infusion 400 units/h for 4 h then 300 units/h for 4 h then 200 units/h intravenously, adjusted to target anti-Xa levels 0.5–0.8 anti-Xa U/mL
Bivalirudin	Omit the bolus. Infuse at a rate of 0.15–0.20 mg/kg/h intravenously
	Target aPTT 1.5–2.5 times patient's baseline aPTT
Fondaparinux	Dose by weight
	50 kg: 5.0 mg subcutaneously daily
	50–100 kg: 7.5 mg subcutaneously daily
	>100 kg: 10 mg subcutaneously daily

[a]Danaparoid was withdrawn from US market in 2002 by the manufacturer (Linkins et al. 2012)

Platelet transfusion is reserved for patients who are bleeding or patients who require invasive procedures with a high risk of bleeding (Linkins et al. 2012).

Baseline platelet counts are taken prior to initiating heparin. Platelet count monitoring should be performed every 2–3 days from day 4 to day 14 (or until heparin is stopped, whichever is first) for patients considered to have a risk of HIT of more than 1 %, e.g., cardiac and orthopedic surgery patients (Linkins et al. 2012). The American College of Chest Physicians recommends that platelet counts need not be monitored when the risk of HIT is less than 1 % (Linkins et al. 2012).

If a previous exposure to heparin has occurred within the past 100 days, the platelet count should be repeated 24 h later as HIT can develop rapidly.

Reexposure to Heparins

Although there is no evidence to suggest that patients with a prior history of HIT have an amnestic response to heparin reexposure,[9] reexposure to heparin should be avoided in most patients because (1) there is evidence to suggest that the longer the reexposure to heparins, the higher the likelihood of recurrence of HIT antibodies; (2) thrombosis may precede a drop in platelet count; and (3) of the established efficacy and safety of alternative anticoagulants (Linkins et al. 2012).

The diagnosis of HIT is challenging, yet over the years, there has been a change from lack of recognition of this prothrombotic syndrome to overdiagnosis because of the increased awareness and concern of the risk of limb or life-threatening thrombosis. Vigilance, the use of probability scores, and laboratory testing should decrease the risk of exposing patients unnecessarily to costly direct thrombin inhibitors with their associated risk of major hemorrhage and allow for the prompt diagnosis of patients with true HIT so that initiation of appropriate therapy is not delayed.

Cross-References

▶ Anticoagulation/Antiplatelet Agents and Trauma
▶ DVT, as a Complication
▶ Pulmonary Embolus
▶ Thromboembolic Disease
▶ Venous Thromboembolism Prophylaxis and Treatment Following Trauma

References

Cuker A, Arepally G, Crowther MA, Rice L, Datko F, Hook K, Propert KJ, Kuter DJ, Ortel TL, Konkle BA, Cines DB (2010) The HIT Expert Probability (HEP) Score: a novel pre-test probability model for heparin-induced thrombocytopenia based on broad expert opinion. J Thromb Haemost 8(12):2642–2650

Levine RL, McCollum D, Hursting MJ (2006) How frequently is venous thromboembolism in heparin-treated patients associated with heparin-induced thrombocytopenia? Chest 130(3):681–687

Linkins LA, Dans AL, Moores LK, Bona R, Davidson BL, Schulman S, Crowther M, American College of Chest Physicians (2012) Treatment and prevention of heparin-induced thrombocytopenia: antithrombotic therapy and prevention of thrombosis, 9th ed: American College of Chest Physicians Evidence-Based Clinical Practice Guidelines. Chest 141(2 Suppl):e495S–e530S

Lubenow N, Hinz P, Thomaschewski S, Lietz T, Vogler M, Ladwig A, Jünger M, Nauck M, Schellong S, Wander K, Engel G, Ekkernkamp A, Greinacher A (2010) The severity of trauma determines the immune response to PF4/heparin and the frequency of heparin-induced thrombocytopenia. Blood 115(9):1797–1803

Martel N, Lee J, Wells PS (2005) Risk for heparin-induced thrombocytopenia with unfractionated and low-molecular-weight heparin thromboprophylaxis: a meta-analysis. Blood 106(8):2710–2715

Morris TA, Castrejon S, Devendra G, Gamst AC (2007) No difference in risk for thrombocytopenia during treatment of pulmonary embolism and deep venous thrombosis with either low-molecular-weight heparin or unfractionated heparin: a metaanalysis. Chest 132(4):1131–1139

Warkentin TE (2011) How I, diagnose and manage HIT. Hematol Am Soc Hematol Edu Program 2011:143–149

Warkentin TE (2012) HITlights: a career perspective on heparin-induced thrombocytopenia. Am J Hematol 87(Suppl 1):S92–S99

Warkentin TE, Greinacher A (2007) So, does low-molecular-weight heparin cause less heparin-induced thrombocytopenia than unfractionated heparin or not? Chest 132(4):1108–1110

Warkentin TE, Roberts RS, Hirsh J, Kelton JG (2003) An improved definition of immune heparin-induced thrombocytopenia in postoperative orthopedic patients. Arch Intern Med 163(20):2518–2524

Heparin-Induced Thrombocytopenia (HIT)

▶ Heparin-Induced Thrombocytopenia

Heparin-Induced Thrombocytopenia and Thrombosis (HITT)

▶ Heparin-Induced Thrombocytopenia

Hepatic and Biliary Injuries

Brian P. Smith
Perelman School of Medicine, University of
Pennsylvania, Philadelphia, PA, USA

Synonyms

Hepatic trauma; Liver trauma

Definition

Hepatic and biliary injuries can occur from any form of trauma including blunt and penetrating mechanisms. They occur when these structures are physically disrupted, resulting in parenchymal contusions, hematomas, or lacerations. Injuries to these organs most commonly result in direct hemorrhage or disruptions of the normal production and flow of bile.

Liver injuries occur in 5 % of patients with blunt trauma to the abdomen (Malhotra et al. 2000), and most of these injuries can be managed without operation. There is a high rate of concomitant injuries, and the overall mortality rate among these patients ranges from 10 % to 15 % (Malhotra et al. 2000; Richardson et al. 2000). Of these patients, one-quarter of the deaths are early, directly resulting from hepatic hemorrhage. Therefore, optimal management of hepatic trauma is based on careful selection of nonoperative versus operative management as well as prompt operative or interventional management to effect rapid control of hemorrhage.

The severity of liver injury is graded by the Organ Injury Scale. Except for the highest grades of liver injury, nonoperative management is the mainstay of therapy for patients who are hemodynamically stable and have no peritoneal signs or other indication for operative intervention. The failure rate of nonoperative management increases with liver injury grade. The overall success rate of nonoperative management is high because in most series, the majority of liver injuries are lower grade. For higher-grade injuries, nonoperative management should be considered a "trial," in order to encourage a prompt change to operative or interventional management when appropriate.

Most hemodynamically stable blunt trauma patients undergo computed tomography (CT), which has high accuracy in diagnosis of liver injury. CT findings of hepatic injury include liver parenchymal hypoperfusion, subcapsular hematoma, intravenous contrast extravasation ("blush"), and intrahepatic pseudoaneurysms. Hemoperitoneum may also be present. The indications for hepatic angiography and embolization remain controversial. In many centers, hepatic angiography and embolization remains a primary therapy for patients who are hemodynamically stable with IV contrast extravasation on CT (Misselbeck et al. 2009). Other centers may base the decision on a combination of liver injury grade and CT findings.

Patients with liver injury and signs of shock that are refractory to resuscitation should undergo emergency laparotomy to control hemorrhage. Exploration should be preceded (but not delayed) by large-bore intravenous access and mobilization of resuscitative resources such as a massive transfusion strategy with near-equal replacement of blood cells, plasma products, and platelets. Tranexamic acid (TXA) should be considered in hemodynamically unstable patients with suspected blood loss and transfusion requirements. Liver anatomy can be highly variable (Peitzman and Marsh 2012). The mobilization of additional experienced surgeons is encouraged, as the operative management of severe liver injuries requires judgment, meticulous exposure, and knowledge of hepatic anatomy.

The first step of controlling liver hemorrhage is reducing and compressing the fractured area. This is achieved with minimal (if any) formal mobilization. The surgeon should use two hands to restore the normal positioning of the injured liver, thereby apposing injured liver surfaces. This is buttressed with firm packing of dry laparotomy sponges. Pressure must be enough to arrest venous bleeding but not so great as to compress the inferior vena cava and prevent adequate cardiac preload (Peitzman and Marsh 2012). If bleeding persists despite adequate packing, then the surgeon must control vascular inflow to the liver using the Pringle maneuver (Kozar et al. 2011). The surgeon should initially encircle the porta hepatis with the thumb and forefinger (Pringle 1908). The pars flaccida of the hepatogastric ligament is divided, and the porta hepatis is occluded with an atraumatic clamp, vessel loop, or Rummel tourniquet.

Bleeding that stops with application of a Pringle maneuver is highly suggestive of a hepatic arterial or portal venous injuries. The wound should be explored and bleeding sources controlled with direct repair or ligation. Techniques such as finger fracture or linear stapling can be used to extend the injury. However, this approach should only be used to the extent of hemorrhage control. For hemorrhage that is controlled with packing, anatomic or non-anatomic resection is typically not indicated at index operation. Application of the Pringle maneuver should be restricted to short intervals if possible to minimize hepatic ischemic time. However, the optimal time of portal triad occlusion remains unknown, particularly among bleeding patients with liver injuries. As such, rapid identification and control of bleeding is paramount.

Bleeding that continues despite portal triad occlusion suggests hepatic venous injury. Several techniques to control these injuries have been described. Direct repair necessitates exposure of the injury. This is achieved by division of the falciform ligament to the suprahepatic inferior vena cava. The surgeon should then dissect the diaphragmatic attachments of the left or right hemiliver based on the suspected source of hemorrhage. The left hepatic vein is exposed by first dividing the gastrohepatic ligament. The left lateral segment is then retracted inferiorly, and the left triangular ligament is divided with electrocautery or scissors. This allows an assistant to pull the left lobe medially, dropping the gastroesophageal junction down, elevating the caudate lobe, and exposing the confluence of the IVC and left hepatic vein. Much of this venous confluence will be intrahepatic.

If bleeding is suspected from the right or middle hepatic veins, exposure should occur from the right side. The right hemiliver is retracted inferiorly, and the right triangular ligament is incised at the most lateral aspect. This dissection is carried medially, dividing the anterior and posterior leaflets of the coronary ligaments. The liver is then elevated anterior and toward the patient's left side, exposing the right kidney and adrenal gland. These structures are dropped posteriorly. At this point the surgeon must take great care to avoid injury to the short hepatic veins that drain directly from the liver into the IVC.

Intraparenchymal hepatic venous injuries that are not accessible with liver mobilization and exposure of the hepatic veins are particularly challenging. Atriocaval shunting of the retrohepatic IVC is well described, but it is rarely employed in clinical practice. Similarly, venovenous bypass in the setting of total hepatic vascular occlusion has been described but in practice is logistically challenging, and data regarding efficacy and outcomes in trauma is lacking. In practice, the most effective operative management is damage control extensive perihepatic packing to restore normal anatomy supplemented with immediate postoperative angioembolization. The management of complex hepatic injuries is likely to evolve as hybrid operating rooms and endovascular techniques are incorporated into the trauma surgery armamentarium.

Damage control surgery remains the technique of choice for trauma patients with exsanguinating abdominal injuries (Rotondo et al. 1993). Therefore injury severity must be recognized early, and efforts should be made to truncate the operation when bleeding is controlled and contamination is minimized. The optimal timing of repeat laparotomy is unknown, but the patient should be resuscitated such that hypothermia, coagulopathy, and acidosis have all been reversed (Kozar et al. 2011). At such time, all packs should be gently removed, and tissue viability should be assessed. For nonviable hepatic tissue, non-anatomic resection using finger fracture and linear stapler techniques is associated with improved outcomes (Polanco et al. 2008; Kozar et al. 2011). Endo GIA staplers are oftentimes helpful when anatomy makes utilization of standard staplers difficult. Topical hemostatic agents and the argon beam coagulator are useful adjuncts for operative control of bleeding.

Allogenic liver transplantation is unlikely to become a viable option for the management of severe liver injuries in the foreseeable future. Although it has been performed for severely injured patients when conventional techniques fail to control the liver injuries, in a case series, the overall mortality rate was greater than 40 %, with 25 % of patients requiring a repeat transplant surgery (Kaltenborn et al. 2013).

Tract injuries of the liver, such as those caused by gunshot or stab wounds, create a unique circumstance in that external compression might fail to tamponade the bleeding. In these circumstances, tractotomy might not be possible based on the length, depth, and trajectory of the wound. Such injuries may be amenable to balloon or plug tamponade devices. Balloon tamponade devices are made by passing a red rubber catheter into a large Penrose drain. The free end of the Penrose drain is ligated, and the end that accepts the red rubber catheter is tied around the catheter itself, allowing instillation of water, saline, or contrast agent into the Penrose. The devise is passed through the tract and then inflated, thereby exerting circumferential tamponade along the length of the wound (Parks et al. 1999). Similarly, plugs can be made from numerous surgical materials such as collagen, Gelfoam, Vicryl, etc. that can be useful for occluding wounds. Omental pedicle flaps might provide similar effects with more favorable biologic profiles.

Complications after liver trauma can be particularly challenging to manage and occur in three major forms: hepatic necrosis, bile leak, and organ space surgical site infection (or abscess). These complications have been associated with increasing injury severity, hepatic angioembolization, and presence of concomitant hollow visceral injuries.

Hepatic necrosis has been associated with fever, leukocytosis, abnormal liver function tests, and abnormal liver synthetic function. The optimal treatment for hepatic necrosis is unknown. Some surgeons argue that sterile necrosis (in the setting of sufficient residual liver parenchyma) poses minimal danger to the patient. Small areas of liver necrosis can be managed expectantly. Large areas of compromised liver often require operative debridement or percutaneous drainage. In addition to liver parenchyma, the gallbladder is at risk for ischemia and necrosis if its arterial supply (based on the right hepatic artery) is ligated or embolized. Some surgeons have advocated preemptive cholecystectomy among these patients, but the optimal timing of that procedure is unknown.

Bile leaks occur in 10–15 % of patients with liver injuries. Hepatobiliary iminodiacetic acid (HIDA) scanning is the study of choice to rule out bile leak. Its negative predictive value approaches 100 %, but its specificity has been called into question. Treatment of posttraumatic bile leak varies greatly by institution and location of the leak. Techniques include open exploration, laparoscopic washout and drainage, percutaneous drainage, endoscopic retrograde cholangiography (ERCP) with sphincterotomy and stenting, pharmacotherapies, and observation. Early wide drainage of liver injuries has also proven useful in the diagnosis of posttraumatic bile leak. Although drains help to control bile peritonitis, the efficacy of drains in expediting closure of bile leaks is unknown.

Bile that is in communication with the pleural space must be drained. Most biliary-pleural fistulae can be successfully treated with tube thoracostomy and antibiotic therapy. Many surgeons advocate the use of ERCP sphincterotomy and stenting if a biliary leak is demonstrated. Other surgeons have reported favorable outcomes with a thoracoscopic approach for biliary-pleural fistulae, but high-quality data regarding complications and outcomes are lacking. Bronchobiliary fistulae should be managed early with surgical exploration because of the high rate of morbidity and mortality. In such cases, the subdiaphragmatic space should also be explored and well drained.

Abscesses develop in 5–10 % of patients with liver injuries, with higher rates among patients with penetrating trauma and coincident hollow visceral injuries. Most of these infections are effectively treated with percutaneous drainage and culture-guided antibiotic therapy. More severe infections, however, especially those associated with hepatic necrosis, require operative debridement and drainage.

Isolated non-iatrogenic extrahepatic bile duct injuries are exceedingly rare. Bile duct injuries that do occur are often found in combination with major injuries to the pancreas, duodenum, and IVC that require operative exploration. This constellation of injuries is frequently lethal, and survivor morbidity is extremely high. Nevertheless, early recognition and diagnosis of these injuries is crucial to their management. Intraoperative interrogation of the common bile duct is best achieved with cholangiography, most commonly through the gallbladder (or cystic duct stump if cholecystectomy is performed). Occasionally, cholangiography can be performed in a retrograde fashion through the ampulla of Vater. This should be reserved for patients with preexisting duodenal injuries. Intentional duodenostomy for purposes of retrograde cholangiography is not recommended.

Bile duct injuries that are discovered at the index operation should be repaired if patient physiology permits. Partial injuries can be repaired over a T tube if the blood supply is sufficient and the anastomosis is tension-free. Complete transections should be reconstructed with a choledochoduodenostomy or a choledochojejunostomy. These can be time-consuming reconstructions, however; and the resuscitation of the injured patient must take priority. Many of these patients are better served with ligation of the proximal and distal bile duct injuries, with temporary external biliary drainage via a cholecystostomy tube. Delayed definitive reconstruction can be performed at a later date. Alternatively, if an injury is not defined and the operation needs to be truncated, the area can be widely drained, and interrogated during subsequent operation or with imaging such as magnetic resonance cholangiopancreatography (MRCP).

If the injury complex does not mandate laparotomy as the first-line management and there is clinical suspicion of bile leak, patients should undergo HIDA scan followed by MRCP or ERCP if the bile ducts warrant further study. These injuries can most often be managed with endoscopic techniques and percutaneous drainage of biloma.

Cross-References

► Adjuncts to Transfusion: Antifibrinolytics
► Coagulopathy
► Compressible Hemorrhage
► Damage Control Surgery
► Debridement
► Hemobilia
► Hemorrhage
► Hemorrhagic Shock
► Hepatic Failure
► Imaging of Abdominal and Pelvic Injuries
► Massive Transfusion
► Shock Management in Trauma

References

Kaltenborn A, Reichert B, Bourg CM, Becker T, Lehner F, Klempnauer J, Schrem H (2013) Long-term outcome analysis of liver transplantation for severe hepatic trauma. J Trauma Acute Care Surg 75(5):864–869

Kozar RM, Feliciano DV, Moore EE, Moore FA, Cocanour CS, West MA, Davis JW, McIntyre RC Jr (2011) Western Trauma Association/critical decisions in trauma: operative management of blunt hepatic trauma. J Trauma 71(1):1–5

Malhotra AK, Fabian TC, Croce MA, Gavin TJ, Kudsk KA, Minard G, Pritchard FE (2000) Blunt hepatic injury: a paradigm shift from operative to nonoperative management in the 1990s. Ann Surg 231(6):804–813

Misselbeck TS, Teicher EJ, Cipolle MD, Pasquale MD, Shah KT, Dangleben DA, Badellino MM (2009) Hepatic angioembolization in trauma patients: indications and complications. J Trauma 67(4):769–773

Parks RW, Chrysos E, Diamond T (1999) Management of liver trauma. Br J Surg 86(9):1121–1135

Peitzman AB, Marsh JW (2012) Advanced operative techniques in the management of complex liver injury. J Trauma Acute Care Surg 73(3):765–770

Polanco P, Leon S, Pineda J, Puyana JC, Ochoa JB, Alarcon L, Harbrecht BG, Geller D, Peitzman AB (2008) Hepatic resection in the management of complex injury to the liver. J Trauma 65(6):1264–1270

Pringle JH (1908) Notes on the arrest of hepatic hemorrhage due to trauma. Ann Surg 48:541–549

Richardson JD, Franklin GA, Lukan JK, Carrillo EH, Spain DA, Miller FB, Wilson MA, Polk HC Jr, Flint LM (2000) Evolution in the management of hepatic trauma: a 25 year perspective. Ann Surg 232(3):324–330

Rotondo MF, Schwab CW, McGonigal MD, Phillips GR 3rd, Fruchterman TM, Kauder DR, Latenser BA, Angood PA (1993) 'Damage control': an approach for improved survival in exsanguinating penetrating abdominal injury. J Trauma 35(3):375–382

Hepatic Failure

Nazia Selzner
University of Toronto, Toronto, ON, Canada

Synonyms

Acute liver failure; Fulminate hepatitis

Definition

Acute liver failure (ALF) is an uncommon condition in which rapid deterioration of liver function results in altered mentation, i.e., hepatic encephalopathy (HE), jaundice, and coagulopathy (usually an international normalized ratio (INR) >1.5) in individuals without known preexisting liver disease (cirrhosis). ALF often affects young people and carries a very high mortality. The time interval of onset of symptoms like jaundice and the appearance of encephalopathy led to several definitions of ALF as "hyperacute," "acute," and "subacute" liver failure referring to a jaundice-to-encephalopathy interval of 0–7, 8–28, and 29–84 days, respectively. The incidence of ALF has been estimated at 2,800 cases per year in the United States or approximately 3.5 deaths per million population. It remains one of the most challenging medical emergencies, because of the multi-organ nature and rapid progression of the disease, the need for multidisciplinary supportive interventions, and the requirement for the clinician to prompt the transfer of these patients to centers with intensive care unit and a liver transplantation center. Despite advances in supportive care, spontaneous survival without orthotopic liver transplantation (OLT) is as low as 20 %; therefore, early recognition and prompt transfer of potential transplant candidates to tertiary centers with intensive care and liver transplantation expertise are vital.

Preexisting Condition

The most prominent causes of ALF include drug-induced liver injury, viral hepatitis, autoimmune liver disease, mushroom poisoning (*Amanita phalloides*), and shock or hypoperfusion; many cases (>15 %) have no discernible cause. Etiology of ALF provides one of the best indicators of prognosis and also dictates specific management options (Khashab et al. 2007).

Drug-Induced Liver Disease
One of the most common causes of FHF is a substance that by itself is cytotoxic or after metabolizing is able to trigger a cascade of cytotoxic and/or autoimmune phenomena. The most common drug is acetaminophen (either as an overdose or in medicinal quantities) accounting for the majority of drug-induced ALF (at least in the United States and United Kingdom) (Bower et al. 2007). Many other prescription and over-the-counter medications have been associated with acute liver injury and liver failure. These include anti-inflammatories, anticonvulsants, antibiotics as well as certain herbal preparations, and weight-loss agents. A careful drug history should include listing of all agents taken, the time period involved, and the quantity or dose ingested. Determination of a particular medication as the cause of ALF is a diagnosis of exclusion.

Mushroom Poisoning
Mushroom poisoning (usually Amanita phalloides) may cause ALF, and the initial history should always include inquiry concerning recent mushroom ingestion. This diagnosis should be suspected in patients with a history of severe gastrointestinal symptoms (nausea, vomiting, diarrhea, abdominal cramping), which occur within hours to a day of ingestion. If these effects are present, it may be early enough to treat patients with gastric lavage and activated charcoal via nasogastric tube.

Viral Hepatitis
ALF occurs in less than 5 % of viral hepatitis infections, and hepatitis B accounts for the

majority of cases. Hepatitis E virus-induced ALF is uncommon in Western countries, but accounts for sporadic and major epidemics of viral hepatitis in the developing world, particularly in pregnant women (India, Pakistan, Mexico, Central Asia, Southeast Asia, Russia, and North Africa) and in travelers returning from these areas. Other viruses causing ALF include herpes simplex virus (HSV), varicella zoster virus, cytomegalovirus, Epstein–Barr virus, parvovirus B19, and yellow fever virus. These viruses generally lead to ALF in the setting of immune compromise or pregnancy, but cases in immunocompetent individuals have been reported.

Other Causes of ALF

Acute fatty liver of pregnancy (AFLP) and the HELLP syndrome (hemolysis, elevated liver enzymes, low platelets) are part of a spectrum of the same disease process. ALF presents during the third trimester but may in some rare cases occur postpartum.

ALF from autoimmune hepatitis occurs in patients with unrecognized preexisting disease. Serum autoimmune antibodies may be absent, and in this situation, liver biopsy may be helpful in establishing the diagnosis.

Wilson disease is another uncommon cause of ALF due to an autosomal recessive disorder of copper metabolism. The diagnosis of ALF from Wilson disease is often difficult because the usual diagnostic features may be absent, for example, Kayser–Fleischer rings are absent in up to 50 % of patients. Serum ceruloplasmin will be normal in 15 % of patients, and low ceruloplasmin levels can be seen in ALF from other causes. However, Wilson disease–ALF is often accompanied by a Coombs-negative hemolytic anemia, severe hyperbilirubinemia, moderate elevations in aminotransferases (<500 IU/l), and high serum and urinary copper concentration.

The most common form of hypoxic liver injury is "shock liver" seen after episodes of systemic hypotension or a low blood-flow state. The prognosis depends upon the patient's underlying disease state, and shock liver per se is rarely fatal. Conditions, which result in more severe vascular obstruction, are more likely to lead to ALF and death. These include Budd–Chiari syndrome, sinusoidal obstruction syndrome (venoocclusive disease) due to medications or herbs, and malignancies involving the liver (i.e., lymphoma).

Clinical Features

The initial clinical presentation of ALF may be nonspecific and may include anorexia, fatigue, nausea, abdominal pain, jaundice, and fever before progressing to HE (Bernal et al. 2010). The development of HE is the hallmark of fulminant hepatic failure. In contrast to the patient with chronic liver disease, the evolution to grade III/IV HE is a grave prognostic sign as this group is at risk of intracranial hypertension (ICP) and subsequent herniation of the brainstem structures may lead to irreversible brain injury that would not be corrected with liver transplantation. Clinical signs suggestive of increasing ICP include worsening of HE, systemic hypertension and bradycardia, altered pupillary reflexes, and decerebrate rigidity. All of these clinical signs occur late in the clinical course, when therapeutic interventions may be ineffective, and this has led to the direct monitoring of ICP in patients with ALF.

Application

Patient Management

Although patients with ALF represent a heterogeneous group, they have consistent clinical features which include acute loss of hepatocellular function, the systemic inflammatory response, and multi-organ system failure. No single therapy has yet been found to improve the outcome of all patients with ALF, with the possible exception of NAC (Craig et al. 2010). Since there is no proven therapy for ALF in general, management consists of intensive care support after treatments for specific etiologies have been initiated. A patient with onset of grade III/IV HE warrants admission to an intensive care unit since the condition may deteriorate quickly.

Careful attention must be paid to fluid management, hemodynamics, metabolic parameters, as well as management of infection. Coagulation parameters, complete blood counts, serum glucose, and arterial blood gas should be checked frequently.

Hepatic Encephalopathy

Lactulose can be administered at the onset of HE; however, its ongoing use is not recommended due to its potential for gaseous distension of the bowel that could present technical difficulties during liver transplantation (Trotter 2009). Patients should be positioned with the head elevated at 30°. Frequent neurological evaluation for signs of ICH, such as pupillary size and reactivity, posturing, and changes in peripheral reflexes, should be conducted. As patients progress to grade III/IV encephalopathy, intubation and mechanical ventilation are mandatory.

Management of Elevated Intracranial Pressure (ICP)

The use of ICP monitoring devices in patients with ALF remains controversial, and practices vary among different centers because of the lack of consensus over treatment goals, the associated risks of bleeding and infection, and the lack of randomized trial data supporting improved survival. The rationale for the insertion of an ICP monitor is to improve the early recognition of ICH so that corrective therapy can be initiated as well as assessment of the cerebral perfusion pressure (CPP; calculated as mean arterial pressure [MAP] minus ICP) can be performed, in order to avoid hypoperfusion of the brain (Lee et al. 2011). The goal in management of ICH is therefore to lower ICP (generally to <20 mmHg) while preserving CPP (generally to >60 mmHg). If ICH develops, intravenous osmotic agents such as mannitol or barbiturates such as thiopentone are often transiently effective in decreasing cerebral edema. Limited evidence supports the use of hypertonic saline chloride, propofol sedation, and indomethacin. Some groups have reported the use of moderate hypothermia (32–33 °C) to reduce ICP as a bridge to transplantation. However, the benefit of this strategy has not been studied in a controlled trial and has not been shown to improve transplant-free survival.

Infection

Impaired level of consciousness with associated risk of aspiration, the insertion of intravenous and urinary catheter, the loss of hepatic Kupffer cell functions, as well as other factors contribute to the high rate of bacterial and fungal infection in patients with ALF which may preclude liver transplantation. Broad-spectrum intravenous antibacterial therapy reduces the incidence of infection and should be started as soon as patients are admitted to the ICU. Close surveillance for infection should be maintained in all ALF patients with frequent chest radiographs and cultures of blood, urine, and sputum.

Coagulopathy

ALF is characterized by prolongation of prothrombin time and quantitative and qualitative platelet dysfunction, hypofibrinogenemia, and reductions in coagulation factors II, V, VII, and X. This is due both to the impaired production of the clotting factors by the liver and to increased consumption related to disseminated intravascular coagulation. However, despite the severity of the coagulopathy, clinically significant spontaneous bleeding is relatively unusual in ALF, and the prophylactic administration of large volumes of fresh frozen plasma (FFP) in ALF is unnecessary, interferes with prognostic scoring systems, and may worsen cerebral edema or volume overload. Therefore, transfusions of FFP, platelet, and cryoprecipitate should be reserved for use in actively bleeding patients or prior to planned invasive procedures.

Hemodynamic Disturbances and Renal Dysfunction

Hemodynamic disturbances with low systemic vascular resistance, increased cardiac output, and hypotension occur frequently in patients with ALF and contribute to low peripheral tissue oxygenation and multi-organ system failure. Hypotensive patients with ALF should be resuscitated with normal saline first and changed to half-normal saline containing sodium bicarbonate if acidotic, before consideration of the use of vasopressors. There are no studies that define the optimal vasopressor regimen for use in hypotensive patients with ALF. The general consensus appears to be that norepinephrine may best augment peripheral organ perfusion while minimizing tachycardia and preserving splanchnic (thereby hepatic) blood flow.

Acute renal failure is a frequent complication in patients with ALF. Etiology of renal failure in this setting is multifactorial and may be related to hemodynamic alterations or acute tubular necrosis. The frequency of renal failure may be even greater with acetaminophen overdose as acetaminophen may cause direct nephrotoxicity. Careful attention should be given to avoid nephrotoxic agents such as nonsteroidal drugs (NSAID), aminoglycosides, and contrast agents. Prompt treatment of sepsis and maintenance of adequate hemodynamic are also recommended. Renal replacement therapy is frequently required for management of renal failure seen in these patients. Hypophosphatemia is associated with renal failure in ALF and may also be linked to hepatic regeneration; persistently elevated phosphate levels may reflect failure of this regenerative process and have been associated with a poorer prognosis in acetaminophen-induced ALF.

Hypoglycemia

Reduced hepatic glycogen stores and hyperinsulinemia contribute to hypoglycemia, which complicates up to 40 % of ALF cases. Continuous glucose administration is frequently required. Hypoglycemia should be managed with continuous glucose infusions, since symptoms may be obscured in the presence of encephalopathy.

Etiology-Specific Therapies

N-acetylcysteine (NAC) is the specific antidote for acetaminophen-induced ALF. Administration of NAC is recommended in any case of ALF in which acetaminophen overdose is suspected. NAC should be given as early as possible but may still be of value 48 h or more after ingestion. It has been proven to have few side effects, essentially nausea and vomiting. Controversy exists over when to stop the use of NAC, whether

a standard 72-h period is optimal or should be continued until liver chemistry values have improved. NAC is also often administered in ALF of non-acetaminophen etiology as it may improve outcomes in these cases.

There is no specific treatment for acute liver failure due to hepatitis A. In patients with ALF due to hepatitis B, the use of Lamivudine or other more potent nucleoside/nucleotide analogues has not been shown to improve prognosis. For other viruses such as herpesviruses, specific antiviral therapy should be administered (Larson 2010).

Early delivery is recommended in cases of ALF related to pregnancy for both safety of the fetus and treatment for the disease process itself. Close postpartum observations of both mother and infant are important to detect any hemorrhagic complications or clinical or biochemical deterioration, which can occasionally necessitate emergency liver transplantation.

Corticosteroids have not been proven as effective treatment in ALF due to autoimmune hepatitis. They might increase the risk of sepsis, particularly fungal sepsis, which may preclude liver transplantation.

Isolated cases report the successful use of plasmapheresis and chelation therapy in the treatment of fulminant Wilson's disease, although these remain a bridge to transplantation rather than definitive therapies.

Prognosis

The decision to list an ALF patient for liver transplantation should balance the inherent risks associated with delaying listing against the potential for spontaneous recovery with medical therapy alone. Multiple prognostic models have been proposed to help determine the likelihood of spontaneous survival. Many of these models, however, are methodologically flawed as unblinded, retrospective, and subject to bias.

The most widely applied prognostic system is the King's College Hospital criteria (KCH Criteria), developed from a retrospective cohort of nearly 600 patients. These criteria incorporate both the etiology of ALF and clinical/biochemical parameters of disease. In a meta-analysis of studies using the KCH Criteria, the pooled sensitivity and specificity were 68–69 % and 82–92 %, respectively. Other widely used model is the Clichy criteria, which are based on the measurement of factor V levels. The Clichy criteria were developed in a cohort of French patients with acute hepatitis B virus infection. A serum factor V level of <20 % in patients younger than 30 years or <30 % in any patient with grades 3–4 HE predicted mortality with a positive predictive value of 82 % and a negative predictive value of 98 %. Serum lactate has also been proven to be an independent predictor of poor outcome in acetaminophen-induced ALF. MELD (Model for End-Stage Liver Disease) score, which is used for organ allocation in chronic liver disease, is not used in patients with ALF.

Liver Transplantation

Emergency orthotopic liver transplantation for ALF is the only treatment to date to alter substantially the mortality resulting from the condition. Patient survival following liver transplantation for ALF is generally poorer than that in those transplanted for chronic liver failure, usually in the order of 65–80 % at 1 year. However, following the first year, this trend has reversed and ALF patients have a better long-term survival. The majority of deaths occurs within the first 1–3 months following transplantation and is usually secondary to neurological complications or sepsis.

Cross-References

▶ Coagulopathy
▶ ICU Management
▶ Systemic Inflammatory Response Syndrome

References

Bernal W, Auzinger G, Dhawan A et al (2010) Acute liver failure. Lancet 376:190–201
Bower WA, Johns M, Margolis HS et al (2007) Population-based surveillance for acute liver failure. Am J Gastroenterol 102:2459–2463
Craig DGN, Lee A, Hayes PC et al (2010) The current management of acute liver failure. Aliment Pharmacol Ther 31:345–358
Khashab M, Tector AJ, Kwo PY (2007) Epidemiology of acute liver failure. Curr Gastroenterol Rep 9:66–73
Larson AM (2010) Diagnostic and management of acute liver failure. Curr Opin Gastroenterol 26:214–221
Lee W, Larson AM, Stravitz T (2011) AASLD position paper: the management of acute liver failure; update. Hepatology 2011:1–22
Trotter JF (2009) Practical management of acute liver failure in the intensive care unit. Curr Opin Crit Care 15:163–167

Hepatic Trauma

▶ Hepatic and Biliary Injuries

Heterotopic Bone Formation

▶ Heterotopic Ossification

Heterotopic Ossification

Khanjan H. Nagarsheth
R Adams Cowley Shock Trauma Center,
University of Maryland School of Medicine,
Baltimore, MD, USA

Synonyms

Heterotopic bone formation; HO

Definition

Heterotopic ossification (HO) is the presence of bone formation in soft tissues and can be a complication of traumatic wounds. This condition was reported during World War I in soldiers who had experienced significant spinal cord injury (SCI) (Dejerne and Ceilier 1918). HO can be confused with both dystrophic calcification and calcium deposition associated with calciphylaxis. Early on, the overlying soft tissue will also often display signs of rubor, dolor, calor, and tumor (redness, pain, heat, and swelling), which can be confused with osteomyelitis or a soft tissue infection and make the diagnosis difficult. Later HO can lead to joint immobility and ankylosis.

The underlying cause of HO can be broadly broken up into two categories, acquired and idiopathic (Shehab et al. 2002). The acquired form is more common and can occur after sustaining musculoskeletal or soft tissue trauma. This can be further subdivided based on anatomic location. Posttraumatic myositis ossificans occurs in the soft tissues adjacent to long bone fractures. Posttraumatic neurogenic HO occurs after trauma to the nervous system and is not necessarily associated with soft tissue injury. There have also been reports of HO occurring after serious burn and scald injuries and desquamation from toxic epidermal necrolysis (Gibson and Poduri 1997).

In the literature, the incidence of HO is noted to vary with the type of trauma that preceded it. In patients who had a closed head injury, the incidence of HO is 10–20 %. In patients with SCI, the incidence of HO is reported as 20–30 % and these patients also have a 35 % chance of limited joint mobility. Of these patients that develop limited joint mobility, 10 % will also have ankylosis and develop contractures (Shehab et al. 2002).

Preexisting Condition

Typically HO will begin to manifest and appear between 3 to 12 weeks after trauma. The major concern with HO is loss of joint mobility and loss of function (Sawyer et al. 1991). Other complications that can occur include pressure necrosis and ulceration of soft tissue as well as chronic pain from peripheral nerve entrapment.

As mentioned earlier, HO is bone formation in the soft tissue and very often, this occurs as a result of trauma. In the literature, there have been several mechanisms for why HO could occur. The crux of what needs to occur for HO to exist is a method of changing mesenchymal cells into osteogenic cells in the soft tissues. One mechanism proposed for this phenomenon is presence of a morphogenetic protein with the ability to facilitate this cellular change. This protein, known as bone morphogenic protein, is found in normal bone and believed to be released after trauma in response to venous stasis and inflammation (Urist et al. 1978). Other work has shown that patients who develop HO have higher levels of osteoblast-stimulating factors than patients with similar injury patterns who did not have HO (Kurer et al. 1992). Factors that also lead to HO formation include hypercalcemia, tissue hypoxia, prolonged immobilization, remobilization, and imbalance between parathyroid hormone (PTH) and calcitonin production.

Pathophysiology

Histologically, HO is identified by cellular fibrous proliferation and the presence of osteoid and primitive bone. These areas show calcification peripherally such that a radiopaque rim is seen around a radiolucent center. This also helps differentiate HO from malignancies like osteosarcoma (Shehab et al. 2002). On the outside of HO, one will find mature lamellar bone surrounded by attenuated and compacted muscular and fibrous tissues.

Although there is no perfect test to be used for early detection of HO, there are a few laboratory studies that could be helpful adjuncts in identifying HO in patients who are deemed clinically high risk for its development. Alkaline phosphatase is a hydrolase enzyme that is responsible for dephosphorylating many types of molecules. In humans, alkaline phosphatase is found in highest concentrations in the liver and biliary tree, in the kidney, bones, and the placenta. In patients with HO, the alkaline phosphatase level is elevated to 3.5 times the normal value at 10 weeks post injury and returns to normal by 18 weeks post injury (Orzel and Rudd 1985). Another laboratory study that may be useful is 24-h urine excretion of prostaglandin E_2 (PGE_2). PGE_2 is felt to possibly be responsible for stimulating differentiation of progenitor cells responsible for HO formation. This is also why indomethacin, a nonsteroidal anti-inflammatory drug (NSAID), has been proposed and used to slow the progression of HO (Schurch et al. 1997).

Application

Imaging

Radiographs can be obtained that reveal radiopaque calcification peripherally with central radiolucency. Unfortunately, conventional x-rays will usually only display these calcifications 6–9 weeks after initial trauma, whereas three-phase bone scintigraphy will detect HO formation at about 2–3 weeks after initial injury. This modality is widely regarded as the most sensitive. On bone scan, the abnormal signal present from HO will remain elevated for about 6–12 months and will then again return to baseline. Computed tomography (CT) scan and magnetic resonance imaging (MRI) have also been used to identify HO. On MRI, the most common finding for HO is a rim of low signal intensity (Shehab et al. 2002).

Treatment

HO is not without complications and morbidity. As noted earlier, pressure ulceration, infection, nerve entrapment, and loss of function can all be associated with HO. Physical therapy is the initial treatment of choice when encountering HO, so as to prevent loss of function and movement. The problem with this method of treatment is the possibility of exacerbating the injuries that lead to HO formation. It was also mentioned that one of the prevailing theories about HO formation was the inciting effects of PGE2. Treatment with an NSAID, such as indomethacin, has been advocated. There has been experience with radiation therapy for the prevention and treatment of HO. Some work has also recommended the use of radiation therapy in conjunction with indomethacin in order to prevent HO formation (Knelles et al. 1997). This has been seen usually in the setting of total hip arthroplasty but has also been applied in trauma patients after acetabular repair. The standard treatment dose has been a single treatment with 7 Gy of radiation. This is typically in patients who have contraindications to indomethacin, as many trauma patients do, and people who have a history of forming HO (Knelles et al. 1997).

There have been attempts to stage the maturity of HO after its formation. This is done in order to reduce the complications of surgery and reduce intraoperative hemorrhage. There exist certain recommended time frames for when to surgically remove HO based on its etiology. For example, one should wait 6 months to remove HO as a result of musculoskeletal trauma, 1 year after SCI, and 18 months after TBI. Serial perioperative nuclear medicine bone scans have been used to stage HO formation and determine maturity. A decreasing ratio of HO to normal bone is indicative of maturity and associated with decreased morbidity for HO resection.

According to Shehab et al., the ideal candidate for surgical resection of HO will have no joint pain or swelling, normal laboratory results including alkaline phosphatase, and mature HO as indicated by nuclear medicine bone scintigraphy (Shehab et al. 2002).

Summary

HO formation is complication noted in patients after sustaining significant musculoskeletal trauma, SCI, or TBI. The diagnosis of HO can be difficult to make as it mimics cellulitis and is associated with acute inflammation. The exact pathogenesis of HO has not yet been completely elucidated, but there are many promising theories that attempt to explain this occurrence at a cellular level. Currently, the best imaging modality is bone scintigraphy although CT scanning is proving to be a useful adjunct in preoperative planning. Nonoperative therapies such as indomethacin and other NSAIDs are available and have varying degrees of success. Surgery should be timed and performed in such a way that the HO is mature as this will reduce intraoperative morbidity and blood loss. HO continues to be an area of interest and research in the posttrauma patient.

Cross-References

▶ Contractures

References

Dejerne A, Ceilier A (1918) Para-osteo-arthropathies des paraplegiques par lesion medullaire; etude clinique et radiographique. Ann Med 5:497

Gibson CJ, Poduri KR (1997) Heterotopic ossification as a complication of toxic epidermal necrolysis. Arch Phys Med Rehabil 78:774–776

Knelles D, Barthel T, Karer A et al (1997) Prevention of heterotopic ossification after total hip replacement: a prospective, randomized study using acetyl salicylic acid, indomethacin and fractional or single dose irradiation. J Bone Joint Surg Br 79:596–602

Kurer MH, Khoker MA, Dandona P (1992) Human osteoblast stimulation by sera from paraplegic patients with heterotopic ossification. Paraplegia 30:165–168

Orzel JA, Rudd TG (1985) Heterotopic bone formation: clinical, laboratory and imaging correlation. J Nucl Med 26:125–132

Sawyer JR, Myers MA, Rosier RN, Puzas JE (1991) Heterotopic ossifiction: clinical and cellular aspects. Calcif Tissue Int 49:208–215

Schurch B, Capaul M, Vallotton MB, Rossier AB (1997) Prostaglandin E$_2$ measurements: their value in the early diagnosis of heterotopic ossification in spinal cord injury patients. Arch Phys Med Rehabil 78:687–691

Shehab D, Elgazzar AH, Collier BD (2002) Heterotopic ossification. J Nucl Med 43:346–353

Urist MR, Nakagawa M, Nakata N, Nogami H (1978) Experimental myositis ossificans: cartiledge and bone formation in muscle in response to diffusible bone matrix-derived morphogen. Arch Pathol Lab Med 102:312–316

High Powered

▶ Cavitation
▶ High-Velocity

High Velocity

▶ Cavitation

High-Frequency Ventilation

▶ Mechanical Ventilation, High-Frequency Oscillation

High-Velocity

Craig D. Silverton[1] and Paul Dougherty[2]
[1]Department of Orthopedic Surgery, Henry Ford Hospital, Detroit, MI, USA
[2]Department of Orthopedic Surgery, University of Michigan, Ann Arbor, MI, USA

Synonyms

Ballistics; Cavitation; High powered; Muzzle velocity; Speed

Definition

Velocity of a projectile or bullet is usually measured in ft/s or m/s. The two most common descriptions of velocity are high and low velocity relating to rifle (>2,500 ft/s) or handgun (<1,000 ft/s). These two arbitrary numbers cover the majority of handgun and rifle calibers but leave projectiles traveling in the 1,000–2,500 ft/s open for interpretation as to whether they are truly low or high velocity by definition (Fackler 1988). High velocity is a ill defined term which in wound ballistics is meant to imply greater tissue damage associated with center fire rifle bullet wounds when compared with those of a handgun. Velocity was and is a relative term and high velocity was considered about 1,600 fps during the late 19th century but today the threshold has moved up to 2,500 fps (Fig. 1 and 2).

Most handgun calibers are low velocity and most rifle calibers are high velocity according to the definition. However, the wounding potential of many handgun calibers (357 magnum, 44 magnum) approaches rifle ballistics. A 240 grain bullet traveling at 1,550 ft/s (44 magnum) creates a larger permanent and temporary cavity compared to a 158 grain bullet traveling at 850 ft/s (38 special).

In contrast is the rifle bullet traveling at less than 2,000 ft/s with 400 grains of lead that creates

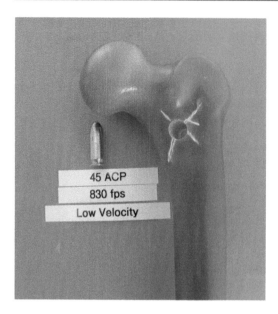

High-Velocity, Fig. 1 The slow moving 45 ACP pistol caliber usually creates a smaller temporary and permanent cavity through soft tissue and bone

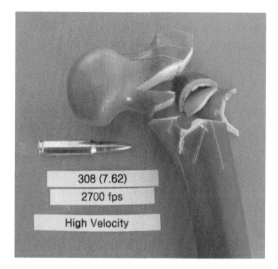

High-Velocity, Fig. 2 The fast moving 308. rifle caliber creates devastating effects to both soft tissue and bone

a devastation permanent and temporary cavity despite its comparatively lower rifle velocity.

One cannot just look at velocity of a bullet to determine the wounding effects. It is just one of many variables that determines the overall wound channel (Belkin 1978).

In comparing the velocity of common calibers and projectiles, it must be emphasized that these are muzzle velocities and not impact velocities. The farther one is from the target, the lower the impact velocity. Eventually all high-velocity projectiles become low velocity somewhere along their flight path. The overall distance traveled by a projectile is governed by the size of the bullet, composition, powder, rotational and vertical velocity, as well as the humidity and air density.

In the treatment of low- or high-velocity wounds, one should concern themselves with actual wound itself and not be swayed by the history as most patients have no idea as to the actual weapon they were shot with (Peters and Sebourn 1996). Wounds should be debrided of necrotic tissue (permanent cavity) only and all viable tissue (temporary cavity) should be left intact. The old adage that high-velocity wounds need major debridement has been shown to be more harmful in many cases as the temporary cavities in most cases seem to heal without additional debridement required. In summary, ballistic wounds should be treated based on their appearance and not on the velocity of the weapon they were fired from.

Cross-References

▶ Cavitation
▶ Debridement
▶ Explosion
▶ Fragment Injury
▶ Mortars
▶ Spalling

References

Belkin M (1978) Wound ballistics. Prog Surg 16:7–2

Fackler ML (1988) Wound ballistics. A review of common misconceptions. JAMA 259:2730–2736

Peters CE, Sebourn CL (1996) Wound ballistics of unstable projectiles. Part II: temporary cavity formation and tissue damage. J Trauma 40:S16–S21

High-Velocity Trauma

▶ Military Trauma, Anesthesia for

HI-MAP

▶ Ultrasound in the Trauma and ICU Setting

Hindfoot Injury

▶ Calcaneus Fractures

Hip Dislocations

▶ Pediatric Fractures About the Hip

Hip Dislocations and Fracture-Dislocations

Fernando Serna
Orthopedic Trauma Surgeon, Department of
Orthopedics, Mayo Clinic Health System,
Eau Claire, WI, USA

Synonyms

Acetabulum fracture-dislocation; Femoral head
fracture-dislocation; Pelvis fracture-dislocation;
Proximal femur fracture-dislocation

Definition

Hip dislocations and fracture-dislocations are
injuries that most often result from high-energy
traumatic mechanisms of injury in which the
femoral head is dislocated from the acetabulum
with or without an associated fracture of the
proximal femur or pelvis/acetabulum. Hip dislocations are also a known complication of hip
arthroplasty (or replacement) surgery, but discussion of this is outside the scope of this text.

Anatomy and Physiology

The femoroacetabular joint is classified as a true
ball-and-socket joint and, as such, has a great
degree of inherent bony stability with a vacuum-
suction fit. As with all articular surfaces, the acetabular socket and femoral head are covered with
articular cartilage to allow for smooth, low friction
motion. Added to this bony stability are several
soft tissue stabilizing factors such as (1) an acetabular labrum to deepen the socket, (2) a ligament
between the femoral head and the acetabulum
(ligamentum teres), (3) a complex series of ligaments that contribute to the hip joint capsule, and
(4) a large number of muscles that cross the hip
joint. This all allows for a very stable joint capable
of powerful range of motion in nearly all planes.
Normal hip motion is generally described as flexion greater than 90°, abduction to 45°, extension
past neutral, and internal and external rotation
(measured at 90° of flexion) of 15 and 45°, respectively. Underlying anatomic variations can result
in more or less motion, and conditions such as
femoroacetabular impingement (FAI) can lead to
pain and impaired function, but discussion of these
is outside of the scope of this text.

An important consideration in fracture and dislocation injuries of the hip joint is the tenuous
blood supply to the femoral head. Femoral head
perfusion is provided predominantly by the
ascending branches of the medial femoral circumflex artery (which forms an extracapsular anastomotic ring with a smaller contribution from the
lateral femoral circumflex artery) which penetrate
the capsule at the intertrochanteric line and course
proximally. There is a small contribution from the
artery of the ligamentum teres, but this contribution, while larger during growth and development,
diminishes with age. Therefore, intracapsular fractures and injuries that cause gross disruption of the
vascular anatomy (such as dislocations) impart
a risk of avascular necrosis secondary to impaired

H

perfusion. Immediate ischemia at the time of injury as well as progressive and delayed arterial damage may both play a role (Yue et al. 1996). This underscores the need for urgent reduction of the hip joint when dislocations and fracture-dislocations occur.

There are also several large neurovascular structures that traverse the hip joint. These structures can be damaged or affected directly by these injuries to the joint or can occur iatrogenically. The femoral nerve, artery, and vein lie anteriorly, but more often affected is the sciatic nerve – with its separate tibial and peroneal contributions – which lies posterior to the hip. While not common, acute nerve palsies can occur with these injuries and must be recognized and treated appropriately. This is achieved through prompt reduction, direct protection, and often careful observation and expectant management.

Mechanisms of Injury

Traumatic hip dislocations and fracture-dislocations most commonly result from high-energy mechanisms of injury such as motor vehicle/cycle collisions, falls from height, direct blunt force trauma, and high-energy twisting or torquing forces across the hip joint. However, such injuries can be seen in the setting of minor trauma in patients with lesser bone quality (e.g., elderly, malnourished, vitamin deficient, and patients chronically taking certain classes of medications such as corticosteroids and antiepileptics).

When determining the forces necessary to create such an injury, one must look at the most common injury patterns: posterior and anterior dislocations.

Posterior injuries (>90 %) result from an axial loading injury to the femur (i.e., knee striking the dashboard) with the hip in varying degrees of flexion. The degree of flexion often determines the associated injury patterns. Pure dislocations are associated with an axial load while in a position of deep flexion and adduction. Shallower degrees of flexion with more neutral abduction pose more risk of associated injury or fracture of the proximal femur or acetabulum.

Anterior injuries (<10 %) result from a forceful abduction-external rotation force through the femur (i.e., leg being torqued and rotated sideways). The femoral head will lie either superior to the pelvic brim (anterior-superior dislocation) or inferiorly and trapped in or below the obturator foramen (anterior-inferior dislocation).

Diagnosis

Patients with injuries from high-energy mechanisms will often present as trauma activations to treating facilities, and standard ACLS protocol care should be instituted. These injuries are often discovered as part of the primary survey, and protocol radiographic images should be obtained as the standard of care (e.g., AP chest and AP pelvis radiographs). Although radiographic findings can be subtle, with fine details of the injury often difficult to appreciate on plain films, a standard AP radiograph of the pelvis will reveal the injury to a skilled observer. The femoral head will not be contained within the acetabulum, and there may or may not be an associated fracture (most commonly of the actetabulum). In certain instances (if positioned posterior or anterior to the acetabulum), the femoral head may appear located, but comparison to the other side reveals a slight difference in the size of the femoral head, as it lies more anterior or posterior relative to the film cartridge.

Clinically, the lower extremity is often positioned characteristically dependent on the direction of dislocation. Posterior dislocations present with rigid and painful hip flexion, adduction, internal rotation, and compensating knee flexion, while anterior dislocations often present with rigid and painful hip extension, abduction, and external rotation. A full survey should be performed, as there is a significant association with other-system trauma and other injuries of the musculoskeletal system. A 95 % associated injury rate has been reported in the setting of hip dislocations; therefore, a general surgery/trauma evaluation is recommended for all hip dislocation patients (Hak and Goulet 1999). Consistent with the mechanism of injury, knee symptoms or clinical findings have been reported in up to 85 % of hip injury patients, and 75 % had other associated injuries (Tabuenca and Truan 2000). For the injured extremity, particular focus should be given to assessing for open injuries, as well as circulation and perfusion status, and, if possible, volitional motor and sensory function.

A hip dislocation is a true emergency, and urgent reduction should be the first treatment priority once other life-threatening injuries or illnesses have been appropriately assessed for and managed. Advanced imaging studies – such as CT and MRI – do have a role but are often performed once the dislocation has been reduced to assess for congruency, tissue or fragment interposition, injury details (i.e., associated fracture patterns, size and location of fragments, etc.), and preoperative planning. MRI scans can reveal labral and other soft tissue trauma but has not been shown to be effective in the diagnosis or treatment of acute hip dislocations.

Multiple classification schemes exist for these injuries and are largely based on two main factors: direction of dislocation (anterior or posterior) and the presence of associated fractures (Thompson and Epstein 1951; Epstein 1973). The AO/OTA classification scheme is the most comprehensive but is most useful for research purposes such as data reporting and comparing groups of patients from different studies.

Treatment

Dependent on the injury type (with or without an associated fracture), the first step taken once the diagnosis is made is often an attempted closed reduction under sedation or anesthesia. Muscle paralysis is beneficial, but not necessary, and conscious sedation can be an acceptable means of anesthesia. However, attempting a reduction with inadequate anesthesia can result in increased discomfort for the patient and provider, further damage to the bony and soft tissue anatomy, and muscle spasms making the index attempt and future attempts more difficult.

It is generally accepted that a hip dislocation is an emergency, and reduction should be obtained as soon as possible to decrease the risk of developing avascular necrosis, traumatic arthrosis, and other complications. While exact timing to reduction is controversial with no universally agreed-upon limits reported in the literature, it is generally accepted that earlier is better. There are reports in the literature to support this: a 20 times increased risk of avascular necrosis was demonstrated in a pediatric population with dislocations reduced after more than 6 h (Mehlman et al. 2000), and a better prognosis has been demonstrated in dislocations and fracture-dislocations reduced within 12 h (Sahin et al. 2003).

There are multiple well-documented reduction maneuvers, with the goal of each to gently manipulate the lower extremity with varying amounts of axial traction, abduction or adduction, and internal or external rotation to allow for a smooth and atraumatic reduction. Most require more than one provider, but single-provider techniques have been shown to be successful.

If successful, a repeat pelvis radiograph should be obtained with the patient still anesthetized to assess for successful reduction and radiographic congruency. The hip should also be tested for stability by taking the hip through a range of motion examination and evaluating for subluxation or recurrent dislocation. Stability may be difficult to assess in the presence of certain fracture patterns. Special radiographic views of the hip (Judet views) are then obtained to further assess the bony anatomy and are particularly useful for evaluating acetabular fractures. A follow-up CT scan should be obtained for those reasons discussed in the section above. If there is no reason for further intervention, the patient should be placed into a knee immobilizer (aids in preventing hip flexion), abduction pillow placed while in bed, hip precautions, and allowed protected weight-bearing with crutches or a walker. Orthopedic follow-up is recommended, and consultation should be sought if there is any question of congruency, tissue interposition, or associated fractures.

Associated fractures may or may not require operative stabilization, and interposed fragments can pose a risk of continued instability or damage to the articular cartilage. The involved lower extremity may require traction as a temporizing measure to help preserve joint health until definitive stabilization can be undertaken.

The Unstable Hip

Most hip dislocations are stable once reduced. Recurrent instability is often due to an associated fracture and may require operative stabilization. Injuries to or inadequate healing of soft tissues can also be a cause of instability and may require repair. MRI is beneficial in establishing these diagnoses.

The Irreducible Dislocation

Multiple unsuccessful reduction attempts should not be performed, and orthopedic consultation should be obtained, if not done so already. These patients generally require urgent operative stabilization from the direction of dislocation. A final attempt at closed reduction under general anesthesia may be indicated, if prior attempts were done under lesser sedation. Irreducible injuries portend poor results (McKee et al. 1998).

Associated Fractures

Closed treatment may not be indicated in patients with certain associated fractures, such as femoral neck fractures. Reduction attempts may result in displacement of non-displaced fractures or may be nearly impossible with already-displaced fractures. Pediatric patients with open physes also require further evaluation prior to any attempted closed treatment. Prompt operative stabilization may be indicated in these situations.

Outcomes

Outcomes vary widely from painless, normal function to severe pain and early degeneration. Associated fractures are associated with poorer results. Avascular necrosis occurs in up to 20 % of cases, posttraumatic arthrosis have been reported in up to 24 % of uncomplicated or simple injuries, and up to 88 % in those with associated acetabular fractures (Upadhyay et al. 1983). The most common nerve injury associated with hip dislocation is sciatic nerve palsy (most commonly of the peroneal nerve) and has been documented in up to 10–15 % of patients with hip dislocations (Upadhyay and Moulton 1981). The nerve can be stretched, compressed, or transected, and recovery rates with reduction have been reported as complete in 40 % and partial in 25–35 %. If no recovery is noted at 6–8 weeks, further evaluation and treatment may be indicated. Patients are at high risk for venous thromboembolism; therefore, pharmacologic prophylaxis is indicated and they should be mobilized as early as possible.

Summary

Hip dislocation injuries often result from high-energy mechanisms and can be simple or complex (often with an associated fracture). Treatment focuses on prompt diagnosis and successful treatment of these injuries through a variety of means, from closed reduction to prompt operative stabilization, dependent on the severity and characteristics of the injury. There are significant rates of associated injuries, posttraumatic arthrosis, and neurovascular injury, and outcomes vary widely across the spectrum of these injuries.

Pearls

- Hip dislocations and fracture-dislocations are orthopedic emergencies, requiring prompt diagnosis and treatment.
- There is a high rate of associated other-system injury.
- Closed reduction under sedation or general anesthesia is often the first treatment priority.
- Operative stabilization may be required for associated fractures, irreducible injuries, and unstable or incongruent reductions.
- Outcomes vary widely, and there are high rates of associated neurovascular injury and posttraumatic arthrosis.

Cross-References

- ► ABCDE of Trauma Care
- ► Acetabulum Fractures
- ► Damage Control Orthopedics
- ► Motor Vehicle Crash Injury
- ► Pelvis Fractures

References

Epstein HC (1973) Traumatic dislocation of the hip. Clin Orthop Relat Res 92:116–142

Hak DJ, Goulet JA (1999) Severity of injuries associated with traumatic hip dislocation as a result of motor vehicle collisions. J Trauma 47:60–63

McKee MD, Garay ME, Schemitsch EH, Kreder HJ, Stephen DJ (1998) Irreducible fracture-dislocation of the hip: a severe injury with a poor prognosis. J Orthop Trauma 12(4):223–229

Mehlman CT, Hubbard GW, Crawford AH et al (2000) Traumatic hip dislocation in children: long-term follow-up of 42 patients. Clin Orthop Rel Res 376:68–79

Sahin V, Karakas ES, Aksu S et al (2003) Traumatic dislocation and fracture-dislocation of the hip: a long-term follow-up study. J Trauma Acute Care Surg 54(3):520–529

Tabuenca J, Truan JR (2000) Knee injuries in traumatic hip dislocation. Clin Orthop Rel Res 377:78–83

Thompson VP, Epstein HC (1951) Traumatic dislocation of the hip: a survey of two hundred and four cases covering a period of twenty-one years. J Bone Joint Surg Am 33:746–778

Upadhyay SS, Moulton A (1981) The long-term results of traumatic posterior dislocation of the hip. J Bone Joint Surg Br 63:548–551

Upadhyay SS, Moulton A, Srikrishnamurthy K (1983) An analysis of the late effects of traumatic posterior dislocation of the hip without fractures. J Bone Joint Surg Br 65(2):150–152

Yue JJ, Wilbur JH, Lipuma JP et al (1996) Posterior hip dislocations: a cadaveric angiographic study. J Orthop Trauma 10(7):447–454

Hip Fracture

▶ Orthopedic Trauma, Anesthesia for
▶ Proximal Femoral Fractures

Hip Fractures

▶ Falls

Hip Socket Fracture

▶ Acetabulum Fractures

History

▶ Damage Control, History of

History of Trauma Anesthesia and Resuscitation

Anthony L. Kovac
Kasumi Arakawa Professor of Anesthesiology, Department of Anesthesiology, University of Kansas Medical Center, Kansas City, KS, USA

Synonyms

Military history; Shock and resuscitation history; Triage history; War history; Wounded transport history

Definition

The history of trauma anesthesia and resuscitation in Western Civilization includes the treatment of pain, hemorrhagic shock, anesthesia, and surgical developments. War involves infliction of trauma and has contributed to and been the benefit of advancements in anesthesia, critical care, and resuscitation. Trauma to the human anatomy has been similar throughout the ages. The methods of treatment have been different and have evolved from ancient times.

Preexisting Conditions

Greek and Roman Era (500 B.C. to 440 A.D.)

Science and medicine developed through the teachings and writings of physicians and philosophers. Hippocrates (460–377 B.C.) used few drugs (cathartics, sedatives), instead relying on the healing power of nature. He described skull fractures (contrecoup) treated by trepanation. Asclepiades (128–40 B.C.) described tracheostomy as elective treatment for airway obstruction. Bad "humors" were thought to cause disease, leading to the erroneous therapy of purging and bleeding. Plants and herbs containing opium, hemlock, mulberry, and mandrake were used for pain relief. Mandrake's analgesic properties were described by Pliny the Elder (23–70 A.D.). Resuscitation methods included hanging the patient upside down over a barrel or horse's back to stimulate breathing. In "De Medicina," Celsus (25–50 B.C.) described the important use of diet and general care of the patient, as well as treatment for abdominal trauma, head injuries, and fractures.

The Roman army had extensive rules for treatment of wounded soldiers in battle who were cared for in wealthy homes or garrison "infirmaries." Bloodletting was a treatment method. Dioscorides (40–99 A.D.) wrote "De Materia Medica" about herbal medicine and related medicinal substances, such as mandrake's analgesic properties. Galen (130–200 A.D.) studied gladiators' injuries and described use of surgical instruments, wound closure, and bleeding treatment. His influence extended for 1,000 years (Keys 1945; Major 1954; Wilkinson 1993).

Middle Ages (Fifth to Fifteenth Centuries)

Folk healers, physician artists, and barber surgeons gave medical care and treatment. Medical therapy extended from use of herbs and plants to apothecary "medicinal" pharmacy. Pain therapy included use of "drugged" wine, and sea sponges containing fluids of "soporific" plants were also used. The Catholic Church (800 A.D.) was a dominant force. Medical care centered around civilian homes and monasteries, as educated monks gave "hospitality" care. Bloodletting continued as a main treatment for trauma.

Rogerius Salernitanus (1170) of Salerno wrote "Chirurgia Rogerii" (Roger's Surgery), the 1st medieval text on surgery. It described treatment of sword wounds. Roger's pupil, Roland of Parma, reedited "Roger's Practica" in 1250. Another "Cyrurgia" text written by Guy de Chauliac (1363) discussed wound care and opium for pain relief (Keys 1945; Major 1954; Wilkinson 1993).

Renaissance Period (Fourteenth to Seventeenth Centuries)

German surgeon Heinrich von Pfolspeundt (1460) healed wounds by secondary intention and described treatments for arrow and gunshot wounds (GSWs). A "wound drink" was used for anesthesia. Swiss surgeon Paracelsus (1536) described the use of opium and laudanum for pain relief. Refuting "Galenic theory," astringents were used for treatment of hemorrhage in his "Grosse Wundartzney."

Heat was thought necessary to prevent infections. Wounds were cauterized with boiling oil by the English at the battle of Agincourt (1415). Hans von Gersdorff published (1519) his surgery field book. To control bleeding and provide sterility, he recommended pouring boiling oil directly onto the wound. Boiling pitch also was used to control bleeding after amputations. Instead of boiling oil, Ambroise Pare (1570–1590) used simple wound cleaning and antiseptic dressings with ointment mixtures of egg yolk, oil of roses, and turpentine. For analgesia, compression was used (1564) (Keys 1945; Major 1954; Wilkinson 1993).

Seventeenth Century

William Harvey's "De Motu Cordis" (1618) described blood circulation. In Italy, Marco Severino used snow and ice to cause numbness and analgesia (1616). He performed lifesaving tracheostomies during a diphtheria epidemic. Carbon dioxide (CO_2) was described as the "gas sylvestre" by van Helmont in Holland. Major (1667) wrote "Chirurgia Infusoria" and administered intravenous (IV) fluid therapy. Christopher Wren (1665) performed IV injection of fluids and drugs with anesthetic properties. Resuscitation achieved a major advance when Robert Hooke (1642–1727) showed that a dog could be kept alive by artificial ventilation via air bellows to the trachea and lungs. John Mayou (1668) determined that dark venous blood turned red when exposed to air. Monel (1674) determined that hemorrhage could be controlled by the use of tourniquets (Keys 1945; Major 1954; Wilkinson 1993).

Eighteenth Century

Stephan Hales (1677–1761) was 1st to measure blood pressure by inserting a glass tube into a horse's artery observing the rise and fall of blood in the tube (1711). In 1732, mouth-to-mouth air ventilation was used for resuscitation. For newborn resuscitation, Benjamin Pugh (1754) described use of an air pipe inserted into a baby's trachea during breech delivery. Edward Nairne (1760) 1st described the successful use of electricity to defibrillate the heart.

Resuscitation apparatus continued to be developed into the late eighteenth century. Alexander Johnson described techniques to rescue victims from near drowning (1773) and developed a nasal airway (1785). Richard Mead published his treatise (1747) on resuscitation, describing three treatments: (1) indirect body warming, (2) direct application of friction, and (3) blowing tobacco smoke into the victim's rectum. John Hunter (1776) used air bellows with valves for resuscitation in place of mouth-to-mouth ventilation. Charles Kite (1788) developed an airway resuscitation apparatus.

The components of air were discovered: CO_2 by Joseph Black (1757), hydrogen by Henry Cavendish (1766), nitrogen by Daniel Rutherford (1772), and oxygen, independently by Joseph Priestly (1771) and Antoine Lavoisier (1775).

In his treatise (1793) on wound care, John Hunter classified and differentiated high- versus low-velocity injury and treatment of complicated versus simple wounds. Abdominal wounds were treated by conservative therapy. To stop pulmonary hemorrhage, the lung was allowed to collapse. Opium was used for pain relief. At the end of the eighteenth century, general medical care included use of bleeding, purging, and skin cupping (Keys 1945; Major 1954; Wilkinson 1993).

Nineteenth Century

Dominique Jean Larrey (1766–1842), chief surgeon for Napoleon, was the 1st modern military surgeon. An important innovator of battlefield medicine, he was present at Napoleon's campaigns in Italy, Germany, Egypt, Russia, and Waterloo. He was among the 1st to describe "trench foot" (1812). He adapted carriages of the French "flying artillery" as "flying ambulances" to rescue and transfer wounded soldiers at the start and not the end of battle, originating the term "first aid." He established the concept of "triage" care on the basis of urgency and seriousness of injury rather than rank, providing care for his own as well as enemy wounded. He improved the organization and mobility of field hospitals, creating an early form of Mobile Army Surgical Hospital (MASH) units.

Henri Durant (1828–1910), a wealthy Swiss banker and philanthropist, witnessed the Battle of Solferino (June 24, 1859), with 40,000 troops from both sides dead, dying, or wounded. There were no facilities for care of the wounded. Through his efforts, the Geneva Convention signed an agreement (1864) to develop the Red Cross.

Florence Nightingale (1820–1910) revolutionized nursing and patient care in hospitals with her work on sick and wounded British troops in the Crimean War (1854–1856). By instituting sanitary measures, from February to June 1855, the death rate decreased from 42 % to 2 %, respectively.

Joseph Lister (1866) introduced his germ theory and effectiveness of carbolic acid as an antiseptic. Wilhelm Röentgen introduced X-ray into clinical practice (1895). Resuscitation was further developed by the selective use of triage. Cocaine was discovered as a local anesthetic in Austria by Karl Koller (1889). In the USA, cocaine was used for regional anesthesia by William Halstead (1885) and for spinal anesthesia by Leonard Corning (1885).

Michael Faraday (1820–1910) described the soporific effects of sulfuric ether. Horace Wells (1844) introduced N_2O for pain relief in dentistry. In Boston, MA, William Morton (1846) demonstrated the 1st successful use of ether anesthesia for surgery. He was also the first military anesthetist to administer ether at the battles of Fredericksburg (Dec 13, 1862) and the Wilderness (May 5–7, 1864). Julian Chisolm (1861–1865) invented an anesthesia inhaler and described the use of chloroform anesthesia in his "Manual of Military Surgery."

During the Crimean War (1855–1857), the English used chloroform, accounting for a majority of the anesthetic deaths due to respiratory obstruction and anesthesia overdose. To decrease morbidity and mortality related to chloroform, the French used a combination of 1 part chloroform to 4 parts ether.

Chloroform and ether were used during the Franco-Prussian War (1870–1871), Boer War (1899–1901), Spanish-American War (1898), and Russian-Japanese War (1904–1905). Ferdinand Junker designed a "blow over" inhaler (1867). Friedrich von Esmarch's "The Surgeon's Handbook on the Treatment of Wounded in War" (1869) was widely read. He also designed the following: (1) chloroform mask (1869), (2) "triangular-shaped" first aid bandage (1869), and (3) rubber bandage to exsanguinate the limb for bloodless surgery (1873). The "Esmarch bandage" allowed August Bier to invent his technique of IV regional anesthesia (1899).

Toward the end of the nineteenth century, as a therapy for diphtheria in children, the development of laryngoscopes and early techniques of endotracheal intubation were independently introduced by Joseph O'Dwyer of New York (1887), James McEwen of Glasgow, Scotland (1888), and Chevalier Jackson (1910).

Additional advances that helped improve surgical care and decrease morbidity and mortality, pain, and suffering were wound care antiseptic techniques. These included the use of heat, carbolic alcohol, Carrell and Dakin's solutions, blood transfusion, anesthesia, and X-ray. Airway jaw thrust maneuvers and apparatus to relieve an obstructed airway included the Esmarch (1869), Hewitt (1908), Meltzer (1917), Waters (1930), (5) Guedel (1933), Berman (1949), Safar (1957), Brain laryngeal mask (1983), Combitube (1985), and Ovassapian (1987) airways (Keys 1945; Major 1954; Wilkinson 1993).

Application

Twentieth Century: World War I (WWI) (1914–1918)

The modern era of trauma began at the start of the twentieth century with use of premedication, anociassociation theory of George Crile, local anesthesia (procaine, lidocaine), and spinal anesthesia (procaine, stovaine); spinal anesthesia was used infrequently, as hypotension was a problem in trauma patients with hemorrhage and general anesthesia (ether). Major problems contributing

to increased mortality with the use of anesthesia included the following: (1) sepsis, (2) hemorrhagic, and (3) hypovolemic shock, requiring blood and fluid resuscitation.

In WWI, initially general anesthesia included use of chloroform (1914–1916); in later years (1916–1918), ether, N_2O/O_2, and a mixture of alcohol, chloroform, and ether were used. Because of increased morbidity and mortality, chloroform was infrequently used as the only anesthetic during the second half (1916–1918) of WWI. It was quickly realized that wounded soldiers did not easily tolerate chloroform, as they were often anemic, septic, and extremely exhausted. Development of gas gangrene was a major problem. Harvey Cushing (1869–1939) and George Crile (1865–1943) were important physiologic surgeons who furthered the effectiveness and safety of surgery and anesthesia by encouraging use of premedication, regional anesthesia, fluid resuscitation, as well as monitoring and recording of vital signs during surgery. A modified balanced general and regional anesthetic technique using morphine and scopolamine as premedication with N_2O/O_2 for amnesia/oxygenation was popularized by Crile, as part of his theory of anociassociation (1914). Special shock wards were developed.

Karl Landsteiner (1904) demonstrated that blood can be classified into three groups: A, B, and O. At the Surgical Research lab in Dijon, France, Oswald Robertson observed (August 1918) that donor blood mixed with sodium citrate solution could be preserved in a sterile ice box for a month and used at a future time. To find a blood substitute, Bayliss and Hogan (1915) conducted research on acacia and gelatin. Robertson and Cannon (1918) pioneered efforts for the start of the modern "blood bank." Other important individuals contributing to improved anesthesia care during WWI included George Marshall, Agatha Hodgins, Arthur Guedel, and James Gwathmey. During this time, an urgent need was recognized for specially trained anesthesia providers (Courington and Calverley 1986; Metcalfe 2005).

Post-WWI (1918–1941)

Between WWI and WWII, the lessons learned in military anesthesia and resuscitation were introduced into civilian trauma practice. These included development of the uncuffed endotracheal tube (1920) by Ivan Magill and Stanley Rowbotham for head and neck surgery as the field of plastic surgery developed. Magill introduced his "intubating spatula" (1926). Later (1928) Arthur Guedel and Ralph Waters added cuffs to endotracheal tubes, allowing positive pressure ventilation.

IV anesthetics (hexobarbital, sodium pentothal, somnifene, pernocton) were introduced into clinical practice. Inhalation agents were cyclopropane and divinyl ether. Ralph Waters (1921) introduced his "to and fro" inhaler for carbon dioxide absorption during closed circuit anesthesia. General medical improvements included discovery of penicillin by Alexander Fleming (1928) and sulfonamides by Gerhard Domagk (1932). IV fluid therapy became commonplace, with use of plasma, colloids, crystalloid fluids, and blood (Wilkinson 1993; Condon-Rall 1995).

World War II (1941–1945)

Anesthetic agents used during WWII were ether, procaine, and Pentothal. Deaths due to Pentothal occurred among hypovolemic soldiers and sailors at Pearl Harbor in 1941. This led to recognition of the need to titrate drugs such as Pentothal slowly and in small doses. The value of adequate fluid resuscitation and judicious treatment of pain with morphine was also recognized. Pentothal in small IV doses plus N_2O and O_2 were used for most general anesthesia cases. Ether was used for procedures requiring abdominal relaxation. A new inhalation agent was trichloroethylene. Portable anesthesia machines were used by the US military (Ohio Heidbrink) and by the British (Epstein Suffolk Oxford [ESO]).

Henry Beecher (1904–1976) conducted research during WWII on shock, acidosis, and the relationship between shock and blood loss, leading to further development of shock therapy wards which improved trauma outcome. His recommended therapy was rapid evacuation, triage, and resuscitation, followed by surgery. He stressed the need for appropriate resuscitation with the following: (1) whole blood available in operating rooms, (2) recognition of a full

stomach, (3) need to warm patients and avoid hypothermia, and (4) use of O_2 as a form of therapy. He was among the first to describe management of cardiac arrest during surgery using 100 % O_2 and internal cardiac massage (Wilkinson 1993; Condon-Rall 1995).

Post-WWII (1945–1950)

Anesthetics and techniques introduced post-WWII included muscle relaxants, (curare by Griffith in 1939, succinylcholine by Bouet in 1949), local anesthetics (lidocaine by Lofgren in 1943), Miller straight (1941) and Macintosh curved (1943) laryngoscope blades and inhalation agents (halothane by Suckling in 1951). Peter Safar (1924–2003) contributed to resuscitation success through his research and education on CPR, mouth-to-mouth, mouth-to-airway, and other manual ventilation techniques. Anesthesia developed into a specialty post-WWII with development of certified training programs and formation of national and international anesthesia specialty organizations for physicians and nurses (Wilkinson 1993; Condon-Rall 1995).

Korean War (1951–1953)

Research in resuscitation methods and treatment of wounded soldiers were further developed with use of rapid evacuation by helicopters and treatment in MASH units, helping to decrease mortality by 50 % compared to WWII. Blood was a first-line resuscitation fluid. The Korean War saw the first extensive use of the colloid, dextran 70. Agents and techniques successfully used in hypovolemic patients were Pentothal, N_2O/O_2-opioid-muscle relaxant balanced anesthesia, cyclopropane, and regional anesthesia with procaine. Anesthesia post-Korean War included the introduction of the "copper kettle" by Lucian Morris (1952) as a multiuse, easy to use, accurate, inhalation vaporizer. Methoxyflurane and halothane were inhalation agents of choice because they were nonexplosive and provided good muscle relaxation and analgesia (Wilkinson 1993; Condon-Rall 1995).

Vietnam War (1958–1973)

Triage officers selected patients who would best respond to resuscitation. It was believed that

H

a better chance of survival resulted if resuscitation was started in the field and continued into the operating room. Intramuscular morphine was administered by medics in the field. Rapid helicopter transport and Mobile Army Surgical Hospital (MASH) units were key to successful resuscitation. Initial fluid resuscitation of wounded soldiers in shock included use of a venous cutdown. Regional anesthesia was not commonly used because of problems with hemorrhage and sepsis. Most anesthesia was general anesthesia with Pentothal, succinylcholine, endotracheal intubation, N_2/O_2, halothane, methoxyflurane, or diethyl ether performed by nurse anesthetists supervised by anesthesiologists. Ventilators and portable anesthesia machines included the Ohio draw-over vaporizer and the Epstein-Macintosh-Oxford (EMO) inhaler. Following GSWs to the chest, the occurrence of acute adult respiratory distress syndrome (ARDS) was discovered along with "Da Nang Lung."

Post-Vietnam, further research and development with vaporizers and inhalation agents led to the introduction of Ethrane and isoflurane. Propofol was discovered by Kay and Rolly (1977) (Wilkinson 1993; Condon-Rall 1995).

Persian Gulf, Iraqi, and Afghanistan Wars (1990 to Present)

Military medicine adopted civilian methods and advances in anesthesia and critical care for use in wartime. These included new drugs, machines, technology, and techniques. The role of the anesthesia provider expanded to pain management and critical care. Techniques included general anesthesia with inhalation agents, total intravenous anesthesia (TIVA), regional anesthesia, and using IV ketamine as the only anesthetic. Sevoflurane and desflurane were introduced. Massive blood transfusion protocols and "walking" blood banks were developed.

As the ultimate lifesaving method, mobile forward surgical teams (MFST) were used to bring resuscitation and initial care of the injured soldier immediately and directly to the battlefield. Most important, MFSTs were compact, lightweight, portable, and deployable. A draw-over vaporizer

for inhalation agents was used in the MFSTs. In field hospitals, the Penlon Triservice anesthesia machine was used by the UK, and the Drager Narkomed and Ohmeda model 885A by the USA (Wilkinson 1993; Condon-Rall 1995).

Summary

Resuscitation and treatment of the trauma patient has and is continually evolving with adoption of old and existing, as well as development of new techniques from military and civilian arenas. Development of trauma anesthesia and resuscitation in war, military and civilian medicine has been driven by concurrent discoveries and innovations in airway management, control of pain and hemorrhagic shock, triage, transport, and the development of new anesthesia and surgical techniques.

Cross-References

▶ Airway Trauma, Management of
▶ Damage Control Resuscitation, Military Trauma
▶ Disaster Management

References

Condon-Rall ME (1995) A brief history of military anesthesia, ch. 13. In: Zajtchuk R, Grande CM (eds) Anesthesia and perioperative care of the combat casualty. Office of the Surgeon General at TMM Publications, Washington, DC, pp 855–896
Courington FW, Calverley RK (1986) Anesthesia on the Western Front: the Anglo-American experience of World War I. Anesthesiology 65:642–653
Keys TE (1945) The history of surgical anesthesia. Wood Library Museum of Anesthesiology, Park Ridge, IL
Major R (1954) A history of medicine, vol 1 and 2. Charles C. Thomas, Springfield, IL
Metcalfe NJ (2005) Military influence upon the development of anaesthesia from the American Civil War (1861–1865) to the outreach of the first world war. Anaesthesia 60:1213–1217
Wilkinson DJ (1993) The history of trauma anesthesia. In: Grande M (ed) Textbook of trauma anesthesia and critical care. Mosby, St. Louis, MO

HO

▶ Heterotopic Ossification

Hoffman Device

▶ External Fixation

Homemade Bomb

▶ IED (Improvised Explosive Device)

Homicidal Strangulation

▶ Strangulation and Hanging

Homologous Donation

▶ Autologous Donation

Hospice

Young Ho Yun
Department of Medicine, Seoul National
University College of Medicine, Seoul,
South Korea

Synonyms

End-of-life care; Palliative care

Definition

"Hospice" is derived from the Latin *hospes*, a word which served guests and hosts. Hospice is a place or program providing care for the terminally ill. The concept of hospice is believed to have originated in the eleventh century, but many of the foundational principles of modern hospice care were pioneered in the 1950s by Dame Cicely Saunders at St Joseph's Hospice in London. She introduced the notion of "total pain," which included psychosocial and spiritual as well as the physical aspects. Hospice care focuses on the patient rather than the disease, and addresses their fears and concerns with compassionate care (Fallon and O'neill 1998). Additionally, hospice provides people facing a death with symptom management, and emotional, social, and spiritual support tailored to the terminally ill patient's needs and wishes. Hospice care is provided also to the patient's loved ones (National Hospice Palliative Care Organization 2010).

Background

Hospice services are available to patients with any terminal illness or of any age, religion, or race. In the 1970s, cancer patients made up the largest percentage of hospice admissions but, today, cancer diagnoses account for less than half of all hospice admissions. The main noncancer primary diagnoses for patients admitted to hospice were debility unspecified, heart disease, dementia, and lung disease (National Hospice Palliative Care Organization 2010).

Application

Generally, hospice care is provided to patients with terminal illness and a life expectancy of 6 or fewer months. To use hospice, patients must be willing to forgo chemotherapy, use of intensive care unit (ICU), and cardiopulmonary resuscitation (CPR). Therefore, an overview of eligibility requirements in hospice is: (1) life expectancy 6 months or less if the illness runs its usual course, and (2) willingness to accept a palliative plan of care (National Hospice Palliative Care Organization 2010). As a part of the advance care plan, oncologists or hospice care team should

H

determine when to discuss transitions in goals of care and end-of-life (EOL) care with patients or their family members, based on prognosis estimated accurately. Although cancer may follow a variety of trajectories early in the course of disease, many patients with terminal cancer undergo a gradual and predictable loss of function during the last year of life followed by a marked functional decline in the months immediately impending death. Late referral to, and short survival in, a palliative care is a worldwide issue. Introducing hospice in the context of a patient's goals and needs may help patients understand the services available through hospice. Talking with patients about their perceptions of hospice enables providers to address misconceptions early in the process of hospice referral (Finlay and Casarett 2009). The optimal amount of time required for patients to derive maximum benefit from a palliative care is not well established, but at least 2 or 3 months are suggested. In the United States, Medicare patients are eligible for palliative care services if they are terminally ill and expected to live less than 6 months (Morrison and Meier 2004).

Common Care Services

To reduce suffering and to improve quality of life, hospice provides palliative care services, such as medications for pain and symptom management, psychosocial support, respite care, and bereavement services. This care is provided by a multidisciplinary team that includes a physician, nurse, social worker, chaplain, physical/occupational therapist, and volunteers. In detail, multidisciplinary team makes regular visits to assess the patient and provides symptom management, medication and supplies, home health aide services, care planning, 24-h case service, inpatient care as needed, and bereavement support. This care is provided not only in the patient's home but may also be provided in freestanding hospice centers, hospitals, nursing homes, and other long-term care facilities (National Hospice Palliative Care Organization 2010).

Impact of Hospice Care on Survival

Terminally ill cancer patients and their informal caregivers who had EOL discussions with their physicians experienced less aggressive medical care near death and earlier referrals to hospice. Effective palliative and hospice care also appears to result in about half changing their minds about assisted suicide.

In a prospective cohort study with cancer patients immediately after diagnosis of terminal illness, 19 % died within 1 month, while 41.3 % lived for 3 months and 17.7 % lived for 6 months. The median survival time since the cancer was judged terminal was 69 days. Multivariate analysis in this study showed that neither patient awareness of terminal status at baseline nor utilization of a palliative care facility was associated with reduced survival. However, utilization of the ICU was significantly associated with poor survival.

Median survival after determination of terminal status did not differ between cancer types (Yun et al. 2011). Although there is a perception among some health care providers and family caregivers that the decision to forego further curative treatment such as chemotherapy or providing opioids may cause patients to die sooner than they would otherwise, palliative care may actually extend the lives of some patients. In a 2010 study published in the *New England Journal of Medicine*, lung cancer patients receiving early palliative care lived 23.3 % longer than those who delayed with earlier referral to a palliative program, patients may receive care that results in better management of symptoms, leading to stabilization of their condition and prolonged survival (Temel et al. 2010). Patients who refused further chemotherapy and those who were refractory to chemotherapy showed similar survivals, and that may help persuade terminally ill patients to forego aggressive cure-directed therapies. In addition, some family caregivers expect life-sustaining therapy to prolong the life of a dying patient; admission to an ICU or CPR does not prolong survival of EOL patients (Ehlenbach et al. 2009).

Cross-References

▶ Futile Care
▶ Terminal Care

References

Ehlenbach WJ, Barnato AE, Curtis JR, Kreuter W, Koepsell TD, Deyo RA, Stapleton RD (2009) Epidemiologic study of in-hospital cardiopulmonary resuscitation in the elderly. N Engl J Med 361(1):22–31

Fallon M, O'neill B (1998) ABC of palliative care. British Medical Journal Books, Bristol

Finlay E, Casarett D (2009) Making difficult discussion earlier: using prognosis to facilitate transitions to hospice. CA Cancer J Clin 59:250–263

Morrison RS, Meier DE (2004) Palliative care. N Engl J Med 350(25):2582–2590

National Hospice Palliative Care Organization (2010) NHPCO facts and figures: hospice care in America. National Hospice and Palliative Care Organization, Arlington

Temel JS, Greer JA, Muzikansky A et al (2010) Early palliative care for patients with metastatic non-small-cell lung cancer. N Engl J Med 363:733–742

Yun YH, Lee MK, Kim SY, Lee WJ, Jung KH, Do YR, Kim S, Heo DS, Choi JS, Park SY, Jeong HS, Kang JH, Kim SY, Ro J, Lee JL, Park SR, Park S (2011) Impact of awareness of terminal illness and use of palliative care or intensive care unit on the survival of terminally ill patients with cancer: prospective cohort study. J Clin Oncol 29(18):2474–2480

Hospital Corpsman

▶ Corpsman

Hospital Epidemiology

▶ Infection Control

Hospital-Acquired Pneumonia

▶ Ventilator-Associated Pneumonia

House Staff (Interns, Residents, and Fellows)

▶ Postgraduate Education

Howitzer

▶ Mortars

Human Factors

▶ Performance Improvement

Human Fibrinogen Concentrate

▶ Adjuncts to Transfusion: Fibrinogen Concentrate

Hypercapnea

▶ Mechanical Ventilation, Permissive Hypercapnia

Hypercapnia

▶ Mechanical Ventilation, Permissive Hypercapnia

Hypercapnic Acidosis

▶ Mechanical Ventilation, Permissive Hypercapnia

H

Hyperfibrinolysis

▶ Coagulopathy in Trauma: Underlying Mechanisms

Hyperfibrinolysis Management

▶ Cryoprecipitate Transfusion in Trauma

Hyperkalemia

▶ Electrolyte and Acid-Base Abnormalities

Hyperosmolar Therapy

▶ Neurotrauma, Pharmacological Considerations

Hyperreflexivity

▶ Spasticity

Hypertonic

▶ Neurotrauma Management, Osmotherapy

Hypocoaguability

▶ Coagulopathy

Hypoperfusion

▶ Shock

Hypotension

▶ Ultrasound in the Trauma and ICU Setting

Hypothermia

Martin P. Zomaya[1] and Khanjan H. Nagarsheth[2]
[1]Department of General Surgery, Staten Island University Hospital, Staten Island, NY, USA
[2]R Adams Cowley Shock Trauma Center, University of Maryland School of Medicine, Baltimore, MD, USA

Synonyms

Accidental hypothermia; Secondary hypothermia; Systemic hypothermia; Traumatic hypothermia

Definition

Hypothermia is defined in humans as a core body temperature less than 35 °C (95 °F) and can be classified by the degree of change as mild (32.2–35 °C, 90–95 °F), moderate (28–32.2 °C, 82–90 °F), or severe (<28 °C, 82 °F). Hypothermia can be identified as systemic, which is further divided into primary and secondary, or localized, which is seen in frostbite or rapid freeze injury. Primary systemic hypothermia is also known as accidental, nontraumatic hypothermia and is caused by prolonged environmental exposure without proper sheltering or insulation. Secondary systemic hypothermia occurs due to an underlying condition such as trauma, sepsis, advanced age, substance abuse, hypothyroidism, and hypoglycemia. As a part of the traumatic lethal triad, along with acidosis and coagulopathy, hypothermia has been clearly demonstrated to be associated with increased mortality in all trauma patients. At temperatures <34 °C and <32 °C, an increased mortality of 40 % and 100 %, respectively, was reported by Jurkovich (Jurkovich 2011). After review of the National

Trauma Data Bank, Martin revealed that traumatic patients who were admitted with hypothermia had an 11-fold increased risk of mortality and those with severe hypothermia had an associated 40 % mortality consistent with previous studies (Martin et al. 2005).

Preexisting Condition

Pathophysiology
The physiologic changes associated with hypothermia can be divided into what is called the zones of hypothermia. These zones are defined by the degree of hypothermia as follows: safe (>33 °C), transitional (30–33 °C), and danger (<30 °C) zones (Jurkovich 2011). The safe zone is identified by shivering, vasoconstriction, as well as a hyperdynamic cardiovascular, pulmonary, and metabolic response in an effort to increase core temperature. Once in the transitional zone, the cardiovascular response diminishes. The patient gets bradycardic, has a decreased cardiac output, and becomes prone to ventricular dysrhythmia. Their respiratory drive dwindles, shivering stops, and metabolism decreases as hypothermia shifts towards the danger zone causing hypotension, hypoperfusion, and acidosis. Neurologically, there is a progressive loss of reflexes, increased muscular flaccidity, and finally loss of consciousness.

Hypothermia also has a profound effect on the coagulation system as well. In cases where body temperature is less than 34 °C, every 1 °C drop in temperature results in a 10 % decrease in enzymatic activity (Watts et al. 1998). When core temperature falls below 33 °C, enzyme and platelet activity significantly diminishes; possibly playing a role in coagulopathy (Wolberg et al. 2004). Temperatures of less than 32 °C have been shown to inhibit fibrinogen synthesis and prevent the initiation of thrombin generation (Martini 2009).

Application

Diagnostics
Hypothermia can be diagnosed by history and physical assessment alone. Rectal measurement of core body temperature is considered the best way to properly classify the severity of hypothermia. Clinical symptoms may include shivering, tachycardia, tachypnea, weakness, dizziness, or confusion. As shivering diminishes, muscle rigidity increases. Then, bradycardia, hypoventilation, cold diuresis, and lethargy with decreased awareness of the cold occur with temperatures less than 32 °C. In severe hypothermia, patients may be comatose, hypotensive, and oliguric and exhibit cardiac arrhythmias (Hanania and Zimmerman 2005).

Hematocrit is typically increased secondary to decreased plasma volume. Prothrombin time and partial thromboplastin time may be normal since these are measured at 37 °C, but prolonged bleeding time can indicate coagulopathy. Electrolyte derangements are seen more frequently during the rewarming period. Acute hypothermia is hallmarked by hyperglycemia secondary to a catecholamine surge. Moderate and severe hypothermia are associated with respiratory and metabolic acidosis (Hanania and Zimmerman 2005).

Evaluation of an electrocardiogram can reveal J (Osborn) waves during hypothermia. The size of these J waves is proportional to the severity of the hypothermia. An electroencephalogram (EEG) may exhibit abnormalities in moderate hypothermia with a decline in activity during severe hypothermia (Hanania and Zimmerman 2005).

Treatment
Once hypothermia has been diagnosed, the goal is to prevent further heat loss and begin rewarming. Rewarming can be accomplished by passive or active external rewarming and active core rewarming techniques. Passive external rewarming prevents heat loss by removing any cold or wet clothing and applying an insulating material. This gives the patient the ability to rewarm themselves. Active external rewarming methods include the application of warm blankets, heating pads, heated forced air, heating lamps, or warm baths. Active core rewarming methods include the use of heated and humidified oxygen and heated intravenous fluids and blood products to 40 °C. Warm lavage of the peritoneal and chest cavities and

extracorporeal circulatory rewarming can also be used for active core rewarming.

Administering warm fluids prevents further net heat loss, but it takes volumes of more than 10 l of temperatures of more than 40 °C to raise 1 °C (Barthel 2012). Aggressive rewarming with extracorporeal circulation methods can be more efficient, with over ten times the heat transfer rate (Jurkovich 2011). In hypothermic trauma patients, Gentilello and colleagues found that rewarming via extracorporeal circulation significantly decreased early mortality and decreased fluid requirements compared to standard rewarming methods (Gentilello et al. 1997).

Summary

Hypothermia is defined as a core body temperature less than 35 °C (95 °F). Trauma is one of the most common causes of secondary systemic hypothermia. Hypothermic patients have a significantly increased risk of morbidity and mortality when associated with trauma. Hypothermic patients can present with an array of symptoms depending of the severity that ranges from shivering and tachycardia to flaccidness, bradycardia, arrhythmia, and altered mental status. The prevention of heat loss in a traumatic person by minimizing cold exposure is essential. Prompt treatment of hypothermia is imperative with various methods including warming blankets, warm oxygen, heating lamps, heated forced air, warm IV fluids, warm peritoneal and chest lavage, or extracorporeal circulatory warming.

Cross-References

▶ Hypothermia, Trauma, and Anesthetic Management

References

Barthel ER, Pierce JR (2012) Steady-state and time-dependent thermodynamic modeling of the effect of intravenous infusion of warm and cold fluids. J Trauma Acute Care Surg 72(6):1590–1600
Gentilello LM, Jurkovich GJ, Stark MS et al (1997) Is hypothermia in the victim of major trauma protective or harmful? A randomized, prospective study. Ann Surg 226:439–447 (discussion 447–449)
Hanania NA, Zimmerman JL (2005) Hypothermia. In: Hall JB, Schmidt GA, Wood LDH (eds) Principles of critical care, 3rd edn. McGraw-Hill, New York, pp 1679–1686
Jurkovich GJ (2011) Environmental injuries. In: Mulholland MW et al (eds) Greenfield's surgery: scientific principles & practice, 5th edn. Lippincott Williams & Wilkins, Philadelphia, pp 466–485
Jurkovich GJ, Greiser WB, Luterman A et al (1987) Hypothermia in trauma victims: an ominous predictor of survival. J Trauma 27:1019–1024
Martin RS, Kilgo PD, Miller PR et al (2005) Injury-associated hypothermia: an analysis of the 2004 National Trauma Data Bank. Shock 24:114–118
Martini WZ (2009) Coagulopathy by hypothermia and acidosis: mechanisms of thrombin generation and fibrinogen availability. J Trauma 67:202–209
Watts DD, Trask A, Soeken K et al (1998) Hypothermic coagulopathy in trauma: effect of varying levels of hypothermia on enzyme speed, platelet function, and fibrinolytic activity. J Trauma 44:846–854
Wolberg AS, Meng ZH, Monroe DM III et al (2004) A systematic evaluation of the effect of temperature on coagulation enzyme activity and platelet function. J Trauma 56:1221–1228

Hypothermia, Trauma, and Anesthetic Management

J. Seth Jacob
Department of Anesthesiology, Kansas University Medical Center, Kansas City, KS, USA

Synonyms

Body heat loss; Core temperature redistribution; Impaired thermoregulation; Low core temperature

Definition

Patients are considered hypothermic when their core body temperature drops below 35 °C. There are two classifications for hypothermia: traditional and trauma (Table 1). A separate trauma classification was developed due to the recognition that

Hypothermia, Trauma, and Anesthetic Management, Table 1 Classification of hypothermia

	Tradition classification (°C)	Trauma classification (°C)
Mild	32–35	34–36
Moderate	28–32	32–34
Severe	20–28	<32
Profound	14–20	
Deep	<14	

hypothermia is an independent risk factor for morbidity and mortality in the trauma patient (Tsuei and Kearney 2004). Based on the trauma classification of hypothermia, a core body temperature of 34–36 °C is mild, 32–34 °C is moderate, and less than 32 °C is severe.

Preexisting Condition

Acidosis, hypothermia, and coagulopathy are indicators for increased mortality in victims of trauma and are referred to as the "lethal triad" in trauma care. This section will deal with hypothermia, including its causes, physiologic consequences, anesthetic implications, and treatment. Accidental hypothermia should be distinguished from therapeutic hypothermia which is the intentional lowering of body temperature to reduce oxygen consumption and protect end organs from damage.

Numerous factors may contribute to decrease of core temperature in the trauma victim. Environmental exposure, shock, ethanol intoxication, fluid resuscitation, and undressing of the patient during the primary survey in ATLS[TM] contribute to loss of body heat (Tsuei and Kearney 2004; Barash 2009). Patients in shock have decreased oxygen consumption. Oxygen consumption is a source of heat production for the body, and reduced heat production impairs the body's ability to offset heat loss. In addition, thermoregulation is altered as the threshold for shivering and vasoconstriction is lowered (Thorsen et al. 2011). Greater heat loss can be expected in patients with spinal cord injuries, burn injuries, and extensive soft tissue injuries (Barash 2009).

Patients taken to the operating room for treatment of traumatic injuries face multiple sources of heat loss. General anesthesia inhibits thermoregulation. Anesthetic-induced vasodilation causes heat redistribution from the core to periphery of the body. Metabolism and thus heat production decrease. Heat is lost via radiation, conduction, convection, and evaporation from the skin, surgical site, and airway. Administration of cold or room-temperature intravenous fluids further contributes to reductions in patient temperature. Finally, anesthetized patients exhibit lower hypothalamic thresholds for shivering and vasoconstriction in response to decreases in core body temperature (Sessler 2008).

Hypothermia contributes to numerous physiologic disturbances in the trauma patient. For every 1 °C drop in temperature, cerebral blood flow is reduced 6–7 %. Patients with severe hypothermia exhibit loss of deep tendon reflexes as well as loss of pupillary light reflex (Tsuei and Kearney 2004). Cardiac depression, myocardial ischemia, peripheral vasoconstriction, decreased microvascular blood flow, and impaired oxygen delivery to tissues occur. Shivering in response to hypothermia significantly increases oxygen consumption. Moderate hypothermia (28–32 °C) may result in dysrhythmias such as atrial fibrillation. With severe hypothermia (<28 °C), EKG changes such as prolongation of PR, QRS, and QT intervals and J waves (Fig. 1) may be seen. Spontaneous ventricular fibrillation can occur (Barash 2009).

Mild hypothermia results in tachypnea. Progressive respiratory depression occurs with worsening hypothermia due to direct effects on the respiratory centers as well as decreased pCO_2 sensitivity. Mixed respiratory and metabolic acidosis along with hyperglycemia may be seen. Reduced insulin release in addition to reduced glucose consumption contributes to hyperglycemia. Potassium is shifted from extracellular to intracellular compartments with resultant hypokalemia. From a renal standpoint, cold-induced diuresis occurs (Mallet 2002).

With hypothermia, platelets are sequestered in the liver and spleen resulting in lower levels of circulating platelets. Additionally, platelet production of thromboxane B_2 drops with decreasing

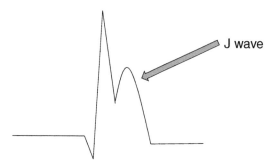

Hypothermia, Trauma, and Anesthetic Management, Fig. 1 Illustration of a J wave

temperature (Mallet 2002). Consequently platelet activity is reduced. When temperature drops below 35 °C, prothrombin time is increased, and below 33 °C activated partial thromboplastin time increases. This occurs as a result of cold-induced reduction of enzymatic activity. Fibrinolysis is increased as well (Tsuei and Kearney 2004).

Application

A number of issues must be considered when proceeding to the operating room with a hypothermic trauma patient. Minimum alveolar concentration is reduced by 5–7 % for each degree decrease in body temperature, so patients may have a reduced anesthetic requirement. Drug metabolism will be decreased, and prolonged duration of action for muscle relaxants and sedatives should be anticipated (Barash 2009). As with all patients undergoing general anesthesia, core body temperature should be monitored. The esophagus, nasopharynx, bladder, pulmonary artery, and tympanic membrane are acceptable sites for core temperature monitoring.

Special consideration is required in evaluating laboratory studies of the hypothermic trauma patient. If blood samples for coagulation studies are not run at the patient's actual body temperature, then the results may underestimate the degree of coagulopathy in a patient with hypothermia-induced coaguloation abnormalities

(Gentilello and Pierson 2001). Platelet count will not account for reduced platelet activity when low body temperature has impaired platelet function. Cold-induced diuresis and increased vascular permeability result in hemoconcentration. There is a 2 % increase in hematocrit for every 1 °C reduction in body temperature. A normal hematocrit may indicate blood loss in the trauma patient with hypothermia (Mallet 2002).

Greater blood loss during the operative course can be expected when a patient is hypothermic. This correlation between blood loss and hypothermia occurs independent of injury severity (Lier et al. 2008). Coagulopathy can exist even in the presence of normal factor and platelet levels. While coagulopathy in trauma is multifactorial, rewarming the patient is an important part of treatment.

During the intraoperative period, further patient heat loss should be prevented and rewarming efforts continued. Increasing room temperature, covering as much of the patient as possible with blankets, and warming intravenous fluids are effective methods for stopping heat loss. Standard fluid warmers can warm fluids at flow rates of up to 150 ml/min. When rapid infusion of large fluid volumes is required, a rapid infuser designed to deliver warmed fluids at higher rates than a standard fluid warmer is necessary. Forced-air and fluid-circulating warming blankets can be used for rewarming. Forced-air blankets are more commonly used and available in operating rooms. Pleural and peritoneal lavage with warm fluids can additionally be used for treating the hypothermic patient. Peritoneal lavage is especially pragmatic in a patient with a laparotomy incision. When rapid rewarming is necessary, continuous arteriovenous rewarming (CAVR) is an effective method. CAVR involves placement of percutanous venous and arterial catheters. Blood is diverted via the arterial catheter through a heat exchanger and then back to the patient via the venous catheter. The tubing used for CAVR systems is heparin bonded eliminating the need for heparinization which is typically undesirable in a trauma patient where bleeding is a major concern.

Hypothermia may be beneficial in certain special circumstances. For instance, mild induced hypothermia (32–35 °C) can be used to treat elevated intracranial pressure (ICP) in patients with severe traumatic brain injury (TBI). A protocol for induced cooling as well as slow rewarming to prevent rebound intracranial hypertension is important for the effective use of this treatment (Urbano and Oddo 2012). It should be noted that while mild induced hypothermia reduces ICP, it is not neuroprotective in itself.

Therapeutic hypothermia is a strategy used across a variety of clinical settings including cardiac and neurosurgical procedures. It has also been used for cardiac arrest patients with spontaneous return of circulation in the postarrest time period. It has potential benefit with injuries resulting in massive uncontrolled hemorrhage. Profound hypothermia (<15 °C) in these circumstances can help prevent ischemia–reperfusion injuries. By inducing hypothermia, transport to the operating room and repair of injuries can be undertaken in patients who would not otherwise survive. This technique is referred to as emergency preservation and resuscitation (EPR). There are many logistical and technical difficulties in inducing profound hypothermia in a patient with massive ongoing hemorrhage. Nonetheless, experimentation with animal models has demonstrated the effectiveness of this technique (Alam 2012). A feasibility trial of EPR involving humans is currently underway: http://clinicaltrials.gov/ct2/show/NCT01042015 ?term=EPR&rank=2.

Development of hypothermia in the trauma patient is multifactorial. It is associated with numerous adverse physiologic consequences and is considered an independent risk factor for mortality (Gentilello et al. 1997; Lier et al. 2008). Alterations in anesthetic requirements, drug metabolism, and the blood's ability to clot should be considered when caring for the hypothermic patient. Prevention of ongoing heat loss and rewarming of the patient are important considerations in the operating room.

Cross-References

- ▶ Acute Coagulopathy of Trauma
- ▶ Blood Component Transfusion
- ▶ Coagulopathy
- ▶ Fluid, Electrolytes, and Nutrition in Trauma Patients
- ▶ General Anesthesia for Major Trauma
- ▶ Hypocoaguability
- ▶ Hypothermia
- ▶ Massive Transfusion
- ▶ Monitoring of Trauma Patients during Anesthesia
- ▶ Multi-trauma, Anesthesia for
- ▶ Operating Room Setup for Trauma Anesthesia
- ▶ Partial Thromboplastin Time
- ▶ Platelets
- ▶ Prothrombin Time
- ▶ Resuscitation Goals in Trauma Patients
- ▶ Spinal Cord Injury, Anesthetic Management for
- ▶ TBI
- ▶ Traumatic Brain Injury, Anesthesia for

References

Alam HB (2012) Translational barriers and opportunities for emergency preservation and resuscitation in severe injuries. Br J Surg 99(Suppl 1):29–39

Barash PG (2009) Clinical anesthesia, 6th edn. Wolters Kluwer Health, Philadelphia

Gentilello LM, Jurkovich GJ et al (1997) Is hypothermia in the victim of major trauma protective or harmful? Ann Surg 226:439–449

Gentilello LM, Pierson DJ (2001) Trauma critical care. Am J Resp Crit Care 163:604–607

Lier H, Krep H et al (2008) Preconditions of hemostasis in trauma: a review. J Trauma Inj Infect Crit Care 65:951–60

Mallet ML (2002) Pathophysiology of accidental hypothermia. QJM 95:775–785

Sessler DI (2008) Temperature monitoring and perioperative thermoregulation. Anesthesiology 109:318–338

Thorsen K, Ringdal KG et al (2011) Clinical and cellular effects of hypothermia, acidosis, and coagulopathy in major injury. Br J Surg 98:894–907

Tsuei BJ, Kearney PA (2004) Hypothermia in the trauma patient. Injury 35:7–15

Urbano LA, Oddo M (2012) Therapeutic hypothermia for traumatic brain injury. Curr Neurol Neurosci Rep 26(7–8):580–591

Hypoxemia, Severe

Christie Lee
Interdepartmental Division of Critical Care,
Department of Medicine, Mount Sinai
Hospital and University Health Network,
Toronto, ON, Canada

Synonyms

Anoxic hypoxia; Arterial desaturation; Hypoxic
hypoxia

Definition

Arterial hypoxemia is classically defined as
a decrease in partial pressure of oxygen that is
less than 60 mmHg in the arterial blood. In most
normal, healthy young people, the PO_2 (partial
pressure of oxygen within the arterial blood) is
95 mmHg, although this decreases with age.
Arterial hypoxemia is important because it can
cause tissue hypoxia – low oxygen content within
tissue or organs. Other causes of tissue hypoxia
can be seen in Table 1.

Most tissue within the body requires oxygen
for survival, growth, and function. Oxygen is
a key component in the production of adenosine
triphosphate (ATP) through a process of oxidative phosphorylation; ATP is the most basic
energy substrate in the body. In the absence of
oxygen, tissue can produce ATP through
a glycolytic pathway; however, the pathway
also produces lactic acid as a by-product and is
an inefficient mechanism for producing ATP.

Oxygen delivery to the tissues is a product of
cardiac output and oxygen content. Oxygen content is dependent on the hemoglobin concentration and its saturation with oxygen (Lumb and
Nunn 2005) with a very small contribution made
by the presence of dissolved oxygen. Oxygen is
poorly soluble in the blood (0.03 mL O_2 per liter
of plasma per mmHg O_2 tension), and the

Hypoxemia, Severe, Table 1 Causes of tissue hypoxia

Anoxic hypoxia	Inadequate oxygen supply to the blood or inadequate ability to oxygenate hemoglobin
Anemic hypoxia	Decreased oxygen content or decreased carrying capacity, i.e., low hemoglobin
Stagnant hypoxia	Inadequate oxygen delivery or blood flow state
Histotoxic hypoxia	Inadequate oxygen utilization by the tissue, i.e., cyanide poisoning

majority of oxygen carried in blood ($\sim$99 %) is
bound by hemoglobin. Oxygen delivery (DO_2)
can be expressed with the following equation:

$$DO_2 = \text{Cardiac Output} \times CaO_2$$

$$DO_2 = \text{Cardiac Output} \times 1.34 \times Hgb \\ \times O_2 \text{ Sat} \times 0.0031 \times PaO_2$$

where DO_2 is oxygen delivery, CaO_2 is arterial
oxygen content, Hgb is hemoglobin content, O_2
Sat is oxygen saturation, and PaO_2 is arterial
partial pressure of oxygen.

The relationship between oxygen saturation
and arterial PO_2 is defined by the oxyhemoglobin
dissociation curve (Fig. 1). Hemoglobin, through
complex conformational changes, has different
affinities for oxygen depending on the number
of molecules being carried (between 1 and 4).
This change in affinity is responsible for the
shape of the oxyhemoglobin dissociation curve.
The curve can shift to the right or left to facilitate
oxygen off-loading. For instance, in the setting of
elevated temperature, increased 2,3-DPG, acidosis, or elevated carbon dioxide, the curve will
shift to the right, decreasing the affinity of hemoglobin for oxygen and increasing unloading of
oxygen to the tissues. From this curve, it is also
important to note that with increases in PaO_2
beyond 60 mmHg, hemoglobin is over 90 % saturated, and further increase in PaO_2 has little
effect in increasing oxygen-carrying capacity;
however, below 60 mmHg, the oxygen saturation
of hemoglobin drops quickly and, as
a consequence, the amount of oxygen delivered.

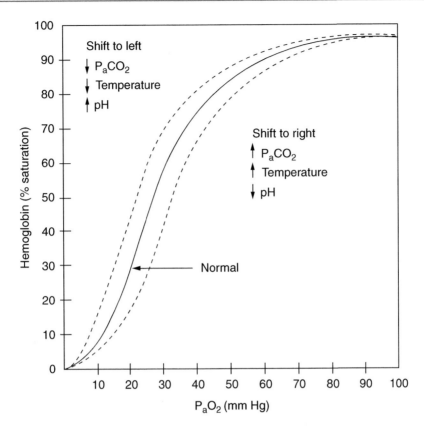

Hypoxemia, Severe, Fig. 1 **Oxyhemoglobin dissociation curve.** The *solid line* depicts the normal relationship between hemoglobin saturation and the PaO2. In cases of increased temperature, acidemia, or 2,3-diphosphoglycerate (2,3-DPG), the curve will shift to the right, suggesting a decrease in affinity for oxygen. A left shift of the curve from normal implies increased affinity for oxygen and less unloading at the tissue level. A left shift can be due to a decrease in temperature and 2,3-DPG or increase in pH

Classification of Hypoxemia

Hypoxemia can be classified into five pathophysiological mechanisms: decreased inspired partial pressure of oxygen, hypoventilation, impaired diffusion, ventilation-perfusion (V/Q) mismatch, and shunt.

Low inspired partial pressure of oxygen is an unusual cause of arterial hypoxemia. In high-altitude settings, the barometric pressure is decreased, while the F_IO_2 remains at 21 %. This would equate to a much lower inspired partial pressure of oxygen (P_IO_2). For example, at the peak of Kilimanjaro (altitude ∼6,000 m), the barometric pressure is approximately 370 mmHg. The P_IO_2 is 78 mmHg. Using the alveolar gas equation, in the absence of compensation, the partial pressure of oxygen within the alveolus (P_AO_2) would be 28. Hyperventilation is often the first adaptation to high-altitude living – this will help to increase the P_AO_2. Chronic inhabitants at high altitude (i.e., Sherpas, Andeans) have evolved over the centuries with changes in the oxygen-hemoglobin curve and position, alterations to mitochondrial function, and changes in capillary density. In the acute hospital setting, low inspired partial pressure of oxygen is an unusual cause of hypoxemia and can almost always be excluded as a cause.

Hypoventilation – an inability to clear carbon dioxide (CO_2) – results in elevation of CO_2 in the blood and acidemia. An elevation in CO_2 affects the delivery of oxygen as well as reducing the P_AO_2. Causes of hypoventilation can include any form of neurological injury from a central (brain and spinal cord) to a peripheral (nerves, neuromuscular junction) problem; it can be caused by pure muscular weakness, chest wall deformities, or upper airway obstruction. Hypoventilation is easily compensated for in the acute hospital setting with some supplemental oxygen; however, the underlying mechanisms should always be elucidated. In an acute setting, it can be easily excluded in the absence of an elevated carbon dioxide level or acidemia.

Impairment in diffusion alone is generally not sufficient to cause acute hypoxemia because the transfer of oxygen across the alveolar-capillary membrane is perfusion limited, rather than diffusion limited. Most hemoglobin molecules become maximally saturated after traversing only 30 % of the capillary length. This means that even in the setting of intrinsic lung disease, there is usually ample time for oxygen to cross the alveolar-capillary membrane. A diffusion abnormality becomes more important when it occurs in conjunction with other processes such as high-cardiac-output states and low mixed venous oxygen saturation.

The most common causes of arterial hypoxemia in the acute care setting are related to V/Q mismatch and venoarterial (right-to-left) shunt. In healthy individuals, ventilation and perfusion throughout the lung are relatively well matched. High-V/Q areas within the lung contribute very little to the overall oxygenation of blood. In the setting of V/Q mismatch, the body attempts to divert blood away from low-V/Q areas to areas with higher ventilation. This is done through a process of hypoxic pulmonary vasoconstriction. In the setting of V/Q mismatch (e.g., pneumonia), hypoxemia can be improved with supplemental oxygen and increase in the total inspired partial pressure of oxygen.

Shunts are essentially areas with very low V/Q. The Thebesian veins and bronchial venous drainage contribute to the normal shunt that is seen within the body. This is also what accounts for the alveolar-arterial (A-a) gradient (see below) that we normally measure. Pathological shunts can be anatomical (i.e., cardiac shunts, pulmonary arterial-venous malformations) or physiological – complete alveolar filling due to either fluid (edema), pus (pneumonia), or blood (hemorrhage, contusions). Hypoxemia due to shunts in general does not improve significantly with supplemental oxygen because the shunted blood is never exposed to the increased F_IO_2, and blood from normal lung units cannot compensate for the decrease in saturation. Most acute cases of hypoxemia present with a combination of V/Q mismatch and shunt.

Preexisting Condition

The pathophysiological classification of hypoxemia is helpful in terms of understanding how a particular disease causes hypoxemia; however, it is often not very useful in trying to make a specific diagnosis.

Causes of Hypoxemia

A more useful method of classifying hypoxemic respiratory failure is structural-anatomical (Table 2). This method is more systematic and can narrow the pathology from the airways, alveoli, interstitium, vasculature, pleura, chest wall, or neurological. This approach can also help the clinician consider a differential diagnosis for hypoxemia.

Diagnosis and Investigation of Hypoxemia

In cases of severe hypoxemia, treatment should be initiated immediately. The diagnosis and investigations should be performed concurrently. All hypoxemic patients should be monitored using a pulse oximeter. The oximeter functions by emitting varying wavelengths of light radiation through the tissue. When it senses pulsatile flow, the oximeter assumes this to be arterial in nature. The saturation of hemoglobin by oxygen is calculated based on the absorption and reflection of two wavelengths; one is reflected by oxyhemoglobin, and the other is reflected by deoxyhemoglobin. The arterial hemoglobin saturation detected by a pulse oximeter is denoted as SpO_2. Pulse

Hypoxemia, Severe, Table 2 Structural classification of hypoxemia[a]

Structure	Possible diagnoses
Airway	Asthma
	Chronic obstructive pulmonary disease (COPD)
	Mucous plugging
	Foreign body/airway obstruction
Air space (alveoli)	Pulmonary edema (cardiogenic)
	Acute lung injury (ALI)
	Acute respiratory distress syndrome (ARDS)
	Pulmonary hemorrhage
	Pneumonia
Interstitium	Pulmonary fibrosis
	Hypersensitivity pneumonitis
	Atypical pneumonia
Vascular	Pulmonary emboli
	Pulmonary hypertension
	Intracardiac or intrapulmonary shunts
Pleura	Pneumothorax
	Pleural effusion (transudative, exudative, or hemorrhagic)
Chest wall	Kyphoscoliosis
	Flail chest
Neurological	Central (ischemic stroke, drugs, spinal cord injury)
	Peripheral (amyotrophic lateral sclerosis, Guillain-Barre syndrome, myasthenia gravis)
	Myopathy (inflammatory myositis, drug-induced)

[a]This is not an exhaustive list—this is only illustrative in nature

oximeters are fairly accurate until the saturation decreases below 80 %. Poor peripheral perfusion, movement, and malpositioning can also affect the measurement. In cases of carbon monoxide poisoning, standard pulse oximeters will not be able to differentiate the presence of carboxyhemoglobin compared with oxygenated hemoglobin. In these cases, use of a CO-oximeter can help with measuring carboxyhemoglobin content.

PaO_2 can be measured through an arterial blood gas analysis. This also yields a direct measurement of the pH and the $PaCO_2$. The percent hemoglobin saturation is calculated from the PaO_2 using the oxygen dissociation curve and assumes a normal P50 and absence of abnormal forms of hemoglobin. The bicarbonate and base excess is also calculated using the measured pH and $PaCO_2$.

Other useful parameters for measuring oxygenation include the alveolar-arterial gradient, which measures the difference between the partial pressure of oxygen within the alveoli and the partial pressure of dissolved oxygen within arterial blood. The (A-a) PO_2 gradient is normally less than 12 mmHg. The P_AO_2 is calculated using the alveolar gas equation:

$$P_AO_2 = F_IO_2(P_{atm} - P_{H_2O}) - (P_ACO_2 \div R) + F,$$

where F_IO_2 is the fraction of inspired oxygen (21 %), P_{atm} is 760 mmHg at sea level, P_{H_2O} is the pressure of water vapor at 37 °C (47 mmHg), P_ACO_2 is the partial pressure of CO_2 in the alveoli (this is assumed to be the same as $PaCO_2$ since the diffusion coefficient of CO_2 is high), R is the respiratory quotient ~ 0.8 in stable states, and F is a factor that we often ignore.

Another useful parameter to measure is the PaO_2/F_IO_2 (P/F) ratio. This is normally over 500 in healthy individuals and, however, in the setting of acute lung injury (ALI), is less than 300, and the diagnosis of acute respiratory distress syndrome (ARDS) is defined as less than 200. A more recent definition of ARDS, the Berlin definition, describes a P/F ratio of 200–300 as mild ARDS, 100–200 as moderate ARDS, and less than 100 as severe ARDS (ARDS Definition Task Force et al. 2012).

In the mechanically ventilated patient, the degree of lung impairment can be assessed based on the mean airway pressure, which also contributes to oxygenation. As a result, the oxygenation index (OI) may be another parameter that can be used to assess the severity of hypoxemia. The oxygenation index can be measured using the following equation:

$$OI = \frac{\text{Mean airway pressure} \times F_IO_2}{PaO_2}$$

where an increase in OI suggests worsening oxygenation.

H

Once hypoxemia has been identified, chest imaging plays a key role in the investigative work-up. This, in addition to an electrocardiogram, routine blood work, serum chemistry, and an arterial blood gas, will help to elucidate the underlying diagnosis. In the setting of a normal chest X-ray and severe hypoxemia, the diagnosis can quickly be narrowed, and the clinician should consider pulmonary embolism or venoarterial shunts as possible diagnoses. Other adjunctive testing can include chest tomography and angiography, echocardiogram, and bronchoscopy. The arterial blood gas (ABG) will also be very useful because it can help to narrow the differential based on the five pathophysiological causes. For instance, in cases of pure hypoventilation, the pCO_2 and pH will be abnormal, but the (A-a) gradient should be normal.

Application

The immediate management of the hypoxemic patient requires supplemental oxygen in order to increase PaO_2 and improve oxygen delivery to tissue. Therapies involving improvements in hemoglobin as well as cardiac output will also help to improve oxygen delivery and, ultimately, tissue perfusion. Ultimately, treatment needs to be geared towards reversal of the underlying pathophysiological mechanism. As mentioned previously, supplemental oxygen will help improve most cases of severe hypoxemia, except in the case of shunt, but supplemental oxygen alone is never sufficient in those patients with severe hypoxemia. Any system that allows entrainment of room air will lead to variability in the delivered F_IO_2 because of high peak inspiratory flows. Venturi masks can provide some consistency; however, the flow rates at high F_IO_2 are often too low for patients with respiratory distress. In the intubated patient, sudden hypoxemia should be evaluated in a systematic way. In particular, tube obstruction or changes in tube positioning must be assessed immediately. Often, use of a suction catheter can quickly eliminate secretions as a primary cause. In acute cases, patients should be disconnected from the ventilator and a trial of manual ventilation be applied. A focused physical can also help to ascertain the presence of an acute pneumothorax or other signs of barotrauma.

In animals, it is well documented that high F_IO_2 can lead to the development of oxygen toxicity. In humans, this phenomenon is thought to be related to the production of oxygen-reactive species and free radicals that can lead to direct toxic effects as well as affect intracellular signaling pathways (Altemeier and Sinclair 2007). Another complication related to high F_IO_2 is absorption atelectasis. In the severely hypoxemic patient, the mixed venous oxygen saturation is often very low. This allows for rapid transfer and binding of oxygen to hemoglobin. In cases where F_IO_2 is high, the absence of nitrogen within the alveolus may lead to atelectasis and volume loss, which may worsen the shunt fraction in a hypoxemic patient.

Lung Open Strategy

In cases where hypoxemia persists despite increased F_IO_2 requirements, application of positive pressure to maintain alveolar lung volume can be beneficial. In the non-intubated patient, positive pressure can be delivered either as a continuous positive airway pressure (CPAP) or as a form of noninvasive ventilation with bi-level positive airway pressure, while in the intubated patient, positive pressure is maintained at end-expiration and is denoted as positive end-expiratory pressure (PEEP). In general, positive pressure can improve V/Q mismatch and oxygenation by increasing the amount of gas in the open alveoli as well as preventing collapse of the alveoli. It can also help to open already collapsed alveoli through recruitment (more below). The increase in lung volume may improve the total lung compliance and decrease work of breathing. In patients with severe hypoxemia that require intubation and mechanical ventilation, a lung-protective strategy incorporating low-tidal-volume ventilation should be utilized. This strategy aims at using a tidal volume of less than 6 ml/kg with plateau pressures of less than

30 cmH$_2$O and accepting higher than normal PaCO$_2$ values as long as the arterial blood pH is greater than 7.15. Compared to previous conventional ventilation strategies with higher tidal volumes of 12 ml/kg and plateau pressures of up to 50 cmH$_2$O, there was a significant improvement in mortality and ventilator-free days (The ARDS Network 2000).

Recruitment Maneuver

Recruitment maneuvers (RM) are performed in the intubated patient with the application of high mean airway pressures, greater than those used to ventilate normal lungs, for a short period of time. The maneuver should be performed in the deeply sedated and/or paralyzed patient. Recruitment maneuvers can be done in various ways but commonly involve the application of a continuous, high, mean airway pressure of between 40 and 50 cmH$_2$O for 40–50 s. RM can be repeated over periodic intervals. Once a RM has been performed, newly opened alveoli should be maintained open with higher PEEP while enabling F$_I$O$_2$ to be reduced to safer levels. Although data from clinical trials is limited, this represents a reasonable form of therapy for the severely hypoxemic patient. Some notable adverse effects can be seen with the application of positive pressure, in particular, the high pressures used in RM. The most common hemodynamic change that is seen is a reduction in mean arterial pressure during the RM. Much of this effect is seen because of increases in intrathoracic pressure and decreases in venous return to the heart. Depending on the pulmonary compliance and capacitance, there may be an initial increase in left ventricular ejection fraction as a result of a sudden increase in blood flow from the pulmonary veins to the left atrium; however, with repeated cardiac cycles, the effect on venous return and preload becomes more substantial.

Patient Positioning

In patients with severe hypoxemia, especially due to acute lung injury or ARDS, ventilation is highest in the ventral surface, while perfusion is increased in the dependent lung zones.

Whether because of obesity, chest wall edema, or increased lung water, there exists a very high pleural pressure gradient from the ventral to dorsal surfaces. In the mechanically ventilated patient, there is increased overdistention anteriorly, while the alveolar units posteriorly are subjected to compressive atelectasis. Prone positioning allows the weight of the abdomen and the heart to be removed, while moving the diaphragm into a more optimal position. Overall, there is improved dorsal lung ventilation, alveolar recruitment through increased functional residual capacity (FRC), redistribution in perfusion, and improvement in chest wall and lung mechanics. Overall, this leads to improvement in V/Q matching, secretion clearance, and redistribution of extravascular lung water. Major adverse effects are related to the risk of equipment dislodgement (endotracheal tubes, central lines, and other monitoring equipment), facial edema, skin breakdown of the forehead or anterior chest, and hemodynamic instability.

Pulmonary Vasodilators

Very little evidence exists for the use of pulmonary vasodilators in the setting of severe hypoxemia. Most vasodilators are inhaled or nebulized and provide local pulmonary vasodilation at sites where ventilation is available. This should lead to improvement in V/Q matching and improved oxygenation. The three most accepted indications are severe hypoxemia, pulmonary hypertension, and right ventricular failure.

The most common inhaled vasodilator is nitric oxide (NO). NO can be delivered at dose between 1 and 40 ppm of NO, although standard starting doses are around 20 ppm. Favorable responses can include greater than or equal to 20 % improvement in P/F ratio when used for hypoxemia, greater than or equal to 15 % decrease in mean pulmonary artery pressure when used for pulmonary hypertension, or greater than or equal to 15 % increase in cardiac output when used for right heart failure. If no improvement is seen, the inhaled NO can be increased by 10 ppm every 15 min to a maximum of 40 ppm. If a favorable response is seen, then the patient should be left on

H

the same dose of NO, and F_IO_2 requirements should be gradually weaned until less than 60 %. If the patient is able to maintain good oxygenation with oxygen requirements of less than 60 %, then the NO can slowly be weaned by 10 ppm every 2–4 h until you reach 20 ppm, then by 1–5 ppm until it is discontinued. If, at any point, there is an unfavorable response, i.e., SpO_2 < 88 % for greater than 5 min, 15 % increase from baseline mean pulmonary artery pressure, or 15 % decrease in cardiac output, then the NO level should be returned to the previous dose. Weaning of inhaled NO should be attempted at least twice a day. NO is very expensive and in a recent meta-analysis was found to have limited benefit in oxygenation and no effect on mortality, but there was an increased risk of developing renal failure (Adhikari et al. 2007). In addition, inhaled NO can be associated with the development of methemoglobinemia as well as requiring some environmental monitoring of reactive NO species. Persistent desaturation of less than 85 % should lead clinicians to consider this and other potential complications.

Inhaled prostaglandins such as epoprostenol are becoming increasingly available. Epoprostenol can be nebulized within the breathing circuit in doses of 5–50 ng/kg/min. Starting doses are generally 50 ng/kg/min for predicted *ideal* body weight; patients are monitored for favorable responses (as described above), then maintained on the current dose. If, at the time of initiation, a favorable response is not seen, then weaning of the epoprostenol should occur by 10 ng/kg/min until off. In cases where a favorable response is noted, as with inhaled NO, attempts should be made to wean the F_IO_2 to less than 60 % while maintaining a SpO_2 greater than or equal to 88 %. Once this is achieved, the epoprostenol can be weaned. The first epoprostenol wean should not be attempted until 12 h after the initiation. Thereafter, weaning should occur at 10 ng/kg/min at a frequency no faster than every 2 h. Abrupt withdrawal can cause rebound pulmonary vasoconstriction, acute V/Q mismatch, hypoxemia, pulmonary hypertension, and right ventricular failure.

If, during the weaning process, any of the following occur, SpO_2 < 88 % for greater than 5 min, 15 % increase from baseline mean pulmonary artery pressure, or 15 % decrease in cardiac output, the weaning process should be stopped and the epoprostenol dose should be returned to the previous dose. Another weaning attempt should not be attempted for at least 12–24 h. Inhaled epoprostenol has no significant toxic metabolites, especially when used in nebulized form. Some common side effects may include flushing, hypotension, headache, nausea/vomiting, chest pain, or dizziness. In patients with a history of reactive airways disease, there may be some airway irritation since the epoprostenol is reconstituted in an alkaline solution, but this is fairly rare.

High-Frequency Oscillatory Ventilation

High-frequency oscillation (HFO) achieves gas exchange through the use of very low tidal volumes and very high frequency delivered around a fixed mean airway pressure. The low tidal volumes are designed to minimize alveolar overdistention and maximize a lung-protective strategy for ventilation. The oscillations are driven by a piston and diaphragm. The mean airway pressure and the F_IO_2 control oxygenation, while the frequency and the amplitude are responsible for ventilation and CO_2 removal. In contrast to standard mechanical ventilation, CO_2 clearance decreases with increased frequency, because as the frequency increases, the tidal volumes become even smaller. The mechanism for oxygenation and ventilation is complex and out of the scope for this entry. The authors suggest the reader to refer to the entry on **Mechanical Ventilation**, **High-Frequency Oscillation** for further information.

Extracorporeal Life Support

Extracorporeal life support (ECLS) or extracorporeal membrane oxygenation (ECMO) is a technique that uses an external circuit to directly oxygenate and remove carbon dioxide from the blood. In most cases, blood is removed via a cannula within a central vein into an extracorporeal circuit. A mechanical pump withdraws the blood into an oxygenator where it runs alongside a membrane. This membrane acts as an interface for gas exchange, and the newly oxygenated blood is then returned to the patient via a central vein. In the past, cannulations were performed at two separate sites; however, newer technology has led to the design of dual-lumen cannula where the cannula is inserted into the internal jugular vein and extends through the right atrium into the inferior vena cava. Venous blood is withdrawn from two ports, one situated in the superior vena cava and the other within the inferior vena cava. The second lumen is the reinfusion lumen with the port directed into the right atrium, directly at the tricuspid valve and into the right ventricle. This reinfusion port delivers oxygenated blood and, when positioned properly, minimizes recirculation. At present, there is very little clinical data on the use of ECMO in severe ARDS. The only modern trial, Conventional Ventilation or ECMO for Severe Adult Respiratory Failure (CESAR trial), randomized patients with severe ARDS to continuing conventional management at a designated treatment center or transfer to a specialized center with standardized mechanical ventilation protocols including consideration for ECMO if necessary (Peek et al. 2009). The primary outcome of death or severe disability at 6 months was seen in 37 % of those patients transferred to a specialized center compared to 53 % in those that received conventional therapy. The important factor to note in this trial is that all transferred patients underwent lung-protective ventilatory strategy and about 75 % underwent ECMO. It is not clear whether the improved mortality was due to improved ventilatory strategies at the specialized centers. This trial clearly demonstrated that transfer to a specialized center improved mortality and not a trial of ECMO compared with standard-of-care mechanical ventilation strategies. A more in-depth review of ECMO can be found in another entry in this textbook under **Extracorporeal Membrane Oxygenation**.

Cross-References

► Acute Respiratory Distress Syndrome (ARDS), General
► Atelectasis
► Extracorporeal Membrane Oxygenation
► Mechanical Ventilation, Conventional
► Mechanical Ventilation, High-Frequency Oscillation
► Mechanical Ventilation, Permissive Hypercapnia
► Oxygen-Carrying Capacity

References

Adhikari NKJ, Burns KEA, Friedrich JO et al (2007) Effect of nitric oxide on oxygenation and mortality in acute lung injury: systematic review and meta-analysis. BMJ 334:779

Altemeier WA, Sinclair SE (2007) Hyperoxia in the intensive care unit: why more is not always better. Curr Opin Crit Care 13:73–78. doi:10.1097/MCC.0b013e32801162cb

ARDS Definition Task Force, Ranieri VM, Rubenfeld GD, Thompson BT, Ferguson ND, Caldwell E, Fan E, Camporota L, Slutsky AS (2012) Acute respiratory distress syndrome: the Berlin definition. JAMA 307:2526–2533

Lumb AB, Nunn JF (2005) Nunn's applied respiratory physiology, 6th edn. Elsevier Butterworth-Heinemann, Oxford

Peek GJ, Mugford M, Tiruvoipati R et al (2009) Efficacy and economic assessment of conventional ventilatory support versus extracorporeal membrane oxygenation for severe adult respiratory failure (CESAR): a multicentre randomised controlled trial. Lancet 374:1351–1363. doi:10.1016/S0140-6736(09)61069-2

The ARDS Network (2000) Ventilation with lower tidal volumes as compared with traditional tidal volumes for acute lung injury and the acute respiratory distress syndrome. The Acute Respiratory Distress Syndrome Network. N Engl J Med 342:1301–1308. doi:10.1056/NEJM200005043421801

Hypoxic Hypoxia

► Hypoxemia, Severe

I

Ice Skating Injuries

▶ Winter Sport Injuries

ICU Acquired Weakness

Barbara Haas[1] and Margaret Herridge[2]
[1]Department of Surgery, University of Toronto, Toronto, ON, Canada
[2]Department of Medicine, University of Toronto, Toronto, ON, Canada

Synonyms

Critical illness myopathy and/or neuropathy; Critical illness neuromyopathy; Intensive care unit-acquired paresis

Definition

ICU-acquired weakness (ICU-AW) is a common and significant complication of critical illness, prolonged mechanical ventilation, and ICU admission. The syndrome of ICU-AW is best characterized as acute neuromuscular dysfunction in critically ill patients for which no other underlying cause other than critical illness can be identified (Stevens et al. 2009; Bolton et al. 1984). Typically, the patient is found to have significant proximal limb or respiratory muscle weakness following prolonged ventilation, sedation, and immobilization. In particular, patients may manifest signs of persisting respiratory failure, despite an absence of radiographic signs of pulmonary abnormalities. On initiation of spontaneous breathing trials, unexplained shallow breathing, tachypnea, tachycardia, and other signs of respiratory distress may occur. Weakness of the respiratory muscles may be further evidenced by decreased maximal inspiratory and expiratory pressures and vital capacity.

ICU-AW refers to a spectrum of nerve and muscle injury that has a multiplicity of underlying physiologic mechanisms. An understanding of these mechanisms, as well as of the means by which ICU-AW is characterized and measured, is critical to understanding potential prevention and treatment strategies.

Incidence

The reported incidence of ICU-AW varies widely in the literature and is dependent on the study population, timing of evaluation, and method of evaluation. In a general medical-surgical ICU patient population, prospective studies have identified the presence of clinically detectable ICU-AW in 25–60 % of patients (De Jonghe et al. 2002; Sharshar et al. 2009). However, the impact of ICU-AW on critically injured patients remains poorly characterized. Patients' underlying injuries, particularly those to the extremities or to the pelvis, may confound the diagnosis of

© Springer-Verlag Berlin Heidelberg 2015
P.J. Papadakos, M.L. Gestring (eds.), *Encyclopedia of Trauma Care*,
DOI 10.1007/978-3-642-29613-0

ICU-AW, since extremity weakness may be missed. Conversely, patients' weakness following injury may be misattributed to their primary injuries, rather than to a complication of their ICU treatment. In addition, patients with severe head injuries, which reduce patients' ability to obey commands and interact appropriately with their caregivers, may complicate the evaluation of patients' motor and sensory function and therefore the diagnosis of ICU-AW.

Etiology

The specific cause of ICU-AW remains unknown. Identified risk factors for ICU-AW include female gender, length of mechanical ventilation, severity of critical illness, multiple organ dysfunction, SIRS, hyperglycemia, hyperosmolality, parenteral nutrition, renal replacement therapy, nondepolarizing neuromuscular blockers, and use of corticosteroids.

Diagnosis

The diagnosis of ICU-AW can be inferred through manual muscle testing, through electrophysiologic studies, or through direct histological examination of muscle or nerve tissue. A variety of methods of diagnosis are cited in the literature; these diagnostic methods vary in their sensitivity, specificity, reliability, ease of implementation, and degree of invasiveness. Importantly, ICU-AW should be considered a diagnosis of exclusion.

The diagnosis of ICU-AW by clinical exam is based on the following: (1) identification of new onset generalized weakness in a critically ill patient with more proximal than distal distribution of weakness, (2) identification of the appropriate setting and risk factors for ICU-AW, (3) exclusion of causes of generalized weakness not related to critical illness, and (4) strength testing (Stevens et al. 2009).

ICU-AW is typically identified among patients with prolonged ICU admissions. Additionally, the presence of known risk factors for ICU-AW, such as severe sepsis, organ failure, hyperglycemia, ongoing inflammation, and use of glucocorticoids, increases the clinical suspicion of ICU-AW. Conversely, early localized or generalized weakness in the severely injured patient must prompt

ICU Acquired Weakness, Table 1 Differential diagnosis of ICU-acquired weakness in the severely injured patient

Pelvic or extremity fracture
Peripheral nerve injury
Spinal cord injury
Vascular injury to the extremities
Compartment syndrome
Rhabdomyolysis
Traumatic brain injury
Preexisting neuromuscular disorder
Medication

a thorough search for a traumatic cause for the patient's clinical findings (Table 1). Beyond vertebral bony injury, spinal cord injury without radiographic abnormality (SCIWORA) must be excluded. Moreover, peripheral nerve injury, in conjunction with head injury or sedation, can result in a confusing clinical picture that may be mistaken for generalized, rather than localized, weakness. For example, if the appropriate mechanism of injury is present, brachial plexus injury or peroneal nerve injury should be considered, particularly in cases of asymmetrical weakness. Peripheral nerve injuries can easily be missed in the trauma bay in a critically injured patient with other life-threatening injuries.

Preexisting Condition

A number of acute myopathies and neuropathies can occur in critically ill patients; though rare, the symptoms associated with these conditions can be incorrectly attributed to ICU-AW. Although rare causes of weakness, such as Guillain-Barré syndrome, may seem less probable in the trauma population, they should nevertheless be considered and excluded. In particular, a history should be sought from family members, scene records, and other medical records that might be suggestive of an acute or chronic neuromuscular disorder that was undiagnosed prior to the patient's injury incident and that may even have contributed to the circumstances of the injury. Rhabdomyolysis as a cause of acute weakness must also be considered, particularly in acutely injured patients with significant crush injuries or those with prolonged immobilization due to orthopedic injuries. Appropriate investigations should be performed where indicated, including neuroimaging, lumbar puncture and CSF analysis, serological analyses, and more invasive neurophysiologic testing.

Clinical Evaluation in ICU-AW

Objective documentation of peripheral muscle weakness is essential to the diagnosis of ICU-AW. A thorough neurological examination of the patient is critical, including an assessment of muscle tone and bulk, level of consciousness, cranial nerve testing, motor strength evaluation, sensory function evaluation, and evaluation of deep tendon reflexes.

The Medical Research Council (MRC) score and handgrip dynamometry are the most commonly cited means of testing and documenting muscle strength in the ICU setting. The MRC score ranges from 5 (normal strength) to 0 (complete paralysis). The MRC sum score accounts for scores from 12 muscle groups in both the upper and lower bodies. A score below 48 is consistent with a diagnosis of ICU-AW and has been used as a cutoff in several prospective studies. Subtle loss of muscle strength, however, may not be detected using the MRC score, resulting in a missed diagnosis of ICU-AW. In addition, MRC demonstrates limited sensitivity and responsiveness over time (Herridge et al. 2012). Most relevant in the severely injured population, however, is the fact that accurate calculation of the MRC score requires an alert and cooperative patient whose movements are not hindered by fracture pain, or by casts or splints. Clearly, these conditions may not be satisfied in injured patients with severe traumatic brain injury or significant orthopedic injuries. For example, in one study examining the feasibility of clinical evaluation in ICU-AW, in a patient population of whom 40 % were trauma patients, MRC score testing could successfully be performed in the ICU for only a minority of patients (Hough et al. 2011).

An alternative to the MRC score is dominant-hand dynamometry, which measures hand strength on a continuous scale. Once again, the ability to evaluate patients for ICU-AW by means of this investigation may be limited in severely injured patients with significant derangements of cognition or with movement limitations secondary to extremity injuries. More importantly, handgrip testing only evaluates strength in distal muscle groups, which are often relatively spared in ICU-AW. As such, hand grip dynamometry may be of limited use in making the diagnosis.

Electrophysiologic Evaluation in ICU-AW

Electrophysiologic testing offers an alternative to clinical testing for the diagnosis of ICU-AW. Proponents of electrophysiologic testing emphasize its efficacy in the obtunded or noncooperative patient; electrophysiologic testing might be particularly useful in the early phases of critical illness or injury when level of consciousness may be decreased due to primary injury or due to sedation.

Nerve conduction studies provide information about the function of the peripheral nervous system. By stimulating peripheral motor and sensory nerves, it is possible to calculate a muscle group's compound muscle action potential (CMAP), which represents the summated response of all stimulated muscle fibers, as well as the sensory nerve action potential (SNAP), which represents the summated response of all stimulated sensory fibers. Stimulation of a nerve fiber at two different points allows for the calculation of nerve conduction velocity. Together, these data provide information about nerve and muscle function, and the mechanism of patients' weakness. In contrast to nerve conduction studies, needle EMG are conducted in cooperative patients who can provide both mild and maximal voluntary muscle contraction. Characteristics of the muscle at rest and during voluntary movement can identify muscle denervation or necrosis and point to the underlying etiology of the patient's clinical findings.

Although advantageous in several respects, electrophysiologic studies also have a number of limitations. Both nerve conduction studies and EMG require trained personnel and specialized equipment and are significantly more invasive than simple clinical strength testing. Moreover, like MRC and hand grip testing, some forms of electrophysiologic testing (e.g., needle EMG) require patients' cooperation. Finally, electrophysiologic testing can be confounded by such factors as tissue edema and limb temperature differences.

In addition to the technical challenges posed by electrophysiologic testing, the clinical utility of these studies has been questioned. For example, in one study examining the incidence of ICU-AW among patients undergoing mechanical ventilation for at least 1 week, 40 % of patients died prior to being evaluable (De Jonghe et al. 2002); diagnosing ICU-AW in the patients that died by means of electrophysiologic testing would likely be of limited clinical utility. Moreover, electrophysiologic abnormalities have been reported in 50–90 % of ICU patients and may not correlate with findings on clinical exam (Bittner et al. 2009; Hund et al. 1996); electrophysiologic abnormalities, in isolation, may therefore be of limited utility. Finally, peripheral edema, which significantly interferes with electrophysiologic testing, is highly prevalent in the severely injured, massively resuscitated trauma population most at risk for ICU-AW.

Electrophysiologic testing should be used in conjunction with clinical history and exam to clarify an otherwise unclear diagnosis, and may be particularly useful in patients with profound paresis or with no clinical improvement over time. In the comatose patient with head injury, electrophysiologic testing may also be useful, since the clinical findings of ICU-AW may otherwise lead clinicians to incorrectly prognosticate the severity a patient's injuries.

Classification of ICU-AW

ICU-AW can broadly be classified as due to either critical illness myopathy (CIM), critical illness polyneuropathy (CIP), or a syndrome that combines features of both CIM and CIP.

Critical Illness Myopathy

Proposed in 2000 by Lacomis and colleagues (2000), the term critical illness myopathy describes a syndrome characterized by flaccid quadriparesis, more prominent in proximal muscle groups compared to distal muscle groups, paired with inability to wean from mechanical ventilation. Facial muscle weakness, with sparing of extraocular muscles, is also common. Notably, sensation is typically spared in the context of CIM. Histologic examination of affected tissues demonstrates myosin loss and myofiber necrosis, with loss of muscle membrane excitability also contributing to patients' clinical and neurophysiologic findings (Lacomis et al. 2000). A number of protein degradation pathways have been implicated in CIM, including the ubiquitin-proteasome-mediated proteolysis, autophagy, calpains, and cathepsins. Critically ill patients also appear to experience a downregulation of genes involved in protein synthesis.

Critical Illness Polyneuropathy

Patients with critical illness polyneuropathy are characterized by sensorimotor findings which include distal muscle weakness or atrophy, reduced or absent deep tendon reflexes, and loss of peripheral sensation. Cranial nerve function is typically preserved. Histologic findings include distal axonal degeneration of both sensory and motor nerve fibers, with absence of demyelination or inflammation (Stevens et al. 2009). Microvascular dysfunction, with local hypoperfusion and acidosis, has been implicated in the development of CIP. Recent immunohistochemical studies of peripheral nerve biopsies from critically ill patients, which demonstrated upregulation of e-selectin in the endothelial cells of epineurial and endoneurial vessels, have implicated endothelial cell activation as an important mechanism in the nerve injury observed in CIP (Fenzi et al. 2003). E-selectin promotes extravasation of activated leukocytes to the endoneurial space, resulting in local tissue injury.

Differentiating CIP and CIM based on history and clinical exam alone can be difficult. Nerve conduction studies and muscle stimulation studies can be helpful in differentiating CIM and CIP. It is important to note, however, that the two conditions often coexist in the same patient, creating a further diagnostic challenge. This combined syndrome is often termed critical illness polyneuromyopathy and may, indeed, be the most common cause of ICU-AW.

Nerve conduction studies in patients with CIP will demonstrate reduced CMAP, reduced SNAP, or both, but normal conduction velocity. Typically, nerve conduction studies will identify relatively normal sensory function in cases of CIM, with motor findings representing the predominant abnormality. As in CIP, conduction velocity in CIM is typically normal. Isolated motor dysfunction may be found in CIP, however, and since the two conditions often coexist, both sensory and motor findings are often seen in the same patient. In contrast to CIP and CIM, traumatic peripheral nerve injuries will result in either a reduced conduction velocity or absent distal conduction response, depending on the degree of injury. Decreased signal amplitude will also be observed 2–3 days after injury occurs (Grant et al. 1999).

EMG findings of CIM include short-duration, low-amplitude motor unit potentials (MUP) with voluntary movement. These findings represent a stable number of motor units available for recruitment, with decreased contractile strength within these muscle units. In contrast, long-duration, high-amplitude, polyphasic MUP are typically seen in CIP, representing a decreased number of motor units available for recruitment, with compensatory increase in the activity of the remaining muscle units. In addition, patients with CIP will demonstrate fibrillation and positive sharp waves at rest. Although somewhat time dependent, EMG following traumatic peripheral nerve injuries will generally result either in normal EMG findings (in the context of neuropraxic injury) or in fibrillations, fasciculations, and positive sharp waves among patients with more severe injuries (Grant et al. 1999).

Patient Outcomes After ICU-AW

Prolonged disability after critical illness has been widely documented. Similarly, disability after severe injury is known to be persistent and profound. Understanding the contribution of ICU-AW to the disability of critically injured patients, many of whom have severe traumatic brain injuries or extremity injuries or who have undergone repeated surgical procedures, is difficult to assess.

The presence of ICU-AW is associated with poorer prognosis among critically ill patients, as compared to patients who do not experience this complication. ICU-AW has been reported as an independent risk factor for failure to wean from mechanical ventilation and appears to be associated with significantly higher inhospital and ICU mortality.

The degree to which survivors of critical illness recover from ICU-AW is unclear. Prospective data suggest that, among patients with ICU-AW, direct measures of muscle strength improve rapidly in a large portion of patients; De Jonghe and colleagues reported a resolution of clinically defined ICU-AW among half of patients within 3 weeks (De Jonghe et al. 2002). It is clear, however, that despite these reports of rapid recovery from ICU-AW based on strength testing, survivors of critical illness experience significant impairment in function and quality of life for prolonged periods after ICU discharge. Specifically, the use of MRC score as a measure of ICU-AW resolution in the study by De Jonghe and colleagues, as opposed to a functional measure of recovery, limits the interpretability of their findings. In contrast, in one large cohort study of patients with acute respiratory distress syndrome, at 1 year following discharge from ICU, survivors were found to have persistent limitations in physical function (6 min walk) and significantly reduced quality of life compared to an age- and sex-matched control population (Herridge et al. 2003). Much of this limitation in function was thought to be attributable to muscle wasting and ICU-AW. At 5 years, the same cohort of patients continued to have significantly reduced ability to exercise, despite the absence of demonstrable weakness on standard physical exam (Herridge et al. 2011).

The impact of ICU-AW on patients' families and caregivers is likely also profound. Im and colleagues demonstrated that, among patients requiring at least 48 h of mechanical ventilation, three quarters required caregiver assistance at the time of hospital discharge (Im et al. 2004).

A third of caregivers reported they had to reduce work hours, and a third reported symptoms consistent with depression. More than half of patients required significant assistance for activities of daily living 1 year after hospital discharge (Chelluri et al. 2004). It is probable that the functional impairment associated with ICU-AW can account for at least some of these findings.

Application

Some degree of nerve injury and muscle proteolysis is an inevitable consequence of critical illness and prolonged ventilation. Histologic studies have demonstrated atrophy and proteolysis in diaphragmatic muscle within hours of onset of mechanical ventilation and diaphragmatic inactivity (Levine et al. 2008). Acknowledging these realities, the treatment and prevention of ICU-AW should begin in the earliest phases of patients' resuscitation and should be an integral component to patients' stay in the intensive care unit. Considerations include avoidance of agents associated with ICU-AW (corticosteroids, neuromuscular blocking agents), the use of ventilation modes which allow the patient to participate in the work of breathing, minimization of sedation, and a focus on early mobility and rehabilitation. One proposed strategy to achieve these goals is the ABCDE bundle, which aims to reduce the incidence of both ICU-AW and delirium among critically ill patients (Vasilevskis et al. 2010). The bundle emphasizes Awakening, Breathing Coordination, Delirium monitoring, and Exercise/Early mobility. Overall, screening for weakness should be a routine component of patients' daily assessment.

Although tight glycemic control has been associated with reduced incidence of ICU-AW in two randomized controlled trials, more recent evidence suggests that tight glycemic control is associated with increased mortality in a mixed medical-surgical ICU population, with no difference in the length of mechanical ventilation.

Multiple protocols for early physical and occupational therapy for mechanically ventilated patients (as early as within the first 72 h of ICU admission) have been described. These protocols emphasize interruption of sedation and either passive or active therapy, based on the patient's abilities. In their study, Pohlman and colleagues report that up to 15 % of mechanically ventilated patients were able to ambulate during the course of their therapy sessions (Pohlman et al. 2010). In a randomized control trial examining the effects of this early mobilization protocol, Schweickert and colleagues demonstrated that early mobilization was associated with a significantly higher probability of independent functional status at hospital discharge as well as significantly lower incidence of delirium, shorter duration of mechanical ventilation, and a nonsignificant reduction in the incidence of ICU-AW (Schweickert et al. 2009). Systematic review of the literature demonstrates that, overall, early mobilization programs are successful in improving patient mobility, but are inconsistent in the outcomes reported. Moreover, the long-term impact of early mobilization programs on patients' functional outcomes remains unknown.

It is important to note, however, that studies examining early mobilization have a number of limitations. First, muscle atrophy and weakness observed in critically ill patients preferentially affects diaphragmatic muscle fibers compared to those of the axial skeleton; early mobility programs are unlikely to ameliorate diaphragmatic dysfunction. Moreover, the described studies predominantly include patients admitted to the intensive care unit for medical, rather than surgical, diagnoses. Early mobilization may be impaired in the trauma ICU, where severe head injuries, extremity injuries, and temporary abdominal closure are commonplace. The benefits of interruption of sedation and tailored therapy programs remain to be investigated in the trauma population. Most importantly, recovery after severe injury and prolonged ICU admission is a complex process. Although patients may experience recovery of muscle strength, multiple other factors may continue to impede their function and impact on their quality of life. Impairment of balance, cognitive impairment, mood disorders, chronic pain, and other issues may complicate functional recovery and must be addressed in order to ensure optimal patient outcomes.

Cross-References

► Activity Restrictions
► ICU Management
► Mechanical Ventilation, Conventional
► Mechanical Ventilation, Weaning
► Physical Therapist
► Sedation, Analgesia, Neuromuscular Blockade in the ICU
► Ventilatory Management of Trauma Patients

References

Bittner EA, Martyn JA, George E, Frontera WR, Eikermann M (2009) Measurement of muscle strength in the intensive care unit. Crit Care Med 37(10 Suppl): S321–S330

Bolton CF, Gilbert JJ, Hahn AF, Sibbald WJ (1984) Polyneuropathy in critically ill patients. J Neurol Neurosurg Psychiatry 47(11):1223–1231

Chelluri L, Im KA, Belle SH et al (2004) Long-term mortality and quality of life after prolonged mechanical ventilation. Crit Care Med 32(1):61–69

De Jonghe B, Sharshar T, Lefaucheur JP et al (2002) Paresis acquired in the intensive care unit: a prospective multicenter study. JAMA 288(22):2859–2867

Fenzi F, Latronico N, Refatti N, Rizzuto N (2003) Enhanced expression of E-selectin on the vascular endothelium of peripheral nerve in critically ill patients with neuromuscular disorders. Acta Neuropathol 106(1):75–82

Grant GA, Goodkin R, Kliot M (1999) Evaluation and surgical management of peripheral nerve problems. Neurosurgery 44(4):825–839, discussion 839–840

Herridge MS, Cheung AM, Tansey CM et al (2003) One-year outcomes in survivors of the acute respiratory distress syndrome. N Engl J Med 348(8):683–693

Herridge MS, Tansey CM, Matte A et al (2011) Functional disability 5 years after acute respiratory distress syndrome. N Engl J Med 364(14):1293–1304

Herridge M, Chu L, Matte A et al (2012) Long-term patient outcomes after prolonged mechanical ventilation: the Towards Recover study. Am J Respir Crit Care Med 185:A2546

Hough CL, Lieu BK, Caldwell ES (2011) Manual muscle strength testing of critically ill patients: feasibility and interobserver agreement. Crit Care 15(1):R43

Hund EF, Fogel W, Krieger D, DeGeorgia M, Hacke W (1996) Critical illness polyneuropathy: clinical findings and outcomes of a frequent cause of neuromuscular weaning failure. Crit Care Med 24(8):1328–1333

Im K, Belle SH, Schulz R, Mendelsohn AB, Chelluri L (2004) Prevalence and outcomes of caregiving after prolonged (> or = 48 hours) mechanical ventilation in the ICU. Chest 125(2):597–606

Lacomis D, Zochodne DW, Bird SJ (2000) Critical illness myopathy. Muscle Nerve 23(12):1785–1788

Levine S, Nguyen T, Taylor N et al (2008) Rapid disuse atrophy of diaphragm fibers in mechanically ventilated humans. N Engl J Med 358(13):1327–1335

Pohlman MC, Schweickert WD, Pohlman AS et al (2010) Feasibility of physical and occupational therapy beginning from initiation of mechanical ventilation. Crit Care Med 38(11):2089–2094

Schweickert WD, Pohlman MC, Pohlman AS et al (2009) Early physical and occupational therapy in mechanically ventilated, critically ill patients: a randomised controlled trial. Lancet 373(9678):1874–1882

Sharshar T, Bastuji-Garin S, Stevens RD et al (2009) Presence and severity of intensive care unit-acquired paresis at time of awakening are associated with increased intensive care unit and hospital mortality. Crit Care Med 37(12):3047–3053

Stevens RD, Marshall SA, Cornblath DR et al (2009) A framework for diagnosing and classifying intensive care unit-acquired weakness. Crit Care Med 37(10 Suppl):S299–S308

Vasilevskis EE, Ely EW, Speroff T, Pun BT, Boehm L, Dittus RS (2010) Reducing iatrogenic risks: ICU-acquired delirium and weakness–crossing the quality chasm. Chest 138(5):1224–1233

ICU Management

Carla J. Wittenberg[1] and Barbara Imhoff[2]
[1]University of California, San Francisco Medical Center, San Francisco, CA, USA
[2]Stanford Hospital and Clinics, Stanford, CA, USA

Synonyms

Critical care; Injured patients; Intensive care unit; Nurse practitioner; Physician assistants; Trauma

Definition

Patients requiring intensive care unit (ICU)-level care are the sickest patients in the hospital.

The authors would like to acknowledge the guidance and assistance of Nicholas M. Perrino, Director of Advanced Practice at Stanford Hospital & Clinics, Stanford, CA, in writing this paper.

They often require life-saving medications, monitoring, and technologies such as ventilators, intracranial pressure monitors, continuous hemodialysis, continuous electrocardiogram monitoring, and frequent radiographic imaging such as CAT scans and MRIs. Medical management of critically ill and traumatically injured patients in an ICU is some of the most scientifically complex, intellectually challenging, and resource-dependent care provided within the hospital. Specialized members of many different healthcare fields are needed to manage each patient's unique combination of life-supporting therapies.

Preexisting Conditions

Traumatically injured patients who enter the ICU are a specialized group of patients with major life- or limb-threatening injuries or burns caused by either preventable traumatic events or natural disasters. Some common causes of traumatic injuries include falls, industrial accidents, motor vehicle crashes, crashes involving bicyclists and pedestrians, gun and knife violence, and fires. These lead to injuries such as penetrating wounds, abdominal injury, burns, near drownings, brain and/or spinal cord injuries, and fractures.

Introduction

One of the specialized areas of care for traumatically injured patients is the intensive care unit where continuity, communication, experience, and evidence-based protocols help to maximize critical care therapies and ultimately save lives. The multidisciplinary team consisting of registered nurses, physicians, nurse practitioners, physician assistants, respiratory therapists, pharmacologists, social workers, case managers, and often many other disciplines must not only strive to provide up-to-date care but must also employ meticulous communication skills. This ICU team succeeds when all members are contributing leaders within their fields of expertise and work together on ever-changing patient care challenges to optimize patient care and patient outcomes.

ICU Management, Table 1 Traditional ICU tasks

24/7 Patient care management
Daily multidisciplinary attending rounds
Obtaining history and performing physical examinations
Diagnosing and treating illnesses
Ordering and interpreting tests
Performing invasive procedures (central line insertion, arterial line insertion, intubations, etc.)
Assessing and implementing nutrition
Collaborating and consulting with the interdisciplinary team, patient, and family
Leading, monitoring, and reinforcing practice guidelines for intensive care unit patients (i.e., central line insertion procedures, infection prevention measures, stress ulcer prophylaxis, etc.)
Data collection
Tracking quality assurance
Performing specialty area consultations
Participating in family conferences
Consulting on transfers and referrals
Educating patients and families regarding anticipated plan of care

Traditional ICU Tasks

The multidisciplinary team in the acute critical care setting is common practice and is used to provide care to the critically ill. Table 1 below delineates many of the traditional tasks in the ICU.

Continuity of Care

A primary critical care team in an academic institution generally consists of an attending faculty physician, a fellow, a resident, and an advanced practice provider. In a nonteaching institution, such as a community hospital the ICU team may consist of only the intensivist attending physician and a team of advanced practice providers (APPs). This team provides 24/7 coverage to meet the high demand for consistent, continuous monitoring and management of critically ill patients.

Many large academic trauma centers are utilizing APPs, made up of nurse practitioners (NPs) and physician assistants (PAs), to augment trauma care (Sherwood 2009). The number of APPs caring for traumatically injured patients has grown over the last several decades along with the scopes of practice for these clinicians. One of the driving factors for this demand-based growth in the United States was the 2003 national mandate to limit medical residents to an 80-h work week (Christmas 2005). Many trauma departments have successfully incorporated nurse practitioners and physician assistants into their trauma teams to effectively care for their injured patients. Often with trauma, ICU, military medic, or prehospital backgrounds, these specialized nonphysician providers have unique perspectives and experience and offer helpful contributions that are different than other medical team members. A small group of research studies looking at the ICU care provided by APPs find that these trauma and critical care specialized nonphysicians are a safe, effective, viable staffing option for maintaining trauma protocols and providing evidence-based ICU care in collaboration with other members of a critical care team.

Substantial evidence shows that continuity of care promotes better outcomes by decreasing medical errors and potentially preventing adverse events when patients are covered by a primary team (Howell 2012). Fragmentation of care has been associated with poor family satisfaction, providing strong evidence that care fragmentation affects an important aspect of the quality of overall care. Length of stay (LOS) increases with fragmentation of care, secondary to inconsistencies with patient management often because of frequently changing providers. ICU provider continuity has been recommended as a measure of high-quality end-of-life care by the Robert Wood Johnson Foundation of Critical Care End-of Life Peer Workgroup which states that "Continuity of care" was identified as one of the seven key domains as quality indicators for measuring end-of-life care in the ICU (Clarke 2003). This is important because the ICU has an average patient mortality rate of 10–29 % (SCCM 2012).

Coordination of Care

The general rule for coordination of care in an ICU primary team starts with providing 24/7 coverage. Team members generally work 12-h rotating shifts and are assigned dedicated patients for whom that team member is responsible for being the "first call" to address patient management issues and emergencies and update the patient or family on plan of care. Members of the team are then responsible to report and keep the attending physician updated with any patient status changes, new patient admissions, and ongoing patient care. The attending intensivist, who is responsible for the global care and management of all the ICU patients, is also responsible for educating the team and providing expert advice on patient care. This defined coordination of care goes hand in hand with continuity of care, promoting improved patient safety, better patient and family satisfaction, with overall care, and improved ICU team satisfaction and lessens the chances of medical error by providing a standardized practice paradigm.

Trauma patients often present challenging medical care situations, as severely injured patients usually have a constellation of injuries where creativity on the part of the ICU team is essential. This can involve patient positioning, transport, procedure prioritization, and challenges to preventing secondary injury, such as, the inability to safely anticoagulate a patient to prevent deep vein thromboses and subsequent pulmonary embolism.

Coordination of care specific to injured patients now most often includes the timely performance of a tertiary trauma survey – a complete head-to-toe physical exam of an injured patient as well as a review of all radiological studies in order to summarize and document all of the patient's injuries. This process is often performed 12–24 h post-injury. Any physical or clinical findings suspicious for additional unknown injuries can be imaged at this time and included in the complete injury list. The tertiary trauma survey injury synopsis is then used as a communication piece for all care providers and most importantly is used to ensure that all necessary consulting services have been involved in the patient's care. This process is the standard of care for not only decreasing missed injuries (Biffl 2003) but also serves as a type of checklist for complex and challenging trauma patients with a constellation of injuries.

Handoff Communication

Each member of the ICU medical team has an essential task of effective communication of all imperative medical information regarding each trauma patient. Throughout the day or night, the flow of communication is important to ensure the patient's needs are being met. With a multidisciplinary team approach, each member of the team holds important information and must continuously evaluate which facts are passed off and to whom. During larger shift changes, this communication sharing becomes even more important as a shift's worth of data must be distilled down to the critical information needed by the next team to effectively and safely care for the patient. Many trauma centers and ICU teams have protocolized ways in which ICU teams sign out to one another by creating a template to follow that helps to prevent error and streamline essential data points.

Another time when important handoff communication takes place is during patient transport into the care of other medical teams such as interventional radiology and the operating room or during transfer to a medical/surgical ward and trauma ward medical team. Trauma APPs, and other experienced providers, can act as communication hubs during these transfers out of, and back to, the ICU.

Debriefing

While nearly all communication in an ICU is critical, knowing how to succinctly describe a patient's condition and plan of care to all participants in the ICU, from patients and their friends and family members to other members of the team, is vital. These members may include registered nurses, intensivists, resident or student physicians, respiratory therapists, physical or occupational therapists, dieticians, social workers, chaplains, and case managers to whom communicating patient status is a valuable skill that not only improves efficiency but is at the core of a unified patient care plan. This communication stream also prevents harmful misunderstandings, medical errors, and frustrating gaps in care.

More formal types of debriefing may include reviews of trauma resuscitations, codes or other unexpected emergencies in the ICU, and formal morbidity and mortality sessions involving traumatically injured ICU patients. Participation by each member of the involved ICU team in these debriefings, whether informal or formal, is

important and helps troubleshoot system weaknesses and areas of strength among the team.

Patient Flow

It is important to facilitate patient flow both into and out of the ICU by prioritization of the patient's medical care needs balanced by resource availability. Traumatically injured patients requiring ICU level care can be identified early on by trauma team members. When a patient meets ICU admission criteria by either life-threatening diagnosis such as intracerebral hemorrhage, unstable organ laceration, critically abnormal lab work such as perturbed coagulation studies, clinical or diagnostic signs of hemorrhage, intubation requiring ventilator management, or the need for close observation, notification of hospital staff involved in triaging ICU beds can occur. With earliest notification to nursing managers and by ICU bed reservation, the patient's arrival to the ICU can be expedited, thereby facilitating optimal medical management of critically injured patients when timing is of the essence. Timely identification of patients who no longer meet ICU level criteria by the ICU team allows them to initiate transfer protocols out of the ICU. This criteria to transfer out of the ICU may include being stabilized, no longer requiring ICU level observation, or by extubation (as examples). Patients may transfer to either a step-down ICU ward or to a medical/surgical trauma care ward.

Transfer Times

Facilitating efficient patient transfers out of the ICU by completing transfer order sets, writing transfer orders, and communicating plans to transfer patients to appropriate staff members in a timely fashion is important. By notifying the bedside nurse, patient, and their family members of the transfer plan, the members of the ICU team can also answer questions and concerns regarding the transfer and proactively address issues (medical, psychosocial, logistical) that may delay the transfer (Christmas 2005).

Impacting Length of Stay

One of the most pervasive ongoing hospital and healthcare initiatives is to decrease all patient's hospital LOS when medically appropriate. This in turn frees up beds and staff to care for other patients, optimizes resource allocation, and reduces healthcare costs to the patient and society as a whole. Decreasing the LOS in an ICU setting also potentially prevents hospital-acquired infections patients may get if they stay longer than what is medically necessary. Many researchers have studied factors that contribute to decreasing LOS and have found that there are staffing, preventative protocols, and goals-of-care decision measures that can positively contribute to patient's efficient ICU stay.

Several studies have found that physician and nursing staff attention and ratios optimize ICU patient care and decrease ICU LOS (Gruenberg 2006). Practices including daily rounding by a full-time intensivist or ICU-trained physician reduce complications and decrease LOS (Gruenberg 2006). Research has also shown that higher registered nurse (RN)-to-patient ratios decreased ICU length of stays and reduced adverse events in the ICU (Thungjaroenkul 2007).

Many ICU working groups have created procedure or care bundles that are evidenced based and have been shown to help prevent the common nosocomial or hospital-acquired infections that increase patient's LOS. These protocols may include sepsis identification and early treatment therapies, ventilator-associated pneumonia (VAP) prevention with oral care policies and protocolized ventilator weaning order sets, sedation and analgesia practices that allow for sedation vacations to decrease prolonged sedation, gastric ulcer prevention, delirium prevention and early identification, aggressive skin care and skin breakdown prevention, and identification and treatment to name a few. Frequently, trauma patients specifically are immobilized and need deep vein thrombosis (DVT) prevention within a specific time frame, and protocols help guide the details of this therapy. These protocols are the onus of all members of the ICU team and often are labor and resource intensive. They involve cost, education, and frequent revisions to remain evidence based and to provide state-of-the-art care.

Finally, communication around the patient's desired medical care and appropriate medical care between ICU teams, patients, and their family members can decrease LOS by clarifying goals of care. When patients have determined their medical directives prior to hospital admission, their care can be aligned with their wishes. This may mean that if a patient or their designated advocate has deemed them do not resuscitate (DNR) or similarly, their care needs may be met more closely on a unit other than the ICU. Palliative care teams and ethics committees can help with challenging patient care scenarios to efficiently determine goals of care for a critical and dying patient, and get them to the most appropriate setting, which may be home with hospice or a hospice care facility.

Improving Hospital Readmission
Readmission into the hospital closely following a hospitalization for a traumatic injury is costly and is often preventable. While some trauma readmissions are planned, for example, to reverse temporary ostomies, to replace bone flaps, or to finalize orthopedic procedures, most are caused by postoperative wound infections and pain (Esposito 2012). Preventing readmissions is a standard of hospital objectives and is the responsibility of the entire healthcare team. By studying institution-specific trends in readmission causes, relevant performance improvement projects can be initiated. The multidisciplinary team can follow a systematic approach to planning an initial hospital discharge by attending to the patient's unique needs of injury-specific education, wound, spine or extremity care, pain management, and, if applicable, anticoagulation therapy. The appropriate discharge destination is critical in ensuring a safe and successful discharge. Case managers and/or social workers can help to match patients with the options open to them in regard to finances, insurance coverage, and area-specific offerings. There is evidence that patients who are discharged home when they cannot afford the medically recommended supervised care such as in a subacute rehab facility are over-represented in readmission groups (Esposito 2012). Creative resource solutions can prevent these readmissions along with possibly allowing this cohort of patients to remain inpatient slightly

beyond the usual pathway to provide them the supervision and care needed in those temperamental early days post-acute injury.

Applications

The current emphasis on national healthcare reform and the business of running a cost-effective hospital continues to challenge ICU teams to provide better more efficient care. When all ICU interdisciplinary team members work together to optimize communication, protocolize pathways to prevent common ICU problems, and embrace evidence-based changes to their care, they can provide the best care to the sickest people. Administrative support of these challenging care areas is critical too in providing leadership and advocacy for these heavily resource-reliant patient care units. The structure of the ICU team must be highly functional and keep abreast of the most current ICU care trends to provide state-of-the-art care for patients whose lives depend on them. Advance practice providers are valuable additions to the ICU team and ultimately maintain excellent patient care, satisfaction, and outcomes (Morris 2012). The ICU and the specialty of critical care practiced there are exciting and challenging, and frequently an area where science, intellect, and creativity intersect.

Cross-References

- ▶ Acute Pain Management in Trauma
- ▶ Advanced Practice Provider Care Delivery Models
- ▶ Delirium as a Complication of ICU Care
- ▶ Discharge Planning
- ▶ End-of-Life Care Communication in Trauma Patients
- ▶ Hemodynamic Monitoring
- ▶ Interdisciplinary Team
- ▶ Mechanical Ventilation, Weaning
- ▶ Nurse Practitioner
- ▶ Physician Assistant
- ▶ Resuscitation Goals in Trauma Patients

- ▶ Sedation, Analgesia, Neuromuscular Blockade in the ICU
- ▶ Teamwork and Trauma Care
- ▶ Trauma Intensive Care Management
- ▶ Venous Thromboembolism Prophylaxis in the Intensive Care Unit
- ▶ Ventilatory Management of Trauma Patients

References

Biffl WL, Harrington DT, Cioffi WG (2003) Implementation of a tertiary trauma survey decreases missed injuries. J Trauma Inj Infect Crit Care 54(1):38–44

Christmas AB, Reynolds J, Hodges S et al (2005) Physician extenders impact trauma systems. J Trauma Inj Infect Crit Care 58(5):917–920

Clarke EB, Curtis JR, Luce JM et al (2003) Robert Wood Johnson foundation critical care end-of-life peer workgroup members. Quality indicators for end-of-life care in the intensive care unit. Crit Care Med 31(9):2255–2262

Esposito TJ, Clark-Kula E, Crowe M et al (2012) Trauma patient unplanned hospital re-admissions. Surg Sci 3:381–388

Gruenberg DA, Shelton W, Rose SL et al (2006) Factors influencing length of stay in the intensive care unit. Am J Crit Care 15:502–509

Howell MD (2012) Intensivist time allocation: economic and ethical issues surrounding how intensivists use their time. Semin Respir Crit Care Med 33(4):401–412

Morris DS, Reilly P, Rohrbach J et al (2012) The influence of unit-based nurse practitioners on hospital outcomes and readmission rates for patients with trauma. J Trauma Acute Care Surg 73(2):474–478

Sherwood KL, Price RR, White TW et al (2009) A role in trauma care for advanced practice clinicians. J Am Acad Phys Assist 22(6):33–37

Society of Critical Care Medicine, SCCM (2012) Critical care statistics in the United States: http://www.sccm.org/SiteCollectionDocuments/StatisticsBroch_d4.pdf

Thungjaroenkul P, Cummings GG, Embleton A (2007) The impact of nurse staffing on hospital costs and patient length of stay: a systematic review. Nurs Econ 25(5):255–265

ICU Psychosis

- ▶ Delirium as a Complication of ICU Care

Idiopathic Pulmonary Arterial Hypertension (iPAH)

▶ Pulmonary Hypertension

IED (Improvised Explosive Device)

Charles A. Frosolone
Medical Department, USS Nimitz CVN-68,
Everett, WA, USA

Synonyms

Antipersonnel landmines; Antitank landmines; Anti-vehicle landmines; Booby trap; Explosive Formed Projectile (EFP) devices; Homemade bomb; Improved explosive devices; Roadside bomb; Roadside explosives and blast mines

Definition

US Department of Defense defines them as *"devices placed or fabricated in an improvised manner incorporating destructive, lethal, noxious, pyrotechnic or incendiary chemicals, designed to destroy, disfigure, distract or harass and often incorporate military stores..."* (NATO 2009; Ramasamy 2009).

IEDs can be sophisticated or quite simple in construction depending on the training and experience of the designer and the materials available. They can be made specifically for use against vehicles and armor or personnel.

For anti-armor explosive formed penetrators (EFP) or shaped charges are constructed that concentrate the blast force or propel a metallic liner at high velocity and are capable of penetrating the protection in vehicles. Antipersonnel IEDs contain fragmentation-generating objects such as nails, ball bearings, or even small rocks to cause wounds.

IEDs are made up of five components: a switch, an initiator, a container, an explosive, and a power source. The switches can be pressure, trip wire, magnetically or remotely activated using wire connection or wireless (often mobile phone activated) methods. Nonmetallic switches are constructed that are undetectable by metal detectors. Suicide bombers can activate them manually. Initiators are blasting caps or can be improvised from flash bulbs or fuses. The containers can be military munitions or as simple as an earthen jar. The charge can be conventional military explosives, commercial explosives, or fabricated from agricultural fertilizer (ammonium nitrate), or combinations of these. The power sources are usually small commercial batteries that can be placed at a distance from the charge again to evade metal detectors. These IEDS can be hidden by the roadside, under the road or paths, or may be delivered by vehicles, personnel (suicide/homicide bombers), animals, or boats. Mostly what this essay covers is fixed roadside bombs and their medical consequences.

Preexisting Condition

IEDs are not new to warfare being first used extensively in World War 2 and since in many "asymmetric" or guerilla type wars or insurgencies including Vietnam, Northern Ireland, and most recently Iraq and Afghanistan.

IEDs in all their forms pose the most prevalent single threat to US and coalition forces operating in both Iraq and Afghanistan. In Iraq, they were the leading cause of death among coalition troops.

In Iraq, explosion was the leading mechanism of injury causing 78 % with IEDs accounting for 38 % (Owens 2008). A higher proportion of IED as cause of injury exists in Afghanistan. The number of IEDs used in Afghanistan had increased by 400 % since 2007 and the number of troops killed by them by 400 %, and those wounded by 700 %.

Prevention: Pre-deployment and ongoing in-theater training of forces in recognition of roadside IEDs has increased awareness and is important in prevention. The detection and inactivation of IEDs has been a focus in these theaters utilizing road clearance teams with specially equipped vehicles, metal detectors for dismounted troops, inactivation of wireless triggering devices by electronic jamming, destruction by roller vehicles, anti-mine-clearing line charges (MCLCs), ever present explosive ordinance disposal teams, and even "sniffer" dogs. Development and fielding of specialized mine-resistant vehicles (MRAPs-mine resistant ambush protected) gives significant protection against many IEDs that escape detection and detonate.

Application

Injury severity and victim outcome from an IED explosion depends on many factors: whether the victim is in a vehicle (mounted) and the type of vehicle, or on foot (dismounted), the type and sophistication of IED, the location of the IED, the power of the explosive charge, distance from the explosion, and care rendered in the field or in hospital.

Injuries from explosions, and thus IEDs, are classified into four categories: primary, secondary, tertiary, and quaternary blast injuries. For a more extensive review of explosion injuries, see the essay in this encyclopedia. To summarize briefly, primary blast injuries occur from an acute overpressure of the air resulting in injury to the air-containing structures in the body, ear, lung, and gut. Secondary blast injuries occur when the victim is struck by objects energized by the explosion, such as parts of the IED or other nearby matter such as rocks resulting in penetrating wounds. Tertiary blast injuries occur when the victim is thrown by the explosion colliding with nearby objects receiving blunt trauma-type injuries. Quaternary blast injuries occur from the thermal effects of the explosion or by chemicals or even biological agents if they are part of the IED.

The injury patterns of particular IEDs and whether the victim is mounted or on foot appear to be different. In a review by Ramasamy (2008) in mounted victims, EFPs were the most common anti-vehicle IEDs. Twenty-two percent of

victims died. Extremity injuries were common in both the survivor and fatalities group and present in 86.7 % of all casualties with multiple injuries, the rule averaging 2–3 injuries per victim. However, in fatalities, the number of injuries per victim averaged 4.6, and injuries to the torso, head, neck, and face were statistically greater in the fatalities. In survivors significant torso injuries were uncommon (most victims were wearing body armor). Ramasamy concluded that there was an "all or nothing" pattern from the EFP blasts due to the focused directional effect of these IEDs. Those receiving fatal injury patterns were in the path of the blast, while those just adjacent to the path received survivable minor injuries. Significant primary blast injuries were very uncommon seen in 3.7 %, and mostly all injuries were due to secondary or tertiary blast effects. Gases from the explosion forced into the compartment of the vehicles caused some quaternary effects.

Currently most coalition forces rarely leave their compounds except in MRAP-type vehicles, and the injury patterns found in them reflect those noted by Ramasamy. The injuries sustained in non-MRAP vehicles are similar, but not "focused" and more devastating and fatal. These injury patterns are still seen in the Afghanistan and Iraqi military and civilians who may travel in non-MRAP-type vehicles.

The injuries in dismounted troops or civilians from roadside IEDs are much more destructive and potentially fatal with multiple amputations very frequent in survivors. Overall, major limb amputation rates for the current US engagement in Afghanistan and Iraq are similar to those of previous conflicts. This must be looked at taking account that in conflicts prior to Vietnam, no vascular reconstruction was done, and it was not widely done early in the Vietnam War (Stansbury 2008).

Nelson at a forward surgery team role 2B noted overall survival of only 50 % for 18 patients suffering close-proximity blast injuries with significant lower-extremity fractures with no active hemorrhage identified at the time of presentation (Nelson 2008). He concluded that close-proximity blast injury leads to severe physical and physiologic effects possibly due to primary blast injury causing autonomic dysfunction as well as secondary and tertiary blast injuries. Ramasamy, however, noted minimal evidence of primary blast effects in his population of mounted troops. Though his number of victims studied was small, in another paper, Nelson noted that sustained hypotension ($p = 0.03$) and presence of two or more factors (three or more long-bone fractures, penetrating head injury, and associated fatalities) were notably associated with mortality ($p = 0.015$). He felt that these were predictive of mortality and could be utilized in triage of mass casualties caused by blast (Nelson 2006).

The majority of current combat extremity injuries are from explosion by secondary and tertiary blast injuries. Explosions can cause fracture, tissue loss, and vascular injury, all of which place the extremities at risk of developing compartment syndrome. As with other explosive weapons, IEDs most commonly wound the extremities with upper and lower limbs affected equally. Studies from the UK and the US Joint Theater Trauma Registries have shown that following explosion, over 70 % of combat wounds are to the extremities, with head and neck injuries accounting for 20–25 % of wounds and with torso injuries seen in less than 10 % of combat casualties. This may be attributed to the effectiveness of the enhanced combat body armor.

The pattern of extremity amputation is typical for primary blast injury to extremities. Hull and Cooper felt that the blast wave itself causes the fractures, and blast wind flailing completes the amputation. The amputations from pure primary blast rarely occur through the joints, but through the long shaft of the upper or lower extremities. Amputation by wind flailing is seen in pilot ejection at high speed, but occurs through the joints. Hull and Cooper (1996) were able to show through computer modeling and animal limb model that the blast wave caused the fracture, the wind flailing the amputation. In the IED-dismounted victim, there also is a major component of secondary (fragmentary) blast injury, and the victim is thrown by the blast wind sustaining tertiary injuries.

Quaternary thermal injuries can complicate the injuries, though usually were not noted to be significant.

The typical injury pattern noted in the author's experience in dismounted IED victims who are close to the blast is mutilating high lower-extremity-completed amputations, often both legs, and an upper-extremity amputation. Truncal injuries are not as common when body armor is worn.

IEDs are a common cause of stable and unstable spinal injuries in the Afghanistan conflict probably due to tertiary blast effects. Spinal immobilization is underutilized in the battlefield care of casualties in the conflict in Afghanistan. This may be a result of tactical limitations, and it is taught in field care courses, like Tactical Combat Casualty Care, that spinal immobilization is not indicated. However, with the mechanism of IED blast, mounted or dismounted, current protocols should continue to emphasize the judicious use of immobilization in these patients (Comstock 2011).

Treatment

The principles of treatment for IED injuries remain the same as for any trauma, identifying and treating immediately life-threatening injuries. This begins on the battlefield with well-trained medic/corpsmen following mnemonic "MARCH" (massive hemorrhage, airway, respiration, circulation (palpable radial pulse hold fluid), hypothermia) utilizing tourniquets for hemorrhage control, compressible hemorrage. The victim is rapidly triaged and if indicated, sent on to the appropriate level of surgical care either a forward surgical team or theater hospital.

At the first level where surgery is available, the concept of damage control is practiced controlling hemorrhage, stopping enteric spillage, and reestablishing circulation. If there are extensive extremity injuries, accent is on saving the limb or maximizing length of the amputation and debridement to decrease infection. The extent of the surgery on the extremities is dictated by the physiologic state of the patient.

Antibiotic prophylaxis is indicated, but is not to replace debridement. Tetanus immunization should be confirmed or administered.

Revascularization is accomplished by temporary shunting and/or definitive vascular repair.

The goal in debridement is to save lives, preserve function, minimize morbidity, and prevent infections. The tissues devitalized by the high explosives form a culture medium for the bacteria introduced with the shell fragments, debris, or pieces of clothing, and all must be removed surgically leaving a clean healthy bed of soft tissue for reconstruction. Copious irrigation should be utilized. Debridement should be done appropriately, but it should be done to maximize extremity length in case of traumatic amputation. Debridement should be done minimally at FSTs (Forward Surgical Teams) if there is prompt evacuation to a higher level of care, theater hospital, to not delay transfer.

With multiple small superficial "peppering" by fragments with no evidence of underlying significant injuries, cleansing of the wounds and antibiotics is usually all that is necessary.

Compartment syndrome should be anticipated and recognized early, and if indicated fasciotomy performed. Fasciotomy should often accompany periods of ischemia with revascularization, temporary shunting, and significant medevac times.

External fixation is the preferred method of fracture stabilization as it facilitates transportation, giving rapid stabilization allowing vascular repair and effective wound care.

Often with IED blasts, the amputation has already taken place. However, sometimes an immediate or early decision between limb reconstruction and amputation must be made. This decision can be a difficult choice between an irreversible loss of limb and an attempt at salvage. It must take into account patient status. The goals in care often might be life over limb. Factors that suggest amputation as therapy are the following: irreparable vascular injury, warm ischemia greater than 8 h, severe crush with minimal remaining viable tissue, a severely damaged limb which may constitute a threat to the patient's life, and even after revascularization the limb remains so severely damaged that function will be less satisfactory than that afforded by a prosthesis. Decision to amputate should be confirmed by a second surgeon if possible, and photo documentation is recommended. It has previously been felt that the presence of an insensate foot at the time of injury indicated an amputation; however, early neurological dysfunction should not be part of the limb salvage decision. There should be no guillotine amputations, and the bone should be cut at the most distal soft tissue levels. There should be no fashioning of flaps at initial debridement.

Mangled extremity severity score (MESS) is a scoring system helpful in deciding whether amputation may be indicated. Brown and Ramasamy (Brown 2009) studying UK casualties injured by ballistic mangled extremity injuries (over half by blasts) demonstrated that the MESS is not predictive of the need for primary amputation in the combat environment. They felt that the factors that should be considered in the initial decision-making are the presence or absence of shock and an ischemic limb.

Another look and debridement is done at 24–72 h and may be repeated many times until all necrotic and/or infected is removed. Closure can be accomplished in a delayed fashion, by skin grafts or flap, and vacuum wound therapy is widely used.

Cross-References

▶ Blast
▶ Blast Lung Injury
▶ Compartment Syndrome, Acute
▶ Compressible Hemorrhage
▶ Damage Control Surgery
▶ Debridement
▶ Explosion
▶ Fragment Injury

References

Brown KV, Ramasamy A, McLeod J, Stapley S, Clasper JC (2009) Predicting the need for early amputation in ballistic mangled extremity injuries. J Trauma 66:S93–S98

Comstock S, Pannell D, Talbot M, Compton L, Withers N (2011) Tien HC spinal injuries after improvised explosive device incidents: implications for tactical combat casualty care. J Trauma 71(5 Suppl 1): S413–S417

Hull JB, Cooper GJ (1996) Pattern and mechanism of traumatic amputations by explosive blast. J Trauma 40(Suppl 3):S198–S205

NATO (2009) Unclassified metrics. Strategic Advisory Group. 9 May, Kandahar

Nelson TJ, Wall DB, Stedje-Larsen ET, Clark RT, Chambers LW, Bohman HR (2006) Predictors of mortality in close proximity blast injuries during operation Iraqi freedom. J Am Coll Surg 202:418–422

Nelson TJ, Clark T, Stedje-Larsen ET, Lewis CT, Grueskin JM, Echols EL, Wall DB, Felger EA, Bohman HR (2008) Close proximity blast injury patterns from improvised explosive devices in Iraq: a report of 18 cases. J Trauma 65:212–217

Owens BT, Kragh JF, Wenke JC, Macaitis J, Wade CE, Holcomb JB (2008) Combat wounds in operation Iraqi freedom and operation enduring freedom. J Trauma 4:295–299

Ramasamy A, Harrison SE, Clasper JC, Stewart MPM (2008) Injuries from roadside improvised explosive devices. J Trauma 65:910–914

Ramasamy A, Hill AM, Clasper JC (2009) Improvised explosive devices: pathophysiology, injury profiles and current medical management. JR Army Med Corps 155(4):265–272

Stansbury LG, Lalliss SJ, Branstette JG, Bagg MR, Holcomb JB (2008) Amputations in U.S. Military personnel in the current conflicts in Afghanistan and Iraq. J Orthop Trauma 22:43–46

IED (Improvised Explosive Device) Trauma

▶ Military Trauma, Anesthesia for

Iliac Vascular Injury

▶ Abdominal Major Vascular Injury, Anesthesia for

Illicit Drug Use

▶ Drug Abuse and Trauma Anesthesia

Imaging

▶ Imaging of CNS Injuries
▶ Imaging of Neck Injuries

Imaging Head & Neck Trauma

▶ Imaging of Neck Injuries

Imaging of Abdominal and Pelvic Injuries

Matthew T. Heller
Department of Radiology, Division of Abdominal Imaging, University of Pittsburgh Medical Center, Pittsburgh, PA, USA

Synonyms

Computed tomography (CT) of abdominal and pelvic injuries; Imaging of abdominal and pelvic trauma

Definition

Imaging of abdominal and pelvic injuries entails the use of various types of radiographic studies to diagnose bodily injuries due to trauma. The general imaging process consists of choosing the most appropriate imaging method, image acquisition, and post-processing and displaying the images on a picture archiving computer system. While ultrasound (US), magnetic resonance imaging (MRI), multi-detector computed tomography (MDCT), and radiography (x-ray) can all be used in the trauma setting, MDCT is the most commonly employed imaging modality due to its speed, reproducibility, spatial resolution, and relative lack of contraindications.

Preexisting Conditions

A key factor in the diagnosis of traumatic injury to the abdomen and pelvis is recognition of the normal appearance of the solid viscera, bowel, and mesentery. The spleen can have a variable appearance on CT, but is best evaluated during the portal venous phase of imaging which occurs approximately 70–80 s after intravenous contrast injection. During the portal venous phase, the splenic parenchyma shows homogeneous enhancement, interrupted only by traversing vessels branching from the hilum. Normal parenchymal vessels are readily identified as enhancing tubular structures that are isodense to the adjacent splenic artery or vein. During the arterial phase of imaging, the splenic parenchyma has a very bizarre, heterogeneous appearance. The arterial phase occurs approximately 30–40 s after intravenous contrast injection and coincides with the time of maximum differentiation between the red and white pulp of the spleen. Therefore, any abnormality perceived during the arterial phase must be corroborated during the portal venous phase. Another potential source of parenchymal ambiguity is the splenic cleft (Fig. 1), most commonly seen as smooth indentation or fissure along the superior pole of the spleen. If not recognized as a normal anatomic variant, a cleft can be potentially confused with a laceration. However, lacerations are typically more irregular and associated with intraparenchymal or perisplenic hematoma. Similarly, the liver contains normally occurring fissures that can potentially be misinterpreted as lacerations. The two most recognizable hepatic fissures are the fissure for the ligamentum venosum, which separates the caudate lobe from the left hepatic lobe, and the fissure for the ligamentum teres, which separates the medial segment from the lateral segment of the left hepatic lobe. Unlike the spleen, the liver parenchyma has a relatively homogeneous appearance during both the arterial and portal venous phases; however, similar to the spleen, hepatic parenchymal injury is best assessed during the portal venous phase of imaging since this is the time of maximum parenchymal enhancement (Soto and Anderson 2012).

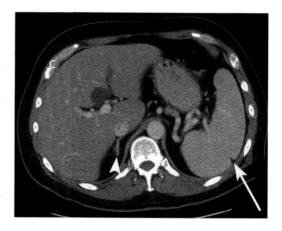

Imaging of Abdominal and Pelvic Injuries, Fig. 1 Splenic cleft. Contrast-enhanced CT shows a cleft (*arrow*) along the posterior margin of the spleen, a normal variant. Note the homogeneous parenchyma of the spleen and liver and a normal-appearing right adrenal gland (*arrowhead*)

During this time, the hepatic and portal veins also show maximum enhancement and are identified as smoothly marginated, tubular structures that are nearly isodense to the abdominal and inferior vena cava. If scanning is performed without the use of intravenous contrast material, unopacified vessels may potentially be confused with parenchymal lacerations if the vessels are not carefully traced to their origins.

In contrast to the relative homogeneity of the splenic and hepatic parenchyma, the pancreas has a more heterogeneous appearance during MDCT due to its lack of an organ capsule (Linsenmaier et al. 2008). Therefore, the undulation of the borders and the intercalation of fat between the acini must be recognized as the normal appearance of the pancreas so that parenchymal injury is not misdiagnosed. The adrenal glands are easily identifiable as inverted V-shaped structures superior to the kidneys. Adrenal adenomas may be occasionally confused with hematoma when sufficiently large and heterogeneous; however, the lack of adjacent fat infiltration and coexisting injury favor the presence of an incidental adenoma. However, while fat infiltration is often an important secondary finding, its presence does not always herald a traumatic injury. An important consideration is the presence of infiltration of the perinephric fat or "perinephric stranding"; infiltration of the perinephric fat is common in patients with advanced age or a variety of kidney diseases and, unless asymmetric, does not usually indicate an acute injury. Similarly, the mesentery may undergo a variable degree of infiltration due to entities such as sclerosing mesenteritis, inflammation, and infection in the absence of trauma.

Finally, evaluating traumatic injury of the stomach, small bowel, and colon is often compromised by the degree of luminal underdistension of these structures. Underdistension results in artifactual wall thickening and may lead to misinterpretation of a focal mural injury or hematoma. The use of secondary signs, such as adjacent extraluminal gas, fluid, or mesenteric hematoma, is helpful when evaluating apparent mural thickening in the setting of trauma (Fang et al. 2006).

Applications

MDCT Technique

MDCT of the abdomen and pelvis is optimized when a bolus of 100–150 mL of intravenous contrast material is administered via a power injector at a rate of 3–5 mL/s. Ideally, the contrast material is injected through a 20-gauge or greater peripheral intravenous catheter followed by a 30–50 mL saline bolus. Oral contrast material is routinely omitted for trauma patients. While there are several variants of trauma imaging protocols, scanning during the portal venous phase is essential; peak visceral enhancement occurs during the portal venous phase and maximizes diagnosis of parenchymal trauma (Soto and Anderson 2012). The addition of arterial phase images have proven beneficial for detecting injuries to the major arteries of the abdomen and pelvis and for detecting vascular injuries of solid viscera such as the spleen, liver, and kidneys (Boscak and Shanmuganathan 2012). Selective inclusion of delayed phase imaging should be obtained in patients suspected of sustaining a urinary tract injury and for further assessment of visceral injuries that involve the vasculature. CT cystography

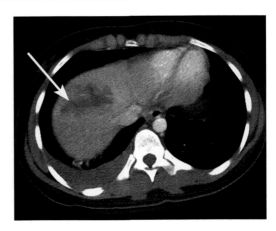

Imaging of Abdominal and Pelvic Injuries, Fig. 2 Liver laceration. Contrast-enhanced CT demonstrates a linear laceration (*arrow*) at the superior margin of the liver

can be performed in cases of suspected bladder injury; this technique consists of instilling approximately 400 mL of diluted iodinated contrast material into the urinary bladder via the existing Foley catheter followed by scanning of the pelvis and creation of reformatted images (Uyeda et al. 2010).

Spleen and Liver

Traumatic injuries to the spleen and liver consist of parenchymal contusions, lacerations, hematomas, active hemorrhage, and vascular injuries (Milia and Brasel 2011). Parenchymal contusions are due to compression of the organ tissue and appear as ill-defined regions of low attenuation or decreased perfusion. On follow-up examinations, contusions become increasingly inconspicuous until complete resolution. Lacerations are due to parenchymal tears and have a variable appearance during MDCT; most lacerations appear as irregular, linear regions of low attenuation (Fig. 2) while others assume a more complex or stellate configuration (Fig. 3) (Soto and Anderson 2012). Lacerations may remain thin and linear while others may be expanded and ovoid due to filling with hematoma. Intraparenchymal hematoma consists of clotted blood of varying age and appears as a heterogeneous collection of high attenuation within the injured organ. The most important splenic and hepatic injuries to

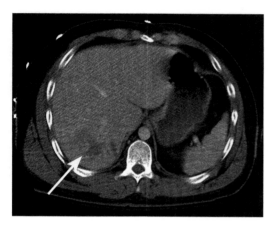

**Imaging of Abdominal and Pelvic Injuries,
Fig. 3** Liver laceration. Contrast-enhanced CT reveals
an irregular, stellate laceration (*arrow*) in the posterior
segment of the liver

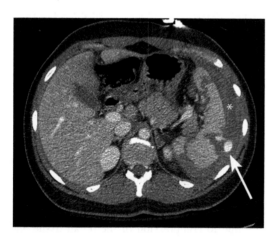

**Imaging of Abdominal and Pelvic Injuries,
Fig. 4** Splenic hemorrhage. Contrast-enhanced CT
shows active hemorrhage (*arrow*) extending from a large
splenic laceration and perisplenic hematoma (*asterisk*)

accurately diagnose during MDCT are active
hemorrhage and vascular injuries as these types
of injuries typically require immediate intervention. Active hemorrhage manifests and an ill-
defined jet or blush of extravasated contrast
material into the injured parenchyma or into the
peritoneal spaces surrounding the viscera (Fig. 4)
(Soto and Anderson 2012). Differentiation of
active hemorrhage from a normal branching
vessel is made by recognizing that active hemorrhage is ill-defined and progressively

accumulates during later phases of imaging
while normal vessels are smoothly marginated
and become less opacified by intravascular contrast material during subsequent imaging.
Another type of vascular injury is traumatic
pseudoaneurysm formation. Pseudoaneurysms
occur when there is focal injury to the vessel
wall without creation of a transmural defect.
Pseudoaneurysms are identified during MDCT
as focal outpouchings of the arterial wall and
are best shown during the arterial phase. Therefore, many MDCT trauma protocols include
biphasic imaging of the abdomen and pelvis to
maximize detection of subtle arterial injury
which may be easily overlooked if only portal
venous phase imaging is performed (Boscak and
Shanmuganathan 2012). Finally, injury of the
biliary system may occur when hepatic lacerations deeply traverse the parenchyma or extend to
the hilum of the liver. Leakage of bile manifests
as low attenuation hepatic fluid or as subhepatic
fluid collections on follow-up examinations.

Bowel and Mesentery

Although bowel and mesenteric injuries constitute are relatively rare, they carry high morbidity
and mortality due to their association with peritonitis and sepsis. Over half of the injuries
affecting hollow viscera involve the small
bowel, most commonly occurring in the proximal
jejunum and distal ileum since these are relative
points of fixation due to strong mesenteric attachments (Atri et al. 2008). After the small bowel,
the colon and stomach are the next most frequently injured hollow viscera. Specific signs of
hollow visceral injury include focal transection of
the wall, pneumoperitoneum, pneumoretro-
peritoneum, and extravasation of oral contrast
material (Fang et al. 2006). More sensitive signs
of hollow visceral trauma include focal
wall thickening, abnormal enhancement of the
bowel wall, increased infiltration ("stranding")
of the adjacent mesentery, and free intraperitoneal fluid. While infiltration of the mesenteric fat
may be due to either bowel injury or primary
mesenteric injury, more specific signs of
mesenteric trauma include mesenteric hematoma, active hemorrhage manifested by

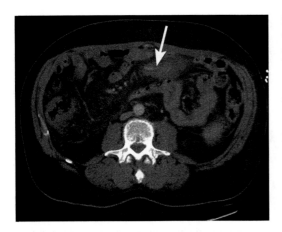

Imaging of Abdominal and Pelvic Injuries, Fig. 5 Mesenteric injury. Contrast-enhanced CT reveals mesenteric hematoma and active bleeding (*arrow*)

peritoneal extravasation of intravascular contrast material (Fig. 5), or abrupt truncation of mesenteric vessels (Atri et al. 2008). In the setting of occult visceral or mesenteric injury, the density of hemoperitoneum can be used to locate the site of injury; the area of most dense hematoma (sentinel clot) is typically located closest to the site of injury (Orwig and Federle 1989).

Adrenal and Kidney

Similar to the spleen and liver, the kidney is subject to contusions, lacerations, hematomas, and vascular injuries. Appreciation of the depth of laceration is a key component to accurate diagnosis since deeper lacerations may traverse the renal collecting system and result in urine leak or urinoma. Therefore, excretory phase imaging is required in all patients in whom perinephric fluid is identified on earlier phases of imaging (Soto and Anderson 2012). While avulsions of the renal pedicle are rare, vascular injuries such as dissection, pseudoaneurysm, and arteriovenous fistula may occur and result in renal ischemia or infarction. Renal ischemia and infarction manifest as decreased or absent perfusion which may be global or geographic. Adrenal trauma is most common on the right and is usually accompanied by injuries to other upper abdominal viscera (Soto and Anderson 2012). Adrenal hematoma commonly appears as

focal high attenuation or glandular enlargement that may extend into the periadrenal or perinephric fat.

Pancreas

The diagnosis of acute pancreatic injuries during initial MDCT can be challenging as the injured pancreas can have a normal appearance for as long as 12 h after the traumatic event (Soto and Anderson 2012). The neck and proximal body of the pancreas are the most commonly injured sites due to the fulcrum effect from the lumbar spine during rapid deceleration (Soto and Anderson 2012). Injuries can be categorized as contusion, laceration, or transection. Parenchymal contusions appear as ill-defined regions of low attenuation, glandular enlargement, or distortion of the normal acinar structures. Focal linear, low attenuation defects are considered as lacerations when superficial but are termed transections when they extend through the entirety of the pancreas. Deep lacerations and transections are associated with disruption of the pancreatic duct; lacerations deeper than 50 % of the pancreatic thickness typically result in ductal injury (Linsenmaier et al. 2008). In equivocal cases, further evaluation with endoscopic retrograde cholangiopancreatography or magnetic resonance imaging is warranted. Nonspecific, secondary signs of pancreatic injury include infiltration of the peripancreatic fat, fluid or hematoma between the pancreas and splenic vein, and thickening of the anterior renal fascia (Linsenmaier et al. 2008).

Pelvis and Retroperitoneum

Acute retroperitoneal injuries with hematoma development are difficult to detect clinically and are not apparent during peritoneal lavage or ultrasound assessment. Due to the potential for large volume blood loss, MDCT plays a critical role in the assessment of retroperitoneal injury. The pelvis is the most common location for extraperitoneal hemorrhage and is commonly associated with pelvic fractures. MDCT provides high sensitivity for the detection of hematoma and allows for accurate determination of its size and extent. The application of MDCT

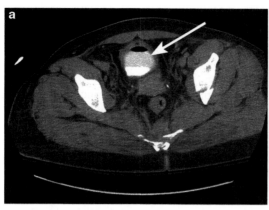
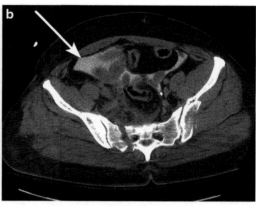

Imaging of Abdominal and Pelvic Injuries, Fig. 6 Intraperitoneal bladder injury. (**a**) Contrast-enhanced CT shows contrast within the urinary bladder lumen (*arrow*) that was instilled during cystography. (**b**) More superiorly, contrast extravasated (*arrow*) from the bladder outlines segments of small bowel, consistent with intraperitoneal bladder rupture

angiography provides high sensitivity and specificity for the detection of active hemorrhage and aids in guiding treatment (Uyeda et al. 2010). Pelvic fractures also place patients at risk for bladder injuries which can be best assessed with CT cystography (Soto and Anderson 2012). Bladder ruptures can be extraperitoneal, intraperitoneal, or combined. Intraperitoneal ruptures are diagnosed when contrast material is extravasated from the urinary bladder and surrounds peritoneal structures such as bowel and mesentery (Fig. 6). Extraperitoneal bladder ruptures are more common and are diagnosed when extravasated contrast fills the perivesical spaces and extends into extraperitoneal soft tissues (Chan et al. 2006).

Summary

Contrast-enhanced MDCT is the best imaging modality to evaluate for traumatic injuries of the abdomen and pelvis. The severity of visceral injuries can be stratified through grading systems such as the one set forth by the American Association for the Surgery of Trauma (AAST). The most important injuries to detect with MDCT are active hemorrhage and ductal disruptions. The speed, reproducibility, and spatial resolution of MDCT allow high sensitivity and specificity for the detection of traumatic injury to the abdomen and pelvis.

Cross-References

▶ Bladder Rupture (Intra/Extraperitoneal)
▶ Motor Vehicle Crash Injury
▶ Seatbelt Injuries
▶ Ultrasound in the Trauma and ICU Setting

References

Atri M, Hanson JM, Grinblat L, Brofman N, Chughtai T, Tomlinson G (2008) Surgically important bowel and/or mesenteric injury in blunt trauma: accuracy of multidetector CT for evaluation. Radiology 249(2):524–533

Boscak A, Shanmuganathan K (2012) Splenic trauma: what is new? Radiol Clin N Am 50(1):105–122

Chan DP, Abujudeh HH, Cushing GL Jr, Novelline RA (2006) CT cystography with multiplanar reformation for suspected bladder rupture: experience in 234 cases. Am J Roentgenol 187(5):1296–1302

Fang JF, Wong YC, Lin BC, Hsu YP, Chen MF (2006) Usefulness of multidetector computed tomography for the initial assessment of blunt abdominal trauma patients. World J Surg 30(2):176–182

Linsenmaier U, Wirth S, Reiser M, Körner M (2008) Diagnosis and classification of pancreatic and duodenal injuries in emergency radiology. RadioGraphics 28(6):1591–1602

Milia DJ, Brasel K (2011) Current use of CT in the evaluation and management of injured patients. Surg Clin N Am 91(1):233–248

Orwig D, Federle MP (1989) Localized clotted blood as evidence of visceral trauma on CT: the sentinel clot sign. Am J Roentgenol 153(4):747–749

Soto JA, Anderson SW (2012) Multidetector CT of blunt abdominal trauma. Radiology 265(3):678–693

Uyeda J, Anderson SW, Kertesz J, Soto JA (2010) Pelvic CT angiography: application to blunt trauma using 64MDCT. Emer Radiol 17(2):131–137

Imaging of Abdominal and Pelvic Trauma

▶ Imaging of Abdominal and Pelvic Injuries

Imaging of Aortic and Thoracic Injuries

Stamatis Kantartzis
Department of Radiology, University of Pittsburgh Medical Center, Pittsburgh, PA, USA

Synonyms

Angiography; Computed tomography (CT); FAST; Fluoroscopy; Magnetic resonance imaging (MRI); Radiography; Radiology; Ultrasound (US)

Definition

A variety of critical and noncritical injuries can occur in the chest. The most common devastating injury is aortic trauma, responsible for one third of blunt traumatic fatalities in a recent study (Teixeira et al. 2011). Damage to the smaller vessels, the heart, the lungs, or the pleura can also result in hemodynamic compromise. Injuries to other thoracic structures, while not immediately life threatening, are nevertheless associated with morbidity and mortality. Although various imaging modalities can play a role in the evaluation of thoracic trauma, computed tomography remains the most useful by virtue of its widespread availability, rapid scan time, and high sensitivity and specificity for various injuries.

Preexisting Condition

Aorta

Aortic injury can be the result of blunt trauma, penetrating trauma, or a combination. Blunt aortic trauma is described as a rapid deceleration which stresses the relatively fixed attachments of the aorta, often in motor vehicle accidents. The most common site of blunt aortic injury is the aortic isthmus (just distal the origin of the left subclavian artery); other sites are the ascending aorta, transverse arch, and diaphragmatic hiatus. Penetrating trauma can occur at any site.

Heart

Penetrating trauma to the heart can result in hemopericardium, the dreaded complication of which is cardiac tamponade. Blunt cardiac trauma has a variety of manifestations including dysfunction, arrhythmia, myocardial infarction, valvular injury, and wall rupture.

Lungs and Pleura

A pneumothorax can be the result of blunt or penetrating trauma to the chest. Blunt trauma resulting in an increase in intrathoracic pressure can rupture alveoli, allowing air to dissect through the interstitium of the lung and eventually through the visceral pleura into the pleural space. Patients with emphysema or cystic lung disease are at especially high risk (Noppen and De Keukeleire 2008).

Penetrating trauma can directly injure the visceral pleura and lacerate the lung, resulting in an air leak into the pleural cavity. Alternatively, it can directly introduce atmospheric air into the pleural cavity through the chest wall and parietal pleura without lung injury or air leak. Tension pneumothorax, the result of a one-way valve mechanism allowing air to progressively accumulate in the pleural space, is a life-threatening manifestation of pneumothorax.

Disruption of pulmonary, chest wall, or mediastinal vessels can result in hematoma formation; with a concomitant pleural injury, a hemothorax will form.

Pulmonary contusions are a common manifestation of blunt trauma to the lungs.

Tracheal or bronchial fracture is a rare injury seen in the setting of deceleration or penetrating trauma. Air escaping through the airway wall may result in a pneumothorax or pneumomediastinum depending on the location of the defect.

Diaphragm

Diaphragmatic rupture can be the result of penetrating trauma from direct injury or from blunt trauma as the result of markedly increased intra-abdominal pressure. Often small injuries will be occult at presentation and manifest later as ventilation mechanics allow abdominal contents to progressively herniate into the chest.

Esophagus

Penetrating trauma to the esophagus puts the patient at risk for mediastinitis as esophageal contents leak into the mediastinum. Rarely, blunt trauma can result in rupture.

Skeleton

Ribs are commonly fractured bones of the thoracic skeleton. Although rarely repaired, fractured ribs should prompt early and adequate pain control to minimize splinting and decrease the risk of pneumonia. A flail chest is classically described as the result of three or more adjacent ribs being fractured in more than one location resulting in an independent segment of chest wall that can alter ventilation mechanics and cause respiratory compromise.

Fractures of the first rib or scapula are associated with high-energy trauma which should prompt the evaluation for additional injuries.

Sternal fractures are commonly seen in motor vehicle collisions as the patient's chest decelerates against the shoulder belt or steering wheel. Sternoclavicular joint injuries can be significant if the clavicle is dislocated posteriorly into the trachea or brachiocephalic vessels.

Application

Radiography

The supine anteroposterior (AP) chest radiograph has become a staple of modern trauma evaluation.

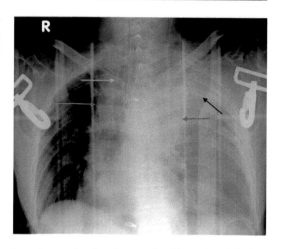

Imaging of Aortic and Thoracic Injuries, Fig. 1 Supine radiograph of the chest showing multiple signs of aortic injury in a patient with aortic rupture: widening of the superior mediastinum (*red arrows*), inferior displacement of the left mainstem bronchus (*green arrow*), and rightward deviation of the trachea and endotracheal tube from hemomediastinum (*blue arrow*) as well as a left apical cap representing extrapleural hematoma (*black arrow*)

Relative to other imaging options, it is inexpensive, easily obtained, and low in radiation dose. Unfortunately, it is also the least sensitive and specific for the detection of injuries. Posteroanterior (PA) and lateral chest radiographs in the upright position are more sensitive for injuries and should be preferred in patients who are ambulatory.

The most common cited sign for aortic injury is an absolute or relative widening of the superior mediastinum. Other radiographic signs include aortic contour abnormalities, depression of the left mainstem bronchus, apical capping, widening of the paraspinal lines, and tracheal or nasogastric tube displacement (Fig. 1). Portable technique and errant positioning of trauma patients makes it difficult to reliably evaluate the width of the superior mediastinum (Kirkham and Blackmore 2007).

A hemopericardium will enlarge the cardiomediastinal silhouette, although cardiomegaly is a more common cause of radiographic abnormality, particularly in older patients. On upright lateral radiographs, soft tissue density separating the pericardial and epicardial fat can often be detected.

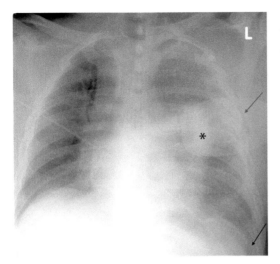

Imaging of Aortic and Thoracic Injuries, Fig. 2 Supine AP chest radiograph revealing the deep sulcus sign of a left pneumothorax (*black arrow*), subcutaneous emphysema (*red arrow*), and a veil-like opacity over the left hemithorax representing a hemothorax layering dependently. Note that the majority of the pulmonary vessels remain distinguishable despite the increased density from the hemothorax; by contrast, the focal area of pulmonary contusion (*asterisk*) obliterates the vessels in the immediate vicinity

Fluids such as blood and air within the pleural cavity will layer by gravity; the ability to detect them is increased when the x-ray beams passing through the patient are oriented parallel to the fluid level. For this reason detecting a pneumothorax or pleural effusion on an anteroposterior film with the patient in the supine position can be challenging. Upright or even decubitus views are far more sensitive (Moskowitz et al. 1973).

Nevertheless, there are imaging features to seek on supine radiographs. A large pneumothorax can form a "deep sulcus sign" as the costophrenic sulcus of the affected side appears to extend more inferiorly. Subcutaneous emphysema is an ancillary finding that should strongly raise the suspicion for underlying pneumothorax. A pleural effusion will result in a veil of increased density of the affected side which does not obscure the pulmonary vessels (Fig. 2). In both cases, comparing the right and left hemithorax for differences can prove helpful.

On upright radiographs, a pneumothorax will typically accumulate at the cupula and should be detected by loss of normal pulmonary vascular markings peripherally, often with a discrete pleural line seen displaced from the chest wall (Fig. 3). A pleural effusion will blunt the costophrenic sulcus when small or form a larger meniscus more superiorly when large. Although the differential densities of water and blood cannot be distinguished by radiography, a pleural effusion, particularly a unilateral one, should be concerning for a hemothorax in a patient presenting with an appropriate trauma mechanism, especially if there are associated ipsilateral traumatic findings such as rib fracture, subcutaneous emphysema, or pneumothorax.

Pneumomediastinum, when large enough, will appear as branching lucent areas; when the air surrounds the great vessels or trachea, it will make the edges of these structures more conspicuous (Fig. 4). Pneumopericardium will conform to the general shape of the pericardial sac including the small recesses superiorly around the great vessels (Fig. 5).

Pulmonary contusions and lacerations will manifest as airspace opacities in the affected lung. As trauma patients often present with concomitant aspiration, the appearance of these opacities remains nonspecific.

Diaphragm rupture is typically left sided, in which cases the gastric bubble or splenic flexure will be displaced superiorly into the chest (Fig. 5). Small diaphragmatic defects can easily be occult on radiography, particularly if only omental fat has herniated without a hollow viscus.

The ribs can be fractured anywhere along their course; depending on the location of the fracture, degree of displacement, positioning of the patient, and quality of the radiographic technique, fractures may not be detected. The costal cartilage anteriorly is radiographically invisible unless densely calcified and thus poorly evaluated.

Sternal fractures are typically not detectable by portable chest radiography. Sternoclavicular dislocation can be detected if the malalignment is significant enough. Radiographic examinations

Imaging of Aortic and Thoracic Injuries,
Fig. 3 Upright PA
radiograph of the chest,
shows the pleural line
(*arrows*) displaced away
from the chest wall as the
result of a pneumothorax.
Note the absent pulmonary
vascular markings
peripherally, most
conspicuous when
comparing the left lung
apex to the right

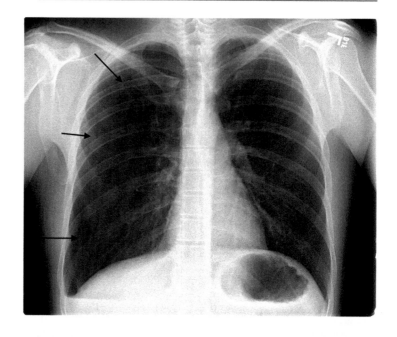

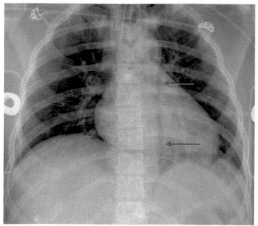

Imaging of Aortic and Thoracic Injuries,
Fig. 4 Supine AP radiograph of the chest demonstrating
streaks of abnormal lucency representing pneumomediastinum, most conspicuous by the outlining of the
descending thoracic aorta (*arrows*)

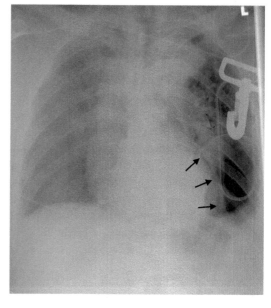

Imaging of Aortic and Thoracic Injuries,
Fig. 5 Figure shows superior herniation of the gastric
bubble into the left chest (*red arrow*) as a result of diaphragmatic rupture. The *black arrows* indicate
pneumopericardium separating the pericardial and epicardial fat

tailored for the evaluation of the sternum or the
sternoclavicular joints will have a higher sensitivity for these injuries than a chest radiograph;
however, if there is a strong clinical concern
despite a negative radiograph, CT should
strongly be considered as patients at risk for sternal fracture or sternoclavicular dislocation are at
high risk of additional thoracic injuries which

will be better detected by CT. Additionally, in
the case of sternoclavicular dislocation, CT can
evaluate for injury to the trachea, great vessels, or
lung by the displaced clavicle.

Computed Tomography

Computed tomography is also readily available in emergency departments. Although it delivers a higher radiation dose to the patient and costs more, it is extremely valuable in the rapid detection and classification of injuries to the chest due to its increased contrast resolution – that is, its ability to distinguish different densities, and, in turn, different anatomic structures.

Multi-slice CT scanners which have been rapidly adopted by emergency departments over the last decade offer increased imaging speed which decreases the chance of respiratory motion artifact and increases the quality of arteriographic studies. Another benefit, decreased slice thickness, yields higher-quality images when the axially-acquired data are reformatted into other anatomic planes.

In the setting of suspected esophageal injury, oral contrast media can be administered prior to the CT scan to aid the diagnosis; however, the dynamic nature of perforations and the supine position of the patient may result in a false-negative result. Fluoroscopy is more sensitive than CT. With either modality, water-soluble contrast media should be used first as barium-containing agents can induce mediastinitis.

Iodinated contrast media is invaluable in the detection of vascular injuries. The remainder of the thorax can be evaluated for trauma without contrast media due to the varying densities of the thoracic organs. Forgoing iodinated contrast media when appropriate spares the patient the inherent risks of renal toxicity and allergic reaction.

Although aortic injuries can be detected in the typical venous phase of imaging, if there is a specific concern of aortic injury, the scan should be performed in the arterial phase. ECG gating can increase the sensitivity for aortic root injury by eliminating motion but usually requires a heart rate under 70 bpm (when prospectively gated) or a higher radiation dose (retrospective gating) and is more technically challenging.

Direct signs of aortic injury on CT are a caliber change, an intramural hematoma, a contour abnormality (pseudoaneurysm), an intimal flap (dissection), or even vessel wall

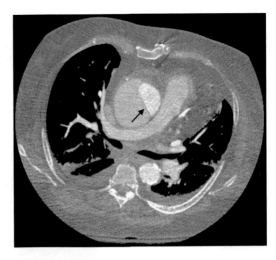

Imaging of Aortic and Thoracic Injuries, Fig. 6 Axial enhanced CT image showing an aneurysmal ascending aorta with an intimal flap (*black arrow*) as well as periaortic hemorrhage (*red arrow*)

disruption and active contrast extravasation into the mediastinum (Figs. 6–8). Indirect signs include mediastinal hemorrhage which will manifest as infiltration of the mediastinal fat planes or a discrete hematoma; injuries to smaller arteries and veins in the chest can also result in mediastinal hemorrhage. Common mimics of periaortic hemorrhage include physiologic fluid in the pericardial recesses surrounding the great vessels and residual thymic tissue.

Intravenous contrast media increases the sensitivity for intimal flap and contour abnormality; aortic caliber and mediastinal hematoma can be assessed on a non-enhanced study.

Pericardial effusions are readily detected by CT as abnormal density interposed between the epicardial and pericardial fat (Fig. 9). Hemopericardium is diagnosed by an increased density of the effusion but should be suspected in any case of penetrating trauma.

Pneumothorax is seen as air in the pleural cavity displacing the lung centrally. The air is typically anterior in the supine patient (Fig. 10); however, small and/or loculated pneumothoraces can be positioned medially, laterally, posteriorly, or even inferiorly (subpulmonic). Similarly, a hemothorax is identified as hyperdense fluid (often >30 Hounsfield units) in the pleural

Imaging of Aortic and Thoracic Injuries,
Fig. 7 Axial unenhanced CT image demonstrating crescentic high density along the left aspect of the descending thoracic aorta (*arrow*) representing intramural hematoma. The window width (*contrast*) of the image was optimized to maximize the conspicuity of the finding. Note the atherosclerotic calcifications along the intima are abnormally displaced away from the adventitia

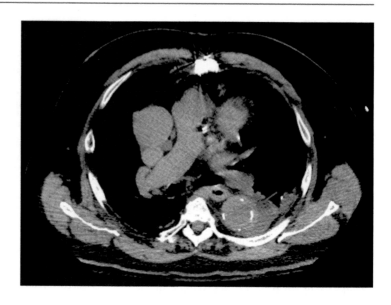

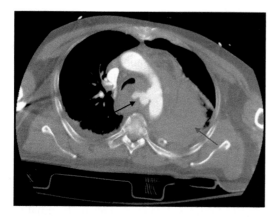

Imaging of Aortic and Thoracic Injuries,
Fig. 8 Enhanced axial CT image showing aortic rupture at the isthmus with active extravasation into the mediastinum (*black arrow*) and hemorrhage displacing and compressing the trachea. Blood dissects laterally into the extrapleural space (*red arrow*). Also evident is a fracture of the thoracic vertebral body at this level

space which typically layers posteriorly but can be positioned elsewhere if loculated.

Pulmonary contusions appear as nonspecific focal airspace consolidation. By imaging alone, it is impossible to diagnose such an abnormality as a contusion with 100 % certainty; however, the diagnosis can be confidently made when the pulmonary abnormalities are focal, unilateral, ill-defined, and adjacent to other traumatic findings

such as chest wall hematomas or rib fractures. When wedge-shaped, bilateral and dependent, aspiration should be favored. When bilateral and diffuse, pneumonia or edema is more likely.

Pulmonary lacerations can present as focal round, discrete collections of air or blood within the lung parenchyma. They may heal as pneumatoceles which are air-containing pseudocysts with a discrete wall.

Pneumomediastinum can be localized or diffuse. In the setting of penetrating trauma to the mediastinum, damage to the esophagus, trachea, or bronchi should be suspected. With blunt trauma, alveolar rupture can allow air to dissect centrally and into the mediastinum, a common phenomenon seen in the atraumatic patient after excessive Valsalva maneuver. Pneumothorax can also dissect into pneumomediastinum. Air can also enter the mediastinum from the neck superiorly or from the retroperitoneum inferiorly.

Occasionally pneumomediastinum can be mistaken for pneumopericardium. The latter is less common due to the smaller plane air must enter to cause it; however, the etiologies are the same. Careful evaluation of the CT images should demonstrate air confining to the pericardial sac (Fig. 11).

CT can detect smaller diaphragm defects than radiography. Axial images will show herniated

Imaging of Aortic and Thoracic Injuries,
Fig. 9 Enhanced axial CT image showing a predominantly posterior and inferior hemopericardium from penetrating trauma to the right ventricle presenting as abnormal density in the pericardial space (*red arrows*). Note the metallic nail fragment (*black arrow*) in the anterior chest wall adjacent to locules of gas

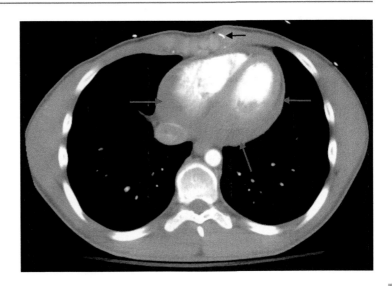

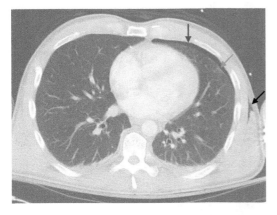

Imaging of Aortic and Thoracic Injuries, Fig. 10 CT image in lung algorithm demonstrating a small left pneumothorax anteriorly (*red arrow*) and subcutaneous emphysema in the lateral chest wall (*black arrow*). The small ground glass opacity in the underlying lingula reflects a contusion (*blue arrow*)

abdominal fat positioned superficial or superior to the diaphragm.

Acute rib fractures manifest as lucent lines or focal angulations through the cortex of a rib in at least one location. Fractures are easier to detect when displaced. Coronal and sagittal reformatted images can be helpful.

As the long axis of the sternum is oriented craniocaudally, a classic transverse sternal fracture can be missed on the axial CT images.

Reformatting the axially acquired images into the sagittal plane increases sensitivity (Fig. 12).

Catheter Aortography

Catheter aortography has been considered the gold standard for the diagnosis of aortic injuries, with a sensitivity of 100 % and specificity of 97 % (Sturm et al. 1990). In unstable patients, it also offers the benefit of endovascular repair at the time of diagnosis. In recent years, however, the prevalence of emergency department CT scanners, the speed at which CT can be performed, and the ability of CT to detect non-aortic injuries have led to a sharp decline in the use of catheter angiography (Demetriades et al. 2008).

Fluoroscopy

Fluoroscopy has a higher sensitivity than CT in diagnosing esophageal injuries due to its higher spatial resolution and its dynamic nature. Unlike CT, it requires a cooperative, responsive patient, ideally one who can stand and move or be moved into multiple obliquities. Oral contrast media is administered and multiple swallows observed in varying projections to assess for any leakage outside of the esophagus. These examinations are initially performed with water-soluble iodinated contrast media as barium-containing agents are associated with mediastinitis. If no leak is detected, the examination can be completed

Imaging of Aortic and Thoracic Injuries, **Fig. 11** CT image in lung windows demonstrating pneumopericardium (*arrow*) outlining the superior aortic and pulmonic recesses of the pericardium

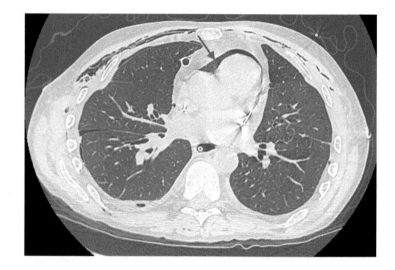

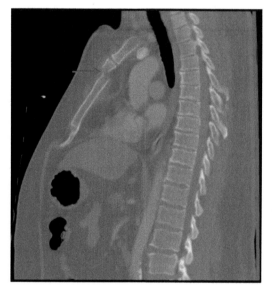

Imaging of Aortic and Thoracic Injuries, Fig. 12 Sagittal image reformatted from axial CT data demonstrating a mildly displaced fracture of the superior sternal body. The sternomanubrial joint just cranial to the fracture remains congruent

with a barium agent which is more easily visualized due to its increased density (Fig. 13).

Ultrasound

Sonography offers a rapid, portable, and relatively inexpensive means of evaluating trauma patients; although it is limited in the diagnoses it can facilitate and is operator dependent.

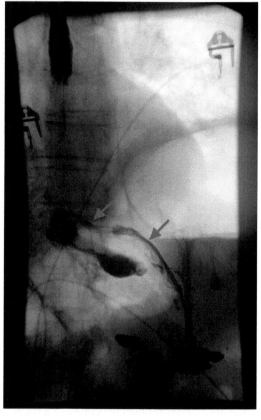

Imaging of Aortic and Thoracic Injuries, Fig. 13 Fluoroscopic image in the left posterior oblique projection after the oral administration of barium demonstrating a large leak (*arrows*) of the distal esophagus extending into the inferior mediastinum and retroperitoneum

Imaging of Aortic and Thoracic Injuries, Fig. 14 Apical sonographic view showing anechoic blood (*arrow*) in the pericardial space surrounding the ventricles

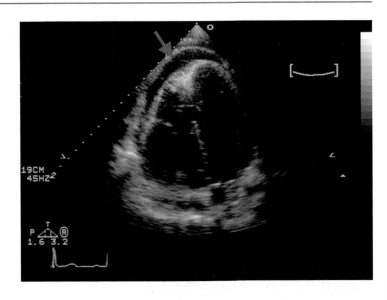

The focused assessment with sonography for trauma (FAST) includes right and left flank windows which should image the posterolateral pleural cavities where anechoic pleural fluid will preferentially collect in the supine patient. Caution should be observed in characterizing the pleural fluid as blood, particularly in a patient with congestive heart failure or other reason for a pleural effusion; the echogenicity of the fluid should not be relied upon.

Pericardial views acquired as part of FAST can assess for a pericardial effusion which will manifest as a hypoechoic or anechoic collection between the visceral and parietal layers of the pericardium (Fig. 14). Unlike radiography or CT, sonography can evaluate for tamponade physiology. The diagnosis of hemopericardium by sonography can significantly decrease the time to surgical repair (Rozycki et al. 1999) when compared to CT. As with pleural effusions, the echogenicity of the fluid may vary.

Extended FAST (eFAST) includes additional views of the pleura to evaluate for pneumothorax. Visualization of sliding pleura and the presence of comet tail artifact together can exclude pneumothorax with a sensitivity that, in experienced hands, approaches that of CT (Rowan et al. 2002).

Transesophageal echocardiography (TEE), when performed by an experienced operator, has sensitivity and specificity for traumatic aortic injury approaching 99 % (Cinnella et al. 2004). Although CT is useful in the diagnosis of concomitant injuries that invariably accompany a patient with aortic trauma, TEE is particularly helpful in providing a diagnosis in the unstable patient who was taken directly to the operating room for exploratory laparotomy or other emergent surgery.

Magnetic Resonance Imaging

MRI is an alternative to computed tomography which does not involve ionizing but is more expensive, more time consuming, and limits access to the patient should a need for resuscitation arise. Additionally, ferromagnetic foreign bodies or implanted surgical devices may pose a risk and can be difficult to reliably screen for in a trauma patient. MRI is best suited to assess a specific organ system rather than screen the entire chest; the heart and aorta are prime targets, whereas the lungs and pleura are poorly evaluated due to the presence of air.

Cross-References

▶ Barotrauma
▶ Cardiac Injuries

► Chest Wall Injury

► Diaphragmatic Injuries

► Echocardiography in the Trauma Setting

► Lung Injury

► Pneumothorax

► Pneumothorax, Tension

► Retained Hemothorax

► Scapula Fractures

► Thoracic Vascular Injuries

► Tracheal and Esophageal Injury

► Ultrasound in the Trauma and ICU Setting

References

Cinnella G, Dambrosio M, Brienza N, Tullo L, Fiore T (2004) Transesophageal echocardiography for diagnosis of traumatic aortic injury: an appraisal of the evidence. J Trauma 57:1246–1255

Demetriades D, Velmahos GC, Scalea TM, Jurkovich GJ, Karmy-Jones R, Teixeira PG, Hemmila MR, O'Connor JV, McKenney MO, Moore FO, London J, Singh MJ, Spaniolas K, Keel M, Sugrue M, Wahl WL, Hill J, Wall MJ, Moore EE, Lineen E, Margulies D, Malka V, Chan LS (2008) Diagnosis and treatment of blunt thoracic aortic injuries: changing perspectives. J Trauma 64:1415–1418

Kirkham JR, Blackmore CC (2007) Screening for aortic injury with chest radiography and clinical factors. Emerg Radiol 14:211–217

Moskowitz J, Platt RT, Schachar R, Mellins M (1973) Roentgen visualization of minute pleural effusion. Radiology 109:33–35

Noppen M, De Keukeleire T (2008) Pneumothorax. Respiration 76:121–127

Rowan KR, Kirkpatrick AW, Liu D, Forkheim KE, Mayo JR, Nicolaou S (2002) Traumatic pneumothorax detection with thoracic US: correlation with chest radiography and CT – initial experience. Radiology 225:210–214

Rozycki GS, Feliciano DV, Ochsner MG, Knudson MM, Hoyt DB, Davis F, Hammerman D, Figueredo V, Harviel JD, Han DC, Schmidt JA (1999) The role of ultrasound in patients with possible penetrating cardiac wounds: a prospective multicenter study. J Trauma 46:543–551

Sturm JT, Hankins DG, Young G (1990) Thoracic aortography following blunt chest trauma. Am J Emerg Med 8:92–96

Teixeira PG, Inaba K, Barmparas G, Georgiou C, Toms C, Noguchi TT, Rogers C, Sathyavagiswaran L, Demetriades D (2011) Blunt thoracic aortic injuries: an autopsy study. J Trauma 70:197–202

Imaging of CNS Injuries

Vikas Agarwal[1] and Ryan T. Fitzgerald[2]
[1]Department of Radiology, Neuroradiology Division, University of Pittsburgh Medical Center, Pittsburgh, PA, USA
[2]Department of Radiology, Neuroradiology Division, University of Arkansas for Medical Sciences, Little Rock, AR, USA

Synonyms

Imaging; Radiology; TBI; Traumatic brain injury

Definition

Prompt recognition and management of the sequelae of TBI traumatic brain injury (TBI) can significantly alter the clinical course and outcome in these patients. Neuroimaging techniques can determine the presence and extent of injury and guide management in the acute setting to prevent secondary injury and significantly reduce morbidity and mortality while reducing hospital stay and health care costs.

Traditionally, the Glasgow Coma Scale (GCS) has been used to clinically divide patients with TBI into minor, mild, moderate, and severe categories (Teasdale and Jennett 1974). TBI can also be classified chronologically into primary and secondary injuries. Primary injuries are defined as those that occur at the moment of impact, while secondary injuries are those that occur after the initial injury as a consequence of physiologic response to injury or complications thereof. Location of injury (intra- and/or extra-axial) and mechanism of injury (penetrating/open, blunt/closed, or blast) can also be used to classify TBI.

Preexisting Condition

The etiology of TBI varies with the age of the patient. In infants, non-accidental trauma (child abuse) is the most common cause whereas falls and sports-related injuries are more common in toddlers and school age children. In adults, motor vehicle accidents are a frequent cause with the elderly population more susceptible to accidental falls.

Extra-Axial Injuries

Skull Injury

The three most common types of skull fractures include linear, depressed, and basilar. Depressed skull fractures are commonly associated with injury involving the underlying brain parenchyma. Basilar skull fractures are important to recognize since they can be associated with injury to vascular structures (internal carotid artery, transverse and sigmoid sinuses, cavernous sinuses), the cranial nerves, and the middle/inner ear structures. Fractures involving the temporal bone are now classified as "otic capsule sparing" and "otic capsule involving" (Little and Kesser 2006). Cerebrospinal fluid leak and the subsequent risk of meningitis are also among the potential complications of basilar skull fracture.

Vascular Injury

The spectrum of traumatic vascular injury includes vessel dissection, pseudoaneurysm formation, complete transaction, or occlusion. These entities are covered in detail in the entry dedicated to Neck Injury.

When laceration of an artery adjacent to a vein occurs in the head, an abnormal communication between the artery and vein can develop and is termed a traumatic arteriovenous fistula (AVF). The classic example is the carotid cavernous fistula (CCF) which results from an injury to the internal carotid artery (ICA) which then directly communicates with the cavernous sinus. Since symptoms related to the CCF (proptosis, ophthalmoplegia with vision loss and facial pain) often present in a delayed fashion, the presence of skull-base fractures involving the carotid canal should raise suspicion. On CT/MRI, there may be lateral bowing of the cavernous sinus,

dilated superior ophthalmic vein, stranding of the retrobulbar fat, enlarged extraocular muscles, and proptosis. Conventional catheter angiography shows early filling of the cavernous sinus during the arterial phase with early venous outflow most commonly to the superior ophthalmic vein.

Epidural Hematoma

Epidural hematomas (EDH) are present in 1–4 % of TBI patients. The epidural space is a potential space located between the dura and the calvarium which can accumulate extravasated blood from injured blood vessels (Zimmerman and Bilaniuk 1982). Epidural hematomas are most commonly arterial in origin (85 %), usually the result of laceration of the middle meningeal artery; however, venous EDHs can occur. An underlying fracture is present in greater than 90 % of cases.

Typically, EDHs will appear as biconvex, hyperdense, extra-axial collections on non-contrast CT examinations (Fig. 1). They do not cross suture lines except at the level of the sagittal suture where dura does not invest the suture due to the presence of the superior sagittal sinus. Unlike subdural hematomas (SDH), an EDH can cross dural reflections such as the falx cerebri or tentorium cerebelli. Mixed density or heterogeneous EDHs have been shown to have a worse prognosis (Pruthi et al. 2009). This is felt to be due to the presence of active bleeding with hypodense areas representing unclotted blood and has been termed the "swirl sign."

Following decompressive craniectomies, small EDHs remote from the surgical site may show dramatic increase in size. This is thought to be related to release of a "tamponade effect" generated by preoperative elevated intracranial pressure.

Subdural Hematoma

Approximately 10–20 % of patients with TBI will have SDH. The subdural space is a potential space located between the inner meningeal layer of the dura and the arachnoid mater. As opposed to EDHs, the majority of SDHs are venous in origin, the result of traumatic injury to bridging

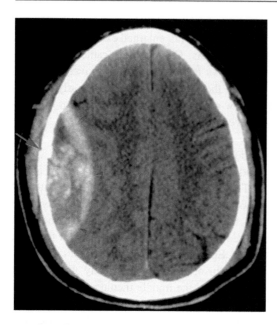

Imaging of CNS Injuries, Fig. 1 Non-contrast head CT in patient after MVA shows high density, biconvex epidural hematoma (*arrowheads*) deep to the parietal skull fracture (*arrow*). Areas of hypodensity within the EDH are likely related to areas of active bleeding

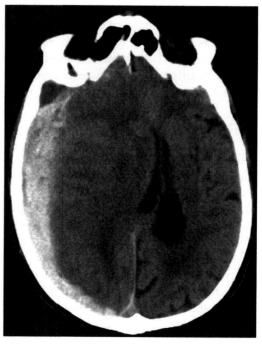

Imaging of CNS Injuries, Fig. 2 Non-contrast CT of elderly female after fall shows large hyperdense extraaxial collection along the right convexity consistent with acute subdural hematoma, causing marked mass effect and right to left midline shift

cortical veins that traverse the subdural space. They are also less frequently associated with skull fractures compared with EDHs.

The majority of SDHs are supratentorial and occur along the cerebral convexities, tentorium cerebelli or falx cerebri. On non-contrast CT, they appear as crescentic extra-axial collections that cross suture lines and often times span the entire hemisphere (Fig. 2). Internal characteristics of SDHs on CT however vary based on whether they are acute, subacute, or chronic. Acute SDH (<1 week) are typically homogenously hyperdense. In cases where there is underlying anemia, acute SDHs can appear iso- or hypointense. Like EDHs, if there is active bleeding, acute SDHs will also appear heterogeneous.

Over time, blood products break down and cellular elements are removed causing a progressive decrease in attenuation. Therefore, subacute SDHs (1–3 weeks) often have internal density on a spectrum that includes an isodense phase. The isodense collection can be difficult to recognize on non-contrast CT. Clues to the presence of an

isodense SDH include white matter buckling, medial displacement of the gray-white junction from the inner table, and presence of mass effect (midline shift, sulcal effacement, compression of ipsilateral ventricle). As the collection ages, it will eventually become homogeneously hypodense. Chronic SDHs (>3 weeks) can sometimes show adhesions and/or membranes producing multiple compartments.

At any point, rebleeding can occur. In the chronic setting, this can have a parfait appearance highlighting the hematocrit effect of denser acute hemorrhage layering dependently.

Subarachnoid Hemorrhage

Subarachnoid hemorrhage (SAH) results from tearing of small cortical vessels, extension of intraparenchymal hemorrhage (IPH) into the subarachnoid space, or extension of intraventricular hemorrhage (IVH) via the fourth ventricular outlet foramina. It is present in approximately

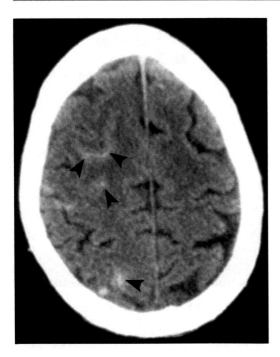

Imaging of CNS Injuries, Fig. 3 Non-contrast head CT in patient following head trauma with high density blood (*arrowheads*) filling the sulci over the right cerebral consistent with subarachnoid hemorrhage

11 % of patients suffering TBI (Greene et al. 1995). Traumatic SAH can lead to vasospasm as well as development of a communicating hydrocephalus.

On non-contrast CT, acute SAH will appear as areas of high attenuation within the subarachnoid spaces which include the basilar cisterns and sulci (Fig. 3). Occasionally, the only clue to presence of SAH is sulcal effacement. As SAH ages, it can be increasingly difficult to detect on CT. MR imaging, in particular FLAIR and/or GRE T2* sequences, is more sensitive for detection of subacute and chronic SAH.

Intraventricular Hemorrhage

IVH results from tearing of subependymal veins along the surface of the ventricles, extension of IPH or SAH into the ventricular system or from direct penetrating injury. IVH occurs in only approximately 1–2 % of patients suffering from TBI, typically those with severe injuries, and is therefore associated with a poor prognosis (Atzema et al. 2006). IVH can lead to ependymal

adhesions and scarring, causing obstruction of the cerebral aqueduct and ultimately non-communicating hydrocephalus.

IVH will appear as high density material within the ventricular system on non-contrast CT. Most commonly, this will be seen as a fluid-fluid level within the dependent portion of the occipital horns of the lateral ventricles.

Intra-axial Injuries

Cerebral Edema

Loss of cerebral autoregulation in TBI can lead to cerebral hyperemia with an overall increase in cerebral blood volume. On non-contrast CT, cerebral hyperemia is seen as the presence of mass effect with relative preservation of gray-white matter differentiation. Over time, cerebral hyperemia may progress to cerebral edema which can be further divided into two major categories: "vasogenic" due to disruption of the blood–brain barrier and accumulation of extracellular water accumulation, and "cytotoxic" due to intracellular water accumulation. Both forms can coexist in TBI patients, with vasogenic edema more prominent in white matter and cytotoxic edema more prominent in gray matter. Non-contrast CT will show compressed ventricles, effaced sulci/cisterns, and loss of gray-white differentiation (Fig. 4).

Cerebral Contusion

Cerebral contusions represent bruises to the brain parenchyma and are the most common form of intra-axial injury in TBI patients. They occur primarily in the cortex but often times will extend into the underlying subcortical white matter. They can occur at a site of direct impact, usually beneath a depressed skull fracture. A coup contusion develops from transient inbending of the calvarium and is not necessarily associated with a fracture. These can occur under the site of impact or in areas of the brain located near bony protuberances on the inside surface of the calvarium under the frontal and temporal lobes and along the roof of the orbit. Contrecoup contusions occur 180° opposite the site of initial head impact.

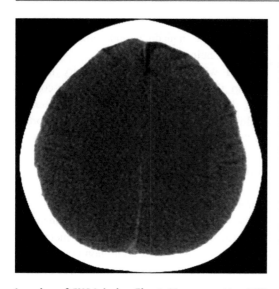

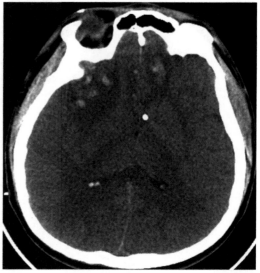

Imaging of CNS Injuries, Fig. 4 Non-contrast head CT in patient 24 h after MVA shows diffuse loss of gray-white matter interface with sulcal and basilar cistern effacement consistent with diffuse cerebral edema

Imaging of CNS Injuries, Fig. 5 23-year-old male in motor vehicle accident. Non-contrast CT shows hemorrhagic contusions anterior inferior frontal lobes, more so on the right than the left. Note surrounding edema resulting in mass effect and ventriculostomy catheter

Acute contusions can be subtle on initial non-contrast CT exams, appearing as patchy ill-defined areas of low attenuation in one of the common locations described above (Fig. 5). As the contusion evolves, vasogenic edema develops and they take on the more classic appearance of solitary or multiple focal areas of low or mixed attenuation with or without tiny areas of increased density representing petechial hemorrhage ("salt and pepper" appearance). Frank hemorrhagic transformation or coalescence of petechial hemorrhages into a hematoma is not uncommon after 24–48 h. Contusions are far more conspicuous on MR imaging and can be used in cases where CT is equivocal and also to better delineate the extent of lesions seen on CT. T2/FLAIR sequences are best for visualizing the edema associated with contusions, and T2* sequences show associated hemorrhagic foci as areas of hypointensity.

Intraparenchymal Hemorrhage

Traumatic IPH can result from rupture of small intraparenchymal blood vessels. In addition, microhemorrhages associated with cortical contusions can coalesce into focal hematomas. IPH are usually more well defined on

non-contrast CT than contusions and tend to have less surrounding edema.

Diffuse Axonal Injury (DAI)

DAI results from rotational acceleration/deceleration forces that exceed the elastic stretching limit for an axon. The result is a spectrum of changes to the axon that depends on the severity of the injury. In the acute phase, injury leads to edema and demyelination. Eventually, disconnection of the axon can occur, resulting in fiber loss (Wallerian degeneration).

Non-contrast CT may initially be normal in the vast majority of the patients subsequently proven to have DAI (50–80 %). Delayed CT scanning may show areas of petechial hemorrhage in characteristic locations (gray-white matter junction, corpus callosum, dorsolateral midbrain) (Fig. 6). Unfortunately, false-negatives with CT are not uncommon (30 %). Therefore, if there is clinical concern for DAI, MRI should be obtained. T2 weighted images will show hyperintense foci in characteristic locations and may be associated with restricted diffusion. Corresponding hypointensity on T2* GRE

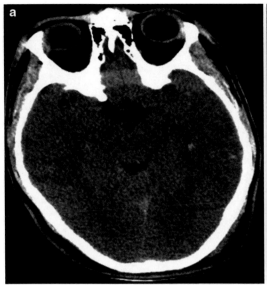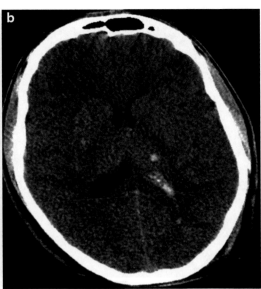

Imaging of CNS Injuries, Fig. 6 28-year-old male in high speed motorcycle accident. (**a–b**) Multiple images from non-contrast CT demonstrate multiple scattered small foci of hemorrhage at the gray-white junction. The overall pattern favors DAI

images will be seen in the presence of hemorrhage (Fig. 7). Often times lesions may only be visible on T2* GRE images.

Application

Skull Radiographs
Conventional radiographs of the skull have little to no role in the evaluation of patients with traumatic brain injuries and have been largely supplanted by computed tomography (CT) (Davis 2007). They may occasionally be used to evaluate position of penetrating objects or radiopaque foreign bodies.

Computed Tomography (CT)
Non-contrast CT is the mainstay for initial assessment of patients with TBI. It is widely available, fast, and compatible with life support devices. CT can accurately identify the presence of hemorrhage, herniation, hydrocephalus, fractures, and radiopaque foreign bodies (Provenzale 2007). A recent study by Stein et al. showed that the cost associated with liberal use of CT head scanning was justified, given the potential consequences of undiagnosed brain injury (Stein et al. 2006). The one drawback to the use of CT is the associated radiation exposure which is especially important in trauma cases where multiple serial examinations may be required.

Magnetic Resonance Imaging (MRI)
MR imaging is generally not utilized in the evaluation of patients with TBI in the acute setting. MR has relatively long imaging times and is incompatible with many trauma-related or other medical devices. It is relatively insensitive for detection of acute subarachnoid hemorrhage (SAH) and is much more sensitive to patient motion than CT. Therefore, MR imaging is best suited for use in the subacute and chronic assessment of TBI as well as a problem-solving tool in cases where neurologic findings are not explained by CT. Advanced MR imaging techniques such as diffusion tensor imaging (DTI) may be able to detect evidence of brain injury in patients with normal conventional MRI exams, thus potentially providing an imaging biomarker of brain injury that can facilitate prognostication and improved understanding of the pathophysiology of TBI (Shenton et al. 2012).

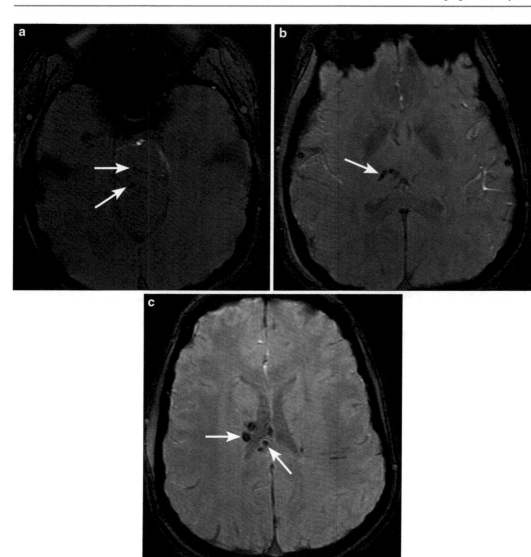

Imaging of CNS Injuries, Fig. 7 29-year-old female involved in high speed motor vehicle accident. (**a–c**) Gradient echo images demonstrate areas of susceptibility (*arrows*) involving the right aspect of the pons, periaqueductal gray matter, right thalamus, and corpus callosum in a pattern consistent with DAI

Cross-References

► Blast
► Brain Death
► Concussion
► Glasgow Coma Scale
► Head Injury
► Imaging of Neck Injuries
► Imaging of Spine and Bony Pelvis Injuries
► Intracranial Hemorrhage
► Intraventricular Hemorrhage
► Subarachnoid Hemorrhage
► Subdural Hematoma
► Traumatic Brain Injury, Mild (mTBI)

References

Atzema C, Mower WR, Hoffman JR et al (2006) Prevalence and prognosis of traumatic intraventricular hemorrhage in patients with blunt head trauma. J Trauma 60:1010–1017

Davis PC (2007) Head trauma. Am J Neuroradiol 28:1619–1621

Greene KA, Marciano FF, Johnson BA et al (1995) Impact of traumatic subarachnoid hemorrhage on outcome in non-penetrating head injury. Part I: a proposed computerized tomography grading scale. J Neurosurg 83:445–452

Little SC, Kesser BW (2006) Radiographic classification of temporal bone fractures: clinical predictability using a new system. Arch Otolaryngol Head Neck Surg 132:1300–1304

Provenzale J (2007) CT and MR imaging of acute cranial trauma. Emerg Radiol 14:1–12

Pruthi N, Balasubramaniam A, Chandramouli BA et al (2009) Mixed-density extradural hematomas on computed tomography-prognostic significance. Surg Neurol 71:202–206

Shenton ME, Hamoda HM, Schneiderman JS et al (2012) A review of magnetic resonance imaging and diffusion tensor imaging findings in mild traumatic brain injury. Brain Imaging Behav 6:103–107

Stein SC, Burnett MG, Glick HA (2006) Indications for CT scanning in mild traumatic brain injury: a cost effectiveness study. J Trauma 61:558–566

Teasdale G, Jennett B (1974) Assessment of coma and impaired consciousness. A practical scale. Lancet 2:81–84

Zimmerman RA, Bilaniuk LT (1982) Computed tomographic staging of traumatic epidural bleeding. Radiology 144:809–812

Imaging of Neck Injuries

Ryan T. Fitzgerald[1] and Vikas Agarwal[2]
[1]Department of Radiology, Neuroradiology Division, University of Arkansas for Medical Sciences, Little Rock, AR, USA
[2]Department of Radiology, Neuroradiology Division, University of Pittsburgh Medical Center, Pittsburgh, PA, USA

Synonyms

Imaging; Imaging head & neck trauma; Penetrating and blunt neck trauma; Radiography; Radiology

Definition

Imaging of neck injuries encompasses all imaging-based methods by which patients with suspected or known traumatic neck injuries may be assessed including plain film radiography, fluoroscopic examinations, computed tomography (CT), magnetic resonance imaging (MRI), and catheter angiography.

Preexisting Condition

Anatomic constraints within the neck result in close proximity of many vital structures. As such, trauma to this region may affect a single or multiple organ systems including injury to the aero-digestive tract, vasculature, and/or spine. Initial assessment of patients with suspected neck injury is aimed at identifying those who are unstable or exhibit clear evidence of vascular or aero-digestive tract injury as these individuals should proceed directly to surgical exploration without delay for imaging evaluation (Inaba et al. 2012). The possibility of cervical spine injury including fracture, dislocation, and/or cervical spinal cord injury should be considered in all cases of significant trauma as such injuries occur in 3–4 % of major trauma victims (Hasler et al. 2012). Traditionally, penetrating injuries are triaged according to the level of entry/exit wound. Injuries involving the neck from the level of the cricoid cartilage to the angle of the mandible (zone II) have traditionally undergone surgical exploration whereas imaging was pursued for injuries more cephalad or caudal to this level (zones I and III). Today, with the increasing availability and speed of imaging, most patients undergo imaging prior to surgery unless expedient treatment is necessary due to poor or declining patient stability.

Vascular and spinal injuries may be clinically occult, often due to the challenges of performing the neurologic exam in altered, sedated, or otherwise uncooperative trauma patients. Occasionally, vascular injuries manifest as a rapidly expanding neck mass; however, such cases are an exception rather than the rule. Most vascular injuries in the neck are not readily detectable on exam but rather clinically suspected based on the mechanism of injury or the presence of neurological deficit suggestive of cerebral infarction. Similarly, spinal

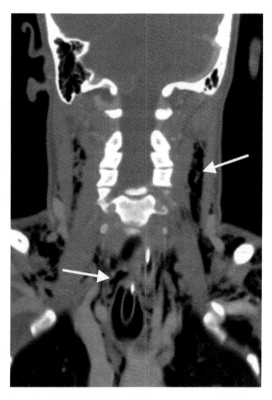

Imaging of Neck Injuries, Fig. 1 Coronal image from a CT angiogram demonstrates extensive soft tissue emphysema throughout the superficial and deep soft tissues of the neck (*arrows*) in a patient with a history of benzodiazepine overdose who was intubated in the field

injuries may manifest clinically; however, even in those with no obvious evidence of cord signs/symptoms, imaging screening for spinal injury is the currently accepted standard of care in patients who have sustained significant trauma.

Injury to the aero-digestive tract may occur as a result of blunt or penetrating trauma to the neck and may also be encountered as an iatrogenic injury related to endotrachael/enteric tube placement (Figs. 1 and 2) Such injuries may be suspected clinically in the presence of crepitus, hemoptysis, stridor, aphonia, loss of laryngeal prominence or hyoid elevation, certain injury patterns such as fracture of the first through third ribs, posterior sterno-clavicular dislocation, and/or detection of soft tissue emphysema on initially screening radiographic studies (Karmy-Jones et al. 2003; Sidell et al. 2011). Ensuring a viable airway is the primary management goal of treating patients with neck injury. Those with clinical signs of airway compromise and rapid decline should undergo emergent surgical tracheotomy. Less critical patients may undergo flexible laryngoscopy for management of the airway at the bedside (Sidell et al. 2011; Duval et al. 2007). Only after an adequate airway has been established should imaging be pursued.

Imaging of Neck Injuries, Fig. 2 Axial image from the same CT angiogram demonstrates focal contour abnormality within the dorso-lateral quadrant of the upper trachea (*arrowhead*) with immediately adjacent paratracheal gas (*arrow*) representing the site of iatrogenic tracheal disruption. Surgical repair of the injured trachea was required

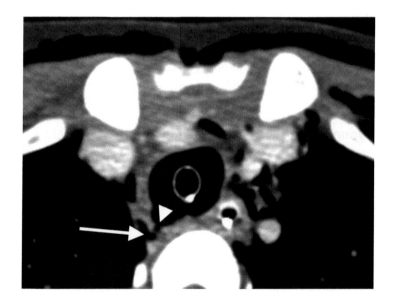

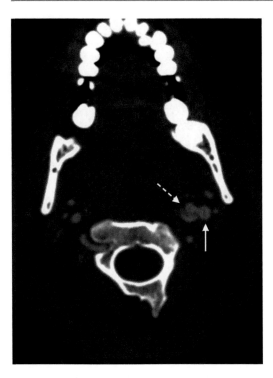

Imaging of Neck Injuries, Fig. 3 Axial CTA image through the neck in a 24-year-old male following blunt motor vehicle trauma shows a psuedoaneurysm (*dashed arrow*) arising from the medial aspect of the cervical left internal carotid artery (*arrow*)

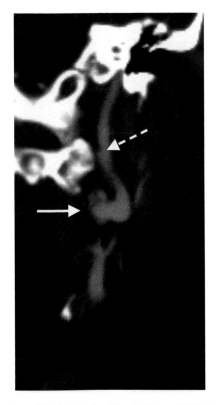

Imaging of Neck Injuries, Fig. 4 Coronal CTA image reveals an intimal dissection flap (*dashed arrow*) distal to the site of pseudoaneurysm formation (*arrow*)

Application

CT angiography (CTA) is recognized as the radiologic examination of choice for the workup of trauma patients with suspected vascular injury in the neck such as dissection or pseudoaneurysm (Figs. 3, 4 and 5). As an initial assessment tool, CTA allows triage toward conservative management versus intervention either endovascular or surgical (Stuhlfaut et al. 2005). As a result, the rate of surgical neck exploration including negative exploration has decreased over the past decade (Woo et al. 2005). Advantages of CT include wide availability, rapid scan times, and high (>95 %) sensitivity and specificity for the detection of clinically significant vascular and aero-digestive tract injuries to the neck (Inaba et al. 2012). Further, CTA of the neck may be performed in conjunction with CT evaluation of

the chest and abdomen, thus negating the need for repeated contrast dosing.

MRI/MRA may also be employed for the detection of carotid and/or vertebral artery dissection with sensitivity and specificity similar to that of CTA (Provenzale and Sarikaya 2009). The choice of imaging modality for potential dissection is thus typically based upon local practice patterns and patient specific factors. Advantages for MRI/MRA include improved detection of small infarctions and diffuse axonal injury when compared to CT. Additionally, for patients suspected of cervical cord injury, MR assessment of the extracranial cerebral vasculature may be included among the sequences acquired during a single although prolonged imaging session. Given the widespread availability of accuracy of noninvasive angiographic techniques, the role of conventional angiography lies mainly in

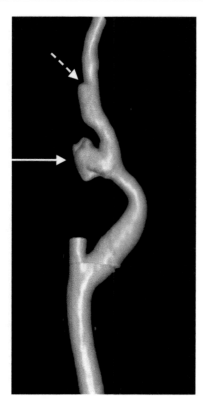

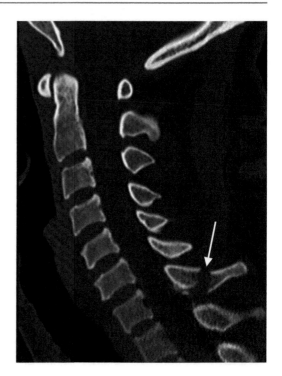

Imaging of Neck Injuries, Fig. 6 Sagittal CT of the cervical spine displays a mild distracted fracture of the C7 spinous process (*arrow*) without malalignment in a 35-year-old patient following a motor vehicle accident. Of note, the intracanalicular contents include the spinal cord that cannot be reliably assessed on this image

Imaging of Neck Injuries, Fig. 5 3D volumetric CTA image of the internal carotid artery with external carotid artery branches removed reveals irregular contour of the ICA pseudoaneurysm (*arrow*). More distally, ICA dissection manifests as focal contour abnormality of the vessel (*dashed arrow*)

cases of equivocal or discrepant results on CTA/ MRA or for those in which high pretest suspicion for injury requiring endovascular intervention demands expedient evaluation and treatment (Provenzale and Sarikaya 2009).

When aero-digestive tract injury is suspected, CT examination of the neck and chest with contrast should be considered the examination of choice for detection and gross localization of the site of aero-digestive tract disruption within the neck and/or chest. Further, CT provides adding benefit of visualization of the vasculature, soft tissues, and osseous structures in the neck. Contrast esophagography, which is regarded as the gold standard radiologic examination for investigation of potential esophageal injury, is often challenging in patients who have sustained significant traumatic injury due to their inability

to cooperate with the exam (Woo et al. 2005). In critically ill and intubated/sedated patients, video-endoscopy often allows detection of hypopharyngeal injuries that are notoriously difficult to identify via contrast esophagography as well as injuries of the cervical esophagus. For those patients who are able to cooperate for contrast fluoroscopic exams, several caveats must be considered. Due to the potential for fibrosing mediastinitis as a sequela of barium extravasation through a thoracic esophageal defect, water-soluble agents such as gastrograffin are used initially. Caution with these agents should be employed in patients at risk for aspiration due to the potential for pneumonitis. Given the improved sensitivity of thicker barium-based agents over water-soluble contrast, many radiologists advance to barium esophagography if no evidence of extravasation is seen with initial water-soluble swallows.

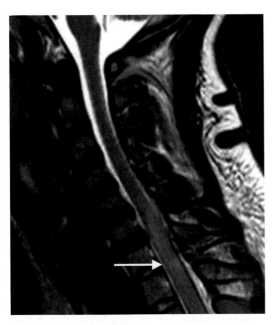

Imaging of Neck Injuries, Fig. 7 Sagittal T2-weighted MR image reveals abnormal cord signal indicative of cord contusion/edema (*arrow*) that was not apparent by CT

Non-enhanced CT of the spine is the current gold standard assessment tool to exclude cervical spine injury following trauma due to its superior depiction of osseous anatomy. In contrast, plain radiography has been shown to detect only 47–60 % of cervical spine fractures and fails to identify up to one third of potentially unstable cervical spine injuries (Hogan et al. 2005). For those with known cervical spine fracture or the clinical finding of spinal cord injury without radiographic abnormality (SCIWORA), MRI provides unparalleled assessment of intracanalicular and paraspinous soft tissues including the intervertebral disks, ligaments, and spinal cord (Figs. 6 and 7). Debate continues regarding the most appropriate management of the obtunded patient or in those otherwise unable to be cleared by neurological examination after negative cervical spine CT (Menaker et al. 2008). Factors include the benefits of early cervical collar removal in those patients whose MRI is negative versus the potential risks involved in transfer of potentially unstable patients to radiology for MR imaging. Multiple groups have examined the necessity of MRI in obtunded

patients and concluded that MRI is not required on a routine basis in these patients (Hogan et al. 2005; Como et al. 2007; Soult et al. 2012). In support of these conclusions, cervical spine CT has negative predictive value of 98.9 % for ligamentous injury and 100 % for unstable cervical spine injury in patients following blunt trauma (Hogan et al. 2005). In contrast, literature also shows that MR of the cervical spine changes the management of 7.9 % of patients with an admission cervical spine CT reported as negative for acute injury (Menaker et al. 2008). Until conclusive data provided by large series is available, decisions regarding the merits of MR in the setting of a negative CT scan may be determined in large part by institutional and individual physician practices.

Cross-References

▶ Airway Anatomy
▶ Airway Assessment
▶ Airway Trauma, Management of
▶ Spinal Shock
▶ Tracheal and Esophageal Injury

References

Como JJ, Thompson MA, Anderson JS et al (2007) Is magnetic resonance imaging essential in clearing the cervical spine in obtunded patients with blunt trauma? J Trauma 63:544–549. doi:10.1097/TA.0b013e31812e51ae

Duval EL, Geraerts SD, Brackel HJ (2007) Management of blunt tracheal trauma in children: a case series and review of the literature. Eur J Pediatr 166:559–563. doi:10.1007/s00431-006-0279-9

Hasler RM, Exadaktylos AK, Bouamra O et al (2012) Epidemiology and predictors of cervical spine injury in adult major trauma patients: a multicenter cohort study. J Trauma Acute Care Surg 72:975–981. doi:10.1097/TA.0b013e31823f5e8e

Hogan GJ, Mirvis SE, Shanmuganathan K, Scalea TM (2005) Exclusion of unstable cervical spine injury in obtunded patients with blunt trauma: is MR imaging needed when multi-detector row CT findings are normal? Radiology 237:106–113. doi:10.1148/radiol.2371040697

Inaba K, Branco BC, Menaker J et al (2012) Evaluation of multidetector computed tomography for penetrating neck injury: a prospective multicenter study. J Trauma Acute Care Surg 72:576–583. doi:10.1097/ TA.0b013e31824badf7, discussion 583–4– quiz 803–4

Karmy-Jones R, Avansino J, Stern EJ (2003) CT of blunt tracheal rupture. AJR Am J Roentgenol 180:1670

Menaker J, Philp A, Boswell S, Scalea TM (2008) Computed tomography alone for cervical spine clearance in the unreliable patient – are we there yet? J Trauma 64:898–903. doi:10.1097/TA.0b013e3181674675, discussion 903–4

Provenzale JM, Sarikaya B (2009) Comparison of test performance characteristics of MRI, MR angiography, and CT angiography in the diagnosis of carotid and vertebral artery dissection: a review of the medical literature. AJR Am J Roentgenol 193:1167–1174. doi:10.2214/AJR.08.1688

Sidell D, Mendelsohn AH, Shapiro NL, St John M (2011) Management and outcomes of laryngeal injuries in the pediatric population. Ann Otol Rhinol Laryngol 120:787–795

Soult MC, Weireter LJ, Britt RC et al (2012) MRI as an adjunct to cervical spine clearance: a utility analysis. Am Surg 78:741–744

Stuhlfaut JW, Barest G, Sakai O et al (2005) Impact of MDCT angiography on the use of catheter angiography for the assessment of cervical arterial injury after blunt or penetrating trauma. Am J Roentgenol 185:1063–1068. doi:10.2214/AJR.04.1217

Woo K, Magner DP, Wilson MT, Margulies DR (2005) CT angiography in penetrating neck trauma reduces the need for operative neck exploration. Am Surg 71:754–758

Imaging of Spine and Bony Pelvis Injuries

Tao Ouyang
Department of Radiology, Penn State Milton S. Hershey Medical Center, Hershey, PA, USA

Definition

There are, most commonly, 12 rib-bearing thoracic vertebrae and five non-rib-bearing lumbar type vertebrae, comprising the thoracic and lumbar spine. The bony pelvis is made up of the sacrum, coccyx, ilium, ischium, and pubis. The ilium, ischium and pubis fuse to form the acetabulum. Injuries to these regions occur frequently due to trauma.

Preexisting Conditions

Thoracic and lumbar spine: Approximately 30,000 spine injuries occur yearly in the United States. Most are due to trauma (motor vehicle collisions, falls, and sport-related injuries). Up to half of spinal injuries produce a neurologic deficit. Indications for imaging remain clinical and include pain, neurologic deficit, altered level of consciousness, and/or high-risk mechanisms of injury. Cervical spine injuries will be discussed in separate entries.

It is useful to think of the spine in Denis' three column model (Wheeless 2013a, b). The anterior column comprises the ALL and the anterior 2/3 of the vertebral body (with some authors using anterior 1/2), the middle column is the posterior 1/3 (or ½) of the vertebral body and the PLL, and the posterior column is everything behind that. A fracture that involves two or more contiguous columns is potentially unstable, thus making the middle column vital to spine stability. More recently, the PLC (posterior ligament complex, consisting of the ligamentum flava, interspinous ligaments, supraspinous ligament, and the facet join capsures) is felt to be a better indicator of stability.

Major fracture types are: compression fracture, burst fracture, Chance fracture, and flexion-dislocation.

Bony pelvis: While pelvic fractures represent only 3 % of all skeletal injuries, they are associated with a high percentage of mortality, from 5 % to 16 %, mostly due to associated internal injuries. Most pelvic fractures are sustained during motor vehicle collisions, motorcycle accidents, pedestrian versus motor vehicle, and falls. Acetabular fractures tend to be caused by similar mechanisms, but especially motor vehicle collisions and motorcycle accidents. Associated significant internal injuries include hemorrhage (potentially active), visceral injury, bladder/urethral injury, nerve injury, and injury to the aorta.

Risk factors for pelvic fractures include: older age, propensity for falls which may indicate frailty, smoking, and low bone mass.

Major types of pelvic fractures are: pelvic ring disruptions, sacral fractures, acetabular fractures, and avulsion injuries.

Imaging of Spine and Bony Pelvis Injuries, Fig. 1 T12 and L1 compression fractures. Sagittal CT reformat shows subtle fractures of T12 and that could easily be missed on radiography (**a**). Axial CT images show that fractures involve the anterior column of the spine (**b** and **c**)

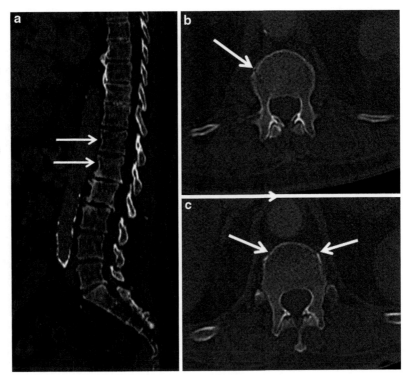

The bony pelvis forms a ring, and therefore, when one fracture occurs, there tends to be a second elsewhere in the ring. Classification of pelvic ring fractures devised by Young and Burgese incorporates mechanism of injury and the direction of the forces:

- Lateral compression injury
- Anterioposterior compression injury
- Vertical shear injury
- Combined
- Open book

Sacral fractures are classified based on zones lateral to, through, and medial to the sacral foramina and central canal, to assist in predicting neurologic injury.

Acetabular fractures are classified by Letournel and Judet into simple and complex patterns, where complex patterns represent combinations of simple fractures. Simple fracture patterns are: posterior wall, posterior column, anterior wall, anterior column, and transverse. Complex fractures are: T-shaped, posterior wall and column, transverse and posterior wall, anterior column and hemi-transverse, and both columns.

Avulsion fractures most commonly occur in skeletally immature athletes, undergoing sudden forceful muscle contraction. They occur at the site of muscle attachments, especially anterior superior iliac spine, anterior inferior iliac spine, ischial tuberosity, and lesser trochanter.

Applications

Thoracic and lumbar spine: Not all trauma patients need imaging. Generally, patients who are awake, alert, without other major non-spinal injury, complaints of spine pain and without pain on physical exam of the spine do not need imaging. Patients with low-energy trauma may be screened with radiography. However, MDCT has been shown to be superior to radiography for detection and characterization of thoracic and lumbar spine fractures. In particular, many simple compression fractures diagnosed on radiography will in fact be burst fractures when seen

Imaging of Spine and Bony Pelvis Injuries, Fig. 2 L1 burst fracture with involvement of the entire vertebral body and extension into the left lamina (**c**). Note the retropulsed fragment which compromises the bony spinal canal and could potentially compress the conus medullaris (**a** and **b**)

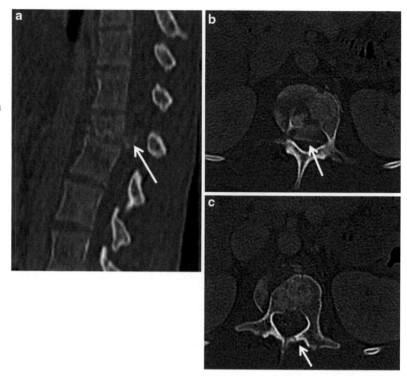

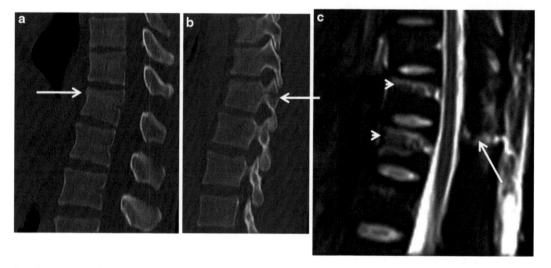

Imaging of Spine and Bony Pelvis Injuries, Fig. 3 T12 Chance fracture. Horizontal fracture through the T12 vertebral body and posterior elements (**a** and **b**), classically seen with motor vehicle trauma involving seat belts. Sagittal T2 MRI of the spine shows marrow edema in T11 and T12, indicating fractures (**c**). Horizontally oriented abnormal signal through the posterior elements is also seen but is more clearly shown by CT. Note that T11 fracture was very subtle on CT but very well seen on MRI

on MDCT (Anderson 2010). Most adult blunt trauma patients will receive a trauma "pan-scan," i.e., CT of the chest, abdomen, and pelvis. Images of the spine reformatted from the body CT can be used to evaluate the spine at no additional radiation or time, and allows for multiplanar reformats which are very useful for detection of subtle fractures, especially those in the horizontal plane. CT images should be viewed in "bone" and "soft tissue" windows, which are specific algorithms optimized for the evaluation of those structures (Figs. 1, 2, and 3).

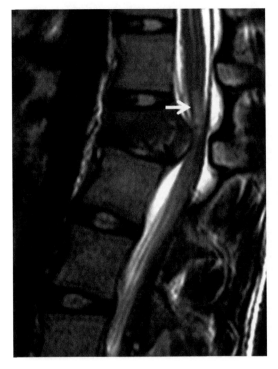

Imaging of Spine and Bony Pelvis Injuries, Fig. 4 L1 burst fracture with conus compression and edema. Note fracture of L1 with wedging of the vertebral body and retropulsion causing severe narrowing of the spinal canal. There is high T2 signal within the conus, indicating edema

MRI is reserved for specific subset of patients, including those with suspected ligamentous injury, a neurologic deficit, or those with high clinical suspicion for injury despite a normal CT. MRI has the unique ability to display cord signal, disk material, epidural structures, and ligamentous structures. However, MRI takes much longer than CT to obtain and may be more challenging for critically injured patients; additionally, MR safety issues can be difficult to resolve in acutely injured patients whose medical history may be sparse (Figs. 4 and 5).

Bony pelvis: Multidetector CT (MDCT) is the preferred modality for evaluation of hemodynamically stable patients with suspected pelvic trauma. Plain radiography of the pelvis is reserved for unstable patients. Most adult blunt trauma patients will receive a trauma "pan-scan," i.e., CT of the chest, abdomen, and pelvis with contrast. This will identify associated soft tissue injuries, including vascular injuries and bladder/urethral injuries. Bony windows of the pelvis can be obtained to evaluate for pelvic fractures. Multiplanar reformats can be made easily on the scanner and 3D reconstructions can be easily made with at scanner or at separate workstation. These reconstructions are potentially useful for treatment planning (Figs. 6, 7, 8, and 9).

There is less of a role for MRI in evaluation of pelvis injuries, with several exceptions. MRI is excellent for visualization of marrow edema, and therefore can identify fractures that are occult on CT. Sacral fractures, especially in patients

Imaging of Spine and Bony Pelvis Injuries, Fig. 5 L1 burst fracture with retropulsion and epidural hematoma. Note the retropulsed bony fragment into the spinal canal (**a**). T1 MRI sequence shows the associated T1 hyperintense epidural hematoma extending from the fractured level down to L2 (**b**)

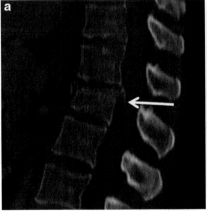
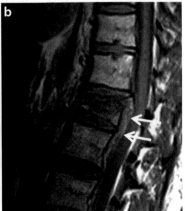

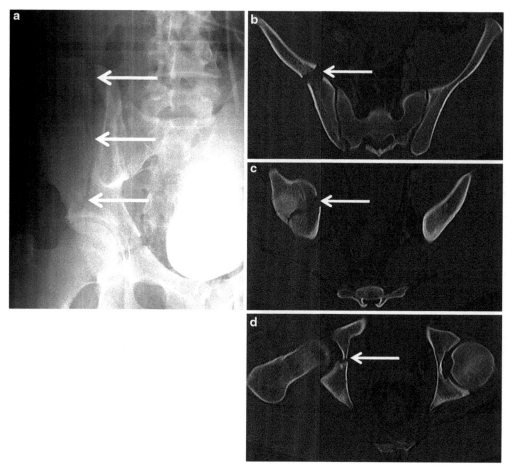

Imaging of Spine and Bony Pelvis Injuries, Fig. 6 Pelvic and acetabular fractures. Radiograph obtained in the trauma bay shows fracture line through the right ilium and extending into the right acetabulum (**a**). Axial CT images better demonstrate the details of the fracture (**b**, **c**, and **d**)

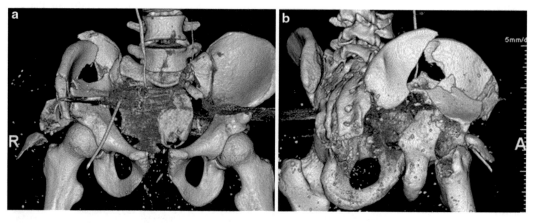

Imaging of Spine and Bony Pelvis Injuries, Fig. 7 Complex pelvic fractures. Three-dimensional reconstructions generated from CT examination can demonstrate extent of fractures and the relationship of fracture fragments and other structures in space (**a** and **b**)

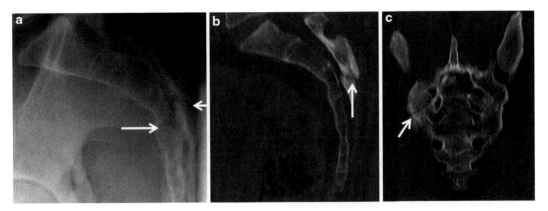

Imaging of Spine and Bony Pelvis Injuries, Fig. 8 Sacral fractures. Lateral radiograph shows cortical irregularity of the sacrum and lucency through the posterior sacral elements (**a**). Sagittal CT images better demonstrate the fracture lines (**b**). Axial CT shows that the fractures extend through neural foramina (**c**)

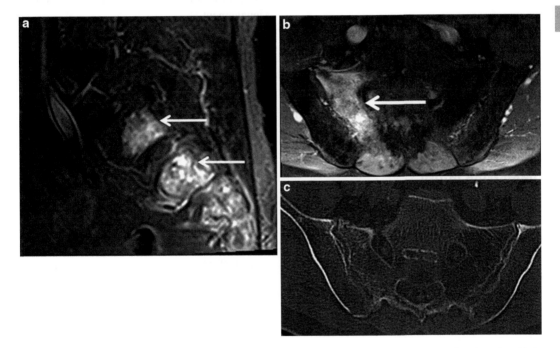

Imaging of Spine and Bony Pelvis Injuries, Fig. 9 Sacral insufficiency fracture. Sagittal STIR MRI sequence through the sacrum shows high signal indicative of marrow edema throughout the right sacrum (**a**), confirmed on axial MRI image (**b**). Note that this is almost imperceptible on CT (**c**). This demonstrates superiority of MRI to detect marrow edema and subtle fractures, especially in patients with reduced bone density

with low bone mass, can be hard to identify on CT in the acute phase, whereas abnormal T2 signal on MRI will be present. MRI is also better at evaluating neural structures in sacral fractures where the neural foramina or central canal is involved. Muscle, tendon/ligamentous, and labral injuries are also better seen on MRI.

Cross-References

▶ Anterior Cord Syndrome
▶ Fracture, Atlas (C1)
▶ Fracture, Axis (C2)
▶ Fracture, Extension Injury
▶ Fracture, Flexion Injury

▶ Fracture, Odontoid
▶ Imaging of Neck Injuries
▶ Posterior Cord Syndrome
▶ Seatbelt Injuries
▶ Spinal Cord Injury

References

Anderson MW (2010) Imaging of thoracic and lumbar spine fractures. Semin Spine Surg 22:8–19
Wheeless C (2013a) Wheeless' textbook of orthopaedics. http://www.wheelessonline.com/ortho/burst_frx_of_spine. Accessed 12 Aug 2013
Wheeless C (2013b) Wheeless' textbook of orthopaedics. http://www.wheelessonline.com/ortho/thoracolumbar_fractures. Accessed 12 Aug 2013

Immediate Postoperative Complications and Their Management

▶ Postoperative Management of Adult Trauma Patient

Immersion Injury

▶ Drowning

Immunomodulation

▶ Nutritional Deficiency/Starvation

Impaired Thermoregulation

▶ Hypothermia, Trauma, and Anesthetic Management

Improved Explosive Devices

▶ IED (Improvised Explosive Device)

Incident Command System

▶ Disaster Management

Incisional Decompression

▶ Escharotomy

Infant Trauma

▶ Pediatric Trauma, Assessment, and Anesthetic Management

Infection Control

Jocelyn A. Srigley[1] and Michael Gardam[2]
[1]University of Toronto, Toronto, ON, Canada
[2]Infection Prevention and Control, University Health Network, Toronto, ON, Canada

Synonyms

Hospital epidemiology; Infection prevention and control; IPAC

Definition

Infection control is the implementation of measures to prevent and control healthcare-associated infections. These measures may include surveillance, policy development, education, and outbreak investigation.

Preexisting Condition

Hospital-acquired infections (HAIs) are a worldwide problem, affecting 3.5–12 % of all hospitalized patients in developed countries, or approximately 7.6 episodes per 100 patients (Clean Care is Safer Care 2011). HAIs result in increased patient morbidity and mortality, prolonged hospital lengths of stay, significant financial losses, and loss of trust in the healthcare system.

Trauma patients are at particularly high risk of HAIs given that they often have disrupted anatomical barriers on presentation to hospital and then they are subjected to invasive interventions such as surgery, intubation and mechanical ventilation, and insertion of intravascular and urinary catheters. These interventions can allow the patient's flora to gain access to normally sterile sites and subsequently cause infections. Trauma patients who develop HAIs have been shown to have an increased risk of mortality (Glance et al. 2011).

HAIs are often caused by antimicrobial resistant organisms (AROs), including methicillin-resistant *Staphylococcus aureus* (MRSA), vancomycin-resistant enterococci (VRE), multidrug-resistant gram-negative organisms (MDRGN), and *Clostridium difficile*, that are frequently resident flora in hospitals. Transmission between patients can occur through either the direct transfer of AROs from patient to patient via healthcare workers or via an intermediate stage of environmental contamination.

It is essential that measures are put in place to prevent ARO transmission and HAIs, particularly in the high-risk setting of acute trauma care and ongoing intensive care unit (ICU) management of trauma patients. The majority of HAIs may be preventable with the implementation of infection control best practice bundles that include the interventions described below (Clean Care is Safer Care 2011).

Application

General Infection Control Measures

There are effective interventions to prevent or at least substantially minimize transmission of AROs, which include standard precautions that are applied to all patient interactions and additional isolation precautions for patients infected or colonized with particular pathogens.

Standard precautions are based on the assumption that all blood and body fluids potentially contain infectious agents, and thus measures should be taken in all patient interactions to reduce the risk of exposure. These precautions include staff hand hygiene, use of personal protective equipment appropriate to the anticipated exposure, and safe handling of needles and other sharps (Siegel et al. 2007). The acute management of a trauma patient carries a risk of exposure to body substances, so healthcare workers should perform a risk assessment in each case and use barrier precautions that may include gowns, gloves, and mouth, nose, and eye protection when there is potential for exposure.

Hand hygiene has been shown to reduce transmission of AROs and is associated with reduced rates of HAIs (Clean Care is Safer Care 2009). Hand hygiene should be performed before and after contact with patients or their environment, before aseptic procedures, after exposures to blood or body fluids, and before donning and after removing gloves. Alcohol-based hand rub (ABHR) is generally considered superior to soap and water washing, except in circumstances where hands are visibly soiled (Clean Care is Safer Care 2009).

Patients known or suspected to have certain infections require additional transmission-based precautions while in hospital (Siegel et al. 2007). Contact precautions are used for patients colonized or infected with AROs, for example MRSA or *Clostridium difficile*, and include the use of gown and gloves for all interactions with patients or their environment. Droplet precautions are required for pathogens transmitted through large respiratory droplets, such as respiratory viruses or *Neisseria meningitidis*. This involves the use of a surgical mask, eye protection, gown, and gloves when within 2 m of the patient. Airborne precautions are necessary for infections such as tuberculosis and varicella virus, which can be transmitted via small particles that remain suspended in the air over long distances. Patients infected with these pathogens require a private room with negative air pressure, and healthcare providers must wear fit-tested N95 respirators while in the room.

Prevention of Specific HAIs

Ventilator-Associated Pneumonia

Trauma patients commonly require intubation in the acute setting, followed by mechanical ventilation during their ICU admission. Ventilator-associated pneumonia (VAP) is one of the most common HAIs and is estimated to occur at a rate of 7.9 episodes (95 % CI 5.7–10.1) per 1,000 ventilator days in high-income countries and at even higher rates in developing countries (Clean Care is Safer Care 2011). VAP generally occurs due to bacterial colonization of the upper airways and aspiration of respiratory secretions, or less commonly through the use of contaminated respiratory equipment (Coffin et al. 2008). There are a number of evidence-based strategies for prevention of VAP that target these mechanisms of disease.

Colonization of the airways can be minimized through use of the oral route for intubation rather than nasotracheal, regular oropharyngeal decontamination with chlorhexidine mouthwash, and avoidance of gastric acid suppression therapy in patients not at high risk for gastrointestinal bleeding. Aspiration can be prevented by maintaining the head of the bed at 30–45° and avoiding supine positioning, using a cuffed endotracheal tube with cuff pressure of at least 20 cm H_2O, draining subglottic secretions, and avoiding gastric overdistension. The risk of equipment contamination can be reduced by minimizing ventilatory circuit changes, maintaining a closed circuit during condensate removal, using sterile water to rinse reusable equipment, and appropriately disinfecting and storing equipment according to the manufacturer's recommendations. ICUs that have implemented these practices have witnessed dramatic reductions in VAP (Marwick and Davey 2009).

Catheter-Related Bloodstream Infections

Trauma patients frequently require a variety of intravascular catheters for monitoring and medication administration. One of the potential complications is catheter-related bloodstream infection (CRBSI), which occurs in developed countries at an incidence of 3.5 episodes

(95 % CI 2.8–4.1) per 1,000 catheter days (Cleaner Care is Safer Care 2011). Research has demonstrated a number of effective strategies to minimize CRBSI risk prior to, during, and after central line insertion (O'Grady et al. 2011).

Prior to insertion, the competency of any healthcare worker to perform this procedure should be assessed and documented. An appropriate insertion site must be chosen, avoiding femoral catheters since they are associated with a significantly increased risk of CRBSI and choosing the subclavian site whenever possible. The catheter chosen for insertion should have the minimum number of ports or lumens required for patient care. Hand hygiene should be performed before insertion, and the insertion site should be disinfected with 2 % chlorhexidine in 70 % alcohol. Full barrier precautions should be used during the procedure, including sterile gloves and gown, surgical mask, and cap. After insertion, the catheter hubs or injection ports should be disinfected with chlorhexidine or 70 % alcohol prior to being accessed. The need for ongoing intravascular access should be assessed daily during ICU rounds, and catheters that are no longer needed should be removed. If CRBSI rates are not decreasing despite implementation of the aforementioned measures, catheters impregnated with antimicrobials or antiseptics can be used for patients who are expected to require the catheter for more than five days.

Catheter-Associated Urinary Tract Infection

Most trauma patients require urinary catheterization at some point during their management, putting them at risk of catheter-associated urinary tract infection (CAUTI). Bacteria from the periurethral area colonize the catheter and then have a direct portal of entry into the bladder. The estimated incidence of CAUTI is 4.1 infections (95 % CI 3.7–4.6) per 1,000 urinary catheter days (Clean Care is Safer Care 2011). The risk of developing CAUTI is approximately 3–7 % per day in a patient with a catheter in situ (Lo et al. 2008).

The primary strategy for CAUTI prevention is to limit the use and duration of catheterization, given the significant daily infection risk (Lo et al. 2008). Each hospital should outline appropriate indications for catheter insertion as well as recommendations for catheter removal. Reminders should be provided to healthcare workers to frequently reassess the need for catheterization and discontinue unnecessary catheters as they may be left in situ more for staff convenience rather than patient need. Silver-coated or other antibacterial catheters may be considered in select situations to decrease bacteriuria, but they have not been shown to reduce the incidence of symptomatic infections and are not recommended for routine use.

Surgical Site and Traumatic Wound Infections

Trauma patients typically present with a variety of wounds related to their initial injury, and they may require surgical management that creates additional incisions. Both the traumatic wounds and the surgical sites may subsequently become infected. Endogenous skin flora often cause surgical site infections (SSI), but the etiology in trauma patients may also include enteric and other endogenous organisms due to penetrating trauma or environmental gram-negative organisms and anaerobes due to exogenous contamination of wounds.

Traumatic wounds should be thoroughly cleansed and debrided to remove foreign material and nonviable tissue. If the patient requires a surgical procedure, standard recommendations for SSI prevention should be followed (Anderson et al. 2008). These include preparation of the surgical site with 2 % chlorhexidine in 70 % alcohol, avoidance of hair removal at the surgical site, hand antisepsis and sterile gown and gloves for all members of the surgical team, surgical mask and cap for anyone in the operating room (OR), limiting traffic in the OR, positive pressure ventilation in the OR with an adequate frequency of air exchanges, and appropriate sterilization of all surgical instruments.

Antimicrobial prophylaxis is recommended for all surgical procedures in which bacterial contamination is possible. The antibiotic should be targeted against the usual pathogens causing SSI for each particular procedure, and it should be administered within 1 h prior to incision (Anderson et al. 2008). Doses may have to be adjusted for larger patients, and drugs may need to be readministered for longer procedures. Broader spectrum therapy may be considered in trauma patients who have dirty wounds potentially contaminated with environmental organisms or penetrating abdominal injuries. The duration of prophylaxis should be limited to 24 h; it has been shown that longer courses do not improve outcomes in trauma patients but increase the risk of resistant infection (Velmahos et al. 2002).

Clostridium difficile Infection

Clostridium difficile infection (CDI) has been increasing in frequency and severity in many areas of the world, making it now one of the most common HAIs (Dubberke et al. 2008). Antibiotic use is the primary risk factor for development of CDI, and most trauma patients receive antibiotics at some point during hospitalization. Thus, appropriate use of antibiotics through the establishment of a stewardship program is a cornerstone of CDI prevention efforts. Antibiotics should be used only when necessary, with as narrow a spectrum and as short a duration as possible. This must be balanced with the need to provide timely and appropriate antibiotic treatment of infections, which has been shown to improve patient outcomes. Each institution can develop an individualized antimicrobial stewardship program that takes into account these two competing goals. Receipt of proton pump inhibitors has also been shown to be an independent risk factor for CDI (Kwok et al. 2012), and as with antibiotics, these should be used only when their benefits outweigh the risks of CDI.

C. difficile can be transmitted between patients via healthcare workers or medical equipment, so patients with suspected or confirmed CDI should be placed in contact precautions as long as they have diarrhea, and their rooms should have dedicated equipment. In vitro studies have shown that alcohol-based hand rubs are not effective against *C. difficile* spores, and some bodies recommend hand hygiene with soap and water rather than ABHR after contact with a *C. difficile* patient or their environment. It is not clear, however, how relevant this is in the clinical setting, and soap and water washing may decrease overall hand hygiene compliance. A sporicidal agent such as 10 % aqueous solution of sodium hypochlorite (household bleach) should be used for environmental cleaning (Dubberke et al. 2008).

Use of Bundles in Infection Control

A bundle is a set of evidence-based interventions that can be implemented simultaneously to improve a particular outcome in patients meeting prespecified criteria. One of the benefits of the bundle approach is that it provides a checklist of procedures to be followed as part of routine practice, as opposed to relying on each individual healthcare worker remembering to implement every step. Well-established bundles exist for prevention of VAP, CRBSI, CAUTI, and SSI, incorporating many of the above-mentioned strategies. Studies have shown these bundles to be successful in preventing HAIs, in some cases reducing incidence to zero (Marwick and Davey 2009).

Implementation

Although the danger of HAIs to patients is well known and there is ample literature proving the effectiveness of control measures to prevent the spread of AROs, healthcare worker compliance with preventative measures is frequently poor (Gardam et al. 2010). HAIs are complex events that have multiple contributing causes, and the role of human psychology and organizational culture is only recently being addressed. The challenge of infection control lies in bringing about change in healthcare culture, which often does not value interventions to prevent HAIs nor acknowledge the link between individual behavior and patient outcomes.

Recently the behavior change technique "Positive Deviance" (PD) has been used to address this issue with some early success (Gardam et al. 2010). PD operates on the premise that solutions to problems already exist among certain members of the affected population. The PD process involves identifying these positive "outliers" and then facilitating the spread of their solutions to others in the group. This represents a significant change from the traditional model of infection control that is based on didactic education and top-down implementation of "best practices." In the PD approach, frontline staff are empowered to implement infection control interventions that are individualized to their particular situation. PD programs have been shown to reduce HAIs and improve hand hygiene in hospitals (Zimmerman et al. 2013). PD and other similar approaches acknowledge the complex challenges of HAI prevention and may help to facilitate lasting behavior and culture change.

Conclusion

HAIs in trauma patients are serious and preventable adverse events. There are effective strategies to reduce ARO transmission and prevent specific HAIs, including standard precautions, additional isolation precautions, and prevention bundles for VAP, CRBSI, CAUTI, SSIs, and CDI. However, it is not enough to merely write policies that contain these strategies; it is also necessary to bring about behavior and culture change so that HAI prevention can be achieved. All members of the healthcare team must be encouraged to take responsibility for their role in patient safety and implement these infection control measures.

Cross-References

▶ Catheter Associated Urinary Tract Infection
▶ Catheter-Related Infections
▶ Central Line Associated Blood Stream Infection
▶ Surgical Site Infections
▶ Ventilator-Associated Pneumonia

References

Anderson DJ, Kaye KS, Classen D, Arias KM, Podgorny K, Burstin H, Calfee DP, Coffin SE, Dubberke ER, Fraser V, Gerding DN, Griffin FA, Gross P, Klompas M, Lo E, Marschall J, Mermel LA, Nicolle L, Pegues DA, Perl TM, Saint S, Salgado CD, Weinstein RA, Wise R, Yokoe DS (2008) Strategies to prevent surgical site infections in acute care hospitals. Infect Control Hosp Epidemiol 29(S1):S51–S61

Clean Care is Safer Care (2009) WHO guidelines on hand hygiene in health care. World Health Organization, Geneva

Clean Care is Safer Care (2011) Report on the burden of endemic health care-associated infection worldwide. World Health Organization, Geneva

Coffin SE, Klompas M, Classen D, Arias KM, Podgorny K, Anderson DJ, Burstin H, Calfee DP, Dubberke ER, Fraser V, Gerding DN, Griffin FA, Gross P, Kaye KS, Lo E, Marschall J, Mermel LA, Nicolle L, Pegues DA, Perl TM, Saint S, Salgado CD, Weinstein RA, Wise R, Yokoe DS (2008) Strategies to prevent ventilator-associated pneumonia in acute care hospitals. Infect Control Hosp Epidemiol 29(S1): S31–S40

Dubberke ER, Gerding DN, Classen D, Arias KM, Podgorny K, Anderson DJ, Burstin H, Calfee DP, Coffin SE, Fraser V, Griffin FA, Gross P, Kaye KS, Klompas M, Lo E, Marschall J, Mermel LA, Nicolle L, Pegues DA, Perl TM, Saint S, Salgado CD, Weinstein RA, Wise R, Yokoe DS (2008) Strategies to prevent *Clostridium difficile* infections in acute care hospitals. Infect Control Hosp Epidemiol 29(S1):S81–S92

Gardam M, Reason P, Rykert L (2010) Healthcare culture and the challenge of preventing healthcare-associated infections. Healthc Q 13:116–120

Glance LG, Stone PW, Mukamel DB, Dick AW (2011) Increases in mortality, length of stay, and cost associated with hospital-acquired infections in trauma patients. Arch Surg 146(7):794–801

Kwok CS, Arthur AK, Anibueze CI, Singh S, Cavallazzi R, Loke YK (2012) Risk of ciostridium difficite infection with acid suppressing drugs and antibiotics. Am J Gastroenterol 107(7):1011–1019

Lo E, Nicolle L, Classen D, Arias KM, Podgorny K, Anderson DJ, Burstin H, Calfee DP, Coffin SE, Dubberke ER, Fraser V, Gerding DN, Griffin FA, Gross P, Kaye KS, Klompas M, Marschall J, Mermel LA, Pegues DA, Perl TM, Saint S, Salgado CD, Weinstein RA, Wise R, Yokoe DS (2008) Strategies to prevent catheter-associated urinary tract infections in acute care hospitals. Infect Control Hosp Epidemiol 29(S1):S41–S50

Marwick C, Davey P (2009) Care bundles: the holy grail of infectious risk management in hospital? Curr Opin Infect Dis 22:364–369

O'Grady NP, Alexander M, Burns LA, Dellinger EP, Garland J, Heard SO, Lipsett PA, Masur H, Mermel LA, Pearson ML, Raad II, Randolph AG, Rupp ME, Saint S, Healthcare Infection Control Practices Advisory Committee (HICPAC) (2011) Guidelines for the prevention of intravascular catheter-related infections. Clin Infect Dis 52:e1–e32

Siegel JD, Rhinehart E, Jackson M, Chiarello L, The Healthcare Infection Control Practices Advisory Committee (2007) Guideline for isolation precautions: preventing transmission of infectious agents in healthcare settings. http://www.cdc.gov/hicpac/pdf/isolation/Isolation2007.pdf. Accessed 6 July 2012

Velmahos GC, Toutouzas KG, Sarkisyan G, Chan LS, Jindal A, Karaiskakis M, Katkhouda N, Berne TV, Demetriades D (2002) Severe trauma is not an excuse for prolonged antibiotic prophylaxis. Arch Surg 137(5):537–541

Zimmerman B, Reason P, Rykert L, Gitterman L, Christian C, Gardan M (2013) Front line ownership-generating a cure mindset for patient safety. Healthcare papers, in press.

Infection Prevention and Control

▶ Infection Control

Inferior Vena Cava Injury

▶ Abdominal Major Vascular Injury, Anesthesia for

Information Disclosure in Trauma

▶ Informed Consent in Trauma

Informational Privacy

▶ Patient Confidentiality

Informed Consent in Trauma

Peter C. W. Loke
Centre for BioMedical Ethics, National University Hospital System, Singapore, Singapore
Mint Medical Centre, Singapore, Singapore
Resolvers Pte Ltd, Singapore, Singapore

Synonyms

Decision making in trauma patients; Information disclosure in trauma

Definition

Informed consent is an individual's autonomous authorization of a medical intervention (or of participation in research); there must be the act of informed and voluntary consent (Beauchamp and Childress 2009, p. 119). Informed consent is also the social rules of consent that maintain that one must obtain a legally or institutionally valid consent from patients (or subjects) before proceeding with diagnostic, therapeutic, or research procedures (Beauchamp and Childress 2009, p. 119).

Background

Requiring consent to treatment arises from respect for autonomy, or the right to self-determination, of a patient. It is a principle recognized in law. In the 1914 case of Schloendorff v. Society of New York Hospital, Judge Cardozo stated that "every person of adult years and sound mind has a right to determine what shall be done with his own body; and a surgeon who performs an operation without his patient's consent commits an assault, for which he is liable in damages."

The Nuremberg trials in the late 1940s, which exposed the human medical experiments in Nazi concentration camps that horrified the world, put the focus firmly on the issue of consent. With the evolution of the concept in the ensuing years, focus has moved from the obligation to disclose information to the quality of the understanding and consent of a patient (Beauchamp and Childress 2009, p. 118).

Application

Trauma is typically sudden and unexpected. A patient being treated for injuries as a result of it can be unconscious and is thus clearly lacking in competence, in which case the usual course for the treating physician is to treat the patient according to the best medical interest of the patient. The usual need for consent to treatment is negated by medical necessity.

Very commonly, however, the trauma patient is not unconscious but in a state of confusion, both in terms of what happened that resulted in the trauma and what needs to be done to stabilize them thereafter. The question of informed consent relating to treatment of such patients becomes a specific concern.

Elements of Informed Consent

Informed consent requires the elements of competence, disclosure, understanding, voluntariness, and consent (Beauchamp and Childress 2009, p. 120). The temptation for intentional nondisclosure and dispensing with informed consent in the trauma patient is high, and indeed, this is accepted in the face of a medical emergency. However, in cases where time is not of the essence or at the point where the patient is stabilized such that he or she is no longer in need of immediate resuscitative treatment, there is the need for informed consent in order to continue with treatment.

Competence

Competence is discussed elsewhere in entry on Refusal of Treatment by Critical Patients. The same considerations apply to competence or otherwise to give informed consent by the trauma patient.

Disclosure

The lack of informed consent is a basis for civil litigation lawsuits against the doctor. This is centered on the failure of a physician either to provide sufficiency of information or to ensure sufficiency of understanding before proceeding with treatment, which results in measurable harm to the patient. Doctors are generally obligated to disclose a core set of information, including (1) facts or descriptions patients usually consider material in deciding whether to refuse consent to the proposed intervention, (2) information the doctor believes to be material, (3) the doctor's recommendation, (4) the purpose of seeking consent, and (5) the nature and limits of consent as an act of authorization (Beauchamp and Childress 2009, p. 121).

There are three possible measures of the-standard for disclosure. They are the professional practice standard, the reasonable patient standard, and the subjective patient standard.

The professional standard is based on the legal standard known as the Bolam test, where a doctor is considered not negligent if he has acted in accordance with the practice accepted as proper by a responsible body of medical men skilled in that particular art. In short, adequate disclosure is achieved when the level of information that is provided is within the boundaries of customary medical practice, and this is according to the practice of the profession.

The reasonable or prudent patient standard requires that a doctor discloses what information or risk that would be expected to affect the judgment of the hypothetical reasonable patient, the information that is needed so the patient can determine for himself or herself as to what course he or she would adopt. While it is a laudable standard, it is difficult to properly define and can result in uncertainty.

The subjective patient standard requires for the doctor to cater information to the individual needs of the specific patient they are providing the information to, especially if the doctor is or should be aware of the patient's informational needs. It is the preferred moral standard, but it is not reasonable to expect a doctor to always fully understand the sometimes whimsical mind of every patient. However, the doctor should always answer any specific question a patient might have.

Understanding

Clinical experience and empirical data indicate that patients and research subjects exhibit a wide variation in their understanding of information about diagnoses, procedure, risks, probable benefits, and prognosis (Beauchamp and Childress 2009, p. 127). This is also dependent on the skill of the doctor in conveying such information in layman's terms and individualizing it to the specific patient. Trauma is an acute condition, so the patient arrives into the healthcare setting unprepared and not having had the opportunity to self-research on their condition and possible treatment options. The trauma would almost inevitably have an impact on the mental state, be it confusion, anxiety, shock, frustration, or even anger, and his or her ability to comprehend is compromised. The patient has then to balance risks against benefits of treatment options, never mind that the treatment required is often an intensive technologically advanced care which is not easily explained.

Information overload is as real a challenge as is insufficient information, and doctors must be mindful that simple terms to them like ruptured spleen or fractured neck of femur might mean nothing to the patient. Information needs to be sufficient and couched in daily language that is as simple as possible.

Challenging as it might be, the doctor should do his or her best to provide information to the patient to enable an autonomous decision for treatment at every appropriate juncture as the condition of the patient evolves.

Voluntariness

A person is said to act voluntarily if he or she wills the action without being under the control of another's influence (Beauchamp and Childress 2009, p. 132). Sometimes, the challenge for the doctor is to balance the need to persuade the patient to undertake a treatment considered to be in his or her best medical interest, without being manipulative or coercive. Doctors can even be subconsciously guilty of such manipulation. Whether information is framed positively or negatively makes a difference: "this operation in my hands has an extremely high level of success" as compared to "the general failure rate of this surgery is in the region of 45 %."

Waiver

Every patient has the autonomous right to relinquish the requirement for informed consent. The patient could delegate such decision-making authority to the doctor, their relative, or indeed anyone they choose. In trauma cases, the likelihood of such delegation is higher. The patient must of course not be incompetent, and delegation should be properly clarified with the patient and clearly documented.

Surrogate Decision Making

The trauma patient is often nonautonomous or doubtfully autonomous. If there is uncertainty as to the competence of the patient and legality of his or her apparent refusal of treatment, the case can be brought to court for authorization to carry out a particular course of action. However, with the urgency of the rapidly evolving condition of a typical trauma patient, this is often not possible. The need for a surrogate decision maker arises.

Three general standards can be employed by the surrogate decision maker.

If there is adequate proof of the wishes of the patient when he or she was competent, for example, if the patient made it very clear he or she does not wish for artificial life-sustaining treatment, this serves as a prior autonomous decision which should be respected.

In substituted judgment, the surrogate decision maker is asked to "don the mental mantle of the incompetent" and make the decision the incompetent person would have made if competent (Beauchamp and Childress 2009, p. 136). This standard of substituted judgment should be used for once-competent patients only if a reason exists to believe that the surrogate decision maker can make a judgment as the patient would have made.

When there is no indication of the patient's preferences, the best interest standard is employed. The surrogate decision maker, who in this case is usually the treating doctor, must determine the highest net benefit among the available treatment options, assigning different weights to interests the patient has in each option and discounting or subtracting inherent risks or costs (Beauchamp and Childress 2009, p. 138). Simply put, the onus is to act for the overall benefit of the patient, based on the medical considerations and, if relevant, other aspects like family wishes and social issues.

Children

The English common law concept of Gillick competence, which applies to children between the ages of 14 and 16 years old, is a good starting point to decide whether a child is fit to give their own consent for treatment. In English law, children above the age of 16 are presumed to be competent to give consent for treatment. The concept in Gillick is that when a child has sufficient maturity and reasoning capability to enable him to understand what is proposed and its implications, he is treated as having the capacity to give a valid consent to medical treatment. The doctor therefore has to assess each individual child for such ability.

For children below the age of 14, they should be given the opportunity to assent to their treatment whenever possible.

The Case for Presumed Consent

As already discussed, the trauma patient is less likely to be able to properly grasp the full extent of their situation, with the implications of the different options for treatment including the no-treatment option. If there are linguistic communication issues between healthcare providers and the patient, this challenge is accentuated. Coupled with that is the urgency for treatment in most trauma patients.

In real life, such considerations could serve to delay treatment, to the detriment of the patient. To simplify matters, the case can be made for presumed consent for the doctor to act in the best interest of the patient in all cases of trauma, at least until the patient is medically stabilized and also clearly more able to make his or her own autonomous decision.

Cross-References

▶ Ethical Issues in Trauma Anesthesia
▶ Refusal of Treatment by Critical Patients
▶ Surrogate, Role in Decision-Making

References

Beauchamp TL, Childress JF (2009) Principles of biomedical ethics, 6th edn. Oxford University Press, New York

Recommended Reading

Adams J, Schmidt T, Sanders A, Larkin GL, Knopp R, The SAEM Ethics Committee (1998) Professionalism in emergency medicine. Acad Emerg Med 5:1193–1199

British Medical Association (2013) Consent tool kit. British Medical Association, London. http://bma.org.uk/practical-support-at-work/ethics/consent-tool-kit. Accessed 6 Mar 2013

Moskop JC (1999) Informed consent in the emergency department. Emerg Med Clin North Am 17(2):327–340

Sanders AB, Derse AR, Knopp R, Malone K, Mitchell J, Moskop JC, Sklar D, Smith J, Jackson Allison E (1991) American college of emergency physicians ethics manual. Ann Emerg Med 20(10):1153–1162

Ingestion or Inhalation of Chemicals

▶ Chemical Burns

Inhalation Injury

▶ Burn Anesthesia

Initial Trauma Assessment

▶ ABCDE of Trauma Care

Initial Trauma Evaluation

▶ ABCDE of Trauma Care

Initial Trauma Resuscitation

▶ ABCDE of Trauma Care

Injured Patients

▶ ICU Management

Injuries in Older Adults

▶ Geriatric Trauma

Injury Databank

▶ Trauma Registry

Injury Database

▶ Trauma Registry

Injury Registries

▶ Trauma Registry

Injury Registry

▶ Trauma Registry

Injury to the Brain

▶ Neurotrauma, Introduction

Innominate Artery

▶ Thoracic Vascular Injuries

Inotropes

▶ Vasoactive Agents in the ICU

Inpatient Management

▶ Trauma Floor Management

INR

▶ International Normalized Ratio

Instrumented Fusion

▶ Cervical Spine Fractures, Indications for Surgery

Insulin

▶ Intensive Insulin Therapy in Surgery/Trauma

Insulin Resistance

▶ Intensive Insulin Therapy in Surgery/Trauma

Intensive Care Unit

▶ Fungal Infections
▶ ICU Management

Intensive Care Unit (ICU) Psychosis

▶ Preventing Delirium in the Intensive Care Unit

Intensive Care Unit-Acquired Paresis

▶ ICU Acquired Weakness

Intensive Insulin Therapy

▶ Intensive Insulin Therapy in Surgery/Trauma

Intensive Insulin Therapy in Surgery/Trauma

Kevin A. Kaucher
Departments of Pharmacy and Emergency
Medicine, Denver Health Medical Center,
Denver, CO, USA

Synonyms

Glucose control; Glycemic control; Insulin;
Insulin resistance; Intensive insulin therapy; Surgery; Trauma

Definition

Intensive insulin therapy (IIT) is defined as the practice of maintaining a patient's blood glucose (BG) between 80 and 110 mg/dL. This goal was established and adopted for use in all critically ill patients requiring intensive care unit (ICU) level of care based on the mortality benefit shown by Van den Berghe et al. (2001). In this study of 1,548 surgical ICU patients, IIT compared to a conventional treatment group (target BG 180–200 mg/dL) significantly reduced overall hospital mortality and morbidity. The results led to a significant paradigm shift in management of hyperglycemia in the ICU. This required the use of insulin infusions and tightly monitored blood glucose levels through the use of titration protocols. However, the results published in 2001 by Van den Berghe have not been reproducible in other patient populations, so extrapolation has been questioned.

Preexisting Condition

Hyperglycemia in the Critically Ill

Hyperglycemia and blood glucose variability is common in the critically ill patient, even without a prior history of diabetes. Hyperglycemia, once defined as a blood glucose level of greater than 200 mg/dL, is thought to be a normal adaptive response to stress in critically ill medical, surgical, trauma, and burn patients. Hyperglycemia in this patient population is likely multifactorial and caused by both intrinsic and extrinsic factors, all causing a disruption of normal pro-inflammatory and anti-inflammatory regulatory processes. Once thought to be protective by increasing substrate for metabolism in glucose-dependent tissues, the benefits of surgery or trauma-induced hyperglycemia were challenged in surgical patients (Van den Berghe et al. 2001). The increase in morbidity and mortality attributed to hyperglycemia led to worldwide adoption of IIT in the ICU.

Insulin Resistance and Inflammatory Effects

During the acute phase of critically ill trauma patients, stress response leads to insulin resistance, glucose intolerance, and hyperglycemia. This is evident by increased levels of circulating cytokines and regulatory hormones such as glucagon, cortisol, growth hormone, and catecholamines. Mediators of the inflammatory response cause upregulation and membrane localization of non-insulin-dependent glucose transporters GLUT-1, GLUT-2, and GLUT-3. The upregulation of interleukin-1 (IL-1) and tumor necrosis factor-α (TNF-α) has also been shown to inhibit insulin release and cause hepatic and peripheral insulin resistance. Impaired glucose uptake and increased hepatic gluconeogenesis and glycogenolysis are also associated with inflammation and stress states. Exogenous catecholamines, dextrose-containing intravenous fluids, and nutritional support combined with the aforementioned factors lead to normal or low insulin levels and impaired counterregulatory systems resulting in stress hyperglycemia (Marik and Raghavan 2004). The effect of this interplay is demonstrated by persistent hyperglycemia throughout a course of patient hospitalization.

The pro-inflammatory effects of hyperglycemia in the critically ill are evident from observed increases in circulating plasma concentrations of reactive oxygen species, interleukin-8, polymorphonuclear leukocytes, and mononuclear cells. Neutrophil function is also inhibited by decreased chemotaxis and increased adherence to the endothelium. The cellular glucose overload resulting in increased oxidative stress leads to mitochondrial dysfunction, inhibition of glycolytic activity, and further cellular toxicity contributing to organ failure. Lipid peroxidation is also increased potentially leading to prothrombotic states. Reduced nitric oxide levels in the setting of acute hyperglycemia can exacerbate low-flow or low-perfusion states further exacerbating organ dysfunction (Marik and Raghavan 2004).

The Anti-inflammatory Effect of Insulin

Insulin also has its own pleiotropic immunomodulating effects which are anti-inflammatory in nature. These effects are likely due to insulin directly causing release of nitric oxide (NO) from endothelium. NO has been shown to downregulate endothelial cell adhesion molecules and pro-inflammatory cytokines such as nuclear factor-kappaB (NF-KB), a transcription factor responsible for regulation of over 150 inflammatory genes including TNF-α, IL-1, IL-6, IL-8, IL-10, and cyclooxygenase-2. These effects in theory are the target of IIT in the critically ill to attenuate the catabolic state of stress and regulate apoptosis, leading to a reduction in morbidity and mortality.

Application

Since the publication of the first study by Van den Berghe in 2001, which showed a significant mortality benefit in cardiothoracic surgery patients receiving IIT, several other studies have evaluated IIT in other populations. Unfortunately, these latter studies have not shown the same benefit or were stopped prematurely due to high protocol variations and hypoglycemia rates. Thus, no randomized controlled study has shown results similar to the Van den Berghe results. The largest and most comprehensive trial, the NICE-SUGAR trial, which enrolled nearly 6,100 patients, showed that tight glucose control was not beneficial and might pose a significant risk of hypoglycemia and death (Finfer et al. 2009). In the NICE-SUGAR trial, tight blood glucose control of 80–108 mg/dL using IIT infusions was compared to a conventional approach of maintaining blood glucose between 140 and 180 mg/dL and showed a significant increase in 90-day mortality with the use of IIT. This study enrolled mixed medical and surgical population across 42 sites. However, in a subset of patients admitted to surgical ICUs for trauma, an odds ratio for death analysis favored intensive control. Thus, clinicians are now left with uncertainty in managing hyperglycemia in a surgical/trauma patient population.

Indications

Surgical/Trauma

Aside from the initial Van den Berghe study in 2001 in a predominantly cardiothoracic surgery patient population, few studies have been done in the surgical or trauma populations to further strengthen the argument that IIT improves outcomes. Krinsley showed similar results to Van den Berghe, but in a mixed medical and surgical population (Krinsley 2004). In this early landmark study, they evaluated an IIT protocol to keep BGs <140 mg/dL, comparing 800 patients pre-protocol implementation to 800 patients post-protocol implementation. Effects seen on organ system dysfunction favored tight glycemic control, with less patients experiencing new-onset renal dysfunction and less patients requiring blood transfusions in the IIT group. However, the rates of ICU-acquired infections were similar between the two groups. Mortality also decreased significantly in the standard of care group as compared with the IIT group. Mean length of stay in the ICU was not significant between the groups. The author therefore concluded similarly to Van den Berghe that protocol-driven IIT reduces mortality and morbidity in the ICU.

A study by Collier et al. prospectively evaluated protocol-driven IIT in their trauma ICU compared to a historical control. Comparing over 800 patients, the investigators found no difference in all-cause mortality or the incidence of pneumonia and surgical site infections. However, in patients who exhibited one BG level ≥150 mg/dL, outcomes were worse for the control group. In this subgroup, mortality was 14.6 % versus 6.1 %, $p = 0.02$, and pneumonia rates were 35.9 % versus 23.3 %, $p = 0.02$, comparing the control to the IIT group (Collier et al. 2005).

In the largest review of a trauma population alone, over 2,000 adult patients were retrospectively analyzed pre- and post-IIT protocol implementation, with a goal BG of 80–110 mg/dL in the latter group (Eriksson et al. 2001). Mortality and hospital length of stay in the pre-IIT group was higher when compared with the post-IIT group. Multivariate analysis identified both mean glucose levels and glycemic variability as independent contributors to the risk of mortality.

Burns

Burn injury typically causes a greater hypermetabolic response when compared to other subsets of trauma. These patients are at the same risk of adverse effects of hyperglycemia such as immune dysfunction, multiorgan failure, and sepsis. Gibson et al. explored the effects of an IIT protocol on a mixed surgical and burn population (Gibson et al. 2009). They found significantly decreased rates of sepsis and mortality among patients that received IIT during the 72 h study period.

Pham et al. also explored the effects of a new IIT protocol used on children admitted to a burn ICU with >30 % total body surface area burns (Pham et al. 2005). When comparing a historical conventional group (goal BG <200 mg/dL) to an IIT group (goal BG 90–120 mg/dL), they found IIT to improve survival and reduce the number of urinary tract infections.

Traumatic Brain Injury

Traumatic brain injury (TBI) is one of the most common causes of death among trauma patients. Hyperglycemia present in patients with TBI has been a strong predictor of poor neurologic outcomes. It may also exacerbate secondary brain injury by disrupting the glucose to glutamate and lactate to pyruvate ratios. Coester et al. examined the effects of IIT on patients presenting with blunt traumatic brain injury (Coester et al. 2010). This study randomized patients to either IIT (goal BG 80–110 mg/dL) or conventional treatment (goal BG <180 mg/dL). The authors reported a higher incidence of hypoglycemia in the IIT group with no prolonged adverse effects noted due to the episodes. They also found no differences in ICU length of stay or sepsis rates between the two groups. Glasgow outcome scale scores, used to assess neurological outcomes, were similar between the two groups. Based on their results, the authors concluded that IIT is not as beneficial in TBI as reported by Van den Berghe so care should be taken to ensure hypoglycemic events do not occur.

Blood Glucose Testing

Various methods of measuring blood glucose exist. Intra-arterial or venous catheters are most accurate but point-of-care bedside devices or glucometers which measure capillary samples are most commonly used. Intra-arterial or venous blood sample from a catheter is also less likely to be contaminated compared to fingerstick methods, however, resulting turnaround time which may take 15–60 min limit their use. Unfortunately, in the setting of critical illness, tissue edema, hypoperfusion, variable volume of blood sample, vasoactive agent use and anemia are all factors that lead to the inaccuracies of the fingerstick methods (Honiden and Inzucchi 2011). In this situation, for example, the fingerstick method tends to overestimate blood glucose values. This is important to note especially in the setting of hypoglycemia where clinical decisions may be delayed based on inaccurate knowledge.

Another method of glucose measurement that will be available for future use is subcutaneous continuous glucose monitoring. These systems are in the beginning phase of use in critically ill patients but have shown significant promise in their reliability and accuracy compared to

standard point-of-care methods or whole blood analysis. Therefore, until accurate continuous glucose monitoring is available, clinicians must know the strengths and weaknesses of each measurement device.

Administration

In the acute phase of critical illness, continuous IV insulin infusions are preferred over subcutaneous insulin therapy. Due to the short half-life and duration of action of regular insulin, the ability to make rapid dose adjustments is crucial to the evolving needs of critically ill patients. With the use of validated written or computerized protocols, insulin infusions have been shown to be the most effective method in achieving specified glucose targets and preventing large fluctuations in glucose levels. This variability has been shown to be an independent risk factor for mortality. Equally important, hypoglycemia should be avoided as this is also an independent risk for mortality. Although the optimal blood glucose range for critically ill patients is yet to be defined, extremes of hypo- or hyperglycemia should be avoided. Upon ICU discharge or when the patient is able to tolerate enteral feeding, conversion to other subcutaneous insulin preparations should be initiated.

Cross-References

▶ Fluid, Electrolytes, and Nutrition in Trauma Patients
▶ Nutritional Support
▶ Trauma Intensive Care Management

References

Coester A, Neumann CR, Schmidt MI (2010) Intensive insulin therapy in severe traumatic brain injury: a randomized trial. J Trauma 68:904–911
Collier B, Diaz J, Forges R et al (2005) The impact of a normoglycemic management protocol on clinical outcomes in the trauma intensive care unit. J Parenter Enteral Nutr 29:353–358
Eriksson EA, Christianson DA, Vanderkolk WE et al (2001) Tight blood glucose control in trauma patients:

who really benefits? J Emerg Trauma Shock 4(3):359–364

Finfer S, Chittock DR, Su SY et al (2009) Intensive versus conventional glucose control in critically ill patients. N Engl J Med 360(13):1283–1297

Gibson BR, Galiatsatos P, Rabiee A et al (2009) Intensive insulin therapy confers a similar survival benefit in the burn intensive care unit to the surgical intensive care unit. Surgery 146:922–930

Honiden S, Inzucchi SE (2011) Glucose controversies in the ICU. Intensive Care Med 26(3):135–150

Krinsley JS (2004) Effect of an intensive glucose management protocol on the mortality of critically ill adult patients. Mayo Clin Proc 79:992–1000

Marik PE, Raghavan M (2004) Stress-hyperglycemia, insulin and immunomodulation in sepsis. Intensive Care Med 30:748–756

Pham TN, Warren AJ, Phan HH et al (2005) Impact of tight glycemic control in severely burned children. J Trauma 59(5):1148–1154

Van den Berghe G, Wouters PJ, Weekers F et al (2001) Intensive insulin therapy in the critically ill patients. N Engl J Med 345(19):1359–1367

Intentional Injury

▶ Interpersonal Violence

Interdisciplinary Team

Douglas Fetkenhour
Department of Physical Medicine and Rehabilitation, University of Rochester School of Medicine, Rochester, NY, USA

Synonyms

Rehabilitation team

Definition

Specialists from different disciplines working together on a common goal.

A fundamental aspect of the rehabilitation process is the interdisciplinary team. It consists of the patient, "physiatrist" (rehabilitation physician), the rehabilitation nurse, physical therapist (PT), occupational therapist (OT), speech-language therapist (SLT), social worker (SW), and recreation therapist (TR).

Patient

The rehabilitation patient is the central component of the interdisciplinary team. They provide the goals, short and long term, for what they are hoping to accomplish through the rehabilitation process. Early goals may reflect basic tasks like climbing several steps into the home or being independent in the bathroom. The later may reflect quality of life goals such as playing with their children on the floor, walking their dog, or attending their daughter's wedding.

Physician

The physiatrist (pronounced "fiz-ee-at-rist") has two main roles: providing medical management to the patient and serving as the interdisciplinary team leader.

Medical management involves treating the patient's medical comorbidities such as pain, diabetes, or heart failure. It also involves diagnosing and treating new conditions such as pulmonary embolism, spasticity, and urinary tract infection. The physiatrist pays particular attention to preventing and treating, if necessary, complications of immobility. These include venous thromboembolism, urinary and bowel incontinence, pressure ulcers, pain, and contracture.

As the interdisciplinary team leader, the physiatrist oversees the plan of care for the interventions provided by the members of the rehab team. They have the responsibility of incorporating the reports from PT, OT, SLT, rehab nursing, neuropsychology, and therapeutic recreation, recommending any modifications to the services being provided. The physiatrist assumes the ultimate responsibility for a safe discharge to the community.

Cross-References

▶ Occupational Therapist
▶ Physical Therapist
▶ Rehabilitation Nursing
▶ Social Worker

Intern

▶ Postgraduate Education

Internal Decapitation

▶ Dislocation, Atlas or Axis

Internal Hemorrhage

▶ Noncompressible Hemorrhage

International Normalized Ratio

Bryan A. Cotton[1] and Laura A. McElroy[2]
[1]Department of Surgery, Division of Acute Care
Surgery, Trauma and Critical Care, University of
Texas Health Science Center at Houston, The
University of Texas Medical School at Houston,
Houston, TX, USA
[2]Department of Anesthesiology, Critical Care
Medicine, University of Rochester Medical
Center, Rochester, NY, USA

Synonyms

INR

Definition

The International Normalized Ratio (INR) is
a standardized measure of the prothrombin time
(PT). The INR is an attempt to control the variation between PT measurements seen in different
regions in the world and even from lab to lab. This
discrepancy arises from different preparations of
tissue factor reagents, primarily thromboplastin
(phospholipids plus tissue factor), supplied by various manufacturers (Kagawa 2002). In 1985, the

International Committee for Standardization in
Hematology (ICSH) and the International Committee on Thrombosis and Hemostasis (ICTH), in
agreement with the World Health Organization
(WHO), published a method of comparing the
activity of manufactured thromboplastin reagents
to a reference preparation labeled British Comparative Thromboplastin BCT/253 (Poller 2004).
This became the INR.

In order for individual laboratories to standardize their PT measurements, thromboplastin manufacturers must provide a calibration number called
the International Sensitivity Index (ISI). The ISI is
derived by an orthogonal regression analysis comparing results from at least 20 normal and 60
stabilized patient PT values using the manufacturers thromboplastin to those of the WHOs International Reference Preparation of thromboplastin
(IRP), which is assigned a value of 1 (van den
Besselaar and Bertina 1993). BCT/253 was the
original IRP. A lower ISI indicates a more sensitive thromboplastin preparation, and the AHA and
NCCLS recommend an ISI < 1.5 to improve precision in INR measurements for patients on "low-
dose" warfarin therapy. Once the ISI is known, the
INR can then be calculated from a ratio of
the individual of interest's PT to an average
of the PT values of at least 20 normal adult subjects
called the MNPT (mean normal PT). The INR
value is thus calculated by the equation

$$INR = [individual\ PT/MNPT]^{ISI}$$

(Riley et al. 2000). Alternatively, in select
populations, the INR can be read from
a nomogram that has been constructed from
known patient ratios and ISI values (Dalere
et al. 1999). Regardless of laboratory or method
used, all practitioners should be aware that error in
any measurement is exponentially increased when
calculating the INR, underscoring the caution that
should be used in interpreting this test (Horsti et al.
2005).

Cross-References

▶ Prothrombin Time

References

Dalere GM, Coleman RW, Lum BL (1999) A graphic nomogram for warfarin dosage adjustment. Pharmacotherapy 19(4):461–467

Horsti J, Uppa H, Vilpo JA (2005) Poor agreement among prothrombin time international normalized ratio methods: comparison of seven commercial reagents. Clin Chem 51(3):553–560

Kagawa K (2002) Prothrombin time and its standardization. Rinsho Byori 50(8):779–785

Poller I (2004) International Normalized Ratios (INR): the first 20 years. J Thromb Haemost 2:849–860

Riley RS, Rowe D, Fisher LM (2000) Clinical utilization of the International Normalized Ratio (INR). J Clin Lab Anal 14(3):101–114

van den Besselaar AM, Bertina RM (1993) Multi-center study of thromboplastin calibration precision: influence of reagent species, composition, and International Sensitivity Index (ISI). Thomb Haemost 69(1):35–40

Interpersonal Violence

Norman Nicolson[1] and Marie Crandall[2]
[1]Northwestern University Feinberg School of Medicine, Chicago, IL, USA
[2]Department of Surgery, Northwestern University Feinberg School of Medicine, Chicago, IL, USA

Synonyms

Abuse; Assault; Harm; Intentional injury; Maltreatment

Definition

Interpersonal violence is a category of behavior by one individual or group that causes injury to another. In general, these behaviors and the injuries they cause are said to be intentional, to distinguish this class of trauma from those caused by unintentional mechanisms such as falls or motor vehicle collisions. Interpersonal violence does not include self-inflicted injuries or suicides, even though these are intentional injuries.

Interpersonal violence may be of interest to practitioners of trauma care for several reasons: It is a mechanism of injury for patients entering the trauma system and a potential target for injury prevention efforts. Information on management of injuries caused by interpersonal violence may be found in other sections of this encyclopedia. This entry will focus on efforts relating to violence prevention, from both a public health perspective and the perspective of the practicing trauma surgeon.

Types of Interpersonal Violence

"Interpersonal violence" is an umbrella term, including a large set of injury-causing behaviors perpetrated by one or more individuals on someone else. Each category of violence may cause a wide range of injuries, from relatively minor scrapes and bruises to lethal gunshot wounds. Although the causes and circumstances of violence are numerous and complex, an understanding of some broad categories may be instructive in considering violence prevention strategies.

Domestic violence refers to interpersonal violence occurring between members of the same household or family, as well as violence in the context of a marriage or other intimate relationship. This category includes several distinct types, including *intimate partner violence, child abuse* and *elder abuse*. Although historically domestic violence has often been assumed to be perpetrated by men on women or children in their household, interpersonal violence in the home can occur in nearly any direction, in many different kinds of relationships (McHugh and Frieze 2006).

Community violence refers to interpersonal violence occurring between friends, acquaintances, or strangers outside the context of a family or intimate relationship. This category may include violence resulting from other criminal activity, but could also occur due to escalation of disagreements between individuals in another context. This category includes *gang violence*, though it is important to note that gang members are at increased risk for becoming victims of violence as well as its perpetrators (Taylor et al. 2008).

Sexual violence refers to interpersonal violence occurring as a result of sexual assault or rape. This category may overlap with those listed above, as sexual violence could occur between intimate partners as well as acquaintances or even complete strangers (Campbell and Wasco 2005). Although sexual violence is most often perpetrated against women, men can be the targets of sexual violence, as well. Patients presenting with injuries resulting from sexual violence may require unique care and follow-up based on their traumatic experience.

Wartime violence is a category of interpersonal violence occurring in the context of a large-scale armed conflict. The victims of wartime violence may be combatants or bystanders, and even trauma surgeons not formally attached to a military service may encounter these patients in the course of their practice. Although not all trauma surgeons will encounter wartime violence, the problem is widespread in many parts of the world.

Preexisting Condition

Epidemiology of Interpersonal Violence

Approximately 50,000 deaths each year in the United States are attributable to violence, with about a quarter to a half of that number specifically attributable to interpersonal violence as opposed to suicide (Karch et al. 2011). Of course, most violent incidents do not result in a death: In 2010, more than 1.5 million nonfatal injuries in the United States were a result of assault, about 5 % of the overall burden of nonfatal injuries (Centers for Disease Control and Prevention 2012). The diversity of causes and contexts of interpersonal violence complicates the epidemiological picture, as well. A return to the previously established categories of interpersonal violence may be helpful.

Domestic violence encompasses many different types of violence and abuse, and each distinct type may present a distinct epidemiological picture. For example, approximately a quarter of intimate relationships have historically involved at least one incident of violence, with between 18 % and 30 % of women being targeted at some point in their lives (McHugh and Frieze 2006). Among US children, there were nearly 125,000 confirmed cases of violent child abuse in 2010, representing about 0.2 % of the child population (Leventhal and Krugman 2012).

Community violence is more difficult to track, since it is a catchall term meant to describe violence not occurring in a home or between family members. Even community violence is rarely committed by strangers: The overwhelming majority of homicides in the United States are perpetrated by individuals known to each other. Only 4.8 % of homicide victims were killed by a previously unknown person, although another 3.6 % of homicides occurred as a result of legal intervention in a crime (Karch et al. 2011).

Sexual violence occurs with alarming frequency. Approximately a quarter of women report either rape or attempted rape in their past, a figure confirmed by multiple research teams (Campbell and Wasco 2005). Although not all victims of rape and sexual assault will have injuries severe enough to be seen by the trauma service, trauma surgeons should be aware of the prevalence of sexual violence and its possible role in many types of intentional injury.

Wartime violence is an important component of the burden of injury worldwide, but its prevalence in a given trauma system is dependent on the political situation in the country or region. The World Health Organization estimated that one fifth of violent deaths in the year 2000 resulted from armed conflict (Brundtland 2002).

In addition to understanding the epidemiology of interpersonal violence in the general population, it is important to understand the higher risks for violent trauma among certain populations. As previously mentioned, membership in a gang increases the risk of violent injury, although this effect may be explained in part by gang members' participation in other high-risk activities (Taylor et al. 2008). As with many other health outcomes, race-related disparities exist in terms of trauma risk and outcome (Harris et al. 2012). Finally, violent trauma itself is a risk factor for future trauma, with one study showing 44 % recurrence of violent trauma within 5 years (Sims et al. 1989).

Application

Prevention of Interpersonal Violence: In-Hospital Approaches

Although many trauma surgeons prefer to focus exclusively on the medical aspects of intentional violent injury, they may be in an ideal position to recognize the underlying issues and help patients to avoid similar outcomes down the line. Specific education on how to address these difficult topics with patients may not be a part of all trauma surgery training programs, and the surgeon may feel uncomfortable in a counseling role for which he or she has not been specifically trained. However, asking a few nonjudgmental questions to give patients the opportunity to discuss their trauma may be enough to get the process started. Surgeons should especially be aware of warning signs of domestic violence, as some patients may be reluctant to admit that they were targeted by a loved one (Mattox et al. 2012).

Prevention of Interpersonal Violence: Public Approaches

Although surgeons do have an important role in recognizing interpersonal violence and helping patients avoid future trauma, the trauma surgeon may often see violently injured patients when it is already too late. Some prevention efforts must begin outside the hospital, to prevent future injuries to those who have not already been targets of violence. These efforts may come from community organizations, law enforcement agencies, or any number of other sources, and may focus on possible victims or even potential perpetrators of interpersonal violence. Some instead spotlight problems of society at large, emphasizing the importance of firearms regulation or media ratings, for example.

Although participation in these violence prevention efforts may not be a part of the trauma surgeon's traditional job description, the medical professionals charged with caring for the violently injured can be a powerful voice at the table. Trauma surgeons may be able to offer data or perspectives on trauma trends in a given area, or participate in establishing public health policy relating to interpersonal violence. Many violence prevention community programs make an explicit commitment to working with hospitals and trauma services, and trauma surgeons can be some of their strongest advocates. In the United States, the National Network of Hospital-based Violence Intervention Programs (nnhvip.org) may help interested trauma surgeons to build relationships with these organizations.

Legal and Ethical Challenges of Interpersonal Violence

Aside from the medical issues relating to the care of the violently injured patient and the challenges of preventing these injuries in the first place, interpersonal violence may pose difficulties in practice due to the victim/attacker dynamic involved. Many states require treating physicians to report suspected abuse, conflicting with the ethical principles of patient autonomy and confidentiality. However, not reporting interpersonal violence likely does a disservice to the patient, who may not receive appropriate follow-up from social services or law enforcement.

Working with law enforcement can present a challenge to the trauma surgeon, as well, since each has different goals in a typical violent injury scenario. The police officer's priority is to prevent future harm by arresting the offender, while the surgeon must focus on saving the life of the victim. These goals will not always conflict, but when disagreements do arise it may be helpful to remember these distinct roles.

Cross-References

▶ Crisis Intervention
▶ Discharge Planning
▶ Fractures
▶ Head Injury
▶ Social Worker

References

Brundtland GH (2002) From the World Health Organization. Violence prevention: a public health approach. J Am Med Assoc 288(13):1580

Campbell R, Wasco SM (2005) Understanding rape and sexual assault: 20 years of progress and future directions. [Review]. J Interpers Violence 20(1):127–131. doi:10.1177/0886260504268604

Centers for Disease Control and Prevention, National Center for Injury Prevention and Control. Web-based Injury Statistics Query and Reporting System. http://www.cdc.gov/injury/wisqars/index.html. Accessed Aug 2012

Harris AR, Fisher GA, Thomas SH (2012) Homicide as a medical outcome: racial disparity in deaths from assault in US Level I and II trauma centers. J Trauma Acute Care Surg 72(3):773–782

Karch DL, Logan J, Patel N (2011) Surveillance for violent deaths–National Violent Death Reporting System, 16 states, 2008. MMWR Surveill Summ 60(10):1–49

Leventhal JM, Krugman RD (2012) "The battered-child syndrome" 50 years later: much accomplished, much left to do. [Historical Article]. J Am Med Assoc 308(1):35–36. doi:10.1001/jama.2012.6416

Mattox KL, Moore EE, Feliciano DV (2012) Trauma, 7th edn. McGraw-Hill Professional, New York

McHugh MC, Frieze IH (2006) Intimate partner violence: new directions. [Review]. Ann N Y Acad Sci 1087:121–141. doi:10.1196/annals.1385.011

Sims DW, Bivins BA, Obeid FN, Horst HM, Sorensen VJ, Fath JJ (1989) Urban trauma: a chronic recurrent disease. J Trauma 29(7):940–946; discussion 946–947

Taylor TJ, Freng A, Esbensen FA, Peterson D (2008) Youth gang membership and serious violent victimization: the importance of lifestyles and routine activities. J Interpers Violence 23(10):1441–1464. doi:10.1177/0886260508314306

Intestinal Epithelial Apoptosis

▶ Gut Mucosal Atrophy

Intestinal Injury

▶ Gastrointestinal Injury, Anesthesia for

Intra/extraperitoneal Bladder Injury

▶ Bladder Rupture (Intra/Extraperitoneal)

Intra-abdominal Hypertension

▶ Abdominal Compartment Syndrome
▶ Abdominal Compartment Syndrome as a Complication of Care

Intra-abdominal Hypertension with Organ Dysfunction

▶ Acute Abdominal Compartment Syndrome in Trauma

Intra-arterial Line

▶ Monitoring of Trauma Patients During Anesthesia

Intra-arterial Shunting

▶ Shunt, Vascular

Intra-articular Fracture of the Distal Tibia

▶ Tibial Pilon Fractures

Intracerebral Hematoma

▶ Traumatic Brain Injury, Intensive Care Unit Management

Intracerebral Hemorrhage

▶ Traumatic Brain Injury, Anesthesia for

Intracranial Hemorrhage

▶ Traumatic Brain Injury, Anesthesia for
▶ Neurotrauma, Anesthesia Management
▶ Neurotrauma, Anticoagulation Considerations

Intracranial Hypertension

▶ Neurotrauma Management, Osmotherapy
▶ Neurotrauma, Multimodal Neuromonitoring

Intracranial Injury

▶ Neurotrauma, Introduction

Intracranial Pressure

▶ Neurotrauma, Pharmacological Considerations
▶ Neurotrauma, Multimodal Neuromonitoring
▶ Traumatic Brain Injury, Intensive Care Unit Management

Intracranial Pressure Monitoring

▶ Neurotrauma, Multimodal Neuromonitoring

Intraluminal Shunting

▶ Shunt, Vascular

Intraoperative Cell Salvage

▶ Autologous Donation

Intraosseous Device

Frank K. Butler
Department of the Army, Committee on Tactical Combat Casualty Care, U.S. Army Institute of Surgical Research, Fort Sam Houston, TX, USA
Department of the Army, Prehospital Trauma Care, Joint Trauma System, U.S. Army Institute of Surgical Research, Fort Sam Houston, TX, USA

Synonyms

IO device

Definition

IV access may be difficult to obtain in casualties who are in shock. It may also be difficult to accomplish for individuals who are not practiced in this skill. Intraosseous (IO) devices offer an alternative route for administering fluids and medications in these situations. The use of intraosseous devices to gain rapid and reliable vascular access was noted by Beekley and his colleagues to one of the significant lessons learned in Afghanistan and Iraq (Beekley et al. 2007).

The Pyng FAST-1 and the EZ-IO have been the most widely used IO devices in the US military to date (Butler et al. 2010). The FAST-1 delivers fluid and medications through the bone marrow of the sternal manubrium. Using the sternal notch as a reference point, an adhesive patch is applied that provides a target area for insertion. The device is then aligned with the target, and firm, steady pressure is applied. This action inserts a small, stainless steel tip connected

---

Frank K. Butler has retired.

to an infusion tube into the marrow of the manubrium. This technique makes the FAST-1 usable in low-light environments. A clear plastic dome attaches via a Velcro ring, keeping the site clean and visible (Butler et al. 2010).

The EZ-IO device has also been gaining increasing acceptance by special operations troops in Iraq and Afghanistan. This device was not originally approved for sternal IO access. This was a problem in that the tibial area initially recommended for the EZ-IO may be injured or missing in combat casualties. The device may now, however, be used on the sternum or at six extremity sites. This device is small, lightweight, and easy to use. Both manual and battery-powered options are available. Disadvantages noted by combat medical personnel with the EZ-IO are the need to protect the infusion needle during transport and significant pain when fluids are administered at tibial sites (Butler et al. 2010). Care must be taken to ensure that the correct site for the IO needle chosen is used.

The intraosseous route of vascular access has been used widely in Iraq and Afghanistan and has proven a valuable option for the combat medic and corpsman (Butler et al. 2007).

Preexisting Condition

Need for vascular access.

Cross-References

▶ Adjuncts to Transfusion: Antifibrinolytics
▶ CASEVAC
▶ Damage Control Resuscitation
▶ Damage Control Resuscitation, Military Trauma
▶ Exsanguination Transfusion
▶ Fluid, Electrolytes, and Nutrition in Trauma Patients
▶ FP24
▶ Hemorrhage
▶ Hemostatic Adjunct
▶ Hypothermia
▶ IED (Improvised Explosive Device)

▶ Monitoring of Trauma Patients During Anesthesia
▶ Packed Red Blood Cells
▶ Plasma Transfusion in Trauma
▶ Rule of Tens
▶ Shock
▶ Shock Management in Trauma
▶ TACEVAC
▶ Tactical Combat Casualty Care
▶ Tranexamic Acid
▶ Whole Blood

References

Beekley AC, Starnes BW, Sebesta JA (2007) Lessons learned from modern military surgery. Surg Clin N Am 87:157–184
Butler FK, Holcomb JB, Giebner SG, McSwain NE, Bagian J (2007) Tactical combat casualty care 2007: evolving concepts and battlefield experience. Milit Med 172(S):1–19
Butler FK, Giebner SD, McSwain N, Salomone J, Pons P (eds) (2010) Prehospital Trauma Life Support Manual. Seventh Edition – Military Version. Mosby JEMS, Elsevier, St. Louis, MO

Intraosseous Vascular Access

▶ Vascular Access in Trauma Patients

Intraparenchymal Hemorrhage

▶ Neurotrauma, Anticoagulation Considerations

Intravascular Shunting (Temporary)

▶ Shunt, Vascular

Intravenous Access (IV)

▶ Vascular Access in Trauma Patients

Intravenous Line

▶ Vascular Access in Trauma Patients

Intraventricular Hemorrhage

▶ Traumatic Brain Injury, Anesthesia for

Intrinsic PEEP

▶ Auto-PEEP

Invasive Catheters

▶ Monitoring of Trauma Patients During Anesthesia

Invasive Mechanical Ventilation

▶ Mechanical Ventilation, Conventional
▶ Ventilatory Management of Trauma Patients

Invasive Positive Pressure Ventilation

▶ Mechanical Ventilation, Conventional

Invasive Ventilation

▶ Mechanical Ventilation, Conventional

IO Device

▶ Intraosseous Device

IPAC

▶ Infection Control

Irreversible Apneic Coma

▶ Brain Death

Irreversible Coma

▶ Brain Death
▶ Neurotrauma, Death by Neurological Criteria

Ischemic Bone Necrosis

▶ Avascular Necrosis of the Femoral Head

Ischemic Contracture

▶ Compartment Syndrome of the Leg

ISR Rule of Tens

▶ Rule of Tens

Joint Contractures

▶ Contractures

Joint Theater Trauma Registry (JTTR)

▶ Joint Trauma Registry
▶ Joint Trauma System (JTS)

Joint Theater Trauma System (JTTS)

▶ Joint Trauma System (JTS)

Joint Trauma Registry

Mary Ann Spott[1] and Donald H. Jenkins[2,3]
[1]U.S. Army Institute of Surgical Research, JBSA Fort Sam Houston, TX, USA
[2]Department of Surgery, Division of Trauma, Critical Care and Emergency General Surgery, Saint Marys Hospital, Rochester, MN, USA
[3]Mayo Clinic, Rochester, MN, USA

Synonyms

Department of Defense Trauma Registry (DoDTR); Joint Theater Trauma Registry (JTTR); Joint Trauma Registry (JTR)

Definition

JTTR – The Joint Theater Trauma Registry is the theater component of the Department of Defense (DoD) Trauma Registry (DoDTR). The DoDTR is the official DoD tri-service trauma registry capturing all battle and non-battle injuries during peacetime and wartime. This is the first comprehensive registry of injury in the combat zone (Eastridge 2009).

A "registry" is a compilation of numerous data points, beginning with essential demographic information about an injured person, such as their name, an identifying patient number, date of birth, age, and gender. Further, it includes significant information about the type of injury sustained, the mechanism of injury (blunt, penetrating, explosion), and the use of injury prevention measures (seat belt, helmet use, protective eyewear, body armor, etc.).

Organ injuries are further documented using an internationally accepted standard classification by degree of organ injury (scale of 0–6) (Champion 2010) ranging from uninjured to organ essentially destroyed with high risk of death conferred. These judgments are made by highly trained professional medical chart abstractors and registrars based upon their review of the medical record (operative notes, CT scan reports, etc.). Combined with essential vital signs, Glasgow coma scale scores and demographics, the registry is used to calculate probability of survival.

© Springer-Verlag Berlin Heidelberg 2015
P.J. Papadakos, M.L. Gestring (eds.), *Encyclopedia of Trauma Care*,
DOI 10.1007/978-3-642-29613-0

Typically, a registry such as this is used primarily for performance improvement purposes and benchmarking. Trends in morbidity and complications can be monitored over time and thresholds set that should cause action to be taken by the trauma team to mitigate further morbidity and mortality (performance improvement) (Eastridge 2006). Regular reports (weekly, monthly, annually, etc.) can also be generated and become an important component, especially in the combat setting, of intelligence gathering (if suddenly casualties' information is entered into the registry showing a new or unprecedented mechanism of injury) (Ennis 2008; Ritenour 2008). Retrospective research can also be generated using an approved methodology and following guidelines by an appropriate Institutional Review Board (Murray 2009; Plotkin 2008; Spinella 2008).

To date, the DoDTR has more than 400 fields of entry on every casualty and well over 25,000 unique records. At each echelon of care, new and updated data is entered and adds to that unique record longitudinally, such that the casualty's entire clinical care is captured across all echelons of care, from care in the field, evacuation, forward surgery, critical care air transport, and care rendered in the continental USA.

Cross-References

▶ Case Fatality Rate (CFR)
▶ Forward Surgical Teams and Echelons of Care

References

Champion HR, Holcomb JB, Lawnick MM, Kelliher T, Spott MA, Galarneau MR, Jenkins DH, West SA, Dye J, Wade CE, Eastridge BJ, Blackbourne LH, Shair EK (2010) Improved characterization of combat injury. J Trauma 68(5):1139–1150. doi:10.1097/TA.0b013e3181d86a0d, PMID:20453770
Eastridge BJ, Jenkins D, Flaherty S, Schiller H, Holcomb JB (2006) Trauma system development in a theater of war: experiences from operation Iraqi freedom and operation enduring freedom. J Trauma 61(6):1366–1372. doi:10.1097/01.ta.0000245894.78941.90, discussion 1372-3 PMID: 17159678
Eastridge BJ, Costanzo G, Jenkins D, Spott MA, Wade C, Greydanus D, Flaherty S, Rappold J, Dunne J, Holcomb JB, Blackbourne LH (2009) Impact of joint theater trauma system initiatives on battlefield injury outcomes. Am J Surg 198(6):852–857. doi:10.1016/j.amjsurg.2009.04.029, PMID:19969141
Ennis JL, Chung KK, Renz EM, Barillo DJ, Albrecht MC, Jones JA, Blackbourne LH, Cancio LC, Eastridge BJ, Flaherty SF, Dorlac WC, Kelleher KS, Wade CE, Wolf SE, Jenkins DH, Holcomb JB (2008) Joint Theater Trauma System implementation of burn resuscitation guidelines improves outcomes in severely burned military casualties. J Trauma 64(Suppl 2): S146–S151. doi:10.1097/TA.0b013e318160b44c discussion S151-2. PMID:18376158
Murray CK, Wilkins K, Molter NC, Yun HC, Dubick MA, Spott MA, Jenkins D, Eastridge B, Holcomb JB, Blackbourne LH, Hospenthal DR (2009) Infections in combat casualties during operations Iraqi and enduring freedom. J Trauma-Inj Infect Crit Care 66(Suppl 4): S138–S144
Plotkin AJ, Wade CE, Jenkins DH, Smith KA, Noe JC, Park MS, Perkins JG, Holcomb JB (2008) A reduction in clot formation rate and strength assessed by thrombelastography is indicative of transfusion requirements in patients with penetrating injuries. J Trauma 64(Suppl 2):S64–S68. doi:10.1097/TA.0b013e318160772d, PMID:18376174
Ritenour AE, Dorlac WC, Fang R, Woods T, Jenkins DH, Flaherty SF, Wade CE, Holcomb JB (2008) Complications after fasciotomy revision and delayed compartment release in combat patients. J Trauma 64(Suppl 2):S153–S161. doi:10.1097/TA.0b013e3181607750, discussion S161-2. PMID:18376159
Spinella PC, Perkins JG, Grathwohl KW, Repine T, Beekley AC, Sebesta J, Jenkins D, Azarow K, Holcomb JB (2008) 31st CSH Research Working Group. Fresh whole blood transfusions in coalition military, foreign national, and enemy combatant patients during operation Iraqi freedom at a U.S. combat support hospital. World J Surg 32(1):2–6. doi:10.1007/s00268-007-9201-5, Epub 2007 Nov 09. PMID:17990028

Joint Trauma Registry (JTR)

▶ Joint Trauma Registry
▶ Joint Trauma System (JTS)

Joint Trauma System (JTS)

Mary Ann Spott[1] and Donald H. Jenkins[2,3]
[1]U.S. Army Institute of Surgical Research,
JBSA Fort Sam Houston, TX, USA
[2]Department of Surgery, Division of Trauma,
Critical Care and Emergency General Surgery,
Saint Marys Hospital, Rochester, MN, USA
[3]Mayo Clinic, Rochester, MN, USA

Synonyms

Department of Defense Trauma Registry
(DoDTR); Department of Defense Trauma
System (DoDTS); Joint Theater Trauma Registry
(JTTR); Joint Theater Trauma System (JTTS);
Joint Trauma Registry (JTR)

Definition

Joint Trauma System (JTS) – the Department of
Defense (DoD) authority for the DoD trauma
system responsible for trauma system development, trauma system performance improvement,
trauma data collection, and trauma registry translational research.

The JTS was a notional creation, first ad hoc
and then formally adopted that had its inception
in 2004 in Iraq. Dr. Brian Eastridge was assigned
as Trauma Director for the U.S. Army 2nd
Medical Brigade in Iraq and gathered Iraq-wide
injury data and created an epidemiologic model
of injury in combat. Under the guidance of
Dr. John Holcomb at the U.S. Army Institute of
Surgical Research (ISR), Eastridge presented his
findings to the Army Surgeon General (SG).
Holcomb combined his own thoughts on his visits
to the Theater of Operations as Trauma Consultant to the SG and proposed a plan to formalize
a trauma system in the combat zone.

While initiating the JTTR (Joint Theater
Trauma Registry), which is the theater
component of the Department of Defense (DoD)

Trauma Registry (DoDTR) at the ISR, Holcomb
petitioned the U.S. Air Force SG to appoint
Dr. Donald Jenkins, serving in theater at the
time at Balad Air Base as trauma director, as
formal inaugural Trauma Director to the Army's
44th Medical Command.

Holcomb was also able to get six Army Nurses
dedicated to this initial project and, in theater from
November 2004 through May of 2005, they created
the first in-theater injury data repository, created
the first JTTR history and physical examination
documentation tool and the first five practice management guidelines for care of the injured combatant. By February of 2005, Dr. Doug Robb, U.S.
Central Command Surgeon, and Holcomb were so
convinced as to the success of the Joint Theater
Trauma System (JTTS) that US CENTCOM formally adopted the concept, expanded it to a truly
tri-service initiative, and applied the principles
developed across the entire CENTCOM Area of
Operations (Eastridge et al. 2009).

Formal training of the JTTS nurses and
subsequent directors was undertaken and a central
Joint Trauma System Office (JTS) was established
by Holcomb at the ISR, with Jenkins as the first
JTS Director and Mary Ann Spott as the first Program Manager. DoD-level funding was obtained,
formal adoption of JTR and JTS across the DoD
ensued, and eventually was adopted as a Defense
Center of Excellence for Trauma and Injury in
2013. Department of Defense Trauma System
(DoDTS) is now applicable across all theaters of
operation, including the continental United States.

As the first comprehensive trauma system and
registry of injury in the combat zone, the JTTR/
JTR/DoDTR allows trends in morbidity and
complications to be monitored over time and
thresholds set that should cause action to be
taken by the trauma team to mitigate further morbidity and mortality (performance improvement)
(Eastridge et al. 2006). Regular reports (weekly,
monthly, annually, etc.) can also be generated and
become an important component, especially in the
combat setting, of intelligence gathering (if suddenly casualties' information is entered into
the registry showing a new or unprecedented

J

mechanism of injury) (Ennis et al. 2008; Ritenour et al. 2008). Retrospective research can also be generated using an approved methodology and following guidelines by an appropriate Institutional Review Board (Murray et al. 2009; Plotkin et al. 2008; Spinella et al. 2008).

To date, the DoDTR, which is the linchpin of the DoDTS, has more than 400 fields of entry on every casualty and well over 40,000 unique records. Further work to better characterize combat-related injury also sets this registry apart from similar civilian registries (Champion et al. 2010). At each echelon of care, new and updated data is entered and adds to that unique record longitudinally, such that the casualty's entire clinical care is captured across all echelons of care, from care in the field, evacuation, forward surgery, critical care air transport, and care rendered in the continental USA.

Cross-References

▶ Joint Trauma Registry

References

Champion HR, Holcomb JB, Lawnick MM, Kelliher T, Spott MA, Galarneau MR, Jenkins DH, West SA, Dye J, Wade CE, Eastridge BJ, Blackbourne LH, Shair EK (2010) Improved characterization of combat injury. J Trauma 68(5):1139–1150. doi:10.1097/TA.0b013e3181d86a0d. PMID:20453770

Eastridge BJ, Jenkins D, Flaherty S, Schiller H, Holcomb JB (2006) Trauma system development in a theater of war: experiences from Operation Iraqi Freedom and Operation Enduring Freedom. J Trauma 61(6):1366–72; discussion 1372–1373. doi:10.1097/01.ta.0000245894.78941.90. PMID:17159678

Eastridge BJ, Costanzo G, Jenkins D, Spott MA, Wade C, Greydanus D, Flaherty S, Rappold J, Dunne J, Holcomb JB, Blackbourne LH (2009) Impact of joint theater trauma system initiatives on battlefield injury outcomes. Am J Surg 198(6):852–857. doi:10.1016/j.amjsurg.2009.04.029. PMID:19969141

Ennis JL, Chung KK, Renz EM, Barillo DJ, Albrecht MC, Jones JA, Blackbourne LH, Cancio LC, Eastridge BJ, Flaherty SF, Dorlac WC, Kelleher KS, Wade CE, Wolf SE, Jenkins DH, Holcomb JB (2008) Joint Theater Trauma System implementation of burn resuscitation guidelines improves outcomes in severely burned military casualties. J Trauma 64(2 Suppl):S146–151; discussion S151–152. doi:10.1097/TA.0b013e318160b44c. PMID:18376158

Murray CK, Wilkins K, Molter NC, Yun HC, Dubick MA, Spott MA, Jenkins D, Eastridge B, Holcomb JB, Blackbourne LH, Hospenthal DR (2009) Infections in combat casualities during Operations Iraqi and Enduring Freedom. J Trauma 66(4 suppl):S138–S144

Plotkin AJ, Wade CE, Jenkins DH, Smith KA, Noe JC, Park MS, Perkins JG, Holcomb JB (2008) A reduction in clot formation rate and strength assessed by thrombelastography is indicative of transfusion requirements in patients with penetrating injuries. J Trauma 64(2 Suppl):S64–S68. doi:10.1097/TA.0b013e318160772d. PMID:18376174

Ritenour AE, Dorlac WC, Fang R, Woods T, Jenkins DH, Flaherty SF, Wade CE, Holcomb JB (2008) Complications after fasciotomy revision and delayed compartment release in combat patients. J Trauma. 64(2 Suppl):S153–161; discussion S161–162. doi:10.1097/TA.0b013e3181607750. PMID:18376159

Spinella PC, Perkins JG, Grathwohl KW, Repine T, Beekley AC, Sebesta J, Jenkins D, Azarow K, Holcomb JB, 31st CSH Research Working Group (2008) Fresh whole blood transfusions in coalition military, foreign national, and enemy combatant patients during Operation Iraqi Freedom at a U.S. combat support hospital. World J Surg 32(1):2–6. doi:10.1007/s00268-007-9201-5. Epub 2007 Nov 09. PMID:17990028

Jugular Venous Oxygen Saturation

▶ Traumatic Brain Injury, Intensive Care Unit Management

Jumped Facets

▶ Dislocation, Facets

Jumper Injuries

▶ Falls from Height

Junctional Pressure Device

▶ Hemostatic Adjunct

K

Kaolin Cephalin Clotting Time

▶ Partial Thromboplastin Time

KccT

▶ Partial Thromboplastin Time

Kidney Failure

▶ Acute Kidney Injury

Kidney Injury

▶ Abdominal Solid Organ Injury, Anesthesia for

Kidney Insult

▶ Abdominal Solid Organ Injury, Anesthesia for

Killed in Action

▶ Case Fatality Rate (CFR)

Knee Dislocations

James Stannard and Shaun Fay Steeby
Department of Orthopaedics, Missouri
Orthopaedic Institute, University Hospital,
University of Missouri, Columbia, SC, USA

Synonyms

Ligamentous knee injury; Multiligamentous knee injury

Definition

Knee dislocations describe an injury pattern where the articulation between the femur and the tibia is disrupted. There are several ligaments both inside and outside the knee capsule, which are essential to the stability of the knee under weight-bearing conditions. When this articulation is disrupted, two or more of these ligaments are disrupted. While knee dislocations are relatively rare, they have a high incidence of associated injuries including damage to surrounding nerves, blood vessels, and bones. They may also have extensive soft tissue injuries. Knee dislocations often present with the articulation in correct alignment, as many will spontaneously reduce shortly after the injury. Because of their association with limb-threatening complications and associated injuries, early diagnosis and

© Springer-Verlag Berlin Heidelberg 2015
P.J. Papadakos, M.L. Gestring (eds.), *Encyclopedia of Trauma Care*,
DOI 10.1007/978-3-642-29613-0

management are essential. It is not uncommon for patients with knee dislocations to report long-term instability, stiffness, and pain.

Preexisting Conditions

Anatomic Considerations

The anterior cruciate ligament (ACL) – resists anterior translation of the tibia with respect to the femur and is usually disrupted in dislocations, although there have been case reports of dislocations occurring with an intact ACL.

The posterior cruciate ligament (PCL) – resists posterior translation of the tibia with relation to the femur and is usually disrupted in dislocations, although there have also been case reports of dislocations with an intact PCL.

The posteromedial corner (PMC) – the most important components are the medial collateral ligament (MCL), posterior oblique ligament, and the semimembranosus.

The posterolateral corner (PLC) – the most important components are the lateral collateral ligament (LCL) or fibular collateral ligament (FCL), the popliteofibular ligament, and the popliteus.

Injury Mechanism

The way in which knee dislocations are sustained is variable and may range from low-velocity to high-energy injuries. Traditionally, most knee dislocations were associated with high-energy trauma including motor vehicle collisions, motorcycle accidents, and falls from a significant height. More recently, the literature documents cases of patients who sustain knee dislocations from standing height falls, particularly in those patients who are morbidly obese. Additionally, subluxation and frank dislocation can occur in a sports setting. While single ligament injuries such as the ACL tear are common in sports, they represent a spectrum of injury which can range from mild ligament sprain to tear. They may include an injury involving one or several ligaments which impart stability to the knee.

Knee Dislocations, Table 1 Schenck classification

Classification	Injury type
KD I	Multiligamentous injury with either cruciate ligament intact
KD II	ACL injury with instability
	PCL injury with instability
	Collateral ligaments intact
KDIIIM	ACL injury with instability
	PCL injury with instability
	Posteromedial corner injury with instability
KDIIIL	ACL injury with instability
	PCL injury with instability
	Posterolateral corner injury with instability
KD IV	ACL injury with instability
	PCL injury with instability
	Posteromedial corner injury with instability
	Posterolateral corner injury with instability
KD V	Periarticular fracture dislocation of the knee

Injury Classification

The Schenck anatomic classification system is the most commonly used system to describe the extent of these injuries (Table 1).

Application

Associated Injuries

Considering that knee dislocations may be related to high-energy trauma, other traumatic injuries such as head injury, major organ damage, and or other musculoskeletal trauma are not uncommon and should always be suspected. Even more common are associated injuries occurring directly in conjunction with the knee dislocation itself.

There are many cartilaginous at risk structures in the knee. Meniscal tears may occur in the setting of traumatic injuries, but are not observed as frequently as one would think. When the tears occur, they are most commonly peripheral and amenable to repair. Contusion and damage to the articular cartilage can occur and may result in areas of full-thickness cartilage loss.

Vascular injuries can be far more devastating. Older literature reports up to 40 % of knee dislocations sustain an injury to the popliteal artery. Contemporary literature suggests an incidence closer to 10 %. The artery's proximity to the joint and anatomic relation to the adductor hiatus and the soleus arch are the predisposing factors increasing the odds of injury. These injuries represent a spectrum and may range from a temporary occlusion that resolves with reduction, vasospasm, or even a tear through the intima or the vessel wall itself. Diligent attention is required to fully evaluate the patient and rule out a vascular injury – ischemia for greater than 8 h is associated with an increased risk of limb loss. Vasospasm or occlusion after intimal tear may occur in a delayed fashion following reduction and initial management; as such, it is essential to continue to monitor vascular status over the first 48 h following dislocation (Stannard et al. 2004).

The incidence of nerve injury varies from 10 % to 35 % within the literature. The most commonly effected nerve is the peroneal nerve which runs with the popliteal artery posterior to the knee joint and then around the fibular neck. The nerve injury may result from hypoxia if there is an associated vascular injury or more commonly is a result of a stretch to the nerve. Tibial nerve injury can occur but is much less frequent.

Fractures may occur to any of the surrounding osseous structures: the tibia, the femur, or the patella. Tibial plateau fractures are by far the most common. Smaller avulsion type fractures are common particularly at the proximal fibula which results in posterolateral instability. Additionally, patients who present with a medial tibial plateau fracture should be evaluated as though they have sustained a knee dislocation, as they carry a higher risk of vascular and ligamentous injury similar to dislocations.

Acute Care

The first step to treating a knee dislocation is always a thorough examination. Patients with knee dislocations often have other associated traumatic injuries, so they should be evaluated using standard advanced trauma life support protocol ensuring that obvious limb deformity does not distract the care provider from assessing airway, breathing, and circulation first and foremost.

The next crucial step is inspection of the affected limb. It is very easy to miss a knee dislocation diagnosis in a trauma patient because there is often no associated deformity. Many will have spontaneously reduced prior to the patient's presentation in the ER, and the only residual signs may be effusion (variable due to capsule tear), ecchymosis, and pain. Less commonly, these injuries may demonstrate gross malalignment and or violation of the nearby soft tissue. A dimple sign may be visualized in patients when the medial femoral condyle has buttonholed through the anteromedial joint capsule – this may indicate an irreducible dislocation (Peskun et al. 2010).

All patients should be evaluated with a thorough vascular exam, which includes palpating for a dorsalis pedis and posterior tibial artery pulse distally along with assessing color, warmth, and capillary refill. An abnormal pulse exam is the best indicator of a vascular injury. Ankle-Brachial Index (ABI) is a commonly accepted reliable test which is performed to assess the perfusion pressure of the lower limb compared to the uninjured upper limb. The ABI is measured using a manual blood pressure cuff applied to the affected limb at the level of the ankle. The cuff is inflated, and a Doppler ultrasound probe is used to determine the systolic pressure in the limb. This value is then divided by the systolic pressure in the patient's upper limb. An ABI of less than 0.9 is worrisome for possible arterial injury or occlusion and can be used as an indicator to pursue more invasive testing such as angiography, CT angiogram, or MR angiography. It should be noted that peripheral vascular disease can also result in an abnormal ABI (Stannard et al. 2004).

Neurologic injury may occur as a result of the trauma itself or may evolve with developing compartment syndrome. Neurologic exam including evaluation of motor and sensory

K

function of the tibial and peroneal nerves should be carefully recorded. Care should be taken to perform serial compartment exams and to maintain a high index of suspicion for the onset of compartment syndrome, which can have devastating consequences if missed.

In order to classify the injury and to determine what sort of reconstructive efforts will be needed to restore stability, a detailed ligamentous exam is required. The ligaments of the knee are most easily examined within the acute period immediately following the accident. A thorough ligament exam should be performed once and in a gentle fashion including a Lachman, anterior and posterior drawer, exam of varus and valgus stress at 30° of flexion, dial test, anterior drawer in external rotation, and an evaluation of the integrity of the extensor mechanism. An MRI is a useful tool in the diagnosis and classification of these injuries when used in conjunction with physical exam (Stannard and Bauer 2012). Recent literature indicates that MRI alone may be interpreted incorrectly, resulting in diagnosis of injuries that are not real and have no associated instability (Stannard and Fanelli 2015).

Initial Management

If the knee is dislocated, it should be reduced as soon as possible. If the vascular exam or ABI are abnormal, vascular consultation and advanced imaging should be obtained. In most cases, the knee is sufficiently stable following reduction with a simple knee immobilizer. Spanning external fixation is reserved for open dislocations, vascular injuries, and knees that redislocate after reduction (Peskun et al. 2010).

Closed reduction is typically undertaken with the aid of conscious sedation and accomplished through gentle traction – countertraction and application of force directed to correct the deformity. Neurovascular examinations should be repeated immediately following reduction and again every 2 h for approximately 48 h. This will allow observation of return of neurologic function from stretch injuries and could help the examiner pick up on any vascular incident such as thrombosis that could occur within this acute window.

Timing of Surgical Intervention

Fracture fixation is typically performed within 1 week of the injury. Each injury is unique, however, and the condition of the soft tissue envelope should be considered when planning surgery. If there is significant soft tissue trauma as evidenced by taut, shiny skin, multiple fracture blisters, or frank open wounds, it may be essential to delay surgical intervention for 1–2 weeks, until the skin is more supple and less inflamed. This is frequently evaluated in terms of whether the skin can wrinkle. This step is crucial to ensure the overlying skin will be able to tolerate an incision.

Ligament reconstruction is typically delayed for 3–4 weeks following the injury. In ideal conditions, the patient may have been working on gentle range of motion in a brace in order to improve postoperative outcomes in terms of maximal flexion and extension.

Operative Considerations

Nonoperative treatment was frequently utilized in the past in the hopes that immobilization would allow enough time for the soft tissues to heal and for scar tissue to form which could restore knee stability. This treatment approach led to high complication rates including residual instability, stiffness, and poor patient satisfaction. Nonoperative management is now reserved only for patients who are not fit enough to tolerate surgery (Peskun et al. 2010). Extensive academic investigation has demonstrated that surgical reconstruction of complex ligamentous knee injuries leads to superior outcomes with regard to stability, motion, and return to work and sport.

It has been shown that the poor vascularity of ligamentous tissue results in poor outcomes when the damaged tissues are surgically repaired. Therefore, reconstruction, and not repair, has become the cornerstone of treatment. There are two kinds of tissue available for reconstruction. Autograft is the patient's own tendinous tissue harvested from a part of the body that is away from the surgical site. Hamstrings and patellar tendon are the most common sites of autograft harvest. Autograft is the preferred graft tissue for single ligament reconstructions in young patients. Allograft is tissue which is harvested from a cadaver and follows strict sterilization protocols. In patients with multiple ligaments that require reconstruction, allograft is usually the most reasonable reconstruction option. This limits morbidity such as weakness or pain at the donor site. Additionally, allograft may be a good option for older, less active patients undergoing single ligament reconstruction, as this patient population has shown similar outcomes with both allograft and autograft.

ACL reconstruction is performed arthroscopically with the intention of recreating the anatomic relationships as close to their native origins and insertions as possible. Multiple options exist including single- or double- bundle reconstruction. Graft fixation may be accomplished with bioabsorbable screw fixation or suspensory fixation (Fanelli et al. 2011).

PCL reconstruction is once again focused on recreating the anatomic origin and insertion in order to mimic the biomechanical constraints imparted by the original ligaments (Fanelli et al. 2011). Surgical techniques include both single- and double- bundle reconstructions; the procedure can be performed using an all-inside arthroscopic technique with specialized drill guides and portals that are designed to create bone tunnels that anatomically recreate the tibial insertion. Another technique involves an open approach to the posterior tibia through a medially based approach. The soft tissue and the neurovascular structures are meticulously protected, while the sulcus in which the PCL inserts on the tibia is directly visualized. A trough is made where a bone block is secured to the posterior tibia, and the graft limbs are passed through the posterior capsule and into the knee joint. The graft limbs are drawn into arthroscopically created anatomic femoral tunnels under the aid of arthroscopic visualization (Stannard and Bauer 2012). Protection of the surrounding neurovascular structures is essential regardless of the technique utilized.

Medial-sided reconstructions are performed in an open fashion. The PMC is complex, and reconstruction involves placing the graft in positions to recreate both the superficial and deep medial collateral ligaments and the posterior oblique ligament.

Lateral-sided reconstruction is also undertaken using an open extra-articular approach. The modified two-tailed graft orientation is designed to recreate not only the lateral collateral ligament but also the popliteus tendon and the popliteofibular ligament. The graft tension is dependent on finding the isometric point.

When tackling reconstruction of multiple ligaments, the order of reconstruction and whether to conduct it in a staged fashion is largely determined by surgeon preference. Some undertake reconstruction of all ligaments simultaneously. It has also been found to be effective to undertake reconstruction of everything except the ACL initially – followed with a staged reconstruction at a later date – coupled with arthroscopic lysis of adhesions (Peskun et al. 2010).

The use of a hinged external fixator is a useful adjunct in surgical treatment as it allows the patient to perform range of motion exercises while providing isometric stability to limit the development of graft laxity.

Rehabilitation

During the postoperative period, a strict rehabilitation protocol is essential to optimize outcomes. Ice should be used at least three times daily to help keep down swelling and improve the patient's comfort level. There are two schools of thought with regard to postoperative motion. Some surgeons prefer to start gentle non-weight-bearing range of motion immediately postoperatively. In these circumstances, a continuous passive motion (CPM) machine is helpful. Some surgeons prefer to delay range of motion acutely. As a general rule, patients should not remain immobilized for more than 4 weeks as prolonged immobilization increases the risk of pain and arthrofibrosis. A stationary bike is a useful tool in improving knee flexion. Isometric quadricep exercises and closed chain strengthening are the key elements of rehab (Stannard and Fanelli 2015).

It is important for the surgeon to understand the timeline of graft incorporation. For the first 3 months, the graft strength diminishes as the tissues begin to be incorporated and the microstructure undergoes reorganization. The grafts are at

K

their weakest 3 months following reconstruction. At 6 months, the grafts have incorporated enough to be of similar strength to native soft tissues.

Outcomes

The complex nature of these injuries imparts a rather high complication rate. Instability of one or more of the reconstructed ligaments is the most common complication following dislocation with and incidence >40 %. Hinged external fixation has been associated with a decrease in this complication. Arthrofibrosis is the 2nd most common complication following knee dislocation. This is commonly treated with manipulation under anesthesia and arthroscopic lysis of adhesions (Stannard and Fanelli 2015).

Patients may experience long-term discomfort ranging from nagging and mild pain to severe disabling pain following knee dislocation and surgical treatment. The literature suggests that 25–68 % patients suffer from some chronic long-term pain.

Studies have shown that most patients are able to return to work following these injuries; however, the severity of the injuries means that some may have to return to a job with lower physical demand (Peskun et al. 2010). Patients who receive treatment of their dislocations acutely are more likely to return to their previous level of work and sport than those who under reconstruction for chronic instability.

Infection and wound healing complications may occur as a result of the injury or the surgical intervention. Open dislocations have up to a 42 % wound infection rate. Reconstruction following knee dislocations has a reported infection rate of up to 12.5 %. Wound healing problems may be more frequent with early surgery and aggressive postoperative motion rehabilitation protocols.

Heterotopic ossification may occur frequently following traumatic dislocation, particularly in cases where the patient had a traumatic brain injury. It occurs most commonly medially and posteriorly.

Posttraumatic osteoarthrosis is likely an underreported complication following dislocation.

Cross-References

▶ ABCDE of Trauma Care
▶ ATV Injuries
▶ Compartment Syndrome of the Leg
▶ Compartment Syndrome, Acute
▶ Damage Control Orthopedics
▶ Distal Femur Fractures
▶ Extremity Injury
▶ Fasciotomy
▶ Femoral Shaft Fractures
▶ High Velocity
▶ Motor Vehicle Crash Injury
▶ Motorcycle-Related Injuries
▶ Open Fractures
▶ Orthopedic Trauma, Anesthesia for
▶ Pedestrian Injuries
▶ Pedestrian Struck
▶ Principles of External Fixation
▶ Tibial Fractures
▶ Vacuum Dressing

References

Fanelli GC, Stannard JP, Stuart MJ, MacDonald PB, Marx RG, Whelan DB, Boyd JL, Levy BA (2011) Management of complex ligamentous knee injuries. Instr Course Lect 60:523–535

Peskun C, Levy B, Fanelli G, Stannard J, Stuart M, MacDonald P, Marx R, Boyd J, Whelan D (2010) Diagnosis and management of knee dislocations. Physician Sports Med 38(4):101–111

Stannard JP, Bauer KL (2012) Current concepts in knee dislocations: PCL, ACL, and medial sided injuries. J Knee Surg 25(4):287–294

Stannard JP, Fanelli G (2015) Chapter 31: Knee dislocations and ligamentous injuries. In: Surgical treatment of orthopaedic trauma, 2nd edn. Thieme, New York/Stuttgart

Stannard JP, Sheils TM, Lopez-Ben RR, McGwin G Jr, Volgas DA (2004) Vascular injuries in knee dislocations: the role of physical exam in determining the need for arteriography. J Bone Joint Surg Am 86A(5):910–915